Stuart & Sundeen's
PRINCIPLES and
PRACTICE of

Psychiatric Nursing

Stuart & Sundeen's PRINCIPLES and PRACTICE of

Psychiatric Nursing

sixth edition

GAIL W. STUART, PhD, RN, CS, FAAN

Center for Health Care Research,

Professor, Colleges of Nursing and Medicine,

Department of Psychiatry and Behavorial Sciences,

Medical University of South Carolina,

Charleston, South Carolina

MICHELE T. LARAIA, PhD, RN, CS

Assistant Professor, Colleges of Medicine and Nursing,

Department of Psychiatry and Behavorial Sciences,

Medical University of South Carolina,

Charleston, South Carolina

with 213 illustrations including 14 in full color

 Mosby

St. Louis Baltimore Boston Carlsbad Chicago Minneapolis New York Philadelphia Portland
London Milan Sydney Tokyo Toronto

Publisher	Sally Schrefer
Editor	Jeff Burnham
Developmental Editor	Linda Caldwell
Associate Developmental Editor	Jeff Downing
Project Manager	Dana Peick
Senior Production Editor	Dottie Martin
Designer	Amy Buxton
Manufacturing Supervisor	Karen Boehme
Cover Art	Jeff and Trisha Wolf, **EFX, Inc.**

sixth edition

Printed in the United States of America

Composition by Clarinda Company
Printing/binding by World Color

Mosby–Year Book, Inc.
11830 Westline Industrial Drive
St. Louis, Missouri 63146

Library of Congress Cataloging-in-Publication Data
Stuart & Sundeen's principles and practice of psychiatric nursing /
  [edited by] Gail W. Stuart, Michele T. Laraia. -- 6th ed.
     p.   cm.
   Rev. ed. of: Principles & practice of psychiatric nursing /
  [edited by] Gail Wiscarz Stuart, Sandra J. Sundeen. 5th ed. c1995.
   Includes bibliographical references and index.
   ISBN 0-8151-2603-4
   1. Psychiatric nursing.   I. Stuart, Gail Wiscarz, 1949-   .
II. Laraia, Michele T.   III. Sundeen, Sandra J., 1940-   .
IV. Principles & practice of psychiatric nursing.
   [DNLM: 1. Psychiatric Nursing--methods. 2. Mental Disorders-
-nursing.   WY 160 S931 1997]
RC440.S795 1997
610.73'68--dc21
DNLM/DLC
for Library of Congress

97-36169
CIP

97   98   99   00   01   /   9 8 7 6 5 4 3 2 1

About the Authors

Dr. Gail Stuart is a tenured professor in the College of Nursing and a professor in the College of Medicine in the Department of Psychiatry and Behavioral Sciences at the Medical University of South Carolina. She received her bachelor of science in nursing degree from Georgetown University, her master of science degree in psychiatric nursing from the University of Maryland, and her doctorate in behavioral sciences from Johns Hopkins University, School of Hygiene and Public Health. She is an American Nurses Association Certified Specialist in psychiatric and mental health nursing, a fellow in the American Academy of Nursing, a member of the American College of Mental Health Administrators, and a former president of the American Psychiatric Nurses Association.

Dr. Stuart's current position at the Medical University of South Carolina is with the Center for Health Care Research where she works as a member of an interdisciplinary research team that focuses on issues of access, resource use, outcomes, and health care delivery systems. She most recently was the administrator and chief executive officer of the Institute of Psychiatry at the Medical University of South Carolina where she was responsible for all clinical, fiscal, and human operations across the continuum of psychiatric care. Dr. Stuart has taught in undergraduate, graduate, and doctoral programs in nursing, and she is also active in clinical practice in the Department of Psychiatry. She serves on numerous academic, pharmaceutical, and governmental boards and represents nursing on a variety of National Institute of Mental Health policy and research panels. Dr. Stuart is a strong advocate for the specialty and is in great demand to speak and consult throughout the United States and Canada. She is a prolific writer and has published numerous articles, textbooks, and media productions. She has received many awards including the American Nurses Association Distinguished Contribution to Psychiatric Nursing–Current Impact on Innovations in Health Care Delivery Systems and Health Policy Award. Dr. Stuart's clinical and research interests involve the study of depression, anxiety disorders, and mental health delivery systems.

Dr. Michele Laraia is an assistant professor in the Colleges of Medicine and Nursing, Department of Psychiatry and Behavioral Sciences, at the Medical University of South Carolina. She received her bachelor of science degree in nursing from D'Youville College in Buffalo, New York, her master of science in nursing degree in psychiatric mental health nursing from the University of Virginia, and her doctorate in public health at the University of South Carolina. Dr. Laraia has more than 25 years' experience in the psychiatric nursing field including teaching, conducting research, and treating persons with psychiatric disorders. Her particular areas of expertise include psychobiology and psychopharmacology for which she has a national reputation in the field. She designed and taught an innovative psychopharmacology course addressing the needs of Advanced Practice Registered Nurses who wished to obtain perspective authority. She has taught psychiatric mental health nursing at the Master's level and holds a joint faculty appointment in the College of Graduate Studies. At the Medical University of South Carolina, Dr. Laraia is involved in informatics and has served in various positions that focus on electronic medical records, networking systems, and patient confidentiality.

Dr. Laraia presents at a variety of psychiatric nursing conferences throughout the country and has published and produced teaching media for the psychiatric nursing specialty. Her clinical practice focuses on persons with depression, panic disorder with agoraphobia, and other anxiety disorders. She conducts research in the fields of Alzheimer's disease, depression, and anxiety disorders and is an investigator for a variety of psychopharmacologic clinical trials. She received the American Psychiatric Nurses Association Award for Excellence in Research and has held several national and local consultant and advisory positions. Most notably, Dr. Laraia chaired the American Nurses Association Psychopharmacology Task Force for Psychiatric Mental Health Nurses.

Contributors

†**Beverly A. Baldwin**, PhD, RN, FAAN
Sonya Ziporkin Gershowitz Professor of Gerontological Nursing,
School of Nursing,
University of Maryland,
Baltimore, Maryland

Carole F. Bennett, MN, RN, CS
Institute of Psychiatry,
Medical University of South Carolina,
Charleston, South Carolina

Sandra E. Benter, DNSc, RN, CS
Psychotherapist and Consultant,
Boca Raton, Florida

Jacqueline C. Campbell, PhD, RN, FAAN
The Anna D. Wolf Endowed Professor,
School of Nursing,
Johns Hopkins University,
Baltimore, Maryland

Carolyn E. Cochrane, PhD, RN, CS
Assistant Professor,
Colleges of Medicine and Nursing;
Associate Clinical Director,
Eating Disorders Program;
Medical University of South Carolina,
Charleston, South Carolina

Victoria Conn, MN, MA, RN
Chair, Curriculum and Training,
National Alliance for the Mentally Ill,
Newtown Square, Pennsylvania

Suzanne D. Friedman, MS, RN, CS
Project Coordinator,
School of Nursing,
University of Maryland,
Baltimore, Maryland

Beth Gage Greco, MSN, RN
Psychiatric Community Health Nurse,
Visiting Nurse Association of Greater Philadelphia,
Philadelphia, Pennsylvania

Christine Cahill Hamolia, MS, RN, CS
Institute of Psychiatry,
Medical University of South Carolina,
Charleston, South Carolina

Patricia E. Helm, MSN, CS
Psychiatric Clinical Specialist,
West Haven Veterans Administration Medical Center,
West Haven, Connecticut

Joan M. Herbert, MS, RN, CS
Administrator,
Institute of Psychiatry,
Medical University of South Carolina,
Charleston, South Carolina

Linda V. Jefferson, PhD, RN, CS, CD
Research Manager,
National Institute of Drug Abuse,
Baltimore, Maryland

Joan Kenerson King, MSN, RN, CS
Director of Mental Health,
Visiting Nurse Association of Greater Philadelphia;
Private Practice,
Paoli and Telford, Pennsylvania

Arthur J. LaSalle, EdD, CCMHC, CSC
Partner, LaSalle Counseling Associates,
Psychotherapist, Consultant, Trainer,
Ellicott City, Maryland

Paula C. LaSalle, MS, RN, CS, CPC
Partner, LaSalle Counseling Associates,
Psychotherapist, Consultant, Trainer,
Elliott City, Maryland

Mary D. Moller, MSN, ARNP, CS
Executive Director,
The Center for Patient and Family Mental Health Education,
Nine Mile Falls, Washington

Millene F. Murphy, PhD, APRN
Associate Professor,
College of Nursing,
Brigham Young University,
Provo, Utah

Linda D. Oakley, PhD, RN
Assistant Professor, School of Nursing,
University of Wisconsin-Madison;
Clinical Specialist in Adult Psychiatric and Mental Health Nursing,
Madison, Wisconsin

---

†Deceased.

Barbara Parker, PhD, RN, FAAN
Professor, School of Nursing,
University of Virginia,
Charlottesville, Virginia

Carol K. Perlin, MS, RN, CS
Director, Division of Patient Access and Emergency Services,
Sheppard Pratt Health System,
Baltimore, Maryland

Susan G. Poorman, PhD, RN, CS
Associate Professor, Department of Nursing,
Community College of Allegheny County–Boyce Campus,
Pittsburgh, Pennsylvania

Victoria A. Queen, MSN, RN, CNA
Standards Coordinator,
DVA Medical Center,
Bay Pines, Florida

Audrey Redston-Iselin, MA, RN, CS
Clinical Specialist, Children's Services,
Soundview Throgs Neck Community Mental Health Center,
Albert Einstein College of Medicine,
Yeshiva University;
Private Practice,
White Plains, New York

Georgia L. Stevens, PhD, RN, CS
Psychotherapist and Consultant,
Adjunct Assistant Professor,
School of Nursing,
Catholic University of America,
Washington, DC

Sandra J. Sundeen, MS, RN, CNAA
Chief, Division of Human Resource Development,
Mental Hygiene Administration,
Maryland Department of Health and Mental Hygiene;
Adjunct Assistant Professor, School of Nursing,
University of Maryland,
Baltimore, Maryland

Nancy K. Worley, PhD, RN
Associate Professor and Department Chair,
College of Nursing,
Medical University of South Carolina;
Associate Chief of Nursing for Research,
Ralph H. Johnson VA Medical Center,
Charleston, South Carolina

Reviewers

Mary E. Allen, PhD, RN, CS
Associate Professor and Division Director,
College of Nursing,
University of Oklahoma,
Oklahoma City, Oklahoma

Charla Mae Andrews, RNC, MS
Instructor,
Spokane Community College;
Staff Nurse,
Sacred Heart Medical Center,
Spokane, Washington

Janette P. Arblaster, RN, MSN
Nursing Instructor,
Pendleton, South Carolina

Sharon E. Beck, DNSc, RN
Assistant Hospital Director,
Nursing Education and Quality Improvement,
Temple University Hospital,
Philadelphia, Pennsylvania

Judith Buchanan, RN, MHSc
Associate Professor,
University of New Brunswick at Saint John;
President,
Canadian Federation of Mental Health Nurses, 1996-1998,
Saint John, New Brunswick, Canada

Karma Castleberry, RN, CS, PhD
Professor,
School of Nursing,
Radford University;
Private Practice,
Radford, Virginia

Rose E. Constantino, PhD, JD, RN, FAAN, BCFF
Associate Professor,
School of Nursing,
University of Pittsburgh,
Pittsburgh, Pennsylvania

Mickie W. Crimone, MS, RN, CS
Nurse Psychotherapist,
Private Practice,
Rockville, Maryland;
The Center for Family Practice,
Bethesda, Maryland

Mary B. Davies, BSN, RN
Resource Nurse,
Healthfront Educational Services, Inc.,
Melrose, Massachusetts

Kathleen Shannon Dorcy, BSN, MN
Lecturer,
University of Washington-Tacoma,
Tacoma, Washington;
Researcher,
Fred Hutchinson Cancer Research Center,
Seattle, Washington

Jacqueline K. Dunn, MS, RN, CS
Clinical Nurse Specialist,
Charlestown Retirement Community;
Staff Nurse,
Sheppard Pratt Health System,
Baltimore, Maryland

Ginger W. Evans, MS, MSN, RN, CS
Assistant Professor,
College of Nursing,
University of Tennessee-Knoxville,
Knoxville, Tennessee

Vicki J. Ferris, MSN, RN
Associate Professor,
School of Nursing,
Central Wyoming College,
Riverton, Wyoming

Edna M. Fordyce, BSNF, MN, EdD
Clinical Specialist and Professor Emeritus,
School of Nursing,
Towson State University,
Towson, Maryland

Rebecca Crews Gruener, MSN, RN
Associate Professor of Nursing,
Louisiana State University-Alexandria,
Alexandria, Louisiana

Lynn E. Hanson, RN, MS
Assistant Professor,
Shepherd College,
Shepherdstown, West Virginia

Arlene N. Hurwitz, RN, PhD
Professor,
City College School of Nursing,
City University of New York,
New York, New York

Susan Kagan, RN, BscN, MeD, EdD
Professor,
Seneca College of Applied Arts & Technology,
Toronto, Ontario, Canada

Barbara J. Limandri, RN, CS, DNSc
Associate Professor,
School of Nursing,
Oregon Health Sciences University;
Psychiatric-Mental Health Nurse Practitioner,
Portland, Oregon

Bernadette Mae Longo, MS, RN, C
Nursing Faculty,
Great Basin College,
Elko, Nevada

Gloria McInnis, MSN, RN, CS
Doctoral Student,
School of Nursing,
Catholic University,
Washington, DC

Mary Love, RN, MSN
Nursing Professor,
Truckee Meadow Community College,
Reno, Nevada

Kenyann Lucas, MS, RN, CS
Associate Professor-ADN,
Texarkana College,
Texarkana, Texas

Susan McCabe, RN, MS, EdD
Assistant Professor,
East Tennessee State University,
Johnston City, Tennessee

Dolores C. Prosser Morris, N, BScN, DEd
Teacher,
Nursing Program,
John Abbott College,
Ste. Anne de Bellevue, Quebec, Canada

Alean Royes, MSN, RN, CS
Faculty/Specialist,
School of Nursing,
The University of Texas at Arlington,
Arlington, Texas

Karen S. Ward, PhD, RN
Associate Professor,
School of Nursing,
Middle Tennessee State University,
Murfreesboro, Tennessee

Student Advisory Panel

Lisa A. Casler
Morehead State University,
Morehead, Kentucky

Karen R. Curtis
California State University-Sacramento,
Sacramento, California

Wendy Harcarik
University of San Francisco,
San Francisco, California

Diane E. Junker
Milligan College,
Milligan College, Tennessee

Kamee Krager
Saint Francis Medical Center College of Nursing,
Peoria, Illinois

Heather Marie Lochtefeld
Tarrant County Junior College,
Fort Worth, Texas

Megan Madden
Marymount University,
Arlington, Virginia

Anita Masiello
Mercer County Community College,
West Windsor, New Jersey

Donna M. Ruppel
Adirondack Community College,
Queensbury, New York

Patricia J. Zubair
California State University-Hayward,
Hayward, California

Preface

Talk about change! Time travelers from other worlds couldn't experience more of a "knowledge warp" than psychiatric nurses live with each day. For that reason, this sixth edition of *Stuart & Sundeen's Principles and Practice of Psychiatric Nursing* is being published a full year ahead of schedule, and I, Gail Stuart, have taken on a new coauthor, Michele Laraia, who is a seasoned navigator in the unfolding landscapes of psychobiology and psychopharmacology. We hope you will travel with us throughout this new edition on the traditional terrain of the printed word and on the exploding frontier of the electronic word, as together we explore the world of psychiatric nursing practice in the new millennium.

There are many reasons why this text has been the leader in its field, and it clearly has an established reputation of being comprehensive, engaging, and futuristic. But both time and knowledge move on. So this new edition builds on its legacy of excellence while launching forward to further define evidence-based psychiatric nursing practice in a rapidly changing health care environment. Thus the sixth edition continues to emphasize the Stuart Stress Adaptation Model, which organizes content based on a holistic biopsychosocial approach to nursing care. It also continues to emphasize the full continuum of care; the broad range of preventive, crisis, and rehabilitative nursing activities; and the strong partnerships psychiatric nurses form with patients and their families. These elements are the foundation of both contemporary and future psychiatric nursing practice. To these elements we have added the latest scientific knowledge on neurobiology and psychopharmacology and new information on managed care, home psychiatric care, and the family's perspective. We have also incorporated the excitement of using the Internet as a learning tool that can rapidly access the most current information because we believe that what we know and how we learn as psychiatric nurses will be radically changed in the years ahead. Our goal with this edition, therefore, is to help psychiatric nurses travel the terrain of the new millennium with state-of-the-art knowledge and competent caring in their work with patients and families.

CONTENT ORGANIZATION

This book is divided into six units. Unit One presents psychiatric nursing principles that are fundamental to practice. First, the contemporary psychiatric nurse's roles and functions are addressed followed by a chapter on therapeutic relationship skills. Conceptual models of psychiatric treatment, including the Stuart Stress Adaptation Model of psychiatric nursing care, are then presented along with separate chapters devoted to the biological, psychological, sociocultural, environmental, and legal-ethical contexts of practice. Finally, separate chapters in this unit focus on the American Nurses Association (ANA) professional practice and performance standards.

Unit Two addresses the continuum of care, including mental health promotion and illness prevention, crisis intervention, and psychiatric rehabilitation. These topics, unique to this textbook, are more important than ever because health care reform focuses on nontraditional settings and a wide range of treatment strategies. A new chapter has also been added on the family's perspective of the continuum of mental health care, further reinforcing the importance of families reflected throughout the text.

Unit Three applies psychiatric nursing principles to specific clinical disorders, based on a continuum of adaptive-maladaptive coping responses, the six-step nursing process, and the Diagnostic and Statistical Manual of Mental Disorders (DSM-IV) and North American Nursing Diagnosis Association (NANDA) diagnoses. There are separate chapters on anxiety, somatoform and sleep, dissociative, mood, psychotic, personality, substance abuse, eating, sexual, and organic mood disorders as well as suicidal behavior. The information in this unit has been completely updated and includes all DSM-IV diagnostic categories.

Unit Four describes various modalities of psychiatric treatment, including chapters on psychopharmacology, somatic therapies, cognitive behavioral therapy, and managing aggressive behavior. Each of these areas is of importance in the field, and together they join with chapters on therapeutic groups and family interventions to round out the repertoire of psychiatric nursing practice.

Unit Five begins with revised chapters on hospital-based and community-based psychiatric nursing care that reflect the most recent developments and current practice in these settings. Also included is a new chapter on home care because health care reform emphasizes the psychiatric nurse's abilities to collaborate, advise, and manage patients in the home.

Unit Six concludes the text with a discussion of the unique issues and concerns in the psychiatric treatment of special populations including revised chapters on children, adolescents, the elderly, survivors of abuse and violence, and patients with HIV/AIDS.

SPECIAL FEATURES

We hope by now your appetite has been stimulated and you are ready to embark with us on this fascinating journey through the art and science of psychiatric nursing. On the way, look for other signposts and special features that we have included to illuminate your journey. Many of the special features listed have been highlighted with a special design or logo to enhance the teaching-learning process.

Your Internet Connection is new to this edition. Each chapter offers you Web sites related to the focus of the chapter that can be accessed on the Internet. In this way, students and faculty can stay current with the latest developments in each content area.

Clinical Examples, highlighted in color, are taken from actual clinical situations. Many of them provide samples of nursing diagnoses related to the particular clinical situation.

Critical Thinking questions, interspersed throughout the narrative of each chapter, challenge students and promote independent clinical reasoning. At the same time, they add interest to the textual information and encourage students to integrate the material with their own understanding of the world and nursing.

Case Studies are in-depth examples of clinical scenarios that discuss each step of the nursing process, providing students with realistic application of the nursing process.

Competent Caring: A Clinical Exemplar of a Psychiatric Nurse is a special box found at the end of chapters in Units Two through Six. In this feature a practicing psychiatric nurse shares clinical experiences and personal insights related to the chapter topic.

Critical Thinking about Contemporary Issues. Every chapter presents a discussion of a current, controversial issue that is related to the chapter's topic and is analyzed from current research findings in the field.

A Patient Speaks and **A Family Speaks** present relevant treatment issues from a patient's and family's point of view, giving students a better understanding of the patient's and family's perspective of the caregiving process.

Patient Education Plans and **Family Education Plans** guide students in educating the patient and the family about important treatment issues.

Nursing Treatment Plan Summaries present care plans based on the major disorders discussed in the book. The care plans include nursing diagnoses, expected outcomes, short-term goals, interventions, and rationales and serve as a guide for students in nursing care related to the treatment of major disorders.

Medical and Nursing Diagnoses and **Detailed Diagnoses** boxes present examples of NANDA diagnoses applicable for a specific disorder and describe the essential features of related DSM-IV diagnoses.

The six steps of the **nursing process** are highlighted with the following special headings as they are discussed in the disorders chapters:

Assessment

Nursing Diagnosis

Outcome Identification

Planning

Implementation

Evaluation

Therapeutic Dialogues provide samples of appropriate verbal therapeutic interactions with patients to educate students about therapeutic communication skills.

Tables and boxes that discuss specific **pharmacology** information emphasize its importance in the treatment of psychiatric illnesses.

Learning objectives and a **topical outline** at the beginning of each chapter inform the students of the basic concepts and organization of the chapter, and a chapter **summary** includes key points at the end of each chapter to help students grasp important concepts.

Key terms are highlighted in color, and many are included in the **glossary** at the back of the book.

Video Resources are provided at the end of chapters for students interested in supplementing their learning with videotaped programs.

Chapter Review Questions have been added to the end of each chapter to help students review important points and master the chapter's content.

TEACHING AND LEARNING PACKAGE
Instructor's Resource Manual and Test Bank

The *Instructor's Resource Manual and Test Bank to Accompany Stuart & Sundeen's Principles and Practice of Psychiatric Nursing* is designed to help you, the instructor, develop lectures, reinforce teaching through classroom and clinical activities, and evaluate student comprehension. This valuable resource manual follows the textbook chapter by chapter and includes critical thinking questions and activities, future research boxes, and learning resources. Adapted outlines for courses of variable durations and transparency masters are also featured. A *Test Bank* containing more than 800 test items in the NCLEX format has also been provided and includes an answer key with correlating page numbers along with the applicable nursing process step and cognitive level of each question.

Transparencies

Mosby's Psychiatric Nursing Transparency Acetates, second edition, provides 48 two-color transparencies that cover a variety of topics in psychiatric nursing, helping to increase understanding through visual learning aids.

Computest 3

Available in IBM 3.5″ and Macintosh, Computest is the computerized version of the *Test Bank* from the *Instructor's Resource Manual.* Complete with an instructional guide, Computest allows users to edit, add, delete, or select questions on the computer.

Finally, we wish to communicate our respect for individuals and the roles they enact, regardless of their gender. To that end, we have attempted to avoid pronouns that express bias and to give recognition and support for the commitment of both men and women to the nursing profession. However, this sometimes creates difficult and tedious language for the reader. Therefore, for clarity and simplicity, the nurse is referred to in the third person, female gender, and the patient in the third person, masculine gender when necessary. It should also be noted that Ms. is used instead of Miss or Mrs. in examples used in the text.

This completes your introduction to the journey that lies ahead. We invite you now to open the pages beneath your fingers and join us in a world of new ideas, challenging beliefs, and expanding competencies. We wish you well and look forward to meeting you in the empowering universe of psychiatric nursing practice.

Gail Wiscarz Stuart
Michele T. Laraia

Contents

UNIT *5 Treatment Settings*

UNIT 6 *Special Populations in Psychiatry*

Color Plates

Stuart & Sundeen's

PRINCIPLES and
PRACTICE of

Psychiatric
Nursing

UNIT 1

Principles of Psychiatric Nursing Care

You are about to begin a voyage to places you have never been before: the world of psychiatric and mental health nursing. In the old days of nursing, students learned about pieces of people—an infected toe, a congested lung, a troubling twitch, or maybe even a broken heart—but pieces nonetheless. Today, students learn about the wholeness of people: a physically ill child struggling for safety in an abusive family, an adolescent coping with eating problems and self-esteem, a young adult grieving over the diagnosis of HIV/AIDS, or an elder confused and disoriented at times but frightened at the thought of going to a nursing home. This is the exciting world of today's psychiatric nurse. It integrates the biological, psychological, sociocultural, environmental, legal, and ethical realities of life and weaves them together in a rich tapestry called psychiatric nursing practice.

This unit introduces you to parts of this world that may be new to you. It will help you explore how patients think, feel, and behave. It will help you learn how to talk with patients and families as partners in the caregiving process. It will suggest that you think about people in terms of their overall functioning and adaptation rather than of the symptoms of their specific illness. Most importantly, it will define for you the responsibilities you have as a professional health-care provider. We hope you are ready to begin your journey, and we wish you curiosity about human nature, openness to new ways of thinking, and delight in the process of learning.

Roles and Functions of Psychiatric Nurses: Competent Caring

Gail W. Stuart

© 1998 M.C. Escher/Cordon Art, Baarn, Holland.

And what they dare to dream of, dare to do. **James Russell Lowell**

LEARNING OBJECTIVES

After studying this chapter the student should be able to:

▼ Describe the evolution of the psychiatric nursing role and functions

▼ Discuss the nature, settings, and functions of contemporary psychiatric nursing practice

▼ Analyze the factors that influence the psychiatric nurse's level of performance

▼ Critique areas of importance for psychiatric nursing's future agenda

TOPICAL OUTLINE

Historical Perspectives
  Role Emergence
  Evolving Functions
Contemporary Practice
  Levels of Prevention
  Continuum of Care
  Competent Caring
Level of Performance
  Laws
  Qualifications
  Practice Setting
  Personal Initiative
Psychiatric Nursing Agenda
  Outcome Evaluation
  Leadership Skills
  Political Action

The function of nursing or caring for the sick has existed since the beginning of civilization. Before 1860 the emphasis in psychiatric institutions was on custodial care, and attendants were hired to maintain control of the patients. Often these attendants were little more than jailers or cellkeepers with little training, and psychiatric care was poor. Nursing as a profession began to emerge in the late nineteenth century, and by the twentieth century it had evolved into a specialty with unique roles and functions.

HISTORICAL PERSPECTIVES

In 1873 Linda Richards graduated from the New England Hospital for Women and Children in Boston. She developed better nursing care in psychiatric hospitals and organized nursing services and educational programs in state mental hospitals in Illinois. For these activities she is called the first American psychiatric nurse. Basic to Richards's theory of care was her statement, "It stands to reason that the mentally sick should be at least as well cared for as the physically sick."[7]

The first school to prepare nurses to care for the mentally ill opened at McLean Hospital in Waverly, Massachusetts, in 1882. It was a 2-year program, but few psychological skills were addressed; the care was mainly custodial. Nurses took care of the patients' physical needs, such as medications, nutrition, hygiene, and ward activities. Until the end of the nineteenth century little changed in the role of psychiatric nurses. They had limited training in psychiatry, and they primarily adapted the principles of medical-surgical nursing to the psychiatric setting. At that time psychological care consisted of kindness and tolerance toward the patients.

One of Linda Richards's more important contributions was her emphasis on assessing both the physical and emotional needs of the patients. In this early period of nursing history, nursing education separated these two needs; nurses were taught either in the general hospital or in the psychiatric hospital. In 1913 Johns Hopkins became the first school of nursing to include a fully developed course for psychiatric nursing in the curriculum. Other schools soon began to do likewise. It was not until the late 1930s that nursing education recognized the importance of psychiatric knowledge in general nursing care for all illnesses (Box 1-1).

An important factor in the development of psychiatric nursing was the emergence of various somatic therapies, including insulin shock therapy (1935), psychosurgery (1936), and electroconvulsive therapy (1937). These techniques all required the medical-surgical skills of nurses. Although these therapies did not help the patient understand one's problems, they did control behavior and make the patient more amenable to psychotherapy. Somatic therapies also increased the demand for improved psychological treatment for patients who did not respond.

As nurses became more involved with somatic therapies,

Box **1-1** *A Nurse Speaks*

We do not hesitate to emphasize the need of some psychiatric training in the life of every nurse who would represent her profession on the basis of modern standards. The psychiatrically trained nurse must remember, on the other hand, that all symptoms are not of mental origin. This fact has been long recognized, so nurses trained in mental hospitals have wisely requested affiliation in general hospitals, thus avoiding the danger of overspecialization. Does it not seem rational, therefore, that the general hospital shall guarantee its nurse an equivalent knowledge of the workings of the patient's mind as the psychiatric nurse has of the workings of his body? Modern psychology reveals the close interrelation of the two; it recognizes the ceaseless interaction of one on the other. Should we not then more consistently work toward the ideal that every hospital shall graduate nurses trained in preventive and curative methods of caring for the inevitably associated physically and mentally ill?

Annie L. Crawford, RN, BS
South Carolina Nurses' Association
Annual Convention Presentation
October 6, 1934

they began the struggle to define their role as psychiatric nurses. An editorial in the *American Journal of Nursing*[8] in 1940 described the conflict between nurses and physicians as nurses tried to implement what they saw as appropriate care for psychiatric patients. This conflict continues to demand attention in current nursing practice (Box 1-2).[18]

The period after World War II was one of major growth and change in psychiatric nursing. Because of the large number of service-related psychiatric problems and the increase in treatment programs offered by the Veterans Administration, psychiatric nurses with advanced preparation were in demand. The content of psychiatric nursing had now become an integral part of the generic nursing curriculum; its principles were applied to other areas of nursing practice, including general medical, pediatric, and public health nursing. By 1947 eight graduate programs in psychiatric nursing had been started.

Role Emergence

The role of psychiatric nursing began to emerge in the early 1950s. In 1947 Weiss[32] published an article in the *American Journal of Nursing* that reemphasized the shortage of psychiatric nurses and outlined the differences between psychiatric and general duty nurses. She described "attitude therapy" as the nurse's directed use of attitudes that contribute to the patient's recovery. In implementing this therapy the nurse observes the patient for small and fleeting changes, demonstrates acceptance, respect, and understanding of the patient, and promotes the patient's interest and participation in reality.

Box **1-2** *A Physician Speaks*

I have spent all of my professional career in close association with, and close dependency on, nurses, and like many of my faculty colleagues, I've done a lot of worrying about the relationship between medicine and nursing.

The doctors worry that nurses are trying to move away from their historical responsibilities to medicine (meaning, really, to the doctors' orders). The nurses assert that they are their own profession, responsible for their own standards, co-equal colleagues with physicians, and they do not wish to become mere ward administrators or technicians

My discovery as a patient is that the institution is held together, *glued* together, enabled to function as an organism, by the nurses and by nobody else.

The nurses make it their business to know everything that is going on. They spot errors before errors can be launched. They know everything written on the chart. Most important of all, they know their patients as unique human beings, and they soon get to know the close relatives and friends. Because of this knowledge, they are quick to sense apprehensions and act on them. The average sick person in a large hospital feels at risk of getting lost, with no identity left beyond a name and a string of numbers on a plastic wristband, in danger always of being whisked off on a litter to the wrong place to have the wrong procedure done, or worse still, *not* being whisked off at the right time. The attending physician or the house officer, on rounds and usually in a hurry, can murmur a few reassuring words on his way out the door, but it takes a confident, competent, and cheerful nurse, there all day long and in and out of the room on one chore or another through the night, to bolster one's confidence that the situation is indeed manageable and not about to get out of hand.

Knowing what I know, I am all for the nurses. If they are to continue their professional feud with the doctors, if they want their professional status enhanced and their pay increased, if they infuriate the doctors by their claims to be equal professionals, if they ask for the moon, I am on their side.

Lewis Thomas, MD
The Youngest Science
New York, 1983, Viking Press

An article by Bennett and Eaton[4] in the *American Journal of Psychiatry* in 1951 identified the following three problems affecting psychiatric nurses:

▼ The scarcity of qualified psychiatric nurses
▼ The under use of their abilities
▼ The fact that "very little real psychiatric nursing is carried out in otherwise good psychiatric hospitals and units"

These psychiatrists believed that the psychiatric nurse should join mental health societies, consult with welfare agencies, work in outpatient clinics, practice preventive psychiatry, engage in research, and help educate the public. They supported the nurse's participation in individual and group psychotherapy and stated, "Despite the fact that most psychiatrists seem to ignore the role of the psychiatric nurse in psychotherapy, all nurses in psychiatric wards do psychotherapy of one kind or another by their contacts with patients."[4] Many of the issues raised in the article were debated years later.

> **?** *Do you think that the problems affecting psychiatric nurses described by Bennet and Eaton in 1951 continue to exist in the specialty today?*

Also in 1951 Mellow[20] wrote of the work she did with schizophrenic patients. She called these activities "nursing therapy." A year later, Tudor[30] published a study in which she described the nurse-patient relationships she established, which were characterized by unconditional care, few demands, and the anticipation of her patients' needs. These articles were some of the earliest descriptions by psychiatric nurses of the nurse-patient relationship and the nature of its therapeutic process.

As nurses engaged in these kinds of activities, many questions arose. Are these activities therapeutic or are they therapy? What is a therapeutic relationship or a one-to-one nurse-patient relationship? How does it differ from psychotherapy? These questions were addressed by Dr. Hildegard Peplau, a dynamic nursing leader whose ideas and beliefs shaped psychiatric nursing.

In 1952 Peplau[25] published a book, *Interpersonal Relations in Nursing,* in which she described the skills, activities, and role of psychiatric nurses. It was the first systematic, theoretical framework developed for psychiatric nursing. Peplau defined nursing as a "significant, therapeutic process." As she studied the nursing process, she saw nurses emerge in various roles: as a resource person; a teacher; a leader in local, national, and international situations; a surrogate parent; and a counselor. She wrote, "Counseling in nursing has to do with helping the patient remember and to understand fully what is happening to him in the present situation, so that the experience can be integrated with rather than dissociated from other experiences in life."[25]

> **?** *Compare the roles of psychiatric nurses identified by Hildegard Peplau in 1952 with your observations of contemporary psychiatric nursing practice.*

Finally, two significant developments in psychiatry in the 1950s also affected nursing's role for years to come. The first was Jones' publication of *The Therapeutic Community: A New Treatment Method in Psychiatry*[12] in 1953. It encouraged using the patient's social environment to provide a therapeutic experience. The patient was to be an active participant in care and become involved in the daily problems of the community. All patients were to help solve problems, plan activities, and develop the necessary rules and regulations. Therapeutic communities became the preferred environment for psychiatric patients.

The second significant development in psychiatry in the early 1950s was the use of psychotropic drugs. With these drugs more patients became treatable, and fewer environmental constraints such as locked doors and straitjackets were required. Also, more personnel were needed to provide therapy, and the roles of various psychiatric practitioners were expanded, including the nurse's role.

Evolving Functions

In 1958 the following functions of psychiatric nurses were described[11]:

▼ Dealing with patients' problems of attitude, mood, and interpretation of reality
▼ Exploring disturbing and conflicting thoughts and feelings
▼ Using the patient's positive feelings toward the therapist to bring about psychophysiological homeostasis
▼ Counseling patients in emergencies, including panic and fear
▼ Strengthening the well part of patients

The nurse-patient relationship was referred to by a variety of terms, including "therapeutic nurse-patient relationship," "psychiatric nursing therapy," "supportive psychotherapy," "rehabilitation therapies," and "nondirective counseling." The distinction between these terms and the exact nature of the nurse's role remained hazy.

Once again Peplau[26] clarified psychiatric nursing's position and directed its future growth. In *"Interpersonal Techniques: The Crux of Psychiatric Nursing,"* published in 1962, she identified the heart of psychiatric nursing as the role of counselor or psychotherapist. Other functions such as mother surrogate, technician, manager, socializing agent, and health teacher were seen as subroles. In her article Peplau differentiated between general practitioners who were staff nurses working on psychiatric units and psychiatric nurses who were specialists and expert clinical practitioners with graduate degrees in psychiatric nursing. Thus, from an undefined role involving primarily physical care, psychiatric nursing was evolving into a role of clinical competence based on interpersonal techniques and use of the nursing process.

In the 1960s the focus of psychiatric nursing began to shift to primary prevention and implementing care and consultation in the community. Representative of these changes was the shift in the name of the field from *psychiatric nursing* to *psychiatric and mental health nursing*. This focus was stimulated by the Community Mental Health Centers Act of 1963, which made federal money available to states to plan, construct, and staff community mental health centers. This legislation was prompted by growing awareness of the value of treating people in the community and

preventing hospitalization whenever possible. It also encouraged the formation of multidisciplinary treatment teams by combining the skills of many professions to alleviate illness and promote mental health. This team approach continues to be negotiated. The issues of territoriality, professionalism, authority structure, consumer rights, and the use of paraprofessionals are still being debated.

The 1970s gave rise to the further development of the specialty. Psychiatric nurses became the pacesetters in specialty nursing practice. They were the first to:

▼ Develop standards and statements on scope of practice
▼ Establish generalist and specialist certification

At this same time, the nursing profession was defining caring as a core element of all nursing practice, and the contributions of psychiatric nurses were embraced by nurses of all specialty groups. Partly as a result of this broader definition of psychiatric nursing and the perceived skills of psychiatric nurses, nursing education reorganized its curriculum and began to integrate psychiatric nursing content into nonpsychiatric courses. This blending of content was evident in the second change in the name of the field in the 1970s from *psychiatric and mental health nursing* to *psychosocial nursing*. The integration of psychiatric nursing content into basic courses became so complete that faculty no longer viewed these areas as psychiatric nursing but saw them as an expanded, more holistic approach to nursing care.[23] At the same time, clinical rotations focusing on the psychiatric illnesses of patients in psychiatric settings were often replaced by clinical rotations integrating psychosocial aspects of the care of physically ill patients in general medical-surgical units. Unfortunately, this trend often did not provide students with an opportunity to care for patients with psychiatric illnesses and learn about new information that was emerging in the field of psychiatry and the broader behavioral sciences.

The 1980s were years of exciting scientific growth in the area of psychobiology. Advancements occurred in five basic areas:

▼ Brain imaging techniques
▼ Neurotransmitters and neuronal receptors
▼ Psychobiology of emotions
▼ Understanding the brain
▼ Molecular genetics related to psychobiology

Although this information explosion advanced knowledge in the field, it lacked integration and was often of limited clinical usefulness. It has also been observed that psychiatric nurses in the 1980s were slow to make the shift away from primarily psychodynamic models of the mind to more balanced psychobiological models of psychiatric care.[1,17]

Psychiatric nurses thus entered the 1990s faced with the challenge of integrating the expanding bases of neuroscience into the holistic biopsychosocial practice of psychiatric nursing. Advances in understanding the relationships of the brain, behavior, emotion, and cognition offered new opportunities for psychiatric nursing.[10] Another issue that

Evolutionary Timeline in Psychiatric Nursing

SOCIAL ENVIRONMENT		PSYCHIATRIC NURSING
	1873	Linda Richards graduated from New England Hospital for Women and Children
	1882	First school to prepare nurses to care for the mentally ill opened at McLean Hospital in Massachusetts
American Journal of Nursing first published	1900	
Florence Nightingale died	1910	
	1913	Johns Hopkins was first school of nursing to include a course on psychiatric nursing in its curriculum
Electroconvulsive therapy developed	1937	
National Mental Health Act passed by Congress, creating National Institute of Mental Health (NIMH) and providing training funds for psychiatric nursing education	1946	
	1950	National League for Nursing (NLN) required that to be accredited schools of nursing must provide an experience in psychiatric nursing
	1952	Hildegard Peplau published *Interpersonal Relations in Nursing*
Maxwell Jones published *The Therapeutic Community*	1953	
Development of major tranquilizers	1954	
Community Mental Health Centers Act passed	1963	*Perspectives in Psychiatric Care* published; *Journal of Psychiatric Nursing and Mental Health Services* published
	1973	*Standards of Psychiatric–Mental Health Nursing Practice* published; certification of psychiatric mental health nurse generalists established by American Nurses' Association (ANA)
Report of the President's Commission on Mental Health	1978	
	1979	*Issues in Mental Health Nursing* published; certification of psychiatric–mental health nurse specialists established by ANA
Nursing: A Social Policy Statement published by ANA	1980	
Mental Health Systems Act passed		
Mental Health Systems Act repealed	1981	
National Center for Nursing Research created in National Institutes of Health (NIH)	1985	*Standards of Child and Adolescent Psychiatric and Mental Health Nursing Practice* published by ANA
	1986	American Psychiatric Nurses Association (APNA) established
	1987	*Archives of Psychiatric Nursing* published; *Journal of Child and Adolescent Psychiatric and Mental Health Nursing* published
	1988	*Standards of Addictions Nursing Practice* published by ANA
	1990	*Standards of Psychiatric Consultation Liaison Nursing Practice* published by ANA
Center for Mental Health Services created	1992	
	1994	Revised *Standards of Psychiatric–Mental Health Clinical Nursing Practice* published by ANA
	1994	*Psychopharmacology Guidelines for Psychiatric–Mental Health Nurses* published by ANA
Revised *Nursing's Social Policy Statement* published by ANA	1995	*Journal of the American Psychiatric Nurses Association (JAPNA)* published

emerged in the 1990s was the importance of sociocultural factors in psychiatric care. Psychiatric nurses also saw the need to become realigned with care and caring, which represent the art of psychiatric nursing and give balance to the science and high technology of current health-care prac-

tices.[16] These changes led to the revision of the *Standards of Psychiatric–Mental Health Clinical Nursing Practice* (see Chapters 10 and 11) in 1994 and the publication of *Psychopharmacology Guidelines for Psychiatric–Mental Health Nurses* (see Chapter 27) in the same year.

The task for psychiatric nurses in the years ahead will be the need for greater differentiation and balance.[27] Psychiatric nursing practice must continue to differentiate between mental health and mental illness, medical and nursing models of care, adaptive and maladaptive responses, and psychiatric and psychosocial problems. For example, the anxiety felt by a patient before surgery is very different from the anxiety experienced by a patient with agoraphobia. Likewise, the care the nurse gives each patient varies based on whether the nurse is prepared to intervene from a psychosocial or psychiatric nursing perspective. As the specialty is able to better differentiate among these phenomena, a balance can be achieved in directing clinical practice, establishing research priorities, and preparing psychiatric nurses for the range of functions they will assume in the next decade.

> **?** *Compare the length of your clinical rotation in psychiatric nursing with your clinicals in medicine, surgery, and pediatrics. Given the high prevalence of mental health problems such as depression and substance abuse, do you feel you have sufficient learning time in psychiatric nursing?*

CONTEMPORARY PRACTICE

Psychiatric nursing is an interpersonal process that promotes and maintains patient behavior that contributes to integrated functioning. The patient may be an individual, family, group, organization, or community. The American Nurses' Association *Statement on Psychiatric–Mental Health Clinical Nursing Practice* defines psychiatric nursing as "a specialized area of nursing practice employing theories of human behavior as its science and purposeful use of self as its art."[2] The Center for Mental Health Services officially recognizes psychiatric nursing as one of the five core mental health disciplines. The other four disciplines are marriage and family therapy, psychiatry, psychology, and social work.

The current practice of psychiatric nursing is based on a number of underlying premises or beliefs. The philosophical beliefs of psychiatric nursing practice on which this text is based are described in Box 1-3. The psychiatric nurse uses knowledge from the psychosocial and biophysical sciences and theories of personality and human behavior. From these sources the nurse derives a theoretical framework on which to base nursing practice. The choice of a conceptual model or theoretical framework is an individual one. Various models of psychiatric treatment are described in Chapter 3. Chapter 4 presents the Stuart Stress Adaptation Model of psychiatric nursing care that is used as the organizing framework for this text.

Finally, the contemporary practice of psychiatric nursing occurs within a social and environmental context[9] (see Critical Thinking about Contemporary Issues). The professional psychiatric nursing role has grown in complexity throughout its history and now must be thought about in a health-care environment in which there is greater consumer responsibility and a broader context of clinician accountability.

Thus the nurse-patient relationship has evolved into a nurse-patient *partnership* that expands the dimensions of

---

Box **1-3** *Philosophical Beliefs of Psychiatric Nursing Practice*

▼ The individual has intrinsic worth and dignity and each person is worthy of respect.

▼ The goal of the individual is one of growth, health, autonomy, and self-actualization.

▼ Every individual has the potential to change.

▼ The person functions as a holistic being who acts on, interacts with, and reacts to the environment as a whole person. Each part affects the total response.

▼ All people have common, basic, and necessary human needs. These include physical needs, safety needs, love and belonging needs, esteem needs, and self-actualization needs.

▼ All behavior of the individual is meaningful. It arises from personal needs and goals and can be understood only from the person's internal frame of reference and within the context in which it occurs.

▼ Behavior consists of perceptions, thoughts, feelings, and actions. From one's perceptions thoughts arise, emotions are felt, and actions are conceived. Disruptions may occur in any of these areas.

▼ Individuals vary in their coping capacities, which depend on genetic endowment, environmental influences, nature and degree of stress, and available resources. All individuals have the potential for both health and illness.

▼ Illness can be a growth-producing experience for the individual.

▼ All people have a right to an equal opportunity for adequate health care regardless of gender, race, religion, ethics, sexual orientation, or cultural background.

▼ Mental health is a critical and necessary component of comprehensive health-care services.

▼ The individual has the right to participate in decision making regarding physical and mental health. The person has the right to self-determination, including the decision to pursue health or illness.

▼ The goal of nursing care is to promote wellness, maximize integrated functioning, and enhance self-actualization. Nursing care is based on health-care needs and expected treatment outcomes mutually determined with individuals, families, groups, and communities.

▼ An interpersonal relationship can produce change and growth within the individual. It is the vehicle for the application of the nursing process and the attainment of the goal of nursing care.

Are Psychiatric Nurses Vulnerable or Valuable in an Era of Health Care Reform?

One question that is often raised when nurses talk about the health care environment is whether psychiatric nurses will be vulnerable to being replaced as expensive and outdated providers or be valued as competent clinicians who can function in a world of changing needs, processes, and structures. Potential areas of vulnerability have been identified and include the following[29]:

▼ Fewer nurses are attracted to psychiatric nursing as compared with other specialty areas.

▼ Content devoted to understanding psychiatric illnesses and working with psychiatric patients in nursing education programs has decreased steadily during the past decade.

▼ Graduate programs are moving toward the preparation of nurse practitioners who have significantly less course work related to the diagnosis and treatment of psychiatric illnesses.

▼ Psychiatric nurses have most often worked in inpatient settings, yet health care reform has stimulated the greater use of community-based settings.

▼ Biopsychosocial skills and expertise of psychiatric nurses are often underused in mental health care systems.

▼ Psychiatric nurses often are viewed as expensive health care providers who can be replaced by two or more less costly personnel.

▼ There are increasing threats to nursing autonomy as state boards of nursing and other regulatory bodies attempt to establish separate advanced practice licensure and examinations, and require advanced practice nurses to be under the full supervision of physicians.

▼ There are few outcome studies that document the nature, extent, and effectiveness of care delivered by psychiatric nurses.

▼ Psychiatric nurses continue to struggle to be perceived as revenue producers and have difficulty receiving direct reimbursement from third-party payers for their services.

▼ Role differentiation for psychiatric nurses based on education and experience is often lacking in the position descriptions, job responsibilities, and reward systems of the health care systems in which they practice.

Each of these issues must be addressed if psychiatric nursing is to continue to develop as a specialty area. Nurses must continue to move into the continuum of care and clearly articulate their skills, functions, and abilities. They must also demonstrate their cost effectiveness and differentiated levels of practice based on education, experience, and credentials. Other strategies that have been suggested are that psychiatric nurses assist in the development of national databases that list and define nursing concerns, continue to develop and use standards and guidelines for clinical practice, and participate in health-care payment reform that results in payment to the most cost-effective qualified provider.[6] Such strategies will position psychiatric nurses as visible, interdependent, central, and collaborating professionals who have much to offer a reformed health care system.

the professional psychiatric nursing role. These elements include *clinical competence, patient-family advocacy, fiscal responsibility, interdisciplinary collaboration, social accountability,* and *legal-ethical parameters* (Fig. 1-1). No longer can psychiatric nurses focus exclusively on bedside care and the immediacy of patient needs. Rather, they must broaden the context of their care and the responsibility and understanding they bring to the caregiving situation. The current practice of psychiatric nursing requires greater sensitivity to the social environment and the advocacy needs of patients and their families. It also mandates thoughtful consideration of complex legal and ethical dilemmas that arise from a delivery system that is focused on the efficiencies of managed care, which can disadvantage and discriminate against those with mental illness. New models of mental health care also require greater skill in interdisciplinary collaboration that is built on the psychiatric nurse's clinical competence and professional self-assertion and balanced by a clear understanding of the costs of psychiatric care in general and psychiatric nursing care in particular. Each of these elements must influence the education, research, and clinical components of contemporary psychiatric nursing practice.

Levels of Prevention

The concepts of primary, secondary, and tertiary prevention provide a framework for discussing contemporary psychiatric nursing practice.

PRIMARY. **Primary prevention** involves lowering the incidence of illness in a community by changing causative factors before they can do harm. It is a concept that precedes disease and is applied to a generally healthy population. It includes health promotion, illness prevention, and protection against disease. Within this area lie many of nursing's independent functions, which are intended to decrease individuals' vulnerability to illness and strengthen their capacity to withstand stressors. Direct nursing care activities in this area include the following:

▼ Teaching about principles of mental health
▼ Effecting changes in living conditions, poverty levels, and education

Fig. 1-1 Elements of the psychiatric nursing role.

▼ Educating consumers in such areas as normal growth and development and sex education

▼ Making appropriate referrals before mental disorder occurs, based on assessment of potential stressors and life changes

▼ Helping patients in a general hospital setting to avoid future psychiatric problems

▼ Working with families to support family members and group functioning

▼ Becoming active in community and political activities related to mental health

SECONDARY. **Secondary prevention** involves reducing illness by early detection and treatment of the problem. Direct nursing care activities in this area include the following:

▼ Intake screening and evaluation services

▼ Home visits for preadmission or treatment services

▼ Emergency treatment and psychiatric services in the general hospital

▼ Creation of a therapeutic milieu

▼ Supervision of patients receiving medication

▼ Suicide prevention services

▼ Counseling on a time-limited basis

▼ Crisis intervention

▼ Psychotherapy with individuals, families, and groups of various ages

▼ Intervention with communities and organizations based on an identified problem

TERTIARY. **Tertiary prevention** involves reducing the residual impairment or disability resulting from an illness. Direct nursing care activities in this area include the following:

▼ Promoting vocational training and rehabilitation

▼ Organizing aftercare programs for patients discharged from psychiatric facilities to ease their transition from the hospital to the community

▼ Providing partial hospitalization options for patients

In addition to direct nursing care functions, psychiatric nurses engage in indirect activities that affect all three levels of prevention. These activities include teaching nursing personnel in various educational programs; administrating in mental health settings; supervising personnel to improve the quality of mental health services; consulting with colleagues, other professionals, consumer groups, community caregivers, and local and national agencies; and researching clinical problems in the field.

> **?** *Where do you think most mental health dollars are spent: primary, secondary, or tertiary prevention activities? Would you change this in any way?*

Continuum of Care

Traditional settings for psychiatric nurses include psychiatric facilities, community mental health centers, psychiatric units in the general hospital, residential facilities, and private practice. With health-care reform, however, alternative

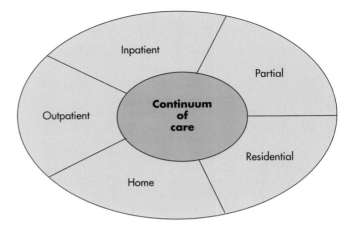

Fig. 1-2   Continuum of mental health care settings.

treatment settings have emerged throughout the continuum of mental health care. Specifically, hospitals are being transformed into integrated clinical systems that provide inpatient care, partial hospitalization or day treatment, residential care, home care, and outpatient or ambulatory care (Fig. 1-2). Current community-based treatment settings have expanded to include foster care or group homes, hospices, visiting nurse associations, home health agencies, emergency departments, nursing homes, shelters, primary care clinics, schools, prisons, industrial settings, managed care facilities, and health maintenance organizations.

The new opportunities for psychiatric nursing practice that are emerging throughout the continuum of mental health care are exciting. However, they require that nurses be proactive in demonstrating their expertise in designing interventions, planning programs, implementing treatment strategies, and managing staff in a variety of traditional and nontraditional settings. Psychiatric nurses who have always worked in inpatient settings may feel a sense of bereavement when they leave the inpatient setting and move into the community.[15] They may also need to learn new skills to make the transition to community-based psychiatric nursing practice.

Psychiatric nurses must also continue to demonstrate flexibility, accountability, and self-direction as they move into these expanding areas of practice. The continuum of care is not only providing new treatment options for patients, but also creating an opportunity for psychiatric nurses to evaluate the full range of their patients' coping responses. With this information, psychiatric nurses can implement primary, secondary, and tertiary prevention functions from a holistic, biopsychosocial perspective.

Competent Caring

There are three domains of contemporary psychiatric nursing practice: **direct care, communication,** and **management.** Within these overlapping domains of practice, the *teaching, coordinating, delegating,* and *collaborating* func-

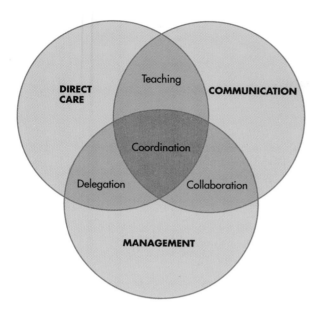

Fig. 1-3 Psychiatric nursing practice.

tions of the role are expressed (Fig. 1-3). Often the communication and management domains of practice are overlooked when discussing the psychiatric nursing role. However, these integrating activities are critically important and very time-consuming aspects of a nurse's role. They are also likely to become even more important in a reformed health-care system that places emphasis on efficient patient triage and management.

It is possible to further delineate the activities engaged in by psychiatric nurses within each of these three domains. Box 1-4 lists the range of specific nursing activities that could be enacted by a psychiatric nurse in each area. Not all nurses participate in all these activities, but they do reflect the current nature and scope of competent caring functions performed by psychiatric nurses. In addition, psychiatric nurses are able to

▼ Make culturally sensitive biopsychosocial health assessments

▼ Design and implement treatment plans for patients and families with complex health problems and comorbid conditions

▼ Engage in case management activities such as organizing, accessing, negotiating, coordinating, and integrating services and benefits for individuals and families

▼ Provide a "health-care map" for individuals, families, and groups to guide them to community resources for mental health, including the most appropriate providers, agencies, technologies, and social systems

▼ Promote and maintain mental health and manage the effects of mental illness through teaching and counseling

▼ Provide care for the physically ill with psychological problems and the psychiatrically ill with physical problems

▼ Manage and coordinate systems of care integrating the needs of patients, families, staff, and regulators

Psychiatric nurses need to be able to articulate both the general and the specific aspects of their practice to patients, families, other professionals, administrators, and legislators. Only when such skills are identified will psychiatric nurses be able to ensure their appropriate roles, adequate compensation for the nursing care provided, and the most efficient use of scarce human resources in the delivery of mental health care.

LEVEL OF PERFORMANCE

The description of psychiatric nursing roles and activities indicates a wide variation in levels of performance. Not all psychiatric nurses can perform each of these functions. Individual nurses have primary responsibility and accountability for their own practice; one aspect of this accountability is that nurses define and adhere to the legitimate scope of their practice. Four major factors—laws, qualifications, setting, and personal initiative—play a part in determining the roles engaged in by each nurse.

Laws

Laws are the primary factor affecting the level of nursing practice. Each state has its own nursing practice act, which regulates entry into the profession and defines the legal limits of nursing practice that must be adhered to by all nurses and addresses aspects of advanced practice.[24] Currently there are three general patterns of nursing practice acts: regulatory acts, expanded definition acts, and delegatory acts. Nurses must be familiar with the nursing practice act of their state and define and limit their practice accordingly.

Qualifications

A nurse's qualifications include education, work experience, and certification. Two levels of psychiatric–mental health clinical nursing practice have been identified[2]:

1. **Psychiatric–Mental Health Registered Nurse (RN)** is a licensed RN who has a baccalaureate degree in nursing and demonstrated clinical skills in psychiatric–mental health nursing exceeding those of a new nurse in the specialty area. Certification is the formal process that validates the nurse's area of clinical expertise. The letter *C* placed after the *RN* (that is, *RN, C*), designates basic level certification status. Many professional nurses who contribute to the care of psychiatric patients have diplomas or associate degrees, are entry-level RNs, or are new to the specialty. These nurses practice in conjunction with psychiatric–mental health registered nurses and are responsible for adhering to the specialty practice standards designated by the profession.

2. **Psychiatric–Mental Health Advanced Practice Registered Nurse (APRN)** is a licensed RN who has a master's degree, at a minimum, and a depth of knowledge of psychiatric nursing theory, supervised clinical practice, and competence in advanced psychiatric nursing skills. Doc-

Box **1-4** *Domains of Psychiatric Nursing Practice*

DIRECT CARE ACTIVITIES

Activity therapy
Advocacy
Aftercare follow-up
Behavioral treatments
Case consultation
Case management
Cognitive treatments
Community assessment
Community education
Compliance counseling
Crisis intervention
Discharge planning
Environmental change
Environmental safety
Family interventions
Group work
Health promotion
Health teaching
High-risk assessment
Holistic interventions
Home visits
Individual counseling
Informed consent acquisition
Intake screening and evaluation
Medication administration
Medication management
Mental health promotion
Mental illness prevention
Milieu therapy
Nutritional counseling
Parent education
Patient triage
Physical assessment
Physiological treatments
Play therapy
Prescription of medications
Providing environmental safety
Psychoeducation
Psychosocial assessment
Psychotherapy
Rehabilitation counseling
Relapse prevention
Research implementation
Self-care activities
Social skills training
Somatic treatments
Stress management
Supporting social systems

COMMUNICATION ACTIVITIES

Clinical case conferences
Developing treatment plans
Documentation of care
Forensic testimony
Interagency liaison
Peer review
Preparing reports
Professional nurse networking
Staff meetings
Transcribing orders
Treatment team meetings
Verbal reports of care

MANAGEMENT ACTIVITIES

Budgeting and resource allocation
Clinical supervision
Collaboration
Committee participation
Community action
Consultation/liaison
Contract negotiation
Coordination of services
Delegation of assignments
Grant writing
Marketing and public relations
Mediation and conflict resolution
Mentorship
Needs assessment and forecasting
Organizational governance
Outcomes management
Performance evaluations
Policy and procedure development
Practice guidelines formulation
Professional presentations
Program evaluation
Program planning
Publications
Quality improvement activities
Recruitment and retention activities
Regulatory agency activities
Risk management
Software development
Staff scheduling
Staff and student education
Strategic planning
Unit governance
Utilization review

torally prepared psychiatric–mental health nurses in advanced practice have both a master's degree and a doctorate in nursing or a related field. The letters *CS*, placed after the *APRN* (that is, *APRN, CS*) designate that the nurse is a *certified specialist* in psychiatric–mental health nursing.

Another qualification is the nurse's work experience. Although work experience does not replace education, it does provide an added and necessary dimension to the nurse's level of competence and ability to function therapeutically.

Practice Setting

Psychiatric nurses may practice in settings that vary widely in purpose, type, location, and administration. They may be employed by an organization or self-employed in private practice.[13] Nurses employed by an organization are paid for their services on a salaried or fee-for-service basis. Most nurses work in such organized settings.[5,21] The administrative policies of these organizations can either foster or limit full use of the psychiatric nurse's potential. Nurses who are self-employed are paid for their services through third-party payment and direct patient fees. Some self-employed advanced practice psychiatric nurses maintain staff privileges with institutional facilities.

The role of a nurse in any psychiatric–mental health setting depends on the following:
▼ Philosophy, mission, values, and goals of the treatment setting
▼ Definitions of mental health and mental illness that prevail in the setting
▼ Needs of the consumers of the mental health services
▼ Number of clinical staff available and the services they are able to provide
▼ Organizational structure and reporting relationships in the setting
▼ Consensus reached by the mental health care providers regarding their respective roles and responsibilities
▼ Resources and revenues available to offset the cost of care needed and provided
▼ Presence of strong nursing leadership and mentorship

A supportive environment for psychiatric nurses is one in which there is open and honest communication among staff, interdisciplinary respect, recognition of nurses' contributions, nursing involvement in decision making about both clinical care and the work environment, delegation of nonessential nursing tasks, opportunity to expand into new roles and responsibilities, and the encouragement of involvement in professional psychiatric nursing activities and organizations.

> **?** *What specific characteristics would you look for in an organization to see whether it promoted professional psychiatric nursing practice?*

Personal Initiative

The personal competence and initiative of the individual nurse determine one's interpretation of the nursing role and the success of its implementation. The importance of this final factor should not be ignored; without a realization of clinical competence and the assumption of professional initiative, the psychiatric nurse's performance is significantly limited.

One strategy for enhancing the personal growth and competence of the psychiatric nurse is the use of support groups. Examples of the purposes and possible activities of a professional support group are described in Table 1-1.

Psychiatric nurses would also benefit from networking. Networks are groups of people drawn together by common concerns to support and help one another. Networks range from informal friendships and small groups providing contacts to larger open groups providing emotional support and local and national organizations representing one's specialty.

Forming networks can help nurses to unite and to value their profession. Networking at the staff nurse level is crucial to the unity and survival of the profession. It would help nurses to care for one another and to influence their work environment. A supportive staff network can extend beyond affirmation of the members and become an influential force in managing daily nursing care.

TABLE **1-1** *Psychiatric Nursing Support Groups*

PURPOSE	RELATED ACTIVITIES
PROVIDE PRACTICAL HELP AND PROFESSIONAL FEEDBACK	Review clinical cases
	Evaluate documentation methods
	Analyze staff interactions and performance
	Develop nursing practice guidelines
	Discuss changes in one's role and work setting
	Describe successful interventions
	Share difficult work experiences
EXCHANGE INFORMATION AND STIMULATE IDEAS	Report on conferences attended
	Distribute articles for reading and discussion
	Update on new developments in psychiatric nursing
	Review nursing practice legislative issues
	Share organizational policies and procedures
	Suggest resources for new information and problem solving

What networks do you have in your life at this time and how do they help you? How might professional networks help you when you graduate?

PSYCHIATRIC NURSING AGENDA

Psychiatric nursing will continue to grow and evolve in the years ahead. There are more than 77,000 registered nurses working in the mental health services in the United States.[28] Health care reform, patient and family needs, scientific developments, economic realities, and societal expectations will shape the future roles and functions of psychiatric nurses. To best meet the challenges of the next decade, psychiatric nurses need to focus their energies on three areas: outcome evaluation, leadership skills, and political action.

Outcome Evaluation

Psychiatric nurses must be able to identify, describe, and measure the effect of the care they provide patients, families, and communities. Psychiatric nursing is largely absent from the numerous published reviews of the cost effectiveness of nursing, and the specialty has found it difficult to articulate the nature and outcomes of psychiatric nursing care.[22] This has made it difficult to justify the need for psychiatric nurses in various treatment settings and to give psychiatric nurses the recognition they deserve.

Outcome studies documenting the quality, cost, and effectiveness of psychiatric nursing practice must become an important part of the psychiatric nursing agenda.[3] These studies should be able to stand up to the scientific review of the broader community of mental health professionals by being methodologically sound, empirically grounded, and replicated across the continuum of psychiatric care settings. The results of these studies can then be used to provide a shared knowledge base, formulate practice guidelines, provide data on clinical course, and better manage treatment outcomes. The nature and process of outcome evaluation are discussed in detail in Chapter 8.

Focusing on ways to critically evaluate the outcomes of psychiatric nursing activities is a task for every psychiatric nurse regardless of role, qualifications, or practice setting. Psychiatric nurse clinicians, educators, administrators, and researchers all must assume responsibility for answering the question, "What difference does psychiatric nurse caring make?"

Leadership Skills

Psychiatric nurses need knowledge and strategies that enable them to exercise leadership and management in their work.[19] Such leadership has an effect on the care patients receive; it also strengthens and expands the contribution of psychiatric nursing to the larger health-care system.

Psychiatric nurses must use their leadership skills and work as change agents to a greater degree than they are doing now. Mental health consumers need adequate, humane, and socially acceptable care. To this end nurses can initiate change; assist by supporting, participating, or implementing change; engage in joint ventures for planned change; and evaluate completed change. To do so, the psychiatric nurse needs to take risks. The nurse must develop the ability to calulate potential risks surrounding the implementation of the change and then decide whether these risks are worth taking.

Another form of leadership is demonstrated by nurses who join their specialty organization. The American Psychiatric Nurses Association (APNA), located in Washington, D.C., is the largest organization of psychiatric nurses in the United States, representing more than 3000 registered nurses in both basic and advanced psychiatric nursing practice. Mental health nurses in Canada belong to the Canadian Federation of Mental Health Nurses. By joining together for a common goal, psychiatric nurses have increased power in the health-care delivery system. Organizations such as APNA can also provide informational networks to psychiatric nurses that are essential for consumer advocacy, continuing education, and effective political action.

Talk with some of the staff nurses who work in psychiatry and ask whether they know about APNA. Are they members? If not, what would it take for them to join?

Political Action

Psychiatric nurses can be significant forces in the process of shaping the future of society. To do so, they must learn to use their power and resources in the political arena—truly one of the most important targets for nursing action. Increasing psychiatric nurses' political awareness and skills is necessary to bring about needed changes in the mental health care delivery system, which is discussed in Chapter 8. Specifically, the political empowerment of nursing involves the development of three dimensions.[14]

▼ Raising consciousness of sociocultural realities
▼ Developing positive self-esteem
▼ Acquiring political skills

These dimensions are overlapping and interactive and form the basis of political action by psychiatric nurses that is respectful of others, confirming of self, and directed toward the common good.

It is essential that psychiatric nurses recognize the value and legitimacy of their own voices. They need to understand the many connections between their work and that of society. This will allow nurses to mobilize their workplaces and effect community and legislative action. To do so effectively, nurses must become educated in legislative and regulatory processes.[31] They need to be involved in political campaigns and testify in legislative hearings.

Psychiatric nurses can then assert their right to an equitable share of the resources, given the value of the services they provide. Passive acceptance of decisions made by legislators, insurers, managed care companies, and other professionals should be replaced with proactive strategies. In this way the psychiatric nursing agenda of the next decade will advance nursing's commitment to caring in a mental health delivery system that is fair, sensitive, and responsible in meeting the biopsychosocial needs of patients, families, and communities.

Summary

1. Psychiatric nursing began to emerge as a profession in the late nineteenth century, and by the twentieth century it had evolved into a specialty with unique roles and functions.
2. Psychiatric nursing is an interpersonal process that promotes and maintains behaviors that contribute to integrated functioning. The patient may be an individual, family, group, organization, or community. The three domains of psychiatric nursing practice are direct care, communication, and management.
3. Four factors that help to determine the level of a psychiatric nurse's performance are the law, the nurse's qualifications, the practice setting, and the nurse's personal initiative.
4. To best meet the challenges of the next decade, psychiatric nurses need to focus their energies on three areas: outcome evaluation, leadership skills, and political action.

your **INTERNET**
connection

American Psychiatric Nurses Association
http://www.apna.org

Canadian Federation of Mental Health Nurses
http://www.iciweb.com/cfmhn

Chapter Review Questions

1. Fill in the blanks.

A. _____ is known as the first American psychiatric nurse.

B. The book *Interpersonal Relations in Nursing* was written by _____.

C. Reducing the residual impairment resulting from an illness is called _____ prevention.

D. The three domains of contemporary psychiatric nursing practice are _____, _____, and _____.

E. The two levels of psychiatric–mental health clinical practice are _____ and _____.

F. The largest organization of psychiatric nurses in the United States is the _____.

2. Identify whether the following statements are true (T) or false (F).

A. ___ The psychiatric nursing role evolved from primarily physical care to clinical competence based on interpersonal techniques and use of the nursing process.

B. ___ Psychiatric nursing was the first specialty to establish generalist (C) and specialty (CS) certification.

C. ___ Reducing illness by early detection and treatment is called primary prevention.

D. ___ Working to support family members at the time of a death is an example of a secondary prevention activity.

E. ___ Intake screening and evaluation services are examples of primary prevention activities.

F. ___ Psychiatric hospitals are being transformed into integrated clinical systems that provide the full continuum of psychiatric care.

G. ___ Each state has its own nursing practice act that regulates entry into the profession and defines the legal limits of nursing practice.

H. ___ Fewer than 50,000 registered nurses work in mental health services in the United States.

I. ___ There are numerous published studies of the nature and outcome of psychiatric nursing care.

3. Provide short answers for the following questions.

A. Why was the development of psychotropic drugs such an important development in the treatment of people with mental illness?

B. List the five core mental health disciplines.

C. Identify the six dimensions of the nurse-patient partnership that characterize today's psychiatric nursing role.

D. Call up APNA on the World Wide Web at **http:/www.apna.org.** Do you think that having information about this nursing organization on the Internet is a service to psychiatric nurses?

REFERENCES

1. Abraham I, Fox J, Cohen B: Integrating the bio into the bio-psychosocial understanding and treating biological phenomena in psychiatric–mental health nursing, *Arch Psychiatr Nurs* 6:296, 1992.
2. American Nurses' Association: *A statement on psychiatric–mental health clinical nursing practice and standards of psychiatric–mental health clinical nursing practice*, Washington, DC, 1994, The Association.
3. Baradell J: Cost-effectiveness and quality of care provided by clinical nurse specialists, *J Psychosoc Nurs* 32:21, 1994.
4. Bennett A, Eaton J: The role of the psychiatric nurse in the newer therapies, *Am J Psychiatry* 108:167, 1951.
5. Betrus P, Hoffman A: Psychiatric–mental health nursing: career characteristics, professional activities, and client attributes of members of the American Nurses' Association Council of Psychiatric Nurses, *Issues Ment Health Nurs* 13:39, 1992.
6. Billings C: Psychiatric–mental health nursing professional progress notes, *Arch Psychiatr Nurs* 7:174, 1993.
7. Doona M: At least as well cared for . . . Linda Richards and the mentally ill, *Image* 16:51, 1984.
8. Editorial, *Am J Nurs* 40:23, 1940.
9. Goering P: Psychiatric nursing and the context of care, *New Dir Ment Health Serv* 58:3, 1993.
10. Hayes A: Psychiatric nursing: what does biology have to do with it? *Arch Psychiatr Nurs* 9:216, 1995.
11. Hays D: Suggested clinical practice of psychiatric nurses recorded in the literature between 1946 and 1958. In *Psychiatric nursing 1946 to 1974: a report on the state of the art*, New York, 1975, American Journal of Nursing Co.
12. Jones M: *The therapeutic community: a new treatment method in psychiatry*, New York, 1953, Basic Books.
13. Lambert V, Lambert C: Advanced practice nurses: starting an independent practice, *Nurs Forum* 31:11, 1996.
14. Mason D, Backer B, Georges C: Toward a feminist model for the political empowerment of nurses, *Image* 23:72, 1991.
15. Massey P: Institutional loss: an examination of a bereavement reaction in 22 mental nurses losing their institution and moving into the community, *J Adv Nurs* 16:573, 1991.
16. McBride A: Psychiatric–mental health nursing in the twenty-first century. In McBride A, Austin J, editors: *Psychiatric–mental health nursing: integrating the behavioral and biological sciences*, Philadelphia, 1996, WB Saunders.
17. McEnany G: Psychobiology and psychiatric nursing: a philosophical matrix, *Arch Psychiatr Nurs* 5:255, 1991.
18. McMahan E, Hoffman K, McGee G: Physician-nurse relationships in clinical settings: a review and critique of the literature, 1966-1992, *Med Care Rev* 51:83, 1994.
19. McNeese-Smith D: The impact of leadership on productivity, *Nurs Econ* 10:393, 1992.
20. Mellow J: Nursing therapy, *Am J Nurs* 68:2365, 1968.
21. Merwin E, Fox J: Cost-effective integration of mental health professions, *Issues Ment Health Nurs* 13:139, 1992.
22. Merwin E, Mauck A: Psychiatric nursing outcome research: the state of the science, *Arch Psychiatr Nurs* 9:311, 1995.
23. Olson T: Fundamental and special: the dilemma of psychiatric–mental health nursing, *Arch Psychiatr Nurs* 10:3, 1996.
24. Pearson L: Annual update of how each state stands on legislative issues affecting advanced nursing practice, *Nurse Pract* 22:18, 1997.
25. Peplau H: *Interpersonal relations in nursing*, New York, 1952, GP Putnam's Sons.
26. Peplau H: Interpersonal techniques: the crux of psychiatric nursing, *Am J Nurs* 62:53, 1962.
27. Pothier P, Stuart G, Puskar K, Babich K: Dilemmas and directions for psychiatric nursing in the 1990s, *Arch Psychiatr Nurs* 4:284, 1990.
28. Redick R et al: *Data highlights on: human resources of mental health organizations: United States, selected years, 1972-1990, Mental Health Statistical Note 216*, Washington, DC, August 1995, Department of Health and Human Services, Center for Mental Health Services.
29. Stuart G: Recent changes and current issues in psychiatic nursing. In McCloskey J, editor: *Current issues in nursing*, St Louis, 1997, Mosby.
30. Tudor G: Sociopsychiatric nursing approach to intervention in a problem of mutual withdrawal on a mental hospital ward, *Psychiatry* 15:193, 1952.
31. Wakefield M: Influencing the legislative process, *Nurs Econ* 8:188, 1990.
32. Weiss MO: The skills of psychiatric nursing, *Am J Nurs* 47:174, 1947.

ANNOTATED SUGGESTED READINGS

*Cohen S et al: Stages of nursing's political development: where we've been and where we ought to go, *Nurs Outlook* 44:259, 1996.
  Provides a framework for the political development of nursing that is useful for analyzing past accomplishments and planning future actions that will enhance nursing and improve health care.
*Dyer J et al: The psychiatric-primary care nurse practitioner: a futuristic model for advanced practice psychiatric-mental health nursing, *Arch Psychiatr Nurs* 11:2, 1997.
  Presents an overview of a graduate program that prepares the psychiatric nurse practitioner for a unique role providing comprehensive health care in both psychiatric and primary care settings.
*Lambert V, Lambert C: Advanced practice nurses: starting an independent practice, *Nurs Forum* 31:11, 1996.
  Thorough and informative discussion of the various elements needed by advanced practice nurses to start an independent practice.
*Lanza M: Power and leadership in psychiatric nursing: directions for the next century, Part I and II, *Perspect Psychiatr Care* 33:5, 1997.
  These timely articles address power and leadership and conclude that empowerment of nursing rests with individuals committed to changing the societal problems holding the profession back.
*McBride A: Psychiatric-mental health nursing in the twenty-first century. In McBride A, Austin J, eds: *Psychiatric-mental health nursing: integrating the behavioral and biological sciences*, Philadelphia, 1996, WB Saunders.
  Highlights the way in which psychiatric nurses are moving toward an agenda for practice that is based on research and scholarship. Advanced reading that makes a unique contribution to the field.
*Merwin E, Mauck A: Psychiatric nursing outcome research: the state of the science, *Arch Psychiatric Nurs* 9:311, 1995.
  Reviews outcome studies in psychiatric nursing conducted between 1989 and 1994. Critiques the state of the science and offers suggestions for improving work in the area.
*Pieranunzi V: The lived experience of power and powerlessness in psychiatric nursing: a Heideggerian hermeneutical analysis, *Arch Psychiatr Nurs* 11:155, 1997.
  The results of this study of the meaning power and powerlessness as they relate to nursing practice will lead nurses to strategies for empowerment of both themselves and their patients.

*Nursing reference.

© 1998 M.C. Escher/Cordon Art, Baarn, Holland.

Therapeutic Nurse-Patient Relationship

Gail W. Stuart

When we treat man as he is, we make him worse than he is. When we treat him as if he already were what he potentially could be, we make him what he should be.
Johann Wolfgang von Goethe

LEARNING OBJECTIVES

After studying this chapter the student should be able to:

▼ State the goals of the therapeutic nurse-patient relationship

▼ Discuss six personal qualities a nurse needs to be an effective helper

▼ Describe the nurse's tasks and possible problems in the four phases of the relationship process

▼ Analyze the levels of communication, two models of the communication process, and therapeutic communication techniques

▼ Describe how the nurse uses each of the responsive dimensions in a therapeutic relationship

▼ Describe how the nurse uses each of the action dimensions in a therapeutic relationship

▼ Define therapeutic impasses and identify nursing interventions to deal with them

▼ Demonstrate increasing effectiveness in using therapeutic relationship skills to produce a therapeutic outcome

TOPICAL OUTLINE

Characteristics of the Relationship
Personal Qualities of the Nurse
  Awareness of Self
  Clarification of Values
  Exploration of Feelings
  Serving as Role Model
  Altruism
  Ethics and Responsibility
Phases of the Relationship
  Preinteraction Phase
  Introductory, or Orientation, Phase
  Working Phase
  Termination Phase
Facilitative Communication
  Verbal Communication
  Nonverbal Communication
  The Communication Process
  Therapeutic Communication Techniques
Responsive Dimensions
  Genuineness
  Respect
  Empathic Understanding
  Development of Empathy
  Concreteness
Action Dimensions
  Confrontation
  Immediacy
  Nurse Self-Disclosure
  Emotional Catharsis
  Role Playing
Therapeutic Impasses
  Resistance
  Transference
  Overcoming Resistance and Transference
  Countertransference
  Boundary Violations
Therapeutic Outcome

he therapeutic nurse-patient relationship is a mutual learning experience and a corrective emotional experience for the patient. It is based on the underlying humanity of nurse and patient, with mutual respect and acceptance of ethnocultural differences. In this relationship the nurse uses personal attributes and clinical techniques in working with the patient to bring about insight and behavioral change.

CHARACTERISTICS OF THE RELATIONSHIP

The goals of a therapeutic relationship are directed toward the patient's growth and include the following:
▼ Self-realization, self-acceptance, and an increased genuine self-respect
▼ A clear sense of personal identity and an improved level of personal integration
▼ An ability to form an intimate, interdependent, interpersonal relationship with a capacity to give and receive love
▼ Improved functioning and increased ability to satisfy needs and achieve realistic personal goals

To achieve these goals, various aspects of the patient's life experiences are explored. The nurse allows the patient to express thoughts and feelings and relates these to observed and reported actions, clarifying areas of conflict and anxiety. The nurse identifies and maximizes the patient's ego strengths and encourages socialization and family relatedness. Together the patient and nurse correct communication problems and modify maladaptive behavior patterns by testing new patterns of behavior and more adaptive coping mechanisms.

In the nurse-patient relationship differing values are respected. The two communicate through a dialogue, or discussion, not a monologue, affirming the patient's reality and worth and allowing the patient to more fully define ego identity. In Box 2-1 Rogers[32] summarizes the characteristics of a helping relationship that facilitate growth. All nurses working with patients may ask themselves these questions; their answers largely determine the progress of the relationship.

The therapeutic nurse-patient relationship is complex.[36] This chapter examines the personal qualities of the nurse as helper, the phases of the relationship, facilitative communication, responsive and action dimensions, therapeutic impasses, and the therapeutic outcome (Fig. 2-1). Each of these factors influences the nurse's effectiveness.

PERSONAL QUALITIES OF THE NURSE

Nurses as helpers must be therapeutic because their goal is to enable the patient to adapt as a unique individual to the stress being experienced. The self is the key helping tool the nurse can use, so self-analysis is the first building block in providing quality nursing care.

Box **2-1** *Characteristics that Facilitate Growth in Helping Relationships*

▼ Can I be in some way that will be perceived by the other person as trustworthy, as dependable, or consistent in some deep sense?
▼ Can I be expressive enough as a person that what I am will be communicated unambiguously?
▼ Can I let myself experience positive attitudes toward this other person—attitudes of warmth, caring, liking, interest, and respect?
▼ Can I be strong enough as a person to be separate from the other?
▼ Am I secure enough within myself to permit him his separateness?
▼ Can I let myself enter fully into the world of his feelings and personal meaning and see these as he does?
▼ Can I be acceptant of each facet of the other person that he presents to me? Can I receive him as he is? Can I communicate this attitude? Or can I only receive him conditionally, acceptant of some aspects of his feelings and silently or openly disapproving of others?
▼ Can I act with sufficient sensitivity in the relationship that my behavior will not be perceived as a threat?
▼ Can I free him from the threat of external evaluation?
▼ Can I meet this other individual as a person who is in the process of *becoming*, or will I be bound by his past and my past?

From Rogers C: *On becoming a person,* Boston, 1961, Houghton Mifflin.

Is it possible that nurses are alienated from their true selves and therefore do not allow patients to express all aspects of themselves? Jourard believes that the socialization process into nursing may destroy the nurse's spontaneity, and that the nurse may become detached from the real self:

Now, if a nurse is afraid or even ignorant of her own self, she is highly likely to be threatened by a patient's real-self expressions. . . . A nurse who is more aware of the breadth and depth of her own real self is in a much better position to empathize with her patients and to encourage (or at least not block) their self-disclosures.[15]

Research suggests some essential qualities needed to help others. These qualities are necessary characteristics for all nurses who wish to be therapeutic. They also help the nurse set goals for future growth.

Awareness of Self

Effective helpers must be able to answer the question, Who am I? Nurses who care for the biological, psychological, and sociocultural needs of patients see a broad range of human experiences; they must learn to deal with anxiety, anger, sadness, and joy in helping patients throughout the health-illness continuum.

Self-awareness is a key component of the psychiatric nursing experience. The nurse's goal is to achieve authentic,

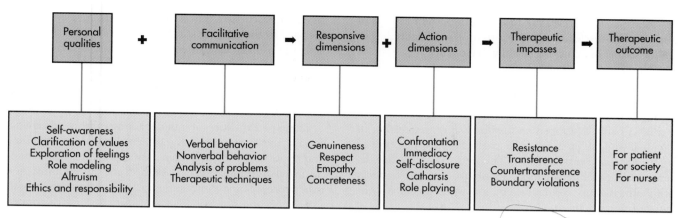

Fig. 2-1   Elements affecting the nurse's ability to be therapeutic.

open, and personal communication. The nurse must be able to examine personal feelings, actions, and reactions. A firm understanding and acceptance of self allow the nurse to acknowledge a patient's differences and uniqueness.

Campbell[5] has identified a holistic nursing model of self-awareness that consists of four interconnected components: psychological, physical, environmental, and philosophical.

▼ The *psychological* component includes knowledge of emotions, motivations, self-concept, and personality. Being psychologically self-aware means being sensitive to feelings and to external elements that affect those feelings.

▼ The *physical* component is the knowledge of personal and general physiology, as well as of bodily sensations, body image, and physical potential.

▼ The *environmental* component consists of the sociocultural environment, relationships with others, and knowledge of the relationship between humans and nature.

▼ The *philosophical* component is the sense of life having meaning. A personal philosophy of life and death may or may not include a superior being, but it does take into account responsibility to the world and the ethics of behavior.

Together these components provide a model that can be used to promote the self-awareness and self-growth of nurses and the patients for whom they care.

INCREASING SELF-AWARENESS. No one ever completely knows the inner self, as shown in the Johari Window (Fig. 2-2). Quadrant 1 is the open quadrant; it includes the behaviors, feelings, and thoughts known to the individual and others. Quadrant 2 is called the blind quadrant because it includes all the things that others know but the individual does not know. Quadrant 3 is the hidden quadrant; it includes the things about the self that only the individual knows. Quadrant 4 is the unknown quadrant, containing aspects of the self unknown to the individual and to others. Taken together, these quadrants represent the total self. The

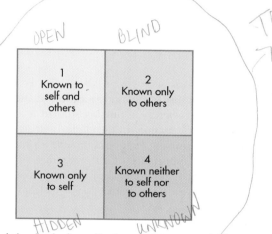

Fig. 2-2   Johari window. Each quadrant, or windowpane, describes one aspect of the self.

following three principles help clarify how the self functions in this representation:

▼ A change in any one quadrant affects all other quadrants.

▼ The smaller quadrant 1, the poorer the communication.

▼ Interpersonal learning means that a change has taken place, so quadrant 1 is larger and one or more of the other quadrants are smaller.

The goal of increasing self-awareness is to enlarge the area of quadrant 1 while reducing the size of the other three quadrants. To increase self-knowledge, it is necessary to **listen to the self.** This means the individual allows genuine emotions to be experienced, identifies and accepts personal needs, and moves the body in free, joyful, and spontaneous ways. It includes exploring personal thoughts, feelings, memories, and impulses.

The next step in the process is to reduce the size of quadrant 2 by **listening to and learning from others.** Knowledge of self is not possible alone. As we relate to others, we broaden our perceptions of self, but such learning requires active listening and openness to the feedback others provide.

The final step involves reducing the size of quadrant 3 by

self-disclosing, or revealing to others important aspects of the self. Self-disclosure is both a sign of personality health and a means of achieving healthy personality.

Compare *A* and *B* of Fig. 2-3. *A* represents a person with little self-awareness whose behaviors and feelings are limited in variety and scope. *B,* however, shows an individual with great openness to the world. Much of this person's potential is being developed and realized. *B* represents an individual who has an increased capacity for experiences of all kinds: joy, hate, work, and love. This person also has few defenses and can interact more spontaneously and honestly with others. This configuration is a worthy goal for the nurse to pursue.

 What does your Johari window look like?

THE NURSE AND SELF-GROWTH. People often assume that because a nursing education includes courses in the behavioral sciences, a nursing student is able to use self in a therapeutic manner in the clinical setting. However, although most nursing textbooks include a paragraph or two stressing the importance of self-awareness in nursing care, the process and components of the nurse's self-growth are seldom described. The patient's self-concept is also often treated in a cursory way. These omissions give an implicit message to the nursing student: Self-analysis is commendable, but a token assessment will do. This message is reinforced by the student's curriculum, which is burdened with tasks and reports that allow little time for quiet thought leading to self-growth.

Nurses need time to explore and define the many facets of their personalities. If nursing does involve perceiving, feeling, and thinking, nursing students should have the time and opportunity to study their own experiences. Authenticity in relationships must be learned and nurses must first experience openness and authenticity in relationships with instructors and supervisors. The student and instructor can participate in a relationship that accepts and respects their individual differences. Instructors can help students by facilitating students' self-awareness, increasing their level of functioning, stimulating more self-direction, and enabling students to cope more effectively with stressors.

Authenticity also involves being open to self-exploration of thoughts, needs, emotions, values, defenses, actions, communications, problems, and goals. Nursing students have many new experiences that provide opportunities for self-learning. Feelings related to these experiences should be focused on and discussed. Students might enter clinical settings with high ideals and unrealistic images. Perhaps they view nurses as all-knowing, all-caring "miracle workers." During initial encounters students may feel fearful, anxious, and inadequate, wondering how a nurse acquires the necessary knowledge. Nursing students might devalue their abilities and feel like an imposition on patients. At another time nurses may identify closely with patients and feel anger at the impersonal system and unresponsive personnel. The feelings involved in all of these situations should be identified, verbalized, and analyzed. Only then can nurses resolve them in a constructive manner.

A career in nursing is not easy if the nurse is still in adolescence. As a nurse the student will be faced with many adult situations, such as disease, bizarre behavior, complex problems, and even death, when most of the student's friends are focusing on youth, enjoyment, and the future. This might alienate the nurse from some friends. Feelings of loneliness and sadness should be shared so that the nurse can work through personal needs.

Throughout the growing process the student needs the support and guidance of a noncritical but challenging instructor. Together they can analyze the student's behavior and the student can assess personal strengths and limitations. Also, it is often helpful to share these experiences with a peer group. Students can empathize, critique, and support each other as they learn more about themselves.

Finally, objective self-examination is not easy or pleasant, particularly when findings conflict with self-ideals. However, like many painful experiences, discovering self-awareness presents a challenge: to accept self-limitations or to change the behaviors that support them.

Fig. 2-3 Johari windows showing varying degrees of self-awareness.

> ? *Think back over the courses you have taken in your nursing program. How much time and emphasis were placed on developing your self-awareness as a person and a nurse?*

Clarification of Values

Nurses should be able to answer the question, What is important to me? Awareness helps the nurse to be honest and to avoid the unethical use of patients to meet personal needs. Nurses should avoid the temptation to use patients for the pursuit of personal satisfaction or security. If nurses do not have sufficient personal fulfillment, they should realize it; their sources of dissatisfaction should then be clarified so that they do not interfere with the success of the nurse-patient relationship.

VALUE SYSTEMS. Values are concepts that are formed as a result of life experiences with family, friends, culture, education, work, and relaxation. The word *value* has positive connotations, because it denotes worth or significance. Yet values also imply negatives. If we value honesty, then it follows that we do not value dishonesty. People are likely to hold strong values related to religious beliefs, family ties, sexual preferences, other ethnic groups, and sex role beliefs.

One of the many challenges facing psychiatric nurses today is the need to provide care for patients from many different ethnocultural backgrounds. Because the goals of treatment are determined greatly by beliefs and values, establishing a therapeutic relationship with patients from different ethnocultural backgrounds requires particular skill and sensitivity (see Chapter 7).

Value systems also provide the framework for many daily decisions and actions. By being aware of their value systems, nurses can identify situations in which value systems are in conflict. Clarification of values also provides some insurance against the tendency to project values onto other people. Many therapeutic relationships test the nurse's values. For example, a patient may describe a sexual behavior that the nurse finds unacceptable; a patient may talk about divorce, whereas the nurse may strongly believe that marriage contracts should not be broken; or a patient may be a "born-again" Christian, but the nurse may not believe in God or religion.

> ? *Can a nurse empathize with and help a patient solve a problem while maintaining personal values that are different from the values of the patient?*

VALUE CLARIFICATION PROCESS. Understanding personal values may be promoted by *value clarification*, which allows individuals to discover their values by assessing, exploring, and determining what those values are and what priority they hold in decision-making processes. Value clarification does not determine what the individual's values should be or what values should be followed. To prevent the imposition of values, value clarification focuses exclusively on the *process* of valuing, or on how people come to have the values they have.

Seven criteria are used to determine a value. These criteria should be considered in relation to a person's strongest value and tested against the person's own definition of a value. The seven criteria are broadly grouped into the three steps listed in Box 2-2.

The three criteria of choosing rely on the person's cognitive abilities, the two criteria of prizing emphasize the emotional or affective level, and the two criteria of acting have a behavioral focus.

A change takes place when certain contradictions are perceived in the person's value system. To eliminate the distress that follows such a realization, the person realigns values to coincide with the new view of self.

THE MATURE VALUING PROCESS. The valuing process in the mature person is complex and the choices are often perplexing and difficult. There is no guarantee that the choice made will prove to be self-actualizing. The valuing process in the mature person has the following characteristics[18]:

▼ It is fluid and flexible, based on the particular moment and the degree to which the moment is enhancing, enriching, and actualizing. Values are continually changing.

▼ The valuing experience is tied to a particular time and experience.

▼ Personal experience provides the value information. Although the person is open to all evidence obtained from other sources, outside evidence is not considered as important as subjective responses. The psychologically mature adult trusts and uses personal wisdom.

▼ In the valuing process the person is open to the immediacy of experience, trying to sense and clarify all its complex meanings. However, the immediate impact of the moment is colored by experiences from the past and conjecture about the future.

Exploration of Feelings

It is often assumed that helping others requires complete objectivity and detachment. This is definitely not true.

Box **2-2** *Steps in the Value Clarification Process*

CHOOSING	1. Freely
	2. From alternatives
	3. After thoughtful consideration of the consequences of each alternative
PRIZING	4. Cherishing, being happy with the choice
	5. Willing to affirm the choice publicly
ACTING	6. Doing something with the choice
	7. Repeatedly, in some pattern of life

Complete objectivity and detachment describe someone who is unresponsive, false, unapproachable, impersonal, and self-alienated—qualities that block the establishment of a therapeutic relationship. Rather, nurses should be open to, aware of, and in control of their feelings so that they can be used to help patients.

The feelings that nurses have serve an important purpose. They are barometers for feedback about themselves and their relationships with others. In helping others, nurses have many feelings: elation at seeing a patient improve, disappointment when a patient regresses, distress when a patient refuses help, anger when a patient is demanding or manipulative, and power when a patient expresses strong dependence on the nurse.

Nurses who are open to their feelings understand how they are responding to patients and how they appear to patients. The nurse's feelings are valuable clues to the patient's problems. For example, despite the patient's statement that "things are going real well," the nurse might perceive a strong sense of despair or anger. So too, the nurse should be aware of the feelings conveyed to the patient. Is the nurse's mood one of hopelessness or frustration? If nurses view feelings as barometers and feedback instruments, their effectiveness as helpers will improve.

Serving as Role Model

Formal helpers have a strong influence on those they help, and nurses function as role models for their patients. Research has shown the power of role models in molding socially adaptive, as well as maladaptive, behavior. Thus a nurse has an obligation to model adaptive and growth-producing behavior. If a nurse has a chaotic personal life, it will show in the nurse's work with patients, decreasing the effectiveness of care. The nurse's credibility as a helper will also be questioned. The nurse may object, saying that it is possible to separate one's personal life from one's professional life, but in caring for patients this is not possible because psychiatric nursing *is* the therapeutic use of self.

However, this is not to imply that the nurse must conform totally to local community norms or must live an idyllic, placid life. What is suggested is that the effective nurse has a fulfilling and satisfying personal life that is not dominated by conflict, distress, or denial, and that the nurse's approach to life conveys a sense of growing and adapting.

 Who have been role models in your life and what qualities did you most admire about them?

Altruism

It is vital for nurses to have an answer to the question, Why do I want to help others? Obviously, an effective helper is interested in people and tends to help out of a deep love for humanity. It is also true that everyone seeks a certain

amount of personal satisfaction and fulfillment from work. The goal is to maintain a balance between these two needs. Helping motives can become destructive tools in the hands of naive or zealous users.

Another danger lies in subscribing to an extreme view of altruism. Altruism is concern for the welfare of others. It does not mean that an altruistic person should not expect adequate compensation and recognition or must practice denial or self-sacrifice. Only if personal needs have been appropriately met can the nurse expect to be maximally therapeutic.

Finally, a sense of altruism can also apply to more general social support and change motives. Activist helpers are needed who are primarily concerned with changing social conditions to meet human welfare needs. One goal of all helping professionals should be to create a people-serving and growth-facilitating society. Thus a legitimate and necessary role for the nurse is to work to change the larger structure and process of society in ways that will promote the individual's health and well-being.

Ethics and Responsibility

Personal beliefs about people and society can serve as conscious guidelines for action. The Code for Nurses reflects common values regarding nurse-patient relationships and responsibilities and serves as a frame of reference for all nurses in their judgments about patient welfare and social responsibility. For psychiatric nurses, decisions are a part of daily functioning. Responsible ethical choice involves accountability, risk, commitment, and justice.

Related to the nurse's sense of ethics is the need to assume responsibility for behavior. This involves knowing limitations and strengths and being accountable for them. As a member of a health care team, the nurse has ready access to the knowledge and expertise of other people; these resources should be used appropriately.

PHASES OF THE RELATIONSHIP

A vital characteristic of the nurse-patient relationship is the sharing of behaviors, thoughts, and feelings. Table 2-1 identifies eight general components of relationships and contrasts social superficiality and therapeutic intimacy with these components. These elements evolve as the nurse moves through the various phases of the therapeutic relationship with the patient. Four sequential phases of the relationship process have been identified: preinteraction phase; introductory, or orientation, phase; working phase; and termination phase. Each phase builds on the preceding one and is characterized by specific tasks.

In the past, when the majority of psychiatric care was delivered in the hospital and patients stayed in inpatient units for weeks or even months, nursing students were able to form long-term relationships with patients and experience each phase of the nurse-patient relationship. With current changes in the delivery of mental health care, however,

TABLE **2-1** *Contrast between Social Superficiality and Therapeutic Intimacy*

COMPONENTS OF RELATIONSHIP	SOCIAL SUPERFICIALITY	THERAPEUTIC INTIMACY
Mutual self-disclosure	Variable	Patient: self-disclosure; nurse: self-disclosure that promotes treatment goals
Focus of conversation	Unknown to participants	Known to nurse and patient
Pertinence of topic	Social, business, generalized, impersonal	Personal and relevant to nurse and patient
Relationship of experiences to topic	Sense of uninvolvement and use of indirect knowledge	Sense of involvement and use of direct knowledge
Time orientation	Past and future	Present
Use of feelings	Mutual sharing of feelings discouraged	Patient sharing of feelings encouraged by nurse
Recognition of individual worth	Not acknowledged	Fully acknowledged
Termination	Open-ended	Specified, agreed upon and honored

Modified from Coad-Denton A: Therapeutic superficiality and intimacy. In Longo D, Williams R, eds: *Psychosocial nursing: assessment and intervention,* New York, 1978, Appleton-Century-Crofts.

nursing students often see patients for only a couple of visits and most often in community settings. Nonetheless, it is important for nurses to understand how nurse-patient relationships progress and the elements that enable them to help patients attain identified treatment outcomes. In addition, as nursing services continue to move into the community and home, nurses are often responsible for caring for many patients over long periods of time. Finally, the elements of a therapeutic nurse-patient relationship apply to all clinical settings. Thus nurses working in medical, surgical, obstetrical, oncology, and other specialty areas also need to understand and be able to use therapeutic nurse-patient relationship skills.

Preinteraction Phase

CONCERNS OF NEW NURSES. The preinteraction phase begins before the nurse's first contact with the patient. The nurse's initial task is one of self-exploration. In the first experience working with psychiatric patients, the nurse brings the misconceptions and prejudices of the general public in addition to feelings and fears common to all novices (Box 2-3). An overriding one usually is anxiety or nervousness, which is common to new experiences of any kind. A related feeling is ambivalence or uncertainty; nurses may see the need for working with these patients but feel unclear about their ability.

The informal nature of psychiatric settings may also threaten the nurse's role identity. A common first reaction among students is a feeling of panic when they realize that they "can't tell the patients from the staff." It is also unsettling for many students to give up their uniforms, stethoscopes, and scissors. Doing so dramatically emphasizes that, in this nursing setting, the most important tools are the ability to communicate, empathize, and solve problems. Without a tangible physical illness to care for, new students are likely to feel acutely self-conscious and hesitant about introducing themselves to a patient and initiating a conversation.

BOX **2-3** *Common Concerns of Psychiatric Nursing Students*

▼ Acutely self-conscious
▼ Afraid of being rejected by the patients
▼ Anxious because of the newness of the experience
▼ Concerned about personally overidentifying with psychiatric patients
▼ Doubtful of the effectiveness of skills or coping ability
▼ Fearful of physical danger or violence
▼ Insecure in therapeutic use of self
▼ Suspicious of psychiatric patients stereotyped as "different"
▼ Threatened in nursing role identity
▼ Uncertain about ability to make a unique contribution
▼ Uncomfortable about the lack of physical tasks and treatments
▼ Vulnerable to emotionally painful experiences
▼ Worried about hurting the patient psychologically

Many nurses express feelings of inadequacy and fears of hurting or exploiting the patient. They worry about saying the wrong thing, which might drive the patient "over the brink;" with their limited knowledge and experience, they doubt that they will be of any value. They wonder how they can help or whether they can really make a difference. Some nurses perceive the plight of psychiatric patients as hopeful; others perceive it as hopeless.

A common fear of nurses is related to the stereotype of psychiatric patients as violent. Because this is the picture portrayed by the media, many nurses are afraid of being physically hurt by a patient's outburst of aggressive behavior. Some nurses fear being psychologically hurt by a patient through rejection or silence. A final fear is related to nurses' questioning their own mental health status. Nurses may fear mental illness and worry that exposure to psychiatric patients might cause them to lose their own grasp on reality. Nurses who are working on their own crises of identity and intimacy may fear overidentifying with patients and using patients to meet their own needs. It has also been noted that students in their psychiatric nursing rotation may use humor as a cognitive coping strategy.[38]

The following clinical example contains many of the feelings and fears expressed by one nursing student in the preinteraction phase of self-analysis, as reported in the notes from her diary of her psychiatric rotation.

Clinical Example When first told that I would have a clinical psychiatric nursing experience, I received this information with a blank mind. Mental overload, denial, repression, or whatever it was made me hear the words but put off dealing with it. Then, when given a chance to sort through my thoughts and feelings, I thought more about what this experience would entail. Having never been personally involved with any people who were psychiatrically ill before, I was unable to rely on past personal experiences. I did, however, have quite a "pseudoknowledge base" from my novels, television, and movie encounters. Do places like the hospitals in *One Flew Over the Cuckoo's Nest* or *Frances* really exist? Was the portrayal of *Sybil* accurate? How could I possibly help someone who has so many problems, like the boy in *Ordinary People*? After all, I have problems myself. I'm afraid these thoughts have raised more questions in me than they have answered.

Three things scare me the most about this experience. First, I feel that the behavior of a psychiatric patient is quite unpredictable. Would they get violent or aggressive without any warning? Would this aggression be directed toward me? If so, would I be hurt? Did I provoke them and was I wrong in my actions that caused this sudden shift?

The second, related to the first, is my feeling of inadequacy. I've been exposed to physically ill people and have learned how to respond to them. But, the psychiatrically ill are almost totally alien to me. How can I help? What if I do, or say, or infer something they could take offense to? Will I have the patience to persevere? I just don't know, and my not knowing makes me even more nervous.

My third fear is how seeing and being in contact with the psychiatrically ill will affect me. Although I know it's not contagious, the more exposure and knowledge I acquire in this area, the more I may begin to doubt my own stability and sanity. I mean, adolescence hasn't been easy for me, and I feel like I'm just now beginning to see things more clearly and feel better about myself. Will this experience stir up any past fears and doubts and, if so, how will I handle it? I am beginning to realize that there is a fine line between health and illness and that the psychiatric patients we'll meet have been unable to gather enough resources from within to cope with their problems. Help, reassurance, and understanding are their needs. I'm hoping I can help them . . . but I'm just not sure.

> **?** *What feelings, fears, and fantasies do you have about working with psychiatric patients?*

SELF-ASSESSMENT. Experienced nurses benefit by analyzing aspects of their practice. They may ask themselves the following questions:

▼ Do I label patients with the stereotype of a group?
▼ Is my need to be liked so great that I become angry or hurt when a patient is rude, hostile, or uncooperative?
▼ Am I afraid of the responsibility I must assume for the relationship, and do I therefore limit my independent functions?
▼ Do I cover feelings of inferiority with a front of superiority?
▼ Do I require sympathy, warmth, and protection so much that I err by being too sympathetic or too protective toward patients?
▼ Do I fear closeness so much that I am indifferent, rejecting, or cold?
▼ Do I need to feel important and keep patients dependent on me?

The self-analysis that characterizes the preinteraction phase is a necessary task. To be effective, nurses should have a reasonably stable self-concept and an adequate amount of self-esteem. They should engage in constructive relationships with others and face reality to help patients do likewise. If they are aware of and in control of what they convey to their patients verbally and nonverbally, nurses can function as role models. To do this, however, some nurses abandon their personal strengths and assume a facade of "professionalism" that alienates their authentic self. This facade immobilizes them and acts as a barrier to establishing mutuality with patients.

Additional tasks of this phase include gathering data about the patient if information is available and planning for the first interaction with the patient. The nursing assessment is begun, but most of the work related to it is accomplished with the patient in the second phase of the relationship. Finally, nurses review general goals of a therapeutic relationship and consider what they have to offer patients.

Introductory, or Orientation, Phase

It is during the introductory phase that the nurse and patient first meet. One of the nurse's primary concerns is to find out why the patient sought help and whether this was voluntary (Table 2-2). Determining the patient's reason directly influences the establishment of mutuality between the nurse and the patient. The reason for seeking help forms the basis of the nursing assessment and helps the nurse to focus on the patient's problem and to determine patient motivation.

FORMULATING A CONTRACT. The tasks in this phase of the relationship are to establish a climate of trust, understanding, acceptance, and open communication and formulate a contract with the patient. Box 2-4 lists the elements of a nurse-patient contract. The contract begins with the introduction of the nurse and patient, exchange of names, and explanation of roles. An explanation of roles includes the responsibilities and expectations of the patient and

TABLE **2-2** *Analysis of Why Patients Seek Psychiatric Help*

REASONS FOR PATIENTS' SEEKING PSYCHIATRIC CARE	APPROPRIATE NURSING APPROACH	SAMPLE RESPONSE
ENVIRONMENTAL CHANGE FROM HOME TO TREATMENT SETTING		
They desire protection, comfort, rest, and freedom from demands of their home and work environments.	Emphasize the ability of the environment to provide protection and comfort while the healing process of the mind occurs.	"Tell me what it was at home/on the job that made you feel so overwhelmed."
NURTURANCE		
They wish for someone to care for them, cure their illnesses, and make them feel better.	Acknowledge their nurturance needs and assure them that help and caring are available.	"I'm here to help you feel better."
CONTROL		
They are aware of their destructive impulses to themselves or others but lack internal control.	Offer sources of internal control such as medication, if prescribed; reinforce external controls available through the staff.	"We're not going to let you hurt yourself. Tell us when these thoughts come to mind and someone will stay with you."
PSYCHIATRIC SYMPTOMS		
They describe symptoms of depression, nervousness, or crying spells, and actively want to help themselves.	Ask for clarification of symptom and strive to understand life experiences of patient.	"I can see that you're nervous and upset. Can you tell me about how things are at home/on the job so I can better understand?"
PROBLEM SOLVING		
They identify a specific problem or area of conflict and express desire to reason it out and change.	Help patient look at problem objectively; use problem-solving process.	"How has drinking affected your life?"
ADVISED TO SEEK HELP		
Family member, friend, or health professional has convinced them to get treatment. They may feel angry, ambivalent, or indifferent.	Confirm facts surrounding seeking of help and set appropriate limits.	"I see that you're angry about being here. I hope that after we talk you might feel differently."

Modified from Burgess A, Burns J: Why patients seek care, *Am J Nurs* 73:314, 1973.

nurse, with a description of what the nurse can and cannot do. This is followed by a discussion of the purpose of the relationship, in which the nurse emphasizes that the focus of it will be the patient and the patient's life experiences and areas of conflict. Because establishing the contract is a mutual process, it is a good opportunity to clarify misperceptions held by either the nurse or patient.

With the "who" and the "why" determined, the "where, when, and how long" are discussed. Where will they meet? How often and how long will the meetings be? The conditions for termination should be reviewed and may include a specified length of time, attainment of mutual goals, or the discharge of the patient from the treatment setting. The issue of confidentiality is an important one to discuss with the patient at this time. Confidentiality involves the disclosure of certain information only to another specifically authorized person (see Chapter 9). This means that information about the patient will be shared only with people who are directly involved in the patient's care in the form of verbal reports and written notes. This is important in providing for the continuity and comprehensiveness of patient care and should be clearly explained to the patient.

Establishing a contract is a mutual process in which the

Box **2-4** *Elements of a Nurse-Patient Contract*

▼ Names of individuals
▼ Roles of nurse and patient
▼ Responsibilities of nurse and patient
▼ Expectations of nurse and patient
▼ Purpose of the relationship
▼ Meeting location and time
▼ Conditions for termination
▼ Confidentiality

patient participates as fully as possible. In some cases, such as with the psychotic or severely withdrawn patient, the patient may be unable to fully participate, and the nurse must take the initiative in establishing the contract. As the patient's contact with reality increases, the nurse should review the elements of the contract when appropriate and strive to attain mutuality.

EXPLORING FEELINGS. Both the nurse and patient may experience some degree of discomfort and nervousness in the introduction phase. The nurse may be well aware of personal anxieties and fears, but the patient's difficulty in receiving help may be overlooked:

▼ It may be difficult to see or admit one's difficulties, first to oneself and then to another.
▼ It is not easy to trust or be open with strangers.
▼ Sometimes problems seem too large, too overwhelming, or too unique to share them easily.
▼ Sharing personal problems with another person can threaten one's sense of independence, autonomy, and self-esteem.
▼ Solving a problem involves thinking about some things that may be unpleasant, viewing life realistically, deciding on a plan of action, and then, most important, carrying out whatever it takes to bring about a change. These activities place great demands on the patient's energy and commitment.

In summary, the tasks of the nurse in the orientation phase of the relationship include the following:

▼ To explore the patient's perceptions, thoughts, feelings, and actions
▼ To identify pertinent patient problems
▼ To define mutual, specific goals with the patient

It is not uncommon for patients to display manipulative or testing behavior during this phase as they explore the nurse's consistency and intent. Patients may also show temporary regressions as reactions to a large amount of self-disclosure in a previous meeting or to the anxiety created by a particular topic.

Finally, nurses need to be flexible in anticipating the length of time required for the orientation phase, particularly for patients who have a serious and persistent mental illness. Nurses might expect that more time will be required for patients who have had many or lengthy hospitalizations in the past.[12] Also, staff changes affect the patient's ability to progress in the therapeutic relationship and should be taken into account when planning nursing care.

> **?** *Talk with a friend or family member who has sought counseling. Why did they do so? Did anything make them uncomfortable about asking for help? What did the clinician do to put them at ease?*

Working Phase

Most of the therapeutic work is carried out during the working phase. The nurse and the patient explore relevant stressors and promote the development of insight in the patient by linking perceptions, thoughts, feelings, and actions. These insights should be translated into action and integrated into the individual's life experiences. The nurse helps the patient to master anxieties, increase independence and self-responsibility, and develop constructive coping mechanisms. Actual behavioral change is the focus of this phase.

Patients usually display resistance behaviors during this

Box 2-5 *Criteria for Determining Patient Readiness for Termination*

▼ The patient experiences relief from the presenting problem.
▼ The patient's functioning has improved.
▼ The patient has increased self-esteem and a stronger sense of identity.
▼ The patient uses more adaptive coping responses.
▼ The patient has achieved the planned treatment outcomes.
▼ An impasse has been reached in the nurse-patient relationship that cannot be worked through.

phase because it encompasses the greater part of the problem-solving process. As the relationship develops, the patient begins to feel close to the nurse and responds by clinging to defensive structures and resisting the nurse's attempts to move forward. An impasse or plateau in the relationship results. Because overcoming resistance behaviors is crucial to the progress of the therapeutic relationship, these behaviors are discussed in greater detail later in this chapter.

Termination Phase

Termination is one of the most difficult but most important phases of the therapeutic nurse-patient relationship. During the termination phase learning is maximized for both the patient and the nurse. It is a time to exchange feelings and memories and to evaluate mutually the patient's progress and goal attainment. Levels of trust and intimacy are heightened, reflecting the quality of the relationship and the sense of loss experienced by both nurse and patient. Box 2-5 lists criteria that can be used to determine whether the patient is ready to terminate.

Although agreement between the patient and the nurse is desirable in deciding when to terminate, this is not always possible. Nonetheless, the nurse's tasks during this phase revolve around establishing the reality of the separation. Together the nurse and the patient review the progress made in treatment and the attainment of specified goals. Feelings of rejection, loss, sadness, and anger are expressed and explored. It may be helpful to prepare the patient for termination by decreasing the number of visits, incorporating others into the meetings, or changing the location of the meetings. The reasons behind a change should be clarified so that the patient does not interpret it as rejection by the nurse. It may also be appropriate to make referrals at this time for continued care or treatment.

It is evident that successful termination requires that the patient work through feelings related to separation from emotionally significant people. The nurse can help by allowing the patient to experience and feel the effects of the anticipated loss, to express the feelings generated by the impending separation, and to relate those feelings to former symbolic or real losses.

REACTIONS TO TERMINATION. Patients may react to termination in a variety of ways. They may deny the separation or deny the significance of the relationship and impending separation, perhaps causing the inexperienced nurse to feel rejected by the patient. Patients may express anger and hostility, either overtly and verbally or covertly through lateness, missed meetings, or superficial talk. These patients may view the termination as personal rejection, which reinforces their negative self-concept. Patients who feel rejected by the nurse may terminate prematurely by rejecting the nurse before the nurse rejects them. It is also common to see the patient regress to an earlier behavior pattern, hoping to convince the nurse not to terminate because of the need for further help.

The nurse should be aware of these possible reactions and discuss them with the patient if they occur. For some patients termination is a critical therapeutic experience because many of their past relationships were terminated in a negative way that left them with unresolved feelings of abandonment, rejection, hurt, and anger. All these patient reactions have a similar goal: to cope with the anxiety about the separation and to delay the termination process.

The patient's response will be significantly affected by the nurse's ability to remain open, sensitive, empathic, and responsive to the patient's changing needs. Helping the patient to work and grow through the termination process is an essential goal of each relationship. It is important that the nurse does not deny the reality of it or allow the patient to repeatedly delay the process. Particularly in this phase of the relationship, as in the orientation phase, the patient will be testing the nurse's judgment, and the issues of trust and acceptance will again predominate.

During the course of the relationship and with the attainment of nursing goals, the nurse and the patient come to realize a growing sense of equality. The impending termination therefore can be as difficult for the nurse as for the patient. Nurses who can begin reviewing their thoughts, feelings, and experiences will be more aware of personal motivation and more responsive to patients' needs.

Learning to bear the sorrow of the loss while working positive aspects of the relationship into one's life is the goal of termination for both the nurse and the patient. At the conclusion of the relationship students can be assisted in guided reflection to gain insight into their psychiatric nursing clinical experience and to better appreciate the roles of psychiatric nurses.[21] The major tasks of the nurse during each phase of the nurse-patient relationship are summarized in Table 2-3.

> **?** *Watch the movies* The Dream Team *and* Awakenings *and discuss how staff-patient relationships are portrayed.*

TABLE **2-3** *Nurse's Tasks in Each Phase of the Relationship Process*

PHASE	TASK
Preinteraction	Explore own feelings, fantasies, and fears
	Analyze own professional strengths and limitations
	Gather data about patient when possible
	Plan for first meeting with patient
Introductory, or orientation	Determine why patient sought help
	Establish trust, acceptance, and open communication
	Mutually formulate a contract
	Explore patient's thoughts, feelings, and actions
	Identify patient's problems
	Define goals with patient
Working	Explore relevant stressors
	Promote patient's development of insight and use of constructive coping mechanisms
	Overcome resistance behaviors
Termination	Establish reality of separation
	Review progress of therapy and attainment of goals
	Mutually explore feelings of rejection, loss, sadness, and anger and related behaviors

FACILITATIVE COMMUNICATION

Communication can either facilitate the development of a therapeutic relationship or serve as a barrier to its development. According to Carkhoff and Truax,[8] "The central ingredient of the psychotherapeutic process appears to be the therapist's ability to *perceive and communicate,* accurately and with sensitivity, the feelings of the patient and the meaning of those feelings."

Every individual communicates constantly from birth until death. All behavior is communication, and all communication affects behavior. This reciprocity is central to the communication process. The relevance of communication to nursing practice is threefold:
▼ Communication is the vehicle for establishing a therapeutic relationship.
▼ Communication is the means by which people influence the behavior of another and thus is critical to the successful outcome of nursing intervention.
▼ Communication is the relationship itself because without it, a therapeutic nurse-patient relationship is impossible.

Verbal Communication

Communication takes place on two levels: verbal and nonverbal. Verbal communication occurs through words, spoken or written. Taken alone, verbal communication can convey factual information accurately and efficiently. It is a less effective means of communicating feelings or nuances of meaning, and it represents only a small segment of total human communication.

Another limitation of verbal communication is that words can change meanings with different cultural groups or subgroups because words have both denotative and connotative meanings. The denotative meaning of a word is its actual or concrete meaning. For example, the denotative meaning of the word *bread* is "a food made of a flour or grain dough that is kneaded, shaped, allowed to rise, and baked." The connotative meaning of a word, in contrast, is its implied or suggested meaning. Thus the word *bread* can conjure up many different connotative or personalized meanings. Depending on a person's experiences, preferences, and present frame of reference, he or she may think of French bread, rye bread, a sesame seed roll, or perhaps pita bread. When used as slang, "give me some bread" may be understood to mean "give me some money." Thus the characteristics of the speaker and the context in which the phrase is used influence the specific meaning of verbal language.

When communicating verbally, many people assume that they are "on the same wavelength" as the listener. But because words are only symbols, they seldom mean precisely the same thing to two people. And if the word represents an abstract idea such as "depressed" or "hurt," the chance of misunderstanding or misinterpretation may be great. In addition, many feeling states or personal thoughts cannot be put into words easily. Nurses should strive to overcome these obstacles by checking their interpretation and incorporating information from the nonverbal level as well.

Finally, today more than ever before nurses need to be prepared to communicate effectively with people from a variety of ethnocultural backgrounds. Sensitivity to several language phenomena may help the psychiatric nurse to establish transcultural psychotherapeutic relationships based on mutual understanding. For example, psychiatric patients may be evaluated in their second language, yet competence in a second language varies depending on the individual and the stage of illness. In addition, cultural nuances may be embedded in language in ways that are not readily conveyed in translation, even when the patient uses similar words in the second language. Patients may also use a second language as a form of resistance in order to avoid intense feelings or conflicting thoughts, and events that may have occurred before a person learned English may not be easily communicated. Finally, the nurse-patient relationship can be affected by the attitudes toward verbalizing thoughts and feelings that are part of the patient's culture.[9,28]

The effective psychiatric nurse uses verbal communication sensitively as a tool to promote mutual respect based on understanding and acceptance of cultural differences. The nurse may also communicate respect for the patient's dialect by adapting to the patient's linguistic style by using fewer words, more gestures, or more expressive facial behaviors.

> **?** *Think of someone you know whose cultural background is different from your own. How does this difference influence your verbal and nonverbal communication?*

Nonverbal Communication

Nonverbal communication includes everything that does not involve the spoken or written word, including all of the five senses. It has been estimated that about 7% of meaning is transmitted by words, 38% is transmitted by paralinguistic cues such as voice, and 55% is transmitted by body cues. Nonverbal communication is often unconsciously motivated and may more accurately indicate a person's meaning than the words being spoken. People tend to verbalize what they think the receiver wants to hear, whereas less acceptable or more honest messages may be communicated simultaneously by the nonverbal route.

TYPES OF NONVERBAL BEHAVIORS. There are various types of nonverbal behaviors. Each of these is greatly influenced by sociocultural background. Following are brief descriptions of five categories of nonverbal communication.

Vocal cues, or paralinguistic cues, include all the nonverbal qualities of speech. Some examples include pitch, tone of voice, quality of voice, loudness or intensity, rate and rhythm of talking, and unrelated nonverbal sounds such as laughing, groaning, and nervous coughing and sounds of hesitation ("um," "uh"). These are particularly vital cues of emotion and can be powerful conveyors of information.

Action cues are body movements, sometimes referred to as kinetics. They include automatic reflexes, posture, facial expression, gestures, mannerisms, and actions of any kind. Facial movements and posture can be particularly significant in interpreting the speaker's mood.

Object cues are the speaker's intentional and nonintentional use of all objects. Dress, furnishings, and possessions all communicate something to the observer about the speaker's sense of self. These cues often are consciously selected by the individual, however, and therefore may be chosen to convey a certain look or message. Thus they can be less accurate than other types of nonverbal communication.

Space provides another clue to the nature of the relationship between two people. It must be examined based on sociocultural norms and customs. The following four zones of space are evident interpersonally in North America:

▼ Intimate space: up to 18 inches. This allows for maximum interpersonal sensory stimulation.
▼ Personal space: 18 inches to 4 feet. This is used for close

relationships and touching distance. Visual sensation is improved over the intimate range.

▼ Social-consultative space: 9 to 12 feet. This is less personal and less dependent. Speech must be louder.

▼ Public space: 12 feet and over. This is used in speech giving and other public occasions.

Observation of seating arrangements and use of space by patients can yield valuable information to the nurse, with implications for both the nurse's assessment of the patient and the way the nursing intervention should be implemented.

Touch involves both personal space and action. It is possibly the most personal of the nonverbal messages. A person's response to it is influenced by setting, cultural background, type of relationship, gender of communicators, ages, and expectations. Touch can express a striving to connect with another person as a way of meeting them or relating to them. It can be a way of expressing or conveying something to another, such as concern, empathy, or caring. Touch can also be used receptively as a way of sensing, perceiving, or allowing someone else to leave an imprint on another person. Finally, there is the concept of *therapeutic touch,* or the nurse's laying hands on or close to the body of an ill person for the purpose of helping or healing. Touch continues to be the imprimatur of nursing and the therapeutic, comforting effects of touch are often overlooked. Thus touch is a universal and basic aspect of all nurse-patient relationships. It is often described as the first and most fundamental means of communication.

INTERPRETING NONVERBAL BEHAVIOR. All types of nonverbal messages are important, but interpreting them correctly can present numerous problems for the nurse. It is impossible to examine nonverbal messages out of context, and sometimes the individual's body reveals a number of different and perhaps conflicting feelings at the same time.

Sociocultural background is also a major influence on the meaning of nonverbal behavior. In the United States, with its diverse ethnic communities, messages between people of different upbringing can easily be misinterpreted. For instance, Arabs tend to stand closer together when speaking, and Orientals tend to touch more; touching in the United States is often minimized because of perceived sexual overtones or because of Puritan heritage. Because the meaning attached to nonverbal behavior is so subjective, it is essential that the nurse check its meaning.

Nurses should respond to the variety of nonverbal behaviors displayed by the patient, particularly voice inflections, body movements, gestures, facial expression, posture, and physical energy levels. Incongruent behavior and contradictory messages are especially significant. The nurse should refer to the specific behavior observed and attempt to confirm its meaning and significance with the patient. If the nurse's words and tone of voice indicate a true attempt at clarification, suggestion, or validation, a defensive reaction usually is not evoked. The nurse may use three kinds of responses to the patient:

1. Questions or statements intended to increase the patient's awareness
2. Content reflections
3. Statements reflecting the nurse's responsiveness

These possible responses are illustrated in the following interaction.

THERAPEUTIC DIALOGUE

PATIENT *(Shifting nervously in his chair, eyes scanning the room and avoiding the nurse) What . . . what do you want to talk about today?*

NURSE RESPONSE #1 *I sense that you are uncomfortable talking to me. Could you describe to me how you are feeling?*

NURSE RESPONSE #2 *You're not sure what we should be talking about, and you want me to start us off?*

NURSE RESPONSE #3 *You look very nervous, and I can feel those same feelings in me as I sit here with you.*

The nurse's first possible response is a reflection and attempt to validate the patient's feelings. The purpose is to communicate to the patient the nurse's awareness of his feelings, to show acceptance of those feelings, and to request that he focus on them and elaborate on them. The nurse's second possible response deals with the content of the patient's message. The nurse is clarifying what the patient is trying to say. The third possible response shares both the nurse's perception of her patient's feelings and the personal disclosure that she has some of those same feelings. This type of response may help the patient feel that the nurse accepts and understands him.

IMPLICATIONS FOR NURSING CARE. Besides responding to patients' nonverbal behavior, nurses should incorporate aspects of it into patient care. For example, patients who resist closeness will be disturbed by entry into their intimate space. The nurse can assess the patient's level of spatial tolerance by observing the distance the patient maintains with other people. The nurse can also be alert to the patient's response during their interaction. If the nurse sits next to the patient on the sofa, does the patient get up and move to a chair? If the nurse moves closer to the patient does the patient move away to reestablish the original space? Sometimes increasing the space between the nurse and an anxious patient can reduce the anxiety enough to allow the interaction to continue. A decrease in the distance the patient chooses to maintain from others may indicate a decrease in interpersonal anxiety.

Territoriality is a concept related to personal distance and personal space. Territoriality is the drive to acquire and defend territory to ensure species survival. Whenever possible, the hospitalized patient should be allowed to control and enjoy personal possessions and private living space, no matter how small or seemingly insignificant. Specifically, patients should be allowed free access to their personal living quarters and, as soon as possible, free access out of doors or at least out of the unit itself. Patients can also be encouraged to wear personal clothing and keep personal items.

Other spatial parameters are also interpersonally significant. Height may communicate dominance and submission. Communication is made easier when both participants are at similar levels. Orientation of the participants' body positions is also significant. Face-to-face confrontation is more threatening than oblique (sideways) body positions. The physical setting also has spatial meaning. A patient may be more comfortable in her own room than in the therapist's office, unless the patient's room is also defined as a bedroom. Control issues are minimized when communication takes place in a neutral area that belongs to neither participant. However, people quickly identify their own turf, even in unfamiliar settings, and then begin to exert ownership rights over this area. A common example of this can be observed in most college classes. At the beginning of the semester, people sit randomly, but the arrangement usually solidifies after a couple of classes. Students then feel vaguely annoyed if they arrive in class to find another person in "their seat." They are experiencing an invasion of personal space. Awareness of a patient's use of space can add a further dimension to the nurse's ability to understand the patient.

Touch also should be used judiciously. Patients who are sensitive to issues of closeness may experience a casual touch as an invasion or an invitation to intimacy, which may be even more frightening. Physical contact with a person of the same gender may be experienced by the patient as a homosexual advance and may precipitate a panic reaction. If procedures requiring physical contact must be carried out, careful explanations should be given both before and during the procedure. In addition, the nurse should always be aware of the potential for touch to be interpreted in a sexual way, thus creating problems related to the sexual conduct of the nurse within the nurse-patient relationship.

Despite these issues, a study on the use of nonprocedural touch shows that it is a significant part of inpatient psychiatric nursing.[37] The researcher found that several elements went into the nurse's decision to touch a patient, such as the patient's age, gender, and needs and the nurse's knowledge of the patient. The nurse's feelings, beliefs, intuition, personal style, and expectations of the nursing role were also considered. Patient needs identified by the nurses included the following:

▼ Establishing contact with the patient
▼ Enhancing communication
▼ Communicating caring, interest, and recognition
▼ Providing reassurance and comfort

Results of this study indicate that touch is a part of psychiatric nursing practice and suggest the importance of studying patients' perceptions of its use and potential benefits and drawbacks.

Finally, nurses must be aware of not only patients' nonverbal cues but also of their own. The nurse's nonverbal cues can communicate interest, respect, and genuineness or disinterest, lack of respect, and an impersonal facade. Affiliative nonverbal behaviors include smiles, positive head nods, gestures, eye contact, and a forward body lean. Nurses need to be aware of a spectrum of nonverbal behaviors in their patients and themselves and incorporate them judiciously into their care.

> **?** *Follow the treatment team making patient rounds and observe body positions. Are staff and patients at eye level? What personal space is maintained? Is touch used at all?*

The Communication Process

Human communication is a dynamic process influenced by the psychological and physiological conditions of the participants. Ruesch[34] has identified three elements of the process: perception, evaluation, and transmission. **Perception** occurs by activation of the sensory end organs of the receiver. The impulse is then transmitted to the brain. Human beings are most reliant on visual and auditory stimuli for communications. Vision is the primary means of perceiving nonverbal communication, and hearing responds primarily to verbal stimuli. However, if one of the primary senses is dysfunctional, the other functional senses accommodate to improve the person's perception. For instance, the deaf person can learn sign language and lip-reading, which rely on vision, to compensate for not being able to hear the verbal component of communication.

When the sensory impulse reaches the brain, **evaluation** takes place. Personal experience is the matrix within which new experience is evaluated. If the person encounters a new experience for which there is no frame of reference, confusion results. Evaluation results in two responses: a cognitive response related to the informational aspect of the message and an affective response related to the relationship aspect of the message. Most messages stimulate both types of responses.

When the evaluation of the message is complete, **transmission** takes place. This is perceived by the sender as feedback, thereby influencing the continued course of the communication cycle. It is impossible not to transmit some kind of feedback. Even lack of any visible response is feedback to the sender that the message did not get through, was considered unimportant, or was an undesirable interruption. Feedback stimulates perception, evaluation, and transmission by the original sender. The cycle continues until the participants agree to end it or one participant physically leaves the setting.

Theoretical models of the communication process show visual relationships more clearly and can aid in finding and correcting communication breakdowns or problems. Two models, the structural and transactional analysis models, are presented, because each gives a valuable but different perspective on the communication process.

STRUCTURAL MODEL. The structural model has five functional components in communication: the sender, the message, the receiver, the feedback, and the context (Fig. 2-4). The **sender** is the originator of the message. The **message** is the information that is transmitted from the sender to the receiver. The **receiver** is the perceiver of the message. The verbal or behavioral response of the receiver is **feedback** to the sender. The fifth structural element of communication is the **context.** This is the setting in which the communication takes place. Knowledge of context is necessary to understand the meaning of the communication. For example, the phrase "I don't understand what you mean" may have different meanings in the context of a classroom or a courtroom. Context involves more than the physical setting for communication, however. It also includes the psychosocial setting, which includes the relationship between the sender and the receiver, their past experiences with each other, their past experiences with similar situations, and cultural values and norms. Consider again the meaning of "I don't understand what you mean" in the following contexts: two college students discussing a philosophy assignment, a wife responding to her husband's accusation of infidelity, and a Japanese tourist asking directions in San Francisco. Although the content of the message is the same, its meaning is different, depending on the context in which the communication takes place.

In the evaluation of the communication process with regard to the five structural elements, specific problems or potential errors become evident (Table 2-4). If the sender is communicating the same message on both the verbal and nonverbal levels, then the communication is **congruent.** However, if the levels are not in agreement, the communication is **incongruent,** which can be problematic.

THERAPEUTIC DIALOGUE

Congruent Communication
VERBAL LEVEL *I'm pleased to see you.*
NONVERBAL LEVEL *Warm tone of voice, continuous eye contact, smile.*

Incongruent Communication
VERBAL LEVEL *I'm pleased to see you.*
NONVERBAL LEVEL *Cold and distant tone of voice, little eye contact, neutral facial expression.*

Incongruent, or double-level, messages produce a dilemma for the listener, who does not know to which level to respond, the verbal or nonverbal. Because both levels cannot be responded to, the listener is likely to feel frustrated, angry, or confused. Obviously, both patients and nurses can display incongruent communication if they are not aware of their internal feeling states and the nature of their communication.

Another problem initiated by the sender is inflexible communication that is either too rigid or too permissive. A rigid approach by the nurse does not allow for spontaneous expression by the patient, nor does it allow the patient to contribute to the flow or direction of the interaction. Exaggerated permissiveness, on the other hand, refers to the lack of a direction and mutuality in the interaction established

Fig. 2-4 Components of communication.

TABLE **2-4** *Problems with the Structural Elements of the Communication Process*

STRUCTURAL ELEMENT	COMMUNICATION PROBLEM	DEFINITION
Sender	Incongruent communication	Lack of agreement between the verbal and nonverbal levels of communication
	Inflexible communication	Exaggerated control or permissiveness by the sender
Message	Ineffective messages	Messages that are not goal directed or purposeful
	Inappropriate messages	Messages not relevant to the progress of the relationship
	Inadequate messages	Messages that lack a sufficient amount of information
	Inefficient messages	Messages that lack clarity, simplicity, and directness
Receiver	Errors of perception	Various forms of listening problems
	Errors of evaluation	Misinterpretation due to personal beliefs and values
Feedback	Misinformation	Communication of incorrect information
	Lack of validation	Failure to clarify and ratify understanding of the message
Context	Constraints of physical setting	Noise, temperature, or various distractions
	Constraints of psychosocial setting	Impaired previous relationship between the communicators

by the nurse. The patient may interpret the nurse's behavior as incompetence or lack of interest.

The message of the communication process can also pose problems. Messages can be ineffective, inappropriate, inadequate, or inefficient. Ineffective messages serve at least to distract and at most to prevent the objectives of the nurse-patient relationship from being met. Inappropriate messages are not relevant to the progress of the relationship. They may include failures in timing, stereotyping the receiver, or overlooking important information. Inadequate messages lack sufficient information. In this case, senders assume that receivers know more than they actually do. Inefficient messages lack clarity, simplicity, and directness. Using more energy than is necessary, these messages confuse or complicate the information.

The third element, the receiver, may experience errors of perception. The receiver may miss nonverbal cues, respond only to content and ignore messages of affect, be selectively inattentive to the speaker's message because of physical or psychological discomfort, be preoccupied with other thoughts, or have a physiological hearing impairment. These errors are problems of listening. The receiver may also have problems in evaluating the message. The meaning of the message may be misinterpreted because the receiver views it in terms of the receiver's value system rather than that of the speaker.

Errors in the feedback element include all of those that apply to the message. Feedback can also convey to the sender incorrect information about the message. Another serious error exists when the receiver fails to use feedback to validate understanding of the message. Although feedback is the last step, it has the potential for correcting previous errors and clarifying the nature of the communication.

The fifth element of context can also contribute to communication problems. The setting may be physically noisy, cold, or distracting to one or both parties. The psychosocial context, or past relationship between the communicators, may be one of mistrust or harbored resentment. This analysis shows the complexity of the communication process. It may seem surprising that successful communication can occur, given all of these vulnerable areas. However, it does occur among people who understand the process and use appropriate techniques.

TRANSACTIONAL ANALYSIS MODEL. Transactional analysis (TA) is the study of the communication or transactions that take place between people; it uncovers the sometimes unconscious and destructive ways ("games") in which people relate to each other. This approach to personality was developed by Berne, a psychiatrist who made transactional analysis a popular theory through his book, *Games People Play: The Psychology of Human Relationships.*[2] It is a method of therapy as well as a model of communication.

The cornerstone of Berne's theory is that each person's personality is made up of three distinct components called

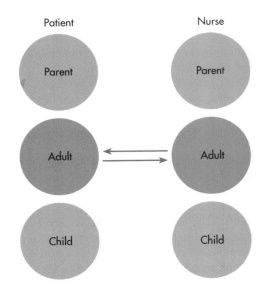

Fig. 2-5   Diagram of complementary transaction.

ego states. An ego state is a consistent pattern of feeling, experiencing, and behaving. The three ego states that make up personality are the parent ego state, adult ego state, and child ego state. It is as though three people reside in each person; the "parent" incorporates all the attitudes and behaviors the individual was taught (directly or indirectly) by parents; the "child" contains all the feelings the individual had as a child; and the "adult" deals with reality in a logical, rational, computerlike manner.

The parent and child ego states are made up of the feelings, attitudes, and behaviors that are remnants of the past but can be reexperienced under certain conditions. The parent ego state consists of all the nurturing, critical, and prejudicial attitudes, behaviors, and experiences learned from other people, especially parents and teachers. The adult ego state is the reality-oriented part of the personality. It gathers and processes information about the world and is objective, emotionless, and intelligent in its approach to problem solving. The child ego state is the feeling part of the personality. In it resides feelings of happiness, joy, sadness, depression, and anxiety.

Berne's model of communication makes it possible to diagram transactions using these ego states. A transaction or communication between two people can be complementary, crossed, or ulterior. In a **complementary transaction** (Fig. 2-5), the arrows in the ego state diagram are parallel, and the communication flows smoothly.

THERAPEUTIC DIALOGUE
Complementary Transaction

PATIENT *I know that when I get mad at my boss, I take it out on my wife and kids.*

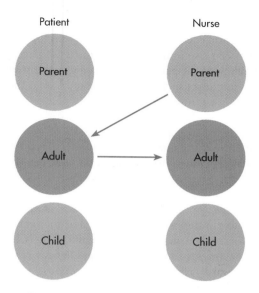

Fig. 2-6 Diagram of a crossed transaction.

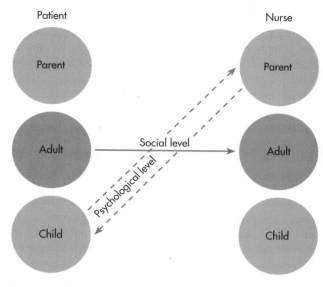

Fig. 2-7 Diagram of an ulterior transaction.

NURSE *Are you ready to think about some other ways you can handle your anger?*

If the arrows in the ego state diagram **cross**, however, communication breaks down (Fig. 2-6).

 THERAPEUTIC DIALOGUE

Crossed Transaction

PATIENT *I know that when I get mad at my boss, I take it out on my wife and kids.*

NURSE *Men always think that's okay, but the women have to suffer for it.*

The third type of transaction is **ulterior** transaction (Fig. 2-7). It takes place on two levels: the social, or overt, level and the psychological, or covert, level. These transactions tend to be destructive because the communicators conceal their true motivations. One of the best known examples of this is the "Why Don't You . . . Yes But" game. This game involves one person asking for a solution to a problem; however, every suggested solution is negated, until the helper is silenced. On the surface, the interaction is two adults problem solving; in reality, one person is using the child ego state to show what a bad parent the other person is.

THERAPEUTIC DIALOGUE

Ulterior Transaction

PATIENT *I know that when I get mad at my boss, I take it out on my wife and kids, but I don't know what else to do.*

NURSE *Do you think you could let your boss know how you're feeling?*

PATIENT *He'll fire me for sure.*

NURSE *Perhaps you could talk it over with someone you work with.*

PATIENT *I don't have time to chat on the job like that. Besides, no one cares about someone else's beefs.*

NURSE *Sometimes physical exercise helps people get rid of their anger. Have you ever tried it?*

PATIENT *Sure. I work out a lot, but it doesn't help.*

NURSE *Perhaps you can explain all this to your family.*

PATIENT *My wife's tired of "all my talk" as she puts it. She says she wants some action.*

The transactional analysis model of communication provides a framework for the nurse to use in exploring the patient's recurrent behaviors, identifying patterns, thinking about causes, and planning alternative ways to respond. Thus nonproductive communication patterns can be stopped and new, healthier, ones learned.

> **?** *Using the transactional analysis model, diagram a recent conversation you have had with a friend, your instructor, and a patient.*

Therapeutic Communication Techniques

There are two basic requirements for effective communication:

▼ All communication must be aimed at preserving the self-respect of both the helper and the helpee

▼ The communication of understanding should precede any suggestions of information or advice giving

These requirements for therapeutic communication make the formation of the nurse-patient relationship and the implementation of the nursing process possible. The collection of data and the planning, implementation, and evaluation activities are carried out *with* the patient, not *for* the patient, when the nurse uses therapeutic communication skills.

Some nurses reject the notion of therapeutic communication techniques because they view them as unnatural, ineffective, or stereotypical. Although simple on the surface, these techniques are difficult and require practice and conscious thought to master. Because they are techniques, they are only as effective as the person using them. If they are worked into existing interpersonal skills, they can enhance the nurse's effectiveness. If they are used as automatic responses and are inappropriate to the nurse's manner of personal expression, they will negate both the nurse's and the patient's individuality and divest them of their dignity.

To ensure that the nurse is using these skills appropriately and effectively, the nurse needs to record interactions with the patient in some way and then analyze them. The nurse should also seek feedback from others. The nurse can benefit from maintaining a diary of thoughts, feelings, and impressions in relation to clinical work. This can prove valuable in working through difficult aspects of termination or counter-transference reactions.

The advantages and disadvantages of the various methods of recording nurse-patient interactions must be considered, along with the nurse's and patient's preferences, before a particular method is chosen. Some form of recording that is as objective and comprehensive as possible is necessary. Only by analyzing the interaction can the nurse evaluate the degree of success in using therapeutic communication techniques.[36] Some of the more helpful techniques are now described.

LISTENING. Listening is essential if the nurse is to reach any understanding of the patient. The only person who can tell the nurse about the patient's feelings, thoughts, and perception of the self in the world is the patient. Therefore the first rule of a therapeutic relationship is to listen to the patient. It is the foundation on which all other therapeutic skills are built.[17,26]

Inexperienced nurses often find it difficult not to talk. This may be caused by their anxiety, the need to prove themselves, or their usual way of social interaction. It is helpful to remember that the patient should be talking more than the nurse during the interaction; the task of the nurse is to listen.

Real listening is difficult. It is an active, not a passive, process. The nurse should give complete attention to the patient and should not be preoccupied. The nurse should suspend thinking of personal experiences and problems and personal judgments of the patient. Listening is a sign of respect for the patient and is a powerful reinforcer. It reinforces verbalization by the patient, without which the relationship could not progress.

BROAD OPENINGS. Broad openings such as "What are you thinking about?," "Can you tell me more about that?,"

and "What shall we discuss today?" confirm the presence of the patient and encourage the patient to select topics to discuss. They can also indicate that the nurse is there, listening to and following the patient. Also serving in this way are acceptance responses such as "I understand," "And then what happened?," "Uh huh," or "I follow you."

RESTATING. Restating is the nurse's repeating of the main thought the patient has expressed. It also indicates that the nurse is listening. Sometimes only a part of the patient's statement is repeated. This technique can serve as a reinforcer or bring attention to something important that might otherwise have been passed over.

CLARIFICATION. Clarification occurs when the nurse attempts to put into words vague ideas or thoughts that are implicit or explicit in the patient's talking. It is necessary because statements about emotions and behaviors are rarely straightforward. The patient's verbalizations, especially if the patient is upset or overwhelmed with feelings, are not always clear and obvious. Nothing should be allowed to pass that the nurse does not hear or understand. Because of this uncertainty, clarification responses often are tentative or phrased as questions such as "I'm not sure what you mean. Are you saying that . . .?" or "Could you go over that again?" This technique is important because two functions of the nurse-patient relationship are to help clarify feelings, ideas, and perceptions and to provide an explicit link between them and the patient's actions.

REFLECTION. Reflection of content is also called **validation;** it lets the patient know that the nurse has heard what was said and understands the content. It consists of repeating in fewer and fresher words the essential ideas of the patient and is like paraphrasing. Sometimes it helps to repeat a patient's statement, emphasizing a key word.

THERAPEUTIC DIALOGUE

PATIENT *When I walked into the room, I felt like I was going to faint. I knew I had tried to do too much too quickly, and I just wasn't ready for it.*

NURSE *You thought you were ready to put yourself to the test, but when you got there, you realized it was too much too soon.*

Reflection of feelings consists of responses to the patient's feelings about the content. These responses let the patient know that the nurse is aware of what the patient is feeling. Broad openings, restatements, clarifications, and reflections of content need not represent empathic understanding. But reflection of feeling signifies understanding, empathy, interest, and respect for the patient. It increases the level of involvement between the nurse and patient.

The purpose of reflecting feelings is to focus on feeling rather than content to bring the patient's vaguely expressed feelings into clear awareness; it helps the patient accept or own those feelings. The steps in reflection of feelings are to determine what feelings the patient is expressing, describe these feelings clearly, observe the effect, and judge by the patient's reaction whether the reflection was correct. Sometimes even inaccurate reflections can be useful because the patient may correct the nurse and state feelings more clearly.

 THERAPEUTIC DIALOGUE

PATIENT *It's not so much that I mind changing jobs. It's just that I let down all the people working for me . . . relying on me.*

NURSE *You feel responsible for your employees and so you're both sad and guilty about what has happened at work.*

PATIENT *Yes—sad, guilty . . . and pretty angry now that we're talking about it.*

Although reflecting techniques are some of the most useful, the nurse can also use them incorrectly. One common error is stereotyping of responses; that is, the nurse begins reflections in the same monotonous way, such as "You think" or "You feel." A second error is in timing. Reflecting back almost everything the patient says provokes feelings of irritation, anger, and frustration in the patient because the nurse appears to be insincere and fails to be therapeutic. Other nurses may have trouble interrupting patients who continue talking in long monologues. Not only is it difficult to capture a feeling after it has passed, but also the nurse is failing to be a responsible, active partner in the relationship. Interruptions may at times be productive and necessary. Another error is inappropriate depth of feeling. The nurse fails by being either too superficial or too deep in assessing the patient's feelings. The final error is use of language that is inappropriate to the patient's sociocultural experience and educational level. Effective language is language that is natural to the nurse and readily understood by the patient.

FOCUSING. Focusing helps the patient expand on a topic of importance. Effectively used, it can help the patient become more specific, move from vagueness to clarity, and focus on reality.

By avoiding abstractions and generalizations, focusing helps the patient face problems and analyze them in detail. It helps a patient talk about life experiences or problem areas and accept the responsibility for improving them. If the goal is to change thoughts, feelings, or beliefs, the patient must first identify and own them.

 THERAPEUTIC DIALOGUE

PATIENT *Women always get put down. It's as if we don't count at all.*

NURSE *Tell me how* you *feel as a woman.*

Encouraging a description of the patient's perceptions, encouraging comparisons, and placing events in time sequence are focusing techniques that promote specificity and problem analysis.

SHARING PERCEPTIONS. Sharing perceptions involves asking the patient to verify the nurse's understanding of what the patient is thinking or feeling. The nurse can ask for feedback from the patient while possibly providing new information. Perception checking can consist of paraphrasing what the patient is saying or doing, asking the patient to confirm the nurse's understanding, and allowing the patient to correct that perception if necessary. Perception checking can also note the implied feelings of nonverbal language. It is best to describe the observed behavior first and then reflect on its meaning.

 THERAPEUTIC DIALOGUE

PATIENT *She was such a good girl . . . and really seemed to care about other people. I don't know what's happened to her . . . what I could have done differently.*

NURSE *You seem to be very disappointed with your daughter, and maybe with yourself. Am I right about that?*

Perception checking is also a way to explore incongruent or double-blind communication. "You're smiling, but I sense that you're really angry with me." Perception checking conveys understanding to the patient and clears up confusing communication.

THEME IDENTIFICATION. Themes are underlying issues or problems experienced by the patient that emerge repeatedly during the course of the nurse-patient relationship. Once the nurse has identified the patient's basic themes, he or she can better decide which of the patient's many feelings, thoughts, and beliefs to respond to and pursue. Important themes tend to be repeated throughout the relationship. They can relate to feelings (depression or anxiety), behavior (rebelling against authority or withdrawal), experiences (being loved, hurt, or raped), or combinations of all three.

SILENCE. Silence on the part of the nurse has varying effects, depending on how the patient perceives it. To a vocal patient, silence on the part of the nurse may be welcome, as long as the patient knows the nurse is listening. When patients pause, they often expect and want the nurse to respond. If the nurse does not, patients may perceive this as rejection, hostility, or disinterest. With a depressed or withdrawn patient, the nurse's silence may convey support, understanding, and acceptance. In this case verbalization by the nurse may be perceived as pressure or frustration.

Silence can prompt the patient to talk. Some introverted people find out that they can be quiet but still be liked. Silence allows the patient time to think and to gain insights. Finally, silence can slow the pace of the interaction. In general, the nurse should allow the patient to break a silence, particularly when the patient has introduced it. Obviously, sensitivity is called for in this regard, and silence should not develop into a contest. However, if the nurse is unsure how to respond to a patient's comments, a safe approach is to maintain silence. If the nurse's nonverbal behavior communicates interest and involvement, the patient often will elaborate or discuss a related issue.

As a general technique, direct questioning has limited usefulness in the therapeutic relationship. Repetitive questioning takes on the tone of an interrogation and negates the element of mutuality. "Why" questions are particularly ineffective and are to be avoided, as are questions that can be answered yes or no. One consequence of it is that patients do not take the initiative and are discouraged or prevented from engaging in the process of exploration.

HUMOR. Humor is a basic part of the personality and has a place within the therapeutic relationship.[4,10,29,31] As a part of interpersonal relationships, it is a constructive coping behavior. By learning to express humor, a patient may be able to learn to express other feelings. As a planned approach to nursing intervention, humor can promote insight by making conscious repressed material. A change in the expression of humor and the quality of interpersonal relationships may be indicators of significant change in the patient.

Humor can serve many functions within the nurse-patient relationship (Box 2-6). These can be either positive or negative. There are no rules for determining how, when, or where humor should be used in the therapeutic relationship. It depends on the nature and quality of the relationship, the patient's receptivity to such themes, and the relevance of the tale or witticism. Some occasions when the use of humor may be of therapeutic value include the following:

▼ When the patient is experiencing mild to moderate levels of anxiety, humor serves as a tension reducer. It is inappropriate if a patient has severe or panic anxiety levels.

▼ When it helps a patient cope more effectively, facilitates learning, puts life situations in perspective, decreases social distance, and is understood by the patient for its therapeutic value. It is inappropriate when it promotes maladaptive coping responses, masks feelings, increases social distance, and helps the individual avoid dealing with difficult situations.

▼ When it is consistent with the social and cultural values of the patient and when it allows the patient to laugh at life, the human situation, or a particular set of stressors. It is inappropriate when it violates a patient's values, ridicules people, or belittles others.

The nurse must also be aware of the dangerous ways it can be used to hide conflicts, ward off anxiety, manipulate the patient, and serve the nurse's own need to be liked and admired. If it is used indiscriminately, humor meets only the nurse's needs and may be destructive to the relationship and frightening to the patient.

INFORMING. Informing, or information giving, is an essential nursing technique in which the nurse shares simple facts with the patient. It is a skill used by nurses in health teaching or patient education, such as in informing a patient when to take medication and about necessary precautions and side effects. Giving information must be distinguished from giving suggestions or advice.

SUGGESTING. Suggesting is the presentation of alternative ideas. As a therapeutic technique, it is a useful intervention in the working phase of the relationship when the patient has analyzed the problem area and is exploring alternative coping mechanisms. At that time, suggestions by the nurse will increase the patient's perceived options.

Suggesting, or giving advice, can also be nontherapeutic. Some patients who seek help expect some pronouncement from the health-care professional on what to do. Likewise, nursing students often perceive their function as giving "common sense" advice. In these instances giving advice shifts responsibility to the nurse and reinforces the patient's dependence.

Another limitation is that the patient may take the nurse's advice and still not have things work out. The patient then returns to blame the nurse for failure. Most commonly, though, patients do not follow the advice offered by others, as in the transactional analysis model. The request for advice is often a child's expression of dependency, and the patient really knows what to do. The nurse who falls into the trap and responds with advice receives the patient's anger and contempt. A more productive strategy is for the nurse to deal with the patient's feelings first—feelings of indecision, dependence, and perhaps fear. Then the request for advice can be looked at and responded to in its proper perspective.

Suggesting is also nontherapeutic if it occurs early in the relationship before the patient has analyzed personal conflicts or if it is a technique the nurse uses frequently. Then it negates the possibility of mutuality and implies that the patient is incapable of assuming responsibility for thoughts and actions. This assumption is also present when suggestion by the nurse is really covert coercion, as the nurse tells patients how they *ought* to live their lives.

The nurse's intent in using the suggesting technique should be to provide feasible alternatives and allow the patient to explore their potential value. The nurse can then focus on helping the patient explore the advantages and disadvantages and the meaning and implications of the alternatives. In this way suggestions can be offered in a nonauthoritarian manner with such phrases as "Some people have tried. . . . Do you think that would work for you?" When using the technique of suggesting, nurses must be

Box **2-6** *Functions of Humor*

▼ Establishes relationships	▼ Expresses emotion
▼ Reduces stress and tension	▼ Facilitates learning
▼ Promotes social closeness	▼ Reinforces self-concept
▼ Provides social control	▼ Voices social conflict
▼ Permits cognitive reframing	▼ Avoids conflict
▼ Reflects social change	▼ Facilitates enculturation
▼ Provides perspective	▼ Instills hope

careful about both the timing of their intervention and their underlying motivation.

The therapeutic communication techniques presented in this chapter are summarized in Box 2-7.

> **?** *Which therapeutic communication techniques listed in Box 2-7 are you skilled in using? Which techniques are more difficult for you?*

RESPONSIVE DIMENSIONS

The nurse must achieve certain skills or qualities to initiate and continue a therapeutic relationship. These skills or qualities incorporate verbal and nonverbal behavior and the attitudes and feelings behind communication. Carkhoff, Berenson, and Truax[6,7,8] have identified specific core conditions for facilitative interpersonal relationships. They broadly divided these conditions into responsive dimensions and action dimensions.

The responsive dimensions include genuineness, respect, empathic understanding, and concreteness. One study suggests that nurses are most skilled in the authoritative interventions of prescribing, informing, and confronting patients and less skilled in the facilitative interventions of drawing out patient's emotions, encouraging their self-exploration, and confirming their self-worth.[22] Another study reports that patients had much anxiety when interacting with psychiatric nurses, although they found them to be friendly and caring. However, they also experienced psychiatric nurses as lacking in empathy and intimacy and thought that they related to patients in stereotypical ways, acting as custodians and enforcers of rules.[25] The helping process can therefore impede the patient's growth rather than enhance it, depending on the level of the nurse's responsive and facilitative skills.

The responsive dimensions are crucial in a therapeutic relationship to establish trust and open communication. The nurse's goal is to gain an understanding of the patient and to help the patient gain self-understanding and insight. These responsive conditions then continue to be useful throughout the working and termination phases.

Genuineness

Genuineness implies that the nurse is an open, honest, sincere person who is actively involved in the relationship. Genuineness is the opposite of self-alienation, which occurs when many of an individual's real, spontaneous reactions to life are suppressed. Genuineness means that the nurse's response is sincere, that the nurse is not thinking and feeling one thing and saying something different. It is an essential quality because nurses cannot expect openness, self-acceptance, and personal freedom in patients if they lack these qualities themselves.

Genuineness does not mean that the nurse must make a complete self-disclosure, but whatever the nurse does show must be real and not merely a "professional" response that has been learned and repeated. Genuineness also does not imply that the nurse will behave in the same way as family, friends, or colleagues. In focusing on the patient, much of the nurse's personal need system is put aside, as well as some of the usual ways of relating to others. Carried to this extreme, genuineness can be destructive and work against the goals of a therapeutic relationship.

Following is an example of genuineness.

🔲 THERAPEUTIC DIALOGUE

PATIENT *I'd like my parents to give me my freedom and let me do my own thing. If I need them or want their advice, I'll ask them. Why don't they trust what they taught me? Why do parents have to make it so hard—like it's all or nothing?*

NURSE *I know what you mean. My parents acted the same way. They offered advice, but what they expected was obedience. When they saw I could handle things on my own and used good judgment, they began to accept me as an individual. There are still times when they slip back into their old ways, but we understand each other better now. Do you think you and your parents need to share more openly and honestly your feelings and ideas?*

Respect

Respect, also called *nonpossessive warmth* or *unconditional positive regard,* does not depend on the patient's behavior. *Caring, liking,* and *valuing* are other terms for respect. The patient is regarded as a person of worth and is respected. The nurse's attitude is nonjudgmental; it is without criticism, ridicule, or reservation. This does not mean that the nurse condones or accepts all aspects of the patient's behavior as desirable or likeable. Patients are accepted for who they are, as they are. The nurse does not demand that the patient change or be perfect to be accepted. Imperfections are accepted along with mistakes and weaknesses as part of the human condition. The inexperienced nurse may have difficulty accepting the patient without transferring feelings about the patient's thoughts or actions. However, acceptance means viewing the patient's actions as coping behaviors that will change as the patient becomes less threatened and learns more adaptive mechanisms. It involves viewing the patient's behavior as natural, normal, and expected, given the circumstances.

Although there should be a basic respect for the patient simply as a person, respect is increased with understanding of the patient's uniqueness. Respect can be communicated in many different ways: by sitting silently with a patient who is crying, by genuine laughter with the patient over a particular event, by accepting the patient's request not to share a certain experience, by apologizing for the hurt unintentionally caused by a particular phrase, or by being open enough to communicate anger or hurt caused by the pa-

Box **2-7** *Therapeutic Communication Techniques*

TECHNIQUE: LISTENING

Definition: An active process of receiving information and examining reaction to the messages received

Example: Maintaining eye contact and receptive nonverbal communication

Therapeutic value: Nonverbally communicates to the patient the nurse's interest and acceptance

Nontherapeutic threat: Failure to listen

TECHNIQUE: BROAD OPENINGS

Definition: Encouraging the patient to select topics for discussion

Example: "What are you thinking about?"

Therapeutic value: Indicates acceptance by the nurse and the value of the patient's initiative

Nontherapeutic threat: Domination of the interaction by the nurse; rejecting responses

TECHNIQUE: RESTATING

Definition: Repeating the main thought the patient expressed

Example: "You say that your mother left you when you were 5 years old."

Therapeutic value: Indicates that the nurse is listening and validates, reinforces, or calls attention to something important that has been said

Nontherapeutic threat: Lack of validation of the nurse's interpretation of the message; being judgmental; reassuring; defending

TECHNIQUE: CLARIFICATION

Definition: Attempting to put into words vague ideas or unclear thoughts of the patient to enhance the nurse's understanding or asking the patient to explain what he or she means

Example: "I'm not sure what you mean. Could you tell me about that again?"

Therapeutic value: Helps to clarify feelings, ideas, and perceptions of the patient and provide an explicit correlation between them and the patient's actions

Nontherapeutic threat: Failure to probe; assumed understanding

TECHNIQUE: REFLECTION

Definition: Directing back the patient's ideas, feelings, questions, or content

Example: "You're feeling tense and anxious and it's related to a conversation you had with your husband last night?"

Therapeutic value: Validates the nurse's understanding of what the patient is saying and signifies empathy, interest, and respect for the patient

Nontherapeutic threat: Stereotyping the patient's responses; inappropriate timing of reflections; inappropriate depth of feeling of the reflections; inappropriate to the cultural experience and educational level of the patient

TECHNIQUE: HUMOR

Definition: The discharge of energy through the comic enjoyment of the imperfect

Example: "That gives a whole new meaning to the word *nervous*," said with shared kidding between the nurse and patient

Therapeutic value: Can promote insight by making conscious repressed material, resolving paradoxes, tempering aggression, and revealing new options, and is a socially acceptable form of sublimation

Nontherapeutic threat: Indiscriminate use; belittling patient; screen to avoid therapeutic intimacy

TECHNIQUE: INFORMING

Definition: The skill of information giving

Example: "I think you need to know more about how your medication works."

Therapeutic value: Helpful in health teaching or patient education about relevant aspects of patient's well-being and self-care

Nontherapeutic threat: Giving advice

TECHNIQUE: FOCUSING

Definition: Questions or statements that help the patient expand on a topic of importance

Example: "I think that we should talk more about your relationship with your father."

Therapeutic value: Allows the patient to discuss central issues and keeps the communication process goal-directed

Nontherapeutic threat: Allowing abstractions and generalizations; changing topics

TECHNIQUE: SHARING PERCEPTIONS

Definition: Asking the patient to verify the nurse's understanding of what the patient is thinking or feeling

Example: "You're smiling but I sense that you are really very angry with me."

Therapeutic value: Conveys the nurse's understanding to the patient and has the potential for clearing up confusing communication

Nontherapeutic threat: Challenging the patient; accepting literal responses; reassuring; testing; defending

TECHNIQUE: THEME IDENTIFICATION

Definition: Underlying issues or problems experienced by the patient that emerge repeatedly during the course of the nurse-patient relationship

Example: "I've noticed that in all of the relationships that you have described, you've been hurt or rejected by the man. Do you think this is an underlying issue?"

Therapeutic value: Allows the nurse to best promote the patient's exploration and understanding of important problems

Nontherapeutic threat: Giving advice; reassuring; disapproving

TECHNIQUE: SILENCE

Definition: Lack of verbal communication for a therapeutic reason

Example: Sitting with a patient and nonverbally communicating interest and involvement

Therapeutic value: Allows the patient time to think and gain insights, slows the pace of the interaction and encourages the patient to initiate conversation, while conveying the nurse's support, understanding, and acceptance

Nontherapeutic threat: Questioning the patient; asking for "why" responses; failure to break a nontherapeutic silence

TECHNIQUE: SUGGESTING

Definition: Presentation of alternative ideas for the patient's consideration relative to problem solving

Example: "Have you thought about responding to your boss in a different way when he raises that issue with you? For example, you could ask him whether a specific problem has occurred."

Therapeutic value: Increases the patient's perceived options or choices

Nontherapeutic threat: Giving advice; inappropriate timing; being judgmental tient. Being genuine with and listening to the patient are also manifestations of respect.

When nurses communicate conditional warmth, they foster feelings of dependency in patients because nurses become the evaluator and superior in the relationship, making mutuality impossible. If dependency feelings arise in patients, nurses can effectively deal with them by acknowledging and exploring these feelings with patients.

> **?** *There is a common expression that "respect needs to be learned." How does this idea affect the lives of psychiatric patients?*

Empathic Understanding

Empathy has been defined by Kalisch[16] as "the ability to enter into the life of another person, to accurately perceive his current feelings and their meanings. It is an essential element of the interpersonal process. When communicated, it forms the basis for a helping relationship between nurse and patient." Rogers[33] described it as "to sense the client's private world as if it were your own, but without losing the 'as if' quality." Rogers believes that a high degree of empathy is one of the most potent factors in bringing about change and learning—"one of the most delicate and powerful ways we have of using ourselves."[32]

Accurate empathy involves more than knowing what the patient means. It also involves sensitivity to the patient's current feelings and the verbal ability to communicate this understanding in a language attuned to the patient. It means frequently confirming with the patient the accuracy of personal perceptions and being guided by the patient's responses. It requires that the nurse lay aside personal views and values to enter another's world without prejudice.

Two types of empathy can be identified in the nursing literature.[1,39,40] The first type is basic empathy. It involves the natural, universal human capacity to feel for others. The second type is trained empathy, which is taught and learned in relation to helping others. Trained empathy is also called clinical empathy or professional empathy. Unfortunately, these two types of empathy are often confused when empathy is discussed in terms of the nurse-patient relationship. For example, it would be important to first assess a baseline of empathic ability in nursing students. After teaching this skill, nursing students can then be assessed for trained empathy and the impact it may have on the outcome of psychiatric nursing care.[19,39]

Development of Empathy

Empathic understanding consists of a number of stages. If patients allow nurses to enter their private world and attempt to communicate their perceptions and feelings, nurses must be receptive to this communication. Next, nurses must understand the patient's communication by putting themselves in the patient's place. Nurses must then step back into their own role and communicate understanding to the patient. It is not necessary or desirable for nurses to feel the same emotion as the patient. Empathy should not be confused with sympathy. Instead, it is an appreciation and awareness of the patient's feelings. A good deal of research has been conducted on empathy. The findings presented in Box 2-8 underscore its importance in counseling.

Rogers[33] expands on the profound consequences empathy can have in promoting constructive learning and change. In the first place, it dissolves the patient's sense of alienation by connecting the patient on some level to a part of the human race. The patient can perceive that "I make sense to another human being . . . so I must not be so strange or alien. . . . And if I am in touch with someone else, I am not so alone." On the other hand, if not responded to empathically, the patient may believe, "If no one understands me, if no one can see what I'm experiencing, then I must be very bad off. . . . I'm sicker than even I thought." Another benefit of empathy is that the patient can feel valued, cared for, and accepted as a person. Then perhaps he or she will come to think, "If this other person thinks I'm worthwhile, maybe I could value and care for myself. . . . Maybe I am worthwhile after all."

EMPATHIC RESPONSES. It is essential that the nurse first provide the contextual base for the relationship through genuineness and unconditional positive regard for the patient. Then the understanding conveyed to the patient through empathy gives him or her personhood or identity. The patient incorporates these aspects into a new, changing self-concept. Once self-concept changes, behavior also changes, thus producing the positive clinical outcome of therapy.

Box **2-8** *Research Findings about Empathy*

- ▼ Empathy is related to positive clinical outcome.
- ▼ The ideal therapist is first of all empathic.
- ▼ Empathy is correlated with self-exploration and self-acceptance.
- ▼ Empathy early in the relationship predicts later success.
- ▼ Understanding is provided by, not drawn from, the therapist.
- ▼ More experienced therapists are more likely to be empathic.
- ▼ Empathy is a special quality in a relationship, and therapists offer more of it than even helpful friends.
- ▼ The better self-integrated the therapist, the higher the degree of empathy.
- ▼ Experienced therapists often fall far short of being empathic. Brilliance and diagnostic perceptiveness are unrelated to empathy.
- ▼ An empathic way of being can be learned from empathic people.

Gazda and co-workers[13] have described the following guidelines for responding with empathy:

▼ Verbal and nonverbal behavior should be focused on by the helper.

▼ The helper should respond in a language and a manner that are easily understood by the patient.

▼ The tone of the helper's response should be similar to that of the patient.

▼ In addition to concentrating on what the patient is expressing, the helper should also be aware of what is not being expressed.

▼ The helper must accurately interpret responses to the patient and use them as a guide in developing future responses.

A nursing study identified specific verbal and nonverbal behaviors that conveyed high levels of empathy to the patient[20]:

▼ Having nurses introduce themselves to patients

▼ Head and body positions turned toward the patient and occasionally leaning forward

▼ Verbal responses to the patient's comments, responses that focus on strengths and resources

▼ Consistent eye contact and response to the patient's nonverbal cues such as sighs, tone of voice, restlessness, and facial expressions

▼ Conveyance of interest, concern, and warmth by the nurse's own facial expressions

▼ A tone of voice consistent with facial expression and verbal response

▼ Mirror imaging of body position and gestures between the nurse and patient

A recent nursing study demonstrated a connection between nurse-expressed empathy and positive patient outcomes.[27] Additional studies are needed in nursing to identify the behavioral indicators and outcomes of this important dimension of nursing care.[1,24]

EMPATHIC FUNCTIONING SCALE. Kalisch[16] devised the Nurse-Patient Empathic Functioning Scale, which describes five categories of empathy. High levels of empathy (categories 3 and 4) communicate "I am with you"; the nurse's responses fit perfectly with the patient's conspicuous current feelings and content. The nurse's responses also serve to expand the patient's awareness of hidden feelings through the use of clarification and reflection. Such empathy is communicated by the language used, voice qualities, and nonverbal behavior, all of which reflect the nurse's seriousness and depth of feeling.

At low levels of empathy (categories 0 and 1), the nurse ignores the patient's feelings, goes off on a tangent, or misinterprets what the patient is feeling. The nurse at this level may be uninterested in the patient or concentrating on the "facts" of what the patient says rather than on current feelings and experiences. The nurse is doing something other than listening, such as evaluating the patient, giving advice,

sermonizing, or thinking about personal problems or needs. A middle level of empathy (category 2) shows that the nurse is making an effort to understand the patient's feelings.

Empathic responses must be properly timed within the nurse-patient relationship. Category 4 responses in the orientation phase may be viewed as too intense and intrusive. Usually a number of category 2 responses are required initially to build an atmosphere of trust and openness. In the later stages of the orientation phase and most particularly in the working phase, categories 3 and 4 responses are appropriate and most effective. Responses from categories 0 and 1 are nontherapeutic at all times and block the development of the relationship.

The various levels of empathy are evident in the following example:

THERAPEUTIC DIALOGUE

PATIENT *I'm really jittery today, and I hope I can get things out right. It started when I saw Bob on Friday, and it's been building up since then.*

NURSE *You're feeling tense and anxious, and it's related to a talk you had with Bob on Friday. (Category 2.)*

PATIENT *Yes. He began putting pressure on me to have sex with him again.*

NURSE *It sounds like you resent it when he pressures you for sex. (Category 3.)*

PATIENT *I do. Why does he think things always have to be his way? I guess he knows I'm a pushover.*

NURSE *It makes you angry when he wants his way even though he knows you feel differently. But you usually give in and then you wind up disappointed in yourself and feeling like a failure. (Category 4.)*

PATIENT *It happens just like that over and over. It's as if I never learn.*

NURSE *So when the incident's all over, you're left blaming yourself and wallowing in self-pity. (Category 4.)*

PATIENT *I guess that's right.*

Finally, sociocultural differences between nurses and patients can be barriers to empathy if nurses are not sensitive to them. Differences in gender, age, income, belief systems, education, and ethnicity can block the development of empathic understanding. However, the greater the nurse's cultural sensitivity and the greater the openness to the world view of others, the greater will be the potential for understanding people.

Identical or similar experiences are not essential for empathy. No man can really experience what it is like to be a woman; no white can experience what it is like to be black. It is not necessary to be exactly like another, but it is desirable for nurses to prepare themselves in any way they can to understand potential patients. It is also important for nurses to realize that empathy can be learned and enhanced in a variety of ways, including staff development programs.

Concreteness

Concreteness involves using specific terminology rather than abstractions when discussing the patient's feelings, experiences, and behavior. It avoids vagueness and ambiguity and is the opposite of generalizing, categorizing, classifying, and labeling the patient's experiences. It has three functions: to keep the nurse's responses close to the patient's feelings and experiences, to foster accuracy of understanding by the nurse, and to encourage the patient to attend to specific problem areas.[8]

The level of concreteness should vary during the various phases of the nurse-patient relationship (Fig. 2-8). In the orientation phase, concreteness should be high; at this time it can contribute to empathic understanding. It is essential for the formulation of specific goals and plans. As patients explore various feelings and perceptions related to their problems in the working phase of the relationship, concreteness should be at a low level to facilitate a thorough self-exploration. At the end of the working phase, when patients are engaging in action, and during the termination phase high levels of concreteness are again desirable.

Concreteness is evident in the following examples:

▌THERAPEUTIC DIALOGUE

Example 1

PATIENT *I wouldn't have any problems if people would quit bothering me. They like to upset me because they know I'm high strung.*

NURSE *What people try to upset you?*

PATIENT *My family. People think being from a large family is a blessing. I think it's a curse.*

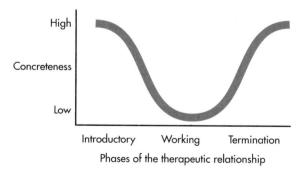

Fig. 2-8 Levels of concreteness in the therapeutic relationship.

NURSE *Could you give me an example of something someone in your family did that upset you?*

Example 2

PATIENT *I don't know what the problem is between us. My wife and I just don't get along anymore. We seem to disagree about everything. I think I love her, but she isn't affectionate or caring—hasn't been for a long time.*

NURSE *You say you're not sure what the problem is, and you think you love your wife. But the two of you argue often and she hasn't given you any sign of love or affection. Have you felt affectionate toward her, and when was the last time you let her know how you felt?*

These four responsive dimensions or conditions—genuineness, respect, empathic understanding, and concreteness—facilitate the formation of a therapeutic relationship. The therapeutic level at which nurses function is unknown at present. Additional research is greatly needed on nurse-patient interactions because there is little empirical evidence on which to base scientific practice in this area.

ACTION DIMENSIONS

Carkhoff[6] identified the action-oriented conditions for facilitative interpersonal relationships as confrontation, immediacy, and therapist self-disclosure. To these will be added the dimensions of catharsis and role playing. The separation of these therapeutic conditions into two groups—the understanding, or responsive conditions and the initiating, or action conditions—is not a distinct separation. To some extent all the dimensions are present throughout the therapeutic relationship. The action dimensions must have a context of warmth and understanding. This is important for inexperienced nurses to remember because they may be tempted to move into high levels of action dimensions without having established adequate understanding, empathy, warmth, or respect. The responsive dimensions allow the patient to achieve insight, but this is not enough. With the action dimensions, the nurse moves the therapeutic relationship upward and outward by identifying obstacles to the patient's progress and the need for both internal understanding and external action.

Confrontation

Confrontation usually implies venting anger and aggressive behavior. However, confrontation as a therapeutic action dimension is an assertive rather than aggressive action. Confrontation is an expression by the nurse of perceived discrepancies in the patient's behavior. Carkhoff[6] identifies three categories of confrontation:

▼ Discrepancy between the patient's expression of what he or she is (self-concept) and what he or she wants to be (self-ideal)

▼ Discrepancies between the patient's verbal self-expression and behavior

▼ Discrepancies between the patient's expressed experience of her- or himself and the nurse's experience of her or him

Confrontation is an attempt by the nurse to make the patient aware of incongruence in his or her feelings, attitudes, beliefs, and behaviors. It may also lead to the discovery of ambivalent feelings in the patient. Confrontation is not limited to negative aspects of the patient. It includes pointing out discrepancies involving resources and strengths that are unrecognized and unused. It requires that the nurse collect sufficient data about the patient's history and accumulate sufficient perceptions and observations of verbal and nonverbal communication so that validation of reality is possible.

The nurse must have developed an understanding of the patient to perceive discrepancies, inconsistencies in word and deed, distortions, defenses, and evasions. The nurse must be willing and able to work through the crisis after confronting the patient. Without this commitment the confrontation lacks therapeutic potential and can be damaging to both nurse and patient. Without question the effects of confrontation are challenge, exposure, risk, and the possibility for growth. The nurse who uses confrontation is modeling an active role to the patient; the nurse is using insight and understanding to remove ambiguity and inconsistency and thus seek deeper understanding.

TIMING IN RELATIONSHIPS. Bromley[3] suggests that before confrontation, nurses should assess the following factors:

▼ The trust level in the relationship
▼ The timing
▼ The patient's stress level
▼ The strength of the patient's defense mechanisms
▼ The patient's perceived need for personal space or closeness
▼ The patient's level of rage and tolerance for hearing another perception

Patients have the capacity to deny or accept nurses' observations, and their response to the confrontation can serve as a measure of its success or failure. Acceptance indicates appropriate timing and patient readiness. Denial serves to allay any threat that the confrontation posed to the patient. It provides nurses with additional information; it tells them that patients are resisting change and are unwilling to enlarge their view of reality at this time.

Confrontation must be appropriately timed to be effective (Fig. 2-9). In the orientation phase of the relationship, the nurse should use confrontation infrequently and pose it as an observation of incongruent behavior. A simple mirroring of the discrepancy between a patient's actions and words is the most nonthreatening type of confrontation. The nurse might say, "You seem to be saying two different things." This type of confrontation closely resembles clarification at this time. Nurses might also identify discrepancies between how they and patients are experiencing their rela-

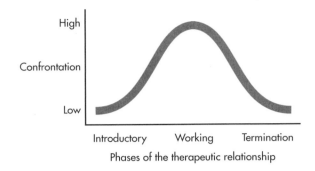

Fig. 2-9 Levels of confrontation in the therapeutic relationship.

tionship, point out unnoticed patient strengths or untapped resources, or provide patients with objective but perhaps different information about their world. Finally, to be effective, confrontation requires high levels of empathy and respect.

In the working phase of the relationship, more direct confrontations may focus on specific patient discrepancies. The nurse may confront the patient with areas of weakness or shortcomings or may focus on the discrepancy between the nurse's perception of the patient and the patient's self-perception. This expands the patient's awareness and helps the patient move to higher levels of functioning. Confrontation is especially important in pointing out when the patient has developed insight but has not changed behavior. This encourages the patient to act in a reasonable and constructive manner, rather than assuming a dependent and passive stance toward life.

Research indicates that effective counselors use confrontation frequently, confronting patients with their assets more often in earlier interviews and with their limitations in later interviews. In the initial interview, these confrontations were based on attempts to clarify the relationship, eliminate misconceptions, give patients more objective information about themselves and their world, and emphasize patient strengths and resources.

Inexperienced nurses often avoid confrontation. It can be nontherapeutic when it is not associated with empathy or warmth or when it is used to vent the nurse's feelings of anger, frustration, and aggressiveness. However, carefully monitored confrontation can be viewed as an extension of genuineness and concreteness. It is a useful therapeutic intervention that can further the patient's growth and progress.

Following are examples of confrontation:

 THERAPEUTIC DIALOGUE

Example 1

NURSE *I see you as someone who has a lot of strength. You've been able to give a tremendous amount of emotional* *support to your children at a time when they needed it very much.*

Example 2

NURSE *You say you want to feel better and go back to work, but you're not taking your medicine, which will help you to do that.*

Example 3

NURSE *The fact that Sue didn't accept your date for Friday night doesn't necessarily mean she never wants to go out with you. She could have had another date or other plans with her family or girlfriends. But if you don't ask her, you'll never find out why she refused you or if she'll accept in the future.*

Example 4

NURSE *You tell me that your parents don't trust you and never give you any responsibility, but each week you also tell me how you stayed out beyond your curfew or had friends over when your parents weren't home. Do you see a connection between the two?*

Example 5

NURSE *We've been talking for 3 weeks now about your need to get out and try to meet some people. We even talked of different ways to do that. But so far you haven't made any effort to join aerobics, take a class, or do any of the other ideas we had.*

> **?** *Your friend tells you that she feels uncomfortable using confrontation with patients. Why do you think this might be and what advice would you give her?*

Immediacy

Immediacy involves focusing on the current interaction of the nurse and the patient in the relationship. It is a significant dimension because the patient's behavior and functioning in the relationship are indicative of functioning in other interpersonal relationships. Most patients experience difficulty in interpersonal relationships; thus the patient's functioning in the nurse-patient relationship must be evaluated. The nurse has the opportunity to intervene directly with the patient's problem behavior, and the patient has the opportunity to learn and change behavior.

Immediacy connotes sensitivity to the patient's feelings and a willingness to deal with these feelings rather than ignore them. This is particularly difficult when the nurse must recognize and respond to negative feelings the patient expresses toward the nurse. The difficulty is compounded by the fact that patients often express these messages indirectly and conceal them in references to other people.

It is not possible or appropriate for the nurse to focus continually on the immediacy of the relationship. It is most appropriate to do so when the relationship seems to be stalled or is not progressing. It is also helpful to look at immediacy when the relationship is progressing particularly well. In both instances the patient is actively involved in describing what is helping or hindering the relationship.

As with the other dimensions, high-level immediacy responses should not be suddenly presented to the patient. The nurse must first know and understand the patient and have developed a good, open relationship. The nurse's initial expressions of immediacy should be tentatively phrased, such as "Are you trying to tell me how you feel about our relationship?" As the relationship progresses, observations related to immediacy can be made more directly, and as communication improves, the need for immediacy responses may decrease.

Following are two examples of immediacy:

▮ THERAPEUTIC DIALOGUE

Example 1

PATIENT *I've been thinking about our meetings, and I'm really too busy now to keep coming. Besides, I don't see the point in them, and we don't seem to be getting anywhere.*

NURSE *Are you trying to say you're feeling discouraged and you feel our meetings aren't helping you?*

Example 2

PATIENT *The staff here couldn't care less about us patients. They treat us like children instead of adults.*

NURSE *I'm wondering if you feel that I don't care about you or perhaps I don't value your opinion?*

Nurse Self-Disclosure

Self-disclosures are subjectively true, personal statements about the self, intentionally revealed to another person. The nurse may share experiences or feelings that are similar to those of the patient and may emphasize both the similarities and differences. This kind of self-disclosure is an index of the closeness of the relationship and involves a particular kind of respect for the patient. It is an expression of genuineness and honesty by the nurse and is an aspect of empathy.

The theoretical and research literature provides significant evidence that therapist self-disclosure increases the likelihood of patient self-disclosure. Patient self-disclosure is necessary for a successful therapeutic outcome. However, the nurse must use self-disclosure judiciously, and this is determined by the quality, quantity, and appropriateness of the disclosures. Criteria for self-disclosure include[35]:

▼ To model and educate
▼ To foster the therapeutic alliance
▼ To validate reality
▼ To encourage the patient's autonomy

The number of self-disclosures appears to be crucial to the success of the therapy. Too few nurse self-disclosures may fail to produce patient self-disclosures, whereas too many may decrease the time available for patient disclosure or may alienate the patient. The problem for the nurse is knowing where the middle ground is. Clinical experience is necessary to determine the optimum therapeutic level.

The appropriateness or relevance of the nurse's self-disclosure is also important. The nurse should self-disclose in response to statements made by the patient. If the nurse's disclosure is far from what the patient is experiencing, it can distract the patient from the problem or cause feelings of alienation. A patient who is experiencing severe anxiety may feel threatened or frightened by the nurse's self-disclosure. In these cases the nurse must be careful not to burden a patient with self-disclosures. Above all, disclosure by the nurse is always for the patient's benefit. The nurse does not disclose to meet personal needs or to feel better. When self-disclosing, the nurse should have a particular therapeutic goal in mind.

Guidelines that nurses can use to evaluate the potential usefulness of their self-disclosure are listed in Box 2-9. These guidelines govern the "dosage" and timing of self-disclosures and help the nurse assess the appropriateness, effectiveness, and anticipated response of the patient to the disclosure.

Self-disclosure by the nurse is evident in the following example:

 THERAPEUTIC DIALOGUE

PATIENT *When he told me he didn't want to see me again, I felt like slapping him and hugging him at the same time. But then I knew the problem was really me and no one could ever love me.*

NURSE *When I broke off with a man I had been seeing, I felt the anger, hurt, and bitterness you just described. I remember thinking I would never date another man.*

In this example the nurse self-disclosed to emphasize that the patient's feelings were natural. She also reinforced the external cause for the separation (boyfriend's decision to leave versus the patient's inadequacy) and implied that, with time, the patient will be able to resolve the loss.

Box **2-9** *Guidelines for Self-Disclosure*

▼ **Cooperation:** Will the disclosure enhance the patient's cooperation, which is necessary to the development of a therapeutic alliance?

▼ **Learning:** Will the disclosure assist the patient's ability to learn about him- or herself, to set short- and long-term goals, and to deal more effectively with life's problems?

▼ **Catharsis:** Will the disclosure assist the patient to express formerly held or suppressed feelings, important to the relief of emotional symptoms?

▼ **Support:** Will the disclosure provide the patient with support or reinforcement for attaining specific goals?

Emotional Catharsis

Emotional catharsis occurs when the patient is encouraged to talk about things that are most bothersome. Catharsis brings fears, feelings, and experiences out into the open so that they can be examined and discussed with the nurse. The expression of feelings can be very therapeutic in itself, even if behavioral change does not result. The previously described responsive dimensions create an atmosphere within the nurse-patient relationship in which emotional catharsis is possible. The patient's responsiveness depends on the confidence and trust the patient has in the nurse.

The nurse must be able to recognize cues from the patient concerning readiness for discussion of problems. It is important that the nurse proceed at the rate chosen by the patient and provide support during discussion of difficult areas. Forcing emotional catharsis on the patient could precipitate a panic episode because the patient's defenses are attacked without sufficient alternative coping mechanisms available.

Patients are often uncomfortable about expressing feelings. Nurses may be equally uncomfortable with expressing feelings, particularly sadness or anger. Nurses often assume that they know the patient's feelings and do not attempt to specifically validate them. The dimensions of empathy and immediacy require the nurse to notice and express emotions. Unresolved feelings and feelings that are avoided can cause stalls or barriers in the nurse-patient relationship. Specific examples are transference and countertransference phenomena, which are discussed later in the chapter.

If patients have difficulty in expressing feelings, nurses may help by suggesting how they or others might feel in the patient's specific situation. Some patients respond directly to the question, "How did that make you feel?" Others intellectualize and avoid the emotional element in their answer. When patients realize they can express their feelings within an accepting relationship, they expand their awareness and potential acceptance of themselves.

The following example illustrates emotional catharsis:

 THERAPEUTIC DIALOGUE

NURSE *How did you feel when your boss corrected you in front of all those customers?*

PATIENT *Well, I understood that he needed to set me straight, and he's the type that flies off the handle pretty easily anyhow.*

NURSE *It sounds like you're defending his behavior. I was wondering how you felt at that moment.*

PATIENT *Awkward . . . uh . . . upset, I guess (pause).*

NURSE *That would have made me pretty angry if it had happened to me.*

PATIENT *Well, I was. But you can't let it show, you know. You have to keep it all in because of the customers. But he can let it out. Oh sure (emphatically)! He can tell me anything he wants. Just once I'd like him to know how I feel.*

Role Playing

Role playing involves acting out a particular situation. It increases the patient's insight into human relations and can deepen the ability to see the situation from another person's point of view. The purpose of role playing is to represent closely real-life behavior that involves individuals holistically, to focus attention on a problem, and to permit individuals to see themselves in action in a neutral situation. It provides a bridge between thought and action in a safe environment in which the patient can feel free to experiment with new behavior. It is a method of learning that makes actual behavior the focus of study; it is action oriented and provides immediately available information. Role playing consists of the following steps:

1. Defining the problem
2. Creating a readiness for role playing
3. Establishing the situation
4. Casting the characters
5. Briefing and warming up
6. Acting
7. Stopping
8. Analyzing and discussing
9. Evaluation

When role playing is used for attitude change, it relies heavily on role reversal. The patient may be asked to assume the role of a certain person in a specific situation or to play the role of someone with opposing beliefs. Role reversal can help a person reevaluate the other person's intentions and become more understanding of the other person's position. After role reversal, patients may be more receptive to modifying their own attitudes.

As a method of promoting self-awareness and conflict resolution, role playing may help the patient experience a situation rather than just talk about it. Role playing can elicit feelings in the patient that are similar to those experienced in the actual situation. It provides an opportunity for insight and for the expression of affect. For these reasons it is a useful method for heightening a patient's awareness of feelings about a situation.

One of the specific ways in which role playing can be used to resolve conflicts and increase self-awareness is through a dialogue that requires the patient to take the part of each person or each side of an argument. If the conflict is internal, the dialogue occurs in the present tense between the patient's conflicting selves until one part of the conflict outweighs the other. If the conflict involves a second person, the patient is instructed to "imagine that the other person is sitting in the chair across from you." The patient is told to begin the dialogue by expressing wants and resentments about the other person. Then the patient changes chairs, assumes the role of the other person, and responds to what was just said. The patient assumes the first role again and responds to the other person. Using dialogue in this way not only serves as practice for the patient in expressing feel-

ings and opinions but also gives a reality base for the probable response from the other party involved in the conflict. This can often remove the barrier that is keeping the patient from making a decision and acting on it.

Role playing is included as an action dimension because it can help the patient develop insight. Nurses need a variety of intervention skills. Role playing can be effective when an impasse has been reached in the patient's progress or when it is difficult for the patient to translate insight into action. In these instances it can reduce tension and give the patient the opportunity to practice or test new behaviors for future use.

Table 2-5 summarizes the responsive and action dimensions for therapeutic nurse-patient relationships. In concluding this section on therapeutic dimensions, it must be emphasized that the nurse's effectiveness is based on openness to learning what works best with particular kinds of patients. Both the use of communication techniques and the therapeutic conditions must be individualized to the nurse's personality and the patient's needs. The nurse must be willing to try other approaches that seem potentially helpful when the current approach seems ineffective at a given time.

THERAPEUTIC IMPASSES

Therapeutic impasses are blocks in the progress of the nurse-patient relationship. They arise for a variety of reasons, but they all create stalls in the therapeutic relationship. Impasses provoke intense feelings in both the nurse and the patient that may range from anxiety and apprehension to frustration, love, or intense anger. Four specific therapeutic impasses and ways to overcome them are discussed here: resistance, transference, countertransference, and boundary violations.

Resistance

Resistance is the patient's attempt to remain unaware of anxiety-producing aspects. It is a natural reluctance or learned avoidance of verbalizing or even experiencing troubled aspects of self. The term *resistance* was initially introduced by Freud to mean the patient's unconscious opposition to exploring or recognizing unconscious or even preconscious material. Primary resistance is often caused by the patient's unwillingness to change when the need for change is recognized. Patients usually display resistance behaviors during the working phase of the relationship, because this phase encompasses the greater part of the problem-solving process.

Resistance may also be a reaction by the patient to the nurse who has moved too rapidly or too deeply into the patient's feelings or who has intentionally or unintentionally communicated a lack of respect. It may also simply be the result of a patient who is working with a nurse who is an inappropriate role model for therapeutic behavior.

TABLE **2-5** *Responsive and Action Dimensions for Therapeutic Nurse-Patient Relationships*

DIMENSION	CHARACTERISTICS
RESPONSIVE DIMENSIONS	
Genuineness	Implies that the nurse is an open person who is self-congruent, authentic, and transparent
Respect	Suggests that the patient is regarded as a person of worth who is valued and accepted without qualification
Empathic understanding	Viewing the patient's world from the patient's internal frame of reference, with sensitivity to the patient's current feelings and the verbal ability to communicate this understanding in a language attuned to the patient
Concreteness	Involves the use of specific terminology rather than abstractions in the discussion of the patient's feelings, experiences, and behavior
ACTION DIMENSIONS	
Confrontation	The expression by the nurse of perceived discrepancies in the patient's behavior to expand self-awareness
Immediacy	Occurs when the current interaction of the nurse and patient is focused on and is used to learn about the patient's functioning in other interpersonal relationships
Nurse self-disclosure	Evident when the nurse reveals personal information, ideas, values, feelings, and attitudes to facilitate the patient's cooperation, learning, catharsis, or support
Emotional catharsis	Takes place when the patient is encouraged to talk about things that are most bothersome
Role playing	The acting out of a particular situation to increase the patient's insight into human relations and deepen the ability to see a situation from another point of view. It also allows the patient to experiment with new behavior in a safe environment

Secondary gain is another cause of resistance. Favorable environmental, interpersonal, and situational changes occur, and material advantages may be secured as a result of the illness. Types of secondary gain include financial compensation, avoiding unpleasant situations, increased sympathy or attention, escape from responsibility, attempted control of people, and lessening of social pressures. Secondary gain can become a powerful force in the perpetuation and propagation of an illness because it makes the environment more comfortable.

Resistance may take many forms. Box 2-10 lists some of the forms of resistance that patients display, as identified by Wolberg.[41]

Transference

Transference is an unconscious response in which the patient experiences feelings and attitudes toward the nurse that were originally associated with significant figures earlier in life. They may be triggered by some superficial similarity, such as a facial feature or manner of speech, or by the patient's perceived similarity of the relationship. These reactions are an attempt to reduce or alleviate anxiety. The outstanding trait defining transference is the inappropriateness of the patient's response in terms of intensity.

Transference reduces self-awareness by helping the patient maintain a generalized view of the world in which all people are seen in similar terms. Thus the nurse may be viewed as an authority figure from the past, such as a parent figure, or as a lost loved object, such as a former spouse. Transference reactions are harmful to the therapeutic process only if they remain ignored and unexamined.

Two types of transference present particular resistances in the nurse-patient relationship. The first is the **hostile transference.** If the patient internalizes anger and hostility, this resistance may be expressed as depression and discouragement. The patient may ask to terminate the relationship on the grounds that there is no chance of getting well. If the hostility is externalized, the patient may become critical, defiant, and irritable and may express doubts about the nurse's training, experience, or personal adjustment. The patient may attempt to compete with the nurse by reading books on psychology and challenging him.

Hostility may also be expressed by the patient in detachment, forgetfulness, irrelevant chatter, or preoccupation with childhood experiences. An extreme form of uncooperativeness and negativism is evident in prolonged silences. Some of the most frustrating moments for the nurse are those spent in total silence with a patient. This is not the therapeutic silence that communicates mutuality and understanding. Rather, it is the silence that seems to be hostile, oppressive, and eternal. It is particularly disturbing for the nurse in the orientation phase, before a relationship has been established. The nurse's task is to understand the meaning of the patient's silence and decide how to deal with it despite feeling somewhat awkward and useless.

A second difficult type of transference is the **dependent reaction transference.** This resistance is characterized by patients who are submissive, subordinate, and ingratiating and who regard the nurse as a godlike figure. The patient overvalues the nurse's characteristics and qualities, and their relationship is in jeopardy because the patient views it

Box **2-10** *Forms of Resistance Displayed by Patients*

▼ Suppression and repression of pertinent information
▼ Intensification of symptoms
▼ Self-devaluation and a hopeless outlook on the future
▼ Forced flight into health where there is a sudden, but short-lived recovery by the patient
▼ Intellectual inhibitions, which may be evident when the patient says she has "nothing on her mind" or that she is "unable to think about her problems" or when she breaks appointments, is late for sessions, or is forgetful, silent, or sleepy
▼ Acting out or irrational behavior

▼ Superficial talk
▼ Intellectual insight in which the patient verbalizes self-understanding with correct use of terminology yet continues destructive behavior, or uses the defense of intellectualization where there is no insight
▼ Contempt for normality, which is evident when the patient has developed insight but refuses to assume the responsibility for change on the grounds that normality "isn't so great"
▼ Transference reactions

as magical. In this reaction the nurse must live up to the patient's overwhelming expectations, which is impossible because these expectations are completely unrealistic. The patient continues to demand more of the nurse, and when these needs are not met, the patient is filled with hostility and contempt.

Overcoming Resistance and Transference

Resistances and transferences can pose difficult problems for the nurse. The psychiatric nurse must be prepared to be exposed to powerful negative and positive emotional feelings coming from the patient, often on a highly irrational basis. The relationship can become stalled and nonbeneficial if the nurse is not prepared to deal with the patient's feelings.

Sometimes resistances occur because the nurse and patient have not arrived at mutually acceptable goals or plans of action. This may occur if the contract was not clearly defined in the orientation stage of the relationship. The appropriate action here is to return to the goals, purposes, and roles of the nurse and patient in the relationship.

Whatever the patient's motivations, the analysis of the resistance or transference is geared toward the patient gaining awareness of these motivations and learning about being completely responsible for all actions and behavior. The first thing the nurse must do is listen. When the nurse recognizes the resistance, clarification and reflection of feeling can be used. Clarification gives the nurse a more focused idea of what is happening. Reflection of content may help patients become aware of what has been going on in their own minds. Reflection of feeling acknowledges the resistance and mirrors it to the patient. The nurse may say, "I sense that you're struggling with yourself. Part of you wants to explore the issue of your marriage and another part says 'No—I'm not ready yet.' "

However, it is not sufficient to merely identify that resistance is occurring. The behavior must be explored and possible reasons for its occurrence analyzed. The depth of exploration and analysis engaged in by nurse and patient is related to the nurse's experience and knowledge base.

Countertransference

Countertransference is a therapeutic impasse created by the nurse's specific emotional response generated by the qualities of the patient. This response is inappropriate to the content and context of the therapeutic relationship or inappropriate in the degree of intensity of emotion. It is transference applied to the nurse. Inappropriateness is the crucial element, as it is with transference, because it is natural that the nurse will have a warmth toward or liking for some patients more than others. The nurse will also be genuinely angry with the actions of certain patients. But in countertransference the nurse's responses are not justified by reality. In this case nurses identify the patient with individuals from their past, and personal needs will interfere with therapeutic effectiveness.

Countertransference reactions are usually of three types:
▼ Reactions of intense love or caring
▼ Reactions of intense disgust or hostility
▼ Reactions of intense anxiety often in response to resistance by the patient

Through the use of immediacy the nurse can identify countertransference in one of its various forms (Box 2-11).

Forms of countertransference occur because the nurse is involved with the patient as a participant observer and is not a detached bystander. These reactions can be powerful tools in exploration and potent instruments for uncovering inner states. They are destructive only if they are brushed aside, ignored, or not taken seriously.

If studied objectively, these reactions can lead to further information about the patient. The ability to remain objective does not mean that the nurse may not at times dislike what the patient says or may not become irritated. The patient's resistance to acquiring insight and transforming it into action and the refusal to change maladaptive and destructive coping mechanisms can be frustrating. But the nurse's capacity to understand personal feelings helps to maintain a working relationship with the patient.

Countertransference may also be manifested as a group phenomenon. Psychiatric staff members can become involved in countertransference reactions when they overreact

Box **2-11** *Forms of Countertransference Displayed by Nurses*

▼ Difficulty empathizing with the patient in certain problem areas
▼ Feelings of depression during or after the session
▼ Carelessness about implementing the contract by being late, running overtime, etc.
▼ Drowsiness during the sessions
▼ Feelings of anger or impatience because of the patient's unwillingness to change
▼ Encouragement of the patient's dependency, praise, or affection
▼ Arguments with the patient or a tendency to push before the patient is ready

▼ Attempts to help the patient in matters not related to the identified nursing goals
▼ Personal or social involvement with the patient
▼ Dreams about or preoccupation with the patient
▼ Sexual or aggressive fantasies toward the patient
▼ Recurrent anxiety, unease, or guilt related to the patient
▼ Tendency to focus on only one aspect or way of looking at information presented by the patient
▼ Need to defend nursing interventions with the patient to others

to a patient's aggressive behavior, ignore available patient data that would promote understanding, or become locked in a power struggle with a patient. Other types of countertransference might include ignoring patient behavior that does not fit the staff's diagnosis, minimizing a patient's behavior, joking about or criticizing a patient, or becoming caught up in intimidation. Although these have been reported as phenomena of group countertransference, they can also illustrate individual countertransference reactions.

The experienced nurse is constantly on the lookout for countertransference, becomes aware of it when it occurs, and holds it in abeyance or uses it to promote the therapeutic goals. In attempting to identify a countertransference, the nurse must apply the same standards of honest self-appraisal personally that are expected of the patient. The nurse should use self-examination throughout the course of the relationship, particularly when the patient attacks or criticizes. The following questions may be helpful:

▼ How do I feel about the patient?
▼ Do I look forward to seeing the patient?
▼ Do I feel sorry for or sympathetic toward the patient?
▼ Am I bored with the patient and believe that we are not progressing?
▼ Am I afraid of the patient?
▼ Do I get extreme pleasure out of seeing the patient?
▼ Do I want to protect, reject, or punish the patient?
▼ Do I dread meeting the patient and feel nervous during the sessions?
▼ Am I impressed by or try to impress the patient?
▼ Does the patient make me very angry or frustrated?

If any of these questions suggests a problem, the nurse should pursue it. What is the patient doing to provoke these feelings? Who does the patient remind me of? The nurse must discover the source of the problem. Because countertransference can be detrimental to the relationship, it should be dealt with as soon as possible. When it is recognized, the nurse can exercise control over it. If the nurse needs help in dealing with countertransference, individual or group supervision can be most beneficial.

PROBLEM PATIENTS. Countertransference problems are most clearly evident when a patient is labeled a "problem patient." Usually such a patient elicits strong negative feelings such as anger, fear, and helplessness and is often described by nurses as manipulative, dependent, inappropriate, and demanding. The label *problem patient* implies that the patient's behavior should change for the sake of the helper rather than for the patient's own benefit. This labeling often causes the patient and nurse to become adversaries, and the nurse avoids contact.

It is more productive for a nurse to view a "problem patient" as one who poses problems for the nurse. This turns the responsibility for action back onto the nurse. It forces the nurse to explore responses to the patient that reinforce the patient's unproductive behavior. In this way the nurse also makes patients responsible for their behavior. By stepping back and reviewing again the patient's needs and problems, the nurse becomes aware of failing to use the responsive dimensions of genuineness, respect, empathic understanding, and concreteness. Without this therapeutic groundwork, a therapeutic outcome is impossible.

Boundary Violations

A final but very important therapeutic impasse is that of boundary violations. These occur when a nurse goes outside the boundaries of the therapeutic relationship and establishes a social, economic, or personal relationship with a patient. As a general rule, whenever the nurse is doing or thinking of doing something special, different, or unusual for a patient, often a boundary violation is involved. A nurse should consider the possibility of a boundary violation if he or she[30]

▼ Receives feedback that his or her behavior is intrusive with patients or their families
▼ Has difficulty setting limits with a patient
▼ Relates to a patient like a friend or family member
▼ Has sexual feelings toward a patient
▼ Feels that he or she is the only one who understands the patient

▼ Receives feedback that he or she is too involved with a patient or family

▼ Feels that other staff are too critical of a particular patient

▼ Believes that other staff members are jealous of his or her relationship with a patient.

Specific examples of possible boundary violations are listed in Box 2-12.

Categorizing boundary violations may be helpful for the psychiatric nurse in examining this issue in greater detail. It is possible to categorize boundary violations under the following categories[11,14]:

▼ **Role boundaries:** These are a core component of the psychiatric nurse's role. They are embodied in the question, Is this what a psychiatric nurse does? Problems with role boundaries require the insight of the nurse and the setting of firm therapeutic limits with the patient.

▼ **Time boundaries:** These address the conditions surrounding the time of day that the nurse implements treatment. Odd and unusual treatment hours that have no therapeutic necessity must be evaluated as potential boundary violations.

▼ **Place and space boundaries:** This issue is related to where treatment actually takes place. An office or hospital unit is the usual locale for most treatment. Treatment out of the office usually merits special scrutiny. Most often treatment over lunch, in the car, or in the patient's home must have a good therapeutic rationale and explicit treatment goals. In an inpatient setting, any time spent by a nurse in a patient's room should be done so only if indicated and with appropriate action taken to respect boundary concerns, such as with the door open and in the presence of other staff.

▼ **Money boundaries:** This issue relates to honoring the compensation for treatment established between the nurse and patient. Bartering or seeing an indigent patient for free should be carefully reviewed for potential boundary violations.

▼ **Gifts and services boundaries:** Gift giving is a controversial issue in nursing (see Critical Thinking about Contemporary Issues). Gifts that are obvious boundary violations place undue obligations on the patient for the benefit of the nurse. Gifts can be divided into five types[23]:

  ▼ Gifts to reciprocate for care given

  ▼ Gifts intended to manipulate or change the quality of care given or the nature of the nurse-patient relationship

  ▼ Gifts given as perceived obligation by the patient

  ▼ Serendipitous gifts or gifts received by chance

  ▼ Gifts given to the organization to recognize excellence of care received

The nurse must carefully consider how to respond to each of these categories based on the intention of the gift and the possibility of boundary violations.

Box **2-12** *Possible Boundary Violations Related to Psychiatric Nurses*

▼ The patient takes the nurse out to lunch or dinner
▼ The professional relationship turns into a social relationship
▼ The nurse attends a party at a patient's invitation
▼ The nurse regularly reveals personal information to the patient
▼ The patient introduces the nurse to family members, such as a son or daughter, for the purpose of a social relationship
▼ The nurse accepts free gifts from the patient's business
▼ The nurse agrees to meet the patient for treatment outside of the usual setting without therapeutic justification
▼ The nurse attends social functions of the patient
▼ The patient gives the nurse an expensive gift
▼ The nurse routinely hugs or has physical contact with the patient
▼ The nurse does business or purchases services from the patient

---

▼ **Clothing boundaries:** This pertains to the nurse's need to dress in an appropriate therapeutic manner. Suggestive or seductive clothing of the nurse is unacceptable and limits should be set on inappropriate dress by patients as well.

▼ **Language boundaries:** This boundary raises questions of when patients should be addressed by their first or last names, the tone that the nurse uses when talking with the patient, and the nurse's choice of words in implementing care. Too familiar, sexual, or leading language constitutes a boundary violation.

▼ **Self-disclosure boundaries:** Inappropriately timed self-disclosure by the nurse and nurse self-disclosure that lacks therapeutic value are suspect for boundary violations, as discussed previously in this chapter.

▼ **Physical contact boundaries:** All physical contact with a patient must be evaluated for possible boundary violations. Sexual contact of any kind is never therapeutic and never acceptable within the nurse-patient relationship.

THERAPEUTIC OUTCOME

The nurse's effectiveness in working with psychiatric patients is related to knowledge base, clinical skills, and capacity for introspection and self-evaluation. The nurse and patient, as participants in an interpersonal relationship, are entwined in a pattern of reciprocal emotions that directly affect the therapeutic outcome. The nurse conveys feelings to the patient. Some of these are in response to the patient; others arise from the nurse's personal life and are not necessarily associated with the patient.

Many painful feelings arise within the nurse because of the nature of the therapeutic process, which can be stressful. These "normal" stresses are caused by a variety of factors.

CRITICAL THINKING *about* *Contemporary Issues*

Is Gift Giving Acceptable Behavior in the Therapeutic Nurse-Patient Relationship?

Gift giving is a controversial issue in nursing. There has been a long-accepted taboo in nursing on accepting gifts from patients. On the other hand, some have questioned the theoretical rationale for this position and suggest that gift giving can sometimes serve discrete therapeutic purposes.[23]

Gifts can take many forms. They can be tangible or intangible, lasting or temporary. Tangible gifts may include such items as a box of candy, a bouquet of flowers, a hand-knit scarf, or a hand-painted picture. Intangible gifts can be the expression of thanks to a nurse by a patient who is about to be discharged or a family member's sense of relief and gratitude at being able to share an emotional burden with another caring person. The underlying element of all of these gifts is that something of value is voluntarily offered to another person, usually to convey gratitude.

Because gifts can be so varied, it is inappropriate to lump them all together and uniformly arrive at an appropriate nursing action. Rather, the nurse's response to gift giving and the role it plays in the therapeutic relationship depends on the timing of the particular situation, the intent of the giver, and the contextual meaning of the giving of the gift. Occasionally it may be most appropriate and therapeutic for the nurse to accept a patient's gift; on other occasions it may be quite inappropriate and detrimental to the relationship.

The timing of the gift giving is an important consideration. In the introductory, or orientation, phase of the relationship, nurses may be asked, "Do you have a cigarette I can borrow?" or "Will you buy me a cup of coffee?" These seemingly minor requests may make the nurse feel uncomfortable refusing them. The nurse may rationalize compliance by thinking that it indicates interest in the patient and may help win his trust. But these responses indicate the nurse's failure to examine the patient's covert, or underlying, need and the nurse's own needs in complying with it. Also, in this early phase of the relationship, the nurse may be the one to initiate gift giving by giving the patient a book, plant, or some other item that expresses interest in the patient.

In the orientation phase of the relationship, gift giving can be detrimental because it often meets personal needs rather than therapeutic goals. The patient may be trying to manipulate the nurse as a way to control the relationship and set interpersonal limits on the level of intimacy that will be allowed. By giving gifts to the patient, the nurse is attempting to relate through objects instead of the therapeutic use of self and is avoiding exploring possible feelings of inadequacy or frustration.

As the relationship progresses, gift giving may take on a different significance. In the working phase, for example, the patient may one day offer to buy the nurse a cup of coffee. This can be an indication of the patient's respect for the nurse and of belief in the mutuality of their work together. As an isolated incident, the nurse's acceptance of it can enhance the patient's confidence, self-esteem, and sense of responsibility.

Gift giving most often arises in the termination phase of the relationship, and it is in this phase that the meaning behind it can be the most complex and difficult to determine. At this time gift giving can be tangible or intangible and can reflect a patient's need to make the nurse feel guilty, delay the termination process, compensate for feelings of inadequacy, or attempt to transform the therapeutic nurse-patient relationship into a social one that can possibly go on indefinitely. The nurse can initiate gift giving for similar reasons. The feelings evoked during the termination process can be very powerful, and they must be acknowledged and explored if termination is to be a learning experience for both participants. If feelings are identified and clarified, then a small gift that reflects gratitude and remembrance can be exchanged, accepted, and valued.

Although it is necessary to be a skilled listener, it is inappropriate for the nurse to discuss personal conflicts or responses, except when they may help the patient. This bottling up of emotions can be painful. The nurse is expected to empathize with the patient's emotions and feelings. At the same time, however, the nurse is expected to retain objectivity and not be caught up in a sympathetic response. This can create a kind of double bind.

Termination poses another stress when the nurse must separate from a patient she has come to know well and care for deeply. It is common to experience a grief reaction in response to the loss. Many nurses find it emotionally draining when a patient communicates a prolonged and intense expression of emotion, such as sadness, despair, or anger. Discomfort also arises when the nurse feels unable to help a patient who is in great distress. Suicide dramatizes this situation. Treating suicidal individuals can arouse intense and prolonged anxiety in the nurse.

The painful nature of these emotional responses makes the practice of psychiatric nursing challenging and stressful.

The therapeutic use of self involves the nurse's total personality, and total involvement is not an easy task. It is essential that the nurse be aware of personal feelings and responses and receive guidance and support.

Summary

1. The therapeutic nurse-patient relationship is a mutual learning experience and a corrective emotional experience for the patient. The nurse uses personal attributes and specified clinical techniques in working with the patient to bring about behavioral change.
2. The following qualities are needed by nurses to be effective helpers: awareness of self, clarification of values, exploration of feelings, ability to serve as a role model, altruism, and a sense of ethics and responsibility.
3. The structural and transactional analysis models were used to examine components of the communication process and to identify common problems. Helpful therapeutic communication techniques were also discussed.

4. The responsive dimensions of genuineness, respect, empathic understanding, and concreteness were presented.
5. The action dimensions of confrontation, immediacy, nurse self-disclosure, catharsis, and role playing stimulate and contribute to patient insight.
6. Therapeutic impasses such as resistance, transference, countertransference, and boundary violations are roadblocks in the progress of the nurse-patient relationship.
7. The therapeutic outcome in working with psychiatric patients is related to the nurse's knowledge base, clinical skills, and capacity for introspection and self-evaluation.

 Video **Resources**

Mosby's Communication in Nursing Video Series:

Basic Principles for Communicating Effectively in Nursing
Communicating with Clients and Colleagues: Effectiveness in the Caring Environment

Communicating with Clients and Colleagues from Different Cultures
Communicating with Difficult Clients and Colleagues
Communicating with Clients with Mental Disorders or Emotional Problems
Communicating Across the Life Span: Children, Families, and the Elderly

your **INTERNET**
connection

National Institute of Mental Health
http://www.nimh.nih.gov

Internet Mental Health
http://www.mentalhealth.com

 Chapter Review Questions

1. **For each of the activities described below, select the correct phase of the therapeutic relationship.**

   Orientation
   Preinteraction
   Termination
   Working

   A. _preinteraction_   Analyze own feelings and fears
   B. _orientation_   Define goals with the patient
   C. _orientation_   Determine why the patient sought help
   D. _termination_   Explore feelings of loss and separation
   E. _working_   Evaluate patient stressors
   F. _orientation_   Formulate a contract
   G. _preinteraction_   Gather data about the patient
   H. _working_   Overcome resistance
   I. _working_   Promote insight and behavioral change
   J. _termination_   Review goal attainment

2. **Fill in the blanks.**

A. When a person sends double messages or verbal and nonverbal messages that do not agree, it is called _incongruent_ communication.

B. Reflection of the content of a patient's communication back to him is called _validation_.

C. The responsive dimension of _empathy_ is the ability to see the patient's world from her point of view and to communicate this to the patient.

D. A _boundary violation_ occurs when a nurse goes outside the limits of the therapeutic relationship and establishes a social, economic, or personal relationship with a patient.

3. **Provide short answers for the following questions.**

A. Identify four guidelines that should be used to evaluate the potential usefulness of nurse self-disclosure.

B. List elements that should be included in a nurse-patient contract.

C. Describe how the items listed apply to a social and a therapeutic relationship.

   Item
   Purpose
      Social _____
      Therapeutic _____
   Use of feelings
      Social _____
      Therapeutic _____
   Content of interaction
      Social _____
      Therapeutic _____
   Confidentiality
      Social _____
      Therapeutic _____
   Termination
      Social _____
      Therapeutic _____

D. Think of a patient you recently cared for as a nurse. Evaluate how well you demonstrated each of the responsive dimensions of the therapeutic nurse-patient relationship described in this chapter.

E. Have you observed any boundary violations among your nursing colleagues? If so, have you talked with them about it? If not, why not?

4. Match the terms in Column A with the correct example in Column B.

Column A	Column B
___Altruism	A. Dependency by a patient on the nurse for getting better and coping with life.
___Catharsis	B. Encouraging a patient to talk about her feelings related to her brother's death.
___Confrontation	C. Having the patient assume the part of her husband when talking with the nurse about her marital problems.
___Countertransference	D. Irritation and disgust evidenced by a nurse toward a patient who is not responding to the treatment plan.
___Resistance	E. Refusal by a patient to discuss early events as they relate to her current depression.
___Role playing	F. Sharing the observation with a patient that he asks to be treated as a responsible adult but he has not been able to keep his last three jobs longer than a month.
___Transference	G. Volunteering to prepare and serve meals at a local homeless shelter.

REFERENCES

1. Alligood M: Empathy: the importance of recognizing two types, *J Psychosoc Nurs* 30:14, 1992.
2. Berne E: *Games people play: the psychology of human relationships,* New York, 1964, Grove Press.
3. Bromley G: Confrontation in individual psychotherapy, *J Psychosoc Nurs Ment Health Serv* 19:15, 1981.
4. Buxman K: Humor in therapy for the mentally ill, *J Psychiatr Nurs Ment Health Serv* 29:15, 1991.
5. Campbell J: The relationship of nursing and self-awareness, *Adv Nurs Sci* 2:15, 1980.
6. Carkhoff R: *Helping and human relations,* vols 1 and 2, New York, 1969, Holt, Rinehart & Winston.
7. Carkhoff R, Berenson B: *Beyond counseling and therapy,* New York, 1967, Holt, Rinehart & Winston.
8. Carkhoff R, Truax C: *Toward effective counseling and psychotherapy,* Chicago, 1967, Aldine Publishing.
9. Cravener P: Establishing therapeutic alliance across cultural barriers, *J Psychosoc Nurs Ment Health Serv* 30:11, 1992.
10. Davidhizar R, Bowen M: The dynamics of laughter, *Arch Psychiatr Nurs* 6:132, 1992.
11. Epstein R: *Keeping boundaries: maintaining safety and integrity in the psychotherapeutic process,* Washington DC, 1994, American Psychiatric Press.
12. Forchuk C: Development of nurse-client relationships: what helps?, *J Am Psych Nurs Assoc* 1:146, 1995.
13. Gazda G et al: *Human relations development: a manual for educators,* Boston, 1971, Allyn & Bacon.
14. Guthiel T, Gabbard G: The concept of boundaries in clinical practice: theoretical and risk-management dimensions, *Am J Psychiatry* 150:188, 1993.
15. Jourard S: *The transparent self,* New York, 1971, Litton Educational Publishing.
16. Kalisch B: What is empathy? *Am J Nurs* 73:1548, 1973.
17. Kemper B: Therapeutic listening, *J Psychosoc Nurs Ment Health Serv* 30:21, 1992.
18. Kirschenbaum H, Simon S, eds: *Readings in values clarification,* Minneapolis, 1973, Winston Press.
19. Mackay R, Hughes J, Carver E, eds: *Empathy in the helping relationship,* New York, 1990, Springer.
20. Mansfield E: Empathy: concept and identified psychiatric nursing behavior, *Nurs Res* 22:525, 1973.
21. McAllister M: The nurse as a tour guide: a metaphor for debriefing students in mental health nursing, *Issues Ment Health Nurs* 16:395, 1995.
22. Morrison P, Burnard P: Students' and trained nurses' perception of their own interpersonal skills: a report and comparison, *J Adv Nurs* 14:321, 1989.
23. Morse J: The structure and function of gift giving in the patient-nurse relationship, *West J Nurs Res* 13:597, 1991.
24. Morse J et al: Exploring empathy: a conceptual fit for nursing practice? *Image J Nurs Sch* 24:273, 1992.
25. Muller A, Poggenpoel M: Patients' internal world experiences of interacting with psychiatric nurses, *Arch Psychiatr Nurs* 10:143, 1996.
26. Nichols M: *The lost art of listening,* New York, 1995, The Guilford Press.
27. Olson J: Relationships between nurse-expressed empathy, patient-perceived empathy and patient distress, *Image* 27:317, 1995.
28. Oquendo M: Psychiatric evaluation and psychotherapy in the patient's second language, *Psychiatr Serv,* 47:614, 1996.
29. Pasquali E: Learning to laugh: humor as therapy, *J Psychosoc Nurs Ment Health Serv* 28:31, 1990.
30. Pilette P, Bereck C, Archber L: Therapeutic management of helping boundaries, *J Psychosoc Nurs* 33:40, 1995.
31. Robinson V: *Humor and the health professions.* Thorofare, NJ, 1991, Slack.
32. Rogers C: *On becoming a person,* Boston, 1961, Houghton Mifflin.
33. Rogers C: Empathic: an unappreciated way of being, *J Counsel Psychol* 5:2, 1975.

34. Ruesch J: *Disturbed communication,* New York, 1972, WW Norton.

35. Stricker G, Fisher M: *Self-disclosure in the therapeutic relationship,* New York, 1990, Plenum Press.

36. Sundeen S et al: *Nurse-client interaction: implementing the nursing process,* ed 6, St Louis, 1998, Mosby.

37. Tommasini N: The use of touch with the hospitalized psychiatric patient, *Arch Psychiatr Nurs* 4:213, 1990.

38. Warner S: Humor: a coping response for student nurses, *Arch Psychiatr Nurs* 5:10, 1991.

39. Wheeler K, Barrett E: Review and synthesis of selected nursing studies on teaching empathy and implication for nursing research and education, *Nurs Outlook* 42:230, 1994.

40. Williams C: Biopsychosocial elements of empathy: a multidimensional model, *Issues Ment Health Nurs* 11:155, 1990.

41. Wolberg L: *The technique of psychotherapy,* ed 4, Orlando Fla, 1988, Grune & Stratton.

Annotated Suggested Readings

Epstein R: *Keeping boundaries: maintaining safety and integrity in the psychotherapeutic process,* Washington, DC, 1994, American Psychiatric Press.

This practical book provides ways for therapists to improve their skills in maintaining therapeutic boundaries by working with patients through continuing self-assessment and education. Highly recommended.

*Hummelvoli J: The nurse-client alliance model, *Perspect Psychiatr Care* 32:12, 1996.

This model compliments the biomedical model and has a holistic, existential basis. It does not try to explain why things happen but rather focuses on helping patients gain insight and access to their subjective experience.

*Nursing reference.

*McAllister M: The nurse as tour guide: a metaphor for debriefing students in mental health nursing, *Issues Ment Health Nurs* 16:395, 1995.

Describes a debriefing learning activity for students after their psychiatric rotation in which they were asked to consider the metaphor "nurse as tour guide" and evaluate how that image could be associated with psychiatric nursing in the agency they had just visited.

Montgomery C: *Healing through communication: the practice of caring,* Newbury Park, Calif, 1993, Safe Publications.

Superb text that examines the concept, manifestations, and effects of caring. Important reading for every nurse.

Nichols M: *The lost art of listening,* New York, 1995, The Guilford Press.

A psychoanalyst and family therapist explain why listening is such a powerful force in our lives, how to listen, how to recognize bad listening habits, and how to really be heard.

Sundeen S et al: *Nurse-client interaction: implementing the nursing process,* ed 6, St Louis, 1998, Mosby.

Describes the nursing process, including concepts relating to self, communication, phases of the nurse-client relationship, and stress and adaptation. A useful reference for developing relationship skills.

Whalley P: Team approach to working through transference and countertransference in a pediatric/psychiatric milieu, *Issues Ment Health Nurs* 15:457, 1994.

Transference issues must be understood to work through the intense pain and anger that often dominate this milieu, and staff must be helped to examine their biases against patients' expressions of anger and hostility.

Willson J, Hobbs H: Therapeutic partnership: a model for clinical practice, *J Psychosoc Nurs* 33:27, 1995

Therapeutic partnership is a highly intense, time-limited, goal-directed involvement that conveys a culture of hope and reinforces shared responsibility, accountability, and decision-making.

Chapter 3

Conceptual Models of Psychiatric Treatment

Gail W. Stuart

© 1998 M.C. Escher/Cordon Art, Baarn, Holland.

Though this be madness, yet there is method in't. **William Shakespeare** Hamlet, Act II

LEARNING OBJECTIVES

After studying this chapter the student should be able to:

▼ Describe the psychoanalytical model, including its view of behavioral deviations, the therapeutic process, and roles of the patient and therapist

▼ Describe the interpersonal model, including its view of behavioral deviations, the therapeutic process, and roles of the patient and therapist

▼ Describe the social model, including its view of behavioral deviations, the therapeutic process, and roles of the patient and therapist

▼ Describe the existential model, including its view of behavioral deviations, the therapeutic process, and roles of the patient and therapist

▼ Describe the supportive therapy model, including its view of behavioral deviations, the therapeutic process, and roles of the patient and therapist

▼ Describe the medical model, including its view of behavioral deviations, the therapeutic process, and roles of the patient and therapist

TOPICAL OUTLINE

Psychoanalytical Model
  View of Behavioral Deviations
  Psychoanalytical Therapeutic Process
  Roles of Patient and Psychoanalyst
  Other Psychoanalytical Theorists
Interpersonal Model
  View of Behavioral Deviations
  Interpersonal Therapeutic Process
  Roles of Patient and Interpersonal Therapist
Social Model
  View of Behavioral Deviations
  Social Therapeutic Process
  Roles of Patient and Social Therapist
Existential Model
  View of Behavioral Deviations
  Existential Therapeutic Process
  Roles of Patient and Existential Therapist
Supportive Therapy Model
  View of Behavioral Deviations
  Supportive Therapeutic Process
  Roles of Patient and Supportive Therapist
Medical Model
  View of Behavioral Deviations
  Medical Therapeutic Process
  Roles of Patient and Medical Therapist

Mental health professionals should base their practice on a conceptual model of psychiatric treatment. A model is a way of organizing a complex body of knowledge, such as concepts related to human behavior. Models help clinicians by suggesting

▼ Reasons for observed behavior
▼ Therapeutic treatment strategies
▼ Appropriate roles for patient and therapist

Models also provide for the organization of data. Organization allows the clinician to measure the effectiveness of the treatment process and facilitates research into human behavior.

This chapter presents an overview of some of the conceptual models used by mental health professionals, including the psychoanalytical, interpersonal, social, existential, supportive, and medical models. Other models often used by nurses are discussed in other chapters of this text including cognitive behavioral (Chapter 30), group (Chapter 31), and family (Chapter 32). Finally, the Stuart Stress Adaptation Model of psychiatric nursing, which is the organizing conceptual framework for this text, is presented in detail in Chapter 4.

PSYCHOANALYTICAL MODEL

Psychoanalytical theory was developed by Sigmund Freud (Fig. 3-1) in the late nineteenth and early twentieth centuries.[8] It focused on the nature of deviant behavior and proposed a new perspective on human development. Many of Freud's ideas were controversial, particularly in the Victorian society of that time. Objective observation of human behavior was a great contribution of the psychoanalysts, as was the identification of a mental structure. Such concepts as id, ego, superego, and ego defense mechanisms are still widely used. Most people also accept the existence of an unconscious level of mental functioning, first introduced by Freud.

View of Behavioral Deviations

Psychoanalysts trace disrupted behavior in the adult to earlier developmental stages. Each stage of development has a task that must be accomplished. If too much emphasis is placed on any stage or if unusual difficulty arises in dealing with the associated conflicts, psychological energy (libido) becomes fixated in an attempt to deal with anxiety.

Psychoanalysts believe that neurotic symptoms arise when so much energy goes into controlling anxiety that it interferes with the individual's ability to function. They believe that everyone is neurotic to some extent. Everyone carries the burden of childhood conflicts and is influenced in adulthood by childhood experiences. Psychoanalysts in training must undergo personal analysis so that their own neurotic behavior does not hinder their objectivity as therapists.

According to psychoanalytic theory, symptoms are sym-

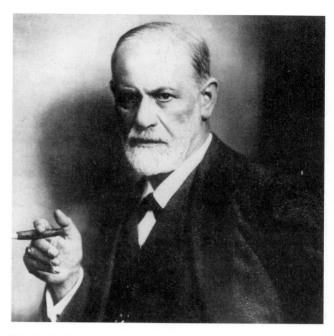

Fig. 3-1 **Sigmund Freud.** (From the Bettman Archive.)

bols of the original conflict. For instance, compulsive hand washing may represent the person's attempt to cleanse the self of impulses that a parent labeled unclean during the anal stage of development. However, the meaning of the behavior is hidden from the conscious awareness of the person, who usually is upset about these uncontrollable feelings.

Freud developed most of his theories around neurotic symptoms. His theory is less well developed in the area of psychosis. However, other psychoanalytical theorists such as Frieda Fromm-Reichmann[9] have successfully worked with patients with psychosis. They believe that the psychotic symptom arises when the ego must invest most or all of the libido to defend against primitive id impulses. This leaves little energy to deal with external reality and leads to the lack of reality testing seen in psychosis.

Psychoanalytical Therapeutic Process

Psychoanalysis uses free association and dream analysis to reconstruct the personality. Free association is the verbalization of thoughts as they occur, without any conscious screening or censorship. Of course, there is always unconscious censorship of thoughts and impulses that threaten the ego. The psychoanalyst searches for patterns in the areas that are unconsciously avoided. Conflictual areas that the patient does not discuss or recognize are identified as resistances. Analysis of the patient's dreams can provide additional insight into the nature of the resistances because dreams symbolically communicate areas of intrapsychic conflict.

The therapist helps the patient recognize intrapsychic conflicts by using interpretation. Interpretation involves explaining to the patient the meaning of dream symbolism and the significance of the issues that are discussed or avoided. However, the process is complicated by transference, which occurs when the patient develops strong positive or negative feelings toward the analyst. These feelings are unrelated to the analyst's current behavior or characteristics; they represent the patient's past response to a significant other, usually a parent. Strong positive transference causes the patient to want to please the therapist and to accept the therapist's interpretations of the patient's behavior. Strong negative transference may impede the progress of therapy as the patient actively resists the therapist's interventions. Countertransference, or the therapist's response to the patient, can also interfere with therapy if the analyst is unaware of it or unable to deal with it.

Because the therapist can temporarily replace the significant other of the patient's early life, previously unresolved conflicts can be brought into the therapeutic situation. These conflicts can be worked through to a healthier resolution and more mature adult functioning. Psychoanalytical therapy is usually long term. The patient is often seen five times a week for several years. This approach is therefore time consuming and expensive.

Roles of Patient and Psychoanalyst

The roles of the patient and the psychoanalyst were defined by Freud. The patient was to be an active participant, freely revealing all thoughts exactly as they occurred and describing all dreams. The patient often lies down during therapy to induce relaxation, which facilitates free association.

The psychoanalyst is a shadow person. The patient is expected to reveal all private thoughts and feelings, and the analyst reveals nothing personal. The analyst usually is out of the patient's sight, to ensure that nonverbal responses do not influence the patient. The analyst keeps his or her verbal responses brief and noncommittal in order to prevent interference with the associative flow. For instance, the analyst might respond with "Uh huh," "Go on," or "Tell me more."

The therapist changes this communication style when interpreting behavior. Interpretations are presented for the patient to accept or reject, but rejections suggest resistance. Likewise, frustration that the patient expresses toward the analyst is interpreted as transference. By the end of therapy, the patient should be able to view the analyst realistically, having worked through conflicts and dependency needs.

> **?** *Do you think that the roles of the patient and psychoanalyst support patient empowerment or patient dependency?*

Box **3-1** *Contemporary Psychoanalytical Theorists*

Erik Erikson[5]: Expanded Freud's theory of psychosocial development to encompass the entire life cycle

Anna Freud[7]: Expanded psychoanalytical theory in the area of child psychology

Melanie Klein[13]: Extended the use of psychoanalytical techniques to work with young children through development of play therapy

Karen Horney[12]: Focused on psychoanalytical theory in terms of cultural and interpersonal factors; rejected Freud's view of feminine sexuality

Frieda Fromm-Reichmann[9]: Used psychoanalytical techniques with psychotic patients

Karl Menninger[15]: Applied the concepts of dynamic equilibrium and coping to mental functioning

Other Psychoanalytical Theorists

Much of Freud's theory is still used by psychotherapists. The theorists who followed him have modified and built on the original psychoanalytical theories.

Box 3-1 lists several contemporary psychoanalytical theorists and a brief statement identifying their major contributions.

INTERPERSONAL MODEL

The theorist most representative of the interpersonal model is Harry Stack Sullivan, a twentieth-century American therapist.[23,24] Attention is also given to the interpersonal nursing theory of Hildegard Peplau[17] (Fig. 3-2). Her work on the psychotherapeutic role of the nurse in the interpersonal relationship is a milestone in the field.

View of Behavioral Deviations

Interpersonal theorists believe that behavior evolves around interpersonal relationships. Whereas Freudian theory emphasizes a person's intrapsychic experience, interpersonal theory emphasizes social or interpersonal experience. Sullivan, like Freud, traces a progression of psychological development. Sullivan's theory states that the person bases behavior on two drives: the drive for satisfaction and the drive for security. Satisfaction includes the basic human drives of hunger, sleep, lust, and loneliness. Security relates to culturally defined needs such as conformity to the social norms and value system of the individual's reference group. Sullivan states that when a person's self-system interferes with the ability to meet the need for satisfaction or security, the person becomes mentally ill.

When Peplau defined nursing as an interpersonal process, she also discussed the importance of basic human needs. Needs must be met if a healthy state is to be achieved and maintained. For Peplau, the two interacting components of health are physiological demands and interpersonal conditions. These may be seen as parallel to the drives

Fig. 3-2   Hildegard E. Peplau. (Courtesy Hildegard E. Peplau.)

of satisfaction and security identified by Sullivan, as evident in the following clinical example.

Clinical Example Ms. Y, an attractive 26-year-old woman, appeared at a psychiatric outpatient clinic requesting therapy. She said, "I can't get close to people." She said that her childhood was happy and that she had loving parents and liked her sister. Her family were devout members of a fundamentalist Protestant church, so most of her activities were church related. She had many friends during childhood and then one close girl friend in early adolescence. She thought that her fear of closeness began when she slept over at her friend's house. During the night her friend began to fondle her in a way that she interpreted as sexual. She became very frightened and felt guilty. She did not tell her parents because of her feelings of guilt and, in fact, had told no one before entering therapy. Although she attended college, she never dated and participated only in superficial social contacts. She realized that this was not healthy young adult behavior and, as the behavior continued into her twenties, Ms. Y decided to seek help.

From an interpersonal perspective, Ms. Y was unable to fulfill her needs for friendship and sexual love. Interpersonal theorists would view the unfulfilled sexual love dynamism as a lack of satisfaction, and her fear that she had deviated from the norm as a lack of security. Her anxiety stemmed from her conviction that her parents would disown her if they heard what had happened. This belief was based on their earlier responses to childhood sexual play.

The therapist decided that Ms. Y first needed to experience intimacy on a nonsexual level. This need was approached in therapy. After Ms. Y began to feel comfortable sharing closeness with the therapist, she gradually explored friendships and later began dating.

Interpersonal Therapeutic Process

The interpersonal therapist, like the psychoanalyst, explores the patient's life history. The crux of the therapeutic process is the corrective interpersonal experience. The idea is that by experiencing a healthy relationship with the therapist, the patient can learn to have more satisfying interpersonal relationships. The therapist actively encourages the development of trust by relating authentically to the patient and sharing feelings and reactions with the patient. The process of therapy is a process of reeducation.

The therapist helps the patient identify interpersonal problems and then encourages attempts at more successful styles of relating. For example, patients often have a fear of intimacy. The therapist allows the patient to become close while showing him or her that there is no threat of sexual involvement. It is believed that closeness within the therapeutic relationship builds trust, facilitates empathy, enhances self-esteem, and fosters growth toward healthy behavior. Peplau[17] describes this process as "psychological mothering," which includes the following steps:

1. The patient is accepted unconditionally as a participant in a relationship that satisfies needs.
2. There is recognition of and response to the patient's readiness for growth, as initiated by the patient.
3. Power in the relationship shifts to the patient, as the patient is able to delay gratification and to invest energy in goal achievement.

Therapy is complete when the patient can establish satisfying human relationships, thereby meeting basic needs. Termination is a significant part of the relationship that must be shared by the therapist and the patient. The patient learns that leaving a significant other involves pain but can also be an opportunity for growth.

> **?** *Do you think that "psychological mothering" promotes maternalism or mutuality in the patient-therapist relationship?*

Roles of Patient and Interpersonal Therapist

The patient-therapist dyad is viewed as a partnership in interpersonal therapy. Sullivan describes the therapist as a "participant observer" whose role is to engage the patient, establish trust, and empathize. There is an active effort to help the patient realize that other people have similar perceptions and concerns. An atmosphere of uncritical acceptance encourages the patient to speak openly. The therapist

Box *3-2* *Interpersonal Nursing Roles Identified by Peplau*

Stranger: the role assumed by both nurse and patient when they first meet

Resource person: provides health information to a patient who has assumed the consumer role

Teacher: helps the patient to grow and learn from experience with the health-care system

Leader: helps the patient to participate in a democratically implemented nursing process

Surrogate: assumes roles that have been assigned by the patient, based on significant past relationships, as in the psychoanalytical phenomenon of transference

Counselor: helps the patient integrate the facts and feelings associated with an episode of illness into the patient's total life experience

interacts as a real person who also has beliefs, values, thoughts, and feelings. The patient's role is to share concerns with the therapist and to participate as fully as possible in the relationship. The relationship itself serves as a model of adaptive interpersonal relationships. As the patient matures in the ability to relate, life experiences with people outside the therapeutic situation are enhanced.

Interpersonal nursing roles have been identified by Peplau[17] and are listed in Box 3-2. These roles may be assumed by the nurse or assigned to others. The therapist helps the patient meet the goals of therapy: need satisfaction and personal growth. In addition, through role performance the nurse also experiences growth and self-discovery. Self-awareness is essential to success as an interpersonal therapist.

SOCIAL MODEL

The two preceding models focused on the individual and intrapsychic processes and interpersonal experiences. The social model moves beyond the individual to consider the social environment as it affects the person and the person's life experience (see Chapter 7). Psychoanalytical theory has been criticized for not extending to other cultures and times. For example, Freud's view of women has been repeatedly challenged, particularly by feminists. Some theorists such as Thomas Szasz[25-27] and Gerald Caplan[3] believe that the culture itself is useful in defining mental illness, prescribing therapy, and determining the patient's future. In addition, the community mental health movement is an example of a government effort to respond to the philosophy of the social theorists (see Chapter 34).

View of Behavioral Deviations

According to the social theorists, social conditions are largely responsible for deviant behavior. Deviance is culturally defined. Behavior considered normal in one cultural setting may be eccentric in another and psychotic in a third. An example is the African exchange student described in the following clinical example.

Clinical Example Early in the fall semester a black male exchange student from Africa was brought to the psychiatric emergency room. He had been walking around the campus carrying a spear and had been apprehended by the university security patrol. His speech was heavily accented and they could not understand his explanation of his behavior. Later evaluation revealed that in his culture one never went walking at night without a spear to defend against attack by wild beasts or hostile neighboring tribes. He was sent back to his dormitory after being convinced that his spear was not appropriate to the culture of the American college campus.

From this point of view Szasz[25] writes of the "myth of mental illness." He believes that society must find a way to manage "undesirables," so it labels them as mentally ill. People who are so labeled usually are unable or refuse to conform to social norms, and their behavior usually leads to confinement. If these people then conform to social expectations, they are considered to have recovered and are allowed to return to the community. Confinement performs the dual function of removing deviant members from the community and exerting social control over their behavior.

Szasz believes that people are responsible for their behavior. The person has control over whether to conform to social expectations. Those labeled as mentally ill may be scapegoats, but they participate in the scapegoating process by inviting it or by allowing it to occur. Szasz objects to describing deviant behavior as illness. He believes that illness can occur and that diseases of the body (such as brain tumors) can influence behavior, but that no physiological disruption can be demonstrated to cause most deviancy. He distinguishes between the biological condition that is central to illness and the social role that is the focus of deviance.

Caplan[3] also has studied deviant behavior from a social perspective. He has extended the public health model of primary, secondary, and tertiary prevention to the mental health field. He has focused particularly on primary prevention because much attention has been given to the secondary and tertiary levels. Lack of understanding of the cause of deviant behavior has hindered the development of primary prevention techniques.

Caplan believes that social situations can predispose a person to mental illness. Such situations include poverty, family instability, and inadequate education. Deprivation throughout the life cycle results in limited ability to cope with stress. The person has few environmental supports. The result is a predisposition to maladaptive coping responses.

> *How do you distinguish between social deviance and psychiatric illness? How do your friends and family define them?*

Social Therapeutic Process

Szasz advocates freedom of choice for psychiatric patients. People should be allowed to select their own therapeutic modalities and therapists. This freedom requires a well-informed consumer who can base this decision on knowledge of available modes of therapy (see Critical Thinking about Contemporary Issues). Szasz does not believe in involuntary hospitalization of the mentally ill. He questions whether any psychiatric hospitalization is truly voluntary. Szasz disapproves of the community mental health movement to place mental health care within the reach of every American. He questions government involvement in what he views as a private concern.

Caplan, on the other hand, supports community psychiatry. He sees the mental health professional as using consultation to combat societal problems. He believes that future psychiatric patients would benefit indirectly from positive social change.

Roles of Patient and Social Therapist

Szasz believes that a therapist can help the patient only if the patient requests help. The patient initiates therapy and defines the problem to be solved. The patient also has the right to approve or reject the recommended therapeutic intervention. Therapy is successfully completed when the patient is satisfied with the changes in his or her life. The therapist collaborates with the patient to promote change. This includes making recommendations about possible means of effecting behavioral change, but it does not include any element of coercion, particularly the threat of hospitalization if the patient does not agree with the therapist's recommendations. The therapist's role also may involve protecting the patient from social demands for coercive treatment.

Caplan believes that society has a moral obligation to provide a wide range of therapeutic services covering all three levels of prevention. The patient has a consumer role and selects the appropriate level of help from a wide array of services. Ideally, effective primary preventive services decrease the need for secondary or tertiary care.

According to this model, therapists may be professionals or nonprofessionals with professional consultation. People such as clergy, police, bartenders, and beauticians can be trained to listen and to refer people who need professional help to appropriate resources. The therapist in the social context is not tied to the office but is involved in the community. Activities may include home visits, lectures to community groups, or consultation with other agencies. The ra-

tionale for this approach is that the more involved therapists are in the community, the greater the impact on the community's mental health. Community involvement also enhances the therapist's understanding of patients who live in that environment.

> *Do you think bartenders and beauticians can be effective therapists? Why or why not?*

EXISTENTIAL MODEL

The existential model focuses on the person's experience in the here and now, with much less attention to the person's past than in other theoretical models.

View of Behavioral Deviations

Existentialist theorists believe that behavioral deviations result when one is out of touch with oneself or the environment. This alienation is caused by self-imposed restrictions. The individual is not free to choose from among all alterna-

TABLE **3-1** *Overview of Existential Therapies*

THERAPY	THERAPIST	PROCESS
Rational-emotive therapy (RET)	Albert Ellis[4]	An active-directive, cognitively oriented therapy. Confrontation is used to force patient to assume responsibility for behavior. Patients are encouraged to accept themselves as they are and are taught to try out new behavior.
Logotherapy	Viktor E. Frank[6]	A future-oriented therapy. The search for meaning (logos) is viewed as a primary life force. Without a sense of meaning, life becomes an "existential vacuum." The aim of therapy is to help patients assume personal responsibility.
Reality therapy	William Glasser[10]	Central theme is the need for identity, which is reached by loving, feeling worthwhile, and behaving responsibly. Patients are helped to recognize life goals and ways in which they keep themselves from accomplishing goals.
Gestalt therapy	Frederick S. Perls[18]	Emphasizes the here and now. The patient is encouraged to identify feelings and become more sensitive to other aspects of existence. Self-awareness is expected to lead to self-acceptance.
Encounter group therapy	Carl Rogers[21,22] (Fig. 3-3)	Focuses on establishing intimate interactions in a group setting. Therapy is oriented to the here and now. The patient is expected to assume responsibility for behavior. Feeling is stressed; intellectualization is discouraged.

tive behaviors. Deviant behavior often is a way of avoiding more socially acceptable or more responsible behavior.

The person who is self-alienated feels helpless, sad, and lonely. Self-criticism and lack of self-awareness prevent participation in authentic, rewarding relationships with others. Theoretically, the person has many choices in terms of behavior. However, existentialists believe that people tend to avoid being real and instead give in to the demands of others.

Existential Therapeutic Process

There are several existential therapies, all of which assume that the patient must be able to choose freely from what life has to offer. Although the approaches are somewhat different, the goal is to return the patient to an authentic awareness of being.

The existential therapeutic process focuses on the encounter. The encounter is not merely the meeting of two or more people; it also involves their appreciation of the total existence of each other. Through the encounter the patient is helped to accept and understand personal history, to live fully in the present, and to look forward to the future. Table 3-1 presents an overview of several existential therapies.

Roles of Patient and Existential Therapist

Existential theorists emphasize that the therapist and the patient are equal in their common humanity. The therapist acts as a guide to the patient, who has gone astray in the search for authenticity. The therapist is direct in pointing out areas where the patient should consider changing, but caring and warmth are also emphasized. The therapist and the patient are to be open and honest. The therapeutic ex-

Fig. 3-3   Carl R. Rogers. (From the Bettman Archive.)

perience is a model for the patient; new behaviors can be tested before risks are taken in daily life.

The patient is expected to assume and accept responsibility for behavior. Dependence on the therapist generally is not encouraged. The patient is treated as an adult. Often, illness is deemphasized. The patient is viewed as a person who is alienated from the self and others but for whom there is hope if he or she trusts the therapist and follows directions. The patient is always active in therapy, working to meet the challenge presented by the therapist.

SUPPORTIVE THERAPY MODEL

Supportive therapy is a newer mode of psychotherapy that is widely used in hospital and community-based psychiatric treatment settings. It differs from other models in that it does not depend on any overriding concept or theory. Instead, it uses many psychodynamic theories to understand how people change. The aims of supportive psychotherapy include the following:

▼ Promote a supportive patient-therapist relationship
▼ Enhance patient's strengths, coping skills, and ability to use coping resources
▼ Reduce the patient's subjective distress and maladaptive coping responses
▼ Help the patient achieve the greatest independence possible based on the specific psychiatric or physical illness
▼ Foster the greatest amount of autonomy in treatment decisions with the patient

Controlled studies have shown supportive therapy to be effective in treating schizophrenia, borderline conditions, and affective, anxiety, posttraumatic stress, eating, and substance abuse disorders, as well as the psychological component of many physical illnesses.[20]

View of Behavioral Deviations

Supportive therapists are psychodynamically based, and they describe behavioral deviations as neurotic, borderline, or psychotic. They believe in the concepts of id, ego, and superego and emphasize the important role of psychological defenses in adaptive functioning.[19] Compared with those of other therapists, however, their focus is more behavior oriented. They emphasize current biopsychosocial coping responses and the person's ability to use available coping resources.

Supportive Therapeutic Process

Supportive therapy is an eclectic form of psychotherapy; that is, it is not based on a particular theory of psychopathology. Rather, it can draw as needed from other models and may address different symptoms with different therapeutic methods. Supportive therapy is equally applicable to high-functioning patients in crisis and low-functioning patients with psychosis or persistent mental illness. Its emphasis is on improving behavior and subjective feelings of distress rather than on achieving insight or self-understanding.

Principles of supportive therapy include the following:

▼ Immediate help to the patient, which may include a variety of treatment modalities
▼ Family and social support system involvement
▼ Focus on the present
▼ Anxiety reduction through supportive measures and medication if necessary
▼ Clarification and problem solving using a variety of approaches including advice, supportive confrontation, limit setting, education, and environmental change

▼ Helping the patient to avoid future crises and seek help early when under stress

Roles of Patient and Supportive Therapist

In supportive therapy the therapist plays an active and directive role in helping the patient improve social functioning and coping skills. The setting for supportive therapy should allow for a moderate to high level of activity by both the patient and the therapist. Communication is seen as an active two-way process, and the use of medications or other therapies is encouraged.

The therapist builds a therapeutic alliance with the patient. Expressing empathy, concern, and nonjudgmental acceptance of the patient are important therapist qualities. The therapist supports the patient's healthy adaptive efforts, conveys a willingness to understand, respects the patient as a unique human being, and takes a genuine interest in the patient's life activities and well-being. The therapist regards the patient as a partner in treatment and encourages the patient's autonomy to make treatment and life decisions. In turn, the patient is expected to show a willingness to talk about life events, accept the therapist's supportive role, participate in the therapeutic program, and adhere to the therapeutic structure.

> **?** *What aspects of supportive therapy are similar to those of the therapeutic nurse-patient relationship? In what ways are they different?*

MEDICAL MODEL

The medical model refers to psychiatric care that is based on the traditional physician-patient relationship. It focuses on the diagnosis of a mental illness, and subsequent treatment is based on this diagnosis. Somatic treatments, including pharmacotherapy and electroconvulsive therapy, are important components of the treatment process. The interpersonal aspect of the medical model varies widely, from intensive insight-oriented intervention to brief sessions involving management of medications.

Much of modern psychiatric care is dominated by the medical model. Other health professionals may be involved in interagency referrals, family assessment, and health teaching, but physicians are seen as the leaders of the team under this model. Elements of other models of care may be used in conjunction with the medical model. For instance, a patient with schizophrenia may be treated with phenothiazine medication. This patient may also be in supportive therapy to develop adaptive social skills.

A positive contribution of the medical model has been the continuous exploration for causes of mental illness using the scientific process. Recently great strides have been made in learning about the functioning of the brain and nervous system (see Chapter 5). This progress has led to greater understanding of the probable physiological components of many behavioral disorders and more effective psychiatric treatment.

> **?** *What problems might the medical model pose for interdisciplinary collaboration in psychiatric treatment?*

View of Behavioral Deviations

The medical model proposes that deviant behavior is a symptom of a central nervous system disorder. As Andreasen writes, "Mental illness is truly a nervous breakdown—a breakdown that occurs when the nerves of the brain have an injury so severe that their own internal healing capacities cannot repair it."[2] She lists several types of brain disorders that could lead to mental illness: loss of nerve cells, excesses or deficits in chemical transmission, abnormal patterns of brain circuitry, problems in the command centers, and disruptions in the movement of messages along nerves.

Currently the exact nature of the physiological disruption is not well understood. It is thought that disorders such as bipolar disorder, major depression, and schizophrenia involve an abnormality in the transmission of neural impulses. It is also thought that this problem occurs at the synaptic level and involves neurochemicals such as dopamine, serotonin, and norepinephrine (see Chapter 5).

Much research into the brain's involvement in emotional response is under way. Another branch of research focuses on stressors and the human response to stress. Researchers are asking, "Why do some people seem to tolerate great stress and continue to function well, whereas others fall apart when a small problem arises?" These researchers suspect that humans have a physiological stress threshold that may be genetically determined. These areas of research may better guide future treatment.

Medical Therapeutic Process

The medical process of therapy is well defined and familiar to most patients. The examination of the patient includes the history of the present illness, social history, medical history, review of body systems, physical examination, and mental status examination. Additional data may be collected from significant others, and medical records are reviewed if available. A preliminary diagnosis is then formulated, pending further diagnostic studies and observation of the patient's behavior. This process may take place on an ambulatory or an inpatient basis, depending on the patient's condition.

The diagnosis is classified according to the *Diagnostic and Statistical Manual of Mental Disorders,* fourth edition (DSM-IV) of the American Psychiatric Association. The names of the illnesses are accompanied by a description of diagnostic criteria, associated general medical and psychiatric features, diagrams showing the longitudinal course of the disorder, and specific gender, age, and cultural aspects of each illness. Changes in the manual reflect changes in the medical model of psychiatric care. DSM-I was first published in 1952,[11] and DSM-IV, published in 1994, is the most up-to-date edition.[1]

After the diagnosis is made, treatment begins. The physician-patient relationship is developed to foster trust in the physician and compliance with the treatment plan. Other health team members may contribute their expertise. Response to treatment is evaluated on the basis of the patient's subjective assessment and the physician's objective observations of symptomatic behavior. Therapy is terminated when the patient's symptoms have remitted. For instance, some people who experience depression may be able to return to their usual lifestyles after a course of medication and supportive therapy. Other patients may require long-term therapy, often including pharmacotherapy and periodic laboratory studies.

Roles of Patient and Medical Therapist

The roles of physician and patient have been well defined by tradition. The physician, as the healer, identifies the patient's illness and formulates a treatment plan. The patient may have some say about the plan, but the physician prescribes the therapy.

The role of the patient involves admitting being ill, which can be a problem in psychiatry. Patients sometimes are not aware of their disturbed behavior and may actively resist treatment. This is not congruent with the medical model. The patient is expected to comply with the treatment program and try to get well. If observable improvement does not occur, caregivers and significant others often suspect that the patient is not trying hard enough. This can be frustrating to a patient who is trying to get well and is disappointed with the lack of progress. The patient also may have difficulty letting people extend care while being self-sufficient.

> **?** *How would each conceptual model described in this chapter view the issue of patient nonadherence to the psychiatric treatment plan?*

Summary

MODEL (MAJOR THEORISTS)	VIEW OF BEHAVIORAL DEVIATION	THERAPEUTIC PROCESS	ROLES OF PATIENT AND THERAPIST
Psychoanalytical (S. Freud, Erikson, A. Freud, Klein, Horney, Fromm-Reichmann, Menninger)	Based on inadequate resolution of developmental conflicts. Ego defenses unable to control anxiety. Symptoms result in effort to deal with anxiety and are related to unresolved conflicts.	Uses techniques of free association and dream analysis. Identifies problem areas through interpretation of patient's resistances and transferences.	Patient verbalizes all thoughts and dreams; considers therapist's interpretations. Therapist remains remote to encourage development of transference and interprets patient's thoughts and dreams.
Interpersonal (Sullivan, Peplau)	Anxiety arises and is experienced interpersonally. Basic fear is fear of rejection. Person needs security and satisfaction that result from positive interpersonal relationships.	Relationship between therapist and patient builds feeling of security. Therapist helps patient experience trusting relationship and gain interpersonal satisfaction.	Patient shares anxieties and feelings with therapist. Therapist uses empathy to perceive patient's feelings, and uses relationship as a corrective interpersonal experience.
Social (Szasz, Caplan)	Social and environmental factors create stress, which causes anxiety and symptoms. Unacceptable (deviant) behavior is socially defined.	Patient helped to deal with social system. May use crisis intervention, environmental manipulation, and social supports.	Patient presents problem to therapist, works with therapist, and uses community resources. Therapist explores patient's social system and resources available.
Existential (Perls, Glasser, Ellis, Rogers, Frankl)	Life is meaningful when the person can fully experience and accept the self. The self can be experienced through authentic relationships with other people.	Person aided to experience authenticity in relationships. Therapy often conducted in groups. Patient encouraged to accept self and to assume control of behavior.	Patient participates in meaningful experiences to learn about real self. Therapist helps patient recognize value of self, clarify realities of situation, and explore feelings.
Supportive therapy (Wermon, Rockland)	Problems are a result of biopsychosocial factors. Emphasis on current maladaptive coping responses.	Reality testing and self-esteem–enhancing measures. Social supports are enlisted and adaptive coping responses are reinforced.	Patient actively involved in treatment. Therapist warm, empathic, and allied with patient.
Medical (Meyer, Kraeplin, Spitzer, Frances)	Behavioral disruptions result from a biological disease process. Symptoms result from a combination of physiological, genetic, environmental, and social factors.	Treatment is related to diagnosis and includes somatic therapies and various interpersonal techniques. Treatment approach adjusted depending on symptomatic response.	Patient complies with prescribed therapy and reports effects of therapy to therapist. Therapist diagnoses illness and prescribes therapeutic approach.

your **INTERNET**
connection

Guide to Psychotherapy
http://www.shef.ac.uk/~psysc/psychotherapy

APA On Line: American Psychiatric Association
http://www.psych.org/main.htm

Chapter Review Questions

1. Match the theorists in Column A with the model of psychiatric treatment in Column B.

Column A	Column B
___Freud	A. Existential
___Rockland	B. Interpersonal
___Rogers	C. Medical
___Spitzer	D. Psychoanalytical
___Sullivan	E. Social
___Szasz	F. Supportive

2. Fill in the blanks.

A. Psychoanalysts believe that behavior problems in adulthood are caused by _____.

B. _____ is the verbalization of thoughts as they occur without any conscious screening or censorship.

C. Interpersonal theorists believe that behavior problems arise from _____.

D. The drives for _____ and _____ are critical to a person's psychological health according to the interpersonal model.

E. Social theorists believe that deviant behavior is caused by _____.

F. The community mental health movement is an example of the _____ model of psychiatric treatment.

G. Existential theorists believe that behavior problems arise when _____.

H. Encounter groups are an example of therapy from the _____ model of psychiatric treatment.

I. Supportive therapy theorists believe that behavior problems arise from _____.

J. In supportive therapy a therapist plays an _____ role and regards the patient as a _____ in the treatment process.

K. Medical model theorists believe that behavior problems arise from _____.

L. A significant contribution of the medical model has been _____.

M. The classification system used in the medical model to diagnose psychiatric illness is the _____.

3. Provide short answers for the following questions.

A. What purposes do dreams serve in psychoanalysis and how are dreams seen by people today?

B. Describe the six nursing roles identified by Peplau.

C. What model of psychiatric treatment do you think is most culture-bound? Which is the most culture-free? Defend your answer.

D. On a scale of 1 to 5, rank order your preference for the five models of psychiatric treatment described in this chapter. Explain your ranking.

References

1. American Psychiatric Association: *Diagnostic and statistical manual of mental disorders,* ed 4, Washington, DC, 1994, The Association.
2. Andreasen NC: *The broken brain,* New York, 1984, Harper & Row.
3. Caplan G: *Principles of preventive psychiatry,* New York, 1964, Basic Books.
4. Ellis A: *Inside rational emotive therapy,* San Diego, 1989, Academic Press.
5. Erikson E: *Childhood and society,* ed 2, New York, 1963, WW Norton.
6. Frankl V: *Man's search for meaning,* New York, 1959, Beacon Press.
7. Freud A: *The ego and the mechanisms of defense,* New York, 1966, International Universities Press.
8. Freud S: In Strachey J, editor: *The standard edition of the complete psychological works of Sigmund Freud,* London, 1953-1974, Hogarth Press.
9. Fromm-Reichmann F: *Principles of intensive psychotherapy,* Chicago, 1950, University of Chicago Press.
10. Glasser W: *Reality therapy: a new approach to psychiatry,* New York, 1965, Harper & Row.
11. Grob G: Origins of DSM-I: a study in appearance and reality, *Am J Psychiatry* 148:421, 1991.
12. Horney K: *The collected works of Karen Horney,* vols 1 and 2, New York, 1937-1950, WW Norton.
13. Klein M: *The psychoanalysis of children,* London, 1949, Hogarth Press.
14. Krupnick J, Pincus H: The cost-effectiveness of psychotherapy: a plan for research, *Am J Psychiatry* 149:1295, 1992.
15. Menninger KA: *The vital balance,* New York, 1963, Viking Press.
16. Olfson M, Pincus H: Outpatient psychotherapy in the United States, I: volume, costs and user characteristics, *Am J Psychiatry* 151:1281, 1994.
17. Peplau HE: *Interpersonal relations in nursing,* New York, 1952, GP Putnam.
18. Perls FS: *In and out of the garbage pail,* Lafayette, Calif, 1969, Real People Press.
19. Rockland L: *Supportive therapy: a psychodynamic approach,* New York, 1989, Basic Books.
20. Rockland L: A review of supportive psychotherapy, 1986-1992, *Hosp Community Psychiatry* 44:1053, 1993.
21. Rogers CR: *Client-centered therapy,* Boston, 1951, Houghton Mifflin.

22. Rogers CR: *Carl Rogers on encounter groups,* New York, 1970, Harper & Row.
23. Sullivan HS: *The interpersonal theory of psychiatry,* New York, 1953, WW Norton.
24. Sullivan HS: *The psychiatric interview,* New York, 1954, WW Norton.
25. Szasz T: *The myth of mental illness,* New York, 1961, Hoeber-Harper.
26. Szasz T: *Insanity: the idea and its consequences,* New York, 1987, Wiley.
27. Szasz T: *A lexicon of lunacy,* New Brunswick, NJ, 1993, Transactional Publishers.

ANNOTATED SUGGESTED READINGS

Albert G: What are the characteristics of effective psychotherapists? The experts speak, *J Practical Psychiatry Behavioral Health* 3:36, 1997.

Important and interesting study. Therapist characteristics found to be the most effective in treatment were the following: flexibility, the ability to create a therapeutic alliance, the ability to create a place of sanctuary, and sensitivity to dynamic issues in patient and self.

Alexander J et al: Determinants of mental health providers' expectations of patients' improvement, *Psychiatr Serv* 48:671, 1997.

Providers' expectations of patients' improvement play an important role in care, and these vary with the characteristics of the provider and the treatment setting. Manipulation of setting characteristics may improve provider expectations of patient improvement.

*Blair T: The placebogenic phenomenon: art in psychiatric nursing, *J Psychosocial Nurs* 34:11, 1996.

*Nursing reference.

Thought-provoking report of how patient perception, beliefs, trust, and expectation and nurse beliefs, nonverbal cues, anticipation, and style have a severely underestimated effect on the efficacy of psychotropic medications, as demonstrated by the 30% to 50% effectiveness of placebos.

Frank J: Psychotherapy: the restoration of morale, *Am J Psychiatry* 131:271, 1974.

Classic article that shares a different view of psychotherapy by describing commonalities of psychotherapeutic rationales and rituals in combating demoralization.

Gabbard G et al: The economic impact of psychotherapy: a review, *Am J Psychiatry* 154:147, 1997

The beneficial effect health care costs of psychotherapy in the treatment of severe mental illness appears to emerge from savings because of reduction in inpatient treatment and decreases in work impairment.

Hoyt M: *Brief therapy and managed care: readings for contemporary practice,* San Francisco, 1995, Jossey-Bass.

Written in workbook style, this book describes the principles and application of brief therapy with useful clinical vignettes. Timely, given the current emphasis on short-term treatment in psychiatry.

Krupnick J et al: The role of the therapeutic alliance in psychotherapy and pharmacotherapy outcome: findings in the National Institute of Mental Health Treatment of Depression Collaborative Research Program, *J Consult Clin Psychol* 64:532, 1996.

The relationship between the therapeutic alliance and treatment outcome was examined. Results indicate that the therapeutic alliance is a common factor with significant influence on outcome.

Rogers P: The therapeutic uses of fairy tale, *Treatment Today* 4:12, 1997.

From a Jungian point of view, fairy tales can be studied as the purest and simplest form of expression of the collective unconscious. They are where the psyche tells its own story and where patients and therapists can relate their life experiences.

© 1998 M.C. Escher/Cordon Art, Baarn, Holland.

The Stuart Stress Adaptation Model of Psychiatric Nursing Care

Gail W. Stuart

Much madness is Divinest Sense—To a discerning eye. **Emily Dickinson**

LEARNING OBJECTIVES

After studying this chapter the student should be able to:

▼ Discuss the theoretical assumptions underlying the Stuart Stress Adaptation Model of psychiatric nursing care

▼ Describe criteria of mental health and dimensions of mental illness in the United States

▼ Analyze the biopsychosocial components of the Stuart Stress Adaptation Model of psychiatric nursing care

▼ Compare coping responses, nursing diagnoses, health problems, and medical diagnoses

▼ Evaluate nursing activities appropriate to the various stages of psychiatric treatment

TOPICAL OUTLINE

Theoretical Assumptions
Describing Mental Health and Illness
  Defining Mental Health
  Dimensions of Mental Illness
Biopsychosocial Components
  Predisposing Factors
  Precipitating Stressors
  Appraisal of Stressor
  Coping Resources
  Coping Mechanisms
Patterns of Response
  Nursing Diagnoses
  Relationship to Medical Diagnoses
  Classifying Mental Disorders
Treatment Stages and Activities

Models serve many purposes. They can help clarify relationships, generate hypotheses, and give perspective to an abstract idea. They also can provide a structure for thinking, observing, and interpreting what is seen. Conceptual nursing models are frames of reference within which patients, their environments and health states, and nursing activities are described. They explain in general terms why individuals respond to stress as they do and help to provide an understanding of the process and desired outcomes of nursing interventions. Psychiatric nurses can enhance their practice if their actions are based on a model of psychiatric nursing care that is inclusive, holistic, and relevant to the needs of patients, families, groups, and communities.

This text is based on the Stuart Stress Adaptation Model of psychiatric nursing care, which integrates biological, psychological, sociocultural, environmental, and legal-ethical aspects of patient care into a unified framework for practice. It was originally developed by Gail Stuart in the 1980s as a synthesis of diverse bodies of knowledge from the perspective of psychiatric nursing and, equally important, as an application of this knowledge to clinical practice. Since then the model has been revised and expanded to include rapidly emerging theoretical and scientific discoveries, as well as a clearer and more complete embodiment of the process, content, and context of contemporary psychiatric nursing care.

THEORETICAL ASSUMPTIONS

The *first assumption* of the Stuart Stress Adaptation Model is that nature is ordered as a social hierarchy from the simplest unit to the most complex (Fig. 4-1). Each level of this hierarchy represents an organized whole with distinctive properties. Each level is also a component of the next higher level, so nothing exists in isolation. Thus the individual is a component of family, group, community, society, and the larger biosphere. Material and information flow across levels, and each level is influenced by all the others. For this reason, one level of organization, such as the individual, cannot be characterized as a dynamic system without incorporating the other levels of the social hierarchy. The most basic level of nursing intervention is the individual level. An exploration of this level must focus on its unique aspects without excluding its relationship to the whole because wholeness is the essence of psychiatric nursing practice.

The *second assumption* of the model is that nursing care is provided within a biological, psychological, sociocultural, environmental, and legal-ethical context. Each of these aspects of care is described in detail in Chapters 5 to 9. The nurse must understand and integrate them in order to provide competent, holistic psychiatric nursing care. Thus the theoretical basis for psychiatric nursing practice is derived from nursing science as well as from the behavioral, social, and biological sciences. The range of theories used by psy-

Fig. 4-1 Levels of organization that make up the social hierarchy.

chiatric nurses includes nursing, developmental psychology, neurobiology, pharmacology, psychopathology, learning, sociocultural, cognitive, behavioral, economic, organizational, political, legal-ethical, interpersonal, group, family, and milieu. Psychiatric nursing practice requires the use of many theories because of the variation in patients' responses, the philosophical backgrounds of psychiatric nurses, and the settings in which nurses work. No one theory is universally applicable to all patients. Rather, the appropriate theory should be selected for its relevance to a particular patient, the presenting problem, and the environment of caregiving.

The *third assumption* of the model is that health/illness and adaptation/maladaptation are two distinct continuums. The health/illness continuum derives from a medical world view. The adaptation/maladaptation continuum derives from a nursing world view. This means that a person with a medically diagnosed illness may be adapting well to it. An example of this is the adaptive coping responses used by some people who have chronic physical or psychiatric illnesses. In contrast, a person without a medically diagnosed illness may have many maladaptive coping responses. This can been seen in the adolescent whose problematic behaviors reflect poor coping responses to the many issues that must be resolved during adolescence. These two continuums thus reflect the complementary nature of the nursing and medical models of practice.

The *fourth assumption* is that the model includes the primary, secondary, and tertiary levels of prevention by describing four discrete stages of psychiatric treatment: crisis, acute, maintenance, and health promotion. For each stage of treatment the model suggests a treatment goal, a focus of the nursing assessment, the nature of nursing interventions, and the expected outcome of nursing care. This aspect of the model is particularly useful in organizing one's practice, as well as in creating a structure for documenting both the process and outcome of psychiatric nursing care. It also embraces the full continuum of psychiatric care and can direct nursing practice in hospital, community, and home settings.

The *fifth assumption* of the Stuart Stress Adaptation Model is that it is based on the use of the nursing process described in Chapter 10 and professional role behavior discussed in Chapter 11. Psychiatric nursing care is provided through assessment, diagnosis, outcome identification, planning, implementation, and evaluation. Each step of the process is critically important, and the nurse assumes full responsibility for all nursing actions implemented and the enactment of a professional nursing role.

In summary, the Stuart Stress Adaptation Model is unique in that it:
▼ Views nature as ordered on a social hierarchy
▼ Assumes a holistic biopsychosocial approach to psychiatric nursing practice
▼ Regards adaptation/maladaptation as distinct from health/illness
▼ Incorporates elements of primary, secondary, and tertiary levels of prevention
▼ Identifies four stages of psychiatric treatment and related nursing activities
▼ Can be used across psychiatric settings throughout the continuum of care
▼ Is based on standards of psychiatric nursing care and professional performance

DESCRIBING MENTAL HEALTH AND ILLNESS

The mental health–mental illness continuum is asymmetrical. The standards of mental health are less clear than those of mental illness. Problems arise with viewing mental health as the average or mean of a group because what is average is not necessarily healthy. It is similarly dangerous to equate social alternatives with illness, such as when an unusual lifestyle is regarded as sick or when aberrant behavior is taken to be a sign of personal abnormality. These problems can be avoided if it is recognized that health/illness and conformity/deviance are independent variables. Combining them generates four patterns: the healthy conformist, the healthy deviant, the unhealthy conformist, and the unhealthy deviant (Fig. 4-2). Psychiatric nurses must carefully consider the meaning of an individual's behavior and its context because it may reflect an adaptation to realistic forces in the individual's life or conformity to group norms.

Defining Mental Health

Mental health is often spoken of as a state of well-being associated with happiness, contentment, satisfaction, achievement, optimism, or hope.[3,9] These are difficult terms to define, and their meanings change by person and life situation. Some have suggested that the idea of any single criterion of mental health should be abandoned because mental health cannot be confined to a simple concept or a single aspect of behavior. Instead, mental health consists of a number of criteria that exist on a continuum with gradients or degrees. These criteria should then be regarded as the optimum of mental health. They are not absolute, however, and each person has limits. Although no one reaches the ideal in all the criteria, most people can approach the optimum.

	Health	Illness
C o n f o r m i t y	Healthy conformist	Unhealthy conformist
D e v i a n c e	Healthy deviant	Unhealthy deviant

Fig. 4-2 Patterns of behavior.

? *Do you think that a person with diabetes that is controlled with medication can still be regarded as healthy? How does this compare with a person who has schizophrenia that is controlled with medication?*

CRITERIA OF MENTAL HEALTH. The following six criteria can be considered to be indicators of mental health:

▼ Positive attitudes toward self
▼ Growth, development, and self-actualization
▼ Integration
▼ Autonomy
▼ Reality perception
▼ Environmental mastery

Positive attitudes toward self include an acceptance of self and self-awareness. A person must have some objectivity about the self and realistic aspirations that necessarily change with age. A healthy person must also have a sense of identity, wholeness, belongingness, security, and meaningfulness.

Growth, development, and self-actualization have been the objects of considerable research. Maslow[11] and Rogers,[16] for example, developed theories on the realization of the human potential. Maslow describes the concept of self-actualization, and Rogers emphasizes the fully functioning person. Both theories focus on the entire range of human adjustment. They describe a self engaged in a constant quest, always seeking new growth, development, and challenges. These theories focus on the total person and whether the person:

▼ Is adequately in touch with the self to free the resources that are there
▼ Has free access to personal feelings and can integrate them with intellectual and cognitive functioning
▼ Is immobilized by inner conflicts and stresses or can interact freely and openly with the environment
▼ Can share with other people and grow from such experiences

Integration is a balance between what is expressed and what is repressed, between outer and inner conflicts and drives, and a regulation of moods and emotions. It includes emotional responsiveness and control and a unified philosophy of life. This criterion can be measured at least in part by the person's ability to withstand stress and cope with anxiety. A strong but not rigid ego enables the person to handle change and grow from it.

Autonomy involves self-determination, a balance between dependence and independence, and acceptance of the consequences of one's actions. It implies that the person is self-responsible for decisions, actions, thoughts, and feelings. Consequently, the person can respect autonomy and freedom in others.

Reality perception is the individual's ability to test assumptions about the world by empirical thought. The men-

tally healthy person can change perceptions in light of new information. This criterion includes empathy or social sensitivity, a respect for the feelings and attitudes of others.

Environmental mastery enables a mentally healthy person to feel success in an approved role in society. The person can deal effectively with the world, work out personal problems, and obtain satisfaction from life. The person should be able to cope with loneliness, aggression, and frustration without being overwhelmed. The mentally healthy person can respond to others, love and be loved, and cope with reciprocal relationships. This individual can build new friendships and have satisfactory social group involvement.

Finally, a person should not be assessed against some vague or ideal notion of health. Rather, each person should be seen in a group context and an individual context. The issue is not how well someone fits an arbitrary sociocultural standard, but rather what is reasonable for a particular person. Is there continuity or discontinuity with the past? Does the person adapt to changing needs throughout the life cycle? Such a view incorporates the concept of psychobiological resilience, which proposes that humans must weather periods of stress and change throughout life.[6] Successfully weathering each period of disruption and reintegration leaves the person better able to deal with the next change.

Dimensions of Mental Illness

Mental disorders are a major contributor to the burden of illness in the United States. Nearly 50% of all people age 15 to 54 have had a psychiatric or substance abuse disorder in their lifetimes, and close to 30% had one of these disorders in the past year (Fig. 4-3). Most importantly, more than half of all lifetime disorders occur in the 14% of the population who have a history of three or more coexisting disorders.[8] This group includes most of the people with severe psychiatric illness and represents a very vulnerable portion of the population. The seriousness and persistence of some disorders cause great strain on affected individuals, their families and communities, and the larger health-care system. Key facts about mental illness prepared by the National Institute of Mental Health[14] are presented in Box 4-1.

Many myths and misunderstandings contribute to the stigmatization of people with mental illness and to their often limited access to health-care services (see Chapter 8). For example, many Americans and policymakers are unaware of a solid body of research that documents the effectiveness of treatment for these illnesses. These studies demonstrate that mental disorders can be diagnosed and treated as effectively as physical illness. However, far too many Americans with severe mental illness and their families find that appropriate treatment is not available to them because they lack insurance coverage or the coverage they have is inequitable and inadequate. For example, private health insurance for mental disorders is often limited to 30 to 60 inpatient days per year, compared with 120 days or unlimited days for physical illnesses. Similarly, Medicare and other in-

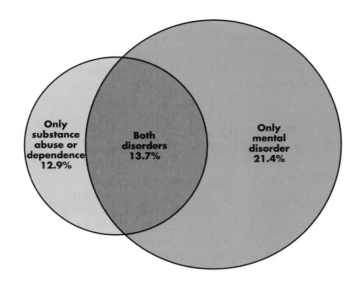

	Lifetime	Past Year
Any Substance Abuse or Mental Disorder	**48.0%**	**29.5%**
Only substance abuse or dependence	12.9	6.6
Only mental disorder	21.4	18.2
Both substance abuse and mental disorder	13.7	4.7

Fig. 4-3 Percentage of population with substance abuse, mental disorder, or both disorders, ages 15 to 54. (Redrawn from Kessler et al: Lifetime and 12-month prevalence of DSM-III-R psychiatric disorders in the US, *Arch Gen Psychiatry* 51:8, 1994.)

surance programs require 50% copayment for outpatient care of mental disorders, compared with 20% copayment for outpatient treatment of physical illnesses.

Fair coverage for Americans with mental illness will result in both human and economic benefits. Millions of Americans will be able to participate more productively at home, at work, and in the community. The enormous but often hidden costs of untreated or undertreated severe mental illness, which are now absorbed by the general health-care system and society at large, can be substantially reduced. Psychiatric nurses should work to make these benefits a reality by supporting national health-care reform initiatives and research funding for the needs of the mentally ill.

> *Identify two key facts about mental illness from Box 4-1 that you did not know. How will these facts change your views about needed health-care reform in this country?*

BIOPSYCHOSOCIAL COMPONENTS

The Stuart Stress Adaptation Model of psychiatric nursing care views human behavior from a holistic perspective that integrates biological, psychological, and sociocultural aspects of care. For instance, a man who has had a myocardial infarction may also be severely depressed because he fears he will lose his ability to work and to satisfy his wife sexu-

ally. He may also have a family history of depression. Likewise, a patient who seeks treatment for a major depression may also have gastric ulcers that are exacerbated by her depression. The holistic nature of psychiatric nursing practice examines all aspects of the individual and his or her environment. The specific biopsychosocial components of the Stuart Stress Adaptation Model are shown in Fig. 4-4.

Predisposing Factors

Predisposing factors are biological, psychological, and sociocultural in nature. They may be seen as conditioning or risk factors that influence both the type and amount of resources the person can use to handle stress. Genetic background, nutritional status, biological sensitivities, general health, and exposure to toxins are examples of **biological** predispositions. **Psychological** factors include intelligence, verbal skills, morale, personality, past experiences, self-concept, motivation, psychological defenses, and locus of control, or a sense of control over one's own fate.

Sociocultural characteristics include age, gender, education, income, occupation, social position, cultural background, religious upbringing and beliefs, political affiliation, socialization experiences, and level of social integration or relatedness. Together these factors provide a link with higher and lower levels of the social hierarchy and a backdrop against which all current experiences are given meaning and value.

Box **4-1** *Key Facts about Mental Illness*

EXTENT AND SEVERITY OF THE PROBLEM

▼ The full spectrum of mental disorders affects 25% of the adult population in a given year. This figure refers to *all* mental disorders and is comparable to rates for "physical disorders" when similarly broadly defined (for example, respiratory disorders affect 50% of adults, and cardiovascular diseases affect 20%).

▼ Severe mental disorders, such as schizophrenia, manic depressive illness and severe forms of depression, panic disorder, and obsessive compulsive disorder:

   Affect 2.8% of the adult population (approximately 5 million people)

   Account for 25% of all Federal disability payments

▼ About 1 in 5 children in the United States under 18 years of age have a mental health problem severe enough to require treatment.

▼ Approximately 18 million people in the United States 18 years of age and older have problems as a result of alcohol use. 10.6 million of these suffer from alcoholism.

▼ An estimated 23 million people in the United States currently use illicit drugs.

▼ At least two thirds of elderly nursing home residents have a diagnosis of a mental disorder, such as major depression.

▼ Nearly one third of the nation's estimated 600,000 homeless people are believed to be adults with severe mental illness.

▼ More than one in four jail inmates has a mental disorder.

▼ 29% of the nation's jails routinely hold people with a mental illness without any criminal charges.

COST OF MENTAL DISORDERS

▼ In 1990 the nation's health-care bill was $670 billion; the direct cost of treating all mental disorders was 10%, or $67 billion.

   $148 billion: total costs (treatment plus indirect costs) of mental disorders in 1990

   $159 billion: total cost of cardiovascular system diseases in 1990

▼ Severe mental disorders: Total direct treatment costs are $20 billion per year plus $7 billion for long-term nursing home care.

   Indirect and related costs bring the total for severe mental disorders to $74 billion per year.

▼ It has been estimated that drug and alcohol abuse contribute to over $163.6 billion in health-care costs, lost productivity, and crime. Estimates of hospital beds occupied by patients whose physical condition is complicated by alcohol and drug problems range from 25% to 50%.

▼ Alcohol or mental illness is involved in 94% of all suicides and suicide ranks as the second leading cause of death among people aged 15-24.

▼ Alcoholism is the third leading cause of illness and disability in the United States and accounts for 10% of all deaths.

TREATMENT EFFICACY

▼ How effective are treatments for severe mental disorders as compared with treatments for physical illness?

Disorder	Treatment Success Rate (%)
Panic	80
Bipolar	80
Major depression	65
Schizophrenia	60
Obsessive compulsive	60
Cardiovascular treatments	
Atherectomy	52
Angioplasty	41

▼ The majority of alcoholics improve through treatment, and evidence suggests that alcoholism treatment is effective in containing costs throughout the health-care system and increasing worker productivity.

REIMBURSEMENT

▼ People who need help often cannot receive it. Approximately 30% of the 2.8 million people with severe mental illness receive active treatment in a given year; 70% to 80% of children needing mental health treatment do not receive appropriate services.

▼ 85% of all drug and alcohol abusers are not in treatment. Only 150,000 of an estimated 1.4 million intravenous drug abusers are currently in treatment.

▼ Under insurance plans offering full, comprehensive, and equitable coverage for mental disorders, the percentage of cost represented by these disorders plateaus at about 10% to 11%.

   Inpatient care for treatment of severe psychiatric disorders has grown less rapidly than inpatient care for all health conditions.

▼ Under health-care reform, making mental health coverage for the severely mentally ill commensurate to other health-care coverage would:

   Add only $6.5 billion in new mental health care costs—10% more than is currently spent

   Produce a 10% decrease in the cost and use of general medical services by people with severe mental disorders

   Yield a $2.2 billion net saving for the United States

From National Advisory Mental Health Council: *Am J Psychiatry* 150:1447, 1993.

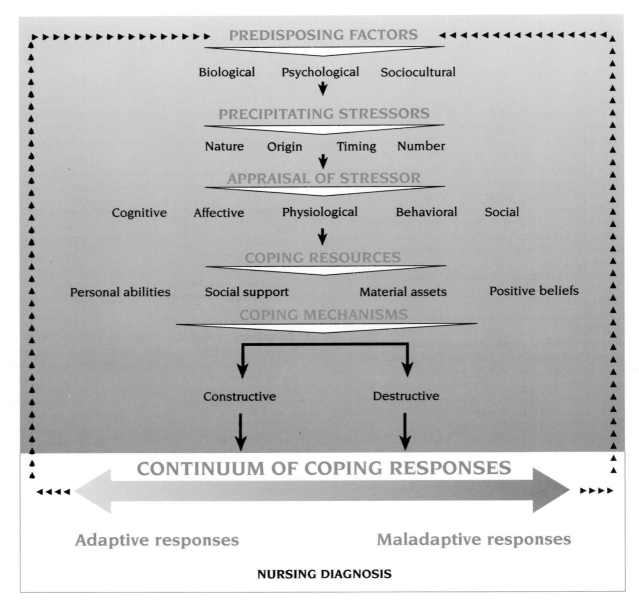

Fig. 4-4 Biopsychosocial components of the Stuart Stress Adaptation Model of psychiatric nursing care.

> **?** *Explain why predisposing factors are also sometimes called risk factors.*

Precipitating Stressors

Precipitating stressors are stimuli that the individual perceives as challenging, threatening, or demanding. They require excess energy and produce a state of tension and stress. They may be biological, psychological, or sociocultural in *nature*, and they may *originate* in the person's internal or external environment. Besides describing the nature and origin of a stressor, it is important to assess the *timing* of the stressor. This timing has many dimensions, such as when the stressor occurred, the duration of exposure to the stressor, and the frequency with which it occurs. A final factor to be considered is the *number* of stressors an individual experiences within a certain period of time because events may be more difficult to deal with when they occur close together.

STRESSFUL LIFE EVENTS. One group of stressors that has received much attention in the health-care literature is stressful life events. The relationship of stressful life events to the cause, onset, course, and outcomes of various psychiatric illnesses, such as schizophrenia, depression, and anxiety, has been the focus of much research.

Recent issues related to life events as stressors focus on the nature of the event and the magnitude of change it represents. Three ways of categorizing events are reported in the literature:

▼ By social activity, which involves family, work, educational, interpersonal, health, financial, legal, or community crises.
▼ By the individual's social field. These events are defined as entrances and exits. An entrance is the introduction of a new person into the individual's social field; an exit is the departure of a significant other from the person's social field.
▼ By relating them to social desirability. In terms of the currently shared values of American society, one group of events can be considered generally desirable, such as promotion, engagement, and marriage. A larger group of events can be viewed unfavorably, such as death, financial problems, being fired, and divorce.

Unfortunately, conclusions about life events are far from definitive. Although they have been correlated with the onset of anxiety and disease symptoms, the methodological and theoretical aspects of research in this area have been the subject of much criticism. Intervening or mediating variables often are not taken into account in the design and execution of studies. Also, the particular events in the scales may not be the most relevant to certain groups, such as students, working mothers, the elderly, the poor, or the persistently mentally ill. Finally, the life-events approach provides no clues to the specific processes by which the events affect physical or mental health.

It may be more helpful, therefore, to suggest that stressful life events act along a continuum to influence the development of psychiatric illness. On one end of the continuum, they may act as triggers to precipitate an illness in people who would have developed the illness eventually for one reason or another. At the other end of the continuum, stressful life events may have a vulnerability effect in depleting an individual's resistance and coping resources and thus greatly advancing or bringing about psychiatric illness.

> **?** *What sociocultural norms and values must be considered in evaluating the impact of potentially stressful life events?*

LIFE STRAINS AND HASSLES. Life-events theory is built on the idea of change. However, much stress arises from chronic conditions such as boredom, continuing family tension, job dissatisfaction, and loneliness. This aspect is reflected in the early work of Pearlin and Schooler,[15] who explored what people considered potential life strains. In their sample of 2300 people 18 to 65 years of age, the following four areas were delineated:

▼ Marital strains
▼ Parental strains associated with teenage and young adult children

▼ Strains associated with household economics
▼ Overloads and dissatisfactions associated with the work role

These findings suggest more long-term life dissatisfactions than major episodic events.

Research indicates that small daily hassles or stresses may be more closely linked to and have a greater effect on a person's moods and health than do major misfortunes.[13] Hassles are irritating, frustrating, or distressing incidents that occur in everyday life. Such incidents may include disagreements, disappointments, and unpleasant surprises such as losing a wallet, getting stuck in a traffic jam, or arguing with a teenage son or daughter. Research suggests that hassles may be better predictors of psychological and physical health than life events. The more frequent and intense the hassles people reported, the poorer their overall mental and physical health. Major events did have some long-term effects, but these effects may be accounted for by the daily hassles they precipitate. A study of the specific hassles and their frequency among people with severe mental illness found that loneliness and boredom were serious concerns. Finances, crime, self-expression, and upward mobility were also important.[17]

A certain amount of stress is necessary for survival, and degrees of it can challenge the individual to grow in new ways. However, too much stress at inappropriate times can place excessive demands on the individual and interfere with integrated functioning. Stress does not reside within the particular life event itself or within the individual. Rather, it is in the interaction between the individual and situation. The questions that emerge are How much stress is too much? and What is a stressful life event? These questions lead the nurse to explore the significance of the event for the individual's value system.

Appraisal of Stressor

Appraisal of a stressor is the processing and comprehension of the stressful situation that takes place on many levels. Specifically, it involves cognitive, affective, physiological, behavioral, and social responses. Appraisal is an evaluation of the significance of an event for a person's well-being. The stressor assumes its meaning, intensity, and importance from the unique interpretation and significance assigned to it by the person at risk.

Cognitive appraisal is a critical part of this model. Monat and Lazarus[13] believe that cognitive factors play a central role in adaptation; they affect the impact of stressful events, the choice of coping patterns used, and the emotional, physiological, and behavioral reactions. Cognitive appraisal mediates psychologically between the person and the environment in any stressful encounter. That is, damage or potential damage is evaluated according to the person's understanding of the situation's power to produce harm and the resources the person has available to neutralize or tolerate the harm.

There are three types of primary cognitive appraisals to stress:

▼ *Harm/loss* that has already occurred
▼ *Threat,* or anticipated or future harm
▼ *Challenge,* in which the focus is placed on potential gain, growth, or mastery rather than on the possible risks

The perception of challenge may play a crucial role in psychological **hardiness** or resistance to stress. This theory proposes that psychologically hardy people are less likely than nonhardy people to fall ill as a result of stressful life events. Three parts of a hardy personality have been described and researched.[10] Hardy people are high in

▼ **Commitment** (the ability to involve oneself in whatever one is doing)
▼ **Challenge** (the belief that change rather than stability is to be expected in life, so events are seen as stimulating rather than threatening)
▼ **Control** (the tendency to feel and believe that they influence events, rather than feeling helpless in the face of life's problems)

From this list one might conclude that stress-resistant people have a specific set of attitudes toward life, an openness to change, a feeling of involvement in whatever they are doing, and a sense of control over events.[7] Such differences in cognitive appraisal affect the person's response to events. Those who view stress as a challenge are more likely to transform events to their advantage and thus reduce their level of stress. With more passive, hostile, avoidant, or self-defeating tactics, the source of stress does not go away. Additional research is needed in this important personality characteristic.[19]

> ? *What is your level of hardiness as measured by the elements of commitment, challenge, and control? How will it influence your effectiveness as a nurse?*

An **affective** response is the arousal of a feeling. In the appraisal of a stressor, the predominant affective response is a nonspecific or generalized anxiety reaction.

This generalized anxiety response becomes expressed as emotions. These may include joy, sadness, fear, anger, acceptance, distrust, anticipation, or surprise. Emotions may be further classified according to type, duration, and intensity, characteristics that change over time and events. For example, when an emotion is prolonged over time, it can be classified as a mood; when prolonged over a longer time, it can be considered an attitude.

Physiological responses reflect the interaction of several neuroendocrine axes involving growth hormone, prolactin, adrenocorticotropic hormone (ACTH), luteinizing and follicle-stimulating hormones, thyroid-stimulating hormones, vasopressin, oxytocin, insulin, epinephrine, norepinephrine, and a variety of other neurotransmitters in the brain. The fight-or-flight physiological response stimulates the sympathetic division of the autonomic nervous system and increases activity of the pituitary-adrenal axis. Additionally, stress has been shown to affect the body's immune system, affecting one's ability to fight disease.

Behavioral responses reflect emotions and physiological changes as well as cognitive analysis of the stressful situation. Caplan[5] described four phases of an individual's responses to a stressful event.

▼ Phase 1 is behavior that changes the stressful environment or enables the individual to escape from it.
▼ Phase 2 is behavior to acquire new capabilities for action to change the external circumstances and their aftermath.
▼ Phase 3 is intrapsychic behavior to defend against unpleasant emotional arousal.
▼ Phase 4 is intrapsychic behavior to come to terms with the event and its sequelae by internal readjustment.

Finally, Mechanic[12] describes three aspects of a person's **social** response to stress and illness. The first aspect is the *search for meaning,* in which people seek information about their problem. This is a prerequisite for devising a coping strategy because only through some idea of what is occurring can a reasonable response be devised.

The second aspect of social response is *social attribution,* in which the person tries to identify the factors that contributed to the situation. Patients who see their problem as resulting from their own negligence may be blocked from an active coping response. They may see their problems as a sign of their personal failure and engage in self-blame and passive, withdrawn behavior. Thus the way cause is viewed by patients and health professionals can greatly affect successful coping.

The third aspect of social response is *social comparison,* in which people compare skills and capacities with those of others with similar problems. A person's self-assessment depends very much on those with whom comparisons are made. The outcome is an evaluation of the need for support from the person's social network or support system. Predisposing factors such as age, developmental level, and cultural background, as well as the characteristics of the precipitating stressor, determine the perceived need for social support.

In summary, the way a person appraises an event is the psychological key to understanding coping efforts and the nature and intensity of the stress response. Unfortunately, many nurses and other health professionals ignore this fact when they presume to know how certain stressors will affect a patient and thus provide "routine" care. Not only does this practice depersonalize the patient, but it also undermines the basis of nursing care. The patient's appraisal of life stressors, with its cognitive, affective, physiological, behavioral, and social components, must be an essential part of the psychiatric nurse's assessment.

> ? *How might social attribution influence a nurse's response to a rape victim, a person with a substance abuse disorder, or a patient with HIV?*

Coping Resources

Coping resources, options, or strategies help to determine what can be done, as well as what is at stake. This component takes into account which coping options are available, the likelihood that a given option will accomplish what it is supposed to, and the likelihood that the person can apply a particular strategy effectively.

Coping resources include economic assets, abilities and skills, defensive techniques, social supports, and motivation. They incorporate all levels of the social hierarchy represented in Fig. 4-1 on p. 67. Relationships between the individual, family, group, and society assume critical importance at this point of the model. Other coping resources include health and energy, positive beliefs, problem solving and social skills, social and material resources, and physical well-being.

Viewing oneself positively can serve as a basis of hope and can sustain a person's coping efforts under the most adverse circumstances. Problem-solving skills include the ability to search for information, identify the problem, weigh alternatives, and implement a plan of action. Social skills facilitate the solving of problems involving other people, increase the likelihood of enlisting cooperation and support from others, and give the individual greater social control. Finally, material assets refer to money and the goods and services that money can buy. Obviously, monetary resources greatly increase a person's coping options in almost any stressful situation.

Knowledge and intelligence are other coping resources that allow people to see different ways of dealing with stress. Finally, coping resources also include a strong ego identity, commitment to a social network, cultural stability, a stable system of values and beliefs, a preventive health orientation, and genetic or constitutional strength.

Coping Mechanisms

It is at this point in the model that coping mechanisms emerge. This is an important time for nursing activities directed toward primary prevention. **Coping mechanisms** can be defined as any efforts directed at stress management. There are three main types of coping mechanisms:

▼ **Problem-focused** coping mechanisms, which involve tasks and direct efforts to cope with the threat itself. Examples include negotiation, confrontation, and seeking advice.

▼ **Cognitively focused** coping mechanisms, by which the person attempts to control the meaning of the problem and thus neutralize it. Examples include positive comparison, selective ignorance, substitution of rewards, and the devaluation of desired objects.

▼ **Emotion-focused** coping mechanisms, by which the patient is oriented to moderating emotional distress. Examples include the use of ego defense mechanisms such as denial, suppression, or projection. A detailed discussion of coping and defense mechanisms appears in Chapter 16.

Coping mechanisms can be constructive or destructive. They are *constructive* when anxiety is treated as a warning

---

CRITICAL THINKING *about* **Contemporary Issues**

How Does Mind-Body Dualism Influence the Way Nurses Think about Patients and Their Illnesses?

In formulating diagnoses, psychiatric nurses must be careful to avoid the mind-body dualism that characterizes the expression, diagnosis, and use of health-care services in the United States.[4] In most other cultures this division between mind and body does not exist. There is a wide range of behavior for expressing emotion and psychological disorders, and in America many people express their distress somatically and attribute their problems to physical illness rather than to psychological, social, or spiritual dilemmas. This can create a variety of problems.

One problem is that nurses can respond to patients' somatic complaints and treat them as problems of physical illness without questioning them about possible psychosocial causes. Many patients often want a somatic explanation and treatment and react with fear or anger to the suggestion that there may be a psychological component to their problem. These patients may receive treatment that results in harm or not receive treatment that is needed for their underlying psychological problem. Conversely, a physical illness with affective or cognitive symptoms might be misdiagnosed and inappropriately treated as a psychological problem. Another mistake is for nurses to believe that if a patient's problem is psychiatric, then physical symptoms can be discounted or ignored.

As a consequence of mind-body dualism, patients are separated according to whether their illnesses are deemed to be psychological or physical. They are then sent to different hospitals and are seen by different kinds of health-care providers. The practical consequence of this dualistic thinking is that it can interfere with a nurse's ability to holistically understand people's reactions to events in their lives and the ways in which they cope and adapt.

---

signal and the individual accepts it as a challenge to resolve the problem. In this respect anxiety can be compared to a fever: Both serve as warnings that the system is under attack. Once used successfully, constructive coping mechanisms modify the way past experiences are used to meet future threats. *Destructive* coping mechanisms ward off anxiety without resolving the conflict, using evasion instead of resolution.

PATTERNS OF RESPONSE

According to the Stuart Stress Adaptation Model, an individual's response to stress is based on specific predisposing factors, the nature of the stressor, the perception of the situation, and an analysis of coping resources and mechanisms. Coping responses of the patient are then evaluated on a continuum of adaptation/maladaptation (see Fig. 4-4). Responses that support integrated functioning are seen as adaptive. They lead to growth, learning, and goal achievement. Responses that block integrated functioning are seen as maladaptive. They prevent growth, decrease autonomy, and interfere with mastery of the environment.

Nursing Diagnoses

Responses to stress, whether actual or potential, are the subject of nursing diagnoses. A **nursing diagnosis** is a clinical judgment about individual, family, or community responses to stress (see Critical Thinking about Contemporary Issues). It is a statement of the patient's nursing problem that includes both the adaptive and maladaptive response and contributing stressors. These responses may be overt, covert, existing, or potential and may lie anywhere on the continuum from adaptive to maladaptive. Formulating the diagnosis and implementing treatment are nursing functions for which the nurse is accountable. Box 4-2 lists the NANDA-approved nursing diagnoses.

Relationship to Medical Diagnoses

Medical diagnosis is the health problem or disease state of the patient. In the medical model of psychiatry these health problems are mental disorders or mental illnesses. It is important for psychiatric nurses to distinguish between nursing and medical models of care, as shown in Fig. 4-5. In particular

▼ Nurses assess *risk factors* and look for *vulnerabilities.*
▼ Physicians assess *disease states* and look for *causes.*
▼ Nursing diagnoses focus on the *adaptive/maladaptive coping continuum of human responses.*
▼ Medical diagnoses focus on the *health/illness continuum of health problems.*
▼ Nursing intervention consists of *caregiving activities.*
▼ Medical intervention consists of *curative treatments.*

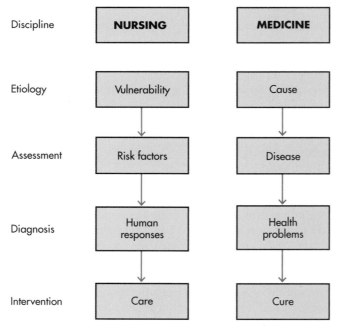

Discipline	**NURSING**	**MEDICINE**
Etiology	Vulnerability	Cause
Assessment	Risk factors	Disease
Diagnosis	Human responses	Health problems
Intervention	Care	Cure

Fig. 4-5 Comparison of nursing and medical models of care.

A nurse may implement the nursing process for maladaptive responses based on the Stuart Stress Adaptation Model whether or not a physician has diagnosed the presence of a psychiatric illness. Also, patients with a persistent psychiatric illness may be adapting well to it. People can successfully adapt to an illness without recovering from it. This is an important aspect of the Stuart Stress Adaptation Model because it suggests that psychiatric nurses can promote their patients' adaptive responses regardless of their health or illness state.[18]

Classifying Mental Disorders

Mental illnesses can be broadly differentiated as neurotic or psychotic. **Neuroses** have the following characteristics:
▼ A symptom or group of symptoms is distressing and is recognized as unacceptable and alien to the individual.
▼ Reality testing is grossly intact.
▼ Behavior does not actively violate gross social norms (although functioning may be significantly impaired).
▼ The disturbance is enduring or recurrent without treatment and is not merely a transitory reaction to stressors.
▼ No demonstrable organic cause or factor is present.

In situations of severest conflict, however, the person may be powerless to cope with the threat by such patterns and may distort reality, as in psychosis. **Psychosis** consists of the following characteristics:
▼ Regressive behavior
▼ Personality disintegration
▼ A significant reduction in level of awareness
▼ Great difficulty in functioning adequately
▼ Gross impairment in reality testing

This last characteristic is critical. When people demonstrate gross impairment in reality testing, they incorrectly evaluate the accuracy of their perceptions and draw incorrect inferences about external reality, even in the face of contrary evidence. Direct evidence of psychosis is the presence of delusions or hallucinations without insight into their pathological nature. Psychotic health problems reflect the most severe level of illness.

Medical diagnoses are classified according to the *Diagnostic and Statistical Manual of Mental Disorders,* fourth edition (DSM-IV), of the American Psychiatric Association.[1] The various illnesses are accompanied by a description of diagnostic criteria, tested for reliability by psychiatric practitioners. DSM-IV uses a multiaxial system that gives attention to various mental disorders, general medical conditions, aspects of the environment, and areas of functioning that might be overlooked if the focus were exclusively on assessing a single presenting problem. The individual thus is evaluated on the following axes:
▼ Axis I: Clinical syndromes
▼ Axis II: Personality disorders
▼ Axis III: General medical conditions
▼ Axis IV: Psychosocial and environmental problems
▼ Axis V: Global assessment of functioning

Box 4-2 *NANDA-Approved Nursing Diagnoses*

Activity intolerance
Activity intolerance, risk for
Adaptive capacity, decreased: intracranial
Adjustment, impaired
Airway clearance, ineffective
Anxiety
Aspiration, risk for
Body image disturbance
Body temperature, altered, risk for
Bowel incontinence
Breastfeeding, effective
Breastfeeding, ineffective
Breastfeeding, interrupted
Breathing pattern, ineffective
Cardiac output, decreased
Caregiver role strain
Caregiver role strain, risk for
Communication, impaired verbal
Community coping, potential for enhanced
Community coping, ineffective
Confusion, acute
Confusion, chronic
Constipation
Constipation, colonic
Constipation, perceived
Coping, defensive
Coping, family: potential for growth
Coping, ineffective family: compromised
Coping, ineffective family: disabling
Coping, ineffective individual
Decisional conflict (specify)
Denial, ineffective
Diarrhea
Disuse syndrome, risk for
Diversional activity deficit
Dysreflexia
Energy field disturbance
Environmental implementation syndrome, impaired
Family processes, altered: alcoholism
Family processes, altered
Fatigue
Fear
Fluid volume deficit
Fluid volume deficit, risk for
Fluid volume excess
Gas exchange, impaired
Grieving, anticipatory
Grieving, dysfunctional
Growth and development, altered
Health maintenance, altered
Health-seeking behaviors (specify)
Home maintenance management, impaired
Hopelessness
Hyperthermia
Hypothermia
Incontinence, functional
Incontinence, reflex
Incontinence, stress
Incontinence, total
Incontinence, urge
Infant behavior, disorganized
Infant behavior, disorganized: risk for
Infant behavior, organized: potential for enhanced
Infant feeding pattern, ineffective
Infection, risk for

Injury, perioperative positioning: risk for
Injury, risk for
Knowledge deficit (specify)
Loneliness, risk for
Management of the therapeutic regimen, community: ineffective
Management of the therapeutic regimen, families: ineffective
Management of the therapeutic regimen, individual: effective
Management of the therapeutic regimen, individuals: ineffective
Memory, impaired
Mobility, impaired physical
Noncompliance (specify)
Nutrition, altered: less than body requirements
Nutrition, altered: more than body requirements
Nutrition, altered: risk for more than body requirements
Oral mucous membrane, altered
Pain
Pain, chronic
Parent/infant/child attachment, altered: risk for
Parental role conflict
Parenting, altered
Parenting, altered, risk for
Peripheral neurovascular dysfunction, risk for
Personal identity disturbance
Poisoning, risk for
Post-trauma response
Powerlessness
Protection, altered
Rape-trauma syndrome
Rape-trauma syndrome: compound reaction
Rape-trauma syndrome: silent reaction
Relocation stress syndrome
Role performance, altered
Self-care deficit, bathing/hygiene
Self-care deficit, dressing/grooming
Self-care deficit, feeding
Self-care deficit, toileting
Self-esteem disturbance
Self-esteem, chronic low
Self-esteem, situational low
Self-mutilation, risk for
Sensory/perceptual alterations (specify) (visual, auditory, kinesthetic, gustatory, tactile, olfactory)
Sexual dysfunction
Sexuality patterns, altered
Skin integrity, impaired
Skin integrity, impaired, risk for
Sleep pattern disturbance
Social interaction, impaired
Social isolation
Spiritual distress (distress of the human spirit)
Spiritual well-being, potential for enhanced
Suffocation, risk for
Swallowing, impaired
Thermoregulation, ineffective
Thought processes, altered
Tissue integrity, impaired
Tissue perfusion, altered (specify type) (renal, cerebral, cardiopulmonary, gastrointestinal, peripheral)
Trauma, risk for
Unilateral neglect
Urinary elimination, altered
Urinary retention
Ventilation, inability to sustain spontaneous
Ventilatory weaning response, dysfunctional (DVWR)
Violence, risk for: directed at others

From *NANDA nursing diagnoses: definitions and classifications, 1997-1998*, Philadelphia, 1997, The Association.

Box **4-3** *Outline for Cultural Formulation in Psychiatric Diagnosis*

Cultural identity of the individual
Cultural explanations of the individual's illness
Cultural factors related to one's psychosocial environment and levels of functioning
Cultural elements of the relationship between the individual and clinician
Overall cultural assessment for diagnosis and care

Axes I-V are presented in Appendix A.

▼ Axes I and II constitute the entire classification of mental disorders plus conditions that are not attributable to a mental disorder that are a focus of attention or treatment.

▼ Axis III allows the clinician to identify any physical disorder potentially relevant to the understanding or treatment of the individual.

▼ Axis IV is for reporting psychosocial and environmental problems that may affect the diagnosis, treatment, and prognosis of mental disorders.

▼ Axis V is for reporting the clinician's judgment of the individual's overall level of functioning. This information is useful in planning treatment, measuring its impact, and predicting outcomes.

Psychiatric nurses use all five axes of the DSM-IV and integrate the axes with related nursing diagnoses.

In addition to Axes I-V, the DSM-IV has an outline for cultural formulation designed to help the clinician in systematically evaluating the person's cultural and social reference group and ways in which the cultural context is relevant to clinical care (see Chapter 7). It is suggested that the clinician provide a narrative summary of the evaluation of the categories listed in Box 4-3. The DSM-IV also includes a list of culture-bound syndromes that are recurrent, locality-specific patterns of aberrant behavior and troubling experiences that may or may not be linked to a particular DSM-IV diagnostic category.[1] Although behaviors related to most DSM-IV categories can be found throughout the world, the particular symptoms, course of illness, and social response are often influenced by cultural factors. In contrast, culture-bound syndromes are generally limited to specific societies or culture areas and are localized, folk, diagnostic categories that give coherent meanings for certain common, patterned, and troubling sets of experiences and observations.

TREATMENT STAGES AND ACTIVITIES

The final aspect of the Stuart Stress Adaptation Model is the integration of the theoretical basis, biopsychosocial components, patterns of response, and nursing activities based on the patient's treatment stage. Once patterns of coping responses have been identified, the nurse determines which treatment stage the patient is in and implements the most appropriate nursing activities.

Fig. **4-6** Psychiatric nursing treatment stages and activities.

The model identifies four possible treatment stages: (1) health promotion, (2) maintenance, (3) acute, and (4) crisis. These stages reflect the range of the adaptive/maladaptive continuum and suggest a variety of nursing activities. For each stage the nurse identifies the treatment goal, focus of the nursing assessment, nature of the nursing intervention, and expected outcome of nursing care (Fig. 4-6).

▼ In the crisis stage of treatment the nursing goal is the stabilization of the patient; the nursing assessment focuses on risk factors that threaten the patient's health and well-being; the nursing intervention is directed toward managing the environment to provide safety; and the expected outcome of nursing care is that no harm will come to the patient or others.

▼ In the acute stage of treatment the nursing goal is for the patient's illness to be placed in remission; the nursing assessment is focused on the patient's symptoms and maladaptive coping responses; the nursing intervention is directed toward treatment planning with the patient and the modeling and teaching of adaptive responses; and the expected outcome of nursing care is symptom relief.

The Stuart Stress Adaptation Model of Psychiatric Nursing Care

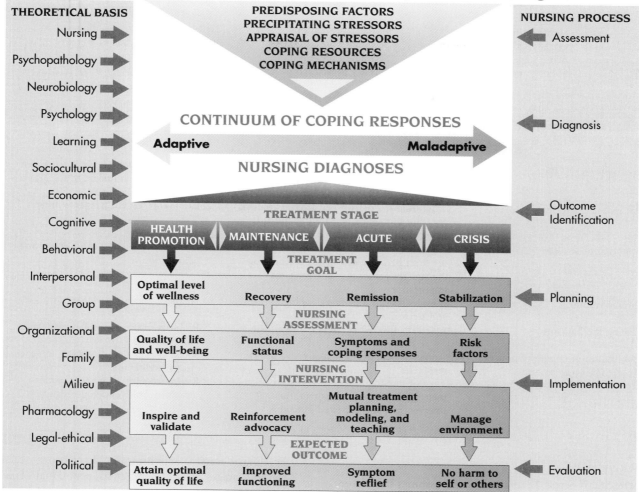

Fig. 4-7 The Stuart Stress Adaptation Model of psychiatric nursing care.

▼ In the **maintenance stage of treatment** the nursing goal is the complete recovery of the patient; the nursing assessment is focused on the patient's functional status; the nursing intervention is directed toward reinforcement of the patient's adaptive coping responses and patient advocacy; and the expected outcome of nursing care is improved patient functioning.

▼ In the **health promotion stage of treatment** the nursing goal is for the patient to achieve the optimal level of wellness; the nursing assessment is focused on the patient's quality of life and well-being; the nursing intervention is directed toward inspiring and validating the patient; and the expected outcome of nursing care is that the patient will attain the optimal quality of life.

This aspect of the model moves the field of psychiatric nursing beyond the usual activities associated with the stabilization of patients in crisis and remission of the acutely ill patient's symptoms. It elaborates nursing responsibilities in the maintenance and health promotion treatment stages as improving patients' functional status and enhancing their

quality of life.[2] These treatment stages are often overlooked in traditional psychiatric nursing practice, yet they are essential aspects of the contemporary psychiatric nursing role. These stages also relate to the levels of prevention in psychiatric care and the clinical chapters of this text, as depicted in Table 4-1.

The synthesis of all of the elements of the Stuart Stress Adaption Model of psychiatric nursing care is depicted in Fig. 4-7. They are also summarized in Table 4-2. Chapters 16 through 26 explore various maladaptive coping responses and related medical diagnoses. The phases of the nursing process are described for patients exhibiting maladaptive responses. Each chapter begins with a continuum of coping responses, followed by a discussion of behaviors, predisposing factors, precipitating stressors, appraisal of stressor, coping resources, coping mechanisms, nursing diagnoses, and related interventions. Through consistent application of the Stuart Stress Adaptation Model, the art and science of psychiatric nursing emerge.

TABLE **4-1** *Stages of Treatment Related to Levels of Prevention and Clinical Chapters of the Text*

STAGE OF TREATMENT	LEVEL OF PREVENTION	CLINICAL CHAPTER(S)
Health promotion stage	Primary prevention	12: Mental Health Promotion
Crisis stage	Secondary prevention	13: Crisis Intervention
Acute stage	Secondary prevention	16-26: Coping Responses
Maintenance stage	Tertiary prevention	14: Psychiatric Rehabilitation

TABLE **4-2** *Summary of the Elements of the Stuart Stress Adaptation Model*

ELEMENT	DEFINITION	EXAMPLES
Predisposing factors	Risk factors that influence both the type and amount of resources the person can elicit to cope with stress	Genetic background, intelligence, self-concept, age, ethnicity, education, gender, belief systems
Precipitating stressors	Stimuli that the person perceives as challenging, threatening, or demanding and that require excess energy for coping	Life events, injury, hassles, strains
Appraisal of stressor	An evaluation of the significance of a stressor for a person's well-being, considering the stressor's meaning, intensity, and importance	Hardiness, perceived seriousness, anxiety, attribution
Coping resources	An evaluation of a person's coping options and strategies	Finances, social support, ego integrity
Coping mechanisms	Any effort directed at stress management	Problem solving, compliance, defense mechanisms
Continuum of coping responses	A range of adaptive or maladaptive human responses	Social changes, physical symptoms, emotional well-being
Treatment stage activities	Range of nursing functions related to treatment goal, nursing assessment, nursing intervention, and expected outcome	Environment management, patient teaching, role modeling, advocacy

Summary

1. The Stuart Stress Adaptation Model assumes that nature is ordered as a social hierarchy, that psychiatric nursing care is provided through the nursing process within a biological, psychological, sociocultural, and legal-ethical context, that health/illness and adaptation/maladaptation are distinct concepts, and that primary, secondary, and tertiary levels of prevention are included in the four discrete stages of psychiatric treatment.

2. Standards of mental health are less clear than those for mental illness. Nearly one of every two people in the United States has had a psychiatric illness or substance abuse disorder in his or her lifetime.

3. The biopsychosocial components of the model include predisposing factors, precipitating stressors, appraisal of stressor, coping resources, and coping mechanisms.

4. Patterns of response include the individual's coping responses, which are the subject of nursing diagnoses, and health problems, which are the subject of medical diagnoses.

5. Psychiatric nursing activities were described for each of the four stages of treatment: crisis, acute, maintenance, and health promotion.

your **INTERNET**
c o n n e c t i o n

Mental Health Net
http://www.cmhcsys.com

Psychlink
http://www.psychlink.com/

Chapter Review Questions

1. Indicate whether the following statements are true (T) or false (F).

A. ___ The standards of mental health are less clear than those of mental illness.

B. ___ Approximately one out of every three people will experience a psychiatric or substance abuse problem in his or her lifetime.

C. ___ The treatment for depression is more effective than that for cardiovascular illness.

D. ___ The parasympathetic division of the autonomic nervous system is stimulated by the fight-or-flight response.

E. ___ A coping mechanism is considered to be constructive when it treats anxiety as a warning signal and the person accepts it as a challenge to solve the problem.

F. ___ Psychotic health problems reflect the most severe level of illness.

2. Fill in the blanks.

A. A person's ability to test assumptions about the world by empirical thought is called _____.

B. The concept of _____ proposes that humans must weather periods of stress and change throughout life.

C. Intelligence, morale, and self-concept are examples of _____ predisposing factors.

D. _____ is when a person tries to identify the unique factors that contributed to one's particular situation.

E. The three types of primary cognitive appraisals to stress are _____, _____, and _____.

F. Personality disorders are identified on Axis _____ of the DSM-IV.

G. Recurrent, locality-specific patterns of aberrant behavior and troubling experience that may or may not be linked to a particular DSM-IV diagnostic category are called _____.

3. Provide short answers for the following questions.

A. Describe the three parts of a hardy personality and the way in which they help a person cope with stress.

B. List the three types of coping mechanisms and give an example of each.

C. Compare the nursing and medical models of care. Which model do you think currently receives more health-care resources, research funding, and professional status? Defend your answer.

D. Identify the four stages of psychiatric treatment and the level of prevention related to each one.

REFERENCES

1. American Psychiatric Association: *Diagnostic and statistical manual of mental disorders,* ed 4, Washington, DC, 1994, The Association.
2. Anthony W: Recovery from mental illness: the guiding vision of the mental health service system in the 1990s, *Psychosoc Rehabil J* 16:11, 1993.
3. Bruckbauer E, Ward S: Positive mental attitude and health: what the public believes, *Image J Nurs Sch* 25:311, 1993.
4. Can your mind heal your body? *Consumer Reports* 58:107, 1993.
5. Caplan G: Mastery of stress: psychosocial aspects, *Am J Psychiatry* 13 8:41, 1981.
6. Dyer J, McGuinness T: Resilience: analysis of concept, *Arch Psychiatr Nurs* 10:276, 1996.
7. Friedman H, VandenBos G: Disease-prone and self-healing personalities, *Hosp Community Psychiatry* 43:1177, 1992.
8. Kessler R et al: Lifetime and 12-month prevalence of DSM-R psychiatric disorders in the United States, *Arch Gen Psychiatry* 51:8, 1994.
9. Lykken D, Tellegen A: Happiness is a stochastic phenomenon, *Psychol Sci* 7:186, 1996.
10. Maddi S, Kobasa S: *Stress and coping: an anthology,* New York, 1991, Columbia University Press.
11. Maslow A: *Motivation and personality,* New York, 1958, Harper & Row.
12. Mechanic D: Illness behavior, social adaptation, and the management of illness, *J Nerv Ment Dis* 165:79, 1977.
13. Monat A, Lazarus R: *Stress and coping,* New York, 1991, Columbia University Press.
14. National Advisory Mental Health Council: Health care reform for Americans with severe mental illnesses, *Am J Psychiatry* 150:1447, 1993.
15. Pearlin LI, Schooler C: The structure of coping, *J Health Soc Behav* 19:2, 1978.
16. Rogers C: *On becoming a person,* Boston, 1961, Houghton Mifflin.
17. Segal S, VanderVoort D: Daily hassles of persons with severe mental illness, *Hosp Community Psychiatry* 44:276, 1993.
18. Stuhlmiller C: The construction of disorders, *J Psychosoc Nurs* 33:20, 1995.
19. Tartasky D: Hardiness: conceptual and methodological issues, *Image J Nurs Sch* 25:225, 1993.

Biological Context of Psychiatric Nursing Care

Michele T. Laraia

© 1998 M.C. Escher/Cordon Art, Baarn, Holland.

We must recollect that all our provisional ideas in psychology will some day be based on an organic substructure. This makes it probable that special substances and special chemical processes control the operation. **Sigmund Freud**

LEARNING OBJECTIVES

After studying this chapter the student should be able to:

▼ Relate the importance of understanding the structure and function of the brain for psychiatric nursing practice

▼ Describe neuroimaging techniques used in psychiatry

▼ Discuss the current status of genetic information related to psychiatric illness

▼ Identify the impact of circadian rhythms on a person's abilities and moods

▼ Describe the new field of psychoimmunology and its implications for psychiatry

▼ Demonstrate the ability to assess patients from a biological perspective

▼ Analyze the clinical implications of recent neuroscientific research related to schizophrenia, mood disorders, panic disorder, and Alzheimer's disease

TOPICAL OUTLINE

Structure and Function of the Brain
Neuroimaging Techniques
Genetics of Mental Illness
Circadian Rhythms
  Sleep
Psychoimmunology
Biological Assessment of the Patient
Biological Components of Mental Illness
  Schizophrenia
  Mood Disorders
  Panic Disorders
  Alzheimer's Disease
Decade of the Brain

Although interest in the brain and human behavior has a history as old as the human race, the twentieth century has witnessed a shift in how science views the brain and behavior, and thus human experience itself. The explosion in knowledge and technology in the neuro-sciences is unprecedented. This is evident in research that focuses on how the brain is structured, how the nervous system functions, how these systems affect health, and how they are affected by disease. Neuroscience research has begun to suggest causes of brain illnesses, interventions to treat these illnesses, and effective preventive measures. The field of neuroscience encompasses many disciplines including anatomy, physiology, biochemistry, genetics, neuroimaging, physics, pharmacology, neurology, neurosurgery, immunology, psychiatry, psychology, electronics, and computer science (Fig. 5-1).

New tools and techniques now help to explain the way in which the brain works and how the brain, mind, and body interact. These technologies, along with standardized behavioral tests, have allowed us to correlate human behavior with specific brain regions, functions, and dysfunctions. A revolution has begun in the study of how the human brain is understood and the way in which mental illness is conceptualized, recognized, and treated.

Psychiatric nursing has a key role to play in this endeavor. Nurses have always been in a pivotal position to integrate theories and technologies with therapeutic interventions and patient-centered approaches. They have demonstrated great ability to do this, for example, in the psychosocial areas of functioning. Psychiatric nurses are using the biological context of psychiatric care to enhance their practice. They must interpret this new biological information and its potential for effective treatments, thus further reinforcing nurses' role as patient advocates and professional colleagues. It is clear that the biological frontier presents great challenges, and if these challenges are accepted, psychiatric nursing can make a significant move forward in further defining the scope of its practice and the outcomes associated with psychiatric nursing care.

STRUCTURE AND FUNCTION OF THE BRAIN

The psychiatric nurse must have a working knowledge of the normal structure and function of the brain, particularly mental functions, just as the cardiac care nurse must know how the heart works. Much is known about various brain structures and how they are linked to some of the symptoms of mental illness. The reader is encouraged to review texts on basic anatomy and physiology or neurophysiology to learn more about these areas.[21] For the purposes of this chapter, a brief review of several key brain regions is presented in Color Plates 1 to 5 on pp. 93-96 and in Box 5-1. This information can be used as a reference for topics discussed in this chapter.

The brain weighs about 3 pounds. It is composed of trillions of groups of cells that have formed structures that have changed over millions of years of evolution. These structures have complex functions and connections to each other that are not fully understood. However, we have some basic information on how these structures function and communicate in health and illness. About 100 billion brain cells form groups of neurons that are arranged in networks. These neurons communicate with each other through neurotransmission, which gives rise to human activity, body functions, consciousness, intelligence, creativity, memory,

Fig. 5-1   The field of neurosciences.

and emotion. Neurotransmission is a key factor in understanding how various regions of the brain function and how biochemical interventions, such as medications, affect brain activity and behavior. There are also chemical messengers called **neurotransmitters.** These are manufactured in the neuron and released from the **axon,** or presynaptic cell membrane, into the **synapse,** which is the space between neurons. From there they are received by the **dendrite,** or postsynaptic membrane, of the next neuron. This neurotransmission process makes communication between brain cells possible (see Color Plate 6 on p. 96).

Like a key inserted into a lock, each of these chemicals fits into specific receptor cells, or proteins, embedded in the membrane of the dendrite, which recognize it. Then one of two things happens: The signal given by the neurotransmitter either excites receiving cells, which causes them to fire and produce an action, or inhibits cells from firing, which modifies the excitability of the receiving cell and stops an action. After release into the synapse and communication with receptor cells, these neurotransmitter chemicals are transported back from the synapse into the axon, where they are stored for reuse or metabolized and inactivated by enzymes. The process of neurotransmitters returning to the presynaptic cell is called **reuptake.**

The **glial cells,** which are support cells that form the **myelin sheaths,** insulate the nervous system. They are thought to remove excess transmitters and ions from the extracellular spaces in the brain, provide glucose to some nerve cells, and direct the flow of blood and oxygen to various parts of the brain.

From this basic explanation it is evident that neurotransmitters perform vital functions in the normal working

Box 5-1 *Structure and Function of the Brain*

CEREBRUM

Largest portion of the brain

Responsible for conscious perception, thought, and motor activity

Governs muscle coordination and the learning of rote movements

Can override most other systems

Divided into two hemispheres, each of which is divided into four lobes

Dominant Hemisphere

Left side is dominant in most people (95% of right-handed and more than 50% of left-handed people)

Responsible for the production and comprehension of language, mathematical ability, and the ability to solve problems in a sequential, logical fashion

Nondominant Hemisphere

Right side is nondominant in most people

Responsible for musical skills, recognition of faces, and tasks requiring comprehension of spatial relationships

Corpus Callosum

Largest fiber bundle in the brain

Connects the two cerebral hemispheres and passes information from one to the other, welding the two hemispheres together into a unitary consciousness, allowing the "right hand to know what the left hand is doing"

Cerebral Cortex

A few millimeters thick and about 2.5 sq. ft. in area

Sheet of gray matter containing 30 billion neurons interconnected by almost 70 miles of axons and dendrites

Forms the corrugated surface of the four lobes of the cerebral hemispheres

Connected to various structures of the brain and has a great deal to do with the abilities we think of as uniquely human, such as language and abstract thinking, as well as basic aspects of perception, movement, and adaptive response to the outside world

Functional areas have been mapped by imaging technology

Damage to certain cortical areas usually results in predictable deficits, depending on the area affected

Frontal Lobes

Aid in planning for the future, motivation, control of voluntary motor function, and production of speech

Play an important part in emotional experience and expression of mood

Parietal Lobes

Reception and evaluation of most sensory information (excluding smell, hearing, and vision)

Central Sulcus

Groove or fissure on the surface of the brain that divides the frontal and parietal lobes

Temporal Lobes

Receive and evaluate olfactory and auditory input and play an important role in memory

Associated with brain functions such as abstract thought and judgment

Lateral Fissure

Separates the temporal lobe from the rest of the cerebrum

Occipital Lobes

Reception and integration of visual input

Clinical example: Aphasia (absent or defective speech or comprehension) results from a lesion in the language areas of the cortex. The several types of aphasia depend on the site of the lesion. Damage to Broca's area, which contains the motor programs for the generation of language, results in expressive, or motor, aphasia, with difficulty producing either written or spoken words but no difficulty comprehending language. Damage to Wernicke's area, which contains the mechanisms for the formulation of language, results in receptive, or sensory, aphasia, where words are produced but their sequence is defective in linguistic content, resulting in paraphasia (word substitutions), neologisms (insertion of new and meaningless words), or jargon (fluent but unintelligible speech), and there is a general deficiency in the comprehension of language. If the lesion occurs in the connection between the two areas, conduction aphasia results, in which a person has poor repetition but good comprehension.

DIENCEPHALON

Constitutes only 2% of the CNS by weight

Has extremely widespread and important connections, and the great majority of sensory, motor, and limbic pathways involve the diencephalon

Thalamus

Composes 80% of the diencephalon

All sensory pathways and many other anatomical loops relay in the thalamus

Takes sensory information and relays it to areas throughout the cortex

Influences prefrontal cortical functions such as affect and foresight

Influences mood and general body movements associated with strong emotions, such as fear or rage

Pineal Gland

Endocrine gland involved in reproductive cycles

During darkness it secretes an antigonadotropic hormone called melatonin, which decreases during light, thus increasing gonadal function

Important in mammals with seasonal sexual cycles, its effects in humans are not yet clear, although tumors of the pineal gland affect human sexual development

May also be involved in the sleep-wake cycle

Hypothalamus

Weighs only 4 g

Major control center for the pituitary gland, for maintaining homeostasis, and regulating autonomic, endocrine, emotional, and somatic functions

Controls various visceral functions and activities involved in basic drives and is very important in a number of functions that have emotional and mood relationships

Directly involved in stress-related and psychosomatic illnesses and with feelings of fear and rage

Regulates feeding and drinking behavior, temperature regulation, cardiac function, gut motility, and sexual activity

Coordinates responses for the sleep-wake cycle to other areas of the body

Contains the mamillary bodies, which are involved in olfactory reflexes and emotional responses to odors

Box **5-1** *Structure and Function of the Brain—cont'd*

BRAINSTEM

Connects the spinal cord to the brain

Location of cranial nerve nuclei

Controls automatic body functions such as breathing and cardiovascular activity

Midbrain

Contains ascending and descending nerve tracks

Visual cortex center

Part of auditory pathway

Regulates the reflexive movement of the eyes and head

Aids in the unconscious regulation and coordination of motor activities

Contains the part of the basal ganglia, the substantia nigra, which manufactures dopamine

Pons

Contains ascending and descending nerve tracks

Relay between cerebrum and cerebellum

Reflex center

Contains the locus ceruleus, which manufactures most of the brain's norepinephrine

Medulla Oblongata

Conduction pathway for ascending and descending nerve tracks

Conscious control of skeletal muscles

Involved in functions such as balance, coordination, and modulation of sound impulses from the inner ear

Center for several important reflexes: heart rate, breathing, swallowing, vomiting, coughing, sneezing

Reticular Formation

Central core of the brainstem

Controls cyclic activities such as the sleep-wake cycle (called the reticular activating system, or RAS)

Plays an important role in arousing and maintaining consciousness, alertness, and attention

Contributes to the motor system, respiration, cardiac rhythms, and other vital body functions

Clinical example: Damage to the RAS can result in coma. General anesthetics function by suppressing this system. It may also be the target of many tranquilizers. Ammonia (smelling salts) stimulate the RAS, resulting in arousal.

BASAL GANGLIA

Several deep gray matter structures that are related functionally and are located bilaterally in the cerebrum, diencephalon, and midbrain

Control muscle tone, activity, and posture

Coordinate large-muscle movements

Major effect is to inhibit unwanted muscular activity

Cause extrapyramidal syndromes when dysfunctional

Clinical example: Parkinson's disease, characterized by muscular rigidity, a slow, shuffling gait, and a general lack of movement, is associated with a dysfunction of the basal ganglia, probably a destruction of the dopamine-producing neurons of the substantia nigra (part of the basal ganglia but located in the midbrain).

LIMBIC SYSTEM

Forms the limbus, or border, of the temporal lobes and is intimately connected to many other structures of the brain

Concerned both with subjective emotional experiences and with changes in bodily functions associated with emotional states

Particularly involved in aggressive, submissive, and sexual behavior, and with pleasure, memory, and learning

Associated with mood, motivation, and sensations, all central to preservation

Clinical example: Klüver-Bucy syndrome develops when the entire limbic system is removed or destroyed. Symptoms include fearlessness and placidity (absence of emotional reactions), an inordinate degree of attention to sensory stimuli (ceaseless and intrusive curiosity), and visual agnosia (the inability to recognize anything).

Hippocampus

Consolidates recently acquired information about facts and events, somehow turning short-term memory into long term

Contains large amounts of neurotransmitters

Clinical example: Surgical removal of the hippocampus results in the inability to form new memories of facts and events (names of new acquaintances, day-to-day events, inability to remember why a task was begun), although long-term memory, intelligence, and the ability to learn new skills are unaffected. A similar memory problem is Korsakoff's syndrome, in which patients have intact intelligence but cannot form new memories. They typically confabulate (make up answers to questions), which occurs when the hippocampus and surrounding areas are damaged by chronic alcoholism. This is also seen in Alzheimer's disease, in which the memory loss is profound, and there is extensive cellular degeneration in the hippocampus.

Amygdala

Generates emotions from perceptions and thoughts (presumably through its interactions with the hypothalamus and prefrontal cortex)

Contains many opiate receptors

Clinical example: Electrical stimulation of the amygdala in animals causes responses of defense, raging aggression, or fleeing. In humans the most common response is fear and its related autonomic responses (dilation of the pupils, increased heart rate, and release of adrenalin). Conversely, bilateral destruction of the amygdala causes a great decrease in aggression, and animals become tame and placid. This is thought to be another kind of memory dysfunction that impairs the ability to learn or remember the appropriate emotional and autonomic responses to stimuli.

Fornix

Two-way fiber system that connects the hippocampus to the hypothalamus

CEREBELLUM

"Little brain"

Full range of sensory inputs finds its way here and in turn projects to various sites in the brainstem and thalamus

Although it is extensively involved with the processing of sensory information, it is also part of the motor system and is involved in equilibrium, muscle tone, postural control, and coordination of voluntary movements

It is thought that, because of connections to other brain regions, the cerebellum may be involved in cognitive, behavioral, and affective functions

Clinical example: The malnutrition often accompanying chronic alcoholism causes a degeneration of the cerebellar cortex, resulting in the anterior lobe syndrome in which the legs are primarily affected, and the most prominent symptom is a broad-based, staggering gait and a general incoordination, or ataxia, of leg movements.

Continued

Box **5-1** *Structure and Function of the Brain—cont'd*

VENTRICLES

Each cerebral hemisphere contains a large cavity, the lateral ventricle

A smaller midline cavity, the third ventricle, is located in the center of the diencephalon, between the two halves of the thalamus

The fourth ventricle is in the region of the pons and medulla oblongata and connects with the central canal of the spinal cord, which extends nearly the full length of the spinal cord

Clinical example: Although the clinical significance of these findings is uncertain, imaging techniques have shown enlargement of the ventricles in many psychiatric disorders, suggesting an atrophy of the many critical structures in the brain with these illnesses

SPINAL FLUID

Cerebral spinal fluid (CSF) is procured from the blood choroid plexuses, located in the ventricles, and fills the ventricles, subarachnoid space (between the brain and the skull), and the spinal cord

CSF bathes the brain with nutrients, cushions the brain within the skull, and exits through the bloodstream

Approximately 140 ml of spinal fluid within the central nervous system travels from its point of origin to the bloodstream at approximately 0.4 ml per minute

Clinical example: Neurotransmitters and their metabolites can be measured in the CSF, plasma, and urine and give an approximation of neurotransmitter production and metabolism in the brain. This provides clues to abnormal neurotransmission in some mental illnesses.

BLOOD-BRAIN AND BLOOD-CSF BARRIERS

Neuronal function requires a microenvironment that is protected from changes elsewhere in the body that may have an adverse effect

Blood-brain and blood-CSF barriers protect the CNS in several ways:

Large molecules, such as plasma proteins, present in the blood are excluded from the CSF and nervous tissue

The brain and spinal cord are protected from neurotransmitters in the blood, such as epinephrine produced by the adrenal gland

Neurotransmitters produced in the CNS are prevented from precipitously leaking into the general circulation

Toxins are excluded either because of their molecular size (too big) or because of their solubility (only substances soluble in water and cell-membrane lipids can pass these barriers), so many drugs are not able to enter the brain and spinal cord

---

brain, and their absence or excess can play a major role in brain disease and behavioral disorders. It is also important to realize that a single neurotransmitter can activate several different subtypes of receptor cells, each located along tracks going to different regions of the brain. Thus one neurotransmitter can have different effects in different areas of the brain. Also, the number of receptors in the brain changes depending on the availability of the neurotransmitter. Nearly all of the known or suspected neurotransmitters fall into one of two categories: small amine molecules (monoamines, acetylcholine, and amino acids) and peptides. These are described in Table 5-1.

One clinical implication of this process is that abnormalities in the structure of the brain or in its activity in specific locations can cause or contribute to psychiatric disorders. For example, a communication problem in one small part of the brain can cause widespread dysfunction. It is also known that the following networks of nuclei that control cognitive, behavioral, and emotional functioning are particularly implicated in psychiatric disorders:

▼ *The cerebral cortex,* which is critical in decision making and higher-order thinking, such as abstract reasoning

▼ *The limbic system,* which is involved in regulating emotional behavior, memory, and learning

▼ *The basal ganglia,* some of which coordinate movement

▼ *The hypothalamus,* which regulates hormones throughout the body and behaviors such as eating, drinking, and sex

▼ *The locus ceruleus,* which manufactures norepinephrine, involved in the body's response to stress

▼ *The raphe nuclei,* made up of serotonin-producing neu-

rons, which regulate sleep and are involved with behavior and mood

▼ *The substantia nigra,* dopamine-producing cells involved in the control of complex movements, thinking, and emotional responses

A second clinical implication is related to the use of psychotropic medications. These can work by blocking the reuptake of neurotransmitters or by decreasing the metabolism of the neurotransmitters, thus allowing more of the neurotransmitter to remain in the synapse. However, unless a medication is specific for the subtype of the receptor involved in the psychiatric symptomatology, it may activate many other receptor subtypes unnecessarily. This lack of specificity is one of the causes of drug side effects. By understanding the biological processes underlying psychiatric symptoms, the psychiatric nurse can select and measure the effects of appropriate medications, maximize positive effects, minimize unwanted effects, and measure and predict outcomes of psychiatric nursing care.

> **?** *How would you respond to a nursing colleague who says that psychiatric nurses do not need to know much about anatomy and physiology because what they do primarily is talk to people?*

NEUROIMAGING TECHNIQUES

Until recently the only way to study the brain was through surgery or autopsy. Brain imaging techniques that have evolved over the past 20 years allow direct viewing of the

TABLE 5-1 *Neurotransmitters and Neuromodulators in the Brain*

Substance	Location	Function
AMINES		

Amines are neurotransmitters that are synthesized from amino molecules such as tyrosine, tryptophan, and histidine. Found in various regions of the brain, amines affect learning, emotions, motor control, and other activities.

Substance	Location	Function
Monoamines		
Norepinephrine (NE)	Derived from tyrosine, a dietary amino acid. Located in the brainstem (particularly the locus ceruleus). *Effect:* Can be excitatory or inhibitory.	Levels fluctuate with sleep and wakefulness. Plays a role in changes in levels of attention and vigilance. Involved in attributing a rewarding value to a stimulus and in the regulation of mood. Plays a role in affective and anxiety disorders. Antidepressants block the reuptake of NE into the presynaptic cell or inhibit monoamine oxidase from metabolizing it.
Dopamine (DA)	Derived from tyrosine, a dietary amino acid. Located mostly in the brainstem (particularly the substantia nigra). *Effect:* Generally excitatory.	Involved in the control of complex movements, motivation, cognition, and regulating emotional responses. Many drugs of abuse (such as cocaine and amphetamines) cause DA release, suggesting a role in whatever makes things pleasurable. Involved in the movement disorders seen in Parkinson's disease and in many of the deficits seen in schizophrenia and other forms of psychosis. Antipsychotic drugs block dopamine receptors in the postsynaptic cell.
Serotonin (5-HT)	Derived from tryptophan, a dietary amino acid. Located only in the brain (particularly in the raphe nuclei of the brainstem). *Effect:* Mostly inhibitory.	Levels fluctuate with sleep and wakefulness, suggesting a role in arousal and modulation of the general activity levels of the CNS, particularly the onset of sleep. Plays a role in mood and probably in the delusions, hallucinations, and withdrawal of schizophrenia. Involved in temperature regulation and the pain-control system of the body. LSD (the hallucinogenic drug) acts at 5-HT receptor sites. Plays a role in affective and anxiety disorders. Antidepressants block its reuptake into the presynaptic cell.
Melatonin	A further synthesis of serotonin produced in the pineal gland. *Effect:* implicated in seasonal affective disorder and the sleep-wake cycle.	Induces pigment lightening effects on skin cells and regulates reproductive function in animals. Role in humans is unclear.
Acetylcholine	Synthesized from choline. Located in the brain and spinal cord but is more widespread in the peripheral nervous system, particularly the neuromuscular junction of skeletal muscle. *Effect:* Can have an excitatory or inhibitory effect.	Plays a role in the sleep-wakefulness cycle. Signals muscles to become active. Alzheimer's disease is associated with a decrease in acetylcholine-secreting neurons. Myasthenia gravis (weakness of skeletal muscles) results from a reduction in acetylcholine receptors.
Amino Acids		
Glutamate	Found in all cells of the body, where it is used to synthesize structural and functional proteins. Also found in the CNS, where it is stored in synaptic vesicles and used as a neurotransmitter. *Effect:* Excitatory.	Overexposure to glutamate can be toxic to neurons and may play a role in brain damage caused by stroke and in some degenerative diseases such as Huntington's disease. Drugs that block glutamate (which are under development) might prevent seizures and neural degeneration from overexcitation.
Gamma-aminobutyric acid (GABA)	A glutamate derivative; most neurons of the CNS have receptors. *Effect:* Major transmitter for postsynaptic inhibition on the CNS.	Drugs that increase GABA function, such as the benzodiazepines, are used to treat anxiety and to induce sleep.
PEPTIDES		

Peptides are chains of amino acids found throughout the body. About 50 have been identified to date, but their role as neurotransmitters is not well understood. Although they appear in very low concentrations in the CNS, they are very potent. They also appear to play a "second messenger" role in neurotransmission; that is, they modulate the messages of the nonpeptide neurotransmitters.

Substance	Location	Function
Endorphins and enkephalins	Widely distributed in the CNS. *Effect:* Generally inhibitory.	The opiates morphine and heroin bind to endorphin and enkephalin receptors on presynaptic neurons, blocking the release of neurotransmitters and thus reducing pain.
Substance P	Spinal cord, brain, and sensory neurons associated with pain. *Effect:* Generally excitatory.	Found in pain transmission pathway. Blocking the release of substance P by morphine reduces pain.

structure and function of the intact, living brain. These techniques not only help in diagnosing some brain disorders but also are important because they can map the regions of the brain and correlate them with function. They are pictures of the working brain. Table 5-2 describes some of the imaging techniques used in brain research, and Color Plates 7 (p. 97) and 10 (p. 99) show positron emission tomography (PET) scans of the normal brain.

Computed tomography (CT) and magnetic resonance imaging (MRI) permit visualization of *brain structures.* They can detect structural abnormalities, changes in the volume of brain tissue, and enlargement of the cerebral ventricles. The function and activity of the brain can be studied using other techniques to determine damage or malfunctioning in specific regions. The techniques that show *brain activity* include brain electrical activity mapping (BEAM), which measures sensory input, PET, and single photon emission computed tomography (SPECT), which permits the study of brain metabolism and cerebral blood flow. PET, SPECT, and the newer functional magnetic resonance imaging (FMRI) techniques can measure the use of glucose and the amount of blood flowing in a region of the brain (regional cerebral blood flow). These are the two basic indicators of brain activity. The more active a region is,

the more blood will flow through it and the more glucose it will use.

When these techniques are coupled with neuropsychological test results, deficits in a person's performance, such as language or cognitive and sensory information processing, can be linked to the activity of the region of the brain responsible for those functions. The remainder of this chapter describes new developments in the understanding of brain structure and function related to psychiatric illness that have been gained from some of these technologies.

GENETICS OF MENTAL ILLNESS

The search for the genes that cause mental illness has been difficult and inconclusive but has stimulated significant scientific, political, and clinical debate (see Critical Thinking about Contemporary Issues). The Human Genome Project, funded by the National Institute of Mental Health, is the largest research project in the history of biology. The only gene that has been linked to any mental illness causes the development of Alzheimer's disease in about 10% of the people with the disorder. Nonetheless, the search for the genes responsible for mental illness has captured the attention of the political, scientific, and lay communities.

Success in the past decade in finding the genes respon-

TABLE **5-2** *Brain Imaging Techniques*

TECHNIQUE	HOW IT WORKS	WHAT IT IMAGES	ADVANTAGES/DISADVANTAGES
Computed tomography (CT)	Series of radiographs that is computer-constructed into "slices" of the brain that can be stacked by the computer, giving a three-dimensional image	Brain structure	Provides clearer pictures of the brain than radiographs alone
Magnetic resonance imaging (MRI)	A magnetic field surrounding the head induces brain tissues to emit radio waves that are computerized for clear and detailed construction of sectional images of the brain	Brain structure; newer functional MRI (FMRI) techniques show brain activity	Avoids the use of harmful radiation, although MRI can be adapted to use radioactive materials also
Brain electrical activity mapping (BEAM)	Uses computed tomographic techniques to display data derived from electroencephalographic (EEG) recordings of brain electrical activity that can be sensory-evoked by specific stimuli, such as a flash of light or a sudden sound, or cognitive-evoked by specific mental tasks	Brain activity/function	Reflects the cumulative activity of broad areas of the brain, usually near the surface, making it difficult to locate areas of possible pathological states
Positron emission tomography (PET)	An injected radioactive substance travels to the brain and shows up as a bright spot on the scan; different substances are taken up by the brain in different amounts depending on the type of tissue and the level of activity	Brain activity/function	Allows the injection of labeled drugs for the study of neurotransmitter receptor activity or concentration in the brain
Single photon emission computed tomography (SPECT)	Similar to PET but uses more stable substances and different detectors to visualize blood flow patterns	Brain activity/function	Useful in diagnosing cerebrovascular accidents and brain tumors

sible for a variety of physical illnesses such as Huntington's disease, cystic fibrosis, breast cancer, and epilepsy has led to the use of similar techniques to search for genetic links to mental illness. However, unlike these physical illnesses, psychiatric illnesses do not appear to be simple Mendelian traits. Several problems with human genetic research have confused the process of genetic discoveries for mental illness.

First, ethical problems are associated with human breeding experiments, so scientists must infer information from animal studies. It is difficult to generalize the interpretation of genetic behavioral links from animals to humans, thus making the interpretation of cognitive and emotional elements extremely difficult. Other factors that make research on the inheritance of mental illness difficult include the following:

▼ The changeable nature of the psychiatric diagnostic classification system
▼ The fact that a gene that sometimes produces a psychiatric disorder may not always do so
▼ The fact that several different genes may be necessary to produce a disorder
▼ The presence of nongenetic factors that may contribute to the development of a disorder

Although the search for the genes of mental illness continues to hold promise, current information regarding the transmission of mental illness is based primarily on investigations into human inheritance. There are three types of studies in this area:

▼ **Adoption studies,** which compare a trait among biological versus adoptive family members or other control groups
▼ **Twin studies,** which compare how often identical twins (who are genetically identical) and fraternal twins (who have the genetic similarity of nontwin siblings) are similar, or concordant, for a trait
▼ **Family studies,** which compare whether a trait is more common among first-degree relatives (parents, siblings, and offspring) than it is among more distant relatives or control groups

The limitation of all of these studies is that they cannot identify a defect of a specific gene.

At this time the clinical implications of genetic information regarding mental illness are not well defined, so only limited information can be provided to patients and their families. The nurse is often in the position to answer questions about the genetics of mental illness, and this information must be conveyed with the highest respect for the patient's and family's autonomy. The nurse can objectively share the results of studies to date while reminding people that this information is preliminary. Referral to a genetic counselor should also be considered when the questions are persistent and complex.

CRITICAL THINKING *about* Contemporary Issues

Are the Mentally Ill Particularly Vulnerable to Attempts at Genetic Engineering?

In Nazi Germany and in the United States during the early twentieth century, people with mental disorders were among the first targets of society's attempt to minimize the transmission of disease-causing genes by reducing or preventing reproduction by people who might be carrying them. People with psychiatric illness were subject to immigration restrictions, involuntary sterilization, and extermination. More sophisticated technology and increased knowledge of genetics have led to speculation about the susceptibility of the mentally ill to future attempts to control their reproductive choices. For example, state sterilization laws still stand, as does the 1927 Supreme Court ruling that such sterilization is constitutional.

Most people believe that eugenics, the science of selective breeding, is not a major concern at this time.[5] Furthermore, current understanding of the cause of psychiatric disorders suggests that they do not have a simple genetic base and that nongenetic factors play an important role. This country's emphasis on human rights also makes eugenics unlikely. However, it is not difficult to see how indirect pressure not to have children may be placed on people who seem to have a greater risk for mental illness and how society may label them as irresponsible or immoral for transmitting illnesses to their children. Given the direct and indirect costs of mental illness to society and the stigma surrounding these disorders, future scientific advances may revive this issue.

? *Do you think there is a gene responsible for alcohol dependency, aggressive behavior, or sexual preference? How would your belief affect the nursing care you give patients?*

CIRCADIAN RHYTHMS

The recognition that human activities and behaviors such as sleeping, eating, body temperature, menses, and mood are cyclical and tend to be correlated with certain external environmental stimuli is not new. Recently, biological research has hypothesized that these body rhythms are governed by internal circadian pacemakers located in specific areas of the brain and that they are subject to change by specific external cues.

Circadian rhythm is like a network of internal clocks that coordinate events in the body according to a 24-hour cycle (Fig. 5-2). This cycle corresponds to the time it takes the earth to spin on its axis, exposing all of life to daily rhythms of light, darkness, and temperature. In turn, these rhythms affect every aspect of health and well-being including lifestyle, sleep, moods, eating, drinking, fertility, and illness.

Because the body's fluids and tissues function according to circadian rhythms, physical and mental abilities and moods may vary widely from one time of day to another. To

Fig. 5-2 The day within: a sample of the body's daily rhythms.

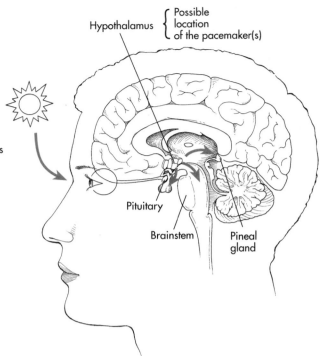

Fig. 5-3 From the sun to the brain.

run according to the 24-hour clock, the circadian system must have a time cue from the external environment. That cue is usually sunlight, which sets the clock and synchronizes the body's complex set of rhythms.

Light enters the retina of the eye, which acts like an antenna of the brain. From the retina, electrical impulses in nerve cells transmit signals of light and dark through special pathways to the hypothalamus and other regions of the brain (Fig. 5-3). Research suggests that one of the most important internal timekeepers is located in the hypothalamus. It consists of two clusters of nerve cells called the suprachiasmatic nuclei (SCN). A direct track leads from the retina to these two clusters of cells, which in turn respond to the light signals from the retina.

The SCN is the pacemaker of circadian rhythm; it sends electrical and chemical messages to other tissues including the hypothalamus, pituitary, pineal gland, and parts of the brainstem. These tissues send hormonal messages to other control systems in the body such as the heart, adrenal glands, liver, kidney, and intestines, keeping them regulated to the internal clock and modulating thoughts, moods, and activities.

Sleep

According to surveys, most people sleep 6 to 9 hours a night, with 8 to 9 hours reported most often. Few people sleep less than 5 or more than 10 hours. Usually people sleep in one nightly phase, although in some cultures and during some times of life a siesta, or afternoon nap, is common. Studies show that the sleep cycle is related to the timing of circadian rhythms, light and darkness, and temperature changes.

Generally, each night a person's sleep passes through a repeated sequence of five stages. The first stage is that of "falling asleep," which is called stage one sleep. A person then progresses into sleep itself (stage two), followed by deep sleep, also called *delta sleep* (stages three and four). Af-

ter a brief return to stage two sleep the person moves into stage five, or rapid eye movement (REM) sleep. Stages two through REM repeat themselves several times a night, with deep sleep becoming briefer in the course of a night and REM sleep becoming progressively longer (see Fig. 19-3).

REM sleep occupies approximately 20% to 25% of the sleep time of adults, stage two about 50%, and stages three and four about 15%. Stages three and four occur primarily in the first half of the sleep period. The lighter stages of sleep and longer REM periods typically occur in the second half. Usually during REM sleep the individual has vivid dreams, and the eyes show bursts of rapid movement beneath the closed lids. Studies show that REM sleep is excessive in depressed people and that dreams may be unusually intense.

PSYCHOIMMUNOLOGY

Evidence from a wide variety of sources suggests that psychosocial factors can have a profound effect on a person's immune system. In particular, psychosocial stressors and the mental state associated with them may depress immune function to the point of enhancing vulnerability to virtually any antigen to which the person is exposed. It is also clear that the central nervous system is involved in mediating any such effects.

Psychoimmunology is a fairly new field that explores the psychological influences on the nervous system's control of immune responsiveness (see Chapter 17). Several diseases commonly encountered by neurologists are thought to have an autoimmune basis. Research has demonstrated the suppression of white blood cell reproduction following sleep deprivation, marathon running, space flight, death of a spouse, and during the course of depression. Another example is that of natural killer cells, which are believed to play a role in tumor surveillance and the control of viral infections.

Identifying a possible role for autoimmunity in the major psychiatric diseases has proved to be more problematic. Narcolepsy, a disease of the central nervous system characterized by excessive daytime drowsiness, appears to be closely linked to the immune system and may offer insights into mechanisms that could apply to some psychiatric disorders.

However, compelling evidence indicates that psychosocial stressors temporarily impair the immune response and thus contribute to the development of a variety of illnesses. Although efforts to relate specific stressors to specific diseases have not generally been successful, stress is recognized as a key to understanding the development and course of many illnesses. Presuming that all people have at least one vulnerable organ in their bodies, a high level of stress may eventually put a person at risk for the breakdown of that organ and the development of clinical symptoms.

BIOLOGICAL ASSESSMENT OF THE PATIENT

Several steps are necessary in the assessment of psychiatric patients from a biological perspective. Brain disorders can be physical or psychiatric and can include many different diagnoses such as stroke, head and spinal cord injury, tumors, multiple sclerosis, alcoholism, and drug addiction. Schizophrenia, depression, anxiety disorders, and Alzheimer's disease are also considered brain disorders, although they are psychiatric in nature. As new understanding has been gained about mind-body connections, it has become clear that symptoms can be assigned more precisely to problems in specific organ systems, including the brain. Thus the ability to screen for undiagnosed physical disorders and distinguish them from psychiatric disorders has important implications for the psychiatric nurse in the assessment of the presenting symptoms, treatment selection, and possible need for referral.

Undiagnosed physical illness, particularly organic brain disorders, can be costly and dangerous if treated incorrectly. For example, it has been estimated that 7% of patients seeking psychiatric help have a physical illness that directly causes psychiatric symptoms and that another 30% have a physical illness that limits functioning and contributes to psychiatric symptomatology.[9] In addition, patients who are psychiatrically ill often have limited access to health-care services because of barriers of availability and associated stigmatization.

These facts make a compelling case for psychiatric nurses to include a thorough biological assessment in their evaluation of psychiatric patients. The psychiatric nurse is well suited to screen for the major signs of physical or organic disorders that may complicate a patient's psychiatric status, to identify physical illnesses that may have been overlooked, or to refer the patient for a thorough medical diagnostic work-up if indicated. In fact, this is one of the unique areas of expertise that the psychiatric nurse brings to the mental health treatment team, and it is essential that psychiatric nurses continue to demonstrate their competence in all aspects of their biopsychosocial assessment.

A complete health-care history of the patient, lifestyle review, physical examination, analysis of laboratory values, and discussion of presenting symptoms and coping responses are essential elements of a baseline biological assessment (Box 5-2). The nurse should be able to perform a basic physical examination to assess for gross abnormalities and be able to interpret the results of more complex physical examinations. Appearance, gait, coordination, bilateral strength, tremors and tics, speech, and symptoms such as headaches, blurred vision, dizziness, vomiting, motor weakness, disorientation, confusion, and memory problems should be assessed in detail.

Obtaining permission from the patient to access other people and documents that will help the nurse and health-care team gain a thorough view of the patient is an important step in the screening process. Particularly when brain disorders, whether physical or psychiatric, are suspected, the nurse should pay close attention to inconsistencies in the patient's account, between those of other people, and in previous health care records. Throughout the course of the screening the nurse should be alert for any indications of head trauma at any time in the patient's life, such as through accidents, fevers, surgery, or seizures.

Only after a patient has been carefully screened can the nurse determine which of the patient's problems are primarily psychiatric and amenable to psychiatric intervention and which may need the attention of a consultant in another specialty. The identified problems that are appropriate for psychiatric intervention then become the target symptoms of specific interventions, and progress toward expected outcomes can be measured throughout the course of treatment.

> **?** *Why is a history of psychiatric medications taken by a patient's first-degree relatives an important part of the psychiatric nurse's biological assessment?*

BIOLOGICAL COMPONENTS OF MENTAL ILLNESS

Our understanding of the biology of mental illness is rapidly expanding. However, the amount of biological information about each psychiatric disorder varies considerably. In addition, what is known about the biology of the various mental illnesses is often incomplete, contradictory, and in-

Box **5-2** *Biological Assessment of the Psychiatric Patient*

HEALTH CARE HISTORY
General Health Care

Regular and specialty health care provider
Frequency of health care visits
Last medical examination and test results
Any unusual circumstances of birth, including mother's preterm
  habits and condition

Hospitalizations and Surgeries

When, why indicated, treatments, outcome

Brain Impairment

Diagnosed brain problem
Head trauma
Details of accidents or periods of unconsciousness for any reason: blows to the head, electrical shocks, high fevers, seizures,
  fainting, dizziness, headaches, falls

Cancer

Full history, particularly consider metastases (lung, breast, mela-
  noma, gastrointestinal tract, and kidney are most likely to
  metastasize)
Results of treatments (chemotherapy and surgeries)

Lung Problems

Details of any condition or event that restricts the flow of air to
  the lungs for more than 2 minutes or adversely affects oxygen
  absorption (the brain uses 20% of the oxygen in the body) such
  as with chronic obstructive pulmonary disease, near drowning,
  near strangulation, high-altitude oxygen deprivation, resuscita-
  tion events

Cardiac Problems

Childhood illnesses such as scarlet or rheumatic fever
History of heart attacks, strokes, or hypertension

Blood Diseases

Anemia resulting in hypoxia
Arteriosclerotic conditions
HIV

Diabetes

Stability of glucose levels

Endocrine Disturbances

Thyroid and adrenal function particularly

Reproductive History
Menstrual History

LIFESTYLE
Eating

Details of unusual or unsupervised diets, appetite, weight
  changes, cravings, and caffeine intake

Medications

Full history of current and past psychiatric medications in self
  and first-degree relatives

Substance Use

Alcohol, drug, and tobacco use

Toxins

Overcome by automobile exhaust or natural gas
Exposure to lead, mercury, insecticides, herbicides, solvents,
  cleaning agents, lawn chemicals

Occupation (current and past)

Chemicals in the workplace (farming, painting)
Work-related accidents (construction, mining)
Military experiences
Stressful job circumstances

Injury

Safe sex practices
Contact sports and sports-related injuries
Exposure to violence or abuse

Impact of culture, race, ethnicity, and gender

PHYSICAL EXAMINATION
Current Health Statistics

Immunizations
Allergies
Last physical examination and Pap smear

Review of Physiological Systems

Integumentary: skin, nails, hair, and scalp
Head: eyes, ears, nose, mouth, throat, and neck
Breast
Respiratory
Cardiovascular
Hematolymphatic
Gastrointestinal tract
Urinary tract
Genital
Neurological
Musculoskeletal
Nutritive
Restorative: sleep and rest
Endocrine
Allergic and immunological

LABORATORY VALUES

Blood, plasma, and serum
Urine
Steroid hormones
Polypeptide hormones
Thyroid hormones
Hematology
Cerebrospinal fluid

PRESENTING SYMPTOMS AND COPING RESPONSES

Description: nature, frequency, and intensity
Threats to safety of self or others
Functional status
Quality of life

conclusive. It is much like finding pieces of a jigsaw puzzle
scattered throughout the house; each piece by itself suggests a glimpse of the overall design, but the full picture
does not emerge until all the pieces are located and then put
together.

In this section of the chapter four major psychiatric disorders are discussed in the context of neurobiological research. These illnesses were selected because of the amount
of biological information available about them. Given the
incomplete state of the science, the discussion walks the

COLOR ATLAS OF PSYCHOBIOLOGY

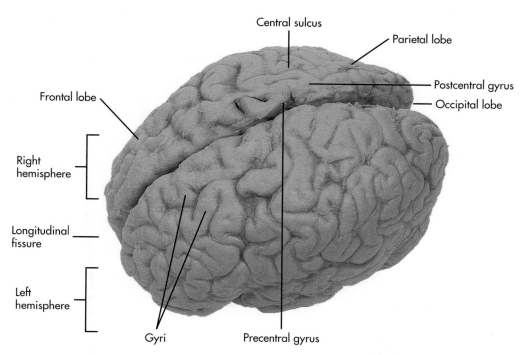

Color Plate 1   **Superior view of the brain.** (From Nolte J, Angevine JB, Jr: *The human brain: in photographs and diagrams,* St Louis, Mosby, 1995.)

Color Plate 2   **Lateral view of the left cerebral hemisphere of the brain.** (From Nolte J, Angevine JB, Jr: *The human brain: in photographs and diagrams,* St Louis, Mosby, 1995.)

A

Cerebrum

Corpus callosum

Diencephalon — Thalamus

Hypothalamus

Brainstem — Midbrain

Pons

Medulla

Cerebellum

B

Color Plate 3 When the brain is cut between the two hemispheres down the middle (a midsagittal section), the main division can be clearly seen in **(A)** an autopsy specimen, **(B)** a magnetic resonance imaging scan, and **(C)** a schematic representation. (**A,** From Nolte J, Angevine JB, Jr: *The human brain: in photographs and diagrams,* St Louis, Mosby, 1995; **B,** from Medical University of South Carolina, Charleston, South Carolina.) *Continued*

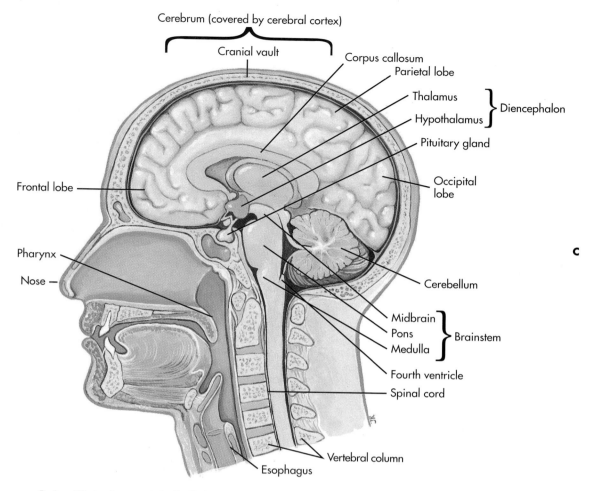

Cerebrum (covered by cerebral cortex)

Cranial vault

Corpus callosum

Parietal lobe

Thalamus ⎫
Hypothalamus ⎬ Diencephalon

Pituitary gland

Occipital lobe

Frontal lobe

Pharynx

Nose

Cerebellum

Midbrain ⎫
Pons ⎬ Brainstem
Medulla ⎭

Fourth ventricle

Spinal cord

Vertebral column

Esophagus

C

Color Plate 3, cont'd   C, Schematic representation of midsagittal section of the brain.

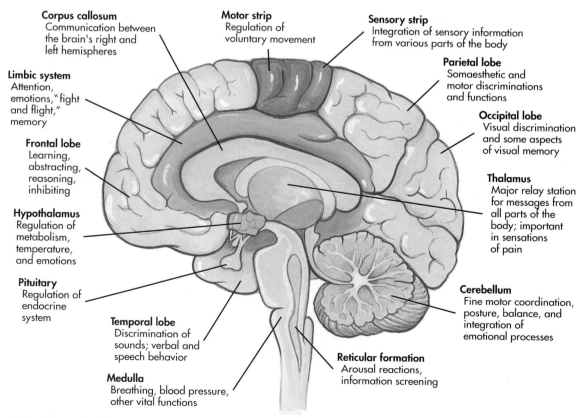

Corpus callosum
Communication between the brain's right and left hemispheres

Motor strip
Regulation of voluntary movement

Sensory strip
Integration of sensory information from various parts of the body

Parietal lobe
Somaesthetic and motor discriminations and functions

Limbic system
Attention, emotions, "fight and flight," memory

Occipital lobe
Visual discrimination and some aspects of visual memory

Frontal lobe
Learning, abstracting, reasoning, inhibiting

Thalamus
Major relay station for messages from all parts of the body; important in sensations of pain

Hypothalamus
Regulation of metabolism, temperature, and emotions

Pituitary
Regulation of endocrine system

Temporal lobe
Discrimination of sounds; verbal and speech behavior

Cerebellum
Fine motor coordination, posture, balance, and integration of emotional processes

Reticular formation
Arousal reactions, information screening

Medulla
Breathing, blood pressure, other vital functions

Color Plate 4   Structure and function of the brain. (From Carson RC, Butcher JN: *Abnormal psychology and modern life,* ed 9, New York, 1992, Harper Collins.)

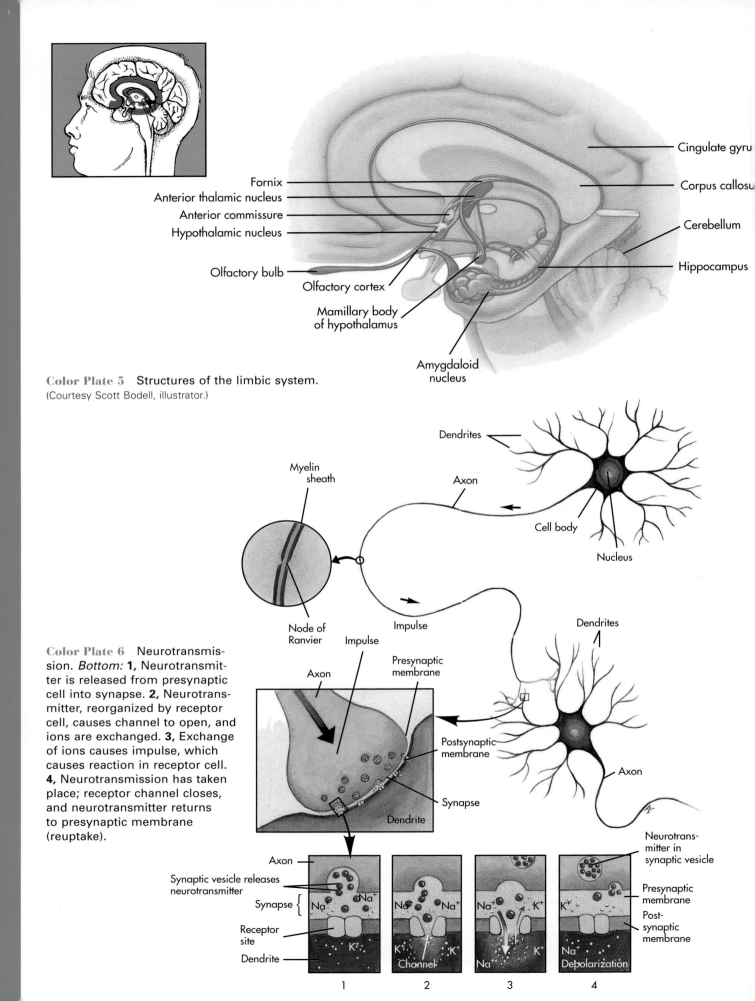

Color Plate 5 Structures of the limbic system.
(Courtesy Scott Bodell, illustrator.)

Cingulate gyru

Corpus callosu

Cerebellum

Hippocampus

Fornix
Anterior thalamic nucleus
Anterior commissure
Hypothalamic nucleus

Olfactory bulb

Olfactory cortex

Mamillary body
of hypothalamus

Amygdaloid
nucleus

Dendrites

Myelin
sheath

Axon

Cell body

Nucleus

Node of
Ranvier

Impulse

Impulse

Dendrites

Axon

Color Plate 6 Neurotransmission. *Bottom:* **1,** Neurotransmitter is released from presynaptic cell into synapse. **2,** Neurotransmitter, reorganized by receptor cell, causes channel to open, and ions are exchanged. **3,** Exchange of ions causes impulse, which causes reaction in receptor cell. **4,** Neurotransmission has taken place; receptor channel closes, and neurotransmitter returns to presynaptic membrane (reuptake).

Axon

Presynaptic
membrane

Postsynaptic
membrane

Synapse

Dendrite

Neurotransmitter in
synaptic vesicle

Axon

Synaptic vesicle releases
neurotransmitter

Synapse

Receptor
site

Dendrite

Presynaptic
membrane

Postsynaptic
membrane

Na   Na⁺

K⁺

Na   Na⁺

K⁺   K⁺

Channel

Na⁺   K⁺

Na⁺   K⁺

K⁺

Na⁺
Depolarization

1   2   3   4

Color Plate 7 Positron emission tomography scan shows varying patterns of glucose consumption during different tasks. The color scale ranges from 2 *(violet)* to 45 *(red)*. **A,** Different kinds of tasks cause increased glucose consumption in distinct areas of the brain. A checkerboard visual stimulus activates the occipital lobes. An auditory stimulus causes increased glucose consumption in the temporal lobes. When an individual is engaged in an active, cognitive task rather than passive perception of stimuli, glucose consumption increases in the frontal lobes. Subjects trying to remember information from a verbal stimulus (a story) show increased glucose consumption in the temporal lobes. Sequential movements of the fingers of the right hand activate motor cortex on the left and the supplementary motor arc *(vertical arrow).* **B,** Increasing complexity of a particular kind of task causes increased glucose consumption in progressively larger areas of the cortex. With the subject blindfolded ("eyes closed"), there is relatively little glucose consumption in the occipital lobes. With the eyes open, looking at a plain white light source activates the primary visual cortex of the occipital lobes. Looking at an outdoor scene ("complex scene") activates the visual association cortex in additional areas of the occipital lobes. **C,** The left hemisphere usually plays a dominant role in language functions, the right hemisphere in musical and certain other functions. When a subject listens simultaneously to a Sherlock Holmes story and a Brandenberg Concerto, both superior temporal lobes and both frontal lobes are activated. Listening to just the story activates predominately the left hemisphere. Musical chords alone activate predominantly the right hemisphere. (**A** and **B,** From Phelps ME, Mazziotta JC: *Science* 228:779, 1985. **C,** Courtesy of Dr. ME Phelps and Dr. JC Mazziotta, University of California School of Medicine.)

Color Plate 8   Computed tomography scans showing enlargement of the lateral cerebral ventricles in a patient with chronic schizophrenia *(right),* as compared with a normal control *(left).*
(From Roberts GS, Leigh PN, Weinberger DR: *Neuropsychiatric disorders,* London, 1993, Mosby-Wolfe.)

Color Plate 9   Magnetic resonance imaging scans through the bodies of the lateral ventricles in a pair of monozygotic twins who are discordant for schizophrenia. Note the increase in the cerebrospinal fluid spaces in the twin with schizophrenia *(right)* as compared with the unaffected twin *(left).* (From Roberts GS, Leigh PN, Weinberger DR: *Neuropsychiatric disorders,* London, 1993, Mosby-Wolfe.)

Color Plate 10 Blood flow demonstrated by a positron emission tomography scan during the performance of the Wisconsin Card Sort Task (a task that activates prefrontal cortex in normal subjects) in a twin with schizophrenia *(right column)* and an unaffected twin *(left column).* The arrows indicate the relatively focused failure of activation in the affected twin compared with the unaffected twin. (From Roberts GS, Leigh PN, Weinberger DR: *Neuropsychiatric disorders,* London, 1993, Mosby-Wolfe.)

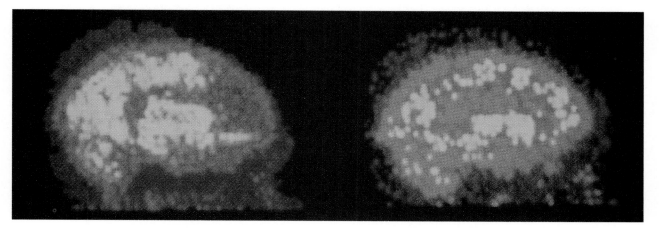

Color Plate 11 Positron emission tomography scans of glucose use in a depressed subject showing frontal hypometabolism *(left),* which improves after treatment with antidepressant medication *(right).* (Courtesy Lewis Baxter, MD, UCLA School of Medicine, Los Angeles.)

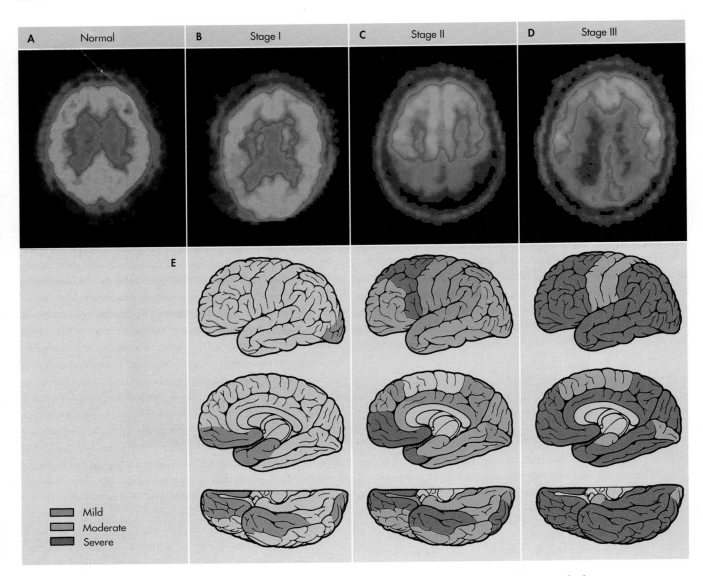

A Normal	B Stage I	C Stage II	D Stage III

E

Mild
Moderate
Severe

Color Plate 12 Pathological spread of Alzheimer's disease as shown by positron emission tomography scans. **A,** Normal brain. **B,** Brain in stage I Alzheimer's disease. **C,** Brain in stage II Alzheimer's disease. **D,** Brain in stage III Alzheimer's disease. **E,** Diagrams show the spread of pathology in Alzheimer's disease. (From Roberts GS, Leigh PN, Weinberger DR: *Neuropsychiatric disorders*, London, 1993, Mosby-Wolfe.)

reader through current areas of biological study related to these disorders and highlights their implications for clinical psychiatric nursing practice. The technologies described are also used in research of many other mental illnesses.

This discussion is intended to expose the reader to emerging knowledge and provide a model that would allow the psychiatric nurse to keep abreast with the biological context of psychiatric nursing care. The psychiatric nurse should become familiar with these research findings and discuss these issues with patients, families, and colleagues. In addition, an overview of biological knowledge related to psychiatric disorders can be found in Chapters 16 to 26.

Schizophrenia

Neuroscientific research continues to make advances in the study of schizophrenia, although the complexity of this disorder and the range of symptoms have made progress slow and research directions unclear. The cause of schizophrenia is unknown, but it is widely believed that at least one biological cause exists. It also appears that schizophrenia is not one but several distinct disorders (see Chapter 21).

GENETICS. There is a 1% lifetime risk of schizophrenia in the general population, except in people with a first-or second-degree relative with the disorder (Table 5-3). The pattern of inherited vulnerability in schizophrenia probably results from the interaction of unknown influences with several genes, which affects the structure and function of the brain. A new hypothesis called trinucleotide repeat amplification—a mutation in which a certain stretch of DNA occurs more than once when genes are copied—could explain some of the differential rates of occurrence of schizophrenia, even among monozygotic twins, who have identical genes but only a 50% concordance rate for the disease. If one child in a family carrying a gene for schizophrenia happens to have more trinucleotide repeats than the others, that child could be pushed over the threshold into mental illness.

BIOCHEMISTRY. Several brain chemicals have been implicated in schizophrenia, but research to date points most strongly to the following:

▼ An excess of the neurotransmitter dopamine
▼ An imbalance between dopamine and other neurotransmitters, particularly serotonin
▼ Problems in the dopamine receptor systems
Several research strategies support the role of dopamine

TABLE **5-3** *Genetic Risk of Schizophrenia*

PERSON AT RISK	PERCENTAGE OF RISK
Monozygotic twin affected	50%
Dizygotic twin affected	15%
Sibling affected	10%
One parent affected	15%
Both parents affected	35%
Second-degree relative affected	2% to 3%
No affected relative	1%

in schizophrenia.[10] For instance, drugs that increase levels of dopamine in the brain can produce psychosis.[3] Drugs that reduce dopamine function have antipsychotic effects as well. This is seen in the antipsychotic drugs that reduce the number of postsynaptic receptors that interact with dopamine.

Some studies have shown an increase in dopamine metabolites and norepinephrine metabolites in the plasma of untreated patients with schizophrenia as compared with normal controls. This implies increased levels of these transmitters in the brain. When patients are treated with haloperidol, a conventional antipsychotic drug, the levels of these transmitters decrease.[11] When patients are treated with atypical antipsychotic drugs, changes in the balance between the dopamine and serotonin systems occur.[12] These strategies suggest that there is an increase of available dopamine and an imbalance between dopamine and other transmitters, particularly serotonin, in people with schizophrenia.

BRAIN IMAGING. Various imaging techniques used in the study of schizophrenia focus on two specific areas of the brain:

▼ The frontal cortex, which appears to be involved in the negative symptoms
▼ The limbic system, which appears to be involved in the positive symptoms of schizophrenia

Although a consistent group of abnormalities seems evident in the brains of schizophrenics, exactly how these and other brain regions interact in the course of schizophrenia still is not understood. Imaging studies may continue to clarify this process and link abnormal brain structure and function with etiology, symptoms, and treatment of schizophrenia (see Color Plates 8 to 10 on pp. 98 and 99).

CT scans have demonstrated enlargement of the ventricles, particularly the lateral ventricle, of patients with chronic schizophrenia. This implies either a lack of brain development or a loss of brain tissue. MRI studies have replicated this finding and have also documented that several brain structures are smaller, such as the hippocampal region (which modulates emotional response and memory) in the limbic system in the temporal lobe of the cerebrum. Although a clear correlation of these findings and clinical symptoms has yet to emerge, there is a trend for large ventricles to be associated with two indicators of poor prognosis: early age of onset and poor premorbid functioning.

For the first time, PET studies have shown functional abnormalities in the brain by documenting activity in various regions of the brain of people who are given psychological tests. For example, the Wisconsin Card Sort Test (a test of working memory and abstract thinking) has been found to activate the cerebral blood flow in the prefrontal cortex in the brains of normal controls and in the nonaffected identical twins of schizophrenics.[17] However, this same region of the brain shows lower metabolism and reduced blood flow (hypofrontality) in schizophrenics, who do worse on this test than normal controls regardless of the length of time they have been ill or whether they have been treated with antipsychotic drugs.

VIRAL PANDEMICS AND SEASON OF BIRTH. Although research in psychoimmunology related to schizophrenia has been difficult to conduct and interpret, some interesting data may be emerging. There is a high rate of births of schizophrenics (approximately 5%) in Europe and the United States in the late winter and early spring, and peaks can be correlated with pandemic viral outbreaks, particularly influenza, that occur during the third to sixth months of gestation.[25] Although this information is inconclusive and is thought to account for a very small percentage of cases, it is helpful in expanding information about the influences of biological and environmental factors on brain development and function.

BIRTH EVENTS. Many attempts have been made to study the influences of maternal nutrition, infection, placental insufficiency, anoxia, hemorrhage, and trauma before or at birth as possible causes of schizophrenia. Much of this research is limited by its retrospective nature because retrieving information about a complex event decades after its occurrence is very difficult. The best studies to date seem to indicate that it is unlikely that these events lead to any significant etiological basis of schizophrenia.

Clinical Implications: Biology of Schizophrenia

Advances in molecular and cellular neurobiology have enabled science to capitalize on a variety of what were originally chance findings. In the early 1950s chlorpromazine was observed to have an antipsychotic effect. Today's technologies show that this effect is caused by dopamine receptor blockade throughout the brain, accounting for the antipsychotic and side effect profiles of the typical antipsychotic drugs. These new technologies have also produced atypical antipsychotic drugs such as clozapine, risperidone, and olanzapine, which specifically block the dopamine receptor implicated in schizophrenia (D2). They also act on other neurotransmitter systems. For these reasons, these drugs avoid some of the usual antipsychotic side effects (see Chapter 27). This research direction continues to bring antipsychotic drugs to market that are more specific in their actions, thus enhancing efficacy while eliminating troublesome and sometimes dangerous side effects.

In the future, brain imaging technologies may direct the clinician to the most appropriate interventions (see Chapter 21), based on the area of the brain specifically involved in each patient's symptomatology. This approach could provide targeted treatment that eliminates the additional costs and adverse effects of strategies that may not be the first line of choice for a patient's particular symptom cluster.

> ? *What would you say to a man and woman who were debating about whether to have children because they both had relatives with schizophrenia?*

Mood Disorders

Biological understanding of mood disorders has advanced in the past several decades. Neuroscientific research has identified biological markers for mood disorders, and psychopharmacological interventions have yielded more specificity and fewer side effects and toxicities than the first-generation antidepressants of 40 years ago.

GENETICS. As in schizophrenia, mood disorders run in families and tend to be inherited. The lifetime risk for mood disorders in the general population is 6%. Family, twin, and adoption studies have documented that the lifetime risk for relatives of people with depression is 20% and 24% for relatives of people with mania. A person with an identical twin with an affective disorder is at highest risk. No clear pattern of genetic mapping for these disorders has been found to date, but preliminary work points to a complex picture of genetic markers. Thus it is unlikely that a single gene causes mood disorders.

BIOCHEMISTRY. Initially it was discovered that drugs such as the tricyclics and monoamine oxidase inhibitors had antidepressant effects, stimulated a manic episode in individuals at risk, and prolonged the activity of norepinephrine (NE). NE is a member of the catecholamine family within the monoamine class of neurotransmitters. These findings led to the catecholamine hypothesis: depression was caused by a shortage of NE, whereas mania was caused by an excess of NE. Current theories of abnormal chemistry in unipolar and bipolar illness have moved beyond the original catecholamine hypothesis to more complex explanations of the biochemistry of mood disorders.

Several findings support the hypothesis that a variety of neurotransmitters are involved in mood disorders. For example, some studies have found that concentrations of serotonin are low in mood disorders, and low concentrations of serotonin have been found in people who commit suicide. In addition, the new class of antidepressants, the selective serotonin reuptake inhibitors (SSRIs), act almost exclusively on the serotonin system, supporting a role for serotonin in mood disorders. Acetylcholine has also been implicated in mood disorders. On the basis of drug effects, some investigators have proposed that too little acetylcholine can cause depression, and too much NE can cause mania, suggesting an imbalance between these two systems as the biological etiology of the mood disorders. Finally, gamma-aminobutyric acid (GABA), an inhibitory neurotransmitter, has a broad range of effects, and it has been proposed that it modulates the other neurotransmitter systems. This is supported by the paradoxical finding that increased GABA activity can have both an antidepressant and an antimanic effect. Thus GABA may play an important role in mood disorders as well.

Another popular biological hypothesis for the development of mood disorders is the dysregulation hypothesis. This theory proposes a more generalized dysfunction in the overall mechanisms that regulate the activities of neurotransmission at the synapse and suggests that clinically effective drugs restore more efficient regulation. Based on available data it has been proposed that decreased activity within the NE-serotonin component of the system is associated with depression, and increased activity of the NE-dopamine component tends to cause mania.[8]

The evolution of biological hypotheses of mood disorders continues to stimulate much research, heated debate, and conflicting theories. This confusion is particularly interesting, given that the pharmacological and somatic treatments of mood disorders have been some of the most effective in the mental health field to date.

> **?** *If depression is partly caused by disturbed biochemistry, does that mean that counseling and psychotherapy are inappropriate treatment strategies?*

BRAIN IMAGING. Imaging research into mood disorders has been largely inconclusive because various studies report contradictory results. This is primarily a result of a lack of standardization of research methodologies between investigators and difficulty in studying fluctuating illnesses. Generally, CT and MRI studies found larger ventricles in patients with affective disorders than in controls, particularly in the temporal horn in the right cerebral hemisphere, and reductions in cortical mass. However, the clinical significance of this finding remains obscure other than for screening for the presence of specific physical illnesses, such as tumors, that manifest as psychiatric illness.[20] One advantage to the use of MRI in affective disorders, however, is that MRI, unlike other scanning techniques, is without radiation risks, so multiple repeat scans of the same patient can be performed. This is of particular importance as MRIs are repeated when the patient shifts mood, starts or stops treatment, or relapses.

PET studies have demonstrated that depressed and manic patients show different metabolism rates and different patterns of cerebral activity from normal controls. In depressed patients, investigators found hypometabolism in the prefrontal cortex of the frontal lobes in scans of glucose use that improved after treatment with antidepressant medication[6] (see Color Plate 11 on p. 99). People with bipolar disorder show a more general decrease in activity involving the whole cortex and the left frontal lobes, although the clinical significance of this finding is also unclear.

In general, studies suggest an association between mood disorders and abnormalities of large regions of the brain, especially the frontal and temporal lobes. An abnormal difference between the left (language and logical thinking) and right (spatial processing) hemispheres is also implied. Although these functions are different, they also overlap and exhibit different levels of activity that appear to be altered in mood disorders. Also, imaging studies have not been well correlated to date with neuropsychiatric testing, and results of the two techniques conflict, suggesting that diverse abnormalities are detected by different methods. Future methods promise to increase the use of imaging techniques as clinical and research tools for understanding affective disorders.

SEASONALITY AND CIRCADIAN RHYTHMS. A variety of studies have linked seasonal variations, such as decreases in the length of daylight hours and wintertime decreases in available sunlight, to such human conditions as mood, sleeping, eating, and energy levels. Seasonal affective disorder (SAD) in particular has been shown to respond to geographical location closer to the equator or to phototherapy (light therapy), although rigorous placebo-controlled research documenting long-term efficacy has not been conducted (see Chapter 28).

The cause of SAD is not fully understood. It is proposed, however, that the neurotransmitter melatonin (a further synthesis of serotonin secreted by the pineal gland), which is secreted with darkness and suppressed with bright light, is implicated in SAD. It is believed that melatonin regulates hypothalamic hormones involved in the generation of circadian rhythms and the synchronization of such rhythms to variations in environmental light in animals.[2] However, it is not clear what role melatonin plays in humans or the effects of changes in melatonin levels on circadian rhythms.

What does appear to be clear is that the sleep cycle is linked to the timing of human circadian rhythms and to malfunctions in the brain's ability to follow environmental cues such as light and darkness, unusual environmental situations such as long, dark winters in northern latitudes, or disturbances in the intensity of the circadian rhythm such as those caused by sleep problems, body temperature changes, mood cycling, and cortisol and thyrotropin abnormalities. The psychiatric nurse should be on the forefront of this research because many patients with psychiatric symptoms suffer from disturbances of biological rhythms.[14]

BIOLOGICAL MARKERS. Perhaps more than in any other psychiatric diagnostic category, investigators have identified biological markers useful in the diagnosis and treatment of mood disorders. Research has identified certain biological markers in depression that are mediated by the hypothalamic-pituitary-adrenal (HPA) axis.[20] For example, in depressed patients sleep electroencephalographs (EEGs) are abnormal, with shortened REM latency experienced by 90% of depressed patients. Normally upon falling asleep the fifth stage of sleep—REM or dream sleep—occurs in 60 to 90 minutes. In depressed patients it occurs in 5 to 30 minutes, thus indicating that there is sleep dysregulation in depression. As a consequence, depressed patients spend less time in the more refreshing slow wave stages of sleep, particularly stages three and four, and more time in REM sleep. This finding may explain why depressed patients complain of feeling tired and unrefreshed after a night's sleep.

Another biological marker is that plasma concentrations of the adrenal hormone cortisol are abnormally high in some depressed patients, and 60% of patients have abnormal results with the dexamethasone suppression test (DST).

In normal controls cortisol levels are flat from late afternoon until 3 or 4 am, when they begin to increase and spike at regular intervals until about noon; then they gradually begin to level out again. In contrast, biologically depressed people have been shown to have erratic cortisol spikes over a 24-hour period.

The DST involves giving a small dose (1 mg) of the synthetic steroid dexamethasone. In normal people this is enough to turn down the pituitary production of adrenocorticotropic hormone (ACTH), thus blunting the adrenal production of cortisol for 24 hours. When plasma cortisol levels are drawn at intervals the next day (usually at 8 am and 4 pm) in depressed people, they escape the cortisol suppression and cortisol levels are high again, an indication of a dysregulation of the HPA axis in depression (Fig. 5-4). The clinical implications of this marker for depression must be assessed cautiously because this technology is not always accurate, but an abnormal DST appears to be a marker for biological depression. As such, positive DST results would support the use of antidepressant medications as a treatment strategy, although negative findings do not necessarily support withholding medication, especially in severe to moderate depression. Finally, a DST retest for a patient at a later time that indicates normal results might be a useful indicator that the biological depression has been corrected.

Finally, two other promising biological markers also deserve mention. The thyroid-stimulating hormone (TSH) response to a thyroid-releasing hormone (TRH) stimulation test is blunted in about 40% of patients with depression, and the growth hormone response to drugs that enhance the norepinephrine system, such as clonidine, is significantly blunted in depressed patients. These and other biological markers continue to stimulate interest from a research perspective and promise to gain in their usefulness in clinical settings as the techniques are improved and their treatment implications are more fully understood.

> ? *What are the implications of being able to identify biological markers for the diagnosis and treatment of depression?*

KINDLING. Animal studies of electrical or chemical kindling and behavioral sensitization have provided clues to the recurrence of mood disorders with increased frequency and intensity over time in some individuals. When an animal's brain is repeatedly stimulated by low-level electrical impulses or low-dose chemicals such as cocaine, the result is an increased responsiveness to stable low doses of the stimulation over time, resulting eventually in seizures. Ultimately the animal becomes so sensitive that seizures occur spontaneously in the absence of the stimulation. This phenomenon is known as kindling. It is theorized that kindling

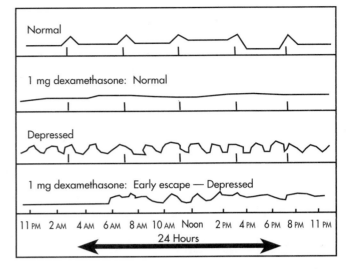

Fig. 5-4 Dexamethasone suppression test and cortisol levels.

underlies the addictive disorders and the cycling and recurrent psychiatric disorders, such as recurrent depression.

According to this theory, first proposed 2 decades ago, early episodes of an illness require precipitating events, but later episodes may occur spontaneously, and repeated exposure to precipitating events may lead to more frequent occurrence of episodes. This sequence is related to the idea that early episodes of mania and depression in humans may be precipitated by psychosocial stresses in vulnerable individuals, but later episodes can occur in the absence of any apparent external stimulus. Episodes may also occur with greater frequency and intensity over time.[15]

Additional evidence of a role for kindling in mood disorders is that the neurotransmitters most implicated in the mood disorders (NE, serotonin, and GABA) inhibit kindling. Also, lithium, an effective treatment for bipolar disorder, blocks behavioral sensitization; carbamazepine, an anticonvulsant effective in the treatment of bipolar disorder, blocks kindling.[8] Thus the effect of the environment on a vulnerable brain is the focus of continued research interest.

BIRTH-COHORT EFFECTS. Rates of depression, mania, and suicide over the past several generations have increased in the United States, Canada, and several European countries. These rates continue to rise as each new birth-cohort ages, even within the general population. Within the at-risk population, the relatives of depressed and manic patients from previous decades are at even greater risk for these illnesses than were the siblings of their affected parents, showing a trend in increased genetic susceptibility in the at-risk population.

Another alarming trend noted in North America and Europe over the past 6 decades is the increase in birth-cohort suicide rates. Suicide rates among 15-to 19-year-olds were 10 times higher for those born in the 1950s than they were for those born in the 1930s. These epidemiological trends point to an unidentified interaction between genes and environment that continues to worsen over the decades.[7]

Birth-cohort studies such as these continue to generate interest in psychiatric and epidemiological arenas and can have very important public health implications. They also underscore the important point that the biological understanding of psychiatric illnesses cannot stand alone as the entire explanation of etiology. Rather, integrated biopsychosocial models and multidimensional treatment strategies are needed. Thus psychiatric nurses must continue to view the person in the context of the environment as well as biologically to understand and treat the individual holistically.

> **?** *What environmental factors might play a role along with genetics in the increased rate of suicide among adolescents in the United States?*

Clinical Implications: Biology of Depression

There are many different pieces to the puzzle of the biology of mood disorders, and an all-inclusive hypothesis has not yet emerged. It is likely, however, that mood disorders occur because integrated control systems are disrupted, as evidenced by the suggestion of an overall dysregulation in neurotransmitter systems and by the fact that the brain mechanisms that control biological rhythms are implicated in mood disorders. What is clear is that the etiologies are diverse, so the treatments must be both diverse and specific to the biopsychosocial context of the individual patient (see Chapter 19).

New information will provide clinicians with more specific drug treatments, again decreasing the cost, time, and adverse effects of treatments that may not be as effective as others for an individual patient. Markers such as the DST may also indicate when abnormal biology has normalized, thus providing more specific information about when treatment can be stopped. Phototherapy may hold promise for those with SAD, and sleep deprivation therapy may produce an antidepressant effect by manipulating a patient's sleep cycle (see Chapter 28).

Panic Disorders

The biological study of anxiety has made significant advances in the past decade, resulting in many important findings that have helped in the understanding and treatment of this universal human experience. In panic disorder, in which the human alarm system seems to be triggered independently from appropriate appraisals of environmental cues, the results of neuroscientific exploration have been impressive. They are also a significant departure from earlier theories that have primarily emphasized psychodynamic causes for the anxiety disorders.

GENETICS. Panic disorder, like schizophrenia and mood disorders, appears to have a genetic component, although there are fewer research data to support this.[18] More family and adoption studies are needed to further document the genetic risk factors for anxiety disorders.

The family studies that have been conducted have found three to four times higher rates of panic disorder among first-degree relatives of people with these disorders than among control populations and the relatives of people with other psychiatric disorders. In addition, these studies distinguish between panic disorder and the other anxiety disorders, suggesting separate mechanisms for the inheritance of each type of anxiety disorder. In families of individuals with both panic disorder and depression, first-degree relatives are at increased risk for panic disorder, depression, and other conditions. The few twin studies that have been conducted show that panic attacks, if not panic disorder, tend to have a genetic component. One early twin study remains the classic in this field and reports a significantly higher concordance for panic disorder in monozygotic than in dizygotic twins, although monozygotic twin concordance was only 31% as compared with 25% in first-degree relatives.[22] Thus genetic factors do not appear to be the only determinant of this disorder.

BIOCHEMISTRY. It is unlikely that any one neurotransmitter system is solely responsible for panic anxiety. The majority of studies to date point to a dysfunction in multiple systems, particularly GABA, norepinephrine, and serotonin regulation and transmission in the development of human anxiety disorders.

The GABA system is a major area of research interest in anxiety and panic disorders because the benzodiazepines are some of the most effective antianxiety drugs and in high doses are effective in treating panic disorder. Benzodiazepines exert their antianxiety effects by increasing the action of the inhibitory neurotransmitter GABA, thus turning down overly active brain cells. Although GABA receptors are located throughout the brain, the areas of the brain where GABA receptors are coupled to benzodiazepine receptors include the hippocampus and the amygdala, both limbic system structures that function as the center of emotions such as rage, arousal, fear, and memory. It is proposed that patients with panic disorder may have a decreased antianxiety ability of the GABA receptors in areas of the limbic system, making them more sensitive to anxiety-producing biological effects.

Panic anxiety is also proposed to be an imbalance between the norepinephrine (NE) system and other transmitter systems, such as serotonin, in the brain. The NE system is thought to mediate the fight-or-flight response. The part of the brain that manufactures NE, the locus ceruleus, is thought to control an active response to anxiety-producing stimuli, and may also play a critical role in responsiveness to changes in the internal and external environment. Neurotransmitter pathways connect the locus ceruleus to other structures of the brain believed to be implicated in anxiety, such as the amygdala, the hippocampus, and the cerebral cortex (the thinking, interpreting, and planning part of the brain).

Medications that decrease the activity of the locus ceruleus (noradrenergic antidepressants agents such as the tricyclics) effectively treat panic disorder. This suggests that panic attacks are at least partly caused by an inappropriate activation of the norepinephrine system in the locus ceruleus and an imbalance between NE and other transmitter systems. Neuroanatomical, neurochemical, neurophysiological, and behavioral studies of the norepinephrine system provide a basis for relating increased activity of this system to the expression of anxiety and fear and to the somatic symptoms and cardiovascular changes that accompany severe anxiety states.

Serotonin has also stimulated research interest in the past several years. It has been proposed that transmission of serotonin in the midbrain may play a role in the etiology of panic attacks, and patients experiencing panic may have hypersensitive serotonin receptors. This notion is supported by the fact that drugs that potentiate the regulation of serotonin, the SSRIs, have been shown to be particularly effective in treating several of the anxiety disorders, notably panic and obsessive-compulsive disorder, implying a major role for serotonin and its relationship with other transmitter systems in the etiology of anxiety disorders. Clinically it has also been documented that many people with panic disorder have noticed the panic effects of caffeine and have limited their ingestion of coffee and chocolate on their own. Caffeine has been shown to provoke panic attacks in people with panic disorder and in normal controls in laboratory challenge studies. Its principal action in the brain is to block the receptors for the inhibitory neurotransmitter adenosine. The role of this transmitter in panic disorder is unclear, however, and more research is needed to define the interaction of all of these biochemical systems in panic disorder.

BRAIN IMAGING. There have been several interesting findings using imaging technologies to study panic disorder (Fig. 5-5). CT and MRI scans consistently provide evidence of brain atrophy or underdevelopment, particularly in the frontal and temporal lobes of people with panic disorder, although the clinical significance of these findings is unclear.

Brain activity is also abnormal in patients with panic disorder. Under normal conditions, cerebral function leads to an increase in metabolic demand, resulting in an increase in cerebral blood flow. Cerebral blood flow studies using PET scans show that, at rest, patients with panic disorder who have panic attacks during lactate infusions have increased cerebral blood flow to the parahippocampal gyrus, an area of the cerebral cortex that is associated with the limbic system. Normal controls and patients with panic disorder who were not sensitive to lactate did not show this effect, suggesting a role for lactate sensitivity as a marker for certain types of panic disorder. Based on these preliminary data, it

has been suggested that a parahippocampal abnormality is involved in a predisposition to panic disorder and that activation of a norepinephrine pathway to the parahippocampal gyrus initiates an attack.[16]

The brainstem reticular formation, with its widespread ascending and descending pathways and functionally specialized groups of neurons, is also associated with the mediation of arousal. Arousal refers to levels of generalized, diffuse activation of the brain and is associated with levels of consciousness and the sleep-wake cycle in humans. Correlations between blood flow to the brainstem and cerebellar regions and various states of arousal have been demonstrated. Reticular neurons affect activity in the regulation of norepinephrine and serotonin.[23] Though still preliminary, this line of research promises to further explain the impact of levels of brain arousal on anxiety states.

It is difficult to draw clinical implications from current findings. More studies are needed to understand structural and functional differences in patients with anxiety and panic disorders and how these changes may affect behavior and ultimately clinical interventions.

> **?** *How would you respond if a patient who is about to have an MRI scan asks you whether the procedure is painful or harmful and how it will be helpful?*

CHALLENGE TESTS AND BASAL PHYSIOLOGY STUDIES. In the past 15 years two basic strategies have been devised to study the biology of panic disorder. The first, provocative challenge testing, is designed to cause panic attacks under controlled conditions so that the biology of the attack can be studied. The administration of chemicals such as lactate or caffeine and inhalants such as carbon dioxide cause panic attacks in vulnerable people. When people with panic disorder are given these challenges,

Fig. 5-5 Nurse preparing a patient for brain scanning. (Courtesy Division of Psychiatric Nursing, Medical University of South Carolina.)

they are more likely to have a panic attack than are normal controls and people with other psychiatric diagnoses. They are also less likely to have another attack when challenged again after adequate treatment with antipanic medications. This strategy may give clues to understanding the mechanism of panic attacks.

The second strategy involves studies of basal physiology, or the nonpanic state (between panic attacks), when the patient is still symptomatic with chronic high levels of anxiety and avoidance behavior. This strategy often leads to a better understanding of which parts of the brain may be important in triggering the panic state. For example, people with panic disorder have been shown to have blunted pituitary hormonal responses to several hypothalamic releasing hormones, suggesting either that the person cannot respond appropriately to stress, thus panic anxiety results, or the pituitary may adapt over time to repeated panic anxiety.

A final interesting physiological finding is that sleep-related panic attacks commonly occur in the transition from stage two to stage three sleep. Panic attacks occur in states of apparent deep relaxation and unconsciousness, rather than during dream (REM) sleep, when it could be suggested that the panic attack was in response to a disturbing dream. This finding further supports a biological component to panic.

Clinical Implications: Biology of Panic Disorder

Although further research is needed to clarify the mechanisms for the cause of anxiety disorders, the clinical significance of the findings to date can be reassuring to patients. Patients can be told, for example, that panic anxiety is a dysregulation in the normal fight-or-flight response. The way in which it is manifested may be the combination of genetic vulnerability and a person's reactions to life's experiences. Perhaps most important, patients should be told that panic disorder usually can be successfully treated by a variety of interventions. This information can give patients a sense of control over its seemingly uncontrollable and debilitating effects. They can then be taught to control their responses to anxiety and to actively participate in treatment in an informed partnership with health-care providers (see

Chapter 16). Finally, the psychiatric nurse can assess symptoms of anxiety disorders and select the most appropriate intervention based on the brain region implicated in the symptom and the treatment most likely to affect the function of that brain region (Table 5-4).

Alzheimer's Disease

The normal aging brain experiences a modest, gradual decline in enzyme activity and levels of selected proteins and neurons in certain brain regions. The aging person may have decreased motor function and flexibility, slowness of movement, and a stooped, shuffling gait. However, changes in the brain appear to have little effect on mental functions such as thinking, except that these functions are slower.

Dementia, a decline of memory and other cognitive functions, is the most disabling psychiatric disorder of adulthood. It is not caused by the normal process of aging but rather appears to have many possible causes, as described in Chapter 23. About 45% of people with dementia are diagnosed with Alzheimer's disease (AD), which is the fourth most common cause of death in the developed world after heart disease, cancer, and stroke. At a cost of $34 billion a year, AD afflicts 4 million people in the United States and results in 100,000 deaths annually. In light of today's aging population, AD has become a major health concern and the target of intensive research efforts nationwide. The causes of AD are not yet known, but a number of risk factors have been associated with it (Box 5-3).

> **?** *Because head injury is a known risk factor for the dementing syndrome, what primary prevention strategies could society take to resolve this problem?*

GENETICS. It was not until 1991 that research in AD showed that genetic mutations cause some cases of AD. In early-onset AD (before age 65) these DNA mutations occur within chromosome 21, the same gene that forms beta-APP (amyloid precursor protein), the substance from which the protein beta-amyloid is made. The normal function of this

TABLE **5-4** *Biological Treatment Model of Panic Disorder*

SYMPTOM	BRAIN REGION	FUNCTION	TREATMENT
Phobic avoidance (a learned phenomenon)	Cerebral cortex (higher brain)	Learning and complex emotion	Desensitization and cognitive restructuring (see Chapter 30)
Anticipatory anxiety (possibly sensitized by hyperventilation)	Limbic lobe (midbrain: rich in neurotransmitter receptors)	Center for human emotions	Relaxation, breathing retraining, desensitization, antipanic medications
Panic attacks	Brainstem (lower brain: includes structures that manufacture neurotransmitters)	Primitive emotion	Antipanic medication (see Chapter 27)

Modified from Gorman JM, Leibowitz MR, Fyer AJ, Stein J: *Am J Psychiatry* 146:2, 1989.

Box **5-3** *Risk Factors for Alzheimer's Disease*

AGE

AD is a disease of old age.

The population prevalence is less than 0.01% at age 45, 2% between age 65 and 70, 5% between 70 and 80, and over 20% at age 85.

AD affects more women than men because women tend to live longer.

An early age of onset (<65) is strongly associated with a positive family history.

FAMILY HISTORY

A positive family history in first-degree relatives is the most persistent positive association for AD.

Approximately 20% of AD cases are thought to be familial.

PARENTAL AGE

Women who bear children before 20 and after 40 years of age have an increased incidence of AD in their offspring.

This group of mothers also has increased risk of premature births, poor maternal fitness, and babies with Down's syndrome.

These findings suggest that children of older parents may have a chromosomal abnormality that makes them more susceptible to AD when they reach old age.

HEAD INJURY

Descriptive reviews of case control studies often report the finding of a history of head injury in some patients with AD.

Support for head injury as a risk factor also comes from evidence that repetitive head trauma is known to cause a dementing syndrome in boxers (dementia pugilistica, or punchdrunk syndrome), which shows the same molecular pathology as AD.

POTASSIUM CHANNEL DYSFUNCTION

One study[4] found that patients with AD, when compared with both control groups and patients with other dementing illnesses, have a potassium (K+) channel dysfunction.

K+ channels change during acquisition of memory in studies of mammals. Thus an abnormal K+ channel may serve as a marker that would distinguish patients with AD from age-matched controls and patients with non-AD neurological and psychiatric disorders.

ENVIRONMENTAL FACTORS

Although there have been anecdotal reports of other factors as risks for AD, systematic evidence is lacking. Some of these include:

Aluminum: ingestion of foods stored in aluminum containers or use of deodorants and hairsprays with aluminum bases

Bloodborne infections: blood transfusions if the blood donor has AD and it is transmitted by an infectious agent

Chemicals: occupational exposure to chemicals

---

protein is not fully understood, but its production is somehow accelerated in AD, and excessive deposits form both the senile plaques clustering outside each affected neuron and amyloid deposits in the walls of cerebral blood vessels. It is probably also related to the production of the neurofibrillary tangles seen within the neurons of patients with AD. Approximately 50% of individuals in each generation of families with this genetic mutation develop AD. Interestingly, AD is also seen in the fourth and fifth decade of life in patients with Down's syndrome, who have three rather than two copies of chromosome 21. Almost all of these patients develop senile plaques, neurofibrillary tangles, and clinical signs of dementia. In late-onset AD (after age 65) some cases have also been linked to chromosome 19 (probably a gene affecting beta-APP metabolism).

Another recent research finding is a link between combinations of a fairly common cholesterol-transporting protein, Apo-E, and AD. Apparently many people with late-onset AD are born with a certain combination of Apo-E that attaches to beta-amyloid, which may pull bits of amyloid from the bloodstream and accumulate it in the brain. Thus developing AD may depend on which combination of Apo-E a person inherits. It remains to be seen whether drugs can be developed that can prevent this form of Apo-E from doing its job.

Although genetics accounts for only a small percentage of AD cases (perhaps 10%) and much of this work is still controversial, these discoveries are landmark scientific achievements. Genetic research in AD continues to be a high funding priority and promises to continue to unlock some of the mysteries of this devastating illness.

BIOCHEMISTRY. Almost every neurotransmitter has been studied and implicated in AD, but the cholinergic hypothesis has commanded much of the attention as an explanation for AD. Disruption of the cholinergic system damages memory in animals and humans. Acetylcholine (ACh) is consistently reduced in AD. ACh is produced in a region of the basal nuclei selectively devastated in AD. It is thought that too little acetylcholine may allow a buildup of amyloid. Although more than a dozen experimental drugs are being tested for efficacy in AD, only a handful have shown promise. Tacrine (Cognex) and donepezil (Aricept), which slow the natural breakdown of acetylcholine, have been approved for use in AD by the Food and Drug Administration.

In addition to cholinergic fibers, noncholinergic, serotonergic, and possibly dopaminergic fibers that innervate hippocampal and cortical areas are all severely affected by the disease. Glutamate and peptide transmitters are also affected in specific brain regions. Although correlations can be drawn between transmitter deficits and pathology and clinical symptoms of AD, they seem to reflect damage specific to affected regions of the brain rather than entire transmitter systems throughout the brain, providing little information about the underlying nature of the disease pro-

TABLE **5-5** *Some Brain Regions Affected by Alzheimer's Disease and Resulting Symptoms*

REGION AFFECTED	FUNCTION	SYMPTOM
Limbic system: hippocampus	Memory, learning, and emotion	First, recent memories fade and then long-standing memories are affected. Symptoms of depression may occur, probably because of damage to the locus ceruleus.
Temporal-parietal-occipital association cortex	Visual impairment, aphasia, apraxia, and agnosia	Increasing difficulty recognizing even familiar faces, places, and objects. The ability to communicate, use and understand language, write, and comprehend reading is lost. Hallucinations and delusions may occur. Seizures may occur.
Prefrontal cortex	Insight, planning, judgment, personality, behavior, and social propriety	Apathy, impaired insight, lack of judgment, concreteness, perseverance, and inefficient problem solving are seen.
Subcortical projections	Memory, learning, and behavior	More research is needed to correlate symptoms with changes seen in these areas, but it is clear that several important transmitter systems are affected: cholinergic basal forebrain, noradrenergic locus ceruleus, serotonergic raphe nuclei, and dopaminergic substantia nigra.
Motor cortex	Movement	Increasing difficulty walking, talking, and swallowing occur later in the disease process.

cess. Another implication is that, unlike the neurochemistry of Parkinson's disease in which one transmitter deficit can be treated effectively by one drug intervention (l-dopa), it seems unlikely that AD can be effectively treated by neurotransmitter replacement therapy alone.

BRAIN IMAGING. PET scans and performance tests indicate that the brains of healthy people in their eighties are almost as active and function nearly as well (although slower) on tests of memory, perception, and language as people in early adulthood.[19] Although diagnostic accuracy for AD requires neuropathological examination at autopsy, skillful neuropsychiatric examinations along with imaging techniques offer 80% to 90% diagnostic accuracy. CT and MRI are useful to rule out space-occupying lesions, infarcts, or infection as causes of dementia but are not specific for the diagnosis of AD. Although patients with early-onset AD may show cortical atrophy and ventricular enlargement with CT or MRI and a marked loss in brain weight, patients with late-onset AD who develop the disease after age 75 usually show only age-related changes. PET scans show a typical pattern of frontal, parietal, and temporal hypometabolism (see Color Plate 12 on p. 100). However, these changes are not specific to AD and thus cannot be used by themselves to make a definitive diagnosis. PET scans and SPECT studies have also shown results that appear to be specific to AD: a localized metabolic deficiency can be seen in the parietal, temporal, and eventually the frontal lobes.[13]

NEUROPATHOLOGICAL CHANGES. It is not known how excessive amyloid protein deposits lead to the plaques and tangles that cause extensive structural and biochemical changes in axons, dendrites, neuronal cell bodies, and glial cells. These changes reduce synaptic function by as much as 40% in affected regions and reduce protein synthesis and cellular processes. However, there is no doubt that this buildup of amyloid protein, combined with the formation of neurofibrillary tangles and other structural changes in neurons, contributes to a progressive breakdown of neuronal circuits necessary for communication in the brain. It is as if the limbic system, particularly the hippocampus and the association cortices (which are affected early in the AD process and are necessary to the organization of mental processes), becomes isolated and out of touch with other brain regions, hence the gradual impairment of memory, judgment, abstraction, and language. Eventually motor and sensory regions are affected also, and the patient with AD becomes totally disabled. Table 5-5 lists some of the affected brain regions and subsequent symptoms.

Clinical Implications: Biology of Alzheimer's Disease

Much research is being focused on understanding the molecular mechanisms underlying dementing diseases so that drugs can be designed to block these processes. In AD, future medications may be able to inhibit the enzymes that release excessive amounts of beta-amyloid protein from beta-APP, preventing it from entering cerebral tissue and causing the inflammatory and neurotoxic responses that result in CNS damage.

At present, although several drugs may lessen some of the disease processes for a time, there is no treatment for AD. Clinical intervention is targeted at differential diagnosis and managing the social and behavioral consequences of the progressive dementia of AD (see Chapters 23 and 38). The Advisory Panel on Alzheimer's Disease suggests minimum curricular requirements for nurses and other healthcare providers for working with patients with AD and their families.[1] An interesting line of nursing research shows that patients with AD who remain at home with a committed and loving caregiver live longer than patients with AD who live in nursing homes.[24] This may have important implications for society regarding the care and support of demented people and their families, as well as the burden and cost of caregiving in this population of extremely ill people.

One remedy to counter the effects of the aging process is to stay physically fit. Older test subjects who regularly do aerobic exercises perform better on cognitive tests than do sedentary people in the same age group. Agents that interfere with the activity of the CNS should also be avoided by older people. This includes alcohol and certain drugs, such as benzodiazepines and other depressants or stimulants of the CNS. People over age 60 are particularly sensitive to these substances and perform poorly on cognitive tests compared with younger people taking the same drugs. It remains to be seen whether early anecdotal reports of therapy with the antioxidant vitamin E or a lifetime of balanced, low-calorie diets have positive effects on mental functions in elderly people.

DECADE OF THE BRAIN

The U.S. Congress has called the 1990s the Decade of the Brain. Advances in the techniques used in the neurosciences, the scientific methodologies used in testing biological hypotheses, and the integration of nonbiological theories and findings in the clinical arena provide the biopsychosocial approach necessary for the study of psychiatric disorders in human beings.

Several well-researched lines of evidence support a biological link to mental illnesses, including the following:

▼ Specific mental disorders can often be differentiated from each other by typical clinical features, epidemiological trends, and symptom presentations.

▼ Exogenous chemicals can produce symptoms of mental illness or exacerbate existing symptoms, thus demonstrating that physical agents can be causative.

▼ A biological cause of psychiatric illness is supported by in vitro simulations of some symptoms that can be replicated, such as the challenge studies in panic disorder.

▼ Genetic studies show that psychiatric disorders are strongly influenced by inheritance: The closer the genetic structure, the more at risk the person is for the disorder.

▼ Many psychiatric disorders have associated biological symptoms or test results, such as altered sleep patterns and failure to suppress cortisol in the dexamethasone suppression test in depression.

▼ Medications can suppress symptoms associated with psychiatric disorders, thus providing chemically mediated relief for many psychiatric illnesses.

As members of the mental health care team, psychiatric nurses are faced with the challenge of integrating the new psychobiology with the long-standing biopsychosocial model of psychiatric nursing care. It is essential that psychiatric nurses make this paradigm shift and combine the enormous amount of information from the neurosciences with that of the other health sciences. They then need to apply this information and provide holistic, effective, and individualized psychiatric nursing care.

Summary

1. Psychiatric nurses must learn about the structure and function of the brain, including the neurotransmission process, to better understand the etiology, course, and most effective treatment strategies for psychiatric illnesses.

2. Brain imaging techniques such as CT, MRI, BEAM, PET, and SPECT allow direct viewing of the brain, which helps in diagnosing some brain disorders and correlating brain structure with function.

3. The search for the gene or genes that carry mental illness has been difficult and inconclusive to date but is a promising field for future research.

4. Circadian rhythm is like a network of internal clocks that time and coordinate events within the body including lifestyle, sleep, moods, eating, drinking, fertility, and illness according to a 24-hour cycle.

5. Psychoimmunology is a new field that explores the influence of psychosocial factors on the nervous system's control of immune responses.

6. Psychiatric nurses need to be able to obtain a thorough history, perform a basic physical examination, and interpret the results of laboratory tests to screen for signs of physical disorders and refer to specialists as indicated.

7. The clinical implications of neuroscientific research were discussed in relation to schizophrenia, mood disorders, panic disorder, and Alzheimer's disease.

8. The 1990s have been called the Decade of the Brain, and psychiatric nurses are faced with the challenge of integrating the latest neuroscientific information into the biopsychosocial model of psychiatric nursing care.

your **INTERNET**
c o n n e c t i o n

Brainscape
http://beast.cbmv.jhu.edu:8000/research/brain/brain.htm

Neurosciences on the Internet
http://www.lm.com/~nab

Chapter Review Questions

1. Match the terms in Column A with the best description from Column B.

Column A	Column B
___Tryptophan	A. Homeostasis
___PET	B. May underlie cyclical disorders
___Eugenics	C. Space between brain cells
___Synapse	D. Dream sleep
___REM	E. Manufactures norepinephrine
___Hippocampus	F. Cause panic attacks under controlled conditions
___DST	G. Neurotransmitter precursor
___Locus ceruleus	H. Functional neuroimaging technique
___Basal ganglia	I. Movement
___Challenge tests	J. Selective breeding
___Kindling	K. Memory
___Hypothalamus	L. Biological marker for depression

2. Fill in the blanks.

A. The microenvironment that protects the CNS from large molecules, toxins, and peripheral chemicals is the _____ and _____ barriers.

B. Communication between neurons in the brain is called _____.

C. The scientific field made up of many disciplines that has revolutionized our understanding of mental illness is called _____.

D. The network of internal clocks that time and coordinate events within the body according to a 24-hour cycle is called _____.

E. Rates of depression, mania, and suicide in the United States, Canada, and Europe have been rising within certain age groups over the past several generations, in the general population as well as in at-risk populations. This trend is called a _____.

3. Identify whether the following statements are true (T) or false (F).

A. ___ The gene for Alzheimer's disease is currently implicated in 90% of cases.

B. ___ Family, adoption, and twin studies suggest that the pattern of inherited vulnerability to mental illness probably results from the interaction of genes as well as the environment.

C. ___ The catecholamine hypothesis is now the most recent and dominant explanation for the mood disorders.

D. ___ Brain imaging techniques have generally found smaller ventricles in some people with schizophrenia, depression, and anxiety disorders than in nonaffected people.

E. ___ When neurotransmission has taken place, the process by which neurotransmitters travel from the synapse into the presynaptic axon is called reuptake.

4. Provide short answers for the following questions.

A. Briefly describe the role of each of the following components in brain communication:
Axon
Dendrite
Receptor cell
Autoregulation
Reuptake
Enzymatic degradation

B. Discuss how the limbic system is involved in feelings, emotion, and self-preservation.

C. List the stages of sleep and define REM latency and decreased REM latency.

D. How is challenge testing useful in the study of panic disorder?

References

1. Advisory Panel on Alzheimer's Disease: *Second report of the Advisory Panel on Alzheimer's Disease,* DHHS Pub. No. (ADM) 91-1791, Washington, DC, 1991, US Government Printing Office.
2. Betrus P, Elmore S: Seasonal affective disorder: part I. A review of the neural mechanisms for psychosocial nurses, *Arch Psychiatr Nurs* 5:357, 1991.
3. Carpenter WT, Buchanan RW: Medical progress: schizophrenia, *N Engl J Med* 330:10:681-690, 1994.
4. Etcheberrigaray R, Ito E, Oka K, Tofel-Grehl B, Gigson E: Potassium channel dysfunction in fibroblasts identifies patients with Alzheimer's disease, *Proc Natl Acad Sci U S A* 90:8209, 1993.
5. Garver K, Garver B: Eugenics: past, present, and future, *Am J Hum Genet* 49:1109, 1991.
6. George MS, Ketter TA, Post RM: Prefrontal cortex dysfunction in clinical depression, *Depression* 2:59-72, 1994.
7. Gershon ES, Rieder RO: Major disorders of mind and brain, *Sci Am* 267:133, 1992.
8. Goodwin W, Jamison K: *Manic depressive illness,* New York, 1990, Oxford University Press.
9. Holmes C: *Recognizing brain dysfunction: a guide for mental health professionals,* Brandon, Vt, 1992, Clinical Psychology Publishing Company.
10. Joyce J: The dopamine hypothesis of schizophrenia: limbic interactions with serotonin and norepinephrine, *Psychopharmacology* 112:516, 1993.

11. Kapur S, Remington G, Jones C, Wilson A, DaSilva J, Houle S, Zipursky R: High levels of dopamine D_2 receptor occupancy with low-dose haloperidol treatment: a PET study, *Am J Psychiatry* 153:7:948-950, 1996.
12. Kronig MH, Munne RA, Szymanski S, Safferman AZ, Pollack S, Cooper T, Kane JM, Lieberman JA: Plasma clozapine levels and clinical response for treatment-refractory schizophrenic patients, *Am J Psychiatry* 152:179-182, 1995.
13. Margolin R: Neuroimaging. In Sadovoy J, Lazarus L, Jarvik L, editors: *Comprehensive review of geriatric psychiatry,* Washington, DC, 1993, American Psychiatric Press.
14. McEnany G: Rhythm and blues revisited: biological rhythm disturbances in depression, *J Am Psych Nurs Assoc* 2:1:15-22, 1996.
15. Post R, Weiss S: Nonhomologous animal models of affective illness: clinical relevance of sensitization and kindling. In Koob G, Ehlers C, Kupfer D, editors: *Animal models of depression,* Boston, 1989, Birkhauser.
16. Reiman E: PET, panic disorder, and normal anticipatory anxiety. In Ballenger J, editor: *Frontiers of clinical neuroscience,* vol 8, *Neurobiology of panic disorder,* New York, 1990, Alan R Liss.
17. Roberts GW, Leigh PN, Weinberger DR: *Neuropsychiatric Disorders,* London, 1993, Wolfe.
18. Robins L, Regier D: *Psychiatric disorders in America: the Epidemiology Catchment Area Study,* New York, 1991, Free Press.
19. Selkoe D: Aging brain, aging mind, *Sci Am* 267:135, 1992.
20. Thase M, Frank E, Kupfer D: Biological processes in major depression. In Beckman E, Leber W, editors: *Handbook of depression,* ed 2, New York, 1993, Guilford Press.
21. Thibodeau G, Patton K: *Anatomy and physiology,* ed 2, St Louis, 1993, Mosby.
22. Torgesen S: Twin studies in panic disorder. In Ballenger J, editor: *Neurobiology of panic disorder,* New York, 1990, Alan R Liss.
23. Wilson W, Mathew R: Cerebral blood flow and metabolism in anxiety disorders. In Hoehn-Saric R, McLeod DR, editors: *Biology of anxiety disorders,* Progress in Psychiatry Series no. 36, Washington, DC, 1993, American Psychiatric Press.
24. Wright L: *Alzheimer's disease and marriage: an intimate account,* Sage Series in Clinical Nursing Research, Newbury Park, Calif, 1993, Sage Publications.
25. Wright P, Takei N, Rifkin L, Murray RM: Maternal influenza, obstetric complications, and schizophrenia, *Am J Psychiatry* 152:12:1714-1720, 1995.

ANNOTATED SUGGESTED READINGS

Brain imaging and psychiatry, *Harvard Mental Health Letter* 13:1, 1997.
  A simple and informative overview of brain imaging techniques and their role in psychiatry to date.
Casey B et al: Implication of right frontostriatal circuitry in response inhibition and ADHD, *J Am Child Adolesc Psychiatry* 36:374, 1997.
  ADHD children showed differences in the caudate (correlating with abnormal reaction times) and smaller prefrontal cortex volume (correlating with lack of response inhibition) when compared with normal children, implicating a need for more specificity in medication treatments.
Greenfield S: *The human mind explained: an owner's guide to the mysteries of the mind,* New York, 1996, Henry Holt and Company.
  Richly informative case histories that illustrate dysfunction and examples from everyday life. Contains many graphics. A must for everyone with a brain, from the layperson to the nurse.

Harasty J et al: Language-associated cortical regions are proportionally larger in the female brain, *Arch Neurol* 54:171, 1997.
  Interesting findings demonstrate that in two language-associated regions of the brain and not in nonlanguage areas, women's brains are 20% to 30% larger than men's, perhaps accounting for the fact that women show better verbal fluency and verbal memory than men.
Hublin C et al: Prevalence and genetics of sleepwalking: a population-based twin study, *Neurology* 48:177, 1997.
  This study documented that sleep walking is more than 50% genetically based in children and more than 33% in adults. The concordance rate for sleep walking is 55% among identical twins and 35% in fraternal twins.
*Hudak C, Gallo B: Quick review of neurodiagnostic testing, *Am J Nurs* 97:16cc, 1997.
  Provides a succinct summary of the most common neurodiagnostic tests, how they work, why they are used, nursing implications, and what a patient needs to be taught.
*Keltner N: The basal ganglia and movement disorders, *Perspect Psychiatr Care* 32:30, 1996.
  Overview of the structure and function of the basal ganglia, including their role in movement, reward, cognition, and their disorders.
Koslow S et al: *The neuroscience of mental health, II: a report on neuroscience research,* US Department of Health and Human Services, Public Health Service, NIH, NIMH, Rockville, Md, 1995.
  Assesses the state of neuroscience research and articulates research directions leading to a complete understanding of the biological mechanisms underlying emotional and behavioral processes. Very informative.
LeDoux J: *The emotional brain: the mysterious underpinnings of emotional life,* New York, 1996, Simon & Shuster.
  Provocative and informative report of research findings and an exploration of the underlying brain mechanisms about little understood human emotions.
Lewis D: Development of the prefrontal cortex during adolescence: insights into vulnerable neural circuits in schizophrenia, *Neuropsychopharmacology* 16:385, 1997.
  Reviews information about developmental refinements in the prefrontal cortex during adolescence that appear to lead to a vulnerability for schizophrenia. A sophisticated but worthwhile read.
Oldham J, Riba M: Psychiatric genetics. In *Review of Psychiatry,* APA Press, 14:339, 1995.
  Gives the reader enough scientific background and current state of the science in this important field to readily understand and place in context new information about genetics as it becomes available.
Purves D et al: *Neuroscience,* Sunderland, Mass, 1997, Sinauer Associates, Inc.
  Richly illustrated with pictures, tables, and graphs, this text builds on basic knowledge and provides a wonderfully comprehensive yet understandable view of how the brain and nervous system function in health and illness.
Schuchter S, Downs N, Zisook S: *Biologically informed psychotherapy for depression,* New York, 1996, The Guilford Press.
  For all psychotherapists at all levels of expertise, this gives many practical examples of how particular points regarding depression as a biological disorder could be presented to a patient.
Transcranial magnetic stimulation, *CNS Spectrum* 2:1, 1997.
  This entire edition addresses TMS, including an overview, its effects on kindling, potential use in the treatment of mood and anxiety disorders, and a review of the biological hypotheses underlying its proposed efficacy. Very informative.

*Nursing reference.

Psychological Context of Psychiatric Nursing Care

Gail W. Stuart

© 1998 M.C. Escher/Cordon Art, Baarn, Holland.

Information is of no value for its own sake, but only because of its personal significance. **Eric Berne**

LEARNING OBJECTIVES

After studying this chapter the student should be able to:

▼ Describe the nature, purpose, and process of the mental status examination

▼ Analyze the observations and clinical implications of each category of the mental status examination

▼ Identify commonly used psychological tests

▼ Discuss the value of behavioral rating scales in psychiatric nursing practice

TOPICAL OUTLINE

Mental Status Examination
  Eliciting Clinical Information
Content of the Examination
  Appearance
  Speech
  Motor Activity
  Interaction during the Interview
  Mood
  Affect
  Perceptions
  Thought Content
  Thought Process
  Level of Consciousness
  Memory
  Level of Concentration and Calculation
  Information and Intelligence
  Judgment
  Insight
  Documenting Clinical Information
  Mini-Mental State
Psychological Tests
Behavioral Rating Scales

Holistic psychiatric nursing care requires the nurse to complete an assessment of the patient's biological, psychological, and sociocultural health status. The assessment of the patient's psychological well-being should include a mental status examination. All nurses, regardless of the clinical setting, should be proficient in administering the mental status examination and be able to incorporate findings from it in the patient's plan of nursing care.

The mental status examination is a cornerstone in the evaluation of any patient with a medical, neurological, or psychiatric disorder that affects thought, emotion, or behavior. It is used to detect changes or abnormalities in a person's intellectual functioning, thought content, judgment, mood, and affect and can be used to identify possible lesions in the brain.[2] The mental status examination is to psychiatric nursing what the physical examination is to general medical nursing.

MENTAL STATUS EXAMINATION

The mental status examination represents a cross-section of the patient's psychological life and the sum total of the nurse's observations and impressions at the moment. It also serves as a basis for future comparison to track the progress of the patient over time. The elements of the examination depend on the patient's clinical presentation as well as his or her educational and cultural background. It includes observing the patient's behavior and describing it in an objective, nonjudgmental manner.

The examination itself is usually divided into several parts. They can be arranged in different ways, as long as the nurse covers all the areas. Much of the information needed for the mental status examination can be gathered during the course of the routine nursing assessment. It should be integrated in the nurse's assessment in a smooth manner. Some parts of the mental status examination are completed through simple observation of the patient, such as by noting the patient's clothing or facial expressions. Other aspects require asking specific questions, such as those related to memory or attention span. Most of all, the nurse should remember that the mental status examination does not reflect how the patient was in the past or will be in the future; it is an evaluation of the patient's current state.

Information obtained during the mental status examination is used along with other objective and subjective data. These include findings from the physical examination, laboratory test results, patient history, description of the presenting problem, and information obtained from family, caregivers, and other health professionals. With these data the nurse is able to formulate nursing diagnoses and design the plan of care with the patient.

> **?** *Do nurses on medical-surgical units routinely assess a patient's psychological status? Explain your findings given the fact that all nurses should be providing holistic, biopsychosocial nursing care.*

Eliciting Clinical Information

The mental status examination requires a clinical rather than social approach to the patient. The nurse listens closely to what is said and reflects on what is not said, structuring the process in a way that allows for broad exploration of many areas for potential problems, as well as for more in-depth exploration of obvious symptoms or maladaptive coping responses. The patient is critically observed. Behaviors that the nurse might not normally attend to in more general situations must be carefully observed and described. Global and judgmental statements are not acceptable.

The skilled nurse attends to both the content and the process of the patient's communication (see Chapter 2). **Content** is the overtly communicated information. **Process** is how the communication occurs and includes feelings, intuition, and behaviors that accompany speech and thought. The content and process may not always be congruent. For example, a patient may deny feeling depressed and yet appear sad and cry. In this case, the stated message does not match the process, and the nurse should record this incongruity.

It is also important for nurses to monitor their feelings and reactions during the mental status examination. A nurse's gut reactions may reflect subtle emotions being expressed by the patient. For example, a depressed patient may make the nurse feel sad, and a hostile patient may make the nurse feel threatened and angry. The nurse's feelings are useful information for the mental status assessment.

The nurse needs to be aware of these feelings and respond in a therapeutic manner toward the patient regardless of such feelings. The nurse should remain calm throughout the interview and simply reflect observations back to the patient. These observations should be related in an objective and nonthreatening manner, as in "You are obviously quite upset about this," or "It seems like you don't feel safe here." By conveying a sense of calm, the nurse also demonstrates being in control, even if the patient is not.

The nurse should try to blend specific questions into the general flow of the interview. For example, questions about orientation, arithmetic problems, or proverbs may be introduced by soliciting patient comments about potential problems with concentration, memory, or understanding of written material. The nurse might then suggest that the patient try answering a few questions to determine whether such problems are evident.

Finally, as with any other skill, nurses need to practice performing the mental status examination to gain proficiency and comfort. The nurse might start by observing a colleague conduct the examination. Videotapes of patient interviews are a particularly effective teaching-learning tool. The nurse should then be observed administering the mental status examination by a colleague or supervisor who can provide helpful feedback and identify ways to further enhance the nurse's competency.

CONTENT OF THE EXAMINATION

The mental status examination includes information in a number of categories (Box 6-1). It is one part of a complete psychiatric nursing assessment tool described in Chapter 10. In completing this examination it is critically important to be aware that sociocultural factors can greatly influence the outcome of the examination (Box 6-2). In addition, biological expressions of psychiatric illness may also be evident during the interview. The content, observations, and some of the clinical implications associated with each category are now described.[8,9]

Appearance

In the mental status examination the nurse takes note of the patient's appearance. This part of the examination is intended to provide an accurate mental image of the patient, as in the following clinical example.

Clinical Example   Mr. W is a middle-aged white man of average weight who appears older than his stated age. He was disheveled, dressed in a torn shirt and jeans, and was unshaven. He was slightly jaundiced and had a prominent red nose and a scar on the left side of his cheek. He sat slumped in the chair and made little eye contact with the interviewer.

Observations   The following physical characteristics should be included in the assessment:
- ▼ Apparent age
- ▼ Manner of dress
- ▼ Cleanliness
- ▼ Posture
- ▼ Gait
- ▼ Facial expressions
- ▼ Eye contact
- ▼ Pupil dilation or constriction
- ▼ General state of health and nutrition

Clinical Implications   Dilated pupils are sometimes associated with drug intoxication, whereas pupil constriction may indicate narcotic addiction. Stooped posture is often seen in depression. Manic patients may dress in colorful or unusual attire.

Speech

Speech is usually described in terms of rate, volume, and characteristics. Rate is the speed of the patient's speech, and volume is how loud a patient talks.

Observations   Speech can be described as follows:
- ▼ Rate: rapid or slow
- ▼ Volume: loud or soft
- ▼ Amount: paucity, muteness, pressured speech
- ▼ Characteristics: stuttering, slurring of words, or unusual accents

---

Box **6-1** *Categories of the Mental Status Examination*

GENERAL DESCRIPTION
Appearance
Speech
Motor activity
Interaction during interview

EMOTIONAL STATE
Mood
Affect

EXPERIENCES
Perceptions

THINKING
Thought content
Thought process

SENSORIUM AND COGNITION
Level of consciousness
Memory
Level of concentration and calculation
Information and intelligence
Judgment
Insight

Box **6-2** *Clinical Judgment or Sociocultural Bias?*

In completing the mental status examination clinicians need to be aware of the possibility of using subconscious and culturally determined criteria when judging a patient. Examples of potential sociocultural clinician bias include the following:
- ▼ How is the manner of dress judged (that is, what is unusual or expected dress)?
- ▼ Do all cultures accept the American norm of direct eye contact?
- ▼ What are the clinician's values about personal hygiene and how do they influence assessment?
- ▼ Do a person's speech and use of language vary based on social class and lifestyle?
- ▼ How does body language and use of personal space vary by ethnicity and social group?
- ▼ Given the fact that 20 to 30 million American adults lack basic educational skills, what is the expected "norm" regarding reading, writing, or problem-solving tasks?
- ▼ How familiar are common proverbs? Which interpretations of them are truly correct?

Clinical Implications Speech disturbances are often caused by specific brain disturbances. For example, mumbling may occur in patients with Huntington's chorea, and slurring of speech in intoxicated patients. Manic patients often show pressured speech, and people suffering from depression often are reluctant to speak.

Motor Activity

Motor activity is concerned with the patient's physical movement.

Observations The nurse should record the following:
▼ Level of activity: lethargic, tense, restless, or agitated
▼ Type of activity: tics, grimaces, or tremors
▼ Unusual gestures or mannerisms: compulsions

Clinical Implications Excessive body movement may be associated with anxiety, mania, or stimulant abuse. Little body activity may suggest depression, organicity, catatonic schizophrenia, or drug-induced stupor. Tics and grimaces may suggest medication side effects (see Chapter 27). Repeated motor movements or compulsions may indicate obsessive-compulsive disorder. Repeated picking of lint or dirt off clothing is sometimes associated with delirium or toxic conditions.

 Which category of psychotropic medications is most often associated with tics and grimaces?

Interaction during the Interview

Interaction describes how the patient relates to the nurse during the interview, as in this clinical example.

Clinical Example The patient was interviewed in her room on the second day of hospitalization. She was a white woman slightly overweight, neatly dressed in jeans and a sweater, and appeared younger than her 36 years of age. Although she was cooperative, her guarded responses to all questions seemed excessively self-centered. She gave the interviewer the feeling that she didn't trust anyone and was preoccupied during the interview. When asked how other people treated her, she responded angrily, "I'd rather not say!"

Because this part of the examination relies heavily on nurses' emotional subjectivity, nurses must carefully examine their responses based on their personal and sociocultural biases. They must guard against overinterpreting or misinterpreting patients' behavior because of social or cultural differences (see Chapter 7).

Observations Is the patient hostile, uncooperative, irritable, guarded, apathetic, defensive, suspicious, or seductive? The nurse may explore this area by asking, "You seem irritated about something. Is that an accurate observation?"

Clinical Implications Suspiciousness may be evident in paranoia. Irritability may suggest an anxiety disorder.

Mood

Mood is the patient's self-report of the prevailing emotional state and reflects the patient's life situation.

Observations Mood can be evaluated by asking a simple, nonleading question such as "How are you feeling today?" Does the patient report feeling sad, fearful, hopeless, euphoric, or anxious? Asking the patient to rate his or her mood on a scale of 0 to 10 can help provide the nurse with an immediate reading. It also can be valuable for comparison of changes that occur during treatment.

If the potential for suicide is suspected, the nurse should inquire about the patient's thoughts about self-destruction (see Chapter 20). Suicidal and homicidal thoughts must be addressed directly. Has the patient felt the desire to harm him- or herself or someone else? Have any previous attempts been made, and if so, what events surrounded the attempts? To judge a patient's suicidal or homicidal risk, the nurse should assess the patient's plans, ability to carry out those plans (such as the availability of guns), the patient's attitude about death, and available support systems, as in the following clinical example.

Clinical Example The patient responded to most of the questions in a flat, dull manner. Although he stated that he felt sad about the recent changes in his life, his lifeless posture and tone of voice did not convey any emotional response. He denied any current suicidal or homicidal plans. He related having made two suicidal gestures in the past year by "taking pills."

Clinical Implications Most people with depression describe feeling hopeless, and 25% of those with depression have suicidal ideation. Suicidal ideation is also common in anxiety disorders and schizophrenia. Elation is most common in mania.

Affect

Affect is the patient's apparent emotional tone. The patient's statements of emotions and the nurse's empathic responses provide clues to the appropriateness of the affect.

Observations Affect can be described in terms of the following:
▼ Range
▼ Duration
▼ Intensity
▼ Appropriateness
Does the patient report significant life events without any emotional response, indicating flat affect? Does the patient's response appear restricted or blunted in some way? Does the patient demonstrate great lability in expression by shifting from one affect to another quickly? Is the patient's response incongruent with speech content? For example,

does the patient report being persecuted by the police and then laugh?

Clinical Implications   Labile affect is often seen in mania, and a flat, incongruent affect is often evident in schizophrenia.

Perceptions

There are two major types of perceptual problems: hallucinations and illusions. **Hallucinations** are defined as false sensory impressions or experiences. **Illusions** are false perceptions or false responses to a sensory stimulus.

Observations   Hallucinations may occur in any of the five major sensory modalities:
▼ Auditory (sound)
▼ Visual (sight)
▼ Tactile (touch)
▼ Gustatory (taste)
▼ Olfactory (smell)

Command hallucinations are those that tell the patient to do something, such as to kill oneself, harm another, or join someone in afterlife. The nurse might inquire about the patient's perceptions by asking "Do you ever see or hear things?" or "Do you have strange experiences as you fall asleep or upon awakening?"

Clinical Implications   Auditory hallucinations are the most common and suggest schizophrenia. Visual hallucinations suggest organicity. Tactile hallucinations suggest organic mental disorder, cocaine abuse, and delirium tremens.

> **?** *You see in the chart that a nursing order has been written placing a patient with command hallucinations on one-to-one observation. What is the rationale for this nursing intervention?*

Thought Content

Thought content is the specific meaning expressed in the patient's communication. It refers to the "what" of the patient's thinking.

Observations   Although the patient may talk about a variety of subjects during the interview, several content areas should be noted in the mental status examination (Box 6-3). They may be complicated and are often concealed by the patient, as in this clinical example.

Clinical Example   The patient's speech was rapid, and he acknowledged feeling as if his thoughts were coming too fast, saying, "My mind is racing ahead." The rapidity of his speech compounded the difficulty understanding him as he quickly moved from one topic to another in what appeared to be an unrelated manner. He denied any visual or auditory hallucinations; however, he believed that he could talk

Box **6-3** *Thought Content Descriptors*

Delusion: false belief that is firmly maintained even though it is not shared by others and is contradicted by social reality
  Religious delusion: belief that one is favored by a higher being or is an instrument of that being
  Somatic delusion: belief that one's body or parts of one's body are diseased or distorted
  Grandiose delusion: belief that one possesses greatness or special powers
  Paranoid delusion: excessive or irrational suspicion and distrust of others, characterized by systematized delusions that others are "out to get them" or spying on them
  Thought broadcasting: delusion about thoughts being aired to the outside world
  Thought insertion: delusion that thoughts are placed into the mind by outside people or influences
Depersonalization: the feeling of having lost self-identity and that things around the person are different, strange, or unreal
Hypochondriasis: somatic overconcern with and morbid attention to details of body functioning
Ideas of reference: incorrect interpretation of casual incidents and external events as having direct personal references
Magical thinking: belief that thinking equates with doing, characterized by lack of realistic relationship between cause and effect
Nihilistic ideas: thoughts of nonexistence and hopelessness
Obsession: an idea, emotion, or impulse that repetitively and insistently forces itself into consciousness, although it is unwelcome
Phobia: a morbid fear associated with extreme anxiety

with God if he needed a consultant on his life situation. He felt this was a special blessing given to him over others.

Tactful questioning by the nurse is needed to explore these areas. Does the patient have recurring, persistent thoughts? Is the patient afraid of certain objects or situations or worry excessively about body and health issues? Does the patient ever feel that things are strange or unreal? Has the patient ever experienced being outside of his or her body? Does the patient ever feel singled out or watched or talked about by others? Does the patient think that thoughts or actions are being controlled by an outside person or force? Does the patient claim to have psychic or other special powers or believe that others can read the patient's mind? Throughout this part of the interview it is important that the nurse obtain information and not dispute the patient's beliefs.

Clinical Implications   Obsessions and phobias are symptoms associated with anxiety disorders. Delusions, depersonalization, and ideas of reference suggest schizophrenia and other psychotic disorders.

Thought Process

Thought process is the "how" of the patient's self-expression. A patient's thought process is observed through speech. The patterns or forms of verbalization rather than the content are assessed.

Observations   A number of problems in a patient's thinking can be assessed (Box 6-4). The nurse might ask questions to evaluate the patient's thought process. Does the patient's thinking proceed in a systematic, organized, and logical manner? Is the patient's self-expression clear? Is it easy for the patient to move from one topic to another?

Clinical Implications   Circumstantial thinking may be a sign of defensiveness or paranoid thinking. Loose associations and neologisms suggest schizophrenia or other psychotic disorders. Flight of ideas indicates mania. Perseveration is often associated with brain damage and psychotic disorders. Word salad represents the highest level of thought disorganization.

Level of Consciousness

Mental status examinations routinely assess a patient's orientation to the current situation. Deciding whether a patient is oriented involves evaluating some basic cognitive functions.

Observations   A variety of terms can be used to describe a patient's level of consciousness, such as *confused, sedated,* or *stuporous.* In addition, the patient should be questioned regarding orientation to time, place, and person.

Typically the nurse can determine this by the patient's answers to three simple questions:

▼ Person: What is your name?
▼ Place: Where are you today (such as in what city or in what particular building)?
▼ Time: What is today's date?

If the patient answers correctly the nurse can note "oriented times three." Level of orientation can be pursued in greater depth, but this area may be confounded by sociocultural factors.

Fully functioning patients may be offended by questions about orientation, so the skilled nurse should integrate questions pertaining to this area in the course of the interview and develop other ways of assessing this category. For example, the nurse could use some of the approaches listed in Box 6-5.

Clinical Implications   Patients with organic mental disorder may give grossly inaccurate answers, with orientation to person remaining intact longer than orientation to time or place. Patients with schizophrenic disorders may say that they are someone else or somewhere else or reveal a personalized orientation to the world.

Memory

A mental status examination can provide a quick screen of potential memory problems but not a definitive answer to whether a specific impairment exists. Neuropsychological assessment is required to specify the nature and extent of memory impairment. Memory is broadly defined as the ability to recall past experiences.

Box **6-4** *Thought Process Descriptors*

Circumstantial: thought and speech associated with excessive and unnecessary detail that is usually relevant to a question, and an answer is ultimately given

Flight of ideas: overproductive speech characterized by rapid shifting from one topic to another and fragmented ideas

Loose associations: lack of a logical relationship between thoughts and ideas that renders speech and thought inexact, vague, diffuse, and unfocused

Neologisms: new word or words created by the patient, often a blend of other words

Perseveration: involuntary, excessive continuation or repetition of a single response, idea, or activity; may apply to speech or movement, but most often verbal

Tangential: similar to circumstantial but the person never returns to the central point and never answers the original question

Thought blocking: sudden stopping in the train of thought or in the middle of a sentence

Word salad: series of words that seem totally unrelated

Box **6-5** *Questions Useful in Determining Orientation*

QUESTIONS RELATED TO TIME
Have you been keeping track of the time lately?
What is the date today? (If patient claims not to recall, ask for an estimate; estimates can help assess level of disorientation.)
What month (or year) is it?
How long have you been here?

QUESTIONS RELATED TO PLACE
There's been a lot happening these past few days (or hours); I wonder if you can describe for me where you are?
Do you recall what city we're in?
What is the name of the building we're in right now?
Do you know what part of the hospital we're in?

QUESTIONS RELATED TO PERSON
What is your name?
Where are you from?
Where do you currently live?
What kinds of activities do you engage in during your free time?
Are you employed? If so, what do you do for a living?
Are you married? If so, what is your spouse's name?
Do you have any children?

Observations The following areas must be tested:

▼ Remote memory: recall of events, information, and people from the distant past

▼ Recent memory: recall of events, information, and people from the past week or so

▼ Immediate memory: recall of information or data to which a person was just exposed

Recall of remote events involves reviewing information from the patient's history. This part of the evaluation can be woven into the history-taking portion of the nursing assessment. This involves asking the patient questions about time and place of birth, names of schools attended, date of marriage, ages of family members, and so forth. The problem with an evaluation of the patient's remote memory is that the nurse is often unable to tell whether the patient is reporting events accurately. This brings about the possibility of *confabulation,* when the patient makes up stories to recount situations or events that cannot be remembered. The nurse may need to call on past records or the report of family or friends to confirm this historical information.

Recent memory can be tested by asking the patient to recall the events of the past 24 hours. A reliable informant may be needed to verify this information. Another test of recent memory is to ask the patient to remember three words (an object, a color, and an address) and then to repeat them 15 minutes later in the interview.

Immediate recall can be tested by asking the patient to repeat a series of numbers either forward or backward within a 10-second interval. The nurse should begin with a short series of numbers and proceed to longer lists.

Clinical Implications Loss of memory occurs with organicity, dissociative disorder, and conversion disorder. Patients with Alzheimer's disease retain remote memory longer than recent memory. Anxiety and depression can impair immediate retention and recent memory.

Level of Concentration and Calculation

Concentration is the patient's ability to pay attention during the course of the interview. Calculation is the person's ability to do simple math. These and other areas of cognitive functioning may vary in expected and unexpected ways (Box 6-6).

Observations The nurse should note the patient's level of distractibility. Calculation can be assessed by asking the patient to do the following:

▼ Count from 1 to 20 rapidly

▼ Do simple calculations, such as 2×3 or $21 + 7$

▼ Serially subtract 7 from 100

If patients have difficulty subtracting 7 from 100, they can be asked to subtract 3 from 20 in the same way. Finally, more functional calculation skills can be assessed by asking practical questions such as "How many nickels are there in $1.35?"

Clinical Implications The clinical implications of this part of the mental status examination must be carefully evaluated. Many psychiatric illnesses impair the ability to concentrate and complete simple calculations. It is particularly important to differentiate between organic mental disorder, anxiety, and depression.

Information and Intelligence

Information and intelligence are controversial areas of assessment, and the nurse should be cautious about judging intelligence after a brief and limited contact typical of the mental status examination (see Critical Thinking about Contemporary Issues). The nurse should also remember that information in this category is highly influenced by sociocultural factors of the nurse, the patient, and the treatment setting.

CRITICAL THINKING *about* Contemporary Issues

Can a Person's Intellectual Functioning Be Validly Assessed in the Mental Status Examination?

The evaluation of a person's intellectual functioning during the mental status examination is a subject of controversy, given the brief nature of the interview and the sociocultural biases that may be brought to it. Nonetheless, knowing a patient's intellectual capacity is important to the nurse in evaluating the patient's coping resources and designing an effective treatment plan.

Furthermore, it has been suggested that there is more than one type of intelligence. Rather, there are seven different types of intelligence.[4]

Linguistic intelligence
Logical-mathematical intelligence
Spatial intelligence
Musical intelligence
Bodily-kinesthetic intelligence
Interpersonal intelligence
Intrapersonal intelligence.

The last two intelligences taken together (interpersonal and intrapersonal) can be described as forming one's personal intelligence or "emotional quotient."[5]

This expanded view of intelligence takes into account the talents people express in the arts, athletics, the ability to work cooperatively with people, and self-definition, as well as the more traditional verbal and mathematical skills usually assessed in standard intelligence tests. For example, a patient may have excellent spatial and mathematical intelligence but may lack formal education and interpersonal intelligence, and thus have difficulty obtaining a job. Such a person could be successful at a job that involved minimal contact with people but close work with designs and visual layouts. Nurses should take a broad approach to the assessment of intellectual functioning. This will allow them to identify the intellectual strengths, skills, and abilities of patients that may otherwise be overlooked.

Box **6-6** *Gender Differences in the Brain*

Women and men differ in physical attributes and in the way they think. The effect of sex hormones on brain organization appears to occur early in life, so the effects of the environment are secondary to the effects of biology. Behavioral, neurological, and endocrinologic studies help explain the processes giving rise to gender differences in the brain. Major gender differences in intellectual functioning seem to lie in patterns of ability rather than in the overall level of intelligence. For example, the problem-solving tasks favoring women and men are shown below.

PROBLEM-SOLVING TASKS FAVORING WOMEN

Women tend to perform better than men on tests of perceptual speed, in which subjects must rapidly identify matching items, as in pairing the house on the far left with its twin:

In addition, women remember whether an object or a series of objects has been displaced or rearranged:

On some tests of ideational fluency, such as those in which subjects must list objects that are the same color, and on tests of verbal fluency, in which participants must list words that begin with the same letter, women also outperform men:

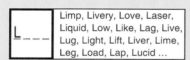

Women do better on precision manual tasks—that is, those involving fine motor coordination—such as placing the pegs in holes on a board:

And women do better than men on mathematical calculation tests:

PROBLEM-SOLVING TASKS FAVORING MEN

Men tend to perform better than women on certain spatial tasks. They do well on tests that involve mentally rotating an object or manipulating it in some fashion, such as imagining turning this three-dimensional object

or determining where the holes punched in a folded piece of paper will fall when the paper is unfolded:

Men also are more accurate than women in target-directed motor skills, such as guiding or intercepting projectiles:

Men do better on disembedding tests, in which they have to find a simple shape, such as the one on the left, hidden within a more complex figure:

And men tend to do better than women on tests of mathematical reasoning:

From Kimura D: *Scientific American* 267:120, 1992 (Jared Schneidman, illustrator).

Observations   The nurse should assess the patient's last grade of school completed, general knowledge, and use of vocabulary. It is also critically important to assess the patient's level of literacy. The ability to conceptualize and abstract can be tested by having the patient explain a series of proverbs. The patient can be given an example of a proverb with its interpretation and then be asked to explain what several proverbs mean. Common proverbs include the following:

▼ When it rains, it pours.
▼ A stitch in time saves nine.
▼ A rolling stone gathers no moss.
▼ The proof of the pudding is in the eating.
▼ People who live in glass houses shouldn't throw stones.
▼ A bird in the hand is worth two in the bush.

Most adults are able to interpret proverbs as symbolic of human behavior or events. However, sociocultural background should be considered when assessing a patient's information and intelligence.

If the patient's educational level is below the eighth grade, asking the patient to list similarities between a series of paired objects may better help the nurse assess the ability to abstract. The following paired objects are often used:

▼ Bicycle and bus
▼ Apple and pear
▼ Television and newspaper

A higher-level reply addresses function, whereas a description of structure indicates more concrete thinking. To assess a patient's general knowledge the nurse can ask the patient to name the last five presidents, the mayor, five large cities, or the occupation of a well-known person.

Clinical Implications   The patient's educational level and any learning disabilities should be carefully evaluated. Mental retardation should be ruled out whenever possible. The patient's level of literacy may be part of a general assessment, but it is also an important factor in any health teaching or didactic information presented to the patient.

Judgment

Judgment involves making decisions that are constructive and adaptive. It involves the ability to understand facts and draw conclusions from relationships.

Observations   Judgment can be evaluated by exploring the patient's involvement in activities, relationships, and vocational choices. For example, is the patient regularly involved in illegal or dangerous activities or engaged in destructive relationships with others? It is also useful to determine whether the judgments are deliberate or impulsive. Finally, several hypothetical situations can be presented for the patient to evaluate:

▼ What would you do if you found a stamped, addressed envelope lying on the ground?
▼ How would you find your way out of a forest in the daytime?

▼ What would you do if you entered your house and smelled gas?
▼ If you won $10,000 what would you do with it?

Clinical Implications   Judgment is impaired in organic mental disorders, schizophrenia, psychotic disorders, intoxication, and borderline or low IQ. It may also be impaired in manic patients and those with personality disorders.

> **?** *What factors would you consider in evaluating the judgment of a man who engages in bungee jumping, rock climbing, and skydiving? How would this compare with a woman who has been in many relationships with abusive men?*

Insight

Insight is the patient's understanding of the nature of the problem or illness.

Observations   It is important for the nurse to determine whether the patient accepts or denies the presence of a problem or illness. In addition, the nurse should ask whether the patient blames the problem on someone else or some external factors. Several questions may help to determine the patient's degree of insight. What does the patient think about the current situation? What does the patient want others, including the nurse, to do about it? The following clinical example illustrates a patient's level of insight.

Clinical Example   The patient described several problems he was having at work. He reluctantly stated that he might have to change, but really thought his difficulties were because of his wife's drinking. He believed he could do nothing until she changed.

Clinical Implications   Insight is impaired in many psychotic illnesses, including organic mental disorder, psychosis, substance abuse, eating disorders, personality disorders, and borderline or low IQ. Whether or not a patient sees the need for treatment also critically affects the therapeutic alliance, setting of mutual goals, implementation of the treatment plan, and future adherence to it.

Documenting Clinical Information

Information from the mental status examination may be recorded in various ways. Some clinicians write a descriptive report such as the one presented in the case study on p. 123. Written reports should be brief, clear, and concise and address all categories of information. Others use an outline format that is completed with short answers. Still others use a format that is compatible with computerized information systems. Regardless of the format, important findings should be documented and verbatim responses by the patient should be recorded whenever they add important information and support the nurse's assessment.

Mini-Mental State

At times it is not practical or desirable to complete a full mental status examination. On these occasions, nurses may find it helpful to use the mini-mental state examination.[3] It is a simplified scored form of the cognitive mental status examination. It consists of 11 questions, requires only 5 to 10 minutes to administer, and can therefore be used quickly and routinely. It is "mini" because it concentrates on only the cognitive aspects of mental functions and excludes questions concerning mood, abnormal psychological experiences, and the content or process of thinking. This examination is reproduced in Box 6-7.

PSYCHOLOGICAL TESTS

Psychological tests are of two types: those designed to evaluate intellectual and cognitive abilities and those designed to describe personality functioning. Commonly used intelligence tests are the Wechsler Adult Intelligence Scale (WAIS) and the Wechsler Intelligence Scale for Children (WISC). Although intelligence tests often are criticized as culturally biased, their ability to determine a person's strengths and weaknesses within the culture provides important therapeutic information.

Material obtained from projective tests reflects aspects of a person's personality function, including reality testing ability, impulse control, major defenses, interpersonal conflicts, and self-concept. A battery of tests is usually administered to provide comprehensive information. The Rorschach Test, Thematic Apperception Test (TAT), Bender Gestalt Test, and Minnesota Multiphasic Personality Inventory (MMPI) are commonly used by the clinical psychologist.

BEHAVIORAL RATING SCALES

The psychological context of psychiatric nursing care goes beyond the important assessment of a patient's mental status. Neither mental health nor mental illness can be mea-

Box **6-7** *Mini-Mental State*

Maximum Score	Score	
		ORIENTATION
5	( )	What is the (year) (season) (date) (day) (month)?
5	( )	Where are we (state) (county) (town) (hospital) (floor)?
		REGISTRATION
3	( )	Name three objects: Give 1 second to say each. Then ask the patient to repeat all three after you have said them. Give 1 point for each correct answer. Then repeat them until the patient learns all three. Count trials and record.
		ATTENTION AND CALCULATION
5	( )	Serial sevens. Give 1 point for each correct. Stop after five answers. Alternatively, spell *world* backwards.
		RECALL
3	( )	Ask for three objects repeated above. Give 1 point for each correct.
		LANGUAGE
9	( )	Name a pencil and watch when pointed to (2 points). Repeat the following, "No ifs, ands, or buts" (1 point). Follow a three-stage command: "Take a paper in your right hand, fold it in half, and put it on the floor" (3 points). Read and obey the following: "Close your eyes" (1 point). Write a sentence (1 point). Copy design (1 point).
Total Score	_____	

From Folstein M, Folstein S, McHugh P: Mini-mental state: a practical method for grading the cognitive state of patients for the clinician, *J Psychiatr Res* 12:189, 1975.

sured directly. Rather, its measurement depends on gathering a number of behavioral indicators of adaptive or maladaptive responses, which together represent the overall concept.

Many behavioral rating scales and measurement tools have been designed to help clinicians do the following:

▼ Measure the extent of the patient's problems
▼ Make an accurate diagnosis
▼ Track patient progress over time
▼ Document the efficacy of treatment

Each of these points is very important to the psychiatric nurse. The knowledge base for psychiatric care is expanding rapidly, and increased emphasis is being placed on clearly describing the nature of the patient's problems and the extent of the patient's progress toward attaining the expected outcomes of treatment.[7] Thus nurses must be able to demonstrate in a valid and reliable way what problems they are treating and what effect their nursing care is having on attaining the treatment goals.

Most psychiatric nurses have not routinely used behavioral rating scales in their practice, and there is little nursing literature on the subject.[1,6] Nonetheless, this is a critical area for contemporary psychiatric nursing practice. Nurses should become familiar with the many standardized rating scales that are available to enhance each stage of the nursing process. Some of the more commonly used behavioral rating scales are listed in Table 6-1. Any of these scales can be used by nurses with training. If the scales are to be used by a group of nurses, such as nurses working together in a specific treatment program or facility, interrater reliability among the nurses should be established.

These tools should not replace required nursing documentation. Rather, they can be used to complement nursing care and provide measurable indicators of treatment outcome. For example, if the nurse is caring for a patient with depression it would be helpful to use one of the depression rating scales with the patient at the beginning of treatment to establish a baseline profile of the patient's symptoms and help confirm the diagnosis. The nurse might then administer the same scale at various times during the course of treatment to measure the patient's progress. Finally, completing the rating scale at the end of treatment would document the efficacy of the care provided.

The increasing focus in health care on high quality, cost containment, and documented effectiveness requires that psychiatric nurses be able to demonstrate the value of the services they provide. The psychological context of psychiatric nursing care suggests the tools and process nurses can use to meet this challenge.

CASE STUDY

Ms. T was a stylishly dressed, neatly groomed, slender woman in apparent good physical health who appeared to be her stated 22 years of age. She was cooperative during the interview but had difficulty expressing herself in specific terms. Her vague responses left the interviewer feeling perplexed about the difficulties she was describing.

The patient was alert and awake and oriented to person, place, and time. Immediate recall and recent memory were intact, demonstrated in her ability to recall three unrelated objects immediately and again in 15 minutes. Some of the historical information given was inconsistent with historical facts reported by her father. Although the vocabulary used by Ms. T and her knowledge of general information was congruent with her twelfth-grade education and past employment, she had difficulty completing the serial sevens but performed serial threes with ease. She stated that she was "nervous," which may be a factor related to performance. She was able to abstract two of three proverbs presented.

Proverb	Interpretation
Don't cry over spilled milk.	"If something happens, then forget about it. Maybe things will get better."
A rolling stone gathers no moss.	"A good person gathers no enemies. If a person stays active, he won't get depressed."

Proverb	Interpretation
People who live in glass houses shouldn't throw stones.	"The glass will break."

Her responses to hypothetical situations were appropriate; however, the manner in which she coped with difficulties at work and home showed impaired judgment about personal issues.

Ms. T's speech was clear, coherent, and of normal rate and tone. Except for the vague, tangential manner in which she discussed her concern for her aunt, her communication was goal directed. There were no apparent delusions, hallucinations, or illusions. She denied any obsessions, compulsions, or phobias.

The central theme during the interview was her fear of being irresponsible and hurting her aunt. Her sadness and concern about her behavior in relation to the aunt pervaded the interview. She appeared nervous (looking away, fidgeting) and cried whenever she talked about her aunt. She described her mood as "low" and rated it as a 4 on a scale of 1 to 10. She denied any suicidal or homicidal ideas or plan previously or at the present time.

Her insight was questionable because she debated her need for treatment, but she agreed to return. She knew that a problem existed but was unaware of the causes of her behavior.

TABLE **6-1** *Behavioral Rating Scales*

CONTENT AREA	SCALE	CONTENT AREA	SCALE
GENERAL HEALTH	MOS Health Survey (SF-36)	**EATING DISORDERS**	Body Attitudes Test Diagnostic Survey for Eating Disorders (DSED) Eating Habits Checklist Eating Behaviors Diary Eating Disorders Inventory 2 (EDI-2)
GENERAL PSYCHIATRIC	Acculturation Scale Assessing Coping Strategies (COPE) Behavior and Symptom Identification Scale (BASIS-32) Brief Symptom Inventory (BSI) Client Satisfaction Questionnaire (CSQ) Clinical Global Impression (CGI) Colorado Client Assessment Record (CCAR) Family Burden Interview Schedule (FBIS) Functional Status Questionnaire (FSQ) General Health Questionnaire (GHQ) Global Assessment Scale (GAS) Global Assessment of Functioning Scale (GAF) NIMH Global Consensus Rating Scales Nurse Observation Scale for Inpatient Evaluation (NOSIE) Quality of Life Interview (QOLI) Service Satisfaction Questionnaire (SSQ-30) Severity of Psychosocial Stressors Scale Symptoms Checklist-90 (SCL-90)	**ORGANIC MENTAL DISORDERS**	Alzheimer's Disease Assessment Scale (ADAS) Cohen-Mansfield Agitation Inventory Blessed Dementia Scale Cornell Scale for Depression in Dementia Face-Hand Test Haycox Dementia Behavioral Scale Memory and Behavior Problems Checklist Neurobehavioral Rating Scale for Dementia (NRS)
		PSYCHOTIC DISORDERS	Andreasen Scale for Assessment of Negative Symptoms (SANS) Andreasen Scale for Assessment of Positive Symptoms (SAPS) Brief Psychiatric Rating Scale (BPRS) Life Skills Profile: Schizophrenia (LSP) Schizophrenia Outcomes Module (SOM) University of Washington Paranoia Scale
AFFECTIVE DISORDERS	Assessment of Suicidal Potentiality Beck Depression Inventory (BDI) Carroll Self-Rating Scale Center for Epidemiologic Studies Depression Scale (CES-D) Depression Outcome Module (DOM) Family Burden Interview Schedule (FBIS) Geriatric Depression Scale (GDS) Hamilton Depression Scale (Ham-D) Inventory for Depressive Symptomatology (IDS) Manic-State Scale Montgomery-Asberg Depression Rating Scale (MADRS) Raskin Depression Scale Young Mania Scale Zung Self-Rating Depression Scale (ZSRDS)	**SUBSTANCE USE DISORDERS**	Addiction Severity Index (ASI) Alcohol Use Scale (AUS) Brief Drug Abuse Screening Test (B-DAST) CAGE Questionnaire Children of Alcoholics Screening Test (CAST) Clinical Institute Withdrawal Assessment-Alcohol, Revised (CIWA-AR) Drug Use Scale (DUS) Michigan Alcoholism Screening Tool (MAST) Substance Abuse Outcome Module (SAOM) Substance Abuse Treatment Schedule (SATS) Treatment Services Review (TSR)
ANXIETY DISORDERS	Beck Anxiety Inventory (BAI) Covi Anxiety Scale Dissociative Experience Scale Dissociative Disorders Interview Schedule (DDIS) Hamilton Rating Scale for Anxiety (Ham-A) Maudsley Obsessional Compulsive Inventory Panic Disorder Outcomes Module (PDOM) Spielberger Anxiety State-Trait Taylor Anxiety Scale Yale-Brown Obsessive Compulsive Scale (YBOCS) Zung Anxiety Scale	**CHILD/ ADOLESCENT**	Behavior Problems Checklist Brief Psychiatric Rating Scale for Children Child Behavior Checklist (CBCL) Children's Global Assessment Scale (CGAS) Competency Skills Questionnaire (CSQ) Conners Parent Rating Scale Home and School Questionnaire Self-Control Rating Scale Yale-Brown Obsessive Compulsive Scale (YBOCS) for Children
		MEDICATION EFFECTS	Abnormal Involuntary Movement Scale (AIMS) Simpson-Angus Extrapyramidal Symptoms Scale

Summary

1. The mental status examination represents a cross-section of the patient's psychological life at that time. It requires that the nurse observe the patient's behavior and describe it in an objective, nonjudgmental manner.

2. The categories assessed in the mental status examination include the patient's appearance, speech, motor activity, mood, affect, interaction during the interview, perceptions, thought content, thought process, level of consciousness, memory, level of concentration and calculation, information and intelligence, judgment, and insight.

3. Psychological tests evaluate intellectual and cognitive abilities and describe personality functioning.

4. Behavioral rating scales help clinicians measure the extent of the patient's problem, make an accurate diagnosis, track patient progress over time, and document the efficacy of treatment. They should be used by psychiatric nurses to complement nursing care and provide measurable indicators of treatment outcome.

your **INTERNET**
c o n n e c t i o n

ERIC Clearinghouse on Assessment and Evaluation
http://ericae2.educ.cua.edu/main.htm

American Psychological Association PsychNET
http://www.apa.org

Chapter Review Questions

1. Match the terms in Column A with the correct description in Column B.

Column A

- C. Affect
- A. Delusion
- E. Flight of ideas
- F. Hallucinations
- B. Illusions
- H. Insight
- D. Loose associations
- G. Mood

Column B

- A. False belief not shared by others or confirmed by reality
- B. False perception or response to a sensory stimulation
- C. Feeling, mood, or emotional tone
- D. Lack of a logical relationship between thoughts and ideas, resulting in unfocused speech
- E. Overproductive speech with rapid shifting of topics and ideas
- F. Perceptual distortion arising from any of the five senses
- G. Self-report by patient of his or her prevailing emotional state
- H. Understanding by the patient of the nature of his or her problem or illness

2. Fill in the blanks.

A. A patient who describes the death of a younger brother without any emotional response is said to have _flat effect_.

B. _Command hallucinations_ are false sensory impressions that tell the patient to do something he would not ordinarily do.

C. The most common type of hallucination involves the sense of _hearing_.

D. When a patient makes up stories in response to questions about situations or events that cannot be remembered it is called _confabulation_.

3. Provide short answers for the following questions.

A. What are the five major categories of information that should be included in a mental status examination?

B. What three questions have been asked when a patient is described as oriented times three?

C. Identify four reasons why psychiatric nurses should use behavioral rating scales in their practice.

REFERENCES

1. Acron S: Use of the brief psychiatric rating scale by nurses, *J Psychosoc Nurs Ment Health Serv* 31:9, 1993.
2. Dilsaver S: The mental status examination, *Am Fam Physician* 41:1489, 1990.
3. Folstein M, Folstein S, McHugh P: Mini-mental state: a practical method for grading the cognitive state of patients for the clinician, *J Psychiatr Res* 12:189, 1975.
4. Gardner H: *Multiple intelligences,* New York, 1993, Basic Books.

5. Goleman D: *Emotional intelligence,* New York, 1995, Bantam.
6. McGorry P, Goodwin R, Stuart G: The development, use, and reliability of the brief psychiatric rating scale (nursing modification): an assessment procedure for the nursing team in clinical and research settings, *Compr Psychiatry* 29:575, 1988.
7. Sederer L, Dickey B: *Outcomes assessment in clinical practice,* Baltimore, 1996, Williams & Wilkins.
8. Sommers-Flanagan J, Sommers-Flanagan R: *Foundations of therapeutic interviewing,* Boston, 1992, Allyn & Bacon.
9. Trzepacz P, Baker R: *The psychiatric mental status examination,* New York, 1993, Oxford University Press.

ANNOTATED SUGGESTED READINGS

*Acron S: Use of the brief psychiatric rating scale by nurses, *J Psychosocial Nurs* 31:9, 1993.
One of the few articles in the field to discuss the use of rating scales by nurses. Describes the BPRS and its use by psychiatric nurses.

*Nursing Reference.

Dunner D: Diagnostic assessment, psychiatric assessment, *Psychiatr Clin North America* 16:431, 1993.
Excellent overview of structured interviews and behavioral rating scales used in psychiatry.
Gardner H: *Multiple intelligences,* New York, 1993, Basic Books.
Reviews the varied human intelligences with the goal of mobilizing the wide range of human abilities and helping people feel more competent. Interesting reading.
Morrison J: *The first interview: a guide to methods and measures,* New York, 1993, The Guilford Press.
Provides a good, clear discussion of interviewing with psychiatric patients.
Sederer L, Dickey B: *Outcomes assessment in clinical practice,* Baltimore, 1996, Williams and Wilkins.
The best text to review outcome and patient satisfaction measures used by psychiatric clinicians in the field. A handy paperback to own, given the importance of this work.
Sommes-Flanagan J, Sommes-Flanagan R: *Foundations of therapeutic interviewing,* Boston, 1992, Allyn & Bacon.
Excellent overview of points to consider when interviewing patients, including the mental status examination.

Sociocultural Context of Psychiatric Nursing Care

Linda D. Oakley

© 1998 M.C. Escher/Cordon Art, Baarn, Holland.

We know what we belong to, where we come from, and where we are going. We may not know it with our brains, but we know it with our roots. **Noel Coward** *This Happy Breed*

LEARNING OBJECTIVES

After studying this chapter the student should be able to:

▼ Describe the qualities of a culturally sensitive psychiatric nurse

▼ Discuss the importance of the sociocultural risk factors of age, ethnicity, gender, education, income, and belief system in developing, experiencing, and recovering from psychiatric disorders

▼ Identify sociocultural stressors that hinder the delivery of psychiatric care

▼ Analyze the impact of sociocultural factors on coping responses

▼ Apply knowledge of sociocultural risk factors to the process of nursing assessment and diagnosis

▼ Discuss the treatment implications of culturally sensitive psychiatric care

TOPICAL OUTLINE

Cultural Sensitivity
Sociocultural Risk Factors
  Age
  Ethnicity
  Gender
  Education
  Income
  Belief System
Sociocultural Stressors
Impact on Coping Responses
Nursing Assessment and Diagnosis
Treatment Implications
  Service Delivery Systems
  Counseling
  Psychobiology

Holistic psychiatric nursing care embraces all aspects of the individual in the assessment, diagnosis, and treatment process. An important element of this holistic perspective is the nurse's sensitivity to the sociocultural context of care. In each interaction with the patient the nurse is aware of the broader world in which the patient lives and knows that perceptions of health and illness, help-seeking behavior, and treatment adherence depend on the patient's beliefs, social norms, and cultural values. Consequently, high-quality psychiatric nursing care must incorporate the unique aspects of the individual into every element of practice and be based on an understanding of the importance of culture, as outlined in Box 7-1. Knowledge of culture and its impact on mental health is gradually

Box *7-1* *The Functions of Culture*

Perception: Perception of reality is based on a cultural interpretation and understanding of events.
Motives: Motives for behavior are conditioned by the values assumed by a culture.
Identity: Individual and group identity is fostered by the oral, written, and social constructs defining a culture.
Values: Concepts of ethics and morality are conditioned by cultural background.
Communication: Language, music, and dance are the external expressions of culture.
Emotions: Emotions are significantly enabled and shaped by cultural ideas, practices, and institutions.

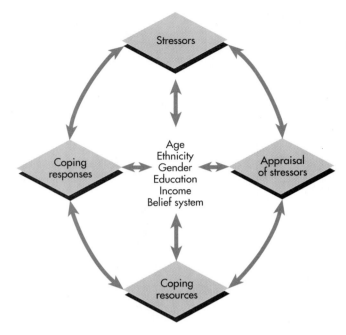

Fig. 7-1 Sociocultural context of psychiatric care.

unfolding, and nurses need to keep abreast of new information and its implications for psychiatric nursing practice.

CULTURAL SENSITIVITY

In recent years greater attention has focused on culturally relevant mental health care.[12,14,22] Nursing expectations are also evolving from a superficial knowledge of differences in age, gender, and ethnic groups to the implementation of culturally sensitive nursing care.[6]

Culturally sensitive nurses have the knowledge and skills to intervene successfully in the lives of patients from culturally diverse backgrounds. As a practice skill, cultural sensitivity is the ability to view each patient as a unique individual, fully considering the patient's cultural experiences within the context of the common developmental challenges faced by all people. The nurse applies this information in nursing interventions that are consistent with the life experiences and cultural values of patients.

Finally, culturally sensitive nurses are in touch with their own personal and cultural experiences. These nurses provide individualized patient care and are aware of actions that may offend a patient who is not a member of the nurses' ethnic, social, or cultural group. The culturally sensitive nurse understands the importance of social and cultural forces, recognizes the uniqueness of the patient, respects nurse-patient differences, and incorporates sociocultural information into psychiatric nursing care.

SOCIOCULTURAL RISK FACTORS

The concept of risk factors is important to understanding how people acquire, experience, and recover from illness. Risk factors are the same as the predisposing factors that nurses assess in the Stuart Stress Adaptation Model of psychiatric nursing (see Chapter 4). Understanding the risk factors involved in health and illness is essential in the prevention, early detection, and effective treatment of physiological illnesses such as cardiac, pulmonary, and hepatic diseases.

Identifying risk factors also is valuable in providing psychiatric care. Risk factors for psychiatric disorders are char-

acteristics of a person that can significantly increase the potential for developing a psychiatric disorder, decrease the potential for recovery, or both. Perhaps the most important outcome of the inclusion of risk or predisposing factors in nursing practice is the development of individualized, culturally sensitive, and socially relevant mental health care.

The sociocultural perspective described in this chapter focuses on age, ethnicity, gender, education, income, and belief systems. No one or two of these factors alone adequately describes the sociocultural context of nursing care; however, together they provide a sociocultural profile of the patient that is essential to psychiatric nursing practice. These risk factors include social norms, cultural beliefs, and personal values, and influence the patient's exposure to stressors, appraisal of stressors, coping resources, and coping responses, as described in the Stuart Stress Adaptation Model (Fig. 7-1).

The sociocultural risk factors of age, ethnicity, gender, education, income, and belief system are predisposing, or conditioning, factors that influence the amount and type of coping resources available to a person. These risk factors do not cause future events. For example, being female may be a predisposing factor for the development of depression, but it does not cause depression. In fact, some of these factors may be a consequence of the illness. For example, being poor may be the result of a substance abuse disorder rather than the cause of it. These risk factors are important because they influence the person's vulnerability to, development of, and recovery from psychiatric disorders. Finally, it is important to realize that these sociocultural risk factors can interact so that different factors become important at different times.

This sociocultural view does not assume that individual members of groups based on age, ethnicity, gender, education, income, or belief systems all have the same risk of developing a psychiatric disorder, nor does it assume that a person's risk of developing a psychiatric disorder is constant. Rather, individual differences between the members of a group and contextual variations in individual risk are key principles of this perspective. Most important, this view does not draw generalizations about groups based on age, ethnicity, gender, education, income, or belief system. Literature that describes and summarizes the values or beliefs of specific populations such as blacks, Hispanics, and Asians often creates new stereotypes, and these generalizations can further depersonalize nursing care. In contrast, the sociocultural view is based on the assessment of risk factors for each person over time as change occurs in the individual and the social environment.

Important health-related differences do exist between various groups in society. Group differences have been reported and examined in relation to a number of physical and psychiatric illnesses.[28] For example, researchers have noted that more females than males are diagnosed and treated for depression regardless of age, ethnicity, education, or income.[11,19] It is not known whether the different prevalence of a psychiatric disorder between groups is an indicator of clinical differences, cultural differences, or both. Specifically, it is not known whether the prevalence of depression among females is greater than that among males because the two groups are clinically different or because females are exposed to more social or cultural stressors that precipitate depression. If the latter were true, it would suggest that if males were exposed to the same stressors and were taught the same coping style as females, the rate of depression for the two groups would be equal.

This example highlights the incorrect assumption that all members of a group behave, think, and feel similarly. Finally, it illustrates the importance of integrating biological, psychological, and cultural contributions to understand more fully the dimensions of mental health and psychiatric illness.

Much research on sociocultural risk factors for psychiatric disorders is relevant to psychiatric nursing practice. However, the scope of the field is beyond that of this chapter, so the reader is referred to other sources for more detailed information.[12,14] Some findings about each risk factor and their possible effects on holistic psychiatric nursing care are described in the following sections. Box 7-2 lists some sociocultural trends and their influences on the health-care system.

> ❓ *Think of a group you belong to based on one of your sociocultural characteristics. What stereotypes exist about this group? Do you fit these stereotypes?*

Box *7-2 Sociocultural Diversity and the Health Care System*

Current U.S. data suggest that the following sociocultural trends will influence the health care system and the way health care is provided:

▼ The population will increase by 60% to almost 400 million by the year 2050.

▼ Growth will be concentrated at the two ends of the age spectrum. By 2050 the population aged 65 and over will more than double, and the population 85 years and older will be the fastest-growing age group.

▼ The U.S. population is becoming more diverse by race and ethnicity. Hispanics will be the largest ethnic group, making up one quarter of the population.

▼ The United States has become a predominantly urban nation, with the population occupying only 2.5% of the land mass.

These trends will have a profound impact on the health care system for the following reasons:

▼ As the aging population grows, there will be an increase in chronic conditions and chronic diseases related to behavior that will exact a greater toll on the health care system.

▼ A rise in the number of young people will bring new waves of problems typically committed by the young, such as murder, rape, robbery, and assault. Almost half of all violent crimes are committed by people under age 24, with those 15 to 19 years of age responsible for most. The overall crime rate has increased 500% since 1960.

▼ Minority populations are currently underserved, a problem that may only intensify. In addition, there is an expected increase in low–birth-weight babies among minority populations.

▼ Minority populations are underrepresented in all health care professions, causing concern about whether health care providers will understand health problems within a cultural context and be able to provide culturally sensitive care.

From *Advances,* Newsletter of the Robert Wood Johnson Foundation, Fall 1993.

Age

It has been reported that the frequency of seeking mental health treatment decreases with age and that help-seeking behavior peaks between 25 and 44 years of age and then declines.[23] A recent review of depression in the elderly revealed the importance of a variety of social factors.[20] Among the elderly the prevalence of depression in women is higher than in men, and elders with high socioeconomic status and levels of education were less likely to be depressed than those with low socioeconomic status and less education. Thus female gender, low income, and less education were identified as risk factors for depression in the elderly.

It was also found that as age increased, the prevalence of depression decreased. Even when compared with younger age groups, elders tended to recover from depression more quickly and were less likely to have a recurrence. Thus younger age emerged as a risk factor for depressive illness, possibly because elders who are socioeconomically stable may also be more resilient because they may have developed effective coping strategies and have less demanding or less stressful social roles than younger adults.[17]

Ethnicity

The term *ethnicity* as used in this chapter includes a person's racial, national, tribal, linguistic, and cultural origin or background. Ethnicity has been shown to influence the development of and recovery from psychiatric disorders. Specifically, significant differences exist in the prevalence of certain disorders among various ethnic groups and in their use of mental health services. For example, the most severe types of psychopathology tend to be diagnosed in black patients, with blacks being underrepresented in affective disorders and overdiagnosed as schizophrenic.[13,32] In addition, blacks, Native Americans, Hispanics, and Asians have higher rates of admission to state and county mental hospitals than to community and private psychiatric hospitals.[21,35]

Regarding the use of mental health services, one study sampled almost 27,000 adults and found that Asians, Hispanics, and whites tended to use outpatient mental health services, whereas blacks tended to use emergency mental health services.[16] Asian, Hispanic, and white females used more services than their male counterparts, thereby improving their probability of recovery. However, the reverse was true for blacks; black males used more mental health services than black females. The authors concluded that because blacks relied on emergency services that are often very brief, they tended to receive less treatment than those in other ethnic groups. In a similar study that included a measure of improvement in patient functioning after treatment, blacks showed the lowest rate of positive treatment outcome despite a high treatment rate and the fact that the patients and providers were members of the same ethnic group.

Recent studies have also examined racial differences in relation to treatment and have found that nonpsychotic black patients had shorter lengths of stay in inpatient facilities than white patients with similar disorders, white patients were more likely to be on one-to-one observational status, and clinicians were more likely to order urine drug screens for black patients with high socioeconomic status than for comparable white patients.[10] It has also been reported that black patients presenting to an emergency service were prescribed more psychiatric medication, receiving more oral doses and more injections of antipsychotic medications and at higher dosages. The tendency to overmedicate black patients was lower, however, when clinicians' efforts to engage the patient in treatment were rated higher.[30] These studies point to the importance of engaging patients from diverse ethnic groups in the treatment process, and the need for clinical skills and training in bridging cultural differences.

How might ethnicity influence the coping responses and the specific symptoms expressed by a patient?

Gender

As a predisposing risk factor, gender is similar to ethnicity in that at first glance there appear to be distinctive male and female patterns of risk. However, when all psychiatric disorders are included, the prevalence of mental illness among males and females is roughly equal.[3] The actual difference between the two groups is in the type of disorder that is most commonly diagnosed. Substance abuse and antisocial personality disorder are the most prevalent psychiatric disorders among males, whereas affective disorders and anxiety disorders are most prevalent among females. In contrast, the prevalence of schizophrenia and manic episodes for males and females is about equal.

These findings support the idea that male and female role socialization in contemporary American society is a significant determinant of the perception of health and illness and that the risk of psychiatric disorders may be sex typed by sociocultural factors. Specifically, it has been proposed that males are taught to aggressively externalize their psychological experiences, whereas females are taught to passively internalize their social experiences.

In a study aimed at measuring gender differences in schizophrenia, the authors found that males and females had the same psychiatric disorder but that for females, conformity to gender roles may have delayed the onset of severe symptoms.[9] Specifically, the mean age of disorder onset was 41 years for females and 31 years for males. This is an important difference because the age of onset is a critical factor in the prognosis for schizophrenia, in that early onset is associated with a longer course of illness and poorer treatment outcome. Thus men have a poorer prognosis for schizophrenia than do women in terms of both symptoms and course of illness. There is also evidence that men face a less tolerant social reaction to functional impairment and may experience greater pressure to assume social responsibilities.[2]

This study also illustrates the interactions of risk factors; gender appears to be significant in the development of schizophrenia, but age seems to be more important than gender in recovery from the illness. A similar relationship between early onset and more difficult course of illness has been reported for male and female depression. Specifically, females develop depression at an earlier age than men do and have longer episodes of depression.[31]

The following clinical example demonstrates the interaction of ethnicity and gender and the way in which they can affect a person's response to stress.

Clinical Example Jose Rodriguez is a 36-year-old Hispanic man. Jose planned to graduate from an MBA program in May and marry his fiancée, Lisa, in June. The couple met in class 2 years ago and have dated for 1 year. Jose visited Lisa's family for the first time during spring break. Lisa's parents are of German descent, and they were shocked when Lisa told them she planned to marry Jose in 3 months. Lisa's father informed her that if she goes through with her wedding plans he will disown her. He said that her mother and brothers agreed with him and that she had to choose between Jose and her family. When she told Jose about her father's reaction he felt they should leave immediately, but Lisa said she could not go with him if it meant going against her family.

Jose drove back to school and on the way was cited twice for speeding. When he returned to his room he spent 2 days alone drinking beer. He did not shave, shower, or change his clothes. On the third day he went out for more beer and as he walked past a group of men, one of them called him a "dirty wetback." When Jose got home he destroyed his room and everything in it, including his completed master's thesis, which he needed to hand in the next day in order to graduate in May.

> **?** *How might a psychiatric nurse's view of gender-appropriate behavior influence one's diagnosis and treatment of male and female patients?*

Education

Mental status examinations are often used to determine diagnosis and treatment for various psychiatric disorders. A study was conducted to compare the scores of black and white patients on the mini-mental state examination in an effort to determine whether education level influenced scores on a measure of dementia.[26] Among both blacks and whites, people with less than an eighth grade education had higher scores for dementia than subjects with ninth grade or higher education. Studies have also reported that education is more important than income in determining use of mental health services. Those with the highest educational level used mental health services most often.

The clinical example that follows illustrates the effect ethnicity, gender, and education can have on a person's ability to interact with others effectively.

Clinical Example Ms. Wong is a 22-year-old Chinese-American woman. She is employed at a university computer center and is a part-time law student. Her roommate is a second-year English major and has an active social life. Because her courses are demanding and her family expects her to be successful, Ms. Wong spends all of her free time studying. While Ms. Wong was studying one Friday afternoon, her roommate came home with several friends, including a young man from Ms. Wong's law class that she thought was very attractive. She was excited about seeing him and acted very friendly toward him until she realized that he was her

roommate's date for the evening. Ms. Wong felt humiliated by her behavior and abruptly left the apartment. As she was leaving, she heard her roommate say, "Now that Miss Perfect is gone, we can party."

Ms. Wong did not know what to do or in whom to confide. She walked around town for hours. Although she was becoming exhausted, she did not stop to rest, eat, or drink. She continued to walk and smiled at the romantic couples she passed but became sad again when they did not smile back at her. Ms. Wong noticed a wig store across the street from where she stood and went in and bought a curly blonde wig that she immediately put on. She wore this wig every day and insisted that everyone call her Patty, her new American name.

Income

The negative effects of poverty on mental health are severe regardless of age, ethnicity, or gender, as evidenced by many community surveys that report a relationship between lower economic status and higher level of psychiatric symptoms and inpatient admissions.[5,25] However, the prevalence of poverty among women, elders, and ethnic minorities is significant. Some researchers believe that the difference in risk for psychiatric disorders between groups is primarily a measure of social stratification and poverty, with those at the bottom facing more daily problems than those at the top.[29] Others suggest that the combination of poverty with other risk factors such as gender and ethnicity predicts both the onset of stress-related psychiatric disorders and the use of mental health services.[4]

The following clinical example describes the effect of ethnicity and income on self-esteem.

Clinical Example John Willis is a 20-year-old black man. He has been looking for work since he graduated from high school 2 years ago and has had several job interviews with local employers. Over the phone, all of these employers seemed very interested in hiring John, but he never received a job offer. Each time he called back after an interview, he was told that the position had been filled and that his application would be kept on file. Last fall, John obtained an interview for an entry-level position at a local bank. He felt that his luck had changed and this would be the perfect job for him.

He arrived early for his interview, and after waiting an hour to meet with the interviewer, John was told that the position had been filled. John was very surprised to hear this. He felt that he had not been treated fairly and that the interviewer just wanted to look him over and decided that he did not like what he saw. John asked the interviewer, "Did the position get filled before or after I got here, or don't you know that either?" The interviewer alerted security and asked John to leave. John was angry and embarrassed and asked the interviewer why he was being treated like a criminal when he came here to apply for a job. Before the interviewer could answer, John left the building. Since then, John has refused to look for work or go to another interview. He has been unemployed for 2 years and continues to live with his parents, sleeping until noon everyday and spending all of his time "hanging out" with his male friends.

> **?** *Most single-parent households in this country are headed by women, and many of them are below the poverty level. How might this affect the mental health of the children living in these homes?*

Belief System

A person's belief system, world view, religion, or spirituality can also have a positive or negative effect on mental health. Human beings in general need to make sense out of and explain their life experiences. This is especially true when they are suffering or in distress. In this quest for meaning, belief systems play a vital role in determining whether a particular explanation and associated treatment plan will have meaning to the patient and others in the patient's social network.[34] The degree of compatibility between the patient's and provider's belief systems often determines the patient's satisfaction with treatment, medication compliance, and treatment outcome.[15]

Adaptive belief system responses can enhance well-being, improve the quality of life, and speed recovery from illness. Maladaptive belief system responses may lead to poor adjustment to changing health status, refusal of necessary treatment, or even self-injury. For example, certain religious belief systems stress avoidance of alcohol, illicit drugs, and cigarette smoking. Spiritually based intervention programs, such as 12-step programs, which encourage the individual to surrender control to an external supreme being, are commonly used treatments for addictive disorders.

> **?** *Think about two patients you took care of last week. Did you discuss with them their belief systems about their health and current illnesses? How might this information have influenced your nursing interventions with them?*

In summary, age, ethnicity, gender, education, income, and belief system are psychiatric disorder risk factors that can increase the likelihood of psychiatric illness and decrease the likelihood of a positive treatment outcome. In particular, age, ethnicity, and gender are powerful risk factors for psychiatric illness when combined with poverty and low education.

SOCIOCULTURAL STRESSORS

Some of the sociocultural stressors that hinder the delivery of psychiatric care are listed in Table 7-1. Disadvantagement

TABLE **7-1** *Sociocultural Stressors*

STRESSOR	DEFINITION
Disadvantagement	The lack of socioeconomic resources that are basic to biopsychosocial adaptation
Stereotype	A depersonalized conception of individuals within a group
Intolerance	Unwillingness to accept different opinions or beliefs from people of different backgrounds
Stigma	An attribute or trait deemed by the person's social environment as unfavorable
Prejudice	A preconceived, unfavorable belief about individuals or groups that disregards knowledge, thought, or reason
Discrimination	Differential treatment of individuals or groups not based on actual merit
Racism	The belief that inherent differences among the races determine individual achievement and that one race is superior

creates profound problems in the prevention, diagnosis, and treatment of psychiatric disorders. In addition to lacking basic resources, people who are poor and poorly educated are often stereotyped in society as freeloaders or lazy. Such people are often the focus of other negative attitudes and behaviors such as intolerance, stigma, prejudice, discrimination, and racism.

For example, consider a woman who is obese. In American society thinness is highly valued and obesity is stigmatized regardless of the person's ethnicity or age. However, obese males are stigmatized less than obese females. Despite the fact that the fashion industry now markets to the "big woman," "big" has yet to become an acceptable standard of femininity in American society. In addition, although obese women and men may encounter the same amount of employment discrimination, obese women are often also viewed as asexual because of their failure to follow the social rule of thinness as a norm of female sexuality. As a result, in comparison to the overweight or obese male, obese females are more likely to be single. Because married and partnered adults consistently report less stress than adults who are single or divorced, it is evident that sociocultural attitudes and values serve as stressors and increase the risk of psychiatric disorders for some individuals.

As another example, consider the impact of racism on people with hypertension, which affects 25% of blacks in the United States. A study aimed at measuring the association between anger and blood pressure reactivity found that anger related to racism increased the systolic and diastolic blood pressures of black students more than anger that was not related to racism.[1] The relationship between racism and psychiatric disorders has not yet been tested, but the relationship between stress and psychiatric disorders has been demonstrated, and for ethnic minorities, racism is a significant sociocultural stressor.[27]

IMPACT ON COPING RESPONSES

The coping responses used by individuals and the ways in which symptoms of mental illness are expressed also vary by culture. Coping responses and the meaning assigned to them are greatly influenced by sociocultural norms, values, beliefs, and expectations. Symptoms that indicate a problem in the context of one group may be tolerated or even ignored by another group for two reasons. First, if a behavior or symptom is widespread, it may be considered normal. Second, if the behavior fits in with social values it may similarly be accepted. For example, hallucinations in Western society are considered a sign of serious illness because the social values emphasize rationality and control. In contrast, visions, hexes, and hearing voices are not necessarily considered signs of psychosis among other cultures, nor is communicating with the dead. In addition, some cultural groups would view symptoms typically associated with mental illness as signs of normality, meanness, laziness, sin, or spiritual distress.

Finally, there are many culture-specific ways of expressing distress. For example, black patients with schizophrenia have been observed to show more anger and suspicion toward others than white patients with schizophrenia. For some black patients, anger and suspicion are coping responses to chronic sociocultural stress. This coping response may be ineffective, however, in that anger and suspicion do not decrease feelings of distress, nor signal to others the need for support.

Box **7-3** *Questions Related to Sociocultural Risk Factors*

AGE
Questions
What is the patient's current stage of development?
What are the developmental tasks of the patient?
Are those tasks age-appropriate for the patient?
What are the patient's attitudes and beliefs regarding the patient's age group?
With what age-related stressors is the patient coping?
What impact does the patient's age have on mental and physical health?

Example
Assessment. Jim is 38 years old and trying to come to terms with balancing his need for intimacy with that of finding his own identity and sense of purpose in life. He describes feelings of anxiety along with waves of hopelessness. He states, "At my age I should stop acting like I'm twenty-something and accept myself, but I just can't seem to do that."
Evaluation. Jim is worried that he will never settle down into an adult lifestyle, but he is more afraid of the high stress and loss of social attractiveness that he associates with being middle-aged.

ETHNICITY
Questions
What is the patient's ethnic background?
What is the patient's ethnic identity?
Is the patient traditional, bicultural, multicultural, or culturally alienated?
What are the patient's attitudes, beliefs, and values regarding his or her ethnic group?
With what ethnicity-related stressors is the patient coping?
What impact does the person's ethnicity have on mental and physical health?

Example
Assessment. Landa is a black woman. She strongly endorses African-American values and considers herself to be culturally traditional. Landa believes that African-American values are superior to Western values and that there would be less poverty and crime in black communities if all black people shared her beliefs. She spends much of her time reading about traditional African ways and has become isolated from her friends and family.
Evaluation. Landa lacks the social support she needs to feel good about her ethnicity without having to idealize or reject members of her own or other ethnic groups. She is having difficulty integrating her values with those of her family and friends.

GENDER
Questions
What is the patient's gender?
What is the patient's gender identity?
How does the patient define gender-specific roles?
What are the patient's attitudes and beliefs regarding males and females and masculinity and femininity?
With what gender-related stressors is the patient coping?
What impact does the person's gender have on mental and physical health?

Example
Assessment. Kelly is male, and enacting the male role is very important to him. As a man, he feels he must provide for his family by working hard, making money, and being smart. Kelly feels that his wife should respect how hard he works and support his plans for providing for her. Recently, he and his wife have had increasing marital conflict. He states "I am doing what is right for both of us. All my wife has to do is help me." Yet Kelly states that his wife does not want him to work 7 days a week and that she does not want to wait until he builds their house before she can go to college. He reports drinking more in the past couple of months and admits that it is difficult for him to express his emotional needs or to respond to those of his wife.
Evaluation. Kelly defines masculinity as authority, and it is extremely important to his self-image. He is unable to express feelings and is struggling to maintain a self-ideal that is in conflict with his wife's needs for her own growth as an individual as well as a spouse.

Continued

NURSING ASSESSMENT AND DIAGNOSIS

Cultural self-awareness is an essential first step for the psychiatric nurse in the delivery of culturally sensitive care.[6,18] To prepare to be culturally responsive to a patient, the nurse should answer the following questions:

▼ What about the patient's appearance or behavior makes me think that what I am seeing or hearing is pathological?

▼ What label am I subconsciously applying to this patient and where did it come from?

▼ What social class am I assuming this patient comes from and what are my prejudices about that group?

▼ What other explanations might account for this patient's unusual behavior?

▼ What personal characteristics of the patient have I noted and what are my positive and negative reactions to those characteristics?

In effect, psychiatric nurses need to qualify their clinical assessments by offering cultural explanations for their patients' behavior and appearance.

Assessment of the patient's sociocultural risk factors and stressors greatly enhances the nurse's ability to establish a therapeutic alliance, identify the patient's problems, and develop a treatment plan that is accurate, appropriate, and culturally relevant. Box 7-3 presents questions the nurse might ask related to each of the risk factors described in this chapter.

A culturally sensitive psychiatric nursing diagnosis takes into account sociocultural risk factors and stressors that af-

---

Box *7-3* *Questions Related to Sociocultural Risk Factors—cont'd*

EDUCATION

Questions

What is the patient's education level?

What were the patient's educational experiences like?

What are the patient's attitudes and beliefs regarding education in general and the patient's own education in particular?

With what education-related stressors is the patient coping?

What impact does the patient's education have on mental and physical health?

Example

Assessment. Ron completed eighth grade and then dropped out of school. He learned to be a plumber by working with a family friend who owned a plumbing business. Recently the friend retired and sold the business to Ron. Ron wants his son to work with him and learn the business, but his son wants to go to college. Ron and his son have been having violent fights about this issue, and Ron has told him, "College is what you do when you don't know anything. Do you think that by going to college you'll be better than me?"

Evaluation. Ron feels bad about his lack of formal education and the negative stereotypes people hold about plumbers. His insecurity makes him unable to support his son's desire to attend college because he fears that his relationship with his son will suffer and that his son will think less of him in the future.

INCOME

Questions

What is the patient's income?

What is the source of the patient's income?

How does the patient describe his or her income group?

What are the patient's attitudes and beliefs regarding personal socioeconomic status?

With what income-related stressors is the patient coping?

What impact does the patient's income have on mental and physical health?

Example

Assessment. Amanda is unemployed. She has always believed that people who are in good health should work; however,

Amanda has never been employed. She married a wealthy, older man when she was 19 years old, and for 10 years he supported her. Then with no warning, her husband left the country with a younger woman and filed for divorce. Amanda states, "He left me. I'm penniless. I'm homeless. I'm nothing." Her family is middle-income and is willing to help her if she gets a job, but she is unwilling to interview for a job because the concept of paid employment conflicts with her self-concept as a wealthy wife.

Evaluation. Amanda's self-concept and self-esteem were based on her marriage and financial status. She never imagined being without these things, and she feels unprepared and resentful of the changes she needs to make.

BELIEF SYSTEM

Questions

What are the patient's beliefs about health and illness?

What was the patient's religious or spiritual upbringing?

What are the patient's current religious or spiritual beliefs?

Who is the patient's regular health-care provider?

With what belief system–related stressors is the patient coping?

What impact does the patient's belief system have on mental and physical health?

Example

Assessment. Xiao believes that illness of the mind is correct punishment. Since her mother's death 2 months ago, she has experienced insomnia, fatigue, and weight loss. She and her mother argued frequently, including the morning her mother had a fatal car accident on her way to work. Xiao now avoids her family and for the last week has been unable to go to work. Xiao states, "I did not love my mother and now I am being punished. No one can help me."

Evaluation. Xiao is unable to resolve her feelings about her mother and to grieve her loss adaptively. She feels guilt about her arguments with her mother and welcomes depression as a correct punishment. Because of this belief, seeking help is unacceptable.

fect the patient's coping responses. Often, nurses exclude sociocultural information in their analysis because they want to avoid stereotyping the patient, feel that the patient's health-care problems are not related to the patient's age, ethnicity, gender, income, education, or belief system, or incorrectly assume that the patient shares their world view. However, sociocultural information must be included in each phase of the nursing process because it has a significant influence on the patient's coping responses. Talking to patients about their sociocultural attitudes, feelings, beliefs, and experiences will not stereotype individuals, but not talking to patients about these important areas of their lives will.

> **?** *Do you think it is possible that two patients displaying the same symptoms could receive two different diagnoses based on the sociocultural factors of age, ethnicity, and gender of either the patient or the clinician?*

TREATMENT IMPLICATIONS

There is growing awareness that the psychotherapeutic treatment process is influenced by the cultural and ethnic context of both the patient and the health-care provider (see Critical Thinking about Contemporary Issues). In terms of treatment planning, it is clear that the psychiatric

---

CRITICAL THINKING *about* **Contemporary Issues**

Should Ethnic Minority Patients Be Treated by White Therapists?

The effectiveness of psychotherapy for ethnic minority patients, especially when treated by white therapists, is controversial. Some researchers and practitioners believe that ethnic minority patients are less likely to benefit from treatment. Others maintain that ethnic minority patients are just as likely as whites to show favorable outcomes from treatment and that studies of ethnic or racial matching of patients have failed to show different outcomes on the basis of the race or ethnicity of the patients and clinicians.

It is likely that ethnicity or race by itself tells very little about the values, attitudes, and experiences of patients and clinicians, who engage in the treatment process.[7] Thus ethnic matches can result in cultural mismatches, as patients and clinicians from the same ethnic group may show markedly different values. Conversely, ethnic mismatches may be cultural matches because patients and clinicians from different ethnic groups may share similar values, lifestyles, and expectations. Thus sociocultural sensitivity includes respect for individual differences regardless of one's age, ethnicity, gender, education, income, or belief system. The consideration of all of these characteristics and the ability to individualize patient care appear to be the best predictors of treatment outcome.

---

nurse needs to be sensitive to sociocultural issues but also must transcend them. Together, the nurse and patient need to agree on the nature of the patient's coping responses, the means for solving problems, and the expected outcomes of treatment. A central responsibility of the nurse is to understand what the illness means to the patient and the way in which the patient's belief system can help to mediate the stressful events or make them easier to bear by redefining them as opportunities for personal growth.

Service Delivery Systems

An important first consideration for effective treatment is the design of a culturally sensitive mental health service delivery system.[8,33] Mental health programs should be based on the assessment of community needs that includes representatives of minority populations in the design, implementation, analysis, and interpretation of needs assessment data. A culturally sensitive mental health care system acknowledges the importance of culture and incorporates this value into all levels of care. To do this requires the assessment of cross-cultural relations, an understanding of the dynamics of cultural differences, an expansion of knowledge about different cultures, and a commitment to adapt services to meet culturally unique needs. In this way, culturally sensitive mental health care (including services for patients who speak languages other than English) provides better access to more appropriate, effective care and the opportunity for improved outcomes.

Specifically, service delivery can be improved through cultural and clinical consultation by experts in the care of nonmainstream populations such as ethnic and cultural minorities and those with physical disabilities. Service use can be improved by the standardization of clinical assessment and treatment guidelines that address patients' cultural issues. In addition, delivery systems should be sensitive to the fact that if a mental health service operates under the auspices of a dominant ethnic, socioeconomic, or religious group, people not of that group may feel uncomfortable or unable to access that service. Staffing has also been shown to affect service use by minorities, and use of racially or ethnically diverse staff who understand the language and culture of patients enhances service use. Finally, an administrative environment must be created that places importance on the role of culture in understanding mental illness and treatment. Criteria should be established that hold clinicians accountable for practicing in culturally appropriate ways and provide them with the necessary tools and training.

Counseling

Culturally responsive counseling strategies should consider ethnic identity and acculturation, family influences, sex-role socialization, religious and spiritual influences, and immigration experiences.[22] In addition, sociocultural differences between the nurse and patient can be a source of misunderstanding by the nurse and resistance by the patient. Alternatively, these differences can serve as a vehicle for discussing important issues in counseling, thereby enriching the experience for both partners in the therapeutic relationship.[2]

Family systems can be major sources of strength for people with mental illness, and nurses should view them as allies and integral components of the treatment process. Families can provide an important economic and emotional buffer against the burden imposed by the patient's illness and give the patient a supportive environment for recovery. Psychoeducational, behavioral, supportive, and family-consultation are the preferred models (see Chapter 32) because they are directly responsive to families' requests for information, support, and techniques for managing their relatives' illnesses.

Religion can also be a core social and spiritual resource.[36] Among blacks, for example, the church often provides collective support, opportunities for self-expression, and the sense of helping others, which can give meaning to life. Supernatural belief systems may also provide a natural support system for mentally ill people, as well as a culturally based way of understanding how the illness fits into the patient's life.

Psychobiology

Sociocultural factors also influence various aspects of psychobiology and psychopharmacology[24] (see Chapters 5 and 27). For example, ethnicity is one of the most important variables that contribute to variations in patients' responses to medications. Racial and ethnic differences in response to psychotropic drugs include the following:

▼ Extrapyramidal effects at lower dosage levels for Asians
▼ Lower effective dosage levels and a lower side-effect threshold for antidepressants among Hispanics
▼ Better response by black patients to phenothiazine and tricyclic antidepressants
▼ Higher red blood cell plasma-lithium ratio in blacks

Gender differences may also result in the need for different doses of psychotropic drugs. For example, women secrete 40% less stomach acid than men. so drugs such as tricyclic antidepressants, benzodiazepines, and certain antipsychotic drugs are more likely to be absorbed before they can be neutralized by the acid, thus requiring a lower dose. In addition, over time, women accumulate more of a drug in their bodies than men because fatty tissue stores psychotropic drugs longest.

Sociocultural characteristics, including belief systems, appear to have a significant impact on treatment compliance, and there may also be normative cultural preferences for the different ways in which medication can be taken. These findings have implications for treatment outcome and reinforce the need for sociocultural sensitivity in planning nursing care.

Equally important is the fact that numerous studies have documented that indigenous systems of health beliefs and practices persist in all societies, including those exposed to modern Western medicine. The nurse should keep in mind that, despite the availability of Western medicine, traditional herbal medicines continue to be used extensively by many different cultural groups living in the United States. Some of these drugs have active pharmacologic properties that may interfere with psychotropic drugs. Clearly the use of alternative healing methods warrants additional research.

Summary

1. The culturally sensitive nurse is one who has the knowledge and skills needed to intervene successfully in the lives of patients from culturally diverse backgrounds.
2. Sociocultural risk factors for psychiatric disorders are predisposing factors that can significantly increase a person's potential for developing a psychiatric disorder, significantly decrease a person's potential for recovery, or both. They include age, ethnicity, gender, education, income, and belief system.
3. A variety of sociocultural stressors hinder the delivery of psychiatric care, including disadvantagement, stereotyping, intolerance, stigma, prejudice, discrimination, and racism.
4. Coping responses and the ways in which symptoms of mental illness are expressed also vary by culture.
5. Assessment of the patient's predisposing sociocultural risk factors and precipitating stressors greatly enhances the nurse's ability to identify the patient's problems and develop a psychiatric nursing treatment plan that is accurate, appropriate, and culturally sensitive.
6. Together, the nurse and patient need to agree on the nature of the patient's coping responses, the means for solving problems, and the expected outcomes of treatment within a sociocultural context.

 Video Resources

Mosby's Community Health Nursing Video Series:
Culture in the Community

Mosby's Communication in Nursing Series:
Communicating with Clients from Different Cultures

your **INTERNET connection**

Wing of Madness: General Mental Health Sources
http://members.aol.com/depress/genment.htm

EthnoMed Ethnic Medicine Guide
http://www.hslib.washington.edu/clinical/ethnomed

Chapter Review Questions

1. Fill in the blanks.

A. _____ are predisposing or conditioning factors that influence the amount and type of coping resources available to a patient.

B. The term _____ is used to describe a person's racial, national, tribal, linguistic, or cultural origin or background.

C. _____ and _____ disorders are the most prevalent psychiatric disorders among males.

D. _____ and _____ disorders are the most prevalent psychiatric disorders among females.

E. The prevalence of _____ and _____ disorders is about equal for males and females.

F. Risk factors are characteristics of an individual that can significantly _____ a person's potential for developing a psychiatric disorder or significantly _____ the potential for recovery, or both.

2. Match each term in Column A with the correct definition in Column B.

Column A	Column B
___Disadvantagement	A. A depersonalized conception of individuals within a group
___Discrimination	B. A preconceived, unfavorable belief about individuals or groups that disregards knowledge, thought, or reason
___Intolerance	
___Prejudice	C. An attribute or trait deemed by the person's social environment as unfavorable
___Racism	
___Stereotype	D. Differential treatment of individuals or groups not based on actual merit
___Stigma	E. The belief that inherent differences among the races determine individual achievement and that one race is superior
	F. The lack of socioeconomic resources that are basic to biopsychosocial adaptation
	G. Unwillingness to accept different opinions or beliefs from people of different backgrounds

3. Provide short answers for the following questions.

A. Define cultural sensitivity.

B. Give an example of how your cultural background influences your perceptions, motives, individual identity, group identity, values, and communication.

C. Think about the facility in which you are having your psychiatric nursing experience. Evaluate whether it meets the criteria of a culturally sensitive mental health delivery system as described in this chapter.

REFERENCES

1. Amstead C et al: Relationship of racial stressors to blood pressure responses and anger expression in black college students, *Health Psychol* 8:541, 1989.
2. Blue H, Gonzalez C: The meaning of ethnocultural difference: its impact on and use in the psychotherapeutic process, *New Dir Ment Health Serv* 55:73, 1992.
3. Bourdon K et al: Estimating the prevalence of mental disorders in US adults from the Epidemiologic Catchment Area Survey, *Public Health Rep* 107:663, 1992.
4. Briones D et al: Socioeconomic status, ethnicity, psychological distress, and readiness to utilize a mental health facility, *Am J Psychiatry* 147:1333, 1990.
5. Bruce M, Takeuchi D, Leaf P: Poverty and psychiatric status: longitudinal evidence from the New Haven Epidemiologic Catchment Area Study, *Arch Gen Psychiatry* 48:470, 1991.
6. Campinha-Bacote J: Transcultural psychiatric nursing: diagnosis and treatment issues, *J Psychosoc Nurs* 32:41, 1994.
7. Carter R: *The influence of race and racial identity in psychotherapy: toward a radically inclusive model,* New York, 1995, Wiley.
8. Casimir G, Morrison B: Rethinking work with multicultural populations, *Community Ment Health J* 29:547, 1993.
9. Castle D, Wessely S, Murray R: Sex and schizophrenia: effects of diagnostic stringency and associations with premorbid variables, *Br J Psychiatry* 162:658, 1993.

10. Chung H, Mahler J, Kakuma T: Racial differences in treatment of psychiatric inpatients, *Psychiatr Serv* 46:586, 1995.

11. Closser M, Blow F: Special populations: women, ethnic minorities, and the elderly, *Psychiatr Clin North Am* 16:199, 1993.

12. Comas-Diaz L, Griffith E: *Clinical guidelines in cross-cultural mental health,* New York, 1988, Wiley.

13. Flaskerud J: Relationship of ethnicity to psychiatric diagnosis, *J Nerv Ment Dis* 180:296, 1992.

14. Gaw A: *Culture, ethnicity, and mental illness,* Washington, DC, 1993, American Psychiatric Press.

15. Giglio J: The impact of patients' and therapists' religious values on psychotherapy, *Hosp Community Psychiatry* 44:768, 1993.

16. Hu T et al: Ethnic populations in public mental health: services choice and level of use, *Am J Public Health* 81:1429, 1991.

17. Huges D, DeMallie D, Blazer D: Does age make a difference in the effect of physical health and social support on the outcome of a major depressive episode? *Am J Psychiatry* 150:728, 1993.

18. Hughes C: Culture in clinical psychiatry. In Gaw A, editor: *Culture, ethnicity, and mental illness,* Washington, DC, 1993, American Psychiatric Press.

19. Jones-Webb R, Snowden L: Symptoms of depression among blacks and whites, *Am J Public Health* 83:240, 1993.

20. Kurlowicz L: Social factors and depression in late life, *Arch Psychiatr Nurs* 7:30, 1993.

21. Lawson W et al: Race as a factor in inpatient and outpatient admissions and diagnosis, *Hosp Community Psychiatry* 45:72, 1994.

22. Lee C, Richardson B: *Multicultural issues in counseling: new approaches to diversity,* Alexandria, Va, 1991, American Association of Counseling and Development.

23. Lewinsohn P et al: Age cohort changes in the lifetime occurrence of depression and other mental disorders, *J Abnorm Psychol* 102:110, 1993.

24. Lin K, Poland R, Nakasaki G: *Psychopharmacology and psychobiology of ethnicity,* Washington, DC, 1993, American Psychiatric Press.

25. Muntaner C et al: Differences in social class among psychotic patients at inpatient admission, *Psychiatr Serv* 46:176, 1995.

26. Murden R et al: Mini-mental state exam scores vary with education in blacks and whites, *J Am Geriatr Soc* 39:149, 1991.

27. Outlaw F: Stress and coping: the influence of racism on the cognitive appraisal processing of African-Americans, *Issues Ment Health Nurs* 14:399, 1993.

28. Regier D et al: The de facto US mental and addictive disorders service system, *Arch Gen Psychiatry* 50:85, 1993.

29. Rogler L, Cortes D: Help-seeking pathways: a unifying concept in mental health care, *Am J Psychiatry* 150:554, 1993.

30. Segal S, Bola J, Watson M: Race, quality of care and antipsychotic prescribing practices in psychiatric emergency services, *Psychiatr Serv* 47:282, 1996.

31. Sorenson S, Ritter C, Aneshensel C: Depression in the community: an investigation into age of onset, *J Consult Clin Psychol* 59:541, 1991.

32. Strakowski S, Shelton R, Kolbrener M: The effects of race and comorbidity on clinical diagnosis in patients with psychosis, *J Clin Psychiatry* 54:96, 1993.

33. Sue S et al: Community mental health services for ethnic minority groups: a test of the cultural responsive hypothesis, *J Consult Clin Psychol* 59:533, 1991.

34. Taggart S: *Living as if: belief systems in mental health practice,* San Francisco, 1994, Jossey-Bass.

35. Wade J: Institutional racism: an analysis of the mental health system, *Am J Orthopsychiatry* 63:536, 1993.

36. Waldfogel S, Wolpe P: Using awareness of religious factors to enhance interventions in consultation-liaison psychiatry, *Hosp Community Psychiatry* 44:473, 1993.

ANNOTATED SUGGESTED READINGS

Comas-Diaz L, Greene B: *Women of color: integrating ethnic and gender identities in psychotherapy,* New York, 1994, The Guilford Press.
   Challenges clinicians to expand beyond traditional psychotherapeutic orientations to integrate realities that enhance effectiveness of mental health services for women of color. A must for all therapists.

*Hales A: West African beliefs about mental illness, *Perspect Psychiatr Care* 32:23, 1996.
   Describes how learning about West Africa's cultural beliefs related to the causes and treatments of mental illness allowed Liberian nursing students to be taught in a way that integrated, rather than dismantled, their cultural beliefs.

Gaw A: *Culture, ethnicity, and mental illness,* Washington, DC, American Psychiatric Press.
   Perhaps the best text available to describe the expression and treatment of mental illness in the context of culture. Highly recommended for all psychiatric nurses.

Gelfand D: *Aging and ethnicity,* New York, 1994, Springer Publishing Company.
   Examines both theory related to ethnicity and aging as well as service delivery issues that emerge from the needs of the ethnic aged. One of the few texts to explore this issue.

Geller J: *Women of the asylum,* New York, 1994, Anchor Books.
   Twenty-six women speak about their experiences while locked behind the walls of psychiatric hospitals between 1840 and 1945. Chilling descriptions of injustice and cultural bias that are part of the history of psychiatric care in this country.

*Mickley J, Carson V, Soeken K: Religion and adult mental health: state of the science in nursing, *Issues Ment Health Nurs* 16:345, 1995.
   A good review of the major empirical data on religion and mental health pertinent to psychiatric nursing. Three areas covered are mental health impact, coping, and aging.

Ruiz P: Issues in the psychiatric care of Hispanics, *Psychiatric Services* 48:539, 1997.
   Reports on Hispanics, the second largest minority group in the United States, who face problems of access to care, high rates of substance abuse and HIV, and shortages of Hispanic psychiatric professionals.

Taggart S: *Living as if: belief systems in mental health practice,* San Francisco, 1994, Jossey-Bass.
   Challenges mental health professionals to rethink their own and their patients' core beliefs in order to provide a rationale for incorporating spiritual and religious belief systems into mental health practices.

*Tuck I: The cultural context of mental health nursing, *Issues Ment Health Nursing* 18:269, 1997.
   Explores the values of psychiatric nursing as found in ANA documents and the congruencies and conflicts of these values with those of the dominant culture in our society. Excellent analysis that includes implications for psychiatric nursing.

*Warren B: Depression, stressful life events, social support, and self-esteem in middle class African American women, *Arch Psychiatr Nurs* 11:107, 1997.
   Nursing research that found that African-American women had a positive relationship between depression and stressful life events and a negative relationship between depression and social support. Self-esteem did not significantly effect depression in this group.

*Nursing reference.

Chapter 8

Environmental Context of Psychiatric Nursing Care

Gail W. Stuart

© 1998 M.C. Escher/Cordon Art, Baarn, Holland.

There is a tide in the affairs of men, Which, when taken at the flood, leads on to fortune; Omitted, all the voyage of their life Is bound in shallows and in miseries. On such a full sea are we now afloat And we must take the current when it serves, Or lose our ventures. **William Shakespeare** Act IV, Scene III, *Julius Caesar*

<table>
<tr><td>

LEARNING OBJECTIVES

After studying this chapter the student should be able to:

▼ Describe the elements of managed care, including characteristics, finances, and government initiatives as they relate to psychiatric care

▼ Discuss problems and opportunities in accessing psychiatric and substance abuse services

▼ Define clinical appropriateness in relation to the issues of medical necessity and the provision of psychiatric services

▼ Identify the purpose and goals of clinical practice guidelines in psychiatric care

▼ Analyze the role of outcome measures in enhancing the quality of psychiatric care

▼ Evaluate issues of accountability in relation to patients, providers, and service settings

▼ Apply knowledge about the environment of psychiatric care to psychiatric nursing practice

</td><td>

TOPICAL OUTLINE

Managed Care
  Defining Characteristics
  Financial Aspects
  Federal and State Initiatives
Access to Services
  Employee Assistance Programs
  Treatment Parity
Clinical Appropriateness
  Medical Necessity
  Carve-Ins and Carve-Outs
Practice Guidelines
  Clinical Pathways
Outcome Measurement
  Quality Report Cards
Accountability Issues
  Patients' Rights
  Provider Concerns
  Service Settings
Impact on Psychiatric Nursing
  Roles in Managed Care
  Evidence-Based Practice
  Threats and Opportunities

</td></tr>
</table>

The interface between mental health care and the environment has become increasingly complex in recent years. In the past, the mental health delivery system had only two components: mental health professionals and patients. Now, however, the system has grown to include six forces, each of which must be taken into account when trying to intervene with any mental health problem (Fig. 8-1).

These groups have related but slightly different interests. Patients are concerned that appropriate services are available when and where needed, and they want to be involved in establishing treatment priorities. The family wants what is best for the patient and is concerned about issues related to quality of life, support, education, and empowerment. The provider has clinical and professional biases. If outside controls must exist, the provider wants them applied fairly, with responsibilities and liabilities clearly defined. Government organizations and other regulators want citizens to have high-quality care at the lowest cost and want providers to be accountable for their care. Reimbursers and insurance companies are concerned about paying for covered services by licensed and credentialed professionals and making a profit. Finally, the courts want to protect patients' constitutional rights regarding access to care and treatment received. The changing priorities and interactions of these six forces affect the quality, availability, and responsiveness of mental health services.

Historically, the mental health delivery system itself has been fragmented along several lines:

Private sector   ⟷   Public sector
Psychiatric illness   ⟷   Substance abuse
Inpatient care   ⟷   Outpatient care
Emotional health   ⟷   Physical health

These divisions have led to the development of many different delivery systems in different settings, using different kinds of clinicians, financed through different types of arrangements, subject to different types of regulations and standards. Currently, these dichotomies are being transformed into a more unified mental health delivery system:

Private sector   ↔ Public sector   ↔ Managed care
Mental illness   ↔ Substance abuse   ↔ Behavioral health
Inpatient care   ↔ Outpatient care   ↔ Continuum of care
Emotional health   ↔ Physical health   ↔ Integrated delivery
                                               systems

These changes are significant and affect every aspect of psychiatric nursing practice. It is essential that nurses understand the environment of mental health care in order to fully perform their duties. This chapter discusses some of the most important elements of the current environment, including managed care, access to services, appropriateness of care, practice guidelines, outcome measurement, and accountability issues, and applies them to psychiatric nursing care.

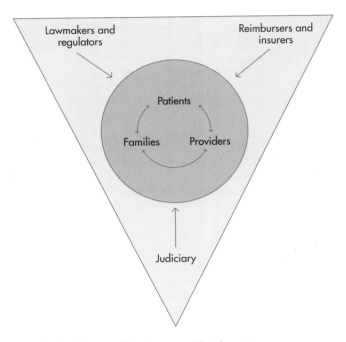

Fig. 8-1   Forces affecting psychiatric care.

MANAGED CARE

Managed care is a reality of the current health-care environment. People use the phrase *managed care* to describe a variety of systems and arrangements for planning, managing, and paying for psychiatric and mental health services. Some of these systems bring rationality and quality to the care setting. Others limit consumer choice and access without appropriate balances. In a well-functioning system of **managed care,** a defined group of people receive treatment services that are clinically necessary, medically appropriate, within defined benefit parameters, for a set amount of time, in compliance with quality standards, and with outcomes that are anticipated and measurable.

At the beginning of 1996 it was estimated that more than 124 million Americans, or 44% of the population, were covered by some type of managed care plan. It is predicted that within the next 10 years, 90% of health care in the United States will be provided in a managed care environment. Managed care is also making headlines because it is driving massive changes in professional practice, the definition of mental disorders, the nature of professional accountability, the allocation of professional resources, and the relationship of mental health professionals to one another.[27] Perhaps the simplest measure of change is that the term *managed care,* as applied to mental and substance abuse disorders, has been replaced by *managed behavioral health care,* which refers to these disorders together as one set of health problems.

TABLE **8-1** *Comparison of Traditional and Managed Care Delivery Systems*

CHARACTERISTIC	TRADITIONAL SYSTEM	MANAGED CARE SYSTEM
Provider focus	Specialized care of individual patient	Total care of member population
Pricing	Separate physician and hospital fee schedules	Discounts, case rate, and capitation
Market share	Number of admissions	Number of covered lives
	Number of procedures	
	Number of visits	
Management focus	High inpatient occupancy rate	Low inpatient occupancy rate
		Correct level of care
Service line	Acute care programs as drivers:	Continuum of care:
	Inconsistent integration	Inpatient
	Physician dependent	Partial hospitalization
	Individual services	Outpatient
		Residential
		Home
Cost management	Payers assume admission rate risk; provider assumes length-of-stay risk	Provider networks assume both admission rate and length-of-stay risk
Costs	Cost per procedure	Cost per life
	Cost per hospitalization	Inpatient days per 1000
		Visits per 1000
Competition	Multiple hospitals for communities	Increased consolidation and network formation as occupancy declines
	Duplication of services and technology	Closure of beds
		Alternative uses of hospitals
Outcomes	Qualitative measures	Quantitative measures
	Reputation	Quality
	Facilities	Cost
Referral base	Focus on high-tech capabilities and separate physician and hospital marketing efforts	Ability to form primary care networks
		Mutual goals/strategies of providers and hospitals

> **?** *Some people support the use of the term* behavioral health care, *believing that it helps to reduce the stigma associated with mental illness. Others oppose the term, believing that it discounts the biological basis of mental disorders. What is your position on this issue?*

Defining Characteristics

As a product of health-care reform, managed care differs in some significant ways from the traditional fee-for-service health-care delivery system. These are outlined in Table 8-1. Each of the characteristics on the left side of the table is described in relation to the traditional fee-for-service health delivery system and a managed care health delivery system. As can be seen from this table, managed care involves a major shift away from the *person-as-customer* to the *population-as-customer*. It also deemphasizes high-cost, episodic inpatient admissions and procedures in favor of creating a full continuum of care and then selecting the correct level of care and treatment setting. Whereas the traditional system fostered duplication of services and technology among hospitals, managed care stimulates the consolidation of services, formation of networks, and use of primary care networks to perform referral and gatekeeping functions.

Each of these characteristics reflects a major change in the delivery of health care in the United States.

A final aspect of managed care is its emphasis on value. *Value* in managed care can be defined as service that yields positive outcomes in the most efficient way. It encompasses the goal of controlling costs while achieving quality outcomes. Value in managed care, therefore, can be represented by the equation

$$\text{Quality/Costs} = \text{Value}$$

Achieving this goal of value requires that a health care organization track costs, measure administrative and clinical processes, measure patient outcomes and satisfaction, and integrate these data to enhance administrative policy and clinical decision making. Each of these elements poses special challenges to health-care professionals and the settings in which they work.

Finally, managed care is not a single entity. Rather, it can assume various forms. The most common are health maintenance organizations (HMOs), preferred provider organizations (PPOs), and point-of-service organizations (POSs). Each of these is described in Box 8-1. *Managed competition* is a purchasing strategy in which managed care organizations contract with several hospitals that provide cost-effective, comprehensive services. Consumers are then in-

Box **8-1** *Types of Managed Care Plans*

Health maintenance organizations (HMOs): HMOs are organized delivery systems that provide care to a defined population, usually for a predetermined fixed amount (capitation rate). Consumers enrolled in HMOs are limited to using HMO providers.

Preferred provider organizations (PPOs): PPOs are plans that contract with a limited number of clinicians, most often physicians, and hospitals that provide care at discounted rates. Members of these plans are given financial incentives to use the preferred providers but are not prevented from using other providers. Insurers or employers select the providers to be included in their preferred plan.

Point-of-service plans (POSs): POSs allow consumers to choose between delivery systems at the time they seek care. In a triple-option plan, for example, people can choose among an HMO, PPO, or fee-for-service plan. Financial incentives are usually provided to encourage people to use the least expensive option.

formed about the hospitals from which they may receive services, even though the facility may not be the patient's preferred choice.

? *One of your nursing colleagues complains that managed care is really only "managed costs." Based on the characteristics of managed care described in this chapter, how might you respond?*

Financial Aspects

One of the major forces that has moved the health-care environment to managed care is the notion that it will reduce health-care costs. It can also shift the financial risk of providing health care from the insurer to the provider. This has implications for patients and clinicians alike. Therefore, it is important for nurses to have a clear understanding of the financial aspects of managed care so that they can base their practice on current economic realities.

In a managed care system there are three major payment mechanisms: discounted fee-for-service, case rate, and capitation. Under a **discounted fee-for-service** payment plan, clinicians are paid for all services that have been authorized and provided to a consumer. The payment rate is discounted or is less than the clinician's standard fee and often includes a provision for a copayment that must be collected from the consumer at the time of each visit. Under a **case rate** system, the clinician is paid a flat fee for a predefined episode of care. The most well-known typical case rate system is Medicare's Diagnostic Related Groups (DRGs). In this instance, Medicare pays a flat fee for a particular hospitalization episode regardless of how many days the person was hospitalized. This system shifts the financial risk to the

provider because the provider receives a flat fee regardless of the actual cost of care. Under a **capitation** system the consumer pays a fixed fee or per-member-per-month (PMPM) premium. In return, the managed care company that receives the PMPM fee agrees to provide all medically necessary health care for all covered people. In this case, most of the financial risk lies with the managed care company, which must deliver all necessary health care within the premiums received by their population pool. HMOs are the best-known examples of capitated payment systems.

Managed care exerts cost control measures through preadmission certification, utilization review, and case management.

▼ **Preadmission certification** takes into account the patient's medical and psychiatric status, level of functioning, socioenvironmental factors, and procedural issues associated with treatment. It is the role of the managed care reviewer to determine the most appropriate form of treatment and the proper treatment setting. In this way, the reviewer monitors issues of cost and quality.

▼ **Utilization review** evaluates the appropriateness and necessity of services and procedures. It is a way of monitoring the care and services administered and it has the most immediate impact on patient care. The patient's treatment plan, diagnostic and therapeutic interventions, and discharge plan are continuously monitored by a third party. Determination for reimbursement of treatment is made by this third party based on current standards of care. The review and approval can be done before providing the services (precertification review), at the time the service is rendered (concurrent review), or after the service has been provided (retrospective review), which may be used to retroactively deny payment.

▼ **Case management** typically is targeted to patients who have treatment complications, have high-expense episodes of care, or who need alternative, less expensive treatments or settings. This often includes those with serious and persistent mental illness. Case management focuses on the achievement of desirable patient outcomes, appropriate lengths of stay, efficient use of resources, and patient involvement and satisfaction.

? *Managed behavioral health-care companies often employ nurses as utilization reviewers and case managers. Identify the special skills and expertise psychiatric nurses can bring to these roles.*

Federal and State Initiatives

Today, the U.S. government is the largest buyer of health care. Through Medicaid and Medicare and numerous other public programs, it is the single most important purchaser of health care in the U.S. It is in this arena that health care reform is being enacted and where the future action will continue. It thus merits review for the impact it is having on psychiatric care.[16]

Medicaid is a health care entitlement program for Aid to Families with Dependent Children (AFDC) recipients; Supplemental Security Income (SSI) recipients; low-income, disabled, elderly people; low-income pregnant women, infants, and children; and medically needy recipients. The serious and persistently mentally ill are often recipients of Medicaid. The states and the federal government share the costs of this program. Although all states are required to provide a basic set of services, other services can be included or excluded at the discretion of the individual state.

Medicaid can give waivers to states to permit them to experiment with alternative delivery systems for the Medicaid population. These waivers can take various forms but the most important one is to let the states contract with providers to provide health care services on a managed care basis. Almost all states that have received waivers provide mental health coverage. The most common approach is to offer acute but limited treatment to all recipients through a basic plan, with a separate plan for people with greater needs. These patients are often assigned to the care of the state mental health department or a private managed care company with which the state has contracted.

These dramatic developments are bringing about major changes in public mental health care that may be as significant as the deinstitutionalization movement of the 1960s and 1970s.[13,25] The introduction of private managed care into the public mental health system involves shifts in responsibility for mental health care, tensions about which populations receive priority for care, and significant changes in the financing and organization of services. Clearly, the prospect of fusing the public and private sectors of mental health care offers both problems and opportunities. If properly managed, however, it can reduce the stigma of mental health care, decrease duplicative administrative costs, and be a first step toward a truly integrated mental health delivery system.

ACCESS TO SERVICES

Access is the degree to which services and information about care are easily obtained and it is an important part of any effective mental health care delivery system. Today, over half of the people who seek health care for mental disorders are treated by primary care practitioners.[10] However, many who need care do not receive it, either from a primary care or specialty provider. It is also known that when access to mental health care is made difficult, the overall costs of general medical care increase because those with behavioral health care problems are frequent users of medical services. For example, people suffering from panic disorder typically are seen by 10 different health-care providers before they are properly diagnosed.

Some access problems apply to the entire health care system, such as the lack of providers in rural areas and care for people who lack health insurance. Other problems are unique to mental health care. These include the stigma associated with seeking care, the lack of knowledge about how to find the right clinician for a highly personal problem, and the lack of general medical settings to adequately respond to mental health and substance abuse disorders. An ideal comprehensive health care system would provide multiple points of entry for treatment, including direct access through self-referral, by a wide variety of providers.

Many controversies exist regarding managed behavioral care. One of the most common is whether patients are granted sufficient access to the care they need. Economic incentives to undertreat may result in denial of care, and managed care companies relate examples of inappropriate care demanded by patients and delivered by providers. Two important balances to offset these problems would be to adequately fund behavioral health care benefits and services and to find ways to measure and reinforce standards for the accessibility, appropriateness, quality, and effectiveness of treatment.[31]

Employee Assistance Programs

Employee assistance programs (EAPs) are worksite-based programs designed to help identify and resolve behavioral, health, and productivity problems that may affect employees' well-being or job performance. Their focus is wide-ranging, covering alcohol and other drug abuse, physical and emotional health, and marital, family, financial, legal, and other personal concerns. As such, they are important points of access to behavioral health care.

EAPs have developed from primarily alcoholism assessment and referral centers to specialized behavioral health programs. Many cost-effectiveness studies document the value of these programs, particularly through their prevention contributions, such as in workplace education, skill development, and policy and environmental changes.[3] Comprehensive EAPs are defined by six major components: identification of problems based on job performance, consultation with supervisors, constructive confrontation, evaluation and referral, liaison with treatment providers, and substance abuse expertise.[34] They thus represent a rich foundation on which other services may be added to promote access to mental health and substance abuse treatment.

Treatment Parity

An analysis of the issue of access in behavioral health care would not be complete without noting that many of the people who need treatment for mental and chemical dependency disorders do not receive it because their insurance policies deny or restrict coverage for the treatment of these illnesses. Historically, insurers and employers have been cautious about offering mental health and substance abuse coverage, often believing that mental disorders were not treatable or were too expensive to treat. In recent years mental health advocates and professionals have placed increased emphasis on parity in insurance coverage between physical and mental health services. There have been some wins and losses in that struggle. A loss for the field was reflected in a new law passed by Congress in 1996. It ended the cash benefits as well as Medicare and Medicaid coverage for people whose disability is based on drug addiction or alcoholism. A win for mental health treatment was the adoption of treatment parity legislation in several states and passage of a national mental health parity bill in the United States in 1996. This bill:

▼ Calls for parity in all health insurance for lifetime and annual caps between physical and mental illness (excluding alcohol and substance abuse) if a plan provides mental health benefits at all (plans are not required to provide such benefits)

▼ Excludes businesses with fewer than 56 employees from the requirement

▼ Is effective January 1, 1998

Ideally, parity would include insurance coverage for mental and addictive disorders that is equal to that provided for any physical disease or illness in terms of service, dollar limits, deductibles, and copayments. Yet many current parity provisions are much narrower.[11] For example, equal coverage may be provided only for medically necessary services to people with severe mental disorders that are biologically based. Even more problematic, the federal parity law allows for the use of a wide range of cost control mechanisms for mental health services, such as higher deductibles or copayments and limits on services or hospital days, that differ from those used for physical health services. In addition, current exemptions in many state insurance regulations may severely limit the number of people covered by parity laws as well as the services they may receive. Finally, parity that covers only "medical treatment" of a particular mental illness may deemphasize or minimize the psychosocial treatments that may be necessary to maintain or preserve a person's functional capacities. Sadly, little attention is given to preventive, rehabilitative, and chronic care services. Thus, although progress is being made in mandating behavioral health benefits, much additional work remains to be done.

? *Do you know what coverage your insurance provides for mental and chemical dependency disorders? Check your policy for inpatient, outpatient, partial hospitalization, and home care benefits. Compare these benefits with those you receive for medical and surgical illnesses. If the coverages are not similar, write a letter bringing this disparity to the attention of your insurance company and requesting a response.*

CLINICAL APPROPRIATENESS

Clinical appropriateness is the degree to which the type, amount, and level of clinical services are delivered to promote the best clinical outcomes. A basic premise of managed behavioral health care is that more is not always better. Specifically, inappropriate hospitalizations not only incur considerable unnecessary costs to the system, but also can harm patients by disrupting their lives through the interruption of work, family, and social functioning, causing them to regress, and recording on their permanent medical record a serious diagnosis that may not have been warranted. In addition, some recent research suggests that although managed care does restrict inpatient psychiatric care, primarily by managing length of stay, it is not associated with higher readmission rates.[2]

In order to meet managed care's criteria of clinical appropriateness, behavioral health care organizations are developing diversified but fully integrated continuums of care by expanding their own services, contracting with other health-care organizations, or affiliating with area providers. These continuums of care must be capable of providing services and alternative levels of care to children, adolescents, adults, and elderly people requiring psychiatric and substance abuse services. The goal is to provide "one-stop shopping" for managed behavioral care and to secure market dominance in a particular geographic area. The levels of care for each stage of treatment expected in an integrated continuum of care are listed in Table 8-2.

Medical Necessity

To comply with issues of clinical appropriateness of care, managed behavioral care companies, government agencies, professional associations, and treatment facilities have each established criteria for the medical necessity of the various levels of care. Criteria are strongest for hospitalization, and there is less consensus regarding outpatient therapy. General criteria for admission to psychiatric services used in one psychiatric setting are presented in Table 8-3. This setting uses additional criteria to assess suicide risk, self-injury risk, assaultiveness, acute psychosis, impaired judgment, substance detoxification, substance abuse rehabilitation, need for electroconvulsive therapy, need for medication monitoring, regulation, initiation or withdrawal, and need for diagnostic evaluation or treatment. In this way, psychiatric facilities can both document and justify the medical appropriateness of the level of psychiatric care selected for a particular patient.

Carve-Ins and Carve-Outs

Another issue debated in the field is how appropriate mental health services can best be provided. Two systems currently exist. The first is the **carve-in,** by which consumers receive services through an integrated care system of both medical/surgical and mental health/substance abuse ser-

Table **8-2** *Levels of Care for each Stage of Treatment in an Integrated Behavioral Continuum of Care*

STAGES OF TREATMENT	CRISIS	ACUTE	MAINTENANCE	HEALTH PROMOTION
GOAL	Stabilization	Remission	Recovery	Optimal level of wellness
EXPECTED OUTCOME	No harm to self or others	Symptom relief	Improved functioning	Attain optimal quality of life
LEVEL OF CARE	▼ Inpatient hospitalization ▼ 24-hour mobile emergency intervention ▼ Crisis stabilization unit and beds ▼ 23-hour observation beds ▼ Outpatient detoxification	▼ Partial hospitalization ▼ Intensive remission-oriented outpatient ▼ Assertive community treatment ▼ Intensive in-home intervention ▼ 23-hour respite beds	▼ Rehabilitative day treatment ▼ Multimodal recovery-oriented outpatient ▼ Relapse prevention ▼ Rehabilitation-oriented residential ▼ Supported independent living	▼ Education ▼ Respite care ▼ Drop-in centers ▼ Peer support ▼ Social activities ▼ School ▼ Employment ▼ Housing

Table **8-3** *General Criteria for Psychiatric Admission across the Continuum of Care*

LEVEL OF CARE			
INPATIENT	**PARTIAL HOSPITALIZATION**	**INTENSIVE OUTPATIENT**	**OUTPATIENT**
Imminent risk for acute medical status deterioration caused by the presence of an active psychiatric or substance abuse condition Unsafe at a less intensive level of service	High risk for acute medical status deterioration caused by the presence of an active psychiatric or substance abuse condition Unsafe at a less intensive level of service Needs intensive therapeutic intervention with physician availability Adequate support system to maintain safety overnight/weekend Reasonable expectation that the patient will form a treatment alliance Unresponsive to treatment or deterioration of usual level of functioning despite participation in a less intensive level of service	Requires frequent therapeutic intervention to improve functioning Unsafe at or inappropriate for a less intensive level of service Adequate support system or coping skills to maintain stability and safety between therapeutic visits Reasonable expectation that the patient will form a treatment alliance Unresponsive to treatment, intensification of symptoms, or deterioration of usual level of functioning despite participation in a less intensive level of service	Outpatient therapy required to alleviate acute symptoms Demonstrates intent to form treatment alliance Adequate support system to maintain safety between therapeutic visits

vices. The second is the behavioral health carve-out, in which mental health and substance abuse benefits are accessed, provided, and otherwise managed separately from medical/surgical care.[25]

Certain advantages and disadvantages are found in both carve-ins and carve-outs. Carve-ins allow all health care to be available at one site of service, which may enable greater access, integration, and coordination of services. The need for this integration is evident from the following facts[28]:

▼ 50% of all mental health care is delivered solely by general practitioners.

▼ 67% of all psychopharmacological drugs are prescribed by general practitioners.

▼ 70% of all primary care visits are primarily for psychosocial concerns.

Primary care is supported in spirit and practice by carve-in arrangements, which also can promote prevention and time-efficient methods of treatment.[7] Carve-ins also have their disadvantages. Some have questioned whether mental health and substance abuse services receive their fair share of resources in benefits, dollars, or services offered. Primary care physicians, who often control access to mental health services, may inappropriately limit care because of their lack of training in behavioral health or because they may be given financial incentives to limit specialty services. In fact, some recent studies have reported that the quality of care given and the clinical outcomes obtained by treating psychological disorders in primary care settings is inadequate.[29,33] Also, payers, consumers, and providers may object to the limitations placed on the choices of mental health clinicians and facilities and to the gatekeeper role of the primary care physician.[15]

Carve-outs also offer both advantages and disadvantages. Although carve-out service delivery models and financial arrangements vary, they generally provide for increased benefits in exchange for following a managed plan of care recommended by a defined panel of behavioral health providers. Advantages to carve-outs are that they typically allow treatment to be provided closer to a person's home or community. They also often demonstrate greater sensitivity and responsiveness to the payer and the consumer and greater expertise in treating mental and chemical dependency disorders, and they may better address the needs of people with serious and persistent mental illness. The disadvantage of carve-outs is the risk of limiting access and undertreatment when the mental health or substance abuse services are capitated. They may also make linkages with primary care clinicians more difficult and discourage collaboration among health-care providers. Finally, consumers may encounter confusing obstacles as they seek to obtain care in two or three systems (general medical, psychiatric, and substance abuse) and among a wide array of health-care providers and sites of service. Thus the dilemma of how to best deliver behavioral health care is far from resolved.

> **?** *One way to provide cost-effective behavioral health care in a primary care setting is to have an advanced practice registered nurse (APRN) in psychiatric and mental health care available on site to work with patients with psychiatric and substance abuse problems. What do you think would be the advantages and disadvantages of such an arrangement?*

PRACTICE GUIDELINES

Another component of the environment of psychiatric care is the development and use of practice guidelines. It is believed that delivery systems that use research-based practice guidelines, and continually improve these guidelines through ongoing outcome research, may be more likely to deliver consistent and high-quality care, and thus have a competitive advantage in some markets. **Practice guidelines** in psychiatric care are strategies for mental health care delivery that are developed to facilitate clinical decision making and provide patients with critical information about their treatment options.[18] The goals of practice guidelines are to:

▼ Document preferred practices
▼ Increase consistency in care
▼ Facilitate outcome research
▼ Enhance the quality of care
▼ Improve staff productivity
▼ Reduce costs

They are given a variety of names in the field, such as *clinical protocols, practice parameters,* and *treatment standards.*

Practice guidelines can be developed in a variety of ways. The best mental health practice guidelines to date are those developed by national policy organizations, such as the depression guidelines developed by the Agency for Health Care Policy and Research (AHCPR). These were based on a scientific review of the available clinical research literature in order to establish which treatments have been documented to be safe and effective for particular conditions. Guidelines have also been developed by professional associations, such as the American Psychiatric Association (Box 8-2), managed care companies, and academic centers using techniques such as expert consensus and data analysis.[9,24]

There is much variability in how guidelines are developed and used. One of the major limitations to their use is that they may not adequately take into account all four variables that influence treatment outcome: patient characteristics, the nature of the therapeutic relationship, treatment interventions, and the placebo effect. Another limitation is that practice guidelines are often developed in isolation by only one discipline and may therefore contain treatment biases reflective of that discipline's model of practice. Box 8-3 lists questions that can be helpful in judging the potential usefulness of a practice guideline. Clearly, practice guidelines are an evolving clinical tool in behavioral health care. As they become more widespread, practice guidelines should grow in sophistication and increase their contribution to quality of care by reducing practice pattern variations.

Box **8-2** *Practice Guidelines Developed by the American Psychiatric Association*

COMPLETED GUIDELINES	
Topic	**When published**
Eating disorders	February 1993
Major depressive disorder	April 1993
Bipolar disorder	December 1994
Substance use disorders	November 1995
Psychiatric evaluation	November 1995
Nicotine dependence	October 1996
Schizophrenia	April 1997
Alzheimer's disease	May 1997
GUIDELINES IN DEVELOPMENT	
Topic	**Anticipated publication**
Panic disorder and related anxiety disorders	November 1997
Delirium	March 1998
Geriatric care	March 1998
Mental retardation	March 1998

▼ Who wrote the guideline? Is it a guild document created by one professional discipline or does it reflect an interdisciplinary point of view?

▼ Who sponsored the guideline? Where did the money come from that supported its creation and distribution?

▼ When was the guideline written? Does it reflect the latest developments in the field?

▼ What methodology was used? Was it based on scientific evidence? Does it differentiate between research findings and clinical opinion?

▼ Do the treatments recommended in the guideline respect consumer rights?

▼ Are the treatments recommended in the guideline affordable and accessible? Can the treatments be provided by a variety of clinicians in various settings or are they limited in some way?

▼ Was the guideline reviewed by a variety of groups, including nurses and consumers?

▼ How does the guideline compare with other guidelines in the field?

Clinical Pathways

Many health-care organizations have undertaken the creation of **clinical pathways,** which identify the key clinical processes and corresponding timelines to which the patient must adhere to achieve standard outcomes within a specified period of time. A clinical pathway is a written plan that serves as a map and timetable for the efficient and effective delivery of health care. Valid clinical pathways are developed over time by a multidisciplinary team.[6] They can be constructed around DSM-IV diagnoses, NANDA diagnoses, clinical conditions, treatment stages, clinical interventions, or targeted behaviors. They are most often used in inpatient settings, serve as a shortened version of the multidisciplinary plan of care for a patient, and require high levels of team cooperation and quality monitoring. Some clinical settings have computerized their paths to enhance the consistency and efficiency of care provided.

The key elements of the clinical pathway are the identification of: a target population; the expected outcome of treatment described in a measurable, realistic, and patient-centered way; specified treatment strategies and interven-

STAGE OF TREATMENT	CRISIS ← - →	ACUTE ← - - →	MAINTENANCE ← - →	HEALTH PROMOTION
Goal	**Stabilization**	**Remission**	**Recovery**	**Optimal level of wellness**
TREATMENT FOCUS	High-risk behaviors	Symptoms and coping responses	Functional status	Quality of life
ASSESSMENTS	Risk factor assessment Nursing assessment	Nursing assessment Medical assessment Supplemental scales	Functional status scale	Well-being scale
EXPECTED OUTCOME	No harm to self or others	Symptom relief	Improved functioning	Optimal quality of life
Consults				
Tests/labs				
Symptom management				
Medications				
Treatments				
Activity				
Safety				
Teaching				
Nutrition				
Discharge planning				

Fig. 8-2   General clinical pathway template for psychiatric care.

tions; and documentation of patient care activities, variances, and goal achievement. The development of a clinical pathway includes reviewing for efficiency and necessity the events that occur when the patient enters the health care facility, and through discharge and aftercare. This includes preadmission work-ups, tests, consultations, treatments, activities, diet, and health teaching.

An example of the format of a general clinical pathway for psychiatric treatment through the four stages of the continuum of care is presented in Figure 8-2. Any stage of psychiatric treatment (crisis, acute, maintenance, or health promotion) identified in this clinical pathway can be singled out and developed in detail. At this time there is great variability in the format and use of clinical pathways in psychiatric care.

> **?** *Many health care providers believe that clinical pathways are more difficult to develop in psychiatry than in other specialty areas. What problems would be particularly challenging in designing clinical pathways for psychiatric treatment?*

OUTCOME MEASUREMENT

Before managed behavioral health care had a name or was a concept for discussion, concerned mental health clinicians were attempting to give the best care possible to their patients. However, they did this most often without reliable data that compared their work with that of others in the field. With the entrance of managed behavioral health care, increasing emphasis was placed on providing the most appropriate care in the most appropriate setting. In order to make decisions about these issues, outcome measurement was needed.

Outcomes are the extent to which services are cost-effective and have a favorable effect on the patient's symptoms, functioning, and well-being. They include all the things that happen to the patient and his or her family while they are in the health care system, such as health status, functional status, quality of life, the presence or absence of illness, type of coping response, and satisfaction with treatment. Outcome evaluation can focus on a clinical condition, an intervention, or a caregiving process. Outcomes that can be examined include clinical, functional, satisfaction, and financial indicators related to the provision of psychiatric care (Box 8-4). The specific purposes of outcome measurement are to:

▼ Evaluate the outcomes of care
▼ Suggest changes in treatment
▼ Evaluate program effectiveness
▼ Profile the practice pattern of providers
▼ Determine the most appropriate level of care
▼ Predict the path of a patient's illness and recovery
▼ Contribute to quality improvement programs

Outcome measurement is no simple task, however. Many scientific and practical problems are involved in knowing what to measure and how to measure it. One of the most difficult aspects is selecting an appropriate scale or measurement tool. The wide variety of rating scales that are commonly used in psychiatry are presented in Chapter 6. Other difficulties encountered in outcome measurement include: the resistance of staff to complete the rating scales; the high rates of spontaneous remission and placebo effect among psychiatric patients; the wide variety of therapeutic approaches and interventions used by mental health clinicians; the many interacting biological, psychological, and sociocultural factors that affect a patient's improvement; the lack of clarity regarding when to measure outcomes (before, during, or after treatment or during long-term follow-up); the validity and reliability problems encountered with patient report and clinical report scales; the lack of correlation between measures of patient satisfaction and clinical assessment of improvement; and the practical problems of administering, collecting, and analyzing the outcome data.[21,23,26] Nonetheless, mental health delivery systems are being asked to provide data regarding the effectiveness of their clinical programs. These data are used to make decisions affecting staffing levels, program development, and financial support.

Box **8-4** *Categories of Outcome Indicators*

CLINICAL OUTCOME INDICATORS
High-risk behaviors
Symptomatology
Coping responses
Relapse
Recurrence
Readmission
Number of treatment episodes
Medical complications
Incidence reports
Mortality

FUNCTIONAL OUTCOME INDICATORS
Functional status
Social interaction
Activities of daily living
Occupational abilities
Quality of life
Family relationships
Housing arrangement

SATISFACTION OUTCOME INDICATORS: Patient and Family Satisfaction with:
Outcomes
Providers
Delivery system
Caregiving process
Organization

FINANCIAL OUTCOME INDICATORS
Cost per treatment episode
Revenue per treatment episode
Length of inpatient stay
Use of health-care resources
Costs related to disability

Clearly, outcome measurement is a critical part of the new environment and it promises to grow in importance.

> **?** *One of your nursing colleagues complains about having to complete clinical rating scales on each new admission. She says she "doesn't have time for such busy-work." How would you respond?*

Quality Report Cards

Another type of outcome measure being developed is related not to the patient, but to the performance of the behavioral health care organization itself. A number of groups are developing standardized report cards on the performance of managed care companies. The Health Plan Employer Data and Information Set (HEDIS) is the most widely used system comparing health plans.[8] However, HEDIS uses only one measure of the quality of behavioral health care: the rate of follow-up after hospitalization for major affective disorder. The American Managed Behavioral Healthcare Association (AMBHA) has developed another set of measures. AMBHA represents managed behavioral health care organizations and their report card is to be used by patients to grade mental health services on three primary indicators: access to care, consumer satisfaction, and quality of care. Finally, at the federal level, the Center for Mental Health Services has also developed a consumer report card for mental health services. These promise to be important aspects of outcome measurement in a managed care environment.

ACCOUNTABILITY ISSUES

Driven by the demand to demonstrate quality and reduce costs, the behavioral health care environment is confronted by new issues of accountability. Areas of concern range from restrictions on patient autonomy in choice of treatment and service setting, to the relationship between the patient and provider, to patient responsibility in complying with treatment recommendations, to the denial, curtailment, or restriction of access to treatment (see Critical Thinking about Contemporary Issues).

Patients' Rights

Central to current debates are questions about the extent to which patients' rights are compromised. With managed care it is clear that limits will be placed on patients' choice of providers, service settings, and sometimes even treatment options. If only a limited number of options are available, patients may be unable to take advantage of newer treatments that could help them. Partly in response to these concerns, a number of different groups have set forth principles for managed mental health care systems. For example, the Center for Mental Health Services has developed a set of principles that emphasizes the need for comprehensive services, continuity of care, and responsiveness to the needs of

---

CRITICAL THINKING *about* Contemporary Issues

Is Managed Care the Devil or Angel of Psychiatric and Mental Health Treatment?

Praise and blame of managed behavioral health care are on the rise across the United States. Public reaction is mixed and the response from mental health professionals is even more conflicted. Proponents of managed care believe that the costs of health care in the United States are enormous, yet many people go without adequate treatment. They propose that managed care can expand access to care, use dwindling resources more responsibly, and reduce the use of unneeded services. Clearly, managed care has demonstrated its ability to control health-care costs. Opponents of managed care raise a number of criticisms. They suggest that managed care could adversely affect the quality of care, limit access to needed care, negatively affect the provider-patient relationship, create problems with informed patient choice, offer unfair benefits and policy coverage, and shift responsibility from the provider to management.[17,22]

Managed care in mental health, as in general health, is neither as good as nor as evil as its advocates or detractors propose. Because it is a reality of the current environment it may be more important to identify ethical principles for its implementation. The following standards have been suggested[4]:

▼ Plans should include a continuum of obligations, with the most intensive care going to those with the most severe but treatable needs.

▼ Limits should be placed on acceptable contractual arrangements between payers and providers, discouraging powerful incentives or coercive practice guidelines.

▼ Constraints should be placed on the amount of information plans collect about enrollees and the uses to which plans put that information.

▼ Plans should be required to provide an adequate amount of information to enrollees.

▼ Plans should allow for greater participation in decision making, such as through the creation of consumer and provider panels.

Managed care is inherently neither good nor bad. The question is how it is used, and every consumer and health-care provider shares responsibility for the answer.

---

service recipients. The principles cover quality of care, consumer participation, accessibility, affordability, linkages and integration, and accountability. Also, a number of mental health organizations, including the American Psychiatric Nurses Association, have endorsed a Bill of Rights for managed care. All of these initiatives reflect a focused effort to protect patients and balance the issues of cost and quality in the current psychiatric care environment.

Provider Concerns

Providers are increasingly aware of their responsibility to provide cost-effective care in an environment of shrinking psychiatric resources. New dilemmas arise for clinicians who must balance a responsibility to both an individual patient and a population of patients. Also, the tension between patient advocacy and resource allocation has been heightened by the introduction of managed care, as providers may feel the need to serve the bottom line of the organization and, in so doing, jeopardize the interests of the patient. Other problems arise when mental health clinicians move from private practice models to become part of networks or organized systems of care. In doing so, they become subject to the review of others, their activities are routinely measured, and they are held accountable for the kind and amount of care they deliver. This is viewed negatively by many mental health professionals, but others see it as a positive trend leading to an overall improvement in behavioral health care services.[30]

Providers also struggle with the ambiguity of many of the rules, regulations, and expectations of this new health care environment.[35] They complain about the overreliance of managed care on treatment protocols that diminish professional judgment and minimize individual patient or clinical factors, and they cite reduced clinician productivity due to administrative burdens and excessive documentation. Even the roles and functions of providers are subject to some confusion, as seen in the example of case managers. From one setting to another the activities, preparation, and expertise of case managers vary greatly.[15] They may fill a cost-containment function, a coordination function, or a direct service delivery function. Some have college or professional degrees; others have little higher education. Finally, the realities of the new environment often escalate conflict among disciplines rather than enhancing interdisciplinary collaboration. This is because as economic resources become scarcer, disciplines revert to protecting and expanding their professional turf as a way of ensuring survival.

> **?** *Many mental health providers and managed care companies are hotly debating which of them should decide what is best for the patient. But where is the patient in all this? Contact a managed care company in your area and ask them how they involve patients in their decision-making processes.*

Service Settings

Service settings may experience the greatest number of challenges to accountability. These challenges can occur on many fronts. For example, mental health facilities have been criticized for denying inpatient care or transferring patients to another facility for economic reasons when it is not in the patient's best interests. Another effect of managed care has been the layoffs of staff and downsizing of inpatient facilities. The resulting shortage of staff and the increased work the remaining staff must assume may adversely affect the care provided. So too, while staff size is decreasing, the severity of inpatients' problems is increasing, thus requiring an adequate number of well-trained staff to deliver quality patient care.

Another challenge arises in the area of information man-

agement. Computerization is radically changing how behavioral health care services are managed and delivered. Computerized patient records provide standardized formats for easier data collection and analysis. Clinical, financial, and administrative information systems are being integrated so that outcomes related to quality and costs of care can be measured. Information system connections are being made between service units within an organization and among organizations, so that for many activities electronic data communication is replacing paper.

This new information technology presents both opportunities and risks. An important accountability issue is confidentiality, appropriate uses of data, and protection of data, particularly in an area as sensitive as psychiatric and substance abuse disorders. Data are being shared within and among organizations, which increases the risk of problems with misrouting, mishandling, misinterpreting, and generally misusing sensitive and potentially stigmatizing data. Many technical measures are being developed to protect patients, but there is also considerable skepticism about their effectiveness. It has been noted that a comprehensive and ongoing strategy is needed to deal with the issues of confidentiality and the appropriate use of data.[36] Such a strategy should address computer security, training, regulation, public information, policies and procedures, data storage and security, informed consent, planning, and locus of responsibility and structure.

Finally, some developments among accrediting organizations may provide incentives for managed care accountability. Examples of such organizations include the Utilization Review Accreditation Committee (URAC), the Joint Commission on Accreditation of Healthcare Organizations (JCAHO), and the National Committee on Quality Assurance (NCQA). The NCQA is an independent, nonprofit HMO accrediting organization composed of independent health care quality experts, employers, labor union officials, and consumers. In 1991 NCQA adopted standards that assess performance in six areas:

▼ Quality improvement and information
▼ Utilization management
▼ Credentialing of providers
▼ Members' rights and responsibilities
▼ Preventive health services
▼ Medical records

NCQA accreditation is designed for most managed care companies. It has the longest track record in managed care and it is required by law in a number of states.

> **?** *Each night, a secretary on your surgical unit pulls up the list of psychiatric patients on his computer. When you ask him about it, he says that he wants to see whether anyone he knows is admitted so that he can visit them. How would you respond to him and what actions would you take?*

IMPACT ON PSYCHIATRIC NURSING

The environment in which psychiatric nurses practice is changing every day. To thrive in this environment, psychiatric nurses must be knowledgeable about current developments and focus their talents on services, programs, and systems of care with patients and families in the center of their vision. They must continue to be patient advocates and help to create an environment that is ethical and respectful of consumers and their psychiatric and mental health needs. There are over 77,000 psychiatric nurses in the United States; working together, they can have a significant impact on the behavioral health care delivery system.

Roles in Managed Care

Nurses bring great value to the managed care arena through their rich blend of skills and expertise. Although there is great variability of nursing activity based on service setting and geographic location, psychiatric nurses have assumed a number of roles:

▼ **Mental health clinician:** Nurses with various backgrounds are currently employed as direct care providers in managed care settings. They function as staff nurses in inpatient and partial hospitalization programs, nurse clinicians in home and community settings, primary care providers, and advanced practice nurses.

▼ **Case manager:** In this role psychiatric nurses assess patient needs, develop treatment plans, allocate resources, and supervise the care given by other providers.

▼ **Evaluation and triage nurse:** Many psychiatric nurses evaluate patients, either in person or over the telephone, and are responsible for triaging the patient to the most appropriate level of care.

▼ **Utilization review nurse:** Many managed care companies employ psychiatric nurses to function as utilization reviewers who review aspects of the patient's care and influence decisions about treatment assignment. In this role they serve as "gatekeepers" to mental health services.

▼ **Patient educator:** Some settings hire nurses with responsibility for patient and family education. This role has grown with the growing emphasis being placed on patient compliance and disease management programs.

▼ **Risk manager:** Nurses who work as risk managers are charged with the task of decreasing the probability of adverse outcomes related to patient care. They engage in identifying risk factors, individual and systemwide problems, corrective actions, and the implementation of strategies to reduce risk.

▼ **Quality improvement officer:** Nurses have assumed primary responsibility for formulating and implementing quality improvement plans for managed care companies. They train other staff on site and synthesize data related to improvement activities across the organization.

▼ **Marketing and development specialist:** Some psychiatric nurses work in the managed care growth areas of marketing and development. In this role they interact with consumers, employers, providers, and regulators and make recommendations for furthering the mission and goals of the managed care organization.

▼ **Corporate manager:** Psychiatric nurses are also present in the boardrooms of some behavioral managed care organizations, where they influence corporate policy and strategic planning.

Evidence-Based Practice

Psychiatric nurses are being asked to describe what they do and how they add value to the health care organization. They should frame their responses with sensitivity to the issues of cost and quality. Nurses need to educate the business community as well as managed care companies on the services they can provide, including prevention and rehabilitation, and the ways in which they deliver high-quality, cost-effective care. An example of how nurses in the North Mississippi Medical Center Home Health Agency did this for their program is presented in Box 8-5. Nurses must then support this position with data from outcome studies that reflect clinical, functional, satisfaction, and financial indicators. This is the essence of evidence-based psychiatric nursing practice.

At this time there are few outcome studies documenting

Box **8-5** *Case Example: Psychiatric Nursing Home Care for a Patient with Chronic Alcohol Abuse and Depression*

PROBLEM: PATIENT FREQUENTLY ADMITTED TO BEHAVIORAL HEALTH FACILITY FOR DEPRESSION AND ALCOHOL WITHDRAWAL SYMPTOMS

According to the patient's physician, every 3 to 6 months this patient was hospitalized for depression, detoxification, and treatment of acute withdrawal symptoms. Patient's average stay was 7 days. The last stay was 12 days.

SOLUTION: HOME CARE TO EDUCATE AND PROVIDE THERAPY AND SUPPORT

Patient had psychiatric nursing home care services for 2 months after one hospitalization and was not readmitted to the hospital again for 6 months. Patient was again referred to home care after this hospitalization and was seen for 18 months. During this time, patient did not have any hospital stays and required no hospital stay during the 6 months following discharge from home care.

Nurses providing home care taught patient about depression, the addiction process, and new ways to cope. They provided supportive psychotherapy to help the patient resolve issues contributing to his depression and develop a more objective view of himself and life situations. With encouragement, the patient became actively involved in a senior citizens' program that provided socialization and a functioning support system.

RESULT

Eighty home care visits over an 18-month period were provided at a cost of $6400 ($80.00 per visit). According to the physician's report of this patient's hospitalization record, he would have averaged four to eight 7-day hospital stays during the past 2 years. The cost for these stays would have been approximately $18,900 to $37,900. Home care provided a savings of $12,500 to $31,500 for this patient.

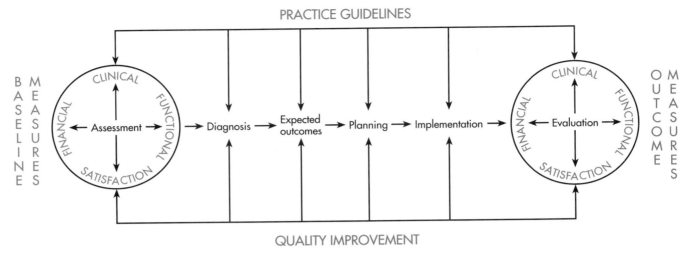

Fig. 8-3 Interaction between the elements of managed care and the nursing process.

the effectiveness of psychiatric nursing care.[19] Programs that psychiatric nurses develop or implement must be clinically practical and incorporate data related to costs as well as quality.[1,12,20,32] The use of measurement or rating scales must be viewed as an essential part of psychiatric nursing practice, and nurses would benefit greatly from mastering the technology that supports this process. Nurses need to research the impact of their activities and control the data set related to nursing outcomes. Finally, nurses need to know how to access, interpret, and use findings from outcome research. Without question, the environment of psychiatric care has changed and so must psychiatric nursing practice.

Threats and Opportunities

Each threat also represents an opportunity. To take advantage of the opportunities, psychiatric nurses must first accept the fact that some form of managed care is here to stay. Nurses need to become knowledgeable about the elements of managed care as it is being enacted in their own communities and across the country. This includes integrating and applying the information to their own practice. For example, Figure 8-3 shows how the characteristics of managed care interact with the activities of the nursing process. Nurses must also master the computer technology and refine their business and accounting skills. In this way, they can use new developments in the environment to deliver better patient care. Finally, the current environment mandates that nurses market their skills in order to be included among the mental health providers of the future.[5]

One fact remains: Throughout all the changes described in this chapter, individuals, families, and communities continue to experience significant emotional problems. Thus, the need for psychiatric nurses as competent and caring professionals will also continue. Nurses must be proactive in realigning their positions within the changing environment. As hospitals downsize, more nurses will be needed in the community and in home settings. Many of the pro-

grams needed by patients in the community have not yet been designed. Psychiatric nurses can assume a leadership role in this new frontier. They must also keep their practice current with the realities of the mental health delivery system, such as by learning new skills in brief therapy, group interventions, psychopharmacology, and disease management.[14] Psychiatric nurses are in an ideal position to work closely with primary care providers to improve access and quality of care for patients with behavioral health problems. Finally, they should continue their commitment to working with underserved populations, the elderly, children, and the serious mentally ill, because they have much to offer to the care and well-being of these vulnerable groups.

Summary

1. The term *managed care* is used to describe a range of health-care arrangements, all focused on value, which is defined as quality divided by costs. Managed care can take a variety of forms and is different from the traditional fee-for-service system in a number of significant ways.

2. Much debate surrounds access to services under managed care. Many people who need behavioral health treatment do not receive it in the United States because their insurance policies deny or restrict coverage for these services.

3. Decisions regarding the clinical appropriateness of care are based on medical necessity and the settings in which care is provided.

4. Practice guidelines are being developed to facilitate clinical decision-making and to provide patients with critical information concerning different treatment options. Clinical pathways identify the key processes and timelines to which a patient must adhere to achieve standard outcomes within a specified period of time.

5. Outcome measurements provide important data about the clinical program and include clinical, functional, satisfaction, and financial indicators. Quality report cards

are being used to measure the performance of the behavioral health care organization.

6. Questions of accountability in the current environment have arisen in relation to patients' rights, provider concerns, and service settings. There are also national standards among accrediting organizations that may provide incentives for managed care accountability.

7. Elements of the environment directly affect psychiatric nursing practice. Nurses must keep abreast of new information and integrate it into practice to provide high-quality, cost-effective care.

your **INTERNET**
connection

Association of Managed Care Providers
http://www.comed.com/amcp/intro.html

Institute for Behavioral Health Care
http://www.ibh.com/

Chapter Review Questions

1. Match each term in Column A with the correct definition in Column B.

Column A

___ Access

___ Clinical pathway

___ Capitation

___ Case rate

___ Clinical appropriateness

___ Outcomes

___ Practice guidelines

___ Utilization review

Column B

A. Degree to which services and information about care are conveniently and easily obtained

B. Degree to which the type, amount, and level of clinical services are delivered to promote positive outcomes for the patient

C. Evaluates the appropriateness and necessity of health-care services and procedures

D. Extent to which services are cost-effective and have a favorable effect on the patient's symptoms, functioning, and well-being

E. Payment system in which the clinic is paid a flat fee regardless of the cost of care

F. Payment system in which the consumer pays a flat fee and in return receives all medically necessary health care

G. Strategies for mental health care delivery that facilitate clinical decision making and provide information to patients about treatment choices

H. Written plan that serves as a map and timetable for the efficient and effective delivery of health care

2. Fill in the blanks.

A. The term _____ is used in managed care to describe the combination of mental and substance abuse disorders.

B. Managed care involves a major shift away from the _____ as customer to the _____ as customer.

C. Value in managed care is defined as _____ divided by _____.

D. Worksite-based programs designed to help identify and facilitate the resolution of behavioral, health, and productivity problems that may adversely affect an employee's well-being or job performance are called _____.

E. The four variables that influence treatment outcome are _____, _____, _____, and _____.

F. The key elements of a clinical pathway include the identification of _____, _____, _____, and _____.

G. The four types of outcome indicators are _____, _____, _____, and _____.

3. Provide short answers for the following questions.

A. Describe the three forms of managed care organizations. If you belong to a managed care organization, identify which type of managed care plan you have.

B. Discuss how stigma associated with substance abuse may have contributed to the law passed in 1996 that ended Medicaid and Medicare coverage for people whose disability is based on drug addiction or alcoholism.

C. Some people believe that we should limit care to people with brain-based mental disorders or the major mental illnesses and not reimburse less serious or minor mental health problems. What position would you take on this issue? Compare this to reimbursement policies for major and minor physical illnesses.

D. Based on your experiences with patients, family, and friends, which system of care delivery for behavioral health services do you think is better: carve-ins or carve-outs?

REFERENCES

1. Baradell J: Clinical outcomes and satisfaction of patients of clinical nurse specialists in psychiatric-mental health nursing, *Arch Psychiatr Nurs* 9:240, 1995.
2. Bezold H, MacDowell M, Kunkel R: Predicting psychiatric length of stay, *Admin Policy Ment Health* 23:407, 1996.
3. Blum T, Roman P: *Cost-effectiveness and preventive implications of employee assistance programs,* Rockville, Md, 1995, US Dept of Health and Human Services, SAMSHA.
4. Boyle P, Callahan D: Managed care in mental health: the ethical issues, *Health Aff* 14:8, 1995.
5. Buerhaus P: Economics of managed competition and consequences to nurses: part II, *Nurs Economics* 12:75, 1994.
6. Bultema J et al: Geriatric patients with depression: improving outcomes using a multidisciplinary clinical path model, *J Nurs Admin* 26:31, 1996.
7. Donaldson M et al, editors: *Primary care: America's health in a new era,* Washington DC, 1996, National Academy Press.
8. Druss B, Rosenheck R: Evaluation of the HEDIS measure of behavioral health care quality, *Psychiatr Serv* 48:71, 1997.
9. Frances A et al: The expert consensus practice guideline project: a new method of establishing best practice, *J Pract Psychiatry Behav Health* 2:295, 1996.
10. Gonzales J, Magruder K, Keith S: Mental disorders in primary care services: an update, *Public Health Rep* 109:251, 1994.
11. Hennessy K, Stephens S: Mental health parity: clarifying our objectives, *Psychiatr Serv* 48:161, 1997.
12. Heyman E, Lombardo B: Managing costs: the confused, agitated, or suicidal patient, *Nurs Econ* 13:107, 1995.
13. Hogan M: Managing the whole system of care, *New Dir Ment Health Serv* 72:13, 1996.
14. Hoyt M: *Brief therapy and managed care,* San Francisco, 1995, Jossey-Bass.
15. Kane C: Deinstitutionalization and managed care: deja vu? *Psychiatr Serv* 46:883, 1995.
16. Mandersheid R, Henderson M: *Federal and state legislative and program directions for managed care: implications for case management,* Rockville, Md, 1995, Center for Mental Health Services.
17. McDaniel C, Erlen J: Ethics and mental health service delivery under managed care, *Issues Ment Health Nurs* 17:11, 1996.
18. McIntyre J, Zarin D, Pincus H: Practice guidelines and outcomes research. In Sederer L and Dickey B, editors: *Outcomes assessment in clinical practice,* Baltimore, Md, 1996, Williams & Wilkins.
19. Merwin E, Mauck A: Psychiatric nursing outcome research: the state of the science, *Arch Psychiatr Nurs* 9:311, 1995.
20. Mitchell A, Reaghard D: Managed care and psychiatric-mental health nursing services: implications of practice, *Issues Ment Health Nurs* 17:1, 1996.
21. Olsen D: Ethical cautions in the use of outcomes for resource allocation in the managed care environment of mental health, *Arch Psychiatr Nurs* 9:173, 1995.
22. Olsen D: Ethical considerations of managed care in mental health treatment, *J Psychosoc Nurs* 32:25, 1996.
23. Pekarik G, Wolff C: Relationship of satisfaction to symptom change, follow-up adjustment, and clinical significance, *Professional Psychology Res Pract* 27:202, 1996.
24. Pigott H: Linking outcomes analysis to critical clinical pathways, *Behav Healthcare Tomorrow* 3:59, 1995.
25. Sederer L, Bennett M: Managed mental health care in the United States: a status report, *Admin Policy Ment Health* 23:289, 1996.
26. Sederer L, Dickey B: *Outcomes assessment in clinical practice,* Baltimore, Md, 1996, Williams & Wilkins.
27. Shore M, Beigel A: Sounding board: the challenges posed by managed behavioral health care, *N Engl J Med* 334:116, 1996.
28. Strosahl K: Mind and body primary mental health care: new model for integrated services, *Behav Healthcare Tomorrow* 4:96, 1996.
29. Tiemens B, Ormel J, Simon G: Occurrence, recognition, and outcome of psychological disorders in primary care, *Am J Psychiatry* 153:636, 1996.
30. Trabin T: Towards greater accountability in behavioral health services: more science, less art? *Behav Healthcare Tomorrow* 3:1, 1995.
31. Trabin T, Freeman M: *Managed behavioral healthcare,* Tiburon, Calif, 1995, Centralink.
32. Tusaie-Mumfrod K, Hahn C: Practical outcome evaluation: patient behavioral health care demonstration project, *Issues Ment Health Nurs* 17:59, 1996.
33. Wells K et al: Use of minor tranquilizers and antidepressant medications by depressed outpatients: results from the Medical Outcomes Study, *Am J Psychiatry* 151:694, 1994.
34. White R et al: New developments in employee assistance programs, *Psychiatr Serv* 47:387, 1996.
35. Wickizer T, Lessler D, Travis K: Controlling inpatient psychiatric utilization through managed care, *Am J Psychiatry* 153:339, 1996.
36. Ziglin A: *Confidentiality and the appropriate uses of data,* Rockville, Md, 1995, Department of Health & Human Services, SAMSHA.

ANNOTATED SUGGESTED READINGS

Institute of Medicine: *Managing managed care: quality improvement in behavioral health,* Washington, DC, 1997, National Academy Press.
>   Provides a framework for the development, use, and evaluation of performance indicators, accreditation standards, and quality improvement mechanisms. A must for providers involved in the purchase and delivery of services within managed care contracts.

Kashner T, Rush A, Altshuler K: Managed care and the focus on outcomes research, *J Pract Psychiatry Behav Health* 3:135, 1997.
>   Discusses how cost outcomes research can help consumers, providers, and health care plan administrators understand how to design more effective psychiatric health benefit packages.

*McDaniel C, Erlen J: Ethics and mental health service delivery under managed care, *Issues Ment Health Nurs* 17:11, 1996.
>   Explores five key ethical issues related to managed care: conflict of interest, confidentiality, patients' rights, underserved populations, and levels of ethical analysis.

New Directions for Mental Health Services, vol 72, 1996.
>   The entire volume of this journal is devoted to managed care, the private sector, and Medicaid mental health and substance abuse services.

Smith G et al: Principles for assessment of patient outcomes in mental health care, *Psychiatr Serv* 48:1033, 1997.
>   Very thorough review of the need for good outcome assessment strategies and a practical guide on the principles that should underlie these assessments.

*Tusaie-Mumford K, Hahn C: Practical outcome evaluation: patient behavioral health care demonstration project, *Issues Ment Health Nurs* 17:59, 1996.
>   A helpful "how to" article describing an interdisciplinary cost-effective outcome evaluation project for inpatient psychiatric units. More research like this is needed in the nursing field.

*Nursing reference.

Legal-Ethical Context of Psychiatric Nursing Care

Gail W. Stuart

© 1998 M.C. Escher/Cordon Art, Baarn, Holland.

Pinel immediately led Couthon to the section for the deranged, where the sight of the cells made a painful impression on him. Couthon asked to interrogate all the patients. From most, he received only insults and obscene apostrophes. It was useless to prolong the interview. Turning to Pinel, Couthon said: "Now, citizen, are you mad yourself to seek to unchain such beasts?" Pinel replied calmly: "Citizen, I am convinced that these madmen are so intractable only because they have been deprived of air and liberty."

Philippe Pinel *Traité Complet du Régime Sanitaire des Aliénés* 56 (1836)

LEARNING OBJECTIVES

After studying this chapter the student should be able to:

▼ Compare and contrast the two types of admission to a psychiatric hospital and the ethical issues raised by commitment

▼ Discuss involuntary community treatment and its implications for improving the care received by psychiatric patients

▼ Analyze the common personal and civil rights retained by psychiatric patients and ethical issues related to them

▼ Identify current legislative initiatives that affect the psychiatric care provided in the United States

▼ Discuss the insanity defense and the psychiatric criteria used in the United States to determine criminal responsibility

▼ Evaluate the rights, responsibilities, and potential conflict of interest that arise from the three legal roles of the psychiatric nurse

TOPICAL OUTLINE

Hospitalizing the Patient
  Voluntary Admission
  Involuntary Admission (Commitment)
  Commitment Dilemma
  Discharge
  Ethical Considerations
Involuntary Community Treatment
Patients' Rights
  Role of Nursing
  Ethical Considerations
  Ethical Dilemmas
Legislative Initiatives
  Omnibus Budget Reconciliation Act
  Protection and Advocacy Act
  Americans with Disabilities Act
  Advanced Directives
Psychiatry and Criminal Responsibility
  Disposition of Mentally Ill Offenders
Legal Role of the Nurse
  Nurse as Provider
  Nurse as Employee
  Nurse as Citizen

The relationship between psychiatry and the law reflects the tension between individual rights and social needs. Both psychiatry and the law deal with human behavior and the relationships and responsibilities that exist among people. Both also play a role in controlling socially undesirable behavior, and together they analyze whether the care psychiatric patients receive is therapeutic, custodial, repressive, or punitive.

Differences also exist between psychiatry and the law. For example, psychiatry is concerned with the meaning of behavior and the life satisfaction of the individual. In contrast, the law addresses the outcome of behavior and the enforcement of a system of rules to encourage orderly functioning among groups of people.

The legal context of care is important for all psychiatric nurses because it focuses concern on the rights of patients and the quality of care they receive.[30] In the past two decades civil, criminal, and consumer rights of patients have been established and expanded through the legal system. Many of the laws vary from state to state, and psychiatric nurses must become familiar with the laws of the state in which they practice. This knowledge enhances the freedom of both the nurse and the patient and ultimately results in better care.

HOSPITALIZING THE PATIENT

Hospitalization can be either traumatic or supportive for the patient, depending on the institution, attitude of family and friends, response of the staff, and type of admission.[16] There are two major types of admission: voluntary and involuntary. Table 9-1 summarizes their distinguishing characteristics.

> **?** *What were your impressions as you walked through the doors of a psychiatric hospital for the first time? How might you use your perceptions and responses to provide better nursing care for patients being admitted for inpatient treatment?*

Voluntary Admission

Under voluntary admission any citizen of lawful age may apply in writing (usually on a standard admission form) for admission to a public or private psychiatric hospital. The person agrees to receive treatment and abide by hospital rules. People may seek help based on their personal decision or the advice of family or a health professional. If someone is too ill to apply but voluntarily seeks help, a parent or legal guardian may request admission. In most states children under the age of 16 years may be admitted if their parents sign the required application form.

Voluntary admission is preferred because it is similar to a medical hospitalization. It indicates that the patient acknowledges problems in living, seeks help in coping with

them, and will probably actively participate in finding solutions. Most patients who enter private psychiatric units of general hospitals do so voluntarily.

When admitted in this way, the patient retains all civil rights, including the right to vote, hold a driver's license, buy and sell property, manage personal affairs, hold office, practice a profession, and engage in a business. It is a common misconception that all admissions to a mental hospital involve the loss of civil rights.

Although voluntary admission is the most desirable, it is not always possible. Sometimes a patient may be acutely disturbed, suicidal, or dangerous to self or others, yet rejects any therapeutic intervention. In these cases involuntary commitments are necessary.

> **?** *Should a psychotic person be allowed to sign forms for voluntary admittance to the hospital? If not, should all voluntary patients be screened for competence before hospitalization?*

Involuntary Admission (Commitment)

In the late 1940s the World Health Organization reported that almost 90% of admissions to state mental hospitals in the United States were involuntary and approximately 10% were voluntary. The trend has shifted to more voluntary admissions. Currently about 73% of the 1.6 million yearly admissions to psychiatric hospitals are voluntary.[31]

Although involuntary commitment has come under intense scrutiny, the United States Supreme Court continues to recognize it based on two legal theories. First, under its police power, the state has the authority to protect the community from the dangerous acts of the mentally ill; and second, under its *parens patriae* powers, the state can provide

TABLE **9-1** *Characteristics of the Two Types of Admission to Psychiatric Hospitals*

	VOLUNTARY ADMISSION	**INVOLUNTARY ADMISSION**
Admission	Written application by patient	Application did not originate with patient
Discharge	Initiated by patient	Initiated by hospital or court but not by patient
Civil rights	Retained fully by patient	Patient may retain none, some, or all, depending on state law
Justification	Voluntarily seeks help	Mentally ill and one or more of the following: Dangerous to self or others Need for treatment Unable to meet own basic needs

care for citizens who cannot care for themselves, such as some mentally ill people.

Almost all states have made dramatic changes in commitment laws in the past 20 years, prompted by two major concerns. The first was the state's need to lessen its role as a major provider of mental health services because of budgetary constraints. The second was greater emphasis on issues of liberty and individual rights and increasing mandated treatment of mentally ill people in the least restrictive settings. As a result of these issues, the police power rationale for civil commitment has been emphasized over the *parens patriae* doctrine, using dangerousness as the standard for commitment. There has also been a trend toward strengthening the requirements for procedural due process for such commitments and the need for proof of mental illness and dangerousness by clear and convincing evidence. However, states with less stringent commitment laws still have higher admission rates to state and county hospitals.[26]

Involuntary commitment means that the patient did not request hospitalization and may have opposed it or was indecisive and did not resist it. The standards for commitment vary among states and reflect the confusion in the medical, social, and legal systems of society. Most laws permit commitment of the mentally ill on the following three grounds:

▼ Dangerous to self or others
▼ Mentally ill and in need of treatment
▼ Unable to provide for own basic needs

Generally, each state identifies which criteria are required and what each criterion means. In addition to people with mental illness, certain states have laws that allow for the involuntary hospitalization of three other groups:

▼ Developmentally disabled (mentally retarded) people
▼ Substance abusers
▼ Mentally disabled minors

THE COMMITMENT PROCESS. State laws vary, but they try to protect the person who is not mentally ill from being detained in a psychiatric hospital against his or her will for political, economic, family, or other nonmedical reasons. Certain procedures are standard. The process begins with a sworn petition by a relative, friend, public official, physician, or any interested citizen stating that the person is mentally ill and needs treatment. Some states allow only specific people to file such a petition. One or two physicians must then examine the patient's mental status; some states require that at least one of the physicians be a psychiatrist.

The decision whether to hospitalize the patient is made next. Precisely who makes this decision determines the nature of the commitment. **Medical** certification means that physicians make the decision. **Court** or **judicial** commitment is made by a judge or jury in a formal hearing. Most states recognize the patient's right to legal counsel, but only about half actually appoint a lawyer for patients if they do not have one. **Administrative** commitment is determined by a special tribunal of hearing officers. The Fourteenth Amendment to the U.S. Constitution protects citizens against infringements on liberty without due process of the law. For this reason medical certification is used rarely, primarily in emergencies, and administrative commitment is subject to judicial review.

If treatment is deemed necessary, the person is hospitalized. The length of hospital stay varies depending on the patient's needs. Fig. 9-1 diagrams the involuntary commitment process. It identifies three types of involuntary hospitalization: emergency, short term, and long term.

> **?** *Most states specify that any physician, not necessarily a psychiatrist, can certify a person for involuntary commitment to a psychiatric hospital. Do you agree with this? What is required by law in your state?*

EMERGENCY HOSPITALIZATION. Almost all states permit emergency commitment for patients who are acutely ill. The goals are primarily intended to control an immediate threat to self or others. In states lacking such a law, police often jail the acutely ill person on a disorderly conduct charge, which is a criminal charge. Such a practice is inappropriate and often harmful to the patient's mental status. Most state laws limit the length of emergency commitment to 48 to 72 hours. Emergency hospitalization allows detainment in a psychiatric hospital only until proper legal steps are taken to provide for additional hospitalization.

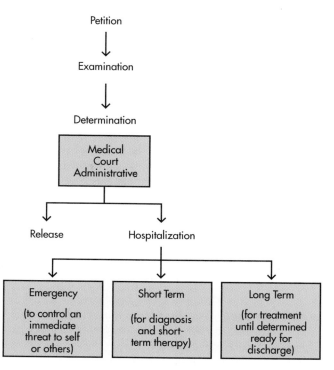

Fig. 9-1 Diagram of the involuntary commitment process.

SHORT-TERM OR OBSERVATIONAL HOSPITALIZATION. This type of commitment is used primarily for diagnosis and short-term therapy and does not require an emergency situation. Again, the commitment is for a specified time that varies greatly from state to state. If at the end of the period the patient is still not ready for discharge, a petition can be filed for a long-term commitment.

LONG-TERM HOSPITALIZATION (FORMAL COMMITMENT). A long-term commitment provides for hospitalization for an indefinite time or until the patient is ready for discharge. Patients in public or state hospitals more often have indefinite commitments than patients in private hospitals. Even when committed, these patients maintain their right to consult a lawyer at any time and to request a court hearing to determine whether additional hospitalization is necessary. The hospital ultimately discharges the patient, however, and a court order is not needed. Periodic reviews for long-term hospitalization may be made every 3, 6, or 12 months.

> **?** *Do you agree with the criteria for committing patients to psychiatric hospitals? How would you assess whether a person met these criteria?*

Commitment Dilemma

In a few states involuntary commitment assumes incompetency and patients lose their civil rights. In those states patients may not be able to make contracts, vote, drive, obtain a professional license, serve on a jury, marry, or enter into civil litigation. In addition, the patient must suffer the stigma attached to the label *committed* in all future activities. Because of the many people affected by involuntary commitment and the loss of personal rights that it can entail, it becomes a matter of great legal, moral, social, and psychiatric significance. In general medicine there is no equivalent loss of individual rights, except for rare cases requiring quarantine for carriers of potentially epidemic diseases.

How ill does a person need to be to merit commitment? It is not necessary to be psychotic, as shown by the number of elderly, addicted, and neurotic patients hospitalized, as well as by the many psychotic people who remain free. Perhaps a person's dangerousness to self or others is a more pertinent consideration. Certainly psychiatric professionals consider hospitalization in this instance as a humanitarian gesture that protects both the individual and society. However, *dangerousness* is a vague term.

> **?** *According to a recent survey commissioned by* Parade *magazine, over 57% of Americans think mentally ill people are more likely to commit acts of violence than other people. How does this compare with the facts? How do the media contribute to this impression of the mentally ill?*

DANGEROUSNESS. Interestingly, courts guard the freedom of people who are mentally healthy but dangerous. For example, after a prison sentence is served, the person is automatically released and can no longer be retained. However, someone who is mentally ill and dangerous can be confined indefinitely. The idea of preventive detention does not exist in most areas of the law because the ability to predict an action does not confer the right to control it in advance. Only illegal acts result in prolonged confinement for most citizens, except the mentally ill.

Most mentally ill people are not dangerous to themselves or others. Studies show that the vast majority of people with serious mental illness are not violent and are no more dangerous than people in the general population. However, a subgroup of such people are more dangerous. Patients in this subgroup display a history of violent behavior, noncompliance with medications, and current substance abuse. These characteristics can serve as predictors of potential violence.[39] It should also be remembered that violent behavior by people with serious mental illness is only one aspect of a larger problem: the failure of public psychiatric services and the deinstitutionalization of the mentally ill without adequate community support. Other aspects of this problem include the large number of mentally ill among the homeless, the large number of mentally ill in jails and prisons, and the revolving door of psychiatric readmissions, in which almost 30% of patients are readmitted within 30 days of discharge, with some patients accumulating more than 100 readmissions.

Another issue is that there are no reliable indicators of dangerousness. Even if some mentally ill people are potentially dangerous, psychiatrists cannot necessarily predict future violence. Psychiatrists often overpredict patients' potential for dangerous acts. This may result from their medical training, which cautions that underdiagnosis is more harmful than overdiagnosis. If psychiatrists underpredict a psychiatric illness and the patient later causes harm, they are held responsible. If they overpredict illness, however, a patient is subjected to treatment unwillingly. Therefore, multidisciplinary teams should be involved in determining dangerousness. It may also be helpful to use the predictors for violence identified above and a clinically based decision-making process that can be validated and evaluated with treatment outcome.[3] Input from those familiar with the patient's home setting and sociocultural background might also improve evaluations.

Five aspects of dangerousness may be useful as a decision-making guide for judges, jurors, probation officers, and mental health professionals[4]:

▼ *Nature of harm or conduct.* Does the person threaten bodily harm, harm to property, or psychological harm?

▼ *Magnitude of the harm.* Does the person threaten murder, assault, or verbal abuse?

▼ *Probability.* How likely is it that the harmful act will occur?

▼ *Imminence.* When will the threatened action take place?

▼ *Frequency.* How often will the threatened action take place? Will it be repeated, or will it be a single act of violence?

The answers to these questions can be very subjective, which suggests that the underlying issue is nonconformity in ways that offend others. In this context, social role becomes important. For example, before the law all men and women are equal, but it is also true that most committed patients are members of the lower classes. Specifically, a recent study reported that the profile of a patient who has the greatest risk for involuntary admission to a psychiatric hospital is a young, unmarried black male who has schizophrenia without comorbid substance abuse.[27] This raises questions regarding the sociocultural context of psychiatric care (see Chapter 7) and the role of mental health professionals as enforcers of social rules and norms. Thus the behavioral standard of dangerousness can change the function of the psychiatric hospital from a place of therapy for mental illness to a place of confinement for offensive behavior.

> **?** *How do you explain the fact that society condones certain kinds of dangerous behavior, such as race car driving, but objects to other kinds?*

FREEDOM OF CHOICE. The legal and psychiatric question thus raised is freedom of choice. Some professionals believe that at certain times the individual cannot be self-responsible. To protect both the patient and society, it is necessary to confine the patient and make decisions for him or her. An example is the suicidal patient. In most states suicide is against the law, so law and psychiatry join to protect the person and help individuals resolve personal conflicts.

How does this compare with cancer or cardiac patients who may reject medical advice and the prescribed treatment? Should society, through law and medicine, attempt to cure these patients against their will? Some clinicians view civil commitment as basically a benevolent system that makes treatment available. They disagree with the assumption that mentally ill people are competent to exercise free will and make decisions in their own best interest, such as whether to take medications or remain outside a hospital. They contend that there are mentally ill people who may not be physically dangerous but still endanger their own prospects for a normal life. Because institutions can protect them and in many cases help them, they think it would be immoral to abolish involuntary civil commitment.

Other clinicians oppose intervention. They favor responsibility for self and the right to choose or reject treatment. If a person's actions violate criminal law, they suggest that the person be punished through the penal system. Currently a middle ground is being sought between meeting the needs of the severely mentally ill and preserving their legal rights and freedom of choice.[23]

> **?** *Who should decide what is in the patient's best interest if a patient is involuntarily committed? Should it be the patient, a family member, a health-care professional, or the judicial system?*

Discharge

The patient who is informally admitted to the hospital can leave at any time, limited only to reasonable hours, such as daytime hours or weekdays. The voluntarily admitted patient can be discharged by the staff when maximum benefit has been received from the treatment. Voluntary patients may also request discharge. Most states require written notice of patients' desire to leave and also that patients sign a form that states they are leaving against medical advice (AMA). This form then becomes part of the patient's permanent record.

In some states voluntarily admitted patients can be released immediately; in others they can be detained 24 to 72 hours after submitting a discharge request. This allows hospital staff time to confer with the patient and family members and decide whether additional inpatient treatment is indicated. If it is and the patient will not withdraw the request for discharge, the family may begin involuntary commitment proceedings, thereby changing the patient's status. Voluntarily admitted patients who leave the hospital before discharge can be brought back only if they agree. Staff often attempt to contact such patients and discuss alternatives. If they refuse to return, either they must be discharged or involuntary commitment procedures must begin.

An involuntarily committed patient has lost the right to leave the hospital when he or she wishes. Short-term and emergency commitments specify the maximum length of detainment. Long-term commitments do not, although the patient's status should be reviewed periodically. The patient may also apply for another commitment hearing. If a committed patient leaves before discharge, the staff has the legal obligation to notify the police and committing courts. Often these patients return home or visit family or friends and can be easily located. The legal authorities then return the patient to the hospital. Additional steps are not necessary because the original commitment is still in effect.

Ethical Considerations

Nurses must analyze their beliefs regarding the voluntary and involuntary hospitalization of psychiatric patients. What should be done if the nonconformist does not wish to change behavior? Do the nonconformists maintain freedom to choose even if their thinking appears to be irrational or abnormal? Is coercion fair? Can social interests be served by less restrictive methods such as outpatient therapy? Nurses are responsible for reviewing commitment procedures in their state and working for necessary clinical, ethical, and legal reforms.

The commitment dilemma exposes current practices and opens areas of controversy for the future. Studies show that more than half of the homeless population have psychiatric or substance abuse disorders. Homeless mentally ill people have a wider array of service needs than homeless people who use only social services. Many seriously mentally ill people cannot obtain or maintain access to community resources such as housing, a stable source of income, or treatment and rehabilitative services. Homeless people lack supportive social networks and underuse psychiatric, medical, and welfare programs. Many avoid the mental health system entirely, often because they are too confused to respond to offers of help. As a consequence, they are often admitted into acute psychiatric hospitals or jailed because of their lack of shelter and other resources, even though such restrictive environments may not best address their psychiatric needs.[41]

Unfortunately, local communities often deny the problem by resisting the establishment of halfway houses or sheltered homes in their neighborhoods. Third-party insurance seldom covers extended outpatient psychiatric care. In today's mobile society, family and friends are often unable to care for the newly discharged patient, who may end up in a boarding house with little to do but watch television.

These issues must be addressed by psychiatric nurses, patients, and citizens across the United States. The value of commitment, goals of hospitalization, quality of life, and rights of patients must be preserved through the judicial, legislative, and health-care systems.

INVOLUNTARY COMMUNITY TREATMENT

There are three major ways in which involuntary community treatment can be provided for those in need: outpatient commitment, preventive commitment, and conditional release from the hospital.[32] These initiatives arose from the mandate to offer psychiatric patients treatment in the least restrictive setting. Geller[12] has proposed 10 guidelines to determine a patient's appropriateness for involuntary outpatient treatment (Box 9-1). They are sequential in that a patient is not evaluated for appropriateness under a guideline unless the criteria for all preceding guidelines have been met. The guidelines also assume that the patient has a serious and persistent mental illness and a history of dangerousness to self or others.

> ? *How might sociocultural factors influence a nurse's interpretation of the guidelines listed in Box 9-1? How might nurses guard against potential bias based on their personal world view?*

Box 9-1 *Guidelines for the Use of Outpatient Commitment*

1. The patient must express an interest in living in the community.
2. The patient must have previously failed in the community.
3. The patient must have that degree of competency necessary to understand the stipulations of his or her involuntary community treatment.
4. The patient must have the capacity to comply with the involuntary community treatment plan.
5. The treatment or treatments being ordered must have demonstrated efficacy when used properly by the patient in question.
6. The ordered treatment or treatments must be such that they can be delivered by the outpatient system, are sufficient for the patient's needs, and are necessary to sustain community tenure.
7. The ordered treatment must be such that it can be monitored by outpatient treatment agencies.
8. The outpatient treatment system must be willing to deliver the ordered treatments to the patient and must be willing to participate in enforcing compliance with those treatments.
9. The public-sector inpatient support system must support the outpatient system's participation in the provision of involuntary community treatment.
10. The outpatient must not be dangerous when complying with the ordered treatment.

From Geller J: On being "committed" to treatment in the community, *Innovations Res* 2:23, 1993.

Outpatient commitment is the process by which the courts can order patients committed to a course of outpatient treatment specified by their clinicians. This type of commitment is an alternative to inpatient treatment for people who meet the involuntary commitment criteria of dangerousness to self or others. A recent survey indicated that 35 states and the District of Columbia have laws permitting outpatient commitment. Georgia, Hawaii, and North Carolina use different criteria for outpatient commitment than for inpatient commitment. In only 12 states and the District of Columbia was use of outpatient commitment rated as common. Reasons for not using it included concerns about civil liberties, liability and financial costs, lack of information and interest, problems with enforcement and ways to deal with lack of compliance, and criteria that are too restrictive.[40] Nonetheless, research suggests that if these problems can be overcome and it is used judiciously, outpatient commitment can be a helpful tool in reducing the rehospitalization rate for people with severe mental illness.[19]

Preventive commitment is a new concept found in only a few states. Preventive commitment permits commitment to outpatient treatment of people who do not yet meet the usual commitment criteria but will do so soon if intervention does not take place. The criterion used for preventive commitment is sometimes called a predicted deterioration standard, in which a person is believed to need treatment to prevent a relapse that would probably result in the person's becoming imminently dangerous.

Conditional release is the third type of involuntary community treatment. It involves continued supervision of a person who has been released from the hospital. It has been available for some time in about 40 states. Under this arrangement, the hospital or court informs the conditionally released person of the conditions for release, such as reporting to a medication clinic. Violation of these conditions usually triggers rehospitalization. In contrast to outpatient commitment, which is designed as an alternative to inpatient commitment, and preventive commitment, which is anticipatory, conditional release is used primarily to see whether the person is able to function in the community under supervision.

Although involuntary community treatment is a potentially useful way for improving treatment compliance and decreasing hospitalizations, it is not widely used. However, it is an interesting approach that merits further research to evaluate its effectiveness.[34]

PATIENTS' RIGHTS

In 1973 the American Hospital Association issued a Patient's Bill of Rights that many hospitals and community-based settings throughout the United States have adopted. These rights were reaffirmed in 1990.[1] Often, they are posted for reading in a location that is easily accessible to patients. In some hospitals they may be given to patients on admission and read or explained to them.

However, this process does not ensure that psychiatric patients know their civil rights. For example, one study reported that reading patients their rights on admission and giving them a copy did not necessarily result in understanding or retaining the information. Two important rights—the right to withdraw from treatment and the right to participate in the development of the treatment plan—were not understood by more than a fourth of the patients in the study.[45] This finding suggests that a change may be needed in how psychiatric patients are informed about their rights and empowered to participate in the treatment process.

> **?** *In your experience, are patients in general hospital settings granted their patient rights? How about patients in psychiatric inpatient units? What specific things could nurses do to see that these rights are honored in all hospitals?*

Although there is great variation among states, psychiatric patients currently have the following rights:
▼ Right to communicate with people outside the hospital through correspondence, telephone, and personal visits

▼ Right to keep clothing and personal effects with them in the hospital
▼ Right to religious freedom
▼ Right to be employed if possible
▼ Right to manage and dispose of property
▼ Right to execute wills
▼ Right to enter into contractual relationships
▼ Right to make purchases
▼ Right to education
▼ Right to habeas corpus
▼ Right to independent psychiatric examination
▼ Right to civil service status
▼ Right to retain licenses, privileges, or permits established by law, such as a driver's or professional license
▼ Right to sue or be sued
▼ Right to marry and divorce
▼ Right not to be subject to unnecessary mechanical restraints
▼ Right to periodic review of status
▼ Right to legal representation
▼ Right to privacy
▼ Right to informed consent
▼ Right to treatment
▼ Right to refuse treatment
▼ Right to treatment in the least restrictive setting
Some of these rights deserve more discussion.

Right to Communicate with People Outside the Hospital

This right allows patients to visit and hold telephone conversations in privacy and send unopened letters to anyone of their choice, including judges, lawyers, families, and staff. Although the patient has the right to communicate in an uncensored manner, the staff may limit access to the telephone or visitors when it could harm the patient or be a source of harassment for the staff. The hospital can also limit the times when telephone calls are made and received and when visitors can enter the facility. On occasions hospital staff have intercepted and destroyed letters presumed to be threatening or abusive. In states where this is not illegal, such activity raises ethical questions of individual freedom and the good of the community.

Right to Keep Personal Effects

The patient may bring clothing and personal items to the hospital, taking into consideration the amount of storage space available. The hospital is not responsible for their safety, and valuable items should be left at home. If the patient brings something of value to the hospital, the staff should place it in the hospital safe or otherwise provide for safekeeping. The hospital staff is also responsible for maintaining a safe environment and should take dangerous objects away from the patient if necessary.

> *How are patients informed of their rights on your psychiatric unit? Talk to some of the patients and see whether they can recall any of the rights that were explained to them.*

Right to Execute Wills

A person's competency to make a will is known as **testamentary capacity**. Patients can make a valid will if the following conditions are met:

▼ They know they are making a will.
▼ They know the nature and extent of their property.
▼ They know who their friends and relatives are and what the relationships mean.

Each of these criteria must be documented for the will to be considered valid. This means that patients must not be mentally confused at the time they sign their will. It does not imply that they must know exact details of their property holdings or specific bank account figures, but they cannot attempt to give away more than they possess. Furthermore, the law requires that patients know who their relatives are but does not require them to bequeath anything to them.

A patient's commitment or a diagnosis of psychosis does not immediately invalidate the will. It is still valid if it was made during a lucid period and the patient met the three criteria. The problem most debated in determining testamentary capacity involves the delusional patient. The important question is whether the false belief or delusion caused the person to dispose of property differently than he or she would have otherwise.

Two or three people must witness the will by watching the patient sign it and watching each other as they sign it. Later a nurse may be summoned to testify to the patient's condition at the time of writing the will. The nurse's testimony should relate to the three competency criteria. Hospital charts and the nurse's notes may also be used in the court proceedings.

Right to Enter into Contractual Relationships

The court considers contracts valid if the person understands the circumstances of the contract and its consequences. Once again, a psychiatric illness does not invalidate a contract, although the nature of the contract and degree of judgment needed to understand it are influencing factors.

INCOMPETENCY. Related to this right is the issue of mental incompetency. Every adult is assumed to be mentally competent, mentally able to carry out personal affairs. To prove otherwise requires a special court hearing to declare an individual **incompetent**. This is a legal term without a precise medical meaning. To prove incompetence, it must be shown that:

▼ The person has a mental disorder
▼ This disorder causes a defect in judgment

▼ This defect makes the person incapable of handling personal affairs

All three elements must be present, and the exact diagnostic label is not important in this case. If a person is declared incompetent, the court will appoint a legal guardian to manage his or her affairs. This often is a family member, friend, or bank executive. Incompetency rulings are most often filed for people with senile dementia, cerebral arteriosclerosis, chronic schizophrenia, and mental retardation.

The legislative trend is to separate the concepts of incompetency and involuntary commitment because the reasons for each are essentially different. Incompetency arises from society's desire to guard its citizens' assets from their inability to understand and transact business. Involuntary commitments are intended to protect patients from themselves (in the case of suicide), protect others from dangerous patients (as in homicide), and administer treatment. However, many states still consider the two equivalent.

If ruled incompetent, a person cannot vote, marry, drive, or make contracts. A release from the hospital does not necessarily restore competency. Another court hearing is required to reverse the previous ruling before the person can once again manage private affairs.

> *How is education provided for emotionally ill children living in your community? Are they mainstreamed in the school system, given special educational resources, or both?*

Right to Education

Many parents exercise this right on behalf of their emotionally ill or mentally retarded children. The U.S. Constitution guarantees this right to everyone, although many states have not provided adequate education to all citizens and are now required to do so.

> *How is the right to education honored in a children's psychiatric inpatient setting? How does this compare with the education provided children in a pediatric hospital?*

Right to Habeas Corpus

Habeas corpus is an important constitutional right patients retain in all states even if they have been involuntarily hospitalized. Its goal is the speedy release of any person who claims being detained illegally. A committed patient may file a writ at any time on the grounds of being sane and eligible for release. The hearing takes place in court, where those who wish to restrain the patient must defend their actions. Patients are discharged if they are judged as sane.

Right to Independent Psychiatric Examination

Under the Emergency Admission Statute, the patient has the right to demand a psychiatric examination by a physician of choice. If this physician determines that the patient is not mentally ill, the patient must be released.

Right to Privacy

The right to privacy implies the person's right to keep some personal information completely secret. **Confidentiality** involves the disclosure of certain information to another person. Every psychiatric professional is responsible for protecting a patient's right to confidentiality, including even the knowledge that a person is in treatment or in a hospital. Revealing such information might damage the patient's reputation or the ability to get or keep a job. The protection of the law applies to all patients. This can create ethical and professional dilemmas, such as the one experienced by the nurse described in this clinical example.

Clinical Example On a Wednesday morning in Springfield, Illinois, a man walked into Lauterbach's Cottage Hardware Store, grabbed an ax, and began swinging. When he left, one person was dead and two others were critically injured. Ten days later, police received a call from Mr. K, who was a patient in the 49-bed psychiatric unit at St. John's Hospital. Mr. K told the police that his roommate at the hospital confessed the crime. However, he didn't know his roommate's name. He asked Nurse M to identify him but she refused to do so because she believed that his name was shielded by a state law guaranteeing the privacy of mental health records. Hospital administrators supported her decision even after she was fined $250 by a county judge for refusing to give the man's name to a grand jury. Nurse M did tell the police that the suspect was not a patient in St. John's at the time of the murder and that he resembled their composite sketch.

The issue of confidentiality is becoming increasingly important.[36] Various agencies require information about a patient's history, diagnosis, treatment, and prognosis, and sophisticated methods for obtaining information through computer systems have been developed. These methods threaten the individual's right to privacy. Clinicians are free from legal responsibility if they release information with the patient's written and signed request. Written consent is desirable for two reasons: It makes clear to both parties that consent has been given, and if questions arise about the consent, a documentary record of it exists. Therefore, it should be made a part of the patient's permanent chart. As a rule, it is best to reveal as little information as possible and discuss with the patient what will be released.

Confidentiality builds on the element of trust necessary in a patient-therapist relationship. Patients place themselves in the care of others and reveal vulnerable aspects of their personal life. In return they expect high-quality care and the protection of their interests. Thus, the patient-therapist relationship is an intimate one that demands trust, loyalty, and privacy.

> **?** One of the adolescent girls on your unit runs away while going to the hospital cafeteria. When you speak to the girl's mother to let her know what has happened, the mother asks you to call the radio and television stations and have them announce it so that the girl can be found. How would you respond to this request?

PRIVILEGED COMMUNICATION. The legal term *privilege* or, more accurately, *testimonial privilege,* applies only in court-related proceedings. It includes communications between husband and wife, attorney and client, and clergy and church member. The right to reveal information belongs to the person who spoke, and the listener cannot disclose the information unless the speaker gives permission. This right protects the patient, who could sue the listener for disclosing privileged information. It also gives the patient the confidence necessary to make a full account of symptoms and conditions so that treatment can be administered.

Testimonial privilege between health professionals and patients exists only if established by law. It varies greatly among professions, even within the same state. A minority of the states allow privilege between nurses and patients. Nurses may also be covered in states that have adopted privileges between psychotherapists and patients. The psychotherapist-patient privilege is usually limited. It applies only when a therapist-patient relationship exists, and only communications of a professional nature are protected. Third persons present during the communication between the therapist and the patient may be required to testify and are not included in privilege.

> **?** What is the law in your state regarding testimonial privilege between nurses and patients? How would you change the law if it does not include nurses?

CIRCLE OF CONFIDENTIALITY. This discussion is summarized in Fig. 9-2. Within the circle, patient information may be shared. Those outside the circle require the patient's permission to receive information. Within the circle are treatment team members, staff supervisors, health care students and their faculty working with the patient, and consultants who actually see the patient. All of these people must be informed about the patient's clinical condition to be able to help. The patient is also inside the circle—an obvious point but one that is often overlooked. The patient can reveal any aspect of his or her life, problems, treatments, and experiences to anyone. This is an important point for the nurse to remember in situations where the requirements of confidentiality are uncertain.

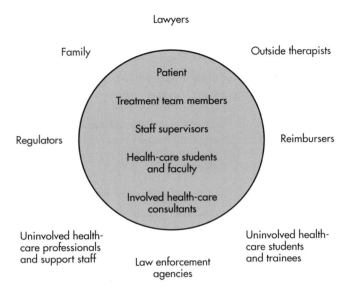

Fig. 9-2 The circle of confidentiality.

Box **9-2** *Exceptions Allowing the Release of Information Without the Patient's Consent*

> ▼ Emergency situations when acting in the patient's best interests
> ▼ Court-ordered evaluations or reports
> ▼ If the patient is incompetent and consent is obtained from a guardian or is not available
> ▼ Commitment proceedings
> ▼ Criminal proceedings
> ▼ Acting to protect third parties
> ▼ Child custody disputes
> ▼ Reports required by state law (contagious diseases, gunshot wounds, child abuse)
> ▼ Patient-litigant exceptions
> ▼ Child abuse proceedings

Many people are outside the circle and these relationships must be carefully considered by the nurse. For example, family members of adult patients are not automatically entitled to clinical information about the patient. Although nurses may wish to engage the family in a therapeutic alliance, it is equally important to remember that information about the patient belongs to the patient. It is essential, therefore, that the nurse first discuss with the patient the benefits of involving the family in the treatment process and obtain clear consent from the patient before doing so. This may create uncomfortable situations for the nurse who is pressured by a family to reveal patient information, but it is a critical aspect of

patient confidentiality and the nurse-patient relationship. Legal representatives, outside or previous therapists, reimbursers or insurance companies, students, health care professionals and support staff not directly involved in the care of the patient, and the police or other law enforcement or regulatory agencies are outside the circle of patient confidentiality. A signed written consent from the patient is required to release information to any of these parties. However, in some situations breaching confidentiality and testimonial privilege is both ethical and legal. These exceptions are listed in Box 9-2.

PATIENT RECORDS. Most treatment facilities keep psychiatric records separately so that they are less accessible than medical records. The law and psychiatric professionals view them as more sensitive than medical records. Many states allow or require that patients have access to their own records. If a patient makes such a request, the clinician should explore the reasons for the request, determine the laws that apply in the particular state, prepare the patient for the review, and be present with the patient to discuss any questions the patient might have. The clinician must not release material from any other sources and must not alter or destroy any part of the record before the patient sees it.

Finally, it is important for the nurse to realize that the physical record itself is the property of the treatment facility or therapist, but the information contained in the record belongs to the patient. Thus, the original record should never be given to the patient; only a copy of it should be provided. A patient's record or chart can be brought into court and its contents used in a lawsuit because privilege does not apply to records or charts.

> **?** *The parents of one of your patients ask for information about their adult son. The patient has been very specific about not wanting to see his family and not wanting them to know anything about his treatment. How would you respond?*

PROTECTING A THIRD PARTY. Another dimension to the concepts of confidentiality and privilege stems from the case of *Tarasoff v. Regents of the University of California et al.*[38] In this case the psychotherapist did not warn Tatiana Tarasoff or her parents that his client had stated he intended to kill Tatiana when she returned from summer vacation. In the lawsuit that followed Tatiana Tarasoff's death, California's Supreme Court decided that the treating therapist has a duty to warn the intended victim of a patient's violence. When a therapist is reasonably certain that a patient is going to harm someone, the therapist has the responsibility to breach the confidentiality of the relationship and warn or protect the potential victim.

Most states now recognize some variation of the duty to warn. This duty obliges the clinician to:

▼ Assess the threat of violence to another
▼ Identify the person being threatened
▼ Implement some affirmative, preventive act

A recent study examined the effects of such warnings on the warned person and the therapeutic relationship. It found that most warnings were issued for patients in inpatient units and emergency rooms. In almost half of the cases the intended victim could not be contacted but the threat was reported to a law enforcement agency. In about three fourths of the cases in which the intended victim was contacted, the person knew of the threat. The most common reaction among those warned was gratitude, and most said that they would take steps to increase their safety. The second most common reaction was denial that the patient would ever hurt them. Clinicians reported that in most cases issuing the warning to an intended victim had a minimal or a positive effect on the psychotherapeutic relationship. The researchers thus concluded that the anticipated negative effects of the *Tarasoff* decision have not materialized.[7]

One of the most problematic areas in which the duty to protect may apply is the protection of sexual partners of people infected with the human immunodeficiency virus (HIV). Laws in some states forbid disclosure of patients' HIV status to sexual partners, whereas others allow it. No statutes mandating disclosure have been enacted, but they appear to be gaining public support.

Right to Informed Consent

Informed consent means that a physician must give the patient a certain amount of information about the proposed treatment and must attain the patient's consent, which must be competent, understanding, and voluntary. The physician should explain the treatment and possible complications and risks. The information to be disclosed in obtaining informed consent is listed in Box 9-3.

The patient must be able to consent and not be a minor or judged legally incompetent. Even if a patient is psychotic, the physician is not relieved from attempting to obtain informed consent for treatment. Psychosis does not necessarily mean that a person is unable to consent to treatment, and many psychotic patients are capable of giving informed consent.[11,15] For patients who are not able to consent and for minors, informed consent should be obtained from a substitute decision maker.

The doctrine of informed consent is consistent with the provision of good clinical care. It allows patients and clinicians to become partners in the treatment process and respects patients' autonomy, needs, and values. Furthermore, informed consent should be viewed as a continuing educational process rather than a procedure performed merely to comply with the law. In obtaining informed

---

Box **9-3** *Obtaining Informed Consent*

INFORMATION TO DISCLOSE

Diagnosis: description of the patient's problem
Treatment: nature and purpose of the proposed treatment
Consequences: risks and benefits of the proposed treatment including physical and psychological effects, costs, and potential resulting problems
Alternatives: viable alternatives to the proposed treatment and their risks and benefits
Prognosis: expected outcome with treatment, with alternative treatments, and without treatment

PRINCIPLES OF INFORMING

Assess the patient's ability to give informed consent.
Simplify the language so that a layperson can understand.
Offer opportunities for the patient and family to ask questions.
Test the patient's understanding after the explanation.
Reeducate as often as needed.
Document all relevant factors, including what was disclosed, the patient's understanding, competency, voluntary agreement to treatment, and the actual consent.

---

consent the clinician should adhere to the principles listed in Box 9-3.

Consent forms usually require the signature of the patient, a family member, and two witnesses. Nurses are often called on to be witnesses. The form then becomes part of the patient's permanent record.

In accordance with this doctrine, informed consent should be obtained for all psychiatric treatments including medication, particularly neuroleptics because of the risk of tardive dyskinesia; somatic therapies, such as electroconvulsive therapy (ECT); and experimental treatments. Whether consent should be obtained for psychotherapy is unclear at present, and other aspects related to obtaining informed consent remain controversial in many states.[42,44]

? *How is informed consent obtained in your psychiatric treatment setting? Ask to observe this process and evaluate it based on the criteria listed in Box 9-3.*

Right to Treatment

Early court cases extended the right to treatment to all mentally ill and mentally retarded people who were involuntarily hospitalized. The courts defined three criteria for adequate treatment:

▼ A humane psychological and physical environment
▼ A qualified staff with a sufficient number of members to administer adequate treatment
▼ Individualized treatment plans

Most important is the requirement for an individualized treatment plan. Failure to provide it means that the patient must be discharged unless he or she agrees to stay voluntarily. This decision was upheld in a recent ruling that revised the standards related to the development of treatment plans, placed more stringent restrictions on the use of seclusion and restraint and ECT, and expanded the definition of a qualified mental health professional.[21]

The right to treatment is not a guarantee of treatment for all patients. It applies only to involuntary or committed patients. In addition, the right to treatment identifies minimal treatment standards, not optimal treatment; it does not guarantee that adequate treatment occurs and it does not require that a range of treatments be available (one treatment choice is adequate). Thus, although much has been gained through this legislation, much remains to be done.

Right to Refuse Treatment

The relationship between the right to treatment and the right to refuse treatment is complex[17] (see Critical Thinking about Contemporary Issues). The right to refuse treatment includes the right to refuse involuntary hospitalization. It has been called the right to be left alone. Some people believe that therapy can control a person's mind, regulate thoughts, and change personality, and the right to refuse treatment

protects the patient. This argument states that involuntary therapy conflicts with two basic legal rights: freedom of thought and the right to control one's life and actions as long as they do not interfere with the rights of others.

In recent years, the number of lawsuits concerning the right to refuse treatment, especially treatment involving psychotropic drugs, has increased. Many states have guidelines for the administration of ECT and psychosurgery; however, the controversy over refusal of medication is a more recent one. Related to this right is the right to refuse experimentation. Any experimental treatment requires the written consent of the patient.

Recently, a group of patients with serious mental illness were surveyed about their experiences and attitudes toward forced psychiatric treatment. The results indicated that at some time during the course of their illness, 57% reported being pressured or forced into hospitalization. In the year before the survey, 30% reported being pressured or forced into taking medication and 26% into attending a therapy or rehabilitation program. The most common type of pressure or force was verbal persuasion. Generally, respondents reported negative effects from forced treatment but about half retrospectively felt that the forced treatment was in their best interest.[18]

This finding suggests that treatment can be successful in a variety of coerced situations and that issues such as degree and source of coercion must be considered. In addition, the following patient factors are believed to predict a positive outcome[13]:

▼ Patients who have the ability to understand the immediate consequences of refusing to comply with treatment even though they may not appreciate the effects of the illness itself.

▼ Patients who value what will be lost if the treatment is refused.

▼ Patients who trust that compliance with treatment will help them avoid negative consequences.

▼ Patients who are able to cooperate at least minimally.

▼ Patients whose problems are psychiatrically treatable.

  FORCING MEDICATIONS. There are many reasons why patients refuse medication. Symptoms such as delusions and denial may cause the refusal, and patients who refuse medication are generally sicker than those who comply.[29] A study of patients' attitudes after involuntary medication suggests that for most patients the decision to refuse medication is a sign of the patient's illness and does not reflect autonomous functioning or consistent beliefs about mental illness or its treatment.[28]

CRITICAL THINKING *about* **Contemporary Issues**

Is the Value of Treatment More Important Than a Person's Right to Liberty?

This question has been debated over the years and is still not resolved for psychiatric patients. The most publicized case examining this issue was that of Billie Boggs, a 40-year-old black woman who lived on the street for a year near a warm-air grate on New York's fashionable Upper East Side and who panhandled money for food. She attracted the attention of a mental health team, who decided to hospitalize her, believing that she was mentally ill and unable to care for herself.

The legal questions raised in this case were whether Billie Boggs was mentally ill and whether she was dangerous. At trial, psychiatrists from one side testified that she was both mentally ill and dangerous. However, psychiatrists who interviewed Boggs after she was hospitalized and had received medication, been bathed, rested, dressed adequately, and fed testified that she was not mentally ill. The questions that emerged were:

  What behavior is socially acceptable?

  How is mental illness determined?

  How is dangerousness defined?

  Although the legal actions proceeded, the hospital discharged Boggs because she refused to accept further antipsychotic medication. The Billie Boggs case has raised more unanswered questions and dramatized the problem of mentally ill street people. What it has not done is address the compelling needs of the chronically mentally ill in this country.

? *Is the refusal of treatment the same as noncompliance? If not, how would you distinguish between them and what nursing intervention would be most appropriate for each?*

Staff members faced with a patient who refuses medication have several options. First, they can offer the patient a lower dosage, or no medication at all. A second option would be to discharge the patient against medical advice if no other staff action can relieve the patient's symptoms and the patient does not meet the criteria for commitment. Another approach would be to have the patient declared incompetent and seek a court order permitting the medication. Similarly, a guardian can consent to medication when the patient's refusal can be shown to result from inability to make a rational decision.

Nurses should judge each situation on a case-by-case basis. The Task Force on Behavior Therapy has examined the issue of coerced treatment and suggested three criteria that may justify it[5]:

▼ The patient must be judged to be dangerous to self or others.

▼ It must be believed by those administering treatment that it has a reasonable chance of benefiting the patient.

▼ The patient must be judged to be incompetent to evaluate the necessity of the treatment.

Even if these three conditions are met, the patient should not be deceived but should be informed regarding what will be done, the reasons for it, and its probable effects.

Nurses are often on the front line in dealing with patients who refuse treatments and medications. It is clear that voluntary patients have the right to refuse any treatment and should not be forcibly medicated except in exceptional situations when the patient is actively violent to self or others and when all less restrictive means have been unsuccessful. The behavior of the patient should be clearly documented and all interventions recorded.

Nurses must know the guidelines identified by the courts and the legislature in the state in which they practice in order to administer medication properly to involuntarily committed patients. Some questions that can help guide the nurse's decision are[24]:

▼ Has the patient been given a psychiatric diagnosis?

▼ Is the treatment consistent with the diagnosis?

▼ Is there a set of defined target symptoms?

▼ Has the patient been informed about the treatment outcome and side effects?

▼ Have medical and nursing assessments been completed?

▼ Are therapeutic effects of treatment being monitored?

▼ Are side effects being monitored?

▼ Is the patient over- or undermedicated?

▼ Is drug therapy being changed too quickly?

▼ Are pro re nata (PRN) and stat doses being used too often?

▼ Is drug therapy being prescribed for an indefinite period of time?

Finally, it is important for the nurse to remember that a therapeutic nurse-patient relationship is critical in working with a patient who refuses to take medication. A positive, caring relationship between the nurse and patient can play a vital role in reversing treatment refusal.

> **?** *Imagine that your mother was admitted to a psychiatric hospital in need of treatment. Once there, however, she refused to take any medication. How would you feel if the staff forced medication on her? How would you feel if they honored her right to refuse treatment? What could you do to help your mother get the treatment she needed?*

Right to Treatment in the Least Restrictive Setting

The right to treatment in the least restrictive setting is closely related to the right to adequate treatment. Its goal is evaluating the needs of each patient and maintaining the greatest amount of personal freedom, autonomy, dignity, and integrity in determining treatment. Table 9-2 presents six clinical dimensions of the concept of restrictiveness in psychiatric nursing. This right applies to both community and noncommunity programs. Greater consideration of this right might limit some of the controversy surrounding commitment and the right to refuse treatment.

> **?** *Which do you think is more restrictive: to be living in the community while actively psychotic or to be involuntarily committed to a psychiatric hospital for treatment?*

TABLE **9-2** *Six Dimensions of the Concept of Restrictiveness*

DIMENSION	COMPONENT
Structural	Type of treatment setting and objective means of physical restraint or limitations on physical freedoms
Institutional policy	Rules, procedures, routines, and regulations for operating the institution and degree of patient involvement in planning
Enforcement	Staff-determined consequences of rule breaking or inability of the patient to leave the setting
Treatment	Use and level of antipsychotic medications and the use of other somatic treatments such as ECT or psychosurgery
Psychosocial atmosphere	Status difference between patients and staff and degrees of staff authoritarianism
Patient characteristics	Patients' ability to manage their care and level of functioning as influenced by the severity of their disorder

From Garritson S: Least restrictive alternatives: ethical considerations, *J Psychosoc Nurs Ment Health Serv* 21:9, 1983.

Another consideration in the right to the least restrictive alternative is that it applies not only to when a person should be hospitalized but also to how a person is cared for. It requires that a patient's progress be carefully monitored so that treatment plans are changed based on the patient's current condition.

Finally, issues related to the use of seclusion and restraints are of particular concern. There must be adequate rationale for the use of these practices. Documentation should include a description of the event that led to seclusion or restraint, alternatives attempted or considered, the patient's behavior while secluded or restrained, nursing interventions, and ongoing evaluation of the patient. It is important to remember that seclusion and restraint must be therapeutically indicated and justified (see Chapter 29).

Role of Nursing

The National League for Nursing in 1977 issued a statement on the nurse's role in patients' rights.[20] It identified respect and concern for patients and competent care as basic rights, along with patients receiving the necessary information to understand their illness and make decisions about their care. The League urged nurses to get involved in ensuring patients' human and legal rights.

The League identified many of the previously mentioned rights, plus the following:

▼ Right to health care that is accessible and meets professional standards, regardless of the setting
▼ Right to courteous and individualized health care that is equitable, humane, and given without discrimination based on race, color, creed, sex, national origin, source of payment, or ethical or political beliefs
▼ Right to information about their diagnosis, prognosis, and treatment, including alternatives to care and risks involved
▼ Right to information about the qualifications, names, and titles of health-care personnel
▼ Right to refuse observation by those not directly involved in their care
▼ Right to coordination and continuity of health care
▼ Right to information on the charges for services, including the right to challenge these charges
▼ Above all, the right to be fully informed about all their rights in all health-care settings

Perhaps the single most important factor is the attitude of mental health professionals. Sensitivity to patients' rights cannot be imposed by the court, the legislature, administrative agencies, or professional groups. If nurses ignore them, implement them casually, or are outwardly hostile about honoring them, patients' rights are an empty legal concept. But if professionals are sensitive to patients' needs in all aspects of their relationships with them, they will secure these human and legal rights.

Ethical Considerations

Ensuring patients' rights is often complicated by ethical considerations. For example, consider the crucial element of power. In the psychiatric setting the nurse can function in many roles, from a custodial keeper of the keys to a skilled therapist. Each of these roles includes a certain amount of power because all nurses have the ability to influence the patient's treatment and serve as the major source of information regarding a patient's behavior. This is particularly true in inpatient settings, in which a nurse and patient spend more time together and the nursing staff is the only group to work a 24-hour day. Nurses also participate in team meetings, individual and group psychotherapy, and behavior modification programs. Finally, nurses can greatly influence decisions about patient medications, such as type, dosage, and frequency.

Many ethical dilemmas arise from health-care professionals' paternalistic attitude toward patients. Paternalism can be defined as deciding what is best for another person without consideration of the person's thoughts or feelings. It occurs when something is done "for the patient's own good" even though the patient would probably disagree with the action. This attitude reduces adult patients to the status of children and interferes with their freedom of action.

The right to treatment also poses several ethical questions. One involves the appropriateness of treatment and whether confinement itself can be therapeutic. A second question deals with the untreatable patient. Should such a patient be released after a certain time? Another problem is the unwilling patient. Might a person refuse treatment and then seek release, claiming that the right to adequate treatment was denied? A more pressing question is whether the public is willing to pay the costs required to provide adequate treatment to the mentally ill in public institutions. In current times of reduced government funds, programs often struggle to survive.

Ethical dilemmas also arise in considering the right to refuse treatment. Does the right apply to all treatments, including medications, or only to those that are hazardous, intrusive, or severe, such as psychosurgery? How can staff meet their obligation for the right to treatment when a patient refuses to be treated? How can refusal, resisting treatment, and noncompliance be differentiated, and does each of these require a different response? There are no solutions to these complex issues, but they concern nurses, who are often responsible for delivering prescribed treatments such as medications.

Finally, the right to treatment in the least restrictive setting raises a number of difficult questions. How do mental health professionals balance human rights with the human needs of patients? Are sufficient funds available to provide adequate supportive care in the community? What happens to chronically ill patients who are not discharged into less restrictive settings? Can community centers provide better care than institutions? How can one counter community resistance to local placement of mentally ill patients? And most important, given economic constraints, how can limited resources be used wisely to provide a full range of mental health services?

Ethical Dilemmas

An ethical dilemma exists when moral claims conflict with one another. It can be defined as:

▼ A difficult problem that seems to have no satisfactory solution

▼ A choice between equally unsatisfactory alternatives

Ethical dilemmas pose such questions as "What should I do?" and "What is the right thing to do?" They can occur both at the nurse-patient-family level of daily nursing care and at the policymaking level of institutions and communities. Although ethical dilemmas arise in all areas of nursing practice, some are unique to psychiatric and mental health nursing. Many of these dilemmas fall under the umbrella issue of behavior control.

At first glance, behavior control may seem a simple issue: Behavior is a personal choice, and any behavior that does not impose on the rights of others is acceptable. Unfortunately, this does not help to address complex situations. For example, a severely depressed person may choose suicide as an alternative to an intolerable existence. On one level, this is an individual choice not directly harming others, yet suicide is forbidden in American society. In many states it is a crime that can be prosecuted. As another example, in some states it is illegal for consenting adults of the same sex to have sexual relations, although it is not illegal for a man to rape his wife. These examples raise difficult questions: When is it appropriate for society to regulate personal behavior? Who will make this decision? Is its goal personal adjustment, personal growth, or adaptation to social norms? And finally, how do we measure the costs and benefits of attempting to control personal freedom in a free society?

One of the most fundamental problems is the blurry line between science and ethics in the field of psychiatry. Theoretically, science and ethics are separate entities. Science is descriptive, deals with what is, and rests on validation; ethics is predictive, deals with what ought to be, and relies on judgment. However, psychiatry is neither purely scientific nor value-free.

Despite these ambiguities, nurses must identify their professional commitment. Are they committed to the happiness of the individual or the smooth functioning of society? Ideally, these values should not conflict, but in reality they sometimes do. The patient's rights to treatment, to refuse treatment, and to informed consent highlight this conflict-of-interest question. Nurses must consider whether they are forcing patients to be socially or politically acceptable at the expense of patients' personal happiness. Nurses

may not be working for either the patient's best interests or their own; they may be acting as agents of society and not be aware of it.

All nurses participate in some therapeutic psychiatric regimens whose scientific and ethical bases are ambiguous. The American health-care system continues to apply a medical model of wellness and illness to human behavior. Wellness is socially acceptable behavior, and illness is socially unacceptable. It becomes critically important for each nurse to analyze such ethical dilemmas as freedom of choice versus coercion, helping versus imposing values, and focusing on cure versus prevention. The nurse must also become active in defining adequate treatment and deciding important resource allocations.

LEGISLATIVE INITIATIVES

The connection between psychiatry and the law is becoming increasingly complex. At present there are simultaneous trends toward adequate treatment of the psychiatrically ill and protection of their constitutional rights. Both trends are occurring at a time of fiscal restraint.

Mental health professionals are concerned about the quantity and quality of psychiatric care. Legal reformers are indignant about perceived violations of patients' rights. Judges are angry that in the day-to-day implementation of the commitment law, their only option is to prosecute the mentally ill defendant. Psychiatric hospitals are understaffed, underfunded, and attacked on all sides for their inability to care for and cure psychiatric patients. Community programs are few and poorly supported, often resulting in deinstitutionalized patients living without treatment in urban ghettos or being treated as criminals. The public is frightened at the thought of psychiatric patients in their neighborhoods. Concerned citizens demand that mental health programs exercise greater control over this population, whom they perceive as dangerous.

Clearly, mechanisms are needed by which patients, families, mental health professionals, attorneys, and concerned citizens can work together to advance mental health care and the rights of all patients. The mentally ill need protection not only of their legal rights but also of their clinical needs and general welfare. No one profession can fulfill all these needs, but increased cooperation among mental health advocates can achieve this goal.

Omnibus Budget Reconciliation Act

Other legislation has also changed the nature of psychiatric care and service delivery in the United States. One major event was passage of the Omnibus Budget Reconciliation Act (OBRA) in 1981. It placed mental health service programs formerly administered by the federal government into alcohol and drug abuse and mental health service block grants to be administered by the states. Overall, this had a negative impact on the quality of mental health services provided throughout the country because each state was able to allocate resources to mental health based on its own priorities and political climate. Although some states made significant progress in developing community-based systems, in most state governments mental health funding was not given high priority.

Since that time, other changes have been mandated through this same annual legislative process. In 1985 the Consolidated OBRA (COBRA) prohibited the transfer of indigent patients with acute medical conditions from general medical hospitals or emergency departments to public psychiatric hospitals that are ill equipped to provide medical care.[9] This measure helped the mentally ill. However, the OBRA passed in 1987 established criteria for Medicaid-or Medicare-certified nursing homes to use in admitting or retaining mentally ill patients. The effect of this law was to continue the trend of shifting costs from federal programs to the states, and it has the potential of increasing homelessness and continuing a pattern of failure to adequately serve patients with severe mental illness.[8]

Protection and Advocacy Act

Under the Protection and Advocacy for Mentally Ill Individuals Act of 1986, all states must designate an agency that is responsible for protecting the rights of the mentally ill. The following three areas of advocacy would help to maximize the fulfillment of patients' rights:

▼ To educate the mental health staff and implement policies and procedures that recognize and protect patients' rights

▼ To establish an additional procedure to permit the speedy resolution of problems, questions, or disagreements that occur based on legal rights

▼ To provide access to legal services when patients' rights have been denied

About 20,000 people were served by the program in 1991 and 1992. The largest category of complaints in those years concerned being able to access psychiatric services. In addition to representing individuals, protection and advocacy programs agencies provide referral and information services, public education, outreach, training, and class-action representation.[22,37] As mental health systems change and more patients are treated in outpatient settings, access to protection and advocacy services for people living in the community will become increasingly important. Advocacy will also be important in ensuring enforcement of new laws and policies affecting psychiatric care and treatment.

Americans with Disabilities Act

The Americans with Disabilities Act (ADA), passed in 1990, protects over 43 million Americans with physical or mental disabilities from discrimination in jobs, public services, and accommodations. It prohibits discrimination against people with physical and mental disabilities in hiring, firing, train-

ing, compensation, and advancement in employment. Employers are prohibited from asking job applicants whether they have a disability, and medical examinations and questions about disability may be required only if the concerns are job related and necessary.[25]

Each of these prohibitions has major implications for people with psychiatric disabilities. However, because the disability is often not obvious, and because of widespread stigma and discrimination, or simply as a statement of self-sufficiency, many people choose not to identify themselves as disabled. If they do, there is concern that employers and co-workers will assume that any work or personal difficulties the person has are related to the psychiatric disability.

Although the act has produced some encouraging advances in job placement, education, and training, the majority of people with psychiatric disabilities remain unemployed or continue to work in sheltered settings. An analysis of nearly 40,000 ADA claims found that 11.4% involved mental illness, with the greatest number of those based on depressive illness. This figure excludes mental retardation. An additional 3.6% filed discrimination claims based on drug or alcohol impairments. The disability most often reported was back problems, which accounted for nearly 20% of claims. Partly because of the ambiguity of the wording of the act, instructions were issued in 1995 to eliminate pregnancy, physical characteristics, common personality traits, cultural and economic disadvantages, a range of sexual disorders, and current illegal drug use.

Unfortunately, a recent study reported that the majority of psychiatric nurses surveyed did not have the knowledge necessary to act as advocates with respect to the ADA. Moreover, few psychiatric nurses in the study had provided patients with ADA information.[43] The act does constitute a cultural as well as legal mandate to include people with disabilities in the social and economic mainstream. It is not likely to totally eliminate the myths, fears, and discrimination faced by people with disabilities, but it does contribute to the educational effort needed to combat widespread biases and misperceptions about people with disabilities, including mental illness.

Advanced Directives

Advanced directives came about as a result of the Patient Self-Determination Act (PSDA) of 1990. They are documents, written while a person is competent, that specify how decisions about treatment should be made if the person becomes incompetent. Use of advanced directives seems particularly appropriate for people with mental illness who may alternate between periods of competence and incompetence. For example, they could formalize a patient's wishes about forced medication or treatment setting.

Some states are already encouraging patients to fill out advanced directive forms.[6] In addition, federal regulations that took effect in 1991 require all facilities that receive Medicare or Medicaid to inform patients, including psychiatric patients, at admission about their rights under state law to sign advanced directives. To date, advanced directives have not had a major impact on psychiatric treatment, but that may change.

> ❓ *Does your psychiatric setting comply with federal law that requires having patients sign advanced directives? If so, talk with some patients and ask them what this document means to them.*

PSYCHIATRY AND CRIMINAL RESPONSIBILITY

The determination of criminal responsibility concerns the accused person's condition when the crime was committed. It has received much public attention as the "insanity defense." This proposes that a person who has committed an act usually considered criminal is not guilty by reason of "insanity." This is a difficult decision to make. Defense attorneys often call on psychiatrists to testify.[33] Nurses are seldom directly involved, but they should understand the law in this area as both citizens and psychiatric professionals.

This defense is based on the humanitarian rationale that people should not be blamed for crimes if they did not know what they were doing or could not help themselves. With the complexity of today's society and judicial system, however, many believe that this defense is being abused, but this belief is not supported by data.[14] Some of the controversy stems from John Hinckley's shooting of President Reagan in 1981, from which he was acquitted by the verdict of "not guilty by reason of insanity." One recent change is the movement away from using the defense "not guilty by reason of insanity" (NGBI) to the more recent "guilty but mentally ill" (GBMI). In addition, most recently three states—Montana, Idaho, and Utah—have abolished the insanity defense completely. Three sets of criteria are used in the United States to determine the criminal responsibility of an offender who is mentally ill: the M'Naghten Test, the Irresistible Impulse Test, and the American Law Institute's Test, the one most often used (Table 9-3).

> ❓ *In the 1994 case of Lorena Bobbitt, who was found not guilty by reason of insanity, the jury concluded that she could not resist the impulse to sever her husband's penis. Mrs. Bobbitt was committed to a psychiatric hospital for observation and was released when she was found not to be psychiatrically ill. Do you agree with the court's decision? Defend your position.*

Disposition of Mentally Ill Offenders

Those found not guilty by reason of insanity (NGBI) are rarely set free. In some states they may be committed at the court's discretion, and in almost a third of the states they are automatically hospitalized. Some offenders are treated in special hospitals, others are sent to state mental hospitals, and still others go to prison treatment facilities. Those found guilty but mentally ill (GBMI) are never freed. Because the insanity defense is used most often in capital offenses, it is usually better to have good security, and penal institutions or maximum security forensic psychiatric hospitals are the best option.

After hospitalization and recovery, the patient may be discharged by the court that ordered the commitment. In other states the governor may discharge the patient. Still others allow the mental institution to make that decision. The major criteria for discharge are that the patient is not likely to repeat the offense and that it is safe to release the patient to the community.

> ❓ *Do you believe in the legal defenses of NGBI and GBMI? What are the pros and cons of each insanity defense?*

LEGAL ROLE OF THE NURSE

Professional nursing practice is not determined by simply following patients' rights. Rather, it is an interplay between the rights of patients, the legal role of the nurse, and concern for high-quality psychiatric care (Fig. 9-3). The psychiatric nurse performs three roles while completing

TABLE **9-3** *Three Sets of Criteria Used to Determine the Criminal Responsibility of a Mentally Ill Offender*

NAME OF TEST	CRITERIA
M'Naghten Test	The person did not know the nature and quality of the act. The person did not know that the act was wrong.
Irresistible Impulse Test	A person is impulsively driven to commit the criminal act with lack of premeditation and a strong urge to do so. This test is usually used with the M'Naghten test.
American Law Institute's Test	A person lacks the capacity to appreciate the wrongfulness of an act or to conform conduct to the requirements of the law. It excludes the sociopath and is the most common criterion for determining criminal responsibility.

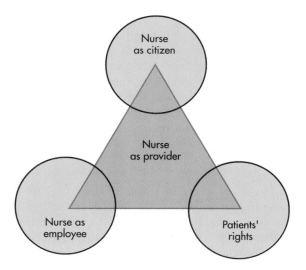

Fig. 9-3 Legal influences on psychiatric nursing practice.

Sexual contact with a patient
Patient suicide
Failure to diagnose
Problems related to electroconvulsive therapy
Misuse of psychoactive prescription drugs
Breach of confidentiality
Failure to refer a patient
False imprisonment in civil commitment
Failure to obtain informed consent
Inadequate supervision of trainees and employees
Failure to warn potential victims
Failure to report abuse

professional and personal responsibilities: provider of services, employee or contractor of services, and private citizen. These roles are simultaneous, and each carries certain rights and responsibilities.

Nurse as Provider

MALPRACTICE. All psychiatric professionals have legally defined duties of care and are responsible for their own work. If these duties are violated, malpractice exists. Malpractice involves the failure of professionals to provide the proper and competent care that is given by members of their profession, resulting in harm to the patient. Nurses are held to national standards of care.

Most malpractice claims are filed under the law of negligent tort. A **tort** is a civil wrong for which the injured party is entitled to compensation. Under the law, individuals are responsible for their own torts, so each nurse can be held responsible in malpractice claims. For this reason, all nurses should carry malpractice liability insurance. Under the law of negligent tort the plaintiff must prove the following:

▼ A legal duty of care existed.
▼ The nurse performed the duty negligently.
▼ Damages were suffered by the plaintiff as a result.
▼ The damages were substantial.

When patients are admitted to a psychiatric hospital, the problems of litigation in connection with their care are many and varied.

LITIGATION. Lawsuits alleging malpractice in psychiatric diagnosis or treatment, once rare, are now increasing. Some of the most common sources of malpractice suits are listed in Box 9-4.[35] Lawsuits against nurses are uncommon. However, they can occur when the nurse errs while acting either dependently or independently.[10] The most common

causes of malpractice suits against psychiatric nurses are negligence in suicide precautions and while assisting in ECT. Box 9-5 describes three recent cases involving psychiatric nurses.

LEGAL RESPONSIBILITIES. The nurse is responsible for reporting pertinent information to co-workers involved in the patient's care. The degree of nursing care depends on the patient's condition, with the seriously ill demanding a higher degree of care to protect them from injury and self-destruction.

Reporting information includes written as well as oral communication, and accurate records are crucial. Box 9-6 lists characteristics of good nursing records. For example, notes that record specific suicidal precautions clarify the nurse's actions. The nurse should also record all patient and family education such as explaining the food precautions needed when taking monoamine oxidase inhibitor (MAOI) medication. Such a note would provide a good defense against a possible lawsuit should the patient violate dietary restrictions and become ill. Accurate reporting is an element of good nursing care that should be completed promptly and thoroughly.

Unlike patients' charts, some hospital records, such as incident reports, are not admissible in court to prove facts but they can cast doubt on the credibility of the involved parties. Currently, more insurance companies are requiring hospitals to keep incident reports, and more state and federal agencies are demanding the right to review them. Because they can be seen and used by so many people, what a nurse writes on an incident report should be carefully considered, and unfounded statements, opinions, interpretations, and vague descriptions should be avoided.

In summary, a psychiatric nurse can follow these preventive measures to avoid possible lawsuits:

▼ Implement nursing care that meets the *Standards of Psychiatric–Mental Health Clinical Nursing Practice* as described by the American Nurses' Association (see Chapters 10 and 11).[2]

Box **9-5** *Selected Litigation Involving Psychiatric Nurses*

CASE 1: *VALENTINE v. STRANGE* (597 F. SUPP. 1316 VA.)

Problem: Nurses were sued when psychiatric patient set self on fire.

Facts: Despite two previous attempts to burn herself, the health-care providers permitted the patient to keep her cigarettes and lighter. Patient subsequently set fire to her clothing and suffered third-degree burns.

Legal lesson: The failure of health-care professionals to take precautions in the face of imminent danger to the life of an involuntarily committed patient constitutes a violation of liberty interests protected by the due process clause of the Fourteenth Amendment.

CASE 2: *DELICATA v. BOURLESSES* (404 N.E. 2ND 667-MASS.)

Problem: Nursing psychiatric assessment disagreed with the psychologist's.

Facts: A nursing assessment indicated that a depressed patient should be closely supervised as potentially suicidal. An evaluation by the staff psychologist advised that suicidal precautions were not necessary. The patient subsequently killed herself in a locked bathroom.

Legal lesson: Medical orders by a staff psychiatrist or an evaluation by a staff psychologist must be questioned when there is a change or deterioration in a patient's condition. Nursing assessments should include the evaluation of such changes in the patient's apparent physical and psychological condition. The responsibility of nursing assessment includes the necessity for making appropriate nursing judgments and implementing nursing actions based on these nursing assessments.

CASE 3: *VATTIMO v. LOWER BUCKS HOSPITAL* (428 A. 2ND 765-PA.)

Problem: Patient required restraint and supervision by psychiatric nurses.

Facts: A patient with a psychotic fascination with fire set fire to his hospital room, resulting in the death of the other occupant. The patient had been diagnosed as a paranoid schizophrenic, and staff had been warned of his preoccupation with fire.

Legal lesson: The hospital was required to exercise reasonable care under the circumstances to restrain, supervise, and protect mentally deficient patients.

Box **9-6** *Characteristics of Good Nursing Records*

Accurate	Factual
Clear	Legible
Complete	Objective
Concise	Relevant
Descriptive	Timely

▼ Know the laws of the specific state, including the rights and duties of the nurse as well as the rights of the patients.

▼ Stay current with advances and new knowledge in the field.

▼ Keep accurate and concise nursing records.

▼ Maintain the confidentiality of patient information.

▼ Maintain current malpractice liability insurance coverage.

▼ Consult a lawyer if any questions arise.

Nurse as Employee

The role of the employee, or contractor of service, is less often studied but also very important. It involves the practitioner's rights and responsibilities in relation to employers, partners, consultants, and other professional colleagues. Professionals often do not know the rights and responsibilities of employees and contractors of service. However, these are the basis of the practitioner's economic security, professional future, and peer relationships.

As employees, nurses have the responsibility to supervise and evaluate those under their authority for the quality of care given. They must also observe their employer's rights and responsibilities to clients and other employees, fulfill the obligations of the contracted service, inform the employer of circumstances and conditions that impair the quality of care, and report negligent care by others. This includes the legal duty to communicate any concerns about other mental health professionals.

> **?** *You have seen a colleague sexually touching a patient on the unit. What should you do based on your legal and professional obligations?*

In return, nurses can expect certain rights from their employer. These include consideration for service, adequate working conditions, adequate and qualified assistance when necessary, documented grievance procedures, and the right to respect all of their other rights and responsibilities.

> **?** *You arrive for work one morning and are told that you and an aide are the only staff assigned to work the day shift on a 25-bed closed psychiatric unit. Based on your legal roles, rights, and responsibilities, how should you respond?*

Nurse as Citizen

The third role that the nurse plays is that of citizen. This role is significant because all other roles, rights, responsibilities, and privileges are based on the inherent rights of citizenship. The U.S. government grants these as inherent: civil rights, property rights, right to protection from harm, right to a good name, and right to due process. These form the foundation for the nurse's other legal relationships. Unfortunately, the best interests of the patient, nurse, and employer do not always coincide. Conflict can occur when, for example, the nurse's right to live and work without threat to personal security is violated by a patient who harms the nurse, as is evident in the following clinical example.

Clinical Example A psychotic patient who has hallucinations that are adequately controlled with psychotropic medications but who refuses to take them was recently admitted to a locked psychiatric unit. Before intervening, the staff considered the following possibilities:

▼ Failing to medicate may deny the patient's right to treatment.

▼ Failing to medicate the patient could have harmful side effects, such as the unnecessary and possibly irreversible continuation of illness.

▼ Failing to medicate the patient may lead to a psychotic episode and result in injury to self, other patients, or the staff.

▼ Failing to medicate the patient may lead to a psychotic episode but no violence.

▼ Medicating the patient in the absence of an emergency situation and without a clear threat of violence violates the patient's right to refuse treatment.

The staff decided not to medicate the patient. When the night nurse checked on the patient in his room that evening, he struck the nurse in the face, resulting in severe bruises and the loss of several teeth. This development leads to new questions:

▼ Was the patient competent and legally liable for his actions?

▼ What were the circumstances of the incident?

▼ Was the nurse sufficiently aware of the potential hazard and, if so, was she responsible for assuming the risk?

▼ Was staffing adequate to discourage, respond to, and control a potentially violent situation?

▼ Was there a provision in the unit for potentially violent patients and, if so, why wasn't it used for this patient?

▼ Was the nurse able to sue the patient for assault and battery?

Obviously, there are no simple or perhaps even equitable solutions to such clinical dilemmas, yet they are real and ever present. All mental health professionals must focus on prevention. This requires a knowledge of legislation, rights, responsibilities, and potential conflicts. In addition, professional nursing judgment requires examining the context of nursing care, the possible consequences of nurses' actions, and practical alternatives. Only then do rights and responsibilities become meaningful.

Summary

1. There are two types of admission to a psychiatric hospital: voluntary and involuntary commitment. Involuntary commitment poses many legal and ethical issues for patients, the law, and psychiatric professionals.

2. Involuntary community treatment mandates a course of outpatient treatment. It can be provided in three ways: outpatient commitment, preventive commitment, and conditional release.

3. Psychiatric patients have a wide variety of personal and civil rights. They should be informed of these rights, and hospitals must honor them. Some of these rights are controversial and create dilemmas for psychiatric nurses.

4. Current legislative initiatives that affect ethical psychiatric care provided in the United States include OBRA, the Protection and Advocacy Act, the Americans with Disabilities Act, and Advanced Directives.

5. Three sets of criteria are used in the United States to determine the criminal responsibility of an offender who is mentally ill: the M'Naghten Test, the Irresistible Impulse Test, and the American Law Institute's Test, which is the one most often used.

6. The psychiatric nurse has three roles in performing professional and personal duties: provider of services, employee or contractor of services, and private citizen.

 Video **Resources**

Mosby's Legal and Ethical Issues in Nursing Video Series:

Ethical Dilemmas and Decision Making
Legal Aspects of Nursing Documentation
Introduction to Legal Issues and Terminology
Minimizing Legal Liability
Patient Self-Determination
The Nurse's Rights as an Employee

your **INTERNET connection**

Bazelon Center for Mental Health Law
http://www.bazelon.org/

Medical-Legal Consulting Institute, Inc.
http://ourworld.compuserve.com/homepages/
Medical_Legal_Consulting

Chapter Review Questions

1. **Identify whether the following statements are true (T) or false (F).**

A. ___ Patients who are voluntarily admitted to a psychiatric hospital retain all civil rights.

B. ___ The *parens patriae* doctrine for civil commitment is currently emphasized over the police power rationale.

C. ___ The profile of the patient at greatest risk for involuntary admission is that of a white, middle-aged woman with depression.

D. ___ People with mental illness are more likely to commit acts of violence than other people.

E. ___ Involuntary community treatment is underused in the current mental health care system.

F. ___ *Incompetent* is a legal term without precise medical meaning.

G. ___ Police and lawyers are always entitled to information about committed psychiatric patients.

H. ___ Information can be released without a patient's consent when it is related to child custody disputes.

I. ___ Patients are allowed to keep their records when they are discharged from treatment.

J. ___ Mental illness is the most commonly reported disability reported under the American Disabilities Act.

K. ___ None of the states in this country have abolished the insanity defense.

2. **Fill in the blanks.**

A. Emergency commitment is usually limited to _____ hours.

B. Psychiatric patients who appear to be prone to violence display a _____, _____, and _____.

C. _____ is the process by which courts can order patients committed to a course of outpatient treatment specified by their clinicians.

D. Informed consent must be _____, _____, and _____.

E. The _____ Act mandates that all states designate an agency that is responsible for protecting the rights of the mentally ill.

F. Documents, written while a person is competent, that specify how decisions about treatment should be made if the person becomes incompetent are called _____.

G. The most commonly used criterion to determine the criminal responsibility of an offender in the United States is the _____.

3. **Provide short answers for the following questions.**

A. List the three grounds that permit commitment or involuntary hospitalization of the mentally ill. Do you believe these are justifiable? Defend your answer.

B. How is confidentiality different from privilege or testimonial privilege? If you were seeing a therapist, would the concept of privileged communication be important to you? Why or why not?

C. What is the duty to warn and how might it affect you first as a nurse and then as a citizen?

D. Describe an ethical dilemma you have experienced in relation to your psychiatric nursing experience and the process you used to choose a course of action.

REFERENCES

1. American Hospital Association: *A patient's bill of rights,* Chicago, 1990, The Association.
2. American Nurses' Association: *Statement on psychiatric–mental health clinical nursing practice and standards of psychiatric–mental health nursing practice,* Washington, DC, 1994, The Association.
3. Anderson J, Eppard J: Clinical decision making during assessment for involuntary psychiatric admission, *Psychiatr Serv* 46:727, 1995.
4. Appelbaum P, Gutheil T: *Clinical handbook of psychiatry and the law,* ed 2, Baltimore, 1991, Williams & Wilkins.
5. Arkin A et al: Behavior modification, *NY State J Med* 76:190, 1976.
6. Backlar P, McFarland B: A survey on use of advance directives for mental health treatment in Oregon, *Psychiatr Serv* 47:1387, 1996.
7. Binder R, McNiel D: Application of the Tarasoff ruling and its effect on the victim and the therapeutic relationship, *Psychiatr Serv* 47:1212, 1996.
8. Eichmann M et al: An estimation of the impact of OBRA-87 on nursing home care in the United States, *Hosp Community Psychiatry* 43:781, 1992.
9. Elliott R: Patient dumping, COBRA, and the public psychiatric hospital, *Hosp Community Psychiatry* 44:155, 1993.
10. Fiesta J: Liability issues: patients with psychiatric problems, *Nurs Management* 22:14, 1991.
11. Galen K: Assessing psychiatric patients' competency to agree to treatment plans, *Hosp Community Psychiatry* 44:361, 1993.
12. Geller J: On being "committed" to treatment in the community, *Innovations Res* 2:23, 1993.
13. Group for the Advancement of Psychiatry: *Forced into treatment: the role of coercion in clinical practice,* Washington, DC, 1994, American Psychiatric Press.

14. Janofsky J et al: Insanity defense pleas in Baltimore City: an analysis of outcome, *Am J Psychiatry* 153:1464, 1996.

15. Janofsky J, McCarthy R, Folstein M: The Hopkins competency assessment test: a brief method for evaluating patients' capacity to give informed consent, *Hosp Community Psychiatry* 43:132, 1992.

16. Joseph-Kinzelman A et al: Clients' perceptions of involuntary hospitalization, *J Psychosoc Nurs* 32:28, 1994.

17. Kapp M: Treatment and refusal rights in mental health: therapeutic justice and clinical accommodation, *Am J Orthopsych* 64:223, 1994.

18. Lucksted A, Coursey R: Consumer perceptions of pressure and force in psychiatric treatments, *Psychiatr Serv* 46:146, 1995.

19. Munetz M et al: The effectiveness of outpatient civil commitment, *Psychiatr Serv* 47:1251, 1996.

20. National League for Nursing: *Nursing's role in patient's rights,* Pub No 11-1671, New York, 1977, The League.

21. News & Notes: Recent court ruling in Alabama's Wyatt case modifies 20-year-old patient care standards, *Hosp Community Psychiatry* 43:851, 1992.

22. Olley M, Ogloff J: Patients' rights advocacy: implications for program design and implementation, *J Ment Health Admin* 22:368, 1995.

23. Parry J: Involuntary civil commitment in the '90s: a constitutional perspective, *Ment Phys Disabil Law Reporter* 18:320, 1994.

24. Rapoport D, Parry J, editors: *The right to refuse antipsychotic medication,* Washington, DC, 1986, The American Bar Association's Commission on the Mentally Disabled.

25. Ravid R, Menon S: Guidelines for disclosure of patient information under the Americans with Disabilities Act, *Hosp Community Psychiatry* 44:280, 1993.

26. Ross R, Rothbard A, Schinnar A: A framework for classifying state involuntary commitment statutes, *Admin Policy Ment Health* 23:341, 1996.

27. Sanguineti V et al: Retrospective study of 2200 involuntary psychiatric admissions and readmissions, *Am J Psychiatry* 153:392, 1996.

28. Schwartz H, Vingiano W, Perez C: Autonomy and the right to refuse treatment: patient's attitudes after involuntary medication, *Hosp Community Psychiatry* 39:1049, 1988.

29. Sheline Y, Beattie M: Effects of the right to refuse medication in an emergency psychiatric service, *Hosp Community Psychiatry* 43:640, 1992.

30. Simon R: *Clinical psychiatry and the law,* ed 2, Washington, DC, 1992, American Psychiatric Press.

31. Simon R: *Psychiatry and law for clinicians,* Washington, DC, 1992, American Psychiatric Association Press.

32. Slobogin C: Involuntary community treatment of people who are violent and mentally ill: a legal analysis, *Hosp Community Psychiatry* 45: 685, 1994.

33. Slovenko R: *Psychiatry and criminal culpability,* New York, 1995, Wiley.

34. Smith C: Use of involuntary outpatient commitment in community care of the seriously and persistently mentally ill patient, *Issues Ment Health Nurs* 16:275, 1995.

35. Smith S: Liability and mental health services, *Am J Orthopsych* 64:235, 1994.

36. Smith-Bell M, Winslade W: Privacy, confidentiality, and privilege in psychotherapeutic relationships, *Am J Orthopsych* 64:180, 1994.

37. Sundram C: Implementation and activities of protection and advocacy programs for persons with mental illness, *Psychiatr Serv* 46:702, 1995.

38. *Tarasoff v Regents of the University of California et al,* 529 p 2d 553.

39. Torrey E: Violent behavior by individuals with serious mental illness, *Hosp Community Psychiatry* 45:7, 1994.

40. Torrey E, Kaplan R: A national survey of the use of outpatient commitment, *Psychiatr Serv* 46:778, 1995.

41. Torrey E et al: Criminalizing the seriously mentally ill: the abuse of jails as mental hospitals, *Innovations Res* 2:11, 1993.

42. Trudeau M: Informed consent: the patient's right to decide, *J Psychosoc Nurs Ment Health Serv* 31:9, 1993.

43. Wasserbauer L: Psychiatric nurses' knowledge of the Americans with Disabilities Act, *Arch Psychiatr Nurs* 10:328, 1996.

44. Weiss F: The right to refuse: informed consent and the psychosocial nurse, *J Psychosoc Nurs Ment Health Serv* 28:25, 1990.

45. Wolpe P, Schwartz S, Sanford B: Psychiatric inpatients' knowledge of their rights, *Hosp Community Psychiatry* 42:1168, 1991.

ANNOTATED SUGGESTED READINGS

Appelbaum P: Managed care and the next generation of mental health law, *Psychiatr Serv* 47:27, 1996.
  Discusses a new paradigm taking shape in response to changes in the organization and financing of mental health care. Issues include benefits, outcomes, databases, privatization, settings, and economic controls.

Benedek E: Emerging issues in forensic psychiatry: from the clinic to the courthouse, *New Directions in Mental Health Services* vol 69, 1996.
  This entire volume addresses issues related to forensic psychiatry. Unfortunately, it lacks a contribution about forensic nursing but is worth reading for the material it presents.

*Peternelj-Taylor C, Johnson C: Custody and caring: clinical placement of student nurses in forensic settings, *Perspectives in Psychiatric Care* 32:23, 1996.
  Reports on a unique clinical placement of nursing students in a forensic setting. Forensic nursing is described as a new and challenging frontier for psychiatric nursing.

Sabin J: What confidentiality standards should we advocate for in mental health care, and how should we do it? *Psychiatr Serv* 48:35, 1997.
  Reviews implications for confidentiality in mental health care environments: office practice, behavioral health care, computerized medical records, and third party utlization review.

*Schauer C: Special report: protection and advocacy: what nurses need to know, *Arch Psychiatr Nurs* 9:233, 1995.
  Discusses the unique role of nurses in advocating and protecting rights of consumers with psychiatric disabilities and identifying and reporting incidents of abuse and neglect.

*Wasserbauer L: Mental illness and the Americans with Disabilities Act: understanding the fundamentals, *J Psychosocial Nurs* 35:22, 1997.
  Reviews specific ADA statutes and definitions and discusses the strengths and limitations of the legislation and the implications for psychiatric nurses and the emotionally and mentally disabled.

Wright E, Pescosolido B, Penslar R: New ethical challenges to mental health services research in the era of community-based care, *J Mental Health Administration* 24:140, 1997.
  Ethical issues such as informed consent of subjects, review by Institutional Review Boards, and the protection of human subjects are discussed in light of the new trend toward community-based research.

*Nursing reference.

© 1998 M.C. Escher/Cordon Art, Baarn, Holland.

Implementing the Nursing Process: Standards of Care

Gail W. Stuart

To be what we are, and to become what we are capable of becoming, is the only end of life.

Robert L. Stevenson FAMILIAR STUDIES OF MEN AND BOOKS

LEARNING OBJECTIVES

After studying this chapter the student should be able to:

▼ Describe the nursing process and the challenges it presents for working with psychiatric patients

▼ Analyze the conditions and behaviors of the psychiatric nurse during the assessment phase of the nursing process

▼ Analyze the conditions and behaviors of the psychiatric nurse during the diagnosis phase of the nursing process

▼ Analyze the conditions and behaviors of the psychiatric nurse during the outcome identification phase of the nursing process

▼ Analyze the conditions and behaviors of the psychiatric nurse during the planning phase of the nursing process

▼ Analyze the conditions and behaviors of the psychiatric nurse during the implementation phase of the nursing process

▼ Analyze the conditions and behaviors of the psychiatric nurse during the evaluation phase of the nursing process

TOPICAL OUTLINE

The Nursing Process
Standard I: Assessment
Standard II: Diagnosis
  Relationship to Medical Diagnosis
Standard III: Outcome Identification
  Specifying Goals
Standard IV: Planning
  Documentation
Standard V: Implementation
  Treatment Stages
Standard VI: Evaluation

The nurse-patient relationship is the vehicle for applying the nursing process. The goal of nursing care is to maximize the patient's positive interactions with the environment, promote a level of wellness, and enhance self-actualization. By establishing a therapeutic nurse-patient relationship and using the nursing process, the nurse strives to promote and maintain patient behavior that contributes to integrated functioning. This is the essence of the nursing therapeutic process and the framework on which this text is based.

The American Nurses' Association defines nursing as "the diagnosis and treatment of human responses to actual or potential health problems."[1] This definition suggests four defining characteristics of nursing: phenomena, theory, actions, and effects. These characteristics reflect the integration of education, practice, and research (Fig. 10-1).

Phenomena refers to the need to understand the full range of human experiences and responses to health and illness. **Theory** is the theoretical basis and conceptual model for psychiatric–mental health nursing practice. **Action** means that the nursing process is a problem-solving process. **Effects** indicates the need for standards of psychiatric nursing practice to evaluate the quality of care provided.

This chapter discusses each component of the therapeutic nursing process in relation to the 1994 American Nurses' Association (ANA) *Standards of Psychiatric–Mental Health Clinical Nursing Practice.*[2] The standards of professional performance are described in Chapter 11.

THE NURSING PROCESS

The nursing process is an interactive, problem-solving process. It is a systematic and individualized way to achieve the outcomes of nursing care.[5] The nursing process respects the individual's autonomy and freedom to make decisions and be involved in nursing care. The nurse and patient emerge as partners in a relationship built on trust and directed toward maximizing the patient's strengths, maintaining integrity, and promoting adaptive responses to stress.

In dealing with psychiatric patients, the nursing process can present unique challenges. Emotional problems may be vague and elusive, not tangible or visible like many physiological disruptions. Emotional problems also can show different symptoms and arise from a number of causes. Similar past events may lead to very different forms of present behavior. Many psychiatric patients are initially unable to describe their problems. They may be withdrawn, highly anxious, or out of touch with reality. Their ability to participate in the problem-solving process may also be limited if they see themselves as powerless victims or if their illness impairs them from fully engaging in the treatment process.

It is essential that the nurse and the patient become partners in the problem-solving process.[18] Nurses may be tempted to exclude patients, particularly if they avoid or resist becoming involved, but this should be avoided for two reasons. First, learning is most effective when patients participate in the learning experience. Second, by including patients as active participants in the nursing process, the nurse helps restore their sense of control over life and their responsibility for action. They reinforce the message that patients, whether they have an acute crisis or a serious and persistent mental illness, can choose either adaptive or maladaptive coping responses.

The phases of the nursing process as described by the *Standards of Psychiatric–Mental Health Clinical Nursing Practice* are assessment, diagnosis, outcome identification, planning, implementation, and evaluation. Validation is part of each step, and all phases may overlap or occur simultaneously. The nursing conditions and nursing behaviors related to each of these phases are shown in Fig. 10-2. Each of these phases as it applies to psychiatric nursing practice is now described.

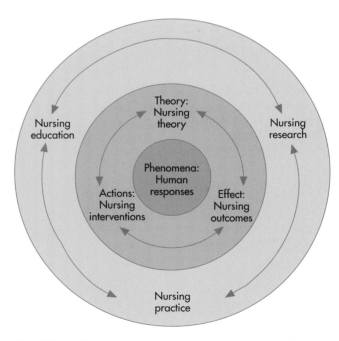

Fig. 10-1 Elements of nursing as an applied science.

> **?** *Some psychotic patients are discouraged and dispirited by their illness. As a result, it may be difficult to engage them in the treatment process. What strategies might you use to connect with these patients and develop a therapeutic alliance with them?*

Assessment

STANDARD I: ASSESSMENT

The psychiatric–mental health nurse collects client health data.

▼ *Rationale*

The assessment interview—which requires linguistically and culturally effective communication skills, interview-

ASSESSMENT

NURSING CONDITIONS
- Self-awareness
- Accurate observations
- Therapeutic communication
- Responsive dimensions of care

NURSING BEHAVIORS
- Establish nursing contract
- Obtain information from patient and family
- Validate data with patient
- Organize data

DIAGNOSIS

NURSING CONDITIONS
- Logical decision making
- Knowledge of normal parameters
- Inductive and deductive reasoning
- Sociocultural sensitivity

NURSING BEHAVIORS
- Identify patterns in data
- Compare data with norms
- Analyze and synthesize data
- Problems and strengths identified
- Validate problems with patient
- Formulate nursing diagnosis
- Set priorities of problems

OUTCOME IDENTIFICATION

NURSING CONDITIONS
- Critical thinking skills
- Partnership with patient and family

NURSING BEHAVIORS
- Hypothesizing
- Specify expected outcomes
- Validate goals with patient

PLANNING

NURSING CONDITIONS
- Application of theory
- Respect for patient and family

NURSING BEHAVIORS
- Prioritize goals
- Identify nursing activities
- Validate plan with patient

IMPLEMENTATION

NURSING CONDITIONS
- Past clinical experiences
- Knowledge of research
- Responsive and action dimensions of care

NURSING BEHAVIORS
- Consider available resources
- Implement nursing activities
- Generate alternatives
- Coordinate with other team members

EVALUATION

NURSING CONDITIONS
- Supervision
- Self-analysis
- Peer review
- Patient and family participation

NURSING BEHAVIORS
- Compare patient's responses and expected outcome
- Review nursing process
- Modify nursing process as needed
- Participate in quality improvement activities

Fig. 10-2   Nursing conditions and behaviors related to psychiatric nursing standards of care.

ing, behavioral observation, database record review, and comprehensive assessment of the client and relevant systems—enables the psychiatric–mental health nurse to make sound clinical judgments and plan appropriate interventions with the client.

▼ *Nursing conditions*

Self-awareness

Accurate observations

Therapeutic communication

Responsive dimensions of care

▼ *Nursing behaviors*

Establish nursing contract

Obtain information from patient and family

Validate data with patient

Organize data

▼ *Key elements*

Identify the patient's reason for seeking help

Assess for risk factors related to the patient's safety including potential for:

    Suicide or self-harm

    Assault or violence

    Substance abuse withdrawal

    Allergic reaction or adverse drug reaction

    Seizure

    Falls or accidents

    Elopement (if hospitalized)

    Physiological instability

Complete a biopsychosocial assessment of patient needs related to this treatment encounter including:

    Patient and family appraisal of health and illness

    Previous episodes of psychiatric care in self and family

    Current medications

    Physiological coping responses

    Mental status coping responses

    Coping resources including motivation for treatment and functional supportive relationships

    Adaptive and maladaptive coping mechanisms

    Psychosocial and environmental problems

    Global assessment of functioning

    Knowledge, strengths, and deficits

In the assessment phase, information is obtained from the patient in a direct and structured manner through observations, interviews, and examinations. An assessment tool or nursing history form can provide a systematic format that becomes part of the patient's written record. This format enables the nurse to assess the patient's level of functioning and serves as a basis for diagnosis, outcome identification, planning, implementation, and evaluation of nursing care. Using a specified data collection format helps ensure that the necessary information is obtained. It also reduces repetition of the patient's medical history and provides a source of information available to all health care team members. The assessment tool the nurse uses to collect data should be derived from a conceptual model of psychiatric nursing.

The nurse should also use the most appropriate psycho-logical assessment tools and behavioral rating scales (see Chapter 6). These can help define current pretreatment aspects of the patient's problems, document the patient's progress over time and the efficacy of the treatment plan, and compare a patient's responses to groups of people with the same illness. This information can help formulate diagnoses and treatment plans, as well as document clinical outcomes of care.

The patient data identified in Standard I relate to all of the components of the Stuart Stress Adaptation Model (Fig. 10-3) used in this text: predisposing factors, precipitating stressors, appraisal of stressor, coping resources, coping mechanisms, and coping responses as described in Chapter 4.

The baseline data should reflect both content and process, and the patient is the ideal source of validation. The nurse should select a private place, free from noise and distraction, in which to interview the patient. Interviewing is a goal-directed method of communication that is required in a formal admission procedure. It should be focused but open ended, progressing from general to specific and allowing spontaneous patient self-expression. The nurse's role is to maintain the flow of the interview and to listen to the verbal and nonverbal messages conveyed by the patient. Nurses must also be aware of their responses to the patient.

Although the patient should be regarded as a source of validation, the nurse should also be prepared to consult with family members or other people knowledgeable about the patient. This is particularly important when the patient is unable to provide reliable information because of the symptoms of the psychiatric illness. The nurse might also consider using a variety of other information sources, including the patient's health care record, nursing rounds, change-of-shift reports, nursing care plan, and evaluation by other health professionals such as psychologists, social workers, or psychiatrists. In using secondary sources, nurses should not simply accept the assessment of another health-care team member. Rather, they should apply the information they obtain to their nursing framework for data collection and formulate their own impressions and diagnoses. This brings another perspective to the work of the health-care team and an unbiased receptivity to patients and their problems.

Nursing Diagnosis

STANDARD II: DIAGNOSIS

The psychiatric–mental health nurse analyzes the assessment data in determining diagnoses.

▼ *Rationale*

The basis for providing psychiatric–mental health nursing care is the recognition and identification of patterns of response to actual or potential psychiatric illnesses and mental health problems.

▼ *Nursing conditions*

Logical decision making

Knowledge of normal parameters

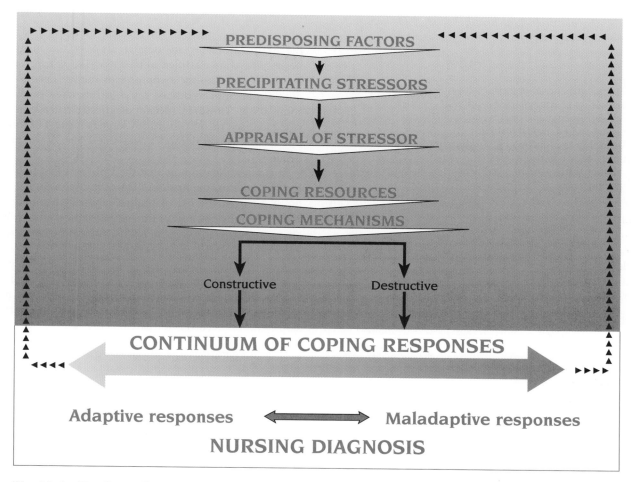

PREDISPOSING FACTORS

PRECIPITATING STRESSORS

APPRAISAL OF STRESSOR

COPING RESOURCES

COPING MECHANISMS

Constructive   Destructive

CONTINUUM OF COPING RESPONSES

Adaptive responses ⟷ Maladaptive responses

NURSING DIAGNOSIS

Fig. 10-3 The Stuart Stress Adaptation Model of psychiatric nursing care.

Inductive and deductive reasoning
Sociocultural sensitivity
▼ *Nursing behaviors*
Identify patterns in data
Compare data with norms
Analyze and synthesize data
Identify problems and strengths
Validate problems with patient
Formulate nursing diagnoses
Set priorities of problems
▼ *Key elements*
Diagnoses should reflect adaptive and maladaptive coping responses based on nursing frameworks such as those of the North American Nursing Diagnosis Association (NANDA).
Diagnoses should incorporate health problems or disease states such as those identified in the *Diagnostic and Statistical Manual of Mental Disorders* (DSM-IV).
Diagnoses should focus on the phenomena of concern to psychiatric–mental health nurses as described in Box 10-1.
After collecting all data, the nurse compares the informa-

tion to documented norms of health and adaptation. Because standards of behavior are culturally determined, the nurse should allow for both the patient's individual characteristics and the larger social group to which the patient belongs.

The nurse then analyzes the data and derives a nursing diagnosis. **A nursing diagnosis is a statement of the patient's nursing problem that includes both the adaptive or maladaptive health response and contributing stressors.** These nursing problems concern aspects of the patient's health that may need to be promoted or with which the patient needs help. The subject of nursing diagnoses therefore is the patient's behavioral response to stress. This response, as represented in Fig. 10-3, may lie anywhere on the coping continuum from adaptive to maladaptive.

According to NANDA, a nursing diagnostic statement ideally consists of three parts:
▼ Health problem
▼ Etiological or contributing factors
▼ Defining characteristics

The defining characteristics are particularly helpful because they reflect the behaviors that are the target of nurs-

Box **10-1** *Psychiatric–Mental Health Nursing's Phenomena of Concern*

ACTUAL OR POTENTIAL MENTAL HEALTH PROBLEMS OF CLIENTS PERTAINING TO:

▼ The maintenance of optimal health and well-being and the prevention of psychobiological illness
▼ Self-care limitations or impaired functioning related to mental and emotional distress
▼ Deficits in the functioning of significant biological, emotional, and cognitive systems
▼ Emotional stress or crisis components of illness, pain, and disability
▼ Self-concept changes, developmental issues, and life process changes
▼ Problems related to emotions such as anxiety, anger, sadness, loneliness, and grief
▼ Physical symptoms that occur along with altered psychological functioning
▼ Alterations in thinking, perceiving, symbolizing, communicating, and decision making
▼ Difficulties in relating to others
▼ Behaviors and mental states that indicate that the patient is a danger to self or others or has a severe disability
▼ Interpersonal, systemic, sociocultural, spiritual, or environmental circumstances or events that affect the mental and emotional well-being of the individual, family, or community
▼ Symptom management, side effects/toxicities associated with psychopharmacological intervention, and other aspects of the treatment regimen

---

From American Nurses' Association: *A statement on psychiatric–mental health clinical nursing practice and standards of psychiatric mental health clinical nursing practice,* Washington, DC, 1994, The Association.

ing intervention. They also provide specific indicators for evaluating the outcomes of psychiatric nursing interventions and for determining whether the expected goals of the nursing care were met.

Psychiatric nurses must continue to define and describe what they do in the psychiatric setting, and this requires the use of nursing diagnoses. Nursing diagnoses pinpoint exactly what nurses treat. When psychiatric nurses name the health responses they treat, they are better able to talk with legislators, reimbursers, administrators, other health-care professionals, patients, families, and even other nurses about the contribution nursing makes to health care.

Relationship to Medical Diagnosis

The relationship between medicine and nursing includes sharing information, ideas, and analyses and developing appropriate care plans for the patient. Interventions are based on the nursing assessment as well as the medical evaluation and ensure a thorough and coordinated plan of treatment.[4] Therefore, while formulating nursing diagnoses and using the nursing process, nurses should also be familiar with medical diagnoses and treatment plans.

Medical diagnosis is the health problem or disease states of the patient. In the medical model of psychiatry, the health problems are mental disorders or mental illnesses. These are classified in the DSM-IV,[3] which comprehensively describes the symptoms of mental disorders but does not attempt to discuss cause or how the disturbances come about. However, specific diagnostic criteria are provided for each mental disorder. Chapters 3 and 4 of this text discuss the medical model and the DSM-IV in greater detail.

It is interesting to note that the DSM was first published in 1952, whereas the first NANDA diagnoses were put forth in 1973. Given the use of multidisciplinary teams in psychiatry and the newness of nursing diagnoses, some psychiatric nurses prefer using the DSM-IV or do not see the relevance of NANDA diagnoses in their practice. However, Malone[10] notes that nurses who opt to use only the DSM-IV do not contribute to public understanding of psychiatric nursing practice, perpetuate the invisibility of nursing to patient care, and invite turf battles with other professions. What is needed is for psychiatric nurses to be familiar with both DSM-IV and NANDA diagnoses and to use both to conceptualize patient problems, needs, and treatment strategies.

? *Some psychiatric nurses have proposed that nursing diagnoses be added as another axis to the DSM-IV. What problems would this create for psychiatric nurses' autonomy, reimbursement for psychiatric nursing services, and interdisciplinary collaboration?*

Outcome Identification

STANDARD III: OUTCOME IDENTIFICATION

The psychiatric–mental health nurse identifies expected outcomes individualized to the client.

▼*Rationale*
Within the context of providing nursing care, the ultimate goal is to influence health outcomes and improve the client's health status.

▼*Nursing conditions*
Critical thinking skills
Partnership with patient and family

▼*Nursing behaviors*
Hypothesizing
Specifying expected outcomes
Validating goals with patient

▼*Key elements*
Outcomes should be mutually identified with the patient.
Outcomes should be identified as clearly and objectively as possible.
Well-written outcomes help nurses determine the effectiveness and efficiency of their interventions.

Before defining expected outcomes, the nurse must realize that patients often seek treatment with goals of their own. These goals may be expressed as relieving symptoms or improving functional ability. Sometimes a patient cannot identify specific goals or may describe them in general terms. Translating nonspecific concerns into specific goal statements is not easy. The nurse must understand the patient's coping responses and the factors that influence them. Some of the difficulties in defining goals are as follows[9]:

▼ The patient may view a personal problem as someone else's behavior. This may be the case of a father who brings his adolescent son in for counseling. The father may view the son as the problem, whereas the adolescent may feel his only problem is his father. One approach to this situation is to focus help on the person who brought the problem into treatment because he "owns" the problem at that moment. The nurse might suggest, "Let's talk about how I could help you deal with your son. A change in your response might lead to a change in his behavior also."

▼ The patient may express a problem as a feeling, such as, "I'm lonely," or "I'm so unhappy." Besides trying to help the patient clarify the feeling, the nurse might ask, "What could you do to make yourself feel less alone and more loved by others?" This helps patients see the connection between actions and feelings and increase their sense of responsibility for themselves.

▼ The patient's problem may be one of lacking a goal or an idea of exactly what is desired out of life. In this case it might be helpful for the nurse to point out that values and goals are not magically discovered but must be created by people for themselves. The patient can then actively explore ways to construct goals or adopt the objectives of a social, service, religious, or political group with whom the patient identifies.

▼ The patient's goals may be inappropriate, undesirable, or unclear. However, the solution is not for the nurse to impose goals on the patient. Even if the patient's desires seem to be against self-interests, the most the nurse can do is reflect the patient's behavior and its consequences. If the patient then asks for help in setting new goals, the nurse can help.

▼ The patient's problem may be a choice conflict. This is especially common if all the choices are unpleasant, unacceptable, or unrealistic. An example is a couple who want to divorce but do not want to see their child hurt or suffer the financial hardship that would result. Although undesirable choices cannot be made desirable, the nurse can help patients use the problem-solving process to identify the full range of alternatives available to them.

▼ The patient may have no real problem but may just want to talk. Nurses must then decide what role to play and carefully distinguish between a social and a therapeutic relationship.

Clarifying goals is an essential step in the therapeutic process. Out of this clarification emerges the mutually agreed on goals on which the patient-nurse relationship is based. A well-intentioned nurse sometimes overlooks the patient's goals and devises a treatment plan leading to an outcome that the nurse believes is better. However, this approach may be a conflict-producing situation that the patient has already experienced. Therefore, the experience of working cooperatively with the nurse to evolve mutually acceptable goals is extremely valuable. If the patient does not share one of the nurse's goals, it may be best to defer it until the patient agrees on its importance.

Specifying Goals

Once goals are agreed on, the nurse must state them explicitly. Box 10-2 lists qualities of well-written outcome criteria. The more specifically the goals of treatment are stated, the more attainable these goals are. These goals also guide later nursing actions and enhance the evaluation of care. Goals should be written in behavioral terms. This means that the verb used to state the objective should represent a behavior that may be observed and should have as few interpretations as possible. Goals should realistically describe what the nurse wishes to accomplish within a specific time span.

> **?** *Review some of the treatment plans in your clinical setting. Are the expected outcomes and short-term goals well written given the qualities listed in Box 10-2?*

Expected outcomes and short-term goals should be developed, with short-term objectives contributing to the longer-term expected outcomes. Following are sample expected outcomes and short-term goals:

Expected outcome: The patient will travel about the community independently within 2 months.

Short-term goals:

▼ At the end of 1 week the patient will sit on the front steps at home.

▼ At the end of 2 weeks the patient will walk to the corner and back home.

▼ At the end of 3 weeks the patient, accompanied by the nurse, will walk around the block.

▼ At the end of 4 weeks the patient will walk around the block alone.

The hierarchy would continue until the desired outcome is achieved. Each goal is stated in terms of observable behavior and includes a period of time in which it is to be ac-

---

Box **10-2** *Qualities of Well-Written Outcome Criteria*

Specific rather than general
Measurable rather than subjective
Attainable rather than unrealistic
Current rather than outdated
Adequate in number rather than too few or too many
Mutual rather than one sided

complished. It also includes any other relevant conditions, such as whether the patient is to be alone or accompanied by the nurse.

Finally, it is important for psychiatric nurses to realize that expected outcomes can be classified into three domains: cognitive, affective, and psychomotor.[14] Correctly identifying the domain of the expected outcome is very important in planning nursing interventions. Some psychiatric nurses assume that the only outcomes necessary are those related to learning new information (cognitive). They forget about the equally important needs of patients to acquire new values (affective) or master new motor skills (psychomotor).

For example, it would be of limited help to teach a patient about medication if the patient did not value taking medications based on a personal belief system or previous life experiences. It would be equally unsuccessful to engage in medication education if the patient did not know how to take public transportation to fill the prescription.

Planning

STANDARD IV: PLANNING

The psychiatric–mental health nurse develops a plan of care that prescribes interventions to attain expected outcomes.

▼*Rationale*

A plan of care is used to guide therapeutic intervention systematically and achieve the expected client outcomes.

▼*Nursing conditions*

Application of theory

Respect for patient and family

▼*Nursing behaviors*

Prioritize goals

Identify nursing activities

Validate plan with patient

▼*Key elements*

The plan of nursing care must always be individualized for the patient.

Planned interventions should be based on current knowledge in the field and contemporary clinical psychiatric–mental health nursing practice.

Planning is done in collaboration with the patient, the family, and the health care team.

Documentation of the plan of care is an essential nursing activity.

One of the most important tasks facing the nurse and patient is to assign priorities to goals. Often, several goals can be pursued simultaneously. Those related to protecting the patient from self-destructive impulses always receive top priority. When identifying expected outcomes and short-term goals, the nurse must keep the proposed time sequence firmly in mind.

Because the nursing care plan is dynamic and should adapt to the patient's coping responses throughout contact with the health care system, priorities are constantly changing. If the focus is always on the patient's behavioral responses, priorities can be set and modified as the patient changes. This personalizes nursing care, and the patient participates in its planning and implementation.

Once the goals are chosen, the next task is to outline the plan for achieving them. The nursing care plan applies theory from nursing and related biological, behavioral, and social sciences to the unique responses of the individual patient. This assumes that as the nurse identifies patient needs, appropriate resources will be consulted. Skilled psychiatric nursing requires a commitment to the ongoing pursuit of knowledge that will enhance professional growth.

The patient's active involvement leads to more successful care plans. After writing a tentative care plan, nurses must validate this plan with the patient. This saves time and effort for them both as they continue to work together. It also communicates to the patient a sense of self-responsibility in getting well. The patient can tell the nurse that a proposed plan is unrealistic regarding financial status, lifestyle, value system, or, perhaps, personal preference. Usually there are several possible approaches to a patient's problem. Choosing the one most acceptable to the patient improves the chances for success.

If a goal answers the question of *what*, the plan of care answers the questions *how* and *why*. The plan chosen obviously depends on the nursing diagnosis, the nurse's theoretical orientation, and the nature of the goals pursued. In general, the goals influence the selection of therapeutic techniques. Failure to reach a goal through one plan can lead to the decision to adopt a new approach or reevaluate the goal. These activities commonly occur in the working phase of the relationship.

Documentation

The Joint Commission on Accreditation of Healthcare Organizations (JCAHO) standards specify that the nursing plan of care must contain the six elements listed in Box 10-3 and that the primary place to document the nursing process is in the patient's health care record.

Psychiatric nurses are beginning to use a variety of formats that often differ from the traditional nursing care

---

Box **10-3** *Essential Elements of the Nursing Plan of Care*

Initial assessment and reassessment

Nursing diagnoses or patient care needs

Interventions identified to meet the patient's nursing care needs

Nursing care provided

Patient's response to and the outcomes of the nursing care provided

Ability of the patient or significant other to manage continuing care needs after discharge plan. Many of these changes have been prompted by changes in the treatment settings and by the advanced computer technology available.

For example, computerized programs have been developed that can provide rapid entry of patient data, retrieve psychiatric treatment plans, and produce a finished document that is clinically useful and highly readable.[16,17] Another advantage of a computerized information system is its ability to store clinical data that can also be used for outcome research, quality improvement activities, and resource management. In addition to computerized plans of care, psychiatric nurses are beginning to use clinical practice guidelines, clinical protocols, teaching protocols, flow sheets, and clinical pathways in their practice settings.[12]

> **?** *What are the potential problems in using computerized patient information systems in psychiatric health care facilities?*

Implementation

STANDARD V: IMPLEMENTATION

The psychiatric–mental health nurse implements the interventions identified in the plan of care.

▼*Rationale*

In implementing the plan of care, psychiatric–mental health nurses use a wide range of interventions designed to prevent mental and physical illness and promote, maintain, and restore mental and physical health. Psychiatric–mental health nurses select interventions according to their level of practice. At the basic level, the nurse may select counseling, milieu therapy, self-care activities, psychobiological interventions, health teaching, case management, health promotion and health maintenance, and a variety of other approaches to meet the mental health needs of patients. In addition to the intervention options available to the basic-level psychiatric–mental health nurse, at the advanced level the certified specialist may provide consultation, engage in psychotherapy, and prescribe pharmacological agents where permitted by state statutes or regulations.

▼*Nursing conditions*

Past clinical experiences
Knowledge of research
Responsive and action dimensions of care

▼*Nursing behaviors*

Consider available resources
Implement nursing activities
Generate alternatives
Coordinate with other team members

▼*Key elements*

Nursing interventions should reflect a holistic, biopsychosocial approach to patient care.

Nursing interventions are implemented in a safe, efficient, and caring manner.

The level at which a nurse functions and the interventions implemented are based on the nursing practice acts in one's state, the nurse's qualifications (including education, experience, and certification), the caregiving setting, and the nurse's initiative.

STANDARD VA: COUNSELING

The psychiatric–mental health nurse uses counseling interventions to help clients improve or regain their previous coping abilities, foster mental health, and prevent mental illness and disability.

STANDARD VB: MILIEU THERAPY

The psychiatric–mental health nurse provides, structures, and maintains a therapeutic environment in collaboration with the client and other health care providers.

STANDARD VC: SELF-CARE ACTIVITIES

The psychiatric–mental health nurse structures interventions around the client's activities of daily living to foster self-care and mental and physical well-being.

STANDARD VD: PSYCHOBIOLOGICAL INTERVENTIONS

The psychiatric–mental health nurse uses knowledge of psychobiological interventions and applies clinical skills to restore the client's health and prevent further disability.

STANDARD VE: HEALTH TEACHING

The psychiatric–mental health nurse, through health teaching, assists clients in achieving satisfying, productive, and healthy patterns of living.

STANDARD VF: CASE MANAGEMENT

The psychiatric–mental health nurse provides case management to coordinate comprehensive health services and ensure continuity of care.

STANDARD VG: HEALTH PROMOTION AND MAINTENANCE

The psychiatric–mental health nurse uses strategies and interventions to promote and maintain mental health and prevent mental illness.

ADVANCED PRACTICE INTERVENTIONS VH–VJ

The following interventions (Vh–Vj) may be performed only by the certified specialist in psychiatric–mental health nursing.

STANDARD VH: PSYCHOTHERAPY

The certified specialist in psychiatric–mental health nursing uses individual, group, and family psychotherapy, child psychotherapy, and other therapeutic treatments to assist patients by fostering mental health, preventing mental illness and disability, and improving or regaining previous health status and functional abilities.

STANDARD VI: PRESCRIPTION OF PHARMACOLOGICAL AGENTS

The certified specialist uses prescription of pharmacological agents in accordance with the state nursing practice act to treat symptoms of psychiatric illness and improve functional health status.

STANDARD VJ: CONSULTATION

The certified specialist provides consultation to healthcare providers and others to influence the plans of care and to enhance the abilities of others to provide psychiatric and mental health care and effect change in systems.

Implementation is the actual delivery of nursing care to the patient and the response to that care. Good planning increases the chances of successful implementation. Such factors as available people, equipment, resources, time, and money must be considered as nursing actions are planned.

The most valid basis for nursing action applies the scientific method to nursing practice.[8] It is also acceptable to use theory selectively from the biological, behavioral, and social sciences. In most situations there is more than one way to accomplish the stated goals. It is helpful when planning care to identify alternative nursing actions that are also appropriate to the goal. If this is done, the nurse is not left floundering if the first approach fails. Considering several alternatives makes the implementation phase of the nursing process highly flexible.

In implementing psychotherapeutic interventions, the nurse helps the psychiatric patient do two things: **develop insight** and **change behavior.** These two areas for nursing intervention correspond with the responsive and action dimensions of the nurse-patient relationship described in Chapter 2. **Insight** is the patient's development of new emotional and cognitive understandings. Often the patient becomes more anxious as defense mechanisms are broken down. This is the time when resistance commonly occurs. But knowing something on an intellectual level does *not* inevitably lead to a change in behavior. Nurses who terminate their interventions at this point are not fully carrying out the therapeutic process to the patient's benefit. An additional step is needed. Patients must decide whether they will revert to maladaptive coping mechanisms, remain in a resisting, immobilized state, or adopt new, adaptive, and constructive approaches to life.

The first step in helping a patient translate insight into action is to build adequate incentives to abandon old patterns of behavior. The nurse should help the patient see the consequences of actions and that old patterns do more harm than good and inflict suffering and pain. The patient will not learn new patterns until the motivation to acquire them is greater than the motivation to retain old ones. The nurse should encourage the patient's desires for mental health, emotional growth, and freedom from suffering. The nurse also should continue to motivate and support patients as they test new behaviors and coping mechanisms. The individual's social support system is vital in this regard. This is relevant to all levels of nursing intervention and all patient populations in all types of settings.

Within the nurse-patient relationship the patient can actively work toward adaptive goals. It is important to allow sufficient time for change. Many of the patient's maladaptive patterns have built up over years; the nurse cannot expect the patient to change them in a matter of days or weeks. Finally, the nurse must help the patient evaluate these new patterns, integrate them into life experiences, and practice problem solving to prepare for future experiences. In this way secondary prevention nursing interventions also fulfill primary and tertiary prevention goals.

The standards of care for implementation are detailed and explicit. The standards identify the range of activities psychiatric nurses use. Information related to each of these implementation standards appears in various chapters throughout this text.

It is evident that psychiatric nurses need to be skilled in biological, psychological, and sociocultural skills to implement these nursing interventions. The current psychiatric population has a higher level of acuity, increased mortality rates, and greater complexity of problems than in the past. Specifically, a large number of people seeking psychiatric treatment have concurrent and often undiagnosed physical illnesses.[7] Thus it is essential that psychiatric nurses stay current with their biomedical as well as psychosocial skill development.[6]

> **?** *Ten years ago, graduating nursing students were advised to work in a medical-surgical setting before going into psychiatry so that they could learn "basic nursing skills." Discuss why this suggestion is no longer valid given contemporary psychiatric patients and the range of treatment settings.*

Treatment Stages

A final issue for the psychiatric nurse to consider in the implementation process is that there are four possible treatment stages:

▼ Health promotion
▼ Maintenance

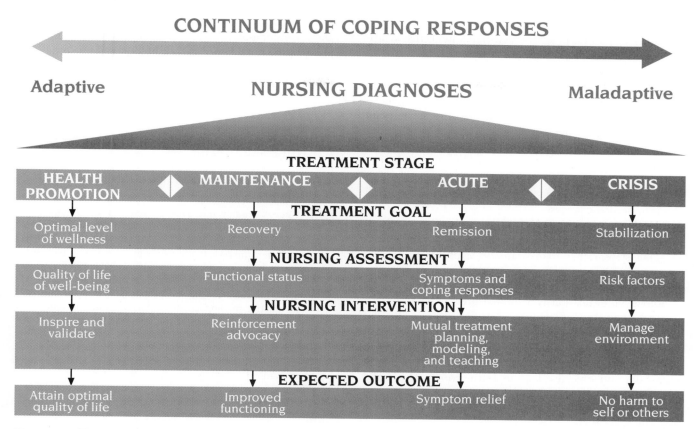

Fig. 10-4 Treatment stages related to implementation of psychiatric nursing care.

▼ Acute
▼ Crisis

These stages reflect the range of adaptive/maladaptive coping responses, and patients can move between these stages at any time. The goal, assessment, intervention, and expected outcome vary with each stage, as seen in Fig. 10-4. It is critically important for psychiatric nurses to determine the patient's stage of treatment and then implement nursing activities that target the treatment goal in the most cost-effective and efficient manner.

Evaluation

STANDARD VI: EVALUATION

The psychiatric–mental health nurse evaluates the client's progress in attaining expected outcomes.

▼*Rationale*

Nursing care is a dynamic process involving change in the client's health status over time, giving rise to the need for new data, different diagnoses, and modifications in the plan of care. Therefore, evaluation is a continuous process of appraising the effect of nursing interventions and the treatment regimen on the client's health status and expected health outcomes.

▼*Nursing conditions*
Supervision
Self-analysis
Peer review
Patient and family participation
▼*Nursing behaviors*
Compare patient's responses and expected outcome
Review nursing process
Modify nursing process as needed
Participate in quality improvement activities
▼*Key elements*
Evaluation is an ongoing process
Patient and family participation in evaluation is essential
Goal achievement should be documented and revisions in the plan of care should be implemented as appropriate

When evaluating care the nurse should review all previous phases of the nursing process and determine whether the expected outcomes for the patient have been met. Key words for the evaluation phase of the nursing process are *mutual, competent, accessible, effective, appropriate, efficient,* and *flexible.* The nurse must make many decisions throughout the process, including the following:

▼ Was my conceptual model appropriate to this patient situation?

▼ Was my data collection adequate and were all relevant coping responses, objective signs, and subjective symptoms identified?

▼ Were my nursing diagnoses accurate and based on the analysis and synthesis of relevant data, the application of theory, and the appropriateness of nursing treatment?

▼ Were the expected outcomes and plan of care relevant and mutual, showing appropriate priorities and the consideration of all realistic alternatives?

▼ Were my nursing interventions effective and efficient in time and energy?

▼ Were the expected outcomes achieved and, if not, did I make needed changes?

▼ Was the patient satisfied with the nursing care received? Often, progress with psychiatric patients is slow and occurs in small steps rather than dramatic leaps. Realizing that progress has been made can produce growth and inspire new enthusiasm in both the patient and the nurse.

Above all, evaluation is a mutual process based on the patient's and family's previously identified goals and level of satisfaction. Patients, families, and psychiatric nurses often have different views of treatment and the effectiveness of care. It is therefore critical that psychiatric nurses have a systematic and objective way to learn from patients and families which aspects of the nursing care provided were helpful, and what additional nursing actions may have further enhanced their well-being.

Finally, evaluation is a continuous, active process that begins early in the relationship and continues throughout. It is an activity that must be documented by psychiatric nurses so that they can demonstrate the value of psychiatric nursing services to consumers, administrators, reimbursers, and other health-care providers (see Critical Thinking about Contemporary Issues). Perhaps more than any other phase of the nursing process, evaluation and outcome measurement will be the key aspects of psychiatric nursing activities in the decade to come.

CRITICAL THINKING *about* *Contemporary Issues*

Does Psychiatric Nursing Care Really Make a Difference?

Most nurses reading this question would automatically and emphatically say, "Yes, of course it does!" But does it really? More specifically, what evidence exists that the care provided by psychiatric nurses actually results in a decrease in patients' symptoms, improvement in patients' functional status, or improved quality of life? What evidence would you provide a hospital administrator who was proposing that all but one of the psychiatric nursing positions on the units be replaced with counselors? How would you convince the director of a community mental health program for the seriously mentally ill that, as a nurse, you should be hired to work with this population rather than the social worker who is also being interviewed?

In fact, very few well-designed psychiatric nursing studies have demonstrated the effectiveness of psychiatric nursing care.[11] Of the hundreds of articles cited in recent reviews, very few psychiatric nursing studies are mentioned.[13,15] It is clear that psychiatric nurses believe they make a valuable contribution to the health care of patients. However, providing the evidence of this contribution remains a challenge for the field.

CASE STUDY

This case study describes the use of the nursing process with a psychiatric patient. It illustrates the interrelationship of the phases of the nurse-patient relationship, the therapeutic dimensions, and the various activities as the nurse works with the patient to foster adaptive coping behavior and more integrated functioning.

Assessment

Ms. G came to the psychiatric outpatient department of the local hospital requesting treatment with a female therapist. The psychiatric nurse specialist agreed to perform the initial screening and evaluation and consider serving as her primary therapist.

To collect the initial data, the nurse followed the admission format required by the department. A description of the presenting problem revealed that Ms. G was a 29-year-old single woman who was neat in appearance and markedly overweight. She reported feelings of "confusion and depression" and said that superficially she appeared "outgoing and friendly and played the role of a clown." In reality, however, she said she had few close friends, felt insecure about herself, felt unsuccessful in her job, and believed she "overanalyzed her problems." She said she had feelings of worthlessness and loss of pleasure in her daily activities on and off for the past 2 years.

Additional information was obtained in other significant areas of her life. Her psychosocial history revealed a disrupted family situation. Her mother died of tuberculosis when she was 11 years of age. Her father, age 73, was alive but had been an alcoholic for as long as Ms. G could remember. She had one sister, age 20, who married at age 16 and was now divorced. She also had one stepsister, age 45, who was married, had two adopted sons, and lived out of state. In giving this family information, Ms. G revealed that her stepsister was her natural mother, but she had continued to call her father's wife "mother." After her "mother" died, her stepsister took over the house. Two years later, however, this stepsister married and moved out of state. Ms. G reported feeling closest to this stepsister and felt abandoned when she left. Ms. G then took charge of the house until age 14, when her father placed her and her younger sister in a group home, where she had difficulty making friends.

She completed high school and college. In college she had four

Continued from previous page

good friends who were all married now. Her only close heterosexual relationship was in high school, and this boyfriend eventually married her best friend. Since that time she had never dated and stated she had no desire to marry.

After college she obtained a job as a "girl Friday" for a law firm and expressed much pleasure with it. She then saw the opportunity to make more money as a waitress and switched jobs. She currently worked at a restaurant, and her schedule involved day and night rotations as well as weekend shifts. She expressed dissatisfaction with many aspects of her job but was unable to identify alternatives. Her goal in life was to have a fulfilling career.

She lived alone. Her best friend was her immediate supervisor at work. She currently had no male friends and only two other female acquaintances.

Pertinent medical history revealed a major weight problem. She was 36 kg (80 pounds) overweight and extremely conscious of it. She viewed her body negatively and believed others were also "repulsed" by her weight. She also recently recovered from infectious hepatitis. She drank an occasional beer when out with friends (once or twice a month), denied any drug use, and smoked three fourths of a pack of cigarettes a day.

Diagnosis

After consultation the psychiatric nurse agreed to work with Ms. G as primary therapist. In the following session they established a contract for working together, and a fee was set. At this time they explored her expressed guilt over seeking help, the reason for her request for a female therapist, their mutual roles, and the confidential nature of the relationship. The nurse also shared with Ms. G the maladaptive coping responses she had noted and the inferences she had made. They discussed these areas, and the following nursing diagnoses were identified:

1. Self-esteem disturbance related to childhood rejection and unrealistic self-ideals, as evidenced by feelings of worthlessness
2. Social isolation related to ambivalence regarding male-female relationships and lack of socialization skills, as evidenced by lack of close friends
3. Altered role performance related to job dissatisfaction with working hours and nature of the work, as evidenced by feeling unsuccessful in her job
4. Body image disturbance related to weight control problem, as evidenced by negative feelings

Ms. G's DSM-IV diagnosis was identified as dysthymia, a mood disorder.

Outcome identification

They mutually agreed to work on her problem areas in weekly therapy sessions. After 3 months they would evaluate the achievement of the following expected outcomes:

1. Ms. G will describe her expectations of the therapeutic process and her commitment to it.
2. Aspects of Ms. G's self-ideal will be identified.
3. Factors influencing her self-concept and negative, stereotyped self-perceptions will be evaluated.
4. Interpersonal relationships will be analyzed to include her patterns of relating, her expectations of others, and specific areas of difficulty.
5. Alternative employment opportunities will be identified.
6. The advantages and disadvantages of a job change will be compared.

Planning

In discussing these areas they agreed that nursing diagnosis 1 was a central one and problems 2, 3, and 4 directly contributed to it. Her coping mechanisms included intellectualization and denial, and she compensated for her self-doubts by an outward appearance that was social, joking, and friendly, yet superficial. The strengths Ms. G brought to the therapy process included her introspective nature and ability to analyze events, her openness to new ideas, the resource people available to her in her immediate environment, and a genuine sense of humor.

Implementation

Because they were in the introductory phase of the relationship, many of the goals involved areas needing further assessment. During this phase of treatment Ms. G displayed much anxiety, testing behavior, and ambivalence, and the nursing actions were focused on promoting respect, openness, and acceptance and minimizing her anxiety. Through the nurse's use of empathic understanding, Ms. G became less jovial and superficial and began to attain some intellectual insight into her behavior. With guidance she began to appraise her own abilities and became more open in expressing feelings.

She feared intimate personal involvement and could not tolerate physical closeness. The nurse incorporated this into nursing actions by initially minimizing confrontation, setting limits on anxiety-producing topics, and arranging the office seating to allow the patient to select her proximity to the nurse.

As they discussed the patient's relationships, the nurse confronted her with the dependent role Ms. G played and the unrealistic expectations she placed on others in the exclusiveness and amount of time she demanded from them. Her pattern of relating was also manipulative in that she elicited a sympathetic response and then used it to meet her own needs. She had great difficulty with mutuality and autonomy in relating to others. She was inexperienced in heterosexual relationships and missed many of the normal adolescent growth experiences in this area. Finally, she had much emotion and fear vested in her family of origin. The only trusting relationship Ms. G could recall was with her stepsister-mother. When this stepsister abruptly left home to marry, Ms. G perceived this as a personal rejection. She had since isolated herself from her family and continued to blame herself for her rejection by others, thus lowering her self-esteem and ability to trust others.

At the end of 2 months Ms. G was being considered for a promotion at work to hostess but, on the basis of an evaluation by her best friend and supervisor, was rejected for it. This precipitated a suicide attempt, which Ms. G revealed at her next regular session. At this point the issue of trust within the relationship became critical, as well as her inability to express anger because she feared rejection. The nurse now began more actively confronting Ms. G in her areas of ambivalence and inconsistency, setting limits on her self-destructive behavior, and suggesting alternatives. Ms. G then revealed that her relationship with her friend-supervisor was also a sexual one, and she expressed fears of homosexuality and loss of identity.

In later sessions Ms. G's relationship with this friend became a critical therapeutic issue because it reflected many of her conflicts. The therapy process presented a threat to the unhealthy parts of this relationship, and during the course of therapy

Continued

Continued from previous page

Ms. G decided she needed to choose between maladaptive behaviors and more growth-producing options.

The nurse-patient relationship had now moved into the working phase, where focus was placed on specifics, and problem-solving activities began. After 3 months the nursing diagnoses were reevaluated to include the following:

1. Potential for self-directed violence related to perceived rejection by friend, as evidenced by suicide attempt
2. Personal identity disturbance related to childhood rejection and unrealistic self-ideals, as evidenced by self statements
3. Social isolation related to inability to trust, lack of socialization skills, and feelings of inadequacy, as evidenced by relationship patterns
4. Powerlessness related to fear of rejection by others, as evidenced by perceived lack of control over life events
5. Altered role performance related to job dissatisfaction with working hours and nature of the work, as evidenced by feeling unsuccessful in her job

At this time the nurse sought consultation as she further evolved her plan of care. Neither medication nor hospitalization was indicated. These formulations were shared with Ms. G, who contracted for safety with the nurse, and together they collaborated about her future progress. They agreed to focus on changing Ms. G's maladaptive behavior by exploring past events and conflicts and helping her learn more productive patterns of living. Ms. G was now ready to commit herself to the work of therapy and interpersonal change, and she began to assume increased responsibility for this therapeutic work.

Because her self-ideal was unrealistically high, specific short-term goals became essential. The nurse's theoretical orientation incorporated the dynamics of Sullivan's and Peplau's interpersonal theories, Beck's cognitive framework, and Glasser's reality therapy. The relationship was focused on through the use of immediacy and became a model for examining many of her conflicts. This proved to be an excellent learning opportunity as Ms. G and the nurse dealt with resistance, transference, and countertransference reactions. During the next couple of months Ms. G made much progress, including the following changes:

1. She moved into an apartment with another girlfriend.
2. She left her previous job and resumed working in an office, where she received more personal satisfaction and a work schedule that allowed her to increase her social activities.
3. She began a diet regimen.
4. She participated in additional activities, such as a dancing class and a health spa.
5. She learned to verbalize her anger more freely with the nurse, friends, and others at work. This included discussing the many relationships in her past that were terminated without her agreement and in which she had internalized her anger.
6. She contacted her stepsister-mother and visited her. This was an important therapeutic goal because it allowed her to review her early experiences and provided her with actual feedback from those involved. Consequently, many of her misperceptions became evident and open to exploration in therapy.
7. She was able to admit her ambivalent feeling about her friend-supervisor and discuss the negative aspects of the relationship. She stopped further sexual contact with her because she felt exploited. Over time, the nature of this relationship changed, and it eventually became a casual acquaintance.
8. She learned about the variety of sexual feelings and responses and saw her needs in this area as appropriate developmental tasks. She became open to evaluating both heterosexual and homosexual expressions of her own sexual feelings.
9. Her perception of personal space changed, and her tolerance for physical closeness increased.
10. She developed new male and female friends and socialized frequently with them.

Evaluation

The terminating phase of the relationship began after about 9 months. At this time Ms. G was independently solving problems and, in therapy, the nurse primarily validated and supported her thinking. She was now receiving and accepting much positive feedback from others, had lost 15 kg (40 pounds), was continuing to diet, was planning future career goals, and had achieved more satisfactory interpersonal relationships with both men and women. The mutual goals for therapy had been met.

Terminating was difficult because of the close, trusting bond that had developed between them. The nurse had feelings of pleasure in Ms. G's growth, as well as personal satisfaction in her effectiveness as therapist. Ms. G openly described her feelings about terminating and raised the question of a possible social relationship between them. Over the course of the sessions she came to realize that the premise of the relationship was therapy and changing individual perceptions or patterns of relating would not be feasible or desirable. Most important, she had control over terminating this relationship and the opportunity to work it through in a positive way.

Summary

1. The nursing process is an interactive, problem-solving process used by the nurse as a systematic and individualized way to fulfill the goal of nursing care.
2. Assessment should reflect content, process, and information about the patient's biopsychosocial world. Data collection is facilitated by a systematic assessment tool that ideally is based on a conceptual model of psychiatric nursing.
3. The nursing diagnosis should include the patient's adaptive or maladaptive health response, defining characteristics of that response, and contributing stressors. Knowledge of both NANDA and DSM diagnoses is needed.
4. Outcome identification involves setting goals that are mutual, congruent, realistic, and appropriately timed.
5. The plan of care should include prioritized nursing diagnoses and expected outcomes, as well as prescribed nursing strategies to achieve those outcomes.
6. Nursing interventions should be directed toward helping

the patient develop insight and resolve problems through carrying out a positive plan of action. Psychiatric nursing practice includes both basic and advanced activities.

7. Evaluation involves reviewing all previous phases of the nursing process and determining the degree to which expected outcomes were attained.

your **INTERNET**
c o n n e c t i o n

American Nurses' Association Nursing World
http://www.ana.org

Canadian Nurses' Association
http://www.cna-nurses.ca

? *Chapter Review Questions*

1. Match the phase of the nursing process identified in Column A with the appropriate nursing behavior in Column B.

Column A	Column B
C Data collection	A. Comparing responses and expected outcome, making modifications as needed
A Evaluation	
B Implementation	B. Considering available resources, generating alternatives, and coordinating with other team members
E Nursing diagnosis	
D Outcome identification	C. Establishing a contract and collecting, validating, and organizing data
F Planning	D. Hypothesizing and validating goals with the patient
	E. Identifying patterns, analyzing, and synthesizing data
	F. Prioritizing goals and identifying nursing activities

2. Fill in the blanks.

Well-written outcome criteria or goals are

A. _specific_ rather than general

B. _measurable_ rather than subjective

C. _attainable_ rather than unrealistic

D. _current_ rather than outdated

E. _adequate_ rather than too few or too many

F. _mutual_ rather than one-sided

G. The three advanced practice interventions for psychiatric nurses are _Rx meds_, _psychotherapy_, and _consultation_.

H. The four stages of psychiatric treatment are _maintenance_, _acute_, _crisis_, and _health promo._.

I. In implementing psychotherapeutic interventions, the nurse helps the patient do two things: _develop insight_ and _Δ behavior_.

J. The _patient_ is the ideal source of validation of data.

3. Provide short answers for the following questions.

A. Identify the four defining characteristics of nursing and relate these to psychiatric nursing.

B. Why is it important for the psychiatric nurse to be knowledgable about DSM-IV diagnoses?

C. Discuss the special problems that can arise in establishing mutual goals when caring for psychiatric patients. How would you deal with them?

D. Do you think that the use of computers in health care dehumanizes it? Explain your position.

REFERENCES

1. American Nurses' Association: *Nursing: a social policy statement,* Kansas City, Mo, 1980, The Association.
2. American Nurses' Association: *A statement on psychiatric–mental health clinical nursing practice and standards of psychiatric–mental health clinical nursing practice,* Washington, DC, 1994, The Association.
3. American Psychiatric Association: *Diagnostic and statistical manual of mental disorders,* ed 4, Washington, DC, 1994, The Association.
4. American Psychiatric Association: Practice guidelines for psychiatric evaluation of adults, *Am J Psychiatry* 152:67, 1995 Supplement.
5. Christensen P, Kenney J: *Nursing process: application of conceptual models,* St Louis, 1995, Mosby.
6. Dunn J: Medical skills and knowledge: how necessary are they for psychiatric nurses? *J Psychosoc Nurs Ment Health Serv* 31:25, 1993.
7. Felker B, Yazel J, Short D: Mortality and medical comorbidity among psychiatric patients: a review, *Psychiatr Serv* 47:1356, 1996.
8. Gross D, Fogg L, Conrad B: Designing interventions in psychosocial research, *Arch Psychiatr Nurs* 7:259, 1993.
9. Krumboltz J, Thorensen C: *Behavioral counseling: cases and techniques,* New York, 1969, Holt, Rinehart & Winston.

10. Malone J: The DSM-III-R versus nursing diagnosis: a dilemma in interdisciplinary practice, *Issues Ment Health Nurs* 12:219, 1991.
11. Merwin E, Mauck A: Psychiatric nursing outcome research: the state of the science, *Arch Psychiatr Nurs* 9:311, 1995.
12. National Quality of Care Forum: Bridging the gap between theory and practice: exploring clinical practice guidelines, *J Qual Improv* 19:384, 1993.
13. Naylor M, Brooten D: The roles and functions of clinical nurse specialists, *Image* 25:73, 1993.
14. Redman B: *The process of patient teaching*, St Louis, 1993, Mosby.
15. Safriet B: Health care dollars and regulatory sense: the role of advanced practice nurses, *Yale J Regulat* 9:419, 1992.
16. Teague D, Laraia M: Success factors for automated systems in the clinical environment: the MUSC experience, *Top Health Inform Management* 14:21, 1994.
17. Weaver R et al: Computerized treatment planning, *Hosp Community Psychiatry* 45:825, 1994.
18. Wilson J, Hobbs H: Therapeutic partnership: a model for clinical practice, *J Psychosoc Nurs* 33:27, 1995.

ANNOTATED SUGGESTED READINGS

American Psychiatric Association: Practice guidelines for psychiatric evaluation of adults, *Am J Psych* 152(Suppl):67, 1995.
    Focuses on the purpose, site, domains, and process of clinical psychiatric evaluations, emergency evaluations, and clinical consultations conducted in inpatient, outpatient, and other settings by psychiatrists.
*Artnak K, Dimmitt J: Choosing a framework for ethical analysis in advanced practice settings: the case for casuistry, *Arch Psychiatr Nurs* 10:16, 1996.
    Advanced reading relating ethical theory to an actual case study in psychiatric nursing.
Eppard J, Anderson J: Emergency psychiatric assessment: the nurse, psychiatrist, and counselor roles during the process, *J Psychosoc Nurs* 33:17, 1995.
    Reports on similarities and differences among nurses, psychiatrists, and counselors in their perceptions of teamwork, responsibility, and role expectation and in connecting with patients in an emergency service.
*Farkas-Cameron M: Clinical supervision in psychiatric nursing, *J Psychosoc Nurs* 33:31, 1995.
    Excellent discussion well worth reading that covers the need for and process of clinical supervision among psychiatric nursing.
Grohol J: *The insider's guide to mental health resources online*, New York, 1997, The Guilford Press.
    For novices and experts, provides step-by-step instructions to the world of mental health resources on the Internet. Saves time and includes insider tips and many relevant addresses.
Guide to behavioral resources on the Internet: A review of mental health and substance abuse web sites, mailing lists, and support forums, New York, 1997, Faulkner & Grau, Inc.
    Detailed information concerning areas of the Internet for the behavioral profession. Includes an introduction to the Internet, a tour of cyberspace, and the future of the 'net for the behavioral health field.
*Hastings C: Perspectives in ambulatory care: the changing multidisciplinary team, *Nurs Econ* 15:106, 1997.
    Reviews the increase in competition for a place on the ambulatory care team in an environment that limits payments and suggests nursing move quickly to assure itself a place.

Keller G: Management for quality: continuous quality improvement to increase access to outpatient mental health services, *Psychiatr Serv* 48:821, 1997.
    Suggests that the use of TQI, with balanced clinical and administrative leadership, can help to forge the needed synthesis of quality and cost in order to improve mental health services.
Kobak K: Computer-administered symptom rating scales, *Psychiatr Serv* 47:367, 1996.
    Computer-administered symptom rating scales are reviewed, the rationale for using them in clinical practice is discussed, and patients' reactions to being interviewed by computer are described.
Kobak K et al: Computerized screening for psychiatric disorders in an outpatient community mental health clinic, *Psychiatr Serv* 48:1048, 1997.
    Computerized and telephone voice response versions of a patient-rated diagnostic screening tool were found to have validity for certain diagnoses over others and good patient acceptance.
*Krch-Cole E et al: Bridging the chasm: incorporating the medically compromised patient into psychiatric practice, *J Psychosoc Nurs* 35:28, 1997.
    Describes the practice challenges facing psychiatric nurses as they provide care to patients who are also medically ill. Includes practical strategies for coping and meeting these challenges.
Lieberman H, Goldberg F, Kaplin G: The CD-ROM as a multipurpose clinical and management tool, *Psychiatr Serv* 48:1014, 1997.
    Outlines the potential for CD-ROM technology to support higher levels of functioning in areas of the service delivery system, such as those related to clinical, adminstration, consumers, and staff.
*Moch S et al: Linking research and practice through discussion, *Image* 29:189, 1997.
    Discussions between nurses in practice and nurses in research were used to foster integration of research into practice. The case study format allows for a rich description of the process and application to the psychiatric nursing setting.
*Poster E, Dee V, Randall B: The Johnson Behavioral Systems Model as a framework for patient outcome evaluation, *J Amer Psychiatr Nurses Association* 3:73, 1997.
    This study shows the importance of having a nursing database within the medical record to be able to measure the effectiveness of nursing interventions on predicted patient outcomes.
*Price J, Stevens H, LaBarre M: Spiritual caregiving in nursing practice, *J Psychosoc Nurs* 33:6, 1995.
    Articulates the lack of attention to spiritual care during nursing assessment, discusses the confusion between spirituality and religiosity, and describes the assimilation of spiritual care in practice.
Walters J, Neugeboren B: Collaboration between mental health organizations and religious institutions, *Psychiatric Rehabilitation Journal* 19:51, 1995.
    Discusses the roles of providers and religious institutions in a collaboration that provides linkages for mental health professionals seeking assistance with mental health service needs.
*Wilson J, Hobbs H: Therapeutic partnership: a model for clinical practice, *J Psychosoc Nurs* 33:27, 1995.
    Describes a model for clinical practice that reinforces shared responsibility, accountability, and decision-making in working with patients and their families.

*Nursing reference.

© 1998 M.C. Escher/Cordon Art, Baarn, Holland.

Actualizing the Psychiatric Nursing Role: Professional Performance Standards

Gail W. Stuart

The professional motive is the desire and perpetual effort to do the thing as well as it can be done, which exists just as much in the Nurse, as in the Astronomer in search of a new star, or in the Artist completing a picture. **Florence Nightingale**

LEARNING OBJECTIVES

After studying this chapter the student should be able to:

▼ Describe how accountability and autonomy relate to the psychiatric nurse's professional role responsibilities

▼ Analyze the conditions and behaviors of the psychiatric nurse related to the quality of care activities

▼ Analyze the conditions and behaviors of the psychiatric nurse related to performance appraisal

▼ Analyze the conditions and behaviors of the psychiatric nurse related to education

▼ Analyze the conditions and behaviors of the psychiatric nurse related to collegiality

▼ Analyze the conditions and behaviors of the psychiatric nurse related to ethics

▼ Analyze the conditions and behaviors of the psychiatric nurse related to collaboration

▼ Analyze the conditions and behaviors of the psychiatric nurse related to research

▼ Analyze the conditions and behaviors of the psychiatric nurse related to resource use

TOPICAL OUTLINE

The standards of care from the American Nurses' Association (ANA) *Standards of Psychiatric–Mental Health Clinical Nursing Practice,* as presented in Chapter 10, describe what the psychiatric nurse does; the standards of professional performance from the same document presented in this chapter describe the context in which the psychiatric nurse performs these activities.[3] Neither set of standards can be taken in isolation; together they complete the picture of contemporary psychiatric nursing practice. They also clarify the many elements that influence the psychiatric nursing role.

ACCOUNTABILITY AND AUTONOMY

Psychiatric nursing is characterized by rules of competency and service. The standards of professional performance apply to self-regulation and accountability for practice by psychiatric nurses, both individually and as a group. They also address issues of professional autonomy and self-definition. As such, the standards of performance are critical.

Accountability means to be answerable to someone for something. It focuses responsibility on the individual nurse for personal actions, or perhaps lack of action. The preconditions of accountability include ability, responsibility, and authority. Accountability also includes formal review processes and an attitude of integrity and vigilance.

Autonomy implies self-determination, independence, and shared power. It is the condition that allows for definition of and control over a work domain. For psychiatric nursing, attaining autonomy means being able to define the domain of nursing and being able to exercise control over psychiatric nursing practice. This idea of shaping destiny, rather than letting outside forces be in control, views power as a positive force that allows nurses to attain goals. It involves a conscious decision to identify objectives, plan strategy, assume responsibility, exercise authority, and be held accountable.

Autonomy has two major interrelated components. The first is **control over nursing tasks,** which means:

▼ Having the opportunity for independent thought and action
▼ Having use of time, skills, and ability by being able to eliminate, refuse, or delegate nonnursing tasks
▼ Having the authority and responsibility for implementing goals related to the quality of care
▼ Being able to initiate changes and innovations in practice

The second component of autonomy is **participation in decision making.** It requires the nurse's participation in the following:

▼ Determining and implementing quality standards
▼ Making decisions affecting each nurse's job context, including salary, staffing, and professional growth
▼ Setting institutional policies, procedures, and goals

This second component of participation in decision making is particularly problematic for nursing. Most nurses are employed in health-care organizations in which authority rests primarily with administrators, physicians, and board members. Furthermore, nurses often are expected to do tasks they are overqualified for, which results in underuse of their many important skills.

Nurses are thus caught in the crossfire. They staff clinical areas around the clock, make important decisions, and shoulder major responsibility for coordinating and managing patient care, but they often lack decision-making authority as to the allocation of resources. Because nurses are usually not compensated on a fee-for-service basis, they are often not seen as a source of revenue by administrators and therefore lack a critical base for power. It is not surprising that if nurses do not have a role in organizational decision making, they will have limited ability to exercise control of their practice.

The full realization of nursing's potential will be obtained through a negotiated process with other health professionals, consumers, and society at large. It requires increased access to resources, demonstration of expertise, and acknowledgment of the skills of nurses by other professionals. Psychiatric nursing is practiced largely in collaboration, coordination, and cooperation with a variety of other professionals working with and on behalf of the patient. As nurses see themselves in a positive way, they will increase their ability to assert themselves, articulate the contributions they make, and function effectively. The conditions and behaviors related to each standard of professional performance are shown in Fig. 11-1. Each of these standards is now discussed.

Quality of Care

STANDARD I: QUALITY OF CARE

The psychiatric–mental health nurse systematically evaluates the quality of care and effectiveness of psychiatric–mental health nursing practice.

▼ *Rationale*
The dynamic nature of the mental health care environment and the growing body of psychiatric nursing knowledge and research enable the psychiatric–mental health nurse to be competent in clinical practice, to continue to develop professionally, and to improve the quality of patient care.

▼ *Nursing conditions*
Personal and professional integrity
Openness to inquiry
Critical thinking skills

▼ *Nursing behaviors*
Identify improvement opportunities
Collect and analyze relevant data
Formulate a planned approach for improvement
Implement suggested changes

▼ *Key elements*
The nurse should be open to critically analyzing the caregiving process.

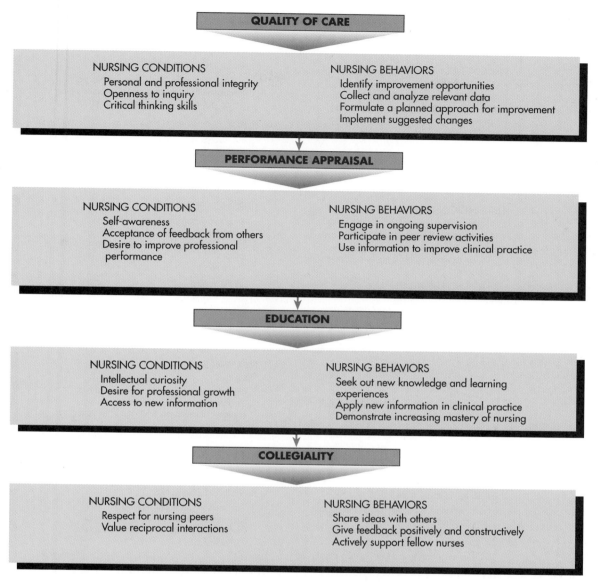

Fig. 11-1   Nursing conditions and behaviors related to the psychiatric nursing standards of professional performance.

Continued

The patient and family should be partners with the nurse in the evaluation of care activities.

Improving the quality of care provided goes beyond discussion and analysis to actually implementing actions that will improve practice.

Psychiatric nurses need to actively participate in the formal organizational evaluation of overall patterns of care through a variety of quality improvement or process improvement activities. In these activities the focus is not on the nurse clinician but on the patient and the overall program of care. The current growth and commitment to critically reviewing health care stems from several sources: consumer demand for high-quality but reasonably priced health care, third-party payer demand for controlled health-care costs, increased professional accountability, and regulatory and federal groups that monitor the quality of care.

The purpose of quality or process improvement programs is to design, implement, evaluate, guide, and modify a process for improving the performance of a health-care organization and to initiate improvement activities. Specific objectives include:

▼ Continuous improvement of customer satisfaction
▼ Continuous improvement of patient outcomes
▼ Efficient use of resources
▼ Adherence to professional and regulatory standards

The successful implementation of such a program re-

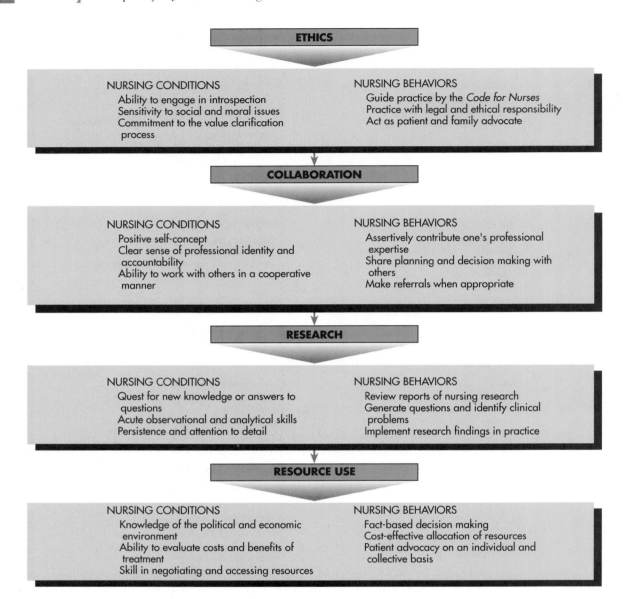

ETHICS

NURSING CONDITIONS	NURSING BEHAVIORS
Ability to engage in introspection	Guide practice by the *Code for Nurses*
Sensitivity to social and moral issues	Practice with legal and ethical responsibility
Commitment to the value clarification process	Act as patient and family advocate

COLLABORATION

NURSING CONDITIONS	NURSING BEHAVIORS
Positive self-concept	Assertively contribute one's professional expertise
Clear sense of professional identity and accountability	Share planning and decision making with others
Ability to work with others in a cooperative manner	Make referrals when appropriate

RESEARCH

NURSING CONDITIONS	NURSING BEHAVIORS
Quest for new knowledge or answers to questions	Review reports of nursing research
Acute observational and analytical skills	Generate questions and identify clinical problems
Persistence and attention to detail	Implement research findings in practice

RESOURCE USE

NURSING CONDITIONS	NURSING BEHAVIORS
Knowledge of the political and economic environment	Fact-based decision making
Ability to evaluate costs and benefits of treatment	Cost-effective allocation of resources
Skill in negotiating and accessing resources	Patient advocacy on an individual and collective basis

Fig. 11-1, cont'd

Fig. 11-2   Quality improvement process.

quires employee empowerment, the removal of barriers, and interdisciplinary teamwork to find new ways to improve existing processes.[6] These processes could affect any of the activities of the health-care organization identified in Table 11-1. Figure 11-2 is a representation of the quality improvement process, which really is the problem-solving process or nursing process applied to making health care processes and outcomes better.

> **?** *Find out about a quality improvement project that is currently under way in your clinical facility. Does it relate to the health-care organization's product, operations, process, or management activities as identified in Table 11-1?*

TABLE **11-1** *Potential Impact of Quality Improvement Projects*

PRODUCT	OPERATIONS	PROCESS	MANAGEMENT
Clinical practice patterns	Information systems	Effectiveness of communication	Commitment to the organization and to high-quality patient care
Patient outcomes	Accuracy and timeliness of information	Information dissemination	Morale
Cost of care	Patient access	Recognition for performance	Team building
Customer satisfaction	Marketing	Employee training and education	Performance evaluation process
Use of human resources	Link between performance and incentives	Medical records	Delivery system integration

Performance Appraisal

STANDARD II: PERFORMANCE APPRAISAL

The psychiatric–mental health nurse evaluates his or her own practice in relation to professional practice standards and relevant statutes and regulations.

▼*Rationale*

The psychiatric–mental health nurse is accountable to the public for providing competent clinical care and has an inherent responsibility as a professional to evaluate the role and performance of psychiatric–mental health nursing practice according to standards established by the profession and regulatory bodies.

▼*Nursing conditions*

Self-awareness

Acceptance of feedback from others

Desire to improve professional performance

▼*Nursing behaviors*

Engage in ongoing supervision

Participate in peer review activities

Use information to improve clinical practice

▼*Key elements*

Supervision should be viewed as an essential and ongoing aspect of one's professional life.

The nurse should strive to grow and develop professional knowledge, skills, and expertise.

Performance appraisal for the psychiatric nurse is generally provided in two forms: administrative and clinical. Administrative performance appraisal involves the review, management, and regulation of competent psychiatric nursing practice. It involves a supervisory relationship in which a nurse's work performance is compared with role expectations in a formal way, such as in a nurse's annual performance evaluation. Administrative performance evaluations should identify areas of competency and areas for improvement. There should also be a method for recognizing quality performance (see Critical Thinking about Contemporary Issues).

Many nursing departments have adopted clinical advancement programs or other formal mechanisms to recognize nursing excellence. Clinical advancement programs have been established to formally validate nurses for in-

CRITICAL THINKING *about* Contemporary Issues

What Kind of Recognition Do Staff Nurses Value?

It is well known that recognition is central to nurses' morale. However, it is less clear what type of recognition is valued and why it is given. A survey asked 239 staff nurses about this issue.[14] They found that verbal feedback was identified as the most meaningful type of recognition. This was followed by letters of praise for performance or achievement, organizational awards, honors or public announcements of outstanding performance, promotion or a prestigious assignment with increased responsibility, being personally thanked and praised during an evaluation, and finally monetary bonuses, salary increases, or gifts.

The main reasons given for receiving recognition included outstanding performance in patient care and positive attitude, followed by demonstrated expertise, willingness to assume extra work, involvement in professional activities, completion of a certification or degree program, and years of service in an organization. Finally, recognition came most often from the head nurse, followed by the nurse administrator, patients and families, coworkers, physicians, and hospital administrators. Studies such as this help to clarify meaningful aspects of administrative performance appraisals and ways to commend nurses for a job well done.

creasing mastery in practice. They allow the nurse to be promoted and economically rewarded for providing direct patient care.[11] Such programs identify levels of professional development in nursing based on increased critical thinking and advanced application of nursing skills (Fig. 11-3). These characteristics result in better care provided by psychiatric nurses throughout their professional career.

Future expectations of psychiatric nursing roles must take into account the diverse education and experiences of psychiatric nurses. Role descriptions and functional assignments must better differentiate among psychiatric nurses based on education, experience, and competency.[13] In addition, responsibilities of psychiatric nurses should clearly reflect their unique knowledge base and biopsychosocial competencies.

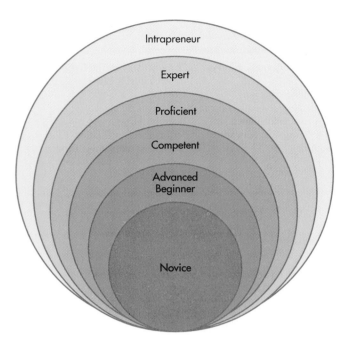

Fig. 11-3 Levels of differentiated nursing practice.

? *One of your nursing colleagues tells you that she thinks nurses' pay should be based on their experience, not their education. After all, she argues, if two nurses do the same job, what does it matter if they have different educational degrees? How would you respond?*

Clinical Supervision

Clinical performance appraisal is guidance provided through a mentoring relationship with a more experienced, skilled, and educated nurse. The professional psychiatric nurse is aware of the need for ongoing mentorship to achieve increasing levels of mastery of psychiatric nursing practice. Clinical supervision not only reviews one's clinical care but also functions as a support system for the nurse, because nurses must care about themselves before being able to care for others.

In many ways the process of supervision parallels the nurse-patient relationship. Both involve a learning process that takes place in the context of a meaningful relationship that facilitates positive change. Self-exploration is a critical element of both. The supervisor should provide the same responsive and action dimensions present in the nurse-patient relationship to help supervised nurses live effectively with themselves and others.

There are four common forms of supervision:

▼ The dyadic, or one-on-one, relationship, in which the supervisor meets the supervisee in a face-to-face encounter
▼ The triadic relationship, in which a supervisor and two

nurses of similar experience and training meet for supervision
▼ Group supervision, in which several supervised nurses meet for a shared session with the supervisory nurse
▼ Peer review, in which nurses meet without a supervisor to evaluate their clinical practice

All four forms have a similar purpose: exploring the problem areas and maximizing the strengths of the supervisees.

PROCESS OF SUPERVISION. The process of supervision requires the nurse to record the interactions with the patient. Both written notes and audio recordings have been used for this purpose, but neither yields as accurate and complete information as that provided by videotape recordings. Videotaped sessions minimize distortion of data. The supervised nurse then analyzes the data, extracts themes, and identifies problems relevant to nursing care. The nurse reviews the literature, draws inferences, evaluates effectiveness, and formulates plans for the next session. In the supervision conference the nurse shares this analysis and receives feedback from the supervisor or peers, if it is a group or peer conference.

Supervision can be seen as a didactic process in which the theory and concepts related to nursing practice are reviewed, or it can be a quasitherapeutic process that explores countertransference problems, attitudes, values, and the nurse's emotional needs and personal biases. A third approach is a process-centered model of supervision that is neither personal therapy nor simply a didactic process of conveying information on theory and technique. In this model the supervisor is an active participant in an affectively charged learning process, the focus of which is learning and personal growth rather than psychotherapy for the supervisee. Problems between the clinician and the supervisor are believed to shed light on problems that exist between the clinician and patient. The very problems experienced in one relationship affect and are reflected in the other relationship.

However, the goal of supervision is not to eliminate these problems, but to use them to achieve greater understanding of the ongoing dynamic processes at work in therapy. The problems become the vehicles through which therapeutic progress may be made. Thus the most effective supervision depends on active insight into the many forces in the parallel processes of therapy and supervision.[8] Finally, it is important to remember that tension in the supervisory relationship is inevitable, but when understood and handled skillfully, it can be very helpful to the clinician's growth.

PURPOSE AND GOALS. Despite its intensity, supervision is not therapy. The essential difference between the two is a difference of purpose. The aim of supervision is to teach psychotherapeutic skills, whereas the goal of therapy is to alter a person's characteristic patterns of coping to function more effectively in all areas of life. The supervisee's problems in the supervisory and therapeutic relationships are dealt with only to the extent that they affect the nurse's ability to learn from the supervisor and be effective with patients. Therefore, the problems are limited in scope and depth; they do not include all other aspects of the supervisee's life. With the resolution of the particular problem, the focus of supervision returns to the teaching of psychotherapeutic skills and their implementation by the nurse. The therapeutic implications for the supervisee are therefore related to the primary goal of supervision: the teaching of psychotherapeutic skills.

Supervision or consultation is necessary for the practicing psychiatric nurse. Although it is crucial for novices, it is equally important for experienced practitioners.[10] Personal limitations create a need for assistance in remaining objective throughout the therapeutic process and the "normal" stresses it presents. Obviously, supervision is only as helpful as the skill of the supervisor, the openness of the supervised nurse, and the motivation of both to learn and grow.

Education

STANDARD III: EDUCATION

The psychiatric–mental health nurse acquires and maintains current knowledge in nursing practice.

▼*Rationale*

The rapid expansion of knowledge pertaining to basic and behavioral sciences, technology, information systems, and research requires a commitment to learning throughout the psychiatric–mental health nurse's career. Formal education, continuing education, certification, and experiential learning are ways the psychiatric–mental health nurse uses to enhance nursing expertise and advance the profession.

▼*Nursing conditions*

Intellectual curiosity

Desire for professional growth

Access to new information

▼*Nursing behaviors*

Seek out new knowledge and learning experiences

Apply new information in clinical practice

Demonstrate increasing mastery of nursing

▼*Key elements*

Professional learning should be regarded as a lifelong process.

The nurse should pursue a variety of educational opportunities.

New knowledge should be translated into professional nursing practice.

The nature of psychiatric care, the mental health delivery system, and the boundaries of nursing are changing rapidly. In addition, the scientific basis for practice is expanding rapidly, and psychiatric nurses need to keep up with this knowledge.

Psychiatric nurses are expected to engage in a continuous learning process to maintain currency with the latest

Archives of Psychiatric Nursing
Journal of the American Psychiatric Nurses Association
Journal of Psychosocial Nursing
and Mental Health Services
Journal of Child and Adolescent Psychiatric Nursing
Issues in Mental Health Nursing
Perspectives in Psychiatric Care

Fig. 11-4 Psychiatric nursing journals.

information in the field. They may do this in the following ways:

▼ Formal educational programs

▼ Continuing education programs

▼ Independent learning activities

▼ Lectures, conferences, and workshops

▼ Credentialing

▼ Certification

Reading journals and textbooks and collaborating with colleagues are other important ways to remain current with expanding areas of knowledge. Fig. 11-4 lists journals that relate to psychiatric nursing practice and are good sources of new information.

The Internet

Perhaps the most exciting new resource for psychiatric nurses is the Internet. This technology allows nurses access to information from around the globe using a desktop or laptop computer, a telephone line, and a modem. Using browser software such as Netscape and Internet Explorer, nurses can receive textual information complemented by sound, video, and graphics on the World Wide Web (WWW), a subset of the Internet that allows the use of multimedia. In addition, the Internet can help nurses communicate through e-mail and network with other nurses through discussion groups or newsgroups.

The number of WWW home pages is growing rapidly, from fewer than 100 sites in 1993 to over half a million in February 1996. These sites offer a wide range of information, from updates on current psychiatric medications to information on various mental disorders to resources on mental health organizations and delivery systems.[15,21] The amount of information available through this technology may revolutionize the way in which psychiatric nurses acquire and maintain current knowledge in nursing practice.

This text facilitates the use of the Internet by providing the addresses of home pages on the WWW that are most relevant to the content of each chapter in the Your Internet Connection feature. Nurses are encouraged to access these resources to further their knowledge and professional growth.

Certification

The certification process is a formal review of clinical nursing practice that has evolved within the American Nurses' Association.[2] The objectives of certification are to

▼ Ensure the public of high-quality care
▼ Provide credentials to expedite employment and third-party reimbursement for services rendered
▼ Expand opportunities for vertical and horizontal mobility and career advancement
▼ Attain greater prestige and peer recognition for achieving clinical expertise
▼ Improve clinical practice

Psychiatric nursing has two levels of certification: the **generalist,** who may be a staff nurse, and the **specialist,** who specializes in either adult or child and adolescent psychiatric nursing. As of 1995 there were 19,145 certified nurse generalists, 6030 certified nurse specialists in adult psychiatric–mental health nursing, and 770 certified nurse specialists in child and adolescent psychiatric–mental health nursing.

To become a **certified generalist** the psychiatric nurse must demonstrate expertise in practice and knowledge of theories concerning personality development and behavior patterns in treating mental illness and the relationship of such treatments to nursing care. Special requirements include

▼ A baccalaureate degree in nursing
▼ Practice as a psychiatric and mental health nurse for a minimum of 1600 hours within 2 of the last 4 years
▼ Current work in psychiatric and mental health nursing for a minimum of 8 hours per week

To become a **certified specialist** the nurse must show a high degree of proficiency in interpersonal skills, the use of the nursing process, and psychological and milieu therapies. Following are five requirements for certification as a specialist in psychiatric and mental health nursing:

▼ Current involvement in psychiatric and mental health nursing practice at least 4 hours per week
▼ A master's or higher degree in nursing, with a specialization in psychiatric and mental health nursing (a nurse may apply for individual consideration if he or she has a master's or higher degree in nursing or a mental health field with a minimum of 24 graduate academic credits in psychiatric and mental health theory and supervised training in two psychotherapeutic treatment modalities)
▼ Experience in at least two different treatment modalities
▼ At least 800 hours of direct patient/client contact in advanced clinical practice of psychiatric and mental health nursing (up to 400 of these hours may be earned through the clinical practicum in a master's program of study)
▼ 100 hours of individual or group clinical consultation/supervision and endorsements from the consultants/supervisors

On successful completion of the certification examination and written documentation, the nurse is identified as certified (C.) if a generalist or as a certified specialist (C.S.) in psychiatric–mental health nursing. Although any specialist nurse may be certified, it is expected that nurses who are self-employed in the practice of psychotherapy will obtain certification to assure the public of their ability to perform as competent nurse psychotherapists.

Collegiality

STANDARD IV: COLLEGIALITY

The psychiatric–mental health nurse contributes to the professional development of peers, colleagues, and others.
▼*Rationale*
The psychiatric–mental health nurse is responsible for sharing knowledge, research, and clinical information with colleagues through formal and informal teaching methods to enhance professional growth.
▼*Nursing conditions*
Respect for nursing peers
Value reciprocal interactions
▼*Nursing behaviors*
Share ideas with others
Give feedback positively and constructively
Actively support fellow nurses
▼*Key elements*
The nurse should regard other nurses as colleagues and partners in caregiving.
Mentorship within nursing is important both to nurses as individuals and to the nursing profession as a whole.

Collegiality is an essential aspect of professional practice. It requires that nurses view their nurse peers as collaborators in the caregiving process who are valued and respected for their unique contributions, regardless of educational, experiential, or specialty background. It suggests that nurses must view themselves as members of an organized professional group or unit and that nurses trust, remain loyal, and demonstrate commitment to other nurses.

Many have observed that nursing, as a profession, has sometimes struggled with this concept. For example, nurses have voiced complaints about "ivory-tower" nurse educators, "nonsupportive" nurse administrators, "nonintellectual" nurse clinicians, and "irrelevant" nurse researchers in the past. Also, psychiatric nurses in various institutions or organizations have had difficulty joining forces and working together on a common psychiatric nursing agenda. However, this intradisciplinary interaction is not consistent with professional performance standards. It has also prevented the profession from acting as a united group in pursuing health care initiatives at local, regional, and national levels.

Nurses need to work together as colleagues to blend their various skills and abilities in creating a better health care system and enhancing the quality and quantity of psychiatric nursing services provided. One specific way to do this is for psychiatric nurses to join a professional nursing organization. The largest psychiatric nursing organization that is open to nursing students and psychiatric nurses of all educational and experiential backgrounds is the American Psychiatric Nurses Association (APNA). The mission and goals of this organization are described in Box 11-1.

> **?** *You approach a colleague about joining the APNA but she tells you that she does not have the money to join a nursing organization. You know that membership in APNA costs less than $2 a week and it includes a subscription to the* Journal of the American Psychiatric Nurses Association. *How would you respond?*

Box **11-1** *Overview of the American Psychiatric Nurses Association (APNA)*

MISSION

To provide leadership to advance psychiatric–mental health nursing practice, improve mental health care for individuals, families, groups, and communities, and shape health policy for the delivery of mental health services.

GOALS

Facilitate the professional development of psychiatric–mental health nurses through programs and services related to the creation, exchange, and engineering of new knowledge and skills

Enhance the quality of care provided by psychiatric–mental health nurses through the promotion of established standards of clinical practice and professional performance

Participate as partners and leaders in the formulation of policies and the design, implementation, and evaluation of delivery systems in psychiatric–mental health care

Represent psychiatric–mental health nursing as a collective and integrated specialty in the professional and public forum of the health-care community

DUES

Regular membership: $100
Student membership: $60

ADDRESS

1200 19th Street NW
Washington, DC 20036-2422
Phone: 202-857-1133
Fax: 202-223-4579
Internet: http:/www.apna.org

Ethics

STANDARD V: ETHICS

The psychiatric–mental health nurse's decisions and actions on behalf of clients are determined in an ethical manner.

▼*Rationale*

The public's trust and its right to humane psychiatric–mental health care are upheld by professional nursing practice. The foundation of psychiatric–mental health nursing practice is the development of a therapeutic relationship with the client. The psychiatric–mental health nurse engages in therapeutic interactions and relationships that support the healing process. Boundaries must be established to safeguard the client's well-being and to prevent the development of intimate or sexual relationships.

▼*Nursing conditions*

Ability to engage in introspection
Sensitivity to social and moral issues
Commitment to the value clarification process

▼*Nursing behaviors*

Guide practice by the Code for Nurses
Practice with legal and ethical responsibility
Act as a patient and family advocate

▼*Key elements*

Nurses should be sensitive to the social, moral, and ethical environment in which they practice.

Patient and family advocacy is a core aspect of nursing practice.

Ethical conduct is essential to the nurse-patient relationship.

Ethical considerations combine with legal and therapeutic issues to affect all aspects of psychiatric nursing practice. The legal-ethical context of psychiatric nursing care is discussed in Chapter 9. Boundary violations related to the nurse-patient relationship are described in Chapter 2.

Ethical Standards

An **ethic** is a standard of behavior or a belief valued by an individual or group. It describes what ought to be, rather than what is—a goal to which an individual aspires. These standards are learned through socialization, growth, and experience. As such, they are not static but evolve to reflect social change.

Groups, such as professions, can also hold a code of ethics. Such a code guides the profession in serving and protecting consumers. It also provides a framework for decision making for members of the profession. Two major purposes for a code of ethics are structuring and sensitizing.[19] Structuring is preventive and aims to restrain impulsive and unethical behavior. Sensitizing is educative, with the goal of raising members' ethical consciousness.

The American Nurses' Association[1] published a code of ethics for nurses (Box 11-2). It emphasizes nurses' accountability for the quality of care they give and their duty to act as patient advocates in ensuring the quality of care given by others. Psychiatric nurses should follow these professional standards as they deliver health care. If nurses know their values and implement them within the framework of the code, they can increase both the quality of the care they give and the satisfaction they receive from practice.

Ethical Decision Making

Ethical decision making involves trying to distinguish right from wrong in situations without clear guidelines.[4]

A decision-making model can help identify factors and principles that affect a decision. Curtin[7] proposed a model for critical ethical analysis (Fig. 11-5) that describes steps or factors that the nurse should consider in resolving an ethical dilemma. The first step is gathering background information to obtain a clear picture of the problem. This includes finding available information to clarify the underlying issues. The next factor is identifying the ethical components or the nature of the dilemma, such as freedom versus coercion or treating versus accepting the right to refuse treatment. The next step is the clarification of the rights and responsibilities of all ethical agents, or those involved in the decision making. This can include the patient, the nurse, and possibly many others, including the patient's family, physician, health-care institution, clergy, social worker, and perhaps even the courts. Those involved may not agree on how to handle the situation, but their rights and duties can be clarified. All possible options must then be explored in light of everyone's responsibilities, as well as the purpose and potential result of each option. This step eliminates alternatives that violate rights or seem harmful. The nurse then engages in the application of principles, which stem from the nurse's philosophy of life and nursing, scientific knowledge, and ethical theory.[9] Ethical theories suggest ways to structure ethical dilemmas and judge potential solutions. Here are four possible approaches:

▼ **Utilitarianism** focuses on the consequences of actions. It seeks the greatest amount of happiness or the least amount of harm for the greatest number, or "the greatest good for the greatest number."

Box **11-2** *American Nurses' Association Code for Nurses*

▼ The nurse provides services with respect for human dignity and the uniqueness of the client unrestricted by considerations of social or economic status, personal attributes, or the nature of health problems.
▼ The nurse safeguards the client's right to privacy by judiciously protecting information of a confidential nature.
▼ The nurse acts to safeguard the client and public when health care and safety are affected by the incompetent, unethical, or illegal practice of any person.
▼ The nurse assumes responsibility and accountability for individual nursing judgments and actions.
▼ The nurse maintains competence in nursing.
▼ The nurse exercises informed judgment and uses individual competence and qualification as criteria in seeking consultation, accepting responsibilities, and delegating nursing activities to others.
▼ The nurse participates in activities that contribute to the ongoing development of the profession's body of knowledge.
▼ The nurse participates in the profession's efforts to implement and improve standards of nursing.
▼ The nurse participates in the profession's efforts to establish and maintain conditions of employment conducive to high-quality nursing care.
▼ The nurse participates in the profession's effort to protect the public from misinformation and misrepresentation and to maintain the integrity of nursing.
▼ The nurse collaborates with members of the health professions and other citizens in promoting community and national efforts to meet public health needs.

From American Nurses' Association: *Code for nurses with interpretive statements*, Kansas City, Mo, 1985, The Association.

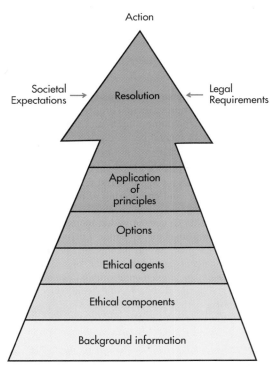

Fig. 11-5 Model for ethical decision making. Societal expectations and legal requirements may sway the resolution of the conflict one way or another. However, the notions of what is legal (or expected) may or may not coincide with what is good, right, or proper. (From Curtin L: A proposed model for critical ethical analysis, *Nurs Forum* 17:12, 1978.)

▼ **Egoism** is a position in which the individual seeks the solution that is best personally. The self is most important, and others are secondary.

▼ **Formalism** considers the nature of the act itself and the principles involved. It involves the universal application of a basic rule, such as "do unto others as you would have them do unto you."

▼ **Fairness** is based on the concept of justice, and benefit to the least advantaged in society becomes the norm for decision making.

The final step is **resolution into action**. Within the context of social expectations and legal requirements, the nurse decides on the goals and methods of implementation. Table 11-2 summarizes these steps and suggests questions nurses can ask themselves in making complex ethical choices in psychiatric nursing practice.

TABLE 11-2 *Steps and Questions in Ethical Decision Making*

STEPS	RELEVANT QUESTIONS
Gathering background information	Does an ethical dilemma exist?
	What information is known?
	What information is needed?
	What is the context of the dilemma?
Identifying ethical components	What is the underlying issue?
	Who is affected by this dilemma?
Clarification of agents	What are the rights of each involved party?
	What are the obligations of each involved party?
	Who should be involved in the decision making?
	For whom is the decision being made?
	What degree of consent is needed by the patient?
Exploration of options	What alternatives exist?
	What is the purpose or intent of each alternative?
	What are the potential consequences of each alternative?
Application of principles	What criteria should be used?
	What ethical theories are subscribed to?
	What scientific facts are relevant?
	What is the nurse's philosophy of life and nursing?
Resolution into action	What are the social and legal constraints and ramifications?
	What is the goal of the nurse's decision?
	How can the resulting ethical choice be implemented?
	How can the resulting ethical choice be evaluated?

? *Think of an ethical problem you have encountered in caring for a psychiatric patient and family. Use the model for ethical decision making to decide on the best course of action.*

Collaboration

STANDARD VI: COLLABORATION

The psychiatric–mental health nurse collaborates with the client, significant others, and health-care providers in providing care.

▼ *Rationale*

Psychiatric–mental health nursing practice requires a coordinated, ongoing interaction between consumers and providers to deliver comprehensive services to the client and the community. Through the collaborative process, different abilities of health-care providers are used to solve problems, communicate, plan, implement, and evaluate mental health services.

▼ *Nursing conditions*

Positive self-concept

Clear sense of professional identity and accountability

Ability to work with others in a cooperative manner

▼ *Nursing behaviors*

Assertively contribute one's professional expertise

Share planning and decision making with others

Make referrals when appropriate

▼ *Key elements*

Respect for others grows out of respect for self.

The nurse should be able to clearly articulate his or her professional abilities and areas of expertise to others.

Collaboration involves the ability to negotiate and formulate new solutions with others.

Collaboration is the shared planning, decision making, problem solving, goal setting, and assumption of responsibilities by individuals who work together cooperatively and with open communication. Three key ingredients are needed for collaboration:

▼ Active and assertive contributions from each person

▼ Receptivity and respect for each person's contribution

▼ Negotiations that build on the contributions of each person to form a new way of conceptualizing the problem

It is important for psychiatric nurses to realize that they have many potential collaborators, including patients and families, interdisciplinary colleagues, and nursing peers (Fig. 11-6). Each of these groups allows the psychiatric nurse an opportunity to problem solve in new ways and thus better plan and implement nursing care.

Interdisciplinary Mental Health Teams

An essential part of contemporary practice is working with other health-care providers. Nurses may be members of three different types of teams: **unidisciplinary**, having all team members of the same discipline; **multidisciplinary**, having members of different disciplines who provide specific services to the patient; and **interdisciplinary**, having members of different disciplines involved in a formal arrangement to provide patient services while maximizing educational interchange. Most organized mental health settings use an interdisciplinary team approach, which requires highly coordinated and often interdependent planning based on the separate and distinct roles of each team member (Table 11-3).

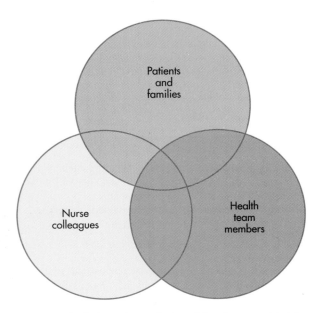

Fig. 11-6 Collaborative relationships for psychiatric nurses.

However, interdisciplinary collaboration does not always proceed smoothly. There are many barriers to interdisciplinary collaboration, including inappropriate education and training of mental health team members, traditional organizational structures, goal and role conflict, competitive and accommodating interpersonal interactions, power and status inequities, and personal qualities of individuals that do not promote shared problem solving. If roles, functions, and channels of communication among the various team members are not clarified and agreed on, confusion, resentment, crossing of boundaries, and inappropriate use of psychiatric team members are likely to result. Steps that can be taken to facilitate the formation of interdisciplinary teams are listed in Box 11-3.

Finally, psychiatric nurses must determine whether they as a group are ready to engage in collaborative practice. Questions that should be considered include the following:

▼ Can psychiatric nurses define, describe, and appropriately defend psychiatric nursing roles and functions?

▼ Is the psychiatric nursing leadership ready for collegial practice?

▼ Are psychiatric nursing roles and functions appropriate for nurses' education, experience, and expertise?

▼ Is nurse staffing appropriate in numbers, patterns, and ratios?

▼ Are inservices, education, credentialing, and certification valued and rewarded?

▼ Are there necessary structural and human support systems?

▼ Are the other disciplines prepared for and supportive of collaboration?

▼ Is the organizational climate conducive to collaboration?

With positive answers to these questions, psychiatric nurses should be able to move forward in implementing collaborative practice.

TABLE **11-3** *Mental Health Personnel, Training, and Roles*

PERSONNEL	TRAINING	ROLE
Psychiatric nurse	Registered nurse (RN) with specialized training in the care and treatment of psychiatric patients. May have an AD, BS, MS, or PhD degree	Accountable for the biopsychosocial nursing care of patients and their milieu
Psychiatrist	Medical doctor with internship and residency training in psychiatry	Accountable for the medical diagnosis and treatment of patients
Social worker	BS, MSW, or PhD degree with specialized training in mental health settings	Accountable for family casework and community placement of patients
Psychologist	PhD or PsyD degree with research and clinical training in mental health	Accountable for psychological assessments and testing
Activity therapist	May have a BS degree with training in mental health settings	Accountable for recreational, occupational, and activity programs
Case worker	Varying degrees of training and usually works under supervision	Accountable for helping patients to be maintained in the community and receive needed services
Substance abuse counselor	Varying degrees of training in alcohol and substance use disorders	Accountable for evaluating and treating patients with substance use problems

? *Most people think that there are more collaborative interdisciplinary relationships in psychiatry than in other specialty areas because of the nature of the work. Others believe that there is more interdisciplinary conflict in psychiatry because roles overlap and boundaries are often unclear. What position would you take on this issue based on your observation of the mental health care team?*

Research

STANDARD VII: RESEARCH

The psychiatric–mental health nurse contributes to nursing and mental health through the use of research.

▼ *Rationale*

Psychiatric–mental health nurses are responsible for contributing to the further development of the field of mental health by participating in research. At the basic level of practice, the psychiatric–mental health nurse uses research findings to improve clinical care and identifies clinical problems for research study. At the advanced level, the psychiatric–mental health nurse engages or collaborates with others in the research process to discover, examine, and test knowledge, theories, and creative approaches to practice.

▼ *Nursing conditions*

Quest for new knowledge or answers to questions
Acute observational and analytical skills
Persistence and attention to detail

▼ *Nursing behaviors*

Review reports of nursing research
Generate questions and identify clinical problems
Implement research findings in practice

Box **11-3** *Steps for Interdisciplinary Team Building*

- ▼ Develop and agree on a team philosophy of care
- ▼ Understand and respect the contributions of each discipline
- ▼ Establish new professional interaction patterns
- ▼ Define disciplinary and individual roles and responsibilities
- ▼ Accept personal and professional changes in authority and status
- ▼ Specify lines of authority and decision making and conflict resolution procedures
- ▼ Accept shared authority and responsibility
- ▼ Communicate regularly, openly, and clearly
- ▼ Use multidisciplinary treatment plans and consolidated charting
- ▼ Strive for consistent leadership and low staff turnover
- ▼ Encourage constant review and exchange of ideas

▼ *Key elements*

Research links nursing theory and practice and is essential to the development of a profession.
Outcome research helps to establish the value of nursing in an era of health-care reform

The relationship between practice, theory, and research is interactive and reciprocal. For theory to be useful, it must have implications for practice, and for practice to be tested and validated, it must be based in theory. Theory that arises out of practice is validated by research, which returns to direct practice and has implications for clinical care.

This cyclical relationship is represented in Fig. 11-7. It shows how the observation of a problem in practice can lead to a more systematic observation and definition of terms, including the nature of the problem and influencing factors. Descriptive and exploratory research can further define a problem. Hypotheses may then be developed concerning relationships between identified variables, which may be tested in correlational or survey research designs. Cause-and-effect relationships between the variables might then be tested in various experiments with natural or controlled settings. Only after establishing cause and effect can specific interventions aimed at changing the clinical problem be prescribed and tested. In this way studies feed knowledge back into practice to improve health care.

This progression of observing from practice, theorizing, testing in research, and subsequently modifying practice must continue to be an essential part of psychiatric nursing. It is important to encourage close collaboration between nurse researchers and nurse clinicians to ensure that the right questions are asked and the right variables are tested.[5] It is also necessary to clearly define how nurses with different educational backgrounds can participate in research. Table 11-4 summarizes the research expectations for nurses based on educational preparation. Finally, one research study on psychiatric nurses' attitudes toward involvement in nursing research found that the three major blocks to clinical nursing research were lack of time, lack of knowledge, and lack of administrative support.[20] They found that positive attitudes toward nursing research were related to nurses' advanced levels of education, although the authors suggested that research skills could be fostered through inservice education classes and individualized learning experiences.

Finally, research is sorely needed on the outcomes of psychiatric nursing intervention to determine its effectiveness and show how psychiatric nurses compare with other mental health care providers.[12] Important data are being accumulated regarding the cost effectiveness of nursing interventions in acute care, chronic care, primary care, and health promotion. One controlled investigation conducted in England demonstrated that community psychiatric nurses' clinical and social care of neurotic patients was comparable with that provided by outpatient psychiatrists.[16]

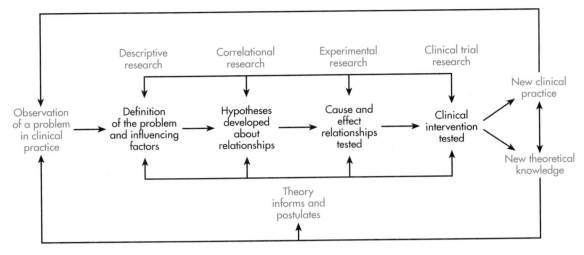

Fig. 11-7 Relationship among practice, theory, and research.

TABLE **11-4** *Nursing Research Participation Based on Education*

EDUCATIONAL PREPARATION	RESEARCH INVOLVEMENT
Associate degree in nursing	Help identify clinical problems in nursing practice, assist in data collection within a structured format, use research findings in practice with supervision
Baccalaureate degree in nursing	Identify clinical problems in need of research, help experienced investigators gain access to clinical sites, influence the selection of appropriate methods of data collection, participate in data collection and implementation of research findings
Master's degree in nursing	Collaborate in proposal development, data collection, data analysis, and interpretation; appraise the clinical relevance of research findings; provide leadership for integrating findings into practice
Doctoral education	Develop nursing knowledge through research and theory development, conduct funded independent research projects, develop and coordinate funded research projects, disseminate research findings to the scientific community

In addition, the patients assigned to the nurses reported greater consumer satisfaction and had higher rates of discharge. Finally, over the whole study period, the care provided by the psychiatric nurses was less expensive. Psychiatric nurses need to undertake and report similar research studies if this specialty area of practice is to survive.

Research on psychiatric nursing has increased in the past decade, and it is obvious that nurses can construct sophisticated designs with both theoretical and practical importance. The clinical problems are numerous, and as nurses gain the skills and experience to validate their work scientifically, they can make a significant contribution to psychiatric theory and practice.

R e s o u r c e   U s e

STANDARD VIII: RESOURCE USE

The psychiatric–mental health nurse considers factors related to safety, effectiveness, and cost in planning and delivering client care.

▼ *Rationale*

The client is entitled to psychiatric–mental health care that is safe, effective, and affordable. As the cost of health care increases, treatment decisions must be made in such a way as to maximize resources and maintain quality of care. The psychiatric–mental health nurse seeks to provide cost-effective, high-quality care by using the most appropriate resources and delegating care to the most appropriate, qualified health-care provider.

▼ *Nursing conditions*

Knowledge of the political and economic environment
Ability to evaluate costs and benefits of treatment
Skill in negotiating and accessing resources

▼ *Nursing behaviors*

Fact-based decision making
Cost-effective allocation of resources
Patient advocacy on an individual and collective basis

▼ *Key elements*

Nurses play a critical role in integrating and coordinating health-care services.

Nurses should be fiscally accountable for the care they provide.

Resources should be allocated based on cost/benefit analyses and documented expected outcomes.

Resource use may be one of the most important aspects of psychiatric nursing practice in the years to come. Discussing the costs and benefits of treatment options with patients, families, providers, and reimbursers will become increasingly important in an era of managed care (see Chapter 8). To fulfill this professional performance standard, psychiatric nurses need to request and obtain both cost and outcome information related to tests, consultations, evaluations, therapies, and continuum of care alternatives. Nurses need to assume an active role in questioning, advising, and advocating for the most cost-effective use of resources.

Psychiatric nurses also need to determine the most appropriate treatment setting for patients given the continuum of psychiatric care. Most recently, the mental health reimbursement system has favored paying for inpatient and acute care. Reimbursement for preventive, early interventions and chronic care has been limited. With managed care, however, this trend is changing and nurses must be aware of all possible treatment options and the advantages and disadvantages of each.[18]

It is also true that the mental health professions previously often acted on professional self-interest rather than on the public interest. This has been a disservice to patients and families of the mentally ill. The time has come for all mental health disciplines to work together in the development of service delivery models that are cost effective and contribute significantly to the quality of life of patients with psychiatric disorders.

Finally, one of the most critical resources in the mental health field is that of psychiatric labor.[17] Because each team member has different competencies, a challenge for the mental health system is to use the best that each discipline has to offer and to develop an integrated set of clinical services that will offer the highest-quality care.

> **?** *Psychiatric nurses must become increasingly cost and outcome conscious. Identify three commonly ordered tests for psychiatric patients. Find out how much they cost and analyze how helpful they are in planning treatment.*

demonstrated by psychiatric nurses both individually and as a group. The standards also relate to professional autonomy and self-definition.

2. Psychiatric nurses need to participate actively in the formal organizational evaluation of overall patterns of care through a variety of quality improvement activities including systems, consumer, and clinical evaluation.

3. Performance appraisal involves administrative review of work performance and clinical supervision of nursing care.

4. Psychiatric nurses are expected to engage in a continual learning process to maintain currency with the latest information in the field.

5. Collegiality requires that psychiatric nurses view their nurse peers as collaborators in the caregiving process who are valued and respected for their unique contributions.

6. Ethical considerations combine with legal and therapeutic issues to affect all aspects of psychiatric nursing practice and require the use of ethical decision making in caring for patients.

7. Collaboration is the shared planning, decision making, problem solving, goal setting, and assumption of responsibilities by people who work together cooperatively and with open communication. Psychiatric nurses collaborate with patients, families, nurse colleagues, and members of the health-care team.

8. Research is an essential professional activity for psychiatric nurses, and additional research is needed on the outcomes of psychiatric nursing intervention to determine its effectiveness.

9. Psychiatric nurses must also evaluate the most appropriate use of resources in the delivery of care. Issues of costs, benefits, outcomes, treatment setting, and appropriate use of mental health care providers must be considered.

your **INTERNET**
c o n n e c t i o n

CIMH: Computers in Mental Health
http://www.ex.ac.uk/cimh/

Mental Health Infosource
http://mhsource.com

Summary

1. The standards of professional performance apply to self-regulation and accountability for practice that must be

Chapter Review Questions

1. Identify whether the following statements are true (T) or false (F).

A. _T._ Adherence to professional and regulatory standards is one of the areas of quality improvement.

B. _F._ An associate degree in nursing qualifies one to become a certified generalist in psychiatric nursing.

C. _T._ The American Psychiatric Nurses Association is the largest specialty organization for psychiatric nurses.

D. _F._ Fairness is the ethical theory that seeks the greatest good for the greatest number.

E. _T._ All nurses, regardless of educational background, can participate in research activities.

F. _F._ There is a large body of research documenting the effectiveness and outcomes of psychiatric nursing care.

2. Fill in the blanks.

A. _Accountability_ focuses responsibility on the individual nurse for personal and professional actions.

B. The condition that allows for definition and control of a work domain and that implies self-determination, independence, and shared power is _autonomy_ .

C. In many ways the supervision process parallels the _nurse-pt. relation._

D. The _Internet_ is technology that allows nurses access to information from around the globe using a computer.

E. The two types of certification in psychiatric nursing are _generalist_ and _specialist_ .

F. An _ethic_ is a standard of behavior or a belief valued by an individual or group that describes what ought to be rather than what is.

G. An _interdisciplinary_ team is one in which members of different disciplines are involved in a formal arrangement to provide patient services while maximizing educational exchange.

3. Provide short answers for the following questions.

A. Describe how the nursing process is similar to the quality improvement process used in health-care organizations.

B. Discuss the differences between clinical supervision and therapy.

C. Access the home pages identified in this chapter and evaluate the information available on these sites.

D. Identify a clinical problem from your own experience. Describe how it might be developed from a research perspective as shown in Figure 11-7.

REFERENCES

1. American Nurses' Association: *Code for nurses with interpretive statements,* Kansas City, Mo, 1985, The Association.
2. American Nurses' Association: *Credentialing in nursing,* Washington, DC, 1993, The Association.
3. American Nurses' Association: *A statement on psychiatric–mental health clinical nursing practice and standards of psychiatric–mental health clinical nursing practice,* Washington, DC, 1994, The Association.
4. Artnak K, Dimmitt J: Choosing a framework for ethical analysis in advanced practice settings: the case for casuistry, *Arch Psychiatr Nurs* 10:16, 1996.
5. Bergman R, Ehrenfeld M, Golander H: Stimulating research thinking: the case for mini-research, *J Psychosoc Nurs* 33:34, 1995.
6. Chamberlain P et al: Innovative culture shock prescribed for health care, *Nurs Outlook* 43:232, 1995.
7. Curtin L: A proposed model for critical ethical analysis, *Nurs Forum* 17:12, 1978.
8. Dombeck M, Brody S: Clinical supervision: a three-way mirror, *Arch Psychiatr Nurs* 9:3, 1995.
9. Duldt B: Integrating nursing theory and ethics, *Perspectives Psychiatr Care* 31:4, 1995.
10. Farkas-Cameron M: Clinical supervision in psychiatric nursing, *J Psychosoc Nurs* 33:31, 1995.
11. Forsey L, Cleland V, Miller B: Job descriptions for differentiated nursing practice and differentiated pay, *J Nurs Admin* 23:33, 1993.
12. Foundation for Health Services Research: *Health outcomes research: a primer,* Washington, DC, 1993, The Association.
13. Glotz N, Johnsen G, Johnson R: Advancing clinical excellence: competency-based patient care, *Nurs Manage* 25:42, 1994.
14. Goode C et al: What kind of recognition do staff nurses want? *Am J Nurs* 1993:64, 1993.
15. Lim R: The Internet: applications for mental health clinicians in clinical settings, training and research, *Psychiatr Serv* 47:597, 1996.
16. Mangen S et al: Cost-effectiveness of community psychiatric nurse or outpatient psychiatrist care of neurotic patients, *Psychol Med* 13:407, 1983.
17. Merwin E, Fox J: Cost-effective integration of mental health professions, *Issues Ment Health Nurs* 13:139, 1992.
18. Mohr W: Values, ideologies and dilemmas: professional and occupational contradictions, *J Psychosoc Nurs* 33:29, 1995.
19. Moore R: Ethics in the practice of psychiatry: origins, functions, models, and enforcement, *Am J Psychiatry* 135:157, 1978.
20. Poster E, Betz C, Randell B: Psychiatric nurses' attitudes toward and involvement in nursing research, *J Psychosoc Nurs Ment Health Serv* 30:26, 1992.
21. Schoech D, Smith K: Use of electronic networking for the enhancement of mental health services, *Behav Healthcare Tomorrow* 4:23, 1995.

Continuum of Care

Continuum. What an interesting word. It means "a series of variations, or a sequence of things in regular order." As such, it is the perfect descriptor of the levels of contemporary psychiatric treatment. The continuum of psychiatric care allows nurses to use the full range of their skills and talents, often in new settings and innovative programs. Perhaps best of all, it provides patients, families, and communities with the healing ability to build competence, resilience, and health rather than merely to treat disability, illness, and disease. It therefore includes working with patients in crisis, acute, maintenance, and health-promotion stages of treatment. Such is the brave new world of psychiatric and mental health nursing.

In this unit you will learn about intervening with primary, secondary, and tertiary prevention activities. You will also hear from family members about their role in the continuum of care. All nurses, regardless of their specialty area, need to know how to promote mental health, intervene with patients and families in crisis, and build rehabilitative functioning in those who are ill. In the future you will use these skills more often than you might ever have imagined, and you will think back to this unit and the information it imparted with greater appreciation for the caregiving continuum.

Mental Health Promotion

Gail W. Stuart

© 1998 M.C. Escher/Cordon Art, Baarn, Holland.

What is this thing called health? Simply a state in which the individual happens transiently to be perfectly adapted to his environment. Obviously, such states cannot be common, for the environment is in constant flux. **H. L. Mencken** *The American Mercury,* March 1930

LEARNING OBJECTIVES

After studying this chapter the student should be able to:

▼ Define primary, secondary, and tertiary prevention

▼ Compare and contrast the medical and nursing models of primary prevention

▼ Assess the vulnerability of various groups to developing maladaptive coping responses

▼ Describe the levels of intervention and activities related to the following primary prevention nursing interventions: health education, environmental change, and supporting social systems

▼ Assess the importance of evaluation of the nursing process when applied to primary prevention

TOPICAL OUTLINE

Conceptualizing Primary Prevention
  Medical Prevention Model
  Nursing Prevention Model
Assessment
Planning and Implementation
  Health Education
  Environmental Change
  Social Support
Evaluation

M ental health promotion and mental illness prevention are important aspects of psychiatric nursing care. In his classic work, *Principles of Preventive Psychiatry,* Caplan[5] applies the three levels of preventive intervention from the public health model to mental illness and emotional disturbance.

▼ **Primary prevention** is lowering the *incidence* of a mental

disorder or reducing the rate at which new cases of a disorder develop.

▼ **Secondary prevention** involves reducing the *prevalence* of a mental disorder by reducing the number of existing cases. Secondary prevention activities include early case finding, screening, and prompt effective treatment.

▼ **Tertiary prevention** activities attempt to reduce the

severity of a mental disorder and associated disability through rehabilitative activities.

The major emphasis in the United States has been on secondary prevention activities or the treatment of mental disorders. This is evident in the allocation of economic resources, the nature of caregiving organizations and institutions, and the activities of mental health professionals. For example, a survey of state mental health authorities focused on the extent to which primary prevention activities were conducted or supported at the state level. All 50 states responded: 7 reported significant involvement in prevention, 7 reported some involvement, and 36 reported none. The authors concluded that although some states are involved in significant prevention activities, few states have made a real commitment to prevention.[9]

CONCEPTUALIZING PRIMARY PREVENTION

Although primary prevention is often described with such slogans as "An ounce of prevention is worth a pound of cure" or "Curing is costly; prevention is priceless," it is only recently emerging as a substantial force in the mental health movement. One of the reasons it is gaining momentum is because of health care reform. As health and mental health care move toward capitated payment and managed care, there is a greater economic incentive to prevent illness rather than treat it.

The reality of this change is evident in two recent reports. The first report was prepared by the National Mental Health Association and 17 national member organizations of the National Prevention Coalition. It recommends five preventive mental health interventions that should be included in a reformed health-care system:

▼ Screening for developmental delays and mental health problems for children and adolescents as part of their regular checkups

▼ Screening for mental health problems in adults as part of routine preventive examinations (for example, to screen for depression, anxiety, or potential suicide)

▼ Counseling for individuals and families in situations that place them at high risk for developing mental or emotional disorders

▼ Home visits and other intensive interventions in high-risk situations involving stress and lack of social support, such as premature births, low-income households, and teenage pregnancies

▼ Self-help groups to assist people confronting health problems, mental health problems, or life situations of stress or change

The second report was issued by the Institute of Medicine in January 1994.[11] It concluded that research on the prevention of mental disorders can play an important role in alleviating the financial and social burdens imposed by these disorders. The report stated that although little evidence exists that any specific mental disorder can be prevented, research aimed at reducing risk factors should be conducted and rigorously evaluated.

The idea of promoting mental health in general is attractive. Promotion sounds optimistic and positive. It is consistent with the idea of self-help and being self-responsible for health. It implies changing human behavior and draws on a holistic approach to health. Also, the ability to prevent the development of a psychiatric illness would reap many benefits for individuals, families, communities, and society. Thus primary prevention activities in psychiatric care have two basic aims[19]:

▼ To help people to avoid stressors or to cope with them more adaptively

▼ To change the resources, policies, or agents of the environment so that they no longer cause stress but rather enhance people's functioning

These are both important functions of contemporary psychiatric nursing practice.

> **?** *The terms* health promotion *and* illness prevention *are often used interchangeably. In what ways do they overlap and how are they different?*

Medical Prevention Model

The medical prevention model focuses on genetic counseling and on biochemical and brain research to discover the specific causes of mental illness. It suggests that primary prevention activities are best focused on illness prevention. This model consists of the following steps:

1. Identify a disease that warrants the development of a preventive intervention program. Develop reliable methods for its diagnosis so that people can be divided into groups according to whether they do or do not have the disease.

2. By a series of epidemiological and laboratory studies, identify the most likely cause of the disease.

3. Launch and evaluate an experimental preventive intervention program based on the results of those studies.

This model has been effective for a broad array of communicable diseases such as smallpox, typhus, malaria, diphtheria, tuberculosis, rubella, and polio and nutritional diseases such as scurvy, pellagra, rickets, kwashiorkor, and endemic goiter. It has also proved useful in a variety of mental disorders caused by poisons, chemicals, licit or illicit drugs, electrolyte imbalances, and nutritional deficiencies. All these diseases have one thing in common: a known necessary, but not always sufficient, causative factor.

> **?** *Identify one psychiatric disorder that would lend itself to the medical prevention model.*

Nursing Prevention Model

The nursing prevention model stresses that mental disorders do not appear to have a single identified precondition and may have causative factors that are multiple, interactive, situational, and sociocultural. They thus require that mental illness prevention be thought of in a more behavioral way as the prevention of problems or maladaptive responses. In this way, many of the services already available in the community can be identified and publicly acknowledged as prevention efforts.

Problems defined in this way can include both single-episode events such as a divorce and long-standing conditions such as marital conflict. They can also reflect either an acute health problem or a chronic health problem. For example, the following categories of problems can arise from alcohol abuse:

▼ Acute health problems such as overdose or delirium tremens
▼ Chronic health problems such as cirrhosis of the liver
▼ Casualties, such as accidents on the road, in the home, or elsewhere, and suicide
▼ Violent crime and family abuse
▼ Problems of demeanor such as public drunkenness and use of alcohol by teenagers
▼ Default of major social roles (work or school and family roles)
▼ Problems of feeling state (demoralization and depression and experienced loss of control)

The nursing prevention model assumes that problems are multicausal, that everyone is vulnerable to stressful life events, and that any disability or problem may arise as a consequence. For example, four vulnerable people can face a stressful life event, such as the collapse of a marriage or the loss of a job. One person may become severely depressed, the second may be involved in an automobile accident, the third may head down the road to alcoholism, and the fourth may develop coronary artery disease. The nursing prevention model does not search for a cause for each problem. Rather, it involves the following steps:

1. Identify a biopsychosocial stressor that appears to have undesirable consequences in a significant proportion of the population. Develop procedures for reliably identifying people who have undergone or are undergoing that stressful experience.
2. By epidemiological and laboratory methods, study the consequences of that stressor and develop hypotheses related to how its negative consequences might be reduced or eliminated.
3. Launch and evaluate experimental preventive intervention programs based on these hypotheses.

The nursing model also includes application of the nursing process, with a focus on the primary prevention of maladaptive coping responses associated with an identified stressor. It thus incorporates the following aspects:

▼ **Assessment:** Identification of a stressor that precipitates maladaptive responses and a target or population group that is vulnerable or at risk for it
▼ **Planning:** Elaboration of specific strategies of prevention and relevant social institutions and situations through which the strategies may be applied
▼ **Implementation:** Application of selected nursing interventions aimed at decreasing maladaptive responses to the identified stressor and enhancing adaptation
▼ **Evaluation:** Determining the effectiveness of the nursing interventions with regard to short-and long-term outcomes, use of resources, and comparison with other prevention strategies

The nursing process can thereby be used in a goal-directed way to decrease the incidence of mental illness and promote mental health.

 Analyze the problem of child abuse from the nursing prevention perspective.

Assessment

Three types of preventive interventions based on target populations have been identified[11]:

▼ *Universal:* targeted to the general population group without consideration of risk factors
▼ *Selective:* targeted to individuals or groups with a significantly higher risk of developing a particular disorder
▼ *Indicated:* targeted to high-risk individuals identified as having symptoms foreshadowing a specific mental disorder or biological markers indicating predisposition for the disorder

A knowledge of normal growth and development is essential for assessing a person's functioning and for intervening with preventive nursing interventions. The nurse should be familiar with normative stages, tasks, and parameters to know what issues the person has faced in the past and what challenges lie ahead. In addition to understanding the person's development, the nurse must know about the family cycle because many nursing interventions are directed at the family, from mobilizing their support of a patient to modifying dysfunctional family patterns.

Assessment in primary prevention therefore involves identifying groups of people who are vulnerable to developing mental disorders or who may display maladaptive coping responses to specific stressors or risk factors. To complete such an assessment, the nurse needs to draw on information generated from theory, research, and clinical practice.

It is also important for the nurse to realize that not all people in these groups are at equal risk. What these groups share is the experience of a life event, stressor, or risk factor that represents a loss of some kind or places an excessive demand on one's ability to cope.[12] The more clearly the subgroup can be defined, the more specifically the prevention strategies can be researched, identified, and implemented.

> *Identify three groups of people vulnerable to the development of psychiatric illness, one based on biological factors, one based on psychological factors, and one based on sociocultural factors.*

Planning

Implementation

Under the sponsorship of the Public Health Service, a national incentive has been undertaken to promote health and prevent disease in this country. The *Healthy People 2000* objectives related to mental health and mental disorders are listed in Box 12-1.[20] A number of potential measures have been identified to meet one of the objectives for the control of stress and violent behavior. These include education, service, and technological and legislative measures as identified in Box 12-2. This list provides the nurse with a good overview of the many areas appropriate for nursing intervention.

In addition, the Stuart Stress Adaptation Model presented in Chapter 4 and represented in Fig. 12-1 is useful for the nurse in planning strategies for primary prevention. It suggests target areas and types of activities that might be useful. If the overall nursing goal is to promote

constructive coping mechanisms and maximize adaptive coping responses, then the model suggests that prevention strategies should be directed toward influencing predisposing factors, precipitating stressors, appraisal of stressors, and coping resources and mechanisms through the following interventions:
▼ Health education
▼ Environmental change
▼ Social support

Because the process depicted in the model is a dynamic one, it is not possible to discretely link a particular strategy with a particular component of the model. Rather, the strategies can affect multiple aspects of a person's life. For example, an environmental change, such as changing jobs, can affect an individual's predisposition to stress, decrease the amount of stress, change the appraisal of the threat, and perhaps increase financial or social coping resources. This interactive effect can thus justify the use of these prevention strategies for vulnerable groups.

Health Education

The health education strategy of primary prevention in mental health involves the strengthening of individuals and groups through **competence building**. It is based on the assumption that many maladaptive responses are the result of a lack of competence, that is, a lack of perceived control over one's own life or effective coping strategies, and the lowered self-esteem that results. Competence building may be the single most important preventive strategy. A competent individual or community is aware of resources and alternatives, can make reasoned decisions about issues, and can cope adaptively with problems.

> ❓ *How is the concept of competency similar to the concept of positive mental health?*

LEVELS OF INTERVENTION. Health education or competence building can be seen as having the following four aspects:
▼ Increasing the individual's or group's awareness of issues and events related to health and illness. Awareness of normal developmental tasks and potential problems is fundamental.
▼ Increasing understanding of the dimensions of potential stressors, possible outcomes (both adaptive and maladaptive), and alternative coping responses.
▼ Increasing knowledge of where and how to acquire the needed resources. Many health professionals assume that this is common knowledge, but for many people it is not.
▼ Increasing the actual abilities of the individual or group. This means improving or maximizing coping skills such as problem-solving skills or interpersonal skills, tolerance of stress and frustration, motivation, hope, self-esteem, and power.

Box **12-1** **Healthy People 2000** *Objectives Related to Mental Health and Mental Disorders*

To reduce mental disorders by the year 2000, objectives target the following:
▼ Reducing suicide
▼ Reducing suicide attempts among children and adolescents
▼ Reducing mental disorders among adults
▼ Reducing adverse health effects from stress
▼ Increasing use of community support programs by people with mental disorders
▼ Increasing use of treatment by people with major depressive disorders
▼ Increasing the proportion of people who seek help for personal and emotional problems
▼ Reducing uncontrolled stress
▼ Increasing appropriate suicide prevention strategies in jails
▼ Increasing the number of workplace stress management programs
▼ Increasing the number of states with mutual help clearinghouses
▼ Increasing routine review of mental functioning by primary care providers for both children and adults

PROGRAMS AND ACTIVITIES. Mental health education can take place in any setting, can have a formal or informal structure, can be directed toward individuals or groups, and can be related to predisposing factors or potential stressors.[16] Health education directed toward strengthening an individual's predisposition to stress can take various forms.[15] Growth groups may be formed for parents that focus on parent-child relations, normal growth and development, or effective methods of child rearing. Groups of children or adolescents can discuss peer relationships, sexuality, or potential problem areas, such as drug abuse or promiscuity. Employee groups can discuss career burnout and related issues. Or a more activity-centered educational program can be initiated, such as Outward Bound, which helps the individual discover that step-by-step competence can be expanded to master new, unexpected, and potentially stressful situations in an adaptive way.

Probably the most common type of health education program is one that helps the individual cope with a specific potential stressor. For example, families about to experience marital separation are vulnerable to emotional problems, physical complaints, and increased use of health care services. Such families may be offered educational and supportive group intervention aimed at enhancing their ability to cope. Education groups can similarly be offered to those experiencing retirement, bereavement, or any other stressful event (see Critical Thinking about Contemporary Issues).

Parent education classes are a well-known example of anticipatory guidance that can be offered to high-risk groups. Although raising children is considered an important responsibility, until recently little attention has been directed to the belief that effective parenting is not an innate ability. Whether nurses subscribe to a specific set of beliefs and strategies for parenting or choose an eclectic approach, the opportunities for promoting mental health abound. Possibly one of the most beneficial results of parent education is the acknowledgment that all parents become frustrated, angry, and ambivalent toward their children. Parent education goes beyond acknowledging feelings and includes learning and practicing alternative ways of interacting with

Box **12-2** *Potential Primary Prevention Measures for the Control of Stress and Violent Behavior*

EDUCATION AND INFORMATION

Increasing public awareness, through planned campaigns using the appropriate media, that stress can be an antecedent of illness and that stress management is an important component of health

Creating new educational pathways for developing enhanced professional skills in biobehavioral fields of medicine and public health

Developing the capacities of health-care professionals in stress diagnosis and management

Helping parents recognize and deal with stress

Training secondary, elementary, and preschool teachers to include discussion of stress recognition and management in school health curricula

Training police to handle calls involving domestic and interpersonal disputes that could lead to violent behavior

Public education, especially for high-risk groups, on steps to take to reduce risks of rape

Training all helping professionals regarding signs that indicate high risk for suicide

Helping the public be aware of indicators of possible suicide

SERVICE

Hotlines for people under acute stress (suicide, child abuse prevention)

Stress management programs in workplaces

Stress management programs targeted to adolescents, parents, and the elderly

Stress appraisal analysis (self-administered or performed by an objective outside source)

Professional and social support systems to assist in resolution of stressful life events, including mutual aid and self-help groups

such as Reach for Recovery, child abusing parents, bereavement groups, and single-parent groups

Information and counseling with regard to leisure and stress-reduction activities, including exercise

A variety of self-help relaxation and biofeedback techniques, which can be individualized to fit a variety of lifestyles and work requirements

Psychophysiological tests to assist employees who are having difficulty adjusting to their work and their coworkers

Support services for inevitable or necessary life change events, especially in relation to death, separation, job changes, and geographic relocation

Domestic crisis teams to defuse domestic disputes

Targeting the above measures to high-risk populations and people with low coping abilities

Evaluating intervention efforts

Follow-up services for people who have attempted suicide

Shelters for abused spouses

Training all health (and other human services, including educational) personnel to be alert to evidence of child abuse

TECHNOLOGY

Actions by employers, labor, and government to reduce stress-creating work environments

Reducing stressful aspects of the environment such as noise pollution and overcrowding

LEGISLATION AND REGULATION

Activities to create employment opportunities for youth

Action to limit the availability of handguns, to reduce homicides and suicides that occur during stressful periods

Strengthening mandatory child abuse reporting laws

Modified from US Department of Health and Human Services: *Healthy people 2000,* Washington, DC, 1990, Public Health Service.

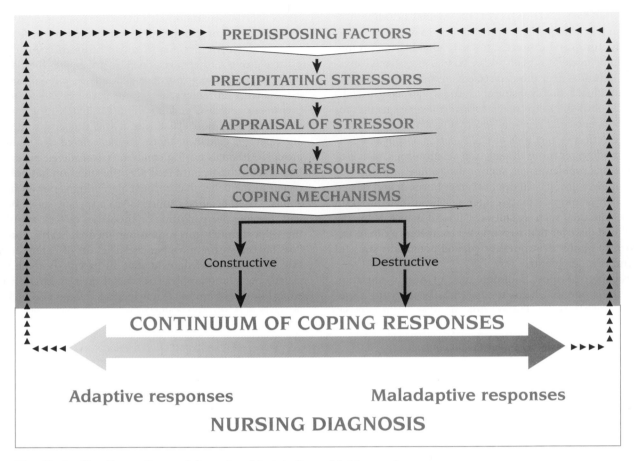

▶▶▶▶▶▶▶▶▶▶▶▶▶▶▶▶ PREDISPOSING FACTORS ◀◀◀◀◀◀◀◀◀◀◀◀◀◀◀◀

PRECIPITATING STRESSORS

APPRAISAL OF STRESSOR

COPING RESOURCES

COPING MECHANISMS

Constructive   Destructive

CONTINUUM OF COPING RESPONSES

Adaptive responses   Maladaptive responses

NURSING DIAGNOSIS

Fig. 12-1   The Stuart Stress Adaptation Model of psychiatric nursing care.

children. During these classes, situations are anticipated, and discussions focus on identifying potential crisis situations and dealing with them through simulated encounters such as role playing. Education for mental health can thus address the needs of both children and parents as family roles shift and respond to societal change.

STIGMA. Finally, health education activities can be directed to the larger community. One way to do this is by changing the attitudes and behavior of health-care providers and consumers. This may involve activities related to dispelling myths and stereotypes associated with vulnerable groups, providing knowledge of normal parameters, increasing sensitivity to psychosocial factors affecting health and illness, and enhancing the ability to give sensitive, supportive, and humanistic health care.

A community-level strategy would be to provide public education on mental health issues and community resources. For example, one study documented that people with mental illnesses have the highest rate of negative portrayal on television.[1] Another study on Americans' attitudes toward mental illness revealed that Americans do not consider themselves well informed about mental illness but do

think they should know more. They are also reluctant to welcome a wide variety of mental health facilities into their communities.[4] Results of these studies suggest that misperceptions regarding vulnerable subgroups of the population must be corrected. They are the result, in part, of the cultural stigma against mental illness that is prevalent in contemporary society.[8]

Stigma, in its original definition, meant a "scar left by a hot iron on the face of an evil doer." Stigma is now defined as a mark of disgrace that is used to identify and separate out people whom society sees as deviant, sinful, or dangerous. For the psychiatrically ill, stigma is a barrier that separates them from society and keeps them apart from others. Patients and their families often report that the diagnosis of a mental illness is followed by increasing isolation and loneliness as family and friends withdraw. Patients feel rejected and feared by others, and their families are met by blame. Stigma against mental illness is clearly a reflection of the cultural biases of contemporary American society that are shared by consumers and health-care providers alike.

The stigma, misunderstanding, and fear surrounding mental illness are related to both the agencies providing

What Is the Future for Children with Mentally Ill Parents?

Living with a mentally ill parent does not necessarily mean that the child will develop the disorder, but it can make growing up more difficult. Although the mechanisms for transmitting psychiatric illness across generations are controversial, many studies support the fact that parental illness affects children. For example, it has been noted that coping with a mentally ill parent may be more difficult than coping with parental loss. These children also feel psychologically vulnerable and fear becoming ill themselves. The major research findings on this topic are as follows:

▼ Children of mentally ill parents are at greater risk for psychiatric and developmental disorders than are children of well parents.

▼ The risk to children is greater if the mother rather than the father is the ill parent.

▼ In studies of depressed versus nondepressed groups, differences in the mother-child interaction are evident as early as 3 months postpartum.

▼ Many children with emotionally disturbed parents do not become disordered themselves. The nature of the parent's illness, the child's genetic and constitutional make-up, the family's functional ability, and the availability of healthy attachment figures all play an important role in the mental health of the child.

The evidence suggests that psychiatric nurses need to focus more attention on the children of mentally ill parents.[2] They should assess parenting problems whenever parents with children at home are hospitalized for psychiatric care.[10] They can also implement psychoeducational, preventive nursing interventions that will enhance mental health in high-risk children and families.[3]

mental health services and the people receiving these services, who are often elderly, poor, or members of social minority groups. Unlike physical illness, which tends to evoke sympathy and the desire to help, mental disorders tend to disturb and repel people. Yet everyone encounters stress, and all people are subject to maladaptive coping responses. Mental health professionals can educate the public that health is a continuum and illness is caused by a complex combination of factors. Consumers must begin to understand that no one is immune from mental illness or emotional problems, and that the fear, anxiety, and even anger we feel about people who suffer these problems may reflect some of our own deepest fears and anxieties.

Have you observed the stigma associated with psychiatric illness in your personal or professional life? If so, what steps have you taken or could you take to overcome it?

Environmental Change

Activities in primary prevention involving environmental change have a social setting focus. They require the modification of an individual's or group's immediate environment or the larger social system. They are particularly appropriate actions when the environment has placed new demands on the person, when it is not responding to the person's developmental needs, and when it provides a diminished level of positive reinforcement.

Various environmental changes may prove to promote mental health, including changes in economic, work, housing, or family situations. **Economically,** resources for financial aid or assistance in budgeting and money management may be obtained. **Work** changes may include vocational testing, guidance, education, or retraining that can result in a change of jobs or careers. It may also mean that an adolescent, a homemaker, or an older adult may be placed in a new career. Changes in **housing** can involve moving to new quarters, which may mean leaving family and friends or returning to them, improvements in existing housing, or the addition or subtraction of coinhabitants, whether they are family, friends, or roommates. Environmental changes that may benefit the **family** include attaining child care facilities, enrolling in a nursery school, grade school, or camp, or obtaining access to recreational, social, religious, or community facilities.

The potential benefit of all of these changes should not be minimized or overlooked by psychiatric nurses. They can promote mental health by increasing coping resources, modifying the nature of stressors, and increasing positive, rewarding, and self-enhancing experiences.

ORGANIZATIONS AND POLITICS. Nurses can also effect environmental changes at a larger organizational and political level. One way is by influencing health care structures and procedures.[6] Nurses might become involved in training community, nonprofessional caregivers to increase the social supports available to vulnerable groups. Another approach would be to stimulate support for women's issues related to mental health, such as through studying the psychology of women; dispelling sex-role stereotypes; promoting feminist therapy; sponsoring programs, conferences, and workshops on women's issues; and recruiting more women into the mental health field.[7]

Obviously, if nurses believe that their profession makes a valuable contribution to health promotion, they should document the cost-effectiveness and quality of nursing care, lobby for greater patient access by nurses, and seek adequate compensation and reimbursement for nursing services. Many of these goals can be obtained if nursing has greater participation in the decision-making structures of health-care institutions, such as hospital boards, advisory groups, health system agencies, and legislative bodies.

Within organizations, environmental change can be achieved through program consultation. Such consultation with a large corporation, for example, may lead to the formulation of more flexible retirement plans or a preretirement counseling program. Involvement in community planning and development can have an impact in many different areas. For instance, a community may be helped to meet the needs of the elderly for educational opportunities, recreational programs, and access to social support networks through telephone or transportation services. Also, the stress associated with environmental pollutants, such as chemicals and radiation, can be addressed.

Some environmental changes require involvement at the national level that may be directed toward the media's portrayal of violence, laws on drunk driving, gun control legislation, access to family planning services, and advocating changes in child-rearing practices, including the provision of day-care centers, flex time, and paternity leave.

Of course, many aspects of the broader social system are in need of change, including racism, sexism, ageism, poverty, and inadequate housing and education. The dilemma is that global problems such as these are too broad, pervasive, and diffuse to be adequately addressed, let alone resolved. For any prevention strategies to be successful in the future, it will be necessary to document the ways in which a particular group is vulnerable to a specific stressor, how the proposed prevention program will be beneficial and cost effective, and the degree to which it succeeds or fails.

> **?** *What legislation in your state is being considered that pertains to mental health care? What is your position on it and how can you influence its chances for passage?*

Social Support

As a primary prevention strategy, supporting social systems does not attempt to remove or minimize the stressor or risk factor. Rather, it is an attempt to strengthen social supports as a way of buffering or cushioning the effects of a potentially stressful event (Box 12-3). It is an important concept for all levels of prevention—primary, secondary, and tertiary—and it has implications for

▼ Encouraging health promotion behavior
▼ Helping people seek assistance earlier
▼ Improving the functioning of the immune system or other biological processes
▼ Reducing the occurrence of potentially stressful events
▼ Fostering the ability to cope with stressful events
▼ Helping one to deal with chronic mental and physical illness

Social support systems can be helpful in emphasizing the strengths of individuals and families and focusing on health rather than illness.[18]

Given the goal that social support systems should be maximized, how can this be achieved? First, how much social support a high-risk group needs must be determined

and compared with the amount of social support available. Although the question is straightforward, it is complicated by the fact that there are multiple determinants of each element. The need for social support is influenced by predisposing factors, the nature of the stressors, and the availability of other coping resources such as economic assets, individual abilities and skills, and defensive techniques. The availability of social supports is similarly influenced by age, gender, socioeconomic status, the nature of the stressor, and the characteristics of the environment. Acute episodic stressors tend to elicit more intense support, whereas in chronic problems, support resources tend to not persist. Also, changes or stressors viewed in a positive way by the individual's social network, such as the birth of a baby or a promotion, may elicit a great deal of support, whereas a negative event, such as a sudden death, may generate little support.

In addition, the quantity and type of social support that meets one need may not meet another. Research suggests that different characteristics of social support may be needed for different stresses. The match between the type and level of social support and the nature of the stressor is important, but not entirely understood.

TYPES OF INTERVENTIONS. Even though many variables related to social support need further study, social support can still be used to design and implement interven-

Box **12-3** *Support System Enhancement*

DEFINITION

Facilitation of support to patient by family, friends, and community

ACTIVITIES

Assess psychological response to situation and availability of support system
Determine adequacy of existing social networks
Identify degree of family support
Identify degree of family financial support
Determine support systems currently used
Determine barriers to using support systems
Monitor current family situation
Encourage the patient to participate in social and community activities
Encourage relationships with people who have common interests and goals
Refer to a self-help group as appropriate
Assess community resource adequacy to identify strengths and weaknesses
Refer to a community-based promotion, prevention, treatment, or rehabilitation program as appropriate
Provide services in a caring and supportive manner
Involve family, significant others, and friends in the care and planning
Explain to concerned others how they can help

From McCloskey J, Bulechek G: *Nursing interventions classification,* St Louis, 1996, Mosby.

tions in primary prevention. Four particular types of interventions are possible.

First, social support patterns can be used to assess communities and neighborhoods to identify problem areas and high-risk groups. Not only will information about the quality of life be gained, but the social isolation of a particular group might become apparent, as well as central individuals who may be enlisted to help develop community-based programs.

A second preventive intervention would be to improve links between community support systems and formal mental health services. Often mental health professionals are not aware of or comfortable with the existence or functioning of community support systems. They should be taught how to use and mobilize community resources and social support systems. All health-care providers need to recognize when patients need social support and to provide them with access to appropriate community support systems.

The third type of intervention is to strengthen natural, existing caregiving networks. Health professionals can provide information and support to informal caregivers in the community, who serve a very important and somewhat different function than more formalized and organized support systems. Informal support systems provide the following:

▼ A natural training ground for the development of problem-solving skills

▼ A medium in which people grow and develop by learning to direct the process of change for themselves

▼ A supportive milieu that capitalizes on the strength of existing ties among people in communities, rather than fragmenting intact social units on the basis of diagnosed needs or specialized services

A fourth possible intervention may be to help the person or group develop, maintain, and use a network. The person may also be encouraged to consider network expansion. This might require health education strategies with the goal of competence building. Alternatively, the network can be influenced more directly. Network therapy involves assembling and mobilizing all the important members of the family's kin and friendship network. The focus is then on tightening social bonds within the network and breaking dysfunctional patterns. For families who are isolated and whose networks are depleted, network members may not be available for such a strategy. In this case, arranging for the use of mutual support groups may be effective.

INFORMAL SUPPORT GROUPS. Numerous informal support groups exist. They may include church groups, civic organizations, clubs, women's groups, or work and neighborhood supports. Self-help groups are becoming more common as members organize themselves to solve their own problems. The members all share a common experience, work together toward a common goal, and use their strengths to gain control over their lives.[13] The processes involved in self-help groups are social affiliation, learning self-control, modeling methods to cope with stress, and acting to change the social environment. Characteristics of self-help groups are listed in Box 12-4.[17]

Self-help groups such as Alcoholics Anonymous, Weight Watchers, Parents Without Partners, Recovery, and Parents Anonymous are familiar to the public. They have demonstrated their ability to help people experiencing psychiatric problems and grief reactions, such as widows and parents of children who died of sudden infant death syndrome. Because self-help groups use a variety of methods and membership criteria, each group should be assessed individually for its general effectiveness and appropriateness for particular individuals and families. Some areas for the nurse to assess before recommending involvement in a self-help group are presented in Box 12-5.

Working with natural, informal support systems should be done cautiously, however, to minimize undesirable consequences. The nurse should attempt to create the least

---

Box **12-4** *Characteristics of Self-Help Groups*

Supportive and educational in nature rather than therapeutic
Based on shared experiences and the fact that the individual is not alone
Focus on a single life-disrupting event
Purpose is to support personal responsibility and change
Anonymous and confidential in nature
Voluntary membership
Members lead the group and implement principles of self-governance
Nonprofit orientation

Box **12-5** *Assessment Guidelines for Self-Help Groups*

QUESTIONS FOR THE GROUP	QUESTIONS FOR THE POTENTIAL MEMBER
What is its purpose?	How does the person feel about attending a self-help group?
Who are the group members and leaders?	How compatible is the group with the individual's approach to the problem?
What are the beneficial aspects of the group?	How accessible is the group to the potential member?
For whom would the group not be suitable?	
What problems are inherent in the group?	
Is the group effective in preventing further emotional distress?	

From Newton G: Self-help groups: can they help? *J Psychosoc Nurs Ment Health Serv* 22:27, 1984.

amount of disruption possible and not to suppress the natural repertoire of helping behaviors of informal caregivers.

If an individual's social support is inadequate, interventions may need to be more direct. To determine what interventions are possible, Norbeck[14] suggests that the following questions be asked:

▼ What is the capacity of the network to change?
  ▼ *Network structure.* Are there people who can be brought into (or back into) the network?
  ▼ *Network functioning.* Can existing network members be helped to provide the kind of support that is needed (for example, by allowing talk about a problematic pregnancy or a loss)?
  ▼ *Network disruption.* Can policies be changed or resources used to minimize network disruption (for example, due to hospitalization at a distant tertiary care facility)?
▼ Does the individual have the interpersonal skills and attitudes required to establish and maintain contact with network members?
▼ Is the individual receptive to using existing self-help or support groups or to having contact with a person who has coped with a similar experience?
▼ If help from the indigenous social support system cannot be made available or acceptable, exactly what support does this person require to cope with the current stressors or illness?
▼ What long-term help would be required to help the individual to establish and maintain an adequate social support network?

Finally, it should be noted that although supporting social supports is an effective intervention, it is not limited to primary prevention activities. Rather, all nurses in all settings can use this strategy as a way of providing holistic care to maximize the health of individuals, families, and groups.

> **?** *Attend one of the self-help groups in your community. Describe the specific ways in which it helped those who attended.*

▼ *Evaluation*

When talking about primary prevention, there is a tendency to think in terms of the total elimination of mental illness and stress. Yet these are not realistic goals and maintaining them can only discourage any possible action. Perhaps it is possible to set goals of reducing suffering and enhancing the capacity to cope, but even these may be unattainable, given that the environment is constantly changing and adaptation is an ongoing challenge. Rather, if the focus is directed toward specific problems of a vulnerable group in society, nursing activity becomes more concentrated and the chance of success increases.

Clearly a need exists for the evaluation of programs in primary prevention. In a world of shrinking resources, only programs with proven effectiveness are likely to be supported in the future. It must be demonstrated that the prevention strategy used has both short-term and long-term effects that benefited the individual and society. Also, it is necessary to determine whether the specific strategy implemented was the most effective, appropriate, and efficient. Considering alternative approaches and comparing clinical and financial outcomes are essential aspects of the evaluation process.

Although preventing all illness is not possible, preventing some particular problems is. But a number of barriers exist that make expansion of primary prevention activities difficult. When faced with a choice, the needs of the ill consistently take precedence over prevention. This holds true for nurses as well as for the larger society. Yet by being more visionary, both groups could benefit greatly. Nursing has long maintained its role in health education and supportive care. If it can document these actions and their effectiveness, it will demonstrate its value as a profession and its importance in promoting the well-being of society.

Summary

1. Caplan's three levels of preventive intervention were described. The major thrust in current psychiatric care is secondary prevention, although primary prevention is beginning to evolve as a major force in the mental health movement.
2. A nursing model for primary prevention was presented that attempts to reduce the incidence of particular stressful life events for vulnerable groups, and it was applied to the nursing process.
3. Assessment in primary prevention was presented as the identification of groups of people who are vulnerable to developing mental disorders or maladaptive coping responses to specific stressors or risk factors.
4. Prevention strategies include health education, environmental change, and social support.
5. In evaluating preventive strategies, one needs to consider specific criteria and use a systematic rating scale of scientific evidence.

your **INTERNET**
connection

Healthy People 2000: Mental Health and Mental Disorders Resource List
http://nhic-nt.health.org/nmp/hp2kpage/6mental2.htm

Health Care Information Resources: Wellness
http://www-hsl.mcmaster.ca/tomflem/well.html

COMPETENT CARING A Clinical Exemplar of a Psychiatric Nurse

Penelope Chase, MSN, MEd, RN, CS

I was changing planes, having just left an inspiring psychiatric clinical nurse specialist conference in Florida, and was on my way to Boston to attend the reunion of my diploma nursing school. I was traveling alone and feeling safe from social interruptions. I was looking forward to some anonymity and a time to reflect and rest.

As I approached the check-in counter of the airport, I saw a young woman sitting nearby in the waiting area. The seats on either side of her were empty except for a soft knapsack on her left. She was wearing the loose-fitting cotton clothing and the nylon-strap sandals that college students often wear. She looked as if she were about to burst into tears or change her mind about being here and dash for the exit. I stopped in my tracks to observe her without being aware of deciding to do so. She turned her head with stiff, slightly jerky movements.

"Responding to internal stimuli," "seizure disorder," "hasn't taken her psychotropic medication" went through my professional mind, while "don't get involved" went through my personal mind, along with, "You're on vacation. Don't mess it up. Relax, you're not the only one who can help." So I went ahead and checked in. I chose to wait in a seat in the row behind the young woman. "She may not be able to ask for help. I should assess further," my professional self reasoned. "Maybe she's not alone. Maybe someone is traveling with her and will be back in a minute."

She compared her ticket information with the boarding announcement and sat back in her seat. A moment later, she shifted in her seat and put her hands over her face. It was then that I noticed that a man, somewhat older than she, seated two rows away and facing her was watching her intensely. My private self was afraid he might be a lonely traveler sizing up a vulnerable young woman that he could take advantage of. I intensified my vigil. I would be her advocate and protector.

I read a bit in my novel, keeping my peripheral vision and ears attuned in her direction. I had difficulty concentrating on my reading because I was constantly interrupted by imposing, opposing thoughts of "Do something" and "Let it be." At one point a uniformed airline employee passed near me on his way out the boarding door. I approached him and said, "I think there's a young lady in trouble here." "I'm a pilot," he replied. "The person you need to talk with is that gentleman at the counter." I wondered what I should do. If I were to say something, the young woman might be embarrassed, delayed, or asked to answer questions that might destroy whatever composure and dignity she was able to preserve. She had not indicated she needed any help . . . yet.

I was still deliberating when my flight was called. The young woman looked at her ticket, got up, and joined the line. I sat and waited until my row number was called. As the flight attendant checked the young woman's boarding pass, she looked carefully at the anguished face, then asked, "Are you okay?" The girl nodded. "Are you sure?" Another nod, but the flight attendant paused in her checking and turned briefly to watch as the girl began down the boarding ramp. It was then that I decided how to resolve my professional-helper's dilemma. I identified myself to the flight attendant as a psychiatric nurse and said that if there were an emergency, they could call on me. "Oh, you noticed her, too," the woman smiled. "Thank you."

I had just gotten settled in my seat when the flight attendant approached me. "I pulled her up in the computer. It's an emergency flight—a death in the family." "Oh," I ventured, the underlying cause of the scenario suddenly becoming clearer in my mind. "Loss and grief are one of my specialties. I'd be happy to sit with her if she'd like, but only if she says she'd like someone with her." I suddenly remembered traveling 450 miles, mostly alone, to my younger brother's funeral.

Within a few minutes the flight attendant returned saying, "She said she'd like that." So, I took my purse and moved toward the back of the plane. As I approached her seat, the young woman looked up at me. I smiled, introduced myself by name, and said I was the person who would sit with her if that would be all right. She nodded assent, managed a wan smile, and said, "Thank you." I was trying to decide what my role would be. This was all happening rather quickly, yet somewhere in my gut or heart I knew it would be okay. I knew I wanted to stay in my role of a psychiatric nurse and a representative of my profession, and I was also aware that in a couple of hours our relationship would be ending. The time limit helped me focus on my goal of simply being available to her as a support.

Realizing that my seat partner was probably in the initial stage of shock in the grief process and thus lacked her usual coping skills, I decided to do a bit of framing for her. "The flight attendant told me you had a death in your family. I'm sorry," I said. "I'm a nurse who works with people who are going through losses. You could talk about it if you want to, or I could just sit here and read my book. It's up to you." I offered her two simple choices.

She sat silently, but with slightly changing facial expressions, and I thought she was getting ready to speak. I focused my attention softly on her and waited. "He wasn't supposed to die. He was going to have chemotherapy," she began. As her story unfolded, I listened, asked clarifying questions occasionally, and acknowledged her words and anguish. In between bits of content, I learned that she was being met by friends of the family and her sister at the airport with a subsequent 45-minute drive until she was in her hometown. At one point she said sadly, "Now he'll never see his grandchildren," and buried her head on my shoulder and sobbed for a little while. After a bit she said, "I think I need to sleep." That sounded like a good idea to me. As she slept, I evaluated what had unfolded and thought about where to go from here. I needed a plan for closure, for termination of the intervention.

I thought of how long she would have to stand in the aisle waiting to get off this big plane. I asked the flight attendant if there were some way the young woman could be one of the first passengers off the plane. We were moved to the first-class section near the door after she awoke. We talked briefly of how she wanted to depart. I let her know I was available to walk off the

Continued

COMPETENT CARING A Clinical Exemplar of a Psychiatric Nurse—cont'd

plane with her if she wanted and that I thought she could manage "just fine" without me, as well. "I'll be all right," she said, giving me a hug as we stood up to disembark. "You don't know how much we appreciate this," the flight attendant said to me with sincere eye contact. I acknowledged her thanks. I motioned for my seat-mate to go ahead of me. As we approached the waiting area, I looked questioningly at her to see how she was managing.

"I've got it," she said, and gave me the thumbs-up sign. I smiled and walked on.

I was met by two classmates and felt clear, reflective, and exhilarated. I felt that my clinical skills had positively influenced the outcome. I felt I had acted in a professionally responsible and caring manner. I felt good about being a psychiatric nurse.

Chapter Review Questions

1. Match each term in Column A with the activity associated with it from Column B.

Column A

___Primary prevention
___Secondary prevention
___Tertiary prevention

Column B

A. Incidence
B. Prevalence
C. Severity

2. Fill in the blanks.

A. The two goals of primary prevention activities are to _____ and _____.

B. The health education strategy of _____ is based on increasing perceived control over one's life, effective coping strategies, and self-esteem.

C. The government document that describes a national incentive to promote health and prevent disease in the United States is called _____.

D. The term used to describe a mark of disgrace that separates out those people that society sees as deviant, sinful, or dangerous is called _____.

E. Becoming involved in health-care organizations and political processes is a nursing intervention related to _____.

F. Social support has important implications for _____ levels of prevention.

3. Provide short answers for the following questions.

A. How do the medical and nursing prevention models differ?

B. Identify and describe three types of primary prevention interventions based on the assessment of targeted populations.

C. Describe the four aspects of health education and give an example of each.

D. Select one specific psychiatric disorder and research the impact of social support on its expression and resolution.

E. Relate one environmental change that would promote the mental health of people living in your community.

REFERENCES

1. American Federation of Television and Radio Artists and the Screen Actors Guild: *Women and minorities in television*, Pennsylvania, 1993, Annenberg School for Communication, University of Pennsylvania.
2. Atkins F: An uncertain future: children of mentally ill parents, *J Psychosoc Nurs Ment Health Serv* 30:13, 1992.
3. Beardslee W et al: Initial findings on preventive intervention for families with parental affective disorders, *Am J Psychiatry* 149:1335, 1992.
4. Borinstein A: Public attitudes toward persons with mental illness, *Health Affairs* Fall 1992, p. 186.
5. Caplan G: *Principles of preventive psychiatry*, New York, 1964, Basic Books.
6. Cohen S et al: Stages of nursing's political development: where we've been and where we ought to go, *Nurs Outlook* 44:259, 1996.
7. Cowan P: Women's mental health issues: reflections on past attitudes and present practices, *J Psychosoc Nurs* 34:20, 1996.
8. Fink P, Tasman A: *Stigma and mental illness*, Washington, DC, 1992, American Psychiatric Press.
9. Goldston S: A survey of prevention activities in state mental health authorities, *Professional Psychol* 26:315, 1991.
10. Mohit D: Management and care of mentally ill mothers of young children: an innovative program, *Arch Psychiatr Nurs* 10:49, 1996.
11. Mrazek P, Haggerty R: *Reducing risks for mental disorders*, Washington, DC, 1994, National Academy Press.
12. Murray J: *Prevention of anxiety and depression in vulnerable groups*, London, 1995, Gaskell.
13. Murray P: Recovery, Inc., as an adjunct to treatment in an era of managed care, *Psychiatr Serv* 47:1378, 1996.
14. Norbeck J: Social support: a model for clinical research and application, *Adv Nurs Sci* 3:42, 1981.

15. Rankin S, Stallings K: *Patient education: issues, principles, practices.* Philadelphia, 1996, Lippincott.
16. Redman B: *The practice of patient education,* ed 8, St Louis, 1993, Mosby.
17. Roots L, Aanes D: A conceptual framework for understanding self-help groups, *Hosp Community Psychiatry* 43:379, 1992.
18. Stewart M: *Integrating social support in nursing,* Newbury Park, Calif, 1993, Sage.
19. Tudor K: *Mental health promotion,* London, 1996, Routledge.
20. US Department of Health and Human Services: *Healthy people 2000,* Washington, DC, 1990, Public Health Service.

ANNOTATED SUGGESTED READINGS

Blumenkrantz D: Fulfilling the promise of children's services: why primary prevention efforts fail and how they can succeed, San Francisco, 1992, Josey Bass.

Uses a series of stories to illustrate key concepts essential for the successful delivery of community-based primary care initiatives.

*Cohen S et al: Stages of nursing's political development: where we've been and where we ought to go, *Nurs Outlook* 44:259, 1996.

Presents four stages of political development of the nursing profession that can help psychiatric nurses in analyzing previous accomplishments and planning future actions.

*Cowan P: Women's mental health issues: reflections on past attitudes and present practices, *J Psychosoc Nurs* 34:20, 1996.

Reviews important issues related to women's mental health and recommends strategies aimed at strengthening women's self-esteem, enhancing problem-solving ability, and reinforcing autonomy and assertiveness skills.

Fink P, Tasman A: *Stigma and mental illness,* Washington, DC, 1992, American Psychiatric Press.

Educates both professionals and the public about the pervasiveness of the stigmatization of mental illness.

*Jewell J, Sullivan E: Application of nursing theories in health education, *J Am Psychiatr Assoc* 2:79, 1996.

*Nursing reference.

Applies the theories of Peplau and Orem to two different health education groups to illustrate the utility of these theories to guide nursing practice.

*Mohit D: Management and care of mentally ill mothers of young children: an innovative program, *Arch Psychiatr Nurs* 10:49, 1996.

Outstanding description of the nature and extent of parenting problems experienced by mentally ill mothers of young children and interventions focused on reducing rehospitalization by decreasing the intensity and duration of maternal role strain.

Mrazek P, Haggerty R: *Reducing risks for mental disorders,* Washington, DC, 1994, National Academy Press.

Important report by the Institute of Medicine that lays a framework for prevention of mental illness and promotion of mental health.

Murray J: *Prevention of anxiety and depression in vulnerable groups,* London, 1995, Gaskell.

Concise review of the theoretical, epidemiological and applied research literature related to preventing anxiety and depression in vulnerable groups.

*Rankin S, Stallings K: Patient education: issues, principles, practices, Philadelphia, 1996, Lippincott.

Excellent overview of the many aspects of patient education. Highly recommended.

*Stewart M: Integrating social support in nursing, Newbury Park, Calif, 1993, Sage.

Excellent discussion of the contribution nurses have made to understanding social support based on research and nursing theory.

Tudor K: *Mental health promotion,* London, 1996, Routledge.

Responds to the forces operating against the promotion of mental health and offers a challenge to the lack of public recognition of mental health promotion. Advanced but important reading for psychiatric nurses.

Crisis Intervention

Sandra E. Benter

Ik ben mij zelf: een licht. Gij vindt
in mij uw eigen lot bepaald.
Blijf aldus niet voor't wezen blind,
dat in mijn schijn U tegenstraalt.

© 1998 M.C. Escher/Cordon Art, Baarn, Holland.

He knows not his own strength that hath not met adversity. **Francis Bacon** OF FORTUNE

Stressful events or crises are a common part of life today. They may be social, psychological or biological in nature, and there is often little that a person can do to prevent their occurrence. Nurses, as the largest group of health care providers, are in an excellent position to help people in times of crisis and promote healthy outcomes. Crisis intervention is a brief, focused, and time-limited treatment strategy that has been shown to be effective in helping people adaptively cope with stressful events. Knowledge of crisis intervention techniques is an important clinical skill of all nurses, regardless of clinical setting or practice specialty.

CONTINUUM OF CRISIS RESPONSES

Adaptive and Maladaptive Crisis Responses

A **crisis** is a disturbance caused by a stressful event or a perceived threat. The person's usual way of coping becomes ineffective in dealing with the threat, causing anxiety. The threat, or precipitating event, can usually be identified. It may have occurred weeks or days ago, and it may or may not be linked in the individual's mind to the crisis state. Precipitating events are perceived losses, threats of losses, or challenges.

After the precipitating event the person's anxiety rises and four phases of a crisis emerge. In the first phase the anxiety activates the person's usual methods of coping. If these do not bring relief and there is inadequate support, the person moves to the second phase, which involves more anxiety because coping mechanisms have failed. In the third phase new coping mechanisms are tried or the threat is redefined so that old ones can work. Resolution of the problem can occur in this phase. However, if resolution does not occur, the person goes on to the fourth phase, in which the continuation of severe or panic levels of anxiety may lead to psychological disorganization. This is discussed in detail in Chapter 16.

In describing the phases of a crisis, it is important to consider the balancing factors identified by Aguilera[1] and shown in Fig. 13-1. These include the individual's perception of the event, situational supports, and coping mechanisms. Successful resolution of the crisis is more likely if the person has a realistic view of the event, if situational supports are available to help solve the problem, and if effective coping mechanisms are present.

The phases of a crisis and the impact of balancing factors are similar to the components of the Stuart Stress Adaptation Model described in Chapter 4. However, by definition, crises are self-limiting. People in crisis are too upset to function at such a high level of anxiety indefinitely. The time needed for resolution, whether it be a positive solution or a state of disorganization, may be 6 weeks or even longer.

It is also important to recognize that periods of intense conflict can result in increased growth, as seen in the continuum of crisis responses (Fig. 13-2). How the crisis is handled determines whether growth or disorganization will result. Growth comes from learning in new situations. People in crisis feel uncomfortable, often reach out for help, and accept help until they feel that their lives are back to normal. The fact that crises can lead to personal growth is important to remember when working with patients in crisis.

> **?** *Think of a crisis you have experienced. Do you feel that the way you handled it made you a better person in some way? If so, how?*

Types of Crises

There are three types of crises: maturational, situational, and adventitious. Sometimes these crises can occur simultaneously. For example, an adolescent who is having difficulty adjusting to a change in role and body image (maturational crisis) may at the same time undergo the stress related to the death of a parent (situational crisis).

MATURATIONAL. Developmental psychology describes a series of steps that must be taken in growing toward maturity. During this process the transitional periods between stages can upset psychological equilibrium.

Maturational crises are developmental events requiring role changes. For example, successful progression from early childhood to middle childhood requires the child to become socially involved with people outside the family. With the move from adolescence to adulthood, financial responsibility is expected. Both social and biological pressures to change can precipitate a crisis.

The nature and extent of the maturational crisis can be influenced by role models, interpersonal resources, and the ease of others in accepting the new role. Positive role models show the person how to act in the new role. Interpersonal resources encourage the trying out of new behaviors to achieve role changes. Other people's acceptance of the new role is also important. The greater the resistance of others, the more stress the person faces in making the changes.

Transitional periods during adolescence, parenthood, marriage, midlife, and retirement are key times for the onset of maturational crises. Some conflicts related to maturational crises are seen in the clinical examples that follow.

Clinical Example Ms. J was a 19-year-old black, single, unemployed woman who came to the mental health clinic a month after the birth of her first child. Ms. J complained of feeling depressed. Her symptoms included difficulty falling asleep, early morning awakening, crying spells, a poor appetite, and difficulty in caring for the baby because of fatigue and apathy. The patient lived with her parents and siblings and had never lived on her own. She had always depended on her mother to take care of her. Her mother worked,

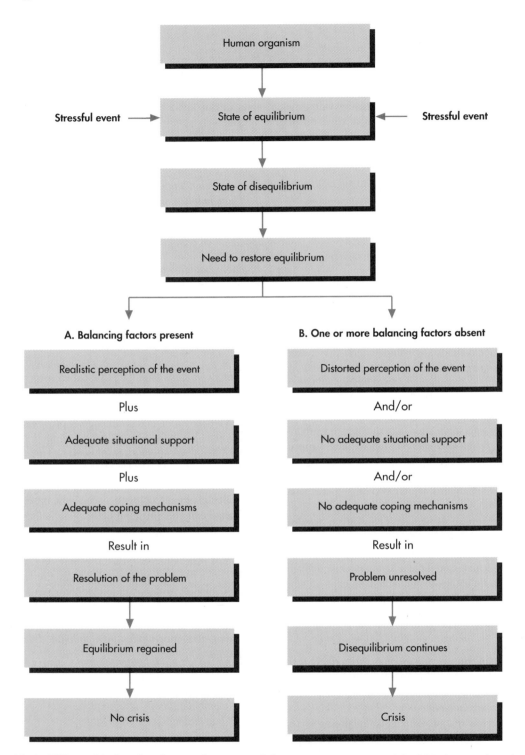

Fig. 13-1 **Effect of balancing factors in a stressful event.** (From Aguilera DC: *Crisis intervention: theory and methodology,* ed 8, St Louis, 1998, Mosby.)

however, and the patient was totally responsible for her daughter's care each day. Also, Ms. J's mother was angry that she had had a child and often refused to care for the baby. The patient's boyfriend, who was the baby's father, had promised to marry her, but he had recently decided he was too young to handle the responsibility of a wife and child. In summary, the young woman who had unmet dependency needs of her own was now a parent and had to meet the dependency needs of her infant. This precipitated a crisis for her.

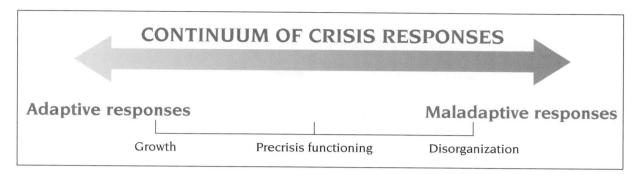

Fig. 13-2 Continuum of crisis responses.

Selected Nursing Diagnoses:

Ineffective individual coping related to birth of a child, as evidenced by feelings of depression

Altered family processes related to birth of a grandchild, as evidenced by lack of family support

Altered parenting related to being a single mother, as evidenced by difficulty caring for her baby

Clinical Example Mr. R was a 67-year-old white, married pharmacist who came to the mental health clinic complaining of anxiety, depression, and insomnia. His symptoms had begun 2 weeks ago when his wife decided that they should move to a retirement community in Florida. He described his wife as a strong, willful woman who was also outgoing and charming and made friends easily. He considered himself a quiet, nervous person who was comfortable only with old friends and his two sons and their families. Mr. R, although at retirement age, had continued to work as a pharmacist, doing relief work for a drugstore chain when the regular pharmacists were absent. In moving to Florida, he would lose his pharmacist's license, which was valid only in his state of residence. He expressed difficulty in making the transition from work to retirement. He had fears of becoming directionless and useless. He was anxious about leaving his sons and his friends. The prospect of complete retirement and moving to another state precipitated his distress.

Selected Nursing Diagnoses:

▼ Relocation stress syndrome related to pending retirement, as evidenced by feelings of anxiety

▼ Altered family processes related to conflict about lifestyle changes, as evidenced by inability to plan future

SITUATIONAL. Situational crises occur when a life event upsets an individual's or group's psychological equilibrium. Examples of situational crises include loss of a job, loss of a loved one, unwanted pregnancy, onset or worsening of a medical illness, divorce, school problems, and witnessing a crime.

The loss of a job can result in financial stress, feelings of inadequacy as a breadwinner, and marital conflict caused by a spouse's anger over the lost job. The loss of a loved one results in bereavement and can also cause financial stress,

change in roles of family members, and loss of emotional support. Homelessness is another possible outcome of the loss of a job or a loved one. The onset or worsening of a medical illness causes anticipatory grief and fear of the loss of a loved one. Again, financial stress and change in roles of family members often occur. Divorce is similar to the stress of the loss of a loved one, except that the crisis can recur with the stress of dealing with the ex-spouse. An unwanted pregnancy is stressful because it requires decisions to be made about whether to complete the pregnancy or to abort it, and whether to keep the baby or place it for adoption. If the pregnancy is aborted or adoption occurs, there can be the need to deal with feelings of grief or anger. If the baby is to be kept, changes in lifestyle are required. School problems can also lead to feelings of inadequacy. Parents often blame themselves or each other, and serious family conflict can result. Finally, being the victim of or witnessing a crime can cause feelings of helplessness, distrust of others, fear, nightmares, and guilt about causing or not stopping the crime.

ADVENTITIOUS. Adventitious crises are accidental, uncommon, and unexpected events. Multiple losses with major environmental changes result. For example, fires, earthquakes, hurricanes, or floods, which disrupt entire communities, are adventitious crises. Recent mass tragedies, which have become all too common, are also examples of adventitious crises and include group kidnappings (the taking of hostages), group killings in the workplace, airplane crashes, riots in cities, and the explosion of bombs in crowded areas.

Unlike maturational and situational crises, adventitious crises do not occur in the lives of everyone. When they do occur, however, they challenge every coping mechanism because of the severity of the stress.[15] During adventitious crises, mental health workers must reach larger numbers of people in crisis states.

Disaster-precipitated emotional problems often surface weeks or even months after the disaster. The symptoms usually occur in roughly five phases, which are described in Table 13-1. If the reconstruction phase does not begin within 6 months after the disaster, the likelihood of lasting psychological problems is greatly increased. The severe psychological stress resulting from adventitious crises is de-

TABLE **13-1** *Five Phases of Human Disaster Response*

PHASE	RESPONSE
Impact	Includes the event itself and is characterized by shock, panic, or extreme fear; the person's judgment and assessment of reality factors are very poor, and self-destructive behavior may be seen.
Heroic	A cooperative spirit exists between friends, neighbors, and emergency teams; constructive activity at this time can help to overcome feelings of anxiety and depression, but overactivity can lead to burnout.
Honeymoon	Begins to appear 1 week to several months after the disaster; the need to help others is sustained, and the money, resources, and support received from various agencies allow life to begin again in the community; psychological and behavioral problems may be overlooked.
Disillusionment	Lasts from about 2 months to 1 year; a time of disappointment, resentment, frustration, and anger; victims often begin to compare their neighbors' plights with their own and may start to resent, envy, or show hostility toward others.
Reconstruction and reorganization	Individuals recognize that they must come to grips with their own problems; they begin to rebuild their homes, businesses, and lives in a constructive fashion; this period may last for years after the disaster.

Data from Frederick C, Garrison J: Disaster and mental health: an overview, *Behav Today* 12:32, 1981.

scribed in a classic work by Terr,[25] who studied 23 child kidnap victims:

> In the town of Chowchilla, California, a school bus containing 26 children and a bus driver was stopped by three masked men and taken over at gunpoint. The captured children were driven around in boarded-over vans for 11 hours and were then transferred to a buried truck trailer. After 16 additional hours, two of the oldest boys dug them out. The children suffered from initial misperceptions, fears of further trauma, and hallucinations. Later they experienced posttraumatic play reenactment, personality changes, repeated dreams, fears of being kidnapped again, and a fear of common mundane experiences.

 Some crises, such as obtaining a divorce, develop over time and are of longer duration. Other crises, such as an earthquake, are sudden and unexpected. How do you think the element of time affects the response to crisis?

Crisis Intervention

Aguilera[1] believes that crisis intervention can offer the immediate help a person in crisis needs. It is an inexpensive, short-term therapy focused on solving the immediate problem, and it is usually limited to 6 weeks. The goal of crisis intervention is for the individual to return to a precrisis level of functioning. Often the person advances to a level of growth that is higher than the precrisis level because new ways of problem solving have been learned.

It is important for the nurse to remember that cultural attitudes strongly influence the communication and response style of the crisis worker. These attitudes are deeply ingrained in the processes of asking for, giving, and receiving help. They also affect the victimization experience, so it is essential to understand and respect the cultural values of the victims. Specific cultural factors to be considered in crisis intervention include the following[5]:
▼ Migration and citizenship status
▼ Gender and family roles
▼ Religious belief systems
▼ Child-rearing practices
▼ Use of extended family and support systems

 Describe how sociocultural factors might affect a woman's decision to seek help after being raped.

Assessment

The first step of crisis intervention is assessment. At this time data about the nature of the crisis and its effect on the patient must be collected. From these data, an intervention plan will be developed.

Although the crisis situation is the focus of the assessment, more significant and long-standing problems may be identified by the nurse. It is important, therefore, to identify which areas can be helped by crisis intervention, and which problems must be referred for further treatment.

During this phase the nurse begins to establish a positive working relationship with the patient. A number of specific areas should be assessed. These balancing factors are important in the development and resolution of a crisis and include the following:
▼ Precipitating event or stressor
▼ Patient's perception of the event or stressor
▼ Nature and strength of the patient's support systems and coping resources
▼ Patient's previous strengths and coping mechanisms

The components of the Stuart Stress Adaptation Model that parallel the balancing factors in crisis intervention are highlighted in Fig. 13-3.

Behaviors

People in crisis experience many symptoms, including those listed in Box 13-1. Sometimes these symptoms can cause further problems. For example, problems at work may lead to loss of a job, financial stress, and lowered self-esteem.

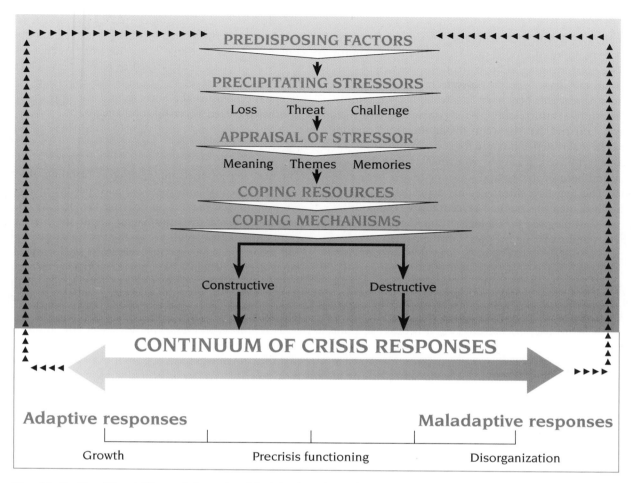

Fig. 13-3 The Stuart Stress Adaptation Model related to crisis responses.

Box **13-1** *Behaviors Commonly Exhibited after a Crisis*

Anger	Headaches	Poor concentration
Apathy	Helplessness	Sadness
Backaches	Hopelessness	School problems
Boredom	Insomnia	Self-doubt
Crying spells	Intrusive thoughts	Shock
Diminished	Irritability	Social withdrawal
sexual drive	Lability	Substance abuse
Disbelief	Nightmares	Suicidal thoughts
Fatigue	Numbness	Survivor guilt
Flashbacks	Overeating or	Work difficulties
Forgetfulness	undereating	

Crises can also be complicated by old conflicts that are brought out by the current problem, making crisis resolution more difficult.

Precipitating Event

To help identify the precipitating event, the nurse should explore the patient's needs, the events that threaten those needs, and the time at which symptoms appear. Four kinds of needs that have been identified are related to self-esteem, role mastery, dependency, and biological function. *Self-esteem* is achieved when the person attains successful social role experience. *Role mastery* is achieved when the person attains vocational, sexual, and family role successes. *Dependency* is achieved when a satisfying interdependent relationship with others is attained. *Biological function* is achieved when a person is safe and life is not threatened.

The nurse determines which needs are not being met by asking the patient to reflect on issues of self-image and self-esteem, the areas of life that are considered a success, the kinds of relationships with others, and the degree of safety and security in life. The nurse looks for obstacles that might interfere with meeting the patient's needs. What recent experiences have been upsetting? What areas of life have had changes?

Coping patterns become ineffective and symptoms appear usually after the stressful incident. When did the patient begin to feel anxious? When did sleep disturbances begin? At what point in time did suicidal thoughts start? If symptoms began last Tuesday, ask what took place in the patient's life on Tuesday or Monday. As the patient connects life events with the breakdown in coping mechanisms, an understanding of the precipitating event can emerge.

Perception of the Event

The patient's perception or appraisal of the precipitating event is very important. What may seem trivial to the nurse may have great meaning to the patient. An overweight adolescent girl may have been the only girl in the class not invited to a dance. This may have threatened her self-esteem. A man with two unsuccessful marriages may have just been told by a girlfriend that she wants to end their relationship; this may have threatened his need for sexual role mastery. An emotionally isolated, friendless woman may have had car trouble and been unable to find someone to give her a ride to work. This may have threatened her dependency needs. A chronically ill man who has had a recent relapse of his illness may have had his need for biological function threatened.

Themes and surfacing memories of the patient give further clues to the precipitating event. Current issues of concern are often connected to past issues. For example, a female patient who talks about the death of her father, which occurred 3 years ago, may, on questioning, reveal a recent loss of a relationship with a male. A patient who talks about feelings of inadequacy he had as a child because of poor school performance may, on questioning, reveal a recent experience in which his feelings of adequacy on his job were threatened. Because most crises involve losses or threats of losses, the theme of loss is a common one. In assessment the nurse looks for a recent event that may be connected to an underlying theme.

Support Systems and Coping Resources

The patient's living situation and supports in the environment must be assessed. Does the patient live alone or with family or friends? With whom is the patient close, and who offers understanding and strength? Is there a supportive clergyman or friend? Assessing the patient's support system is important in determining who should come for the crisis therapy sessions. It may be decided that certain family members should come with the patient so that the family members' support can be strengthened. If the patient has few supports, participation in a crisis therapy group may be necessary so that the support of other group members can be elicited. Assessing the patient's coping resources is also vital in determining whether hospitalization would be more appropriate than outpatient crisis therapy. If there is a high degree of suicidal and homicidal risk along with weak outside resources, hospitalization may be a safer and more effective treatment.

> **?** *Identify people in your social system that you would turn to in a time of crisis. Compare your list with that of a friend.*

Coping Mechanisms

Next, the nurse assesses the patient's strengths and previous coping mechanisms. How has the patient handled other cri-

ses? How were anxieties relieved? Did the patient talk out problems? Did the patient leave the usual surroundings for a period of time to think things out from another perspective? Was physical activity used to relieve tension? Did the patient find relief in crying? Besides exploring previous coping mechanisms, the nurse should also note the absence of other possible successful mechanisms.

Planning and Implementation

The next step of crisis intervention is planning; the previously collected data are analyzed and specific interventions are proposed. Dynamics underlying the present crisis are formulated from the information about the precipitating event. Alternative solutions to the problem are explored, and steps for achieving the solutions are identified. The nurse decides which environmental supports to engage or strengthen and how to do this, as well as which of the patient's coping mechanisms to develop and which to strengthen.

This process is outlined in the Patient Education Plan for coping with crisis. The expected outcome of nursing care is that the patient will recover from the crisis event and return to a precrisis level of functioning. A more ambitious expected outcome would be for the patient to recover from the crisis event to a higher than precrisis level of functioning and improved quality of life.

Nursing interventions can take place on many levels using a variety of techniques. In a classic model, Shields[18] described four levels of crisis intervention that represent a hierarchy from the most basic to the most complex (Fig. 13-4). Each level incorporates the interventions of the preceding level, and the progressive order indicates that the nurse needs additional knowledge and skill for high-level interventions. It is often helpful to consult with others when deciding which approach to use.

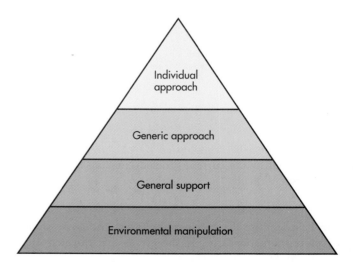

Fig. 13-4 Levels of crisis intervention.

Environmental Manipulation

Environmental manipulation includes interventions that directly change the patient's physical or interpersonal situation. These interventions provide situational support or remove stress. Important elements of this intervention are mobilizing the patient's supporting social systems (see Chapter 12) and serving as a liaison between the patient and social support agencies. For example, a patient who is having trouble coping with her six children may temporarily send several of the children to their grandparents' house. In this situation some stress is reduced. Similarly, a patient having difficulty on his job may take a week of sick leave so that he can be removed temporarily from that stress. A patient who lives alone may move in with his closest sibling for several days. Likewise, involving the patient in family or group crisis therapy provides environmental manipulation for the purpose of providing support.

General Support

General support includes interventions that convey the feeling that the nurse is on the patient's side and will be a helping person. The nurse uses warmth, acceptance, empathy, caring, and reassurance to provide this type of support.

Generic Approach

The generic approach is designed to reach high-risk individuals and large groups as quickly as possible. It applies a specific method to all people faced with a similar type of crisis. The expected course of the particular type of crisis is studied and mapped out. The intervention is then set up to ensure that the course of the crisis results in an adaptive response.

Grief is an example of a crisis with a known pattern that can be treated by the generic approach. Helping the patient to overcome ties to the deceased and find new patterns of rewarding interaction may effectively resolve the grief. Applying this intervention to people experiencing grief, especially with a high-risk group such as families of disaster victims, is an example of the generic approach.

Another example of the generic approach is the use of **debriefing.** Originally a military concept, debriefing can be used as a therapeutic intervention to help people recall events and clarify traumatic experiences.[17] It attempts to place the traumatic event in perspective, allows the individual to relive the event in a factual way, and helps to prevent the maladaptive responses that may result if the trauma is suppressed.

Individual Approach

The individual approach is a type of crisis intervention similar to the diagnosis and treatment of a specific problem in a specific patient. The nurse must understand the specific patient characteristics that led to the present crisis and must use the intervention that is most likely to help the patient develop an adaptive response to the crisis. This type of crisis intervention can be effective with all types of crises. It is particularly useful in combined situational and maturational crises. The individual approach is also beneficial

PATIENT EDUCATION PLAN Coping with Crisis

Content	Instructional Activities	Evaluation
Describe the crisis event	Ask about the details of the crisis event including A timeline of the crisis event Who was affected The events of the crisis Any precipitating events	Patient describes the crisis event in detail
Explore feelings, thoughts, and behaviors related to the crisis event	Determine precrisis level of functioning Discuss patient's perception of the crisis Determine acute and long-term needs, threats, and challenges	Patient discusses precrisis level of functioning and perceptions of the crisis Patient's needs are identified
Identify coping mechanisms	Ask how stressful events have been handled in the past Analyze whether these are adaptive or maladaptive for the current crisis event Suggest additional coping strategies	Patient identifies adaptive coping mechanisms for the current crisis event
Develop a plan for coping adaptively with the crisis event	Reinforce adaptive coping mechanisms and healthy defenses With the patient, construct a coping plan for the aftermath of the crisis event	Patient develops a plan for coping with the crisis event
Assign the patient activities from the coping plan	Review implementation of the coping plan Help patient generalize coping strategies for use in future crisis events	Patient reports satisfaction with coping abilities and level of functioning

when symptoms include homicidal and suicidal risk. In these instances, the nurse should make a formal safety contract in which the patient agrees not to harm himself or herself or others. The individual approach should also be applied if the course of the crisis cannot be determined and to crises that have not responded to the generic approach.

> **?** *How might each level of crisis intervention be used in a high school after a star player of the football team commits suicide?*

Techniques

The nurse uses techniques that are active, focal, and explorative to carry out the interventions. The intervention must be aimed at achieving quick resolution. The nurse also must be active in guiding the crisis intervention through its various steps. A passive approach is inappropriate because of the time limitations of the crisis situation.

The nurse should be creative and flexible, trying many different techniques. Some of these include abreaction, clarification, suggestion, manipulation, reinforcement of behavior, support of defenses, raising self-esteem, and exploration of solutions. A brief description of these techniques is presented.

Abreaction is the release of feelings that takes place as the patient talks about emotionally charged areas. As feelings about the events are realized, tension is reduced. Abreaction is often used in crisis intervention. The nurse encourages abreaction by soliciting the patient's feelings about the specific situation, recent events, and significant people involved in the particular crisis. The nurse asks open-ended questions and repeats the patient's words so that more feelings are expressed. The nurse does not discourage crying or angry outbursts but rather sees them as a positive release of feelings. Only when feelings seem out of control, such as in extreme rage or despondency, should the nurse discourage abreaction and help the patient concentrate on thinking rather than feeling. For example, if a patient angrily talks of wanting to kill a specific person, it is better to shift the focus to a discussion of the consequences of carrying out the act rather than to encourage free expression of the angry feelings.

Clarification is used when the nurse helps the patient to identify the relationship between events, behaviors, and feelings. For example, helping a patient see that it was after he was passed over for a promotion that he thought he was too sick to go to work is clarification. Clarification helps the patient gain a better understanding of feelings and how they lead to the development of a crisis.

Suggestion is influencing a person to accept an idea or belief. In crisis intervention the patient is influenced to see the nurse as a confident, calm, hopeful, empathic person who can help. By believing the nurse can help, the patient may feel more optimistic and less anxious, and may want to please the nurse by getting better.

Manipulation is a technique in which the nurse uses patients' emotions, wishes, or values to their benefit in the therapeutic process. Like suggestion, manipulation is a way of influencing the patient. For example, the nurse may want to point out to the patient who prides himself on his independence that he or she is responsible for much of the work of solving his or her problem.

Reinforcement of behavior occurs when healthy, adaptive behavior of the patient is reinforced by the nurse, who strengthens positive responses made by the patient by agreeing with or complimenting those responses. For example, when a patient who has passively allowed himself to be criticized by his boss states that he asserted himself in a discussion with his boss, the nurse can compliment him on his assertiveness.

Support of defenses occurs when the nurse encourages the use of healthy defenses and discourages those that are maladaptive. Defense mechanisms are used to cope with stressful situations and to maintain self-esteem and ego integrity. When defenses deny, falsify, or distort reality to the point that the person cannot deal effectively with reality, they are maladaptive. The nurse should encourage the patient to use adaptive defenses and discourage those that are maladaptive. For example, when a patient denies the fact that her husband wants a separation despite the fact that he has told her so, the nurse can point out that she is not facing facts and dealing realistically with the problem. This is an example of discouraging the maladaptive use of the defense mechanism of denial. If a patient who is furious with his boss writes a letter to his boss's supervisor rather than assaulting his boss, the nurse should encourage the adaptive use of the defense mechanism of sublimation.

In crisis intervention, defenses are not attacked but rather are more gently encouraged or discouraged. When defenses are attacked, the patient cannot maintain self-esteem and ego integrity. There is also not enough time in crisis intervention to replace the attacked defenses with new ones. Returning the patient to a prior level of functioning is the goal of crisis intervention, not the restructuring of defenses.

Raising self-esteem is a particularly important technique. The patient in a crisis feels helpless and may be overwhelmed with feelings of inadequacy. The fact that the patient has found it necessary to seek outside help may further increase feelings of inadequacy. The nurse should help the patient regain feelings of self-worth by communicating confidence that the patient can participate actively in finding solutions to problems. The nurse should also convey that the patient is a worthwhile person by listening to and accepting the patient's feelings, being respectful, and praising help-seeking efforts.

Exploration of solutions is essential because crisis intervention is geared toward solving the immediate crisis. The nurse and patient actively explore solutions to the crisis. Answers that the patient had not thought of before may become apparent during conversations with the nurse as anxiety decreases. For example, a patient who has lost her job and has not been able to find a new one may become aware of the fact that she knows many people in her field of work whom she could contact to get information regarding the job market and possible openings.

These crisis intervention techniques are summarized in Box 13-2. In addition to using these techniques, Morley,

Messick, and Aguilera[15] listed attitudes that are essential for the crisis worker to have. The crisis worker should see this work as the treatment of choice with people in crisis rather than a second-best treatment. Assessment of the present problem should be viewed as necessary for treatment, but complete diagnostic assessment is unnecessary. The goal and time limitations of crisis intervention should be kept in mind constantly, and unrelated material should not be explored. An active directive role must be taken, and flexibility of approach is essential. If more complex problems are identified that are not suitable for crisis intervention, the patient should be referred for further treatment. Table 13-2 describes interventions for helping individuals and families cope with stress resulting from crisis.

Evaluation

The last phase of crisis intervention is evaluation, when the nurse and patient evaluate whether the intervention re-

Box **13-2** *Techniques of Crisis Intervention*

Technique: **Abreaction**
Definition: The release of feelings that takes place as the patient talks about emotionally charged areas
Example: "Tell me about how you have been feeling since you lost your job."
Technique: **Clarification**
Definition: Encouraging the patient to express more clearly the relationship between certain events
Example: "I've noticed that after you have an argument with your husband you become sick and can't leave your bed."
Technique: **Suggestion**
Definition: Influencing a person to accept an idea or belief, particularly the belief that the nurse can help and that the person will feel better
Example: "Many other people have found it helpful to talk about this and I think you will too."
Technique: **Manipulation**
Definition: Using the patient's emotions, wishes, or values to benefit the patient in the therapeutic process
Example: "You seem to be very committed to your marriage and I think you will work through these issues and have a stronger relationship in the end."
Technique: **Reinforcement of behavior**
Definition: Giving the patient positive responses to adaptive behavior
Example: "That's the first time you were able to defend yourself with your boss and it went very well. I'm so pleased that you were able to do it."
Technique: **Support of defenses**
Definition: Encouraging the use of healthy, adaptive defenses and discouraging those that are unhealthy or maladaptive
Example: "Going for a bicycle ride when you were so angry was very helpful because when you returned you and your wife were able to talk things through."
Technique: **Raising self-esteem**
Definition: Helping the patient to regain feelings of self-worth
Example: "You are a very strong person to be able to manage the family all this time. I think you will be able to handle this situation too."
Technique: **Exploration of solutions**
Definition: Examining alternative ways of solving the immediate problem
Example: "You seem to know many people in the computer field. Could you contact some of them to see whether they might know of available jobs?"

Table **13-2** *Nursing Interventions for Crisis Events*

Target Areas	Nursing Interventions
Basic needs	Provide liaison to social agencies
Physical deficits	Attend to physical emergencies
	Refer to other health-care providers as necessary
PSYCHOLOGICAL EFFECTS	
Shock	Attentive listening to the crisis details
Confusion	Give nurturing support, permit regression
Denial	Permit intermittent denial, identify patient's primary concern
Anxiety	Provide structure, enact antianxiety interventions
Lethargy/heroics	Encourage sublimation and constructive activity
PROTECTIVE FACTORS	
Coping	Encourage patient's favored, adaptive coping mechanisms; emphasize rationalization, humor, sublimation
Self-efficacy	Support patient's previous successes and belief in own abilities, dilute irrational self-doubts, emphasize power of expectations to produce results
Support	Add social supports to the patient's world, provide professional support, refer for counseling when necessary, help patient develop new coping strategies

Modified from Hardin SB: Catastrophic stress. In McBride AB, Austin JK, editors: *Psychiatric–mental health nursing,* Philadelphia, 1996, WB Saunders.

sulted in a positive resolution of the crisis. Specific questions the nurse might ask include the following:

▼ Has the expected outcome been achieved, and has the patient returned to the precrisis level of functioning?
▼ Have the needs of the patient that were threatened by the event been met?
▼ Have the patient's symptoms decreased or been resolved?
▼ Does the patient have adequate support systems and coping resources on which to rely?
▼ Is the patient using constructive coping mechanisms?
▼ Is the patient demonstrating adaptive crisis responses?
▼ Does the patient need to be referred for additional treatment?

The nurse and patient should also review the changes that have occurred. The nurse should give patients credit for successful changes so that they can realize their effectiveness and understand that what they learned from a crisis may help in coping with future crises. If the goals have not been met, the patient and nurse can return to the first step, assessment, and continue through the phases again. At the end of the evaluation process, if the nurse and patient believe referral for additional professional help would be useful, the referral should be made as quickly as possible (see Critical Thinking about Contemporary Issues).

All of the phases of crisis intervention are presented in the Case Study.

SETTINGS FOR CRISIS INTERVENTION

Nurses work in many settings in which they see people in crisis. Hospitalizations are often stressful for patients and their families and are precipitating causes of crises. The patient who becomes demanding or withdrawn or the spouse who becomes bothersome to the nursing staff is a possible candidate for crisis intervention. The diagnosis of an illness, the limitations imposed on activities, and the changes in body image because of surgery can all be viewed as losses or threats that may precipitate a situational crisis. Simply the stress of being dependent on nurses for care can precipitate a crisis for the hospitalized patient.

Nurses who work in obstetric, pediatric, geriatric, or adolescent settings often observe patients or family members undergoing maturational crises. The anxious new mother, the acting-out adolescent, and the newly retired depressed patient are all possible candidates for crisis therapy. If physical illness is an added stress during maturational turning points, the patient is at an even greater risk. Emergency room settings are also flooded with crisis cases. People who attempt suicide, psychosomatic patients, and crime and accident victims are all possible candidates for crisis intervention. If the nurse is not in a position to work with the patient on an ongoing basis, a referral should be made.

Community and home health nurses work with patients in their own environments and can often spot and intervene in family crises. The child who refuses to go to school, the man who refuses to learn how to give himself an insulin

Should Medication Be Included as a Crisis Intervention Treatment for People with Acute Traumatic Stress?

Although people who are experiencing traumatic stress may experience a range of mental health symptoms in the acute phase of the trauma, it is unclear whether all problems share the same biological characteristics. It is also unclear in the initial phases of assessment which symptoms may quickly resolve with crisis intervention and which may endure and ultimately meet criteria for a psychiatric disorder amenable to medication. Should psychopharmacologic agents be offered to victims in the early stages of traumatic stress, which ones would be appropriate, and when in the process of crisis intervention would this be most helpful? Also, are there contraindications for biological interventions under some circumstances?

One might begin this decision-making process by assessing precrisis symptoms (and treatments, if any), history of substance use, family history of psychiatric disorders, and the person's belief system regarding psychiatric medications. Is the symptom already of long duration and, if so, how was it treated in the past? Does the person use substances such as alcohol that could complicate his or her reaction to the crisis or assessment of the crisis impact? If there is a family history of a psychiatric disorder, the person may be at greater risk for developing that or a similar disorder. Psychopharmacological interventions may be inappropriate if many of the symptoms will be short-lived (given the fact that some medications take several weeks to work), if many of the symptoms are natural reactions to trauma rather than symptoms of psychiatric disorders, or if the medications will lead to adverse side effects and possibly stigmatize an already traumatized person.

Some might argue that many medications might blunt, at least initially, the person's cognitive abilities at a time when concentration and problem solving are important, but an important question is whether withholding a treatment from a person who may benefit from it is an ethical decision. Could medication given immediately after exposure to a traumatic event avert a chronic posttraumatic illness? There are no clear-cut answers to these questions, but Kudler and Davidson[11] suggest that crisis clinicians are best guided by a few clinical principles:

▼ What bothers this person the most?
▼ Can this problem be controlled through psychotherapeutic, environmental, or psychopharmacologic interventions?
▼ What treatment is most likely to make this person feel or function better?
▼ Is there a reason *not* to prescribe this particular treatment?

The answers will be governed by a careful assessment of each person's circumstances and a holistic view of the care provided.

injection, and the family with a member dying at home are possible candidates for crisis intervention. Community health nurses are also in an ideal position to evaluate high-risk families such as those with new babies, ill members, recent deaths, and a history of difficulty coping.[6]

Assessment

Mr. A was a 39-year-old, medium-built, casually dressed black man who was referred to the mental health clinic by his primary care provider. The patient came to the center alone. The nurse working with Mr. A collected the following data.

The patient worked in a large naval shipyard that was recently scheduled for closing. It was laying off many workers and reassigning others. One month earlier Mr. A was assigned to an area where he had difficulty 2 years ago. The foreman, the patient believed, was harassing him, as he had done previously. Two weeks ago the patient got angry at the foreman and had thoughts of killing him. Instead, Mr. A became dizzy and his head ached. He requested medical attention but was refused. He then passed out and was taken by ambulance to the dispensary. Since that time Mr. A had a comprehensive physical examination and was found to be in excellent health. He was prescribed diazepam (Valium) on an as-needed basis, which was only slightly helpful. He returned to work for 2 days this week but again felt sick.

Mr. A complained of being depressed, nervous, and tense. He was not sleeping well, was irritable with his wife and children, and was preoccupied with angry feelings toward his foreman. He denied suicidal thoughts but admitted that he felt like killing the foreman. He quickly added that he would really never do anything like that.

He appeared to have good comprehension, above-average intelligence, adequate memory, and some paranoid ideation related to the foreman at work. His thought processes were organized, and there was no evidence of a perceptual disorder. Ego boundary disturbance was evident in the patient's paranoid thoughts. It seemed that the foreman was a difficult man to get along with, but the description of personal harassment seemed distorted.

Mr. A was raised by his parents. His father beat him and his siblings often. His mother was quiet and always agreed with his father. The patient had a younger brother and sister and an older sister. The patient and his brother had always been close. The two of them had stopped their father's beatings by ganging up on him and "psyching him out." As a child, Mr. A hung around with a tough crowd and fought frequently. He believed that he could physically overpower others but tried to keep out of trouble by talking to people rather than fighting.

Mr. A had no psychiatric history. His physical health was excellent and he was taking no medication other than the prescribed Valium. He had a tenth-grade education, and his work record up to this time was good. His interests included bowling and other sports. He had been married for 17 years and had three daughters, ages 16, 13, and 9. Mr. A stated that he had a good relationship with his wife and daughters and that both his wife and his brother were strong supports for him.

His usual means of coping were talking calmly with the threatening party and working hard on his job, at home, and in leisure activities. These coping mechanisms failed to work for him at this time but they had been successful in the past. He had no arrest record and was able to think through his actions rather than act impulsively. Mr. A showed strong motivation for working on his problem. He was reaching out for help and was able to form a therapeutic relationship with the nurse. Although his wife and brother were supportive, he felt a need for outside support because his previous coping skills were not working.

Nursing diagnosis

Mr. A was in a situational crisis. The threat or precipitating stress was his transfer to a former boss, whom he felt was harassing him. The patient's need for role mastery was not being met because he was not feeling successful at his job. Soon after the transfer, Mr. A's usual means of coping became ineffective and he experienced increased anxiety.

His nursing diagnosis was ineffective individual coping related to changes at work, as evidenced by physical complaints of dizziness and tension. His DSM-IV diagnosis was adjustment disorder with mixed anxiety and depressed mood.

Outcome identification and planning

The expected outcome of treatment was for Mr. A to return to his precrisis level of functioning. If possible, he could reach a higher level, having learned new methods of problem solving. The patient showed good potential for growth, and the nurse made a contract with him for crisis intervention. Mutually identified short-term goals included the following:

Mr. A will explore his thoughts and feelings about recent work events.

Mr. A will not harm his boss.

Mr. A will describe coping mechanisms that have been successful for him in the past.

Mr. A will identify three new ways of coping with work stress.

Mr. A will implement two of the new coping strategies.

Mr. A will be free of symptoms and function well at work.

Implementation

The level of intervention used by the nurse was the **individual approach,** which includes the generic approach, general support, and environmental manipulation.

Environmental manipulation involved having the patient remain home from work temporarily. Letters were written by the nurse to his employer explaining Mr. A's absence in general terms. Mr. A was encouraged to talk to his wife about his difficulties so that she could understand his anxiety and provide emotional support.

General support was given by the nurse, who provided an atmosphere of reassurance, nonjudgmental caring, warmth, empathy, and optimism. Mr. A was encouraged to talk freely about the problem, and the nurse assured him that his problem could be solved and that he would be feeling better soon.

The **generic approach** was used to decrease the patient's anxiety and guide him through the steps of problem solving. Levels of anxiety were assessed and ways of reducing anxiety and helping the patient tolerate moderate anxiety were identified. The patient was encouraged to use his anxiety constructively to solve his problem and develop new coping mechanisms.

The **individual approach** was used in assessing and treating the specific problems of Mr. A, who was strongly sensitive to mistreatment as a result of early childhood experiences. His emotional response was to strike out physically, as his father had struck out at him. Intellectually, Mr. A knew this would be disastrous, and his conflict was solved by becoming sick and passing out so that he could not assault his boss. Mr. A's intense anger was recognized and a high priority was placed on channeling the anger in a positive direction. As a way of formalizing this inter-

Continued

Continued from previous page

vention, Mr. A signed a safety contract with the nurse agreeing not to harm himself or others.

The first two meetings were used for data gathering and establishing a positive therapeutic relationship. Through the use of **abreaction** the patient vented angry feelings but did not concentrate on wanting to kill his boss. The nurse used **clarification** to help the patient begin to understand the precipitating event and its effect on him. **Suggestion** was used to allow the patient to see the nurse as one who could help. The nurse told the patient the problem could be worked out by the two of them and that he would soon be feeling better. Mr. A decided to contact several people at work to obtain information about transferring to another department and filing a formal complaint against the foreman. The patient and nurse therefore were **exploring solutions.** The nurse **reinforced** the patient's use of problem solving by telling him that his ideas about alternative solutions were good ones. Throughout these and other sessions the nurse **raised his self-esteem** by communicating her confidence that he could find solutions to his problems. She listened to and accepted his feelings and treated him with respect. By contacting others at work, the patient also found some supportive people.

During the third session the patient described an incident in which he became furious at a worker in an automobile repair shop. The repairs on the patient's car were never right, and the patient kept returning the car there. The patient shoved the worker but limited his physical assault to that. He then felt nervous and jittery. The patient had previously expressed pride in his ability to control his angry feelings and not physically strike out at others. **Manipulation** was used by telling the patient that he showed control in stopping the assault before it had become a full-blown fight and he could continue to do so. Mr. A's ability to honor the safety contract he made with the nurse was also reinforced. During this session the patient spoke of old, angry feelings toward his father. Some of this venting was allowed, but soon thereafter the focus was guided back to the present crisis.

In the fourth session the patient reported no episodes of uncontrollable anger. However, he still put much emphasis on being harassed by others. The nurse questioned the notion that others were out to intentionally harass the patient. Mr. A's defenses were not attacked, but his gross use of projection was discouraged. In the fifth session the patient reported that a car tried to run him off the road. At a red traffic light the patient spoke calmly to the driver and the driver apologized. The nurse **reinforced this behavior** and **supported his use of sublimation** as a defense. Discussion of termination of the therapy was begun.

In the sixth session Mr. A said that things were going well at work and that he would soon be going to a different department. He also talked about a course he had begun at a community college. He showed no evidence of anxiety, depression, or paranoia and thought he didn't need to come back to the mental health clinic.

Evaluation

The interventions resulted in an adaptive resolution of the crisis. The patient's need for role mastery was being met. He was once again comfortable and successful at work. His symptoms of anxiety, paranoia, dizziness, headaches, passing out, and homicidal thoughts had ended. He no longer felt harassed. His original coping mechanisms were again effective. He was talking calmly to people he was having difficulty with, and he was again working hard in a goal-oriented way (his college course). He had learned new methods of coping, which included talking about his feelings to significant others, following administrative or official avenues of protest, and seeking support. The patient and nurse discussed how Mr. A could use the methods of problem solving he had learned from the experience to help cope with future problems. The expected outcome, return to the precrisis level of functioning, had been attained.

It was also recommended to the patient that he engage in psychotherapy so that he could deal with the old angers that continued to interfere with his life. Mr. A refused the recommendation at that time and stated he would contact the clinic if he changed his mind.

Finally, nurses in community mental health centers, departments of psychiatry, managed care clinics, and home health agencies also may see patients in crisis, such as those experiencing depression, anxiety, marital conflict, suicidal thoughts, illicit drug use, and traumatic responses. Crisis intervention can be implemented in any setting and should be a competency skill of all nurses, regardless of specialty area.

MODALITIES OF CRISIS INTERVENTION

Crisis intervention modalities are based on the philosophy that the health-care team must be aggressive and go out to the patients rather than wait for the patients to come to them. Nurses working in these modalities intervene in a variety of community settings, ranging from patients' homes to street corners.

Mobile Crisis Programs

Mobile crisis teams provide front-line interdisciplinary crisis intervention to individuals, families, and communities. The nurse who is a member of a mobile crisis team may respond to a desperate person threatening to jump off a bridge in a suicide attempt, an angry person who is becoming violent toward family members at home, or a frightened person who has barricaded himself in an office building. By defusing the immediate crisis situation, lives can be saved, incarcerations and hospitalizations can be avoided, and people can be stabilized.[12,29]

Mobile crisis programs throughout the country vary in the services they provide and the procedures they use. However, they are usually able to provide on-site assessment, crisis management, treatment, referral, and educational services to patients, families, law enforcement officers, and the community at large.[23]

A 1993 survey of mobile crisis services found that 39 states have implemented mobile crisis services, dispatching teams to a range of settings.[10] Although these services provide favorable outcomes for patients and families and lower hospitalization rates, the survey found that few service systems evaluate the efficiency or cost-effectiveness of these services. Carefully designed studies are needed that specify the target populations, clinical team composition, nature of the mobile intervention, goal of the intervention, cost comparisons with other modalities, and follow-up outcomes. The need for such evaluative research is likely to increase in the emerging managed care environment, in which greater emphasis is placed on the value of services provided.

Group Work

Crisis groups follow the same steps that individual intervention follows. The nurse and group help the patient solve the problem and reinforce the patient's new problem-solving behavior. The nurse's role in the group is active, focal, and present oriented. The group follows the nurse's example and uses similar therapeutic techniques. The group acts as a support system for the patient and is therefore of particular benefit to socially isolated people. Often the way the patient functions in the group suggests the faulty coping pattern that is responsible for the patient's current problem. For example, a patient's interaction with group members may show that he does not appear to listen to anything said by others. This same patient may be in a crisis because his girlfriend left him because she thought he did not care about her thoughts and feelings. The nurse can comment on the faulty coping behavior seen in the group and encourage group discussion about it.

Most crisis groups focus on people who have common traits or stressors. Carter and Brooks[4] described a time-limited school-based group for friends of an adolescent suicide victim. They suggest that the most significant aspects of the group work were the venting of feelings and the support for healthy future responses. Stewart and colleagues[22] described a cognitive social support group that included both didactic and experiential learning activities for adolescents affected by Hurricane Hugo. Brown[2] reported on a hospital-based crisis support group that facilitated grieving following a pregnancy loss. The women and their families shared feelings and received information and support. Other examples of crisis groups include those conducted for families of critically ill patients, children of parents undergoing divorce, and families of hospice patients.

Nurses practicing on acute psychiatric units can use crisis intervention in working with patients and families to prepare for discharge and prevent rehospitalization. With the shortened lengths of hospital stays, crisis intervention is often the treatment of choice. The hospitalization itself may be viewed as an environmental manipulation and part of the crisis intervention.

Telephone Contacts

Crisis intervention is sometimes practiced by telephone rather than through face-to-face contacts. Nurses working for hotlines or those who answer emergency telephone calls may find themselves practicing crisis intervention without visual cues. Referrals for face-to-face contact should be made, but often, because of the patient's unwillingness or inability to cooperate, the telephone remains the only contact. Listening skills must therefore be emphasized in the nurse's role. Most emergency telephone services have extensive training programs to teach this specialized type of crisis intervention. Manuals written for the crisis worker include content such as suicide-potential rating scales, community resources, drug information, guidelines for helping the caller discuss concerns, and advice on understanding the limitations of the crisis worker's role.

Disaster Response

As part of the community, nurses are called on when adventitious crises strike the community. Floods, earthquakes, airplane crashes, fires, nuclear accidents, and other natural and unnatural disasters precipitate large numbers of crises.[28] It is important that nurses in the immediate postdisaster period go to places where victims are likely to gather, such as morgues, hospitals, and shelters. Nursing response after the bombing of the World Trade Center is a good example of such intervention.[21] Later, if Federal Disaster Assistance Centers are established, nurses may assist in the centers. This was a critically important part of nursing intervention in the aftermath of the Oklahoma City bombing.[9] Rather than waiting for people to publicly identify themselves as being unable to cope with stress, it is suggested that nurses work with the American Red Cross, talk to people waiting in lines to apply for assistance, go door-to-door, or, at a relocation site, ask people how they are managing their affairs and explore their reactions to stress.

> **?** *Nurses are often called on to help out in times of disaster. What special needs might nurses have in situations where they are both victims and caregivers?*

Experts in the field of disaster response suggest that organized plans for crisis response be developed and practiced during nondisaster times. For example, one county organized its crisis intervention and disaster services into those that are clinic based, school based, disaster-service based, and ad hoc.[19] The combination of services used depended on the type of disastrous event. For example, the county's community crisis intervention team provided timely services in a school setting following an adolescent's suicide. If the event had been a natural disaster, a comprehensive on-site family community service would have been initiated.

Nurses providing crisis therapy during large disasters use the generic approach to crisis intervention so that as many people as possible can receive help in a short amount of time. Tragedies such as group kidnappings and group killings in communities may affect fewer people and may at times require the individual approach. The nurse may choose to work with families or groups rather than individuals during adventitious crises so that people can gain support from others in their family or community who are undergoing stresses similar to theirs.

A good example of mental health professionals helping victims of an adventitious crisis occurred in Kansas City, Missouri, in the days and weeks following the collapse of the overhead walkways at the Hyatt Hotel. Eight mental health centers in the Kansas City metropolitan area joined to help care for the emotional sufferings of the people involved. The centers formed an unofficial coalition and prepared a joint press release describing the many aspects of the grieving process and publicizing the services they would offer to the survivors of those killed at the hotel, the injured, the observers, and the rescue workers. The services were of three kinds. First, all centers offered phone counseling and support groups free of charge. Second, special services were planned, such as a grief workshop that was attended by about 200 people who had been at the scene. Other related seminars were also held. Third, the centers and media worked together to let the public know about other resources and services as these became available and to reassure people that their strong reactions to the tragedy were normal.

Recently, attention has been focused on offering support and help to the helpers in disasters.[14] Health and mental health professionals who are victims of disasters as well as providers of care during disasters often feel overwhelmed with stress.[27] These care providers describe feelings of concern for both their patients and their own families.[13] Crisis intervention strategies for the caregivers are essential. For example, Stuart and Huggins[24] described the actions that psychiatric nurse administrators used to care for their psychiatric nursing staff, and Stanley[20] reported on a hospital-wide crisis stabilization program that provided large-group debriefing and small-group follow-up sessions for all nursing staff after Hurricane Hugo devastated South Carolina in 1989. Walker and Gatzert-Snyder[26] described the use of debriefing and support groups following the San Francisco earthquake. Hospital nurses who cared for victims of the 1993 New York World Trade Center explosion also held group meetings to help vent their feelings about the tragedy.

Victim Outreach Programs

Violent crime has become a global issue, concerning people in every walk of life and in every country. Many victim outreach programs use crisis intervention techniques to identify the needs of victims and then to connect them with appropriate referrals and other resources.[16] Patient concerns such as the personal meaning of the crime, whom to tell,

and the reaction of others should be discussed. A victim advocate can contact employers regarding the need for temporary time off, can mobilize community resources for food and shelter if necessary, and can arrange for grace periods with debtors to delay payment of bills without penalty until the victim recovers. Although crisis intervention is not considered the appropriate treatment for serious consequences of victimization such as posttraumatic stress disorder (PTSD) or depression, it is very useful as a community support for victims in the immediate aftermath of crime, and may provide an important link for referral for more comprehensive services when needed.[7]

Crisis intervention is successful in the acute phase of rape. It uses an integrated framework of outreach, emergency care, and advocacy assistance. Nurses often work in rape crisis centers, where victims are often seen immediately after the rape. These victims need thorough evaluation, empathic support, information, and help with the legal system. The objectives of crisis intervention are to validate the crisis and criminal nature of the rape, carefully review the details of the rape, identify a supportive social network and self-enhancing ways of solving problems related to the rape and any subsequent events, and identify referral for follow-up of the often prolonged aftermath.[3] Chapter 39 presents more information regarding care of survivors of violence.

Another contemporary issue gaining recognition today is abusive relationships. Whether the victim is a spouse, a child, or an elder, abusive relationships are experienced by people of both genders and of all racial, ethnic, economic, educational, and religious backgrounds. The widespread incidence and complex nature of abusive adult intimate relationships has been well documented. Nurses are often in ideal situations to identify and intervene with these people, most of whom are women. The nurse's validation of and response to people in abusive relationships is one component of a unified community-wide response that is headed by local domestic violence programs in many communities, and is needed in all communities to prevent violence and abuse in the home.[8]

Health Education

Although health education can take place during the entire crisis intervention process, it is emphasized during the evaluation phase. At this time the patient's anxiety has decreased, so better use can be made of cognitive abilities. The nurse and patient summarize the course of the crisis and the intervention to teach the patient how to avoid other similar crises. For example, the nurse helps the patient to identify the feelings, thoughts, and behaviors experienced following the stressful event. The nurse explains that if these feelings, thoughts, and behaviors are again experienced, the patient should immediately become aware of being stressed and take steps to prevent the anxiety from increasing. The nurse then teaches the patient ways to use these newly learned coping mechanisms in future situations.

Nurses are also involved in identifying people who are at high risk for developing crises and in teaching coping strategies to avoid the development of the crises. For example, coping strategies that can be taught include how to request information, access resources, and obtain support.

The public also needs education so that they can identify those needing crisis services, be aware of available services, change their attitudes so that people will feel free to seek services, and obtain information about how others deal with potential crisis-producing problems. For example, a mother who learns about reactions to rape may identify her daughter as a rape victim. She then may take her daughter to the nearest rape crisis center. The mother, in encouraging her daughter to go to the crisis center, tells her daughter that rape is not the fault of the victim, thus enabling her to change her attitude about the rape and feel positive about obtaining outside help. At the center the mother may be given a pamphlet that describes how to help rape victims, which she shares with friends so that they can cope quickly and effectively if their loved ones are raped.

> **?** *Explain how conducting a group on stress management for critical care nurses is an example of health education as crisis intervention.*

The nurse educates the public by participating in programs in the media, by leading or participating in educational groups in the community, and by taking every opportunity to advertise crisis services. For instance, if a nurse is a member of a church group that has developed crisis services, the availability of these services should be shared with school staff members and parent-teacher associations.Nurses, as health-care professionals, have a great opportu-nity to provide health education and crisis intervention, thus preventing mental illness and promoting mental health.

Summary

1. A crisis is a disturbance resulting from a perceived threat that challenges the person's usual coping mechanisms. Crises are a time of increased vulnerability, but they can also stimulate growth. There are three types of crises: maturational, situational, and adventitious.

2. Crisis intervention is a brief, active therapy with the goal of returning the individual to a precrisis level of functioning.

3. In assessing a patient, the nurse should identify the patient's behaviors, precipitating event, perception of the event, support systems and coping resources, and previous strengths and coping mechanisms.

4. The expected outcome of nursing care is that the patient will recover from the crisis event and return to a precrisis level of functioning. Levels of crisis intervention include environmental manipulation, general support, generic approach, and individual approach.

5. The nurse and patient should consider the following factors in evaluating nursing care: the patient's level of functioning, symptoms, coping resources, coping mechanisms, evidence of adaptive coping responses, and need for referral for further treatment.

6. Crisis intervention can be implemented in any setting, including hospitals, clinics, community health centers, and the home. It should be a competency skill of all nurses.

7. New modalities of crisis intervention include mobile crisis programs, group work, telephone contacts, disaster response, victim outreach programs, and health education.

COMPETENT CARING A Clinical Exemplar of a Psychiatric Nurse

Beth Maree, MSN, RN, CS

The mental health center setting presents many challenges, but few are broader in scope and higher in intensity than what I experienced while working there. My client, S, was a 28-year-old, married, unemployed woman with a 4-year-old son. The marriage was interracial, and her husband, 32 years her senior, was terminally ill with cancer. His disease had progressed to the point that he was unable to provide for the family either financially or emotionally. S found herself, for the first time, responsible for the family but without the necessary skills or resources.

At our first meeting, S was an emergency walk-in patient with complaints of anxiety, sadness, tearfulness, lack of appetite, poor impulse control, ambivalent feelings, helplessness, and hopelessness. Upon initial assessment, it was identified that her father was an alcoholic who had been physically abusive to her, her mother, and her siblings. Her mother had fled the home, leaving the children with the father. Both parents later remarried, and S lived with her mother and stepfather, who also was an alcoholic. She-experienced much emotional trauma during her youth and reported having difficulty in dealing with the eventual deaths of her parents and her stepfather. She had been only minimally involved with her siblings, since they were unhappy with the

Continued

COMPETENT CARING A Clinical Exemplar of a Psychiatric Nurse—cont'd

choices she had made in her life. Her identified source of support was her husband, who had promised "to always care for her." S spoke haltingly and was obviously in great distress. During the assessment, she shared that she had abused her own child when he was 6 months old, and she feared losing control again under such extreme stress. This was the precipitating factor for seeking help. S expressed a need to be cared for herself and an inability to cope with the demands of her son and her terminally ill husband.

I knew that much care would be needed for this patient and her family system. I decided that crisis intervention would be my primary strategy to ensure the family's safety. This first meeting was critical for obtaining an accurate assessment, establishing a sound rapport, and developing a plan of action. From here on it would be important for me to maintain a nonjudgmental approach, display empathy, validate concerns, and gain cooperation in establishing safety and ensuring her ongoing involvement in treatment. This could be difficult given the circumstances.

I offered positive reinforcement to S for her courage in admitting past abusive behavior and her recognition of its possible recurrence. The responsibility for reporting information related to abuse was explained to her and framed in a nonpunitive, protective manner. Her reaction of anger and fear was expected and accepted. She was encouraged to vent these feelings. In addition, her expectations of help were discussed and consequences of inadequate actions were explored.

S was able to accept the need to mobilize all available forms of assistance for her and her family as quickly as possible. The Department of Social Services was notified during the first meeting, and a caseworker was assigned to assess the home situation. With help, S was able to identify behavioral cues and situations that evoked her feelings of rage and hopelessness that often led to impulsive acts. She was able to contract for safety until her follow-up appointment and was provided with verbal and written instructions for emergency contacts via the mental health center and Department of Social Services' 24-hour phone line.

S also agreed to ongoing treatment. The targeted problem areas were grief reaction associated with the progressive loss of her husband, combined with few effective coping and parenting skills, dependency issues, and low self-esteem. She had a poor social support network and required mobilization and coordination of many agencies, programs, and professionals to meet her needs and those of her family. In addition to the protective services offered by the Department of Social Services, I enlisted help from the following agencies and professionals:

The mental health center psychiatrist for psychiatric evaluation and follow-up

The patient's medical doctor, with her permission

Family services for formalized parenting classes providing both information and a supportive peer group

Hospice for provision of daily nursing care visits to the husband and teaching S about his case

The youth division of the mental health center to provide evaluation and treatment for her son

Vocational rehabilitation for skill development and exploration of employment opportunities

I also continued as her nurse clinician for crisis intervention and follow-up care. The care I provided during our sessions remained largely supportive and educative. S, with a safety net of resources, began to work on grief and loss issues and related these to feelings of rejection and abandonment from her family of origin. She was allowed to progress through the phases of grief and to develop insight and personal growth at her own pace. Slowly, S began to identify her strengths and set goals. Together we formed a partnership to accomplish these goals with collaboration from the many services now involved in her treatment. My role as coordinator, facilitator, educator, and advocate was to assist S in meeting her goals and improving her self-esteem. In this case the importance of the patient as a human being with dignity and worth was reinforced, and the relationship of the individual to the family and the community was never more apparent.

Termination was the last critical task of our relationship; in this case the termination was twofold. First, her husband died with S at his bedside. She notified me, and support was offered at her request with my quiet presence at his funeral. A home visit was arranged shortly afterward to evaluate her adjustment to her husband's death. Second, due to a change in position, I was no longer able to serve as her clinician. Before I was transferred, S was able to meet her new clinician and establish some rapport with her. This transition went very smoothly, and S became an active, participating member in a strong therapy group. Months later I received a follow-up letter from her in which she expressed a new vision for herself that included assuming responsibility for providing a future for herself and her son. My goal of providing S with a sense of hope and a framework that would support her was accomplished. Looking back on it, I still feel good about what I was able to accomplish as a psychiatric nurse.

 Video Resources

Psychiatric Emergencies Video Series

   Module 1: Crisis Intervention

your **INTERNET**
connection

Crisis Intervention Center
http://www.cris.com/~cicinc

Crisis, Grief, and Healing
http://www.webhealing.com

Chapter Review Questions

1. Match each term in Column A with the correct definition in Column B.

Column A

G. Abreaction
A. Clarification
C. Exploration of solutions
H. Manipulation
E. Raising self-esteem
D. Reinforcement of behavior
F. Suggestion
B. Support of defenses

Column B

A. Encourage the patient to express more clearly the relationship between certain events

B. Encourage the use of healthy, adaptive defenses and discourage those that are unhealthy or manipulative

C. Examining alternative ways of solving the immediate problem

D. Giving the patient positive responses to adaptive behavior

E. Helping the patient to regain feelings of self-worth

F. Influencing an individual to accept an idea or belief (for example, that the nurse can help and the patient will feel better)

G. The release of feelings that takes place as the patient talks about emotionally charged areas

H. Using the patient's emotions, wishes, or values to help the patient in the therapeutic process

2. Fill in the blanks.

A. A disturbance caused by a stressful event or perceived threat to self that challenges the individual's usual coping mechanisms is a ___crisis___.

B. In crisis theory, perceived losses, threats of loss, or challenges that precede the stressor or threat are called ___precipitating events___.

C. Crisis intervention is an active therapy, usually limited in time, with the goal of returning the patient to a ___pre-crisis___ level of functioning.

D. The first step of crisis intervention is ___assessment___.

E. When the nurse teaches the patient or the public principles of crisis intervention and healthy coping mechanisms in times of crisis, he or she is acting in the role of ___educator___.

3. Identify whether the following statements are true (T) or false (F).

A. __T__ When a person's usual way of coping becomes ineffective in dealing with a threat, the result is usually anxiety.

B. __F__ A crisis, by definition, is a chronic, long-term event requiring 12 or more months of treatment.

C. __T__ The fact that crises can lead to personal growth is important to remember when working with patients in crisis.

D. __F__ The patient's perception or appraisal of the precipitating events of a crisis is a relatively unimportant factor in crisis intervention.

E. __F__ The level of crisis intervention designed to reach high-risk individuals and large groups quickly, and that applies specific methods to similar types of crises, is the individual approach. (generic)

4. Provide short answers for the following questions.

A. List the three types of crisis and briefly describe each one.

B. Briefly describe cultural factors to be considered in crisis intervention.

C. Think of a crisis you have experienced in the past year. Identify which of the balancing factors of crisis intervention helped you cope positively with the event and which ones could have helped you even more.

References

1. Aguilera DC: *Crisis intervention: theory and methodology*, ed 7, St Louis, 1994, Mosby.
2. Brown Y: The crisis of pregnancy loss: a team approach to support, *Birth* 19:82, 1991.
3. Burgess AW, Hartman CR: Rape trauma and posttraumatic stress disorder. In McBride AB, Austin JK, editors: *Psychiatric–mental health nursing*, Philadelphia, 1996, WB Saunders.
4. Carter BF, Brooks A: Suicide postvention: crisis or opportunity? *School Counselor* 37:378, 1990.
5. Cohen R: Training mental health professionals to work with families in diverse cultural contexts. In Austin L, editor: *Responding to disaster: a guide for mental health professionals*, Washington, DC, 1992, American Psychiatric Press.
6. England M: Crisis and the filial caregiving situation of African American adult offspring, *Issues Ment Health Nurs* 16:143, 1995.
7. Falsetti SA, Resnick HS: Helping victims of violent crime. In Freedy JR, Hobfoll SE, editors: *Traumatic stress: from theory to practice*, New York, 1995, Plenum Press.
8. Fishwick N: Getting to the heart of the matter: nursing assessment and intervention with battered women in psychiatric mental health settings, *J Am Psychiatr Nurses Assoc* 1:48, 1995.
9. Flynn BW: Thoughts and reflections after the bombing of the Alfred P Murrah Federal Building in Oklahoma City, *J Am Psychiatr Nurses Assoc* 1:166, 1995.
10. Geller J, Fisher W, McDermeit M: A national survey of mobile crisis services and their evaluation, *Psychiatr Serv* 46:893, 1995.

11. Kudler H, Davidson JRT: General principles of biological intervention following trauma. In Freedy JR, Hobfoll SE, editors: *Traumatic stress: from theory to practice,* New York, 1995, Plenum Press.

12. Lamb H et al: Outcome for psychiatric emergency patients seen by an outreach police–mental health team, *Psychiatr Serv* 46:1267, 1995.

13. Laube-Morgan J: The professional's psychological response in disaster: implications for practice, *J Psychosoc Nurs Ment Health Serv* 30:17, 1992.

14. Lesaca T: Symptoms of stress disorder and depression among trauma counselors after an airline disaster, *Psychiatr Serv* 47:424, 1996.

15. Lindemann E: Symptomatology and management of acute grief, *Am J Psychiatry* 101:141, 1944.

16. Morley WE, Messick JM, Aguilera DC: Crisis paradigms of intervention, *J Psychiatr Nurs* 5:537, 1967.

17. Samter J et al: Debriefing: from military origin to therapeutic application, *J Psychosoc Nurs* 31:23, 1993.

18. Shields L: Crisis intervention: implications for the nurse, *J Psychiatr Nurs* 13:37, 1975.

19. Silver T, Goldstein H: A collaborative model of a county crisis intervention team: the Lake County experience, *Community Ment Health J* 28:249, 1992.

20. Stanley SR: When the disaster is over: helping the healers to mend, *J Psychosoc Nurs Ment Health Serv* 28:13, 1990.

21. Steefel L: The World Trade Center disaster: healing the unseen wounds, *J Psychosoc Nurs* 31:5, 1993.

22. Stewart J et al: Group protocol to mitigate disaster stress and enhance social support in adolescents exposed to Hurricane Hugo, *Issues Ment Health Nurs* 13:105, 1992.

23. Stroul BA: *Profiles of psychiatric crisis response systems,* Rockville, Md, 1991, Community Support Program, NIMH.

24. Stuart G, Huggins E: Caring for the caretakers in times of disaster, *J Child Adolesc Psychiatr Nurs* 3:144, 1990.

25. Terr LC: Psychic trauma in children: observations following the Chowchilla school bus kidnapping, *Am J Psychiatry* 138:14, 1981.

26. Walker V, Gatzert-Snyder S: When disaster strikes: the concern of staff nurses, *J Psychosoc Nurs* 29:9, 1991.

27. Waters K, Selander J, Stuart G: Psychological adaptation of nurses post-disaster, *Issues Ment Health Nurs* 13:177, 1992.

28. Weaver JD: *Disasters: mental health interventions,* Sarasota, Fla, 1995, Professional Resource Press.

29. Zealberg J, Santos A, Puckett J: *Comprehensive emergency mental health care,* Dunmore, Pa, 1996, WW Norton.

ANNOTATED SUGGESTED READINGS

*Aguilera D: *Crisis intervention: theory and methodology,* ed 8, St Louis, 1998, Mosby.
Detailed and thorough presentation of crisis theory and methods. A classic in the field.

*Nursing reference.

Chemtob C et al: Postdisaster psychosocial intervention: a field study of the impact of debriefing on psychological distress, *Am J Psychiatry* 154:415, 1997.
Research conducted following a catastrophic natural disaster that showed empirical support for the effectiveness of postdisaster psychological intervention and the feasibility of treatment research in postdisaster environments.

*England M: Crisis and the filial caregiving situation of African American adult offspring, *Issues Ment Health Nurs* 16:143, 1995.
Nursing research on African-American caregivers that documents the long-term impact that crisis experiences can have in one's future coping abilities.

*Flynn BW: Thoughts and reflections after the bombing of the Alfred P Murrah Federal Building in Oklahoma City, *J Am Psychiatric Nurses Assoc* 1:166, 1995.
A nurse's personal account of the intense period in the aftermath of the bombing of the federal building in Oklahoma City. The description of the culture of the city after the bombing is very interesting.

Freedy J, Hobfoll S: *Traumatic stress: from theory to practice,* New York, 1995, Plenum Press.
Translates in a practical way what is known from research about traumatic events and mental health into state-of-the-art prevention, assessment, and treatment activities for mental health clinicians.

*Hoff L: *People in crisis: understanding and helping,* San Francisco, 1995, Jossey-Bass.
Excellent reference on crisis intervention and the role of nurses.

*Ragaisis K: Critical incident stress debriefing: a family nursing intervention, *Arch Psychiatr Nurs* 8:38, 1994.
Uses a case study to describe debriefing and its therapeutic value.

*Steefel L: The World Trade Center disaster: healing the unseen wounds, *J Psychosoc Nurs* 31:5, 1993.
Relates the experiences of several nurses working in local emergency rooms during the World Trade Center bombing and their reactions to the numbers of patients and their needs.

Weaver JD: *Disasters: mental health interventions,* Sarasota, Fla, 1995, Professional Resource Press.
This sensitive and sensible book reviews the history and development of disaster mental health and is a valuable tool for individuals involved in any level of disaster mental health to prepare for the experience, better organize actions, and provide and receive emotional support.

Zealberg J, Santos A, Puckett J: *Comprehensive emergency mental health care,* Dunmore, Penn, 1996, WW Norton.
Outlines current state-of-the-art, community-based, mobile emergency mental health services and treatment. All aspects of the program are described making this a complete training guide for all mental health professionals.

Psychiatric Rehabilitation

Sandra J. Sundeen

© 1998 M.C. Escher/Cordon Art, Baarn, Holland.

> *Of equality—as if it harm'd me giving others the same chances and rights as myself—as if it were not indispensable to my own rights that others possess the same.*
> **Walt Whitman** *THOUGHT*

LEARNING OBJECTIVES

After studying this chapter the student should be able to:

▼ Define tertiary prevention and psychiatric rehabilitation

▼ Assess the behaviors and rehabilitative nursing care needs of people who have serious mental illnesses and how their families and the community respond to their needs

▼ Plan and implement rehabilitative psychiatric nursing interventions with individuals, family members, and communities

▼ Develop a patient education plan to cope with psychiatric illness

▼ Describe approaches to evaluation of psychiatric rehabilitation related to individuals, families, and programs

TOPICAL OUTLINE

Rehabilitation
Assessment
  The Individual
  Specific Populations
  The Family
  The Community
Planning and Implementation
  The Individual
  The Family
  The Community
Evaluation
  Patient Evaluation
  Program Evaluation

The public health model of prevention identifies **tertiary prevention** as the limitation of disability related to an episode of illness. The National Mental Health Advisory Council has addressed the services needed to prevent disability in people who have serious and persistent mental illnesses. "With any illness, but especially with these disorders that endure and disable people, providing the right medication is essential, but not enough. A full range of services attending to rehabilitation, independent living, and enhanced quality of life is needed. Finding ways to improve the standard of care, and ways to provide it through better organization and financing of services is a compelling public health need."[18]

Any episode of illness may involve lasting change in a person's level of functioning. A person who has been seriously ill is more likely to have problems living productively in the community. Hospitalization is especially disruptive, and it is often difficult to adjust after discharge. Nurses must be aware of the total range of patient care needs both during and after hospitalization. The goal of tertiary prevention is to reduce the rate of maladaptive functioning related to mental disorders in a community. Although concepts of tertiary prevention can be applied to anyone who has experienced an episode of illness, they are particularly relevant to those with serious and persistent mental illnesses, sometimes called chronic mental illness. Because of the stigma associated with the term *chronic, serious mental illness* is used in this chapter.

It has been estimated that between 2 and 4 million Americans have serious mental illnesses.[18] Nurses care for people who have serious mental illnesses in a variety of settings: private and public psychiatric hospitals, psychiatric and medical-surgical units in general hospitals, emergency rooms, community-based treatment and rehabilitation programs, and patients' homes. As patients alternate between community-based and hospital-based care, nurses in all settings share responsibility for their care.[22] Knowledge of the special needs and characteristics of this population is important for all nurses.

REHABILITATION

Tertiary prevention is carried out through activities identified as **rehabilitation**. This is the process of helping the person return to the highest possible level of functioning. The goal is to teach "individuals disabled by mental illness to work and live independently, to overcome blocks in both opportunity and motivation, and to follow regimens of living likely to maintain or restore the highest possible level of well-being."[18] In addition, many patients need help developing new skills and finding ways to overcome functional deficits.

Psychiatric rehabilitation grew out of a need to create opportunities for people diagnosed with severe mental illness to live, learn, and work in their own communities. It proposes that mental illnesses should be perceived as a disability. Like people with physical disabilities, people with psychiatric disabilities need a wide range of services, often for extended periods of time. Psychiatric rehabilitation uses a person-centered, people-to-people approach that differs from the traditional medical model of care (Table 14-1).[32] It is supported by the following research findings related to people with long-term mental illness[23]:

▼ They can function in the community with minimal use of inpatient services.

▼ They can be helped to function more successfully in the community with interventions to enhance skills and support.

▼ Measures of skills and support, more than psychiatric diagnoses and symptom patterns, determine how well they function in the community.

▼ Improved functioning in one area of a person's life does not indicate that the other life areas have been similarly improved.

▼ Interventions to develop skills and supports may take time to have an effect on their functioning in the community.

▼ Their typical prognosis may not be increasing deterioration between episodes, but rather stable functioning between episodes, and often gradual improvement over the long term.

TABLE **14-1** *Comparison of Psychiatric Rehabilitation and Traditional Medical Models of Care*

Aspect of Care	Psychiatric Rehabilitation	Traditional Medical Rehabilitation
Focus	Focus on wellness and health, not symptoms	Focus on disease, illness, and symptoms
Basis	Based on person's abilities and functional behavior	Based on person's disabilities and intrapsychic functioning
Setting	Caregiving in natural settings	Treatment in institutional settings
Relationship	Adult-to-adult relationship	Expert-to-patient relationship
Medication	Medicate as appropriate and tolerate some illness symptoms	Medicate until symptoms are controlled
Decision making	Case management in partnership with patient	Physician makes decisions and prescribes treatment
Emphasis	Emphasis on strengths, self-help, and interdependence	Emphasis on dependence and compliance

Anthony[1] has applied the World Health Organization classification of the consequences of disease to psychiatric rehabilitation. According to this model, impairment represents the direct effects of the illness, and dysfunction, disability, and disadvantage are related to its consequences (Table 14-2).

In addition, the following five principles of psychiatric rehabilitation have been identified[27]:

▼ Goals should focus on improving quality of life, as identified by the patient and family.
▼ Rehabilitation takes place in partnership with the disabled person.
▼ Individual differences must be recognized and respected.
▼ Rehabilitation must adjust to the changes people experience over time.
▼ Rehabilitation encompasses all of the services that people need to live successfully in the community.

> **?** *Compare the principles of psychiatric rehabilitation with your knowledge of physical rehabilitation. How do the principles affect nursing intervention?*

Rehabilitative psychiatric nursing must be studied in the contexts of the patient and social system. This requires the nurse to focus on three elements: the individual, the family, and the community. The nursing care of people with serious mental illnesses is related to these three elements and the activities of assessment, intervention, and evaluation.

Assessment

The Individual

Assessment of the need for rehabilitation begins with the initial contact between the nurse and the patient. A comprehensive psychiatric nursing assessment, as described in Chapters 5, 6, 7, and 10, provides information that enables the nurse to help the patient achieve maximum possible functioning. Nurses are expected to identify and reinforce strengths as one means of helping the patient to cope. This is basic to the concept of rehabilitation. Thus good nursing care is really rehabilitative nursing care.

The Stuart Stress Adaptation Model (Fig. 14-1) may be applied within the context of rehabilitative nursing practice. It is important for the nurse to identify stressors that may interfere with the patient's adjustment to a

TABLE **14-2** *The Negative Impact of Severe Mental Illness*

STAGES	DEFINITIONS	EXAMPLES	INTERVENTIONS	RELATIONSHIP TO TREATMENT
Impairment	Any loss or abnormality of psychological, physiological, anatomical structure or function.	In physical disabilities (diabetes is an impairment in physiological function). In psychiatric disabilities (delusions, hallucinations, paranoia in psychological functioning).	Treatment with medication to moderate glucose metabolism; medication to moderate psychiatric symptoms.	Treatment could moderate an impairment.
Dysfunction	Any restriction or lack of ability to perform an activity or task in the manner or within the range considered normal.	In psychiatric disabilities: demonstration of minimal proficiencies in the areas of self-care, social adjustment, or work skills.	Implementation of a rehabilitation program	Treatment may modify the effects of dysfunction.
Disability	Any restriction or lack of ability to perform a role in the manner or within the range that is considered normal.	Severity of disability is defined within the sociocultural context: unemployment, underemployment, homelessness.	Implementation of a rehabilitation program.	Treatment will not change a disability.
Disadvantage	A lack of opportunity for an individual that limits or prevents the performance of an activity or the fulfillment of a role that is normal (depending on age, gender, social, cultural factors) for that individual.	In physical disabilities: inaccessible facilities for wheelchairs. In psychiatric disabilities: stigma and assumptions about rehabilitation potential.	Implementation of a societal rehabilitation and education program on stigma and discrimination.	Treatment will not change a disadvantage.

Modified from Anthony WA: Recovery from mental illness: the guiding vision of the mental health service system in the 1990s, *Psychosoc Rehab J* 16:11-24, 1993. In Palmer-Erbs VK, Anthony WA: Incorporating rehabilitation principles into mental health nursing, *J Psychosoc Nurs* 33(3):36, 1995.

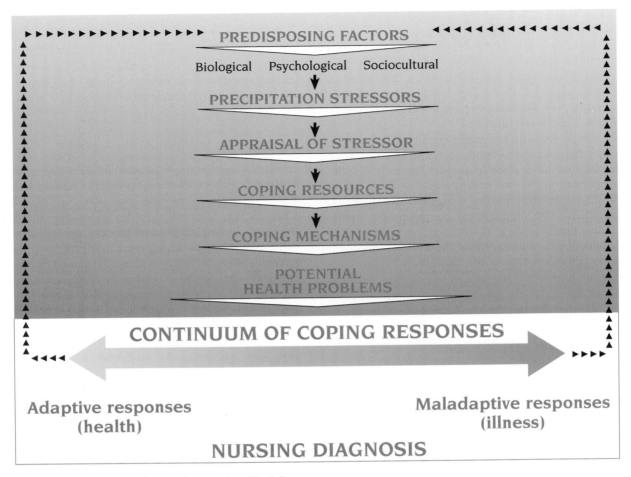

Fig. 14-1 The Stuart Stress Adaptation Model.

health-promoting lifestyle. Nurses need to be aware of patients' perceptions of their experiences. It is also essential to validate each person's response to significant life changes.

When conducting an initial assessment, the nurse needs to think beyond the limits of the patient care setting and try to anticipate the patient's other contacts with the healthcare system. In hospitals this process of discharge planning is expected. Nurses in community settings should also expect patients to progress to other levels of care. Although some people will need long-term outpatient care, others will be discharged from psychiatric care.

CHARACTERISTICS OF SERIOUS MENTAL ILLNESS. People who have serious mental illnesses are likely to have both primary and secondary symptoms. **Primary symptoms** are directly caused by the illness. For example, hallucinations and delusions are primary symptoms of schizophrenia, and elation and hyperactivity are primary symptoms of bipolar disorder. **Secondary symptoms** such as loneliness and social isolation are caused by the person's response to the illness or its treatment.

Behaviors related to primary symptoms may violate so-

cial norms and be considered deviant. Society then tries to protect itself from the person's norm violation. An example of this is community opposition to the establishment of group homes. As this process unfolds, people increasingly identify themselves as mentally ill. They begin to relate to society in terms of this identity rather than others, such as wife, mother, husband, father, or worker.

The person's acceptance of mentally ill status and adjustment to society in terms of this role are accompanied by the secondary symptoms of serious mental illness. A nursing study of the perceptions of people with serious mental illness identified the following themes related to secondary symptoms[34]:

▼ *Stigmatization,* or the sense of being discredited or shamed because of their illness
▼ *Alienation* caused by the outcome of being stigmatized and ostracized
▼ *Loss* of relationships and vocational opportunities
▼ *Distress* caused by the effects of the illness and one's related suffering
▼ *Acceptance* of oneself as having a mental illness and the need for acceptance by others

TABLE **14-3** *Myths and Facts about People with Mental Illness*

MYTHS	FACTS
A person who has been mentally ill can never be normal.	Mental illness is often temporary or episodic. Former mentally ill patients deserve to be judged on their own merits.
Even if some mentally ill people return to normal, chronically mentally ill people remain different—in fact, crazy.	Many people who have chronic mental illnesses have been hospitalized for a long time. After discharge, they must continue to take medication. The combination of the illness and medication side effects may cause them to look or act strange, but the longer they are in the community the more they look like everyone else.
If people who recover from other illnesses can cope on their own, recovered mental patients should be able to do so, too.	Most people who have been through a disabling illness, mental or physical, need rehabilitation. For mentally ill people this is focused on social support.
People with mental illness are unpredictable.	Although some mentally ill people are impulsive and unpredictable when they are actively ill, most are consistent in their behavior when recovered.
Those with schizophrenia or other severe mental disorders must be really crazy.	With appropriate treatment, people who have severe mental disorders tend to be calm and reliable.
Mentally ill people are dangerous.	Patients who have come through mental illness and have returned to the community are more apt to be anxious, timid, and passive. They rarely present a danger to the public.
Recovered mentally ill patients are surely potentially dangerous. They could go berserk at any time.	Most people who are mentally ill never went "berserk" in the first place. Mentally ill patients are more likely to be depressed and withdrawn than wild and aggressive. Most relapses develop gradually.
Anyone who has had shock treatment must really be sick.	Electroconvulsive therapy (ECT) is an effective treatment for serious depression. There is no reason to assume that someone who has received this therapy is sicker than others.
When you learn a person has been mentally ill, you have learned the most important thing about his or her personality.	Every type of disturbance is different in every patient. A recovered patient needs to be viewed as an individual rather than as an anonymous member of a stereotyped group.
You can't talk to someone who has been mentally ill.	Most recovered people who have had mental illnesses are rational and intelligent. Even people with current illnesses are likely to be rational in many ways.
If a former mentally ill patient has a really bad history, there isn't much hope.	Some people may be ill for many years before they receive effective treatment or their condition improves for other reasons. Once recovered, they may remain well for the rest of their lives.
A former mentally ill patient is bound to make a second-rate employee.	Many recovered patients make excellent employees. Some people who are subject to relapses may need to work in a flexible situation.
Perhaps recovered mentally ill patients can work successfully at low-level jobs, but they aren't suited for really important or responsible positions.	The career potentials of recovered mentally ill patients, as with anyone else, depend on the person's talents, abilities, experience, motivation, and health status.
Recovered mentally ill patients have a tough row to hoe, but there's not much that can be done about it.	The way we act toward former mentally ill patients can make all the difference.

From The National Institutes of Mental Health: *The 14 worst myths about recovered mental patients,* DHHS Pub No (ADM) 88-1391, Washington, DC, 1988, DHHS.

BEHAVIORS RELATED TO SERIOUS MENTAL ILLNESS. Surveys have revealed that people with serious mental illnesses are generally unemployed, less educated, less likely to be involved in close relationships, and more likely to live in poverty than their peers.[12] The exact causes of these characteristics have not been identified. Some could be related to primary and secondary symptoms or disabilities of the illness and others to society's reaction to the person with mental illness. Attitudes that could contribute to this reaction are illustrated by the list of myths about people with mental illness compiled by the National Institutes of Mental Health (Table 14-3). None of these myths is true, but they are commonly believed and lead to stigma of people with mental illness. This often prevents people with mental illness from gaining access to needed services and opportunities.

? *Copy the list of myths about mental illness and discuss them with a group of people who have little personal experience with mental illness. Then discuss the list with a small group of people who have a serious mental illness. Compare the responses of the two groups.*

Activities of Daily Living. Activities of daily living (ADL) are the skills that are necessary to live independently, such as housekeeping, shopping, food preparation, money management, and personal hygiene. A major goal of psychosocial rehabilitation is to help the person to develop independent living skills. A national survey of members of the National Alliance for the Mentally Ill (NAMI), a family advocacy group, revealed that 23% of their family members with serious mental illness need help with ADL.[30]

Interpersonal Relations. People who have serious mental illnesses are often described as apathetic, withdrawn, and socially isolated. The existence of interpersonal problems is supported by the very low number of marriages in this population.[12] Previously, it was assumed that relationship problems were a result of prolonged institutional life, which did not encourage close friendships. As more is learned about the nature of neurobiological disorders, it is becoming apparent that these difficulties are more closely related to the primary symptoms of the illness. For instance, depression causes apathy and withdrawal and schizophrenia leads to problems in perceiving and processing communications from others. These behaviors create serious problems in establishing close relationships.

Low Self-esteem. Self-esteem is the feeling of self-worth or regard for oneself. It is difficult to maintain high self-esteem when a person is aware of low achievement compared to cultural expectations. Lack of ability to maintain employment, live independently, marry, and have children all contribute to low self-esteem. People who have serious mental illnesses often feel cheated of the life experiences they expected to enjoy before they became ill. They feel inadequate, especially if they believe that their illness is the result of a personality flaw rather than a physiological disorder.

One mental health professional who also has a serious mental illness describes her experience of being diagnosed with schizophrenia during adolescence[8]:

I was told I had a disease that was like diabetes, and if I continued to take neuroleptic medications for the rest of my life and avoided stress, I might be able to cope. I remember that as these words were spoken to me by my psychiatrist it felt as if my whole teenage world—in which I aspired to dreams of being a valued person in valued roles, of playing lacrosse for the U.S. Women's Team or maybe joining the Peace Corps—began to crumble and shatter. It felt as if these parts of my identity were being stripped from me. I was beginning to undergo that radically dehumanizing and devaluing transformation from being a person to being an illness; from being Pat Deegan to being "a schizophrenic."

Motivation. For many people with serious mental illness, success and greater competence result in increased anxiety, causing regression, rather than in pride and continued progress. Patients attribute their uneasiness with success to fear that it will lead to higher expectations of others that they may not be able to attain. Fear of failure often results in reluctance to try new experiences. This may be perceived by others as lack of motivation. Apparent lack of motivation may also be caused by low energy. This can be related to the biological effect of the illness or to medication. In this case the person may want to be more active but is physically unable.

Strengths. Rehabilitation depends on the control of illness, as well as on the development of health potential by mobilizing strengths. A strength is an ability, skill, or interest that a person has used before. An emphasis on strengths provides hope that improved functioning is possible. Strengths may be related to recreational and leisure activities, work skills, educational accomplishments, self-care skills, special interests, talents and abilities, and positive interpersonal relationships. People with serious mental illness often need help in defining their skills, abilities, and interests as strengths. Low self-esteem may lead them to believe that they have only problems, not strengths.

Nonadherence. Lack of adherence to prescribed treatment is often cited as a behavior of people who have serious mental illnesses. Failure to take medication is a common cause of rehospitalization. It is important to assess the reasons for nonadherence. There may be a denial of the illness or a lack of understanding of the reason for the treatment regimen. Sometimes the person wants to comply but needs help such as transportation to clinic appointments or advice about obtaining a medical assistance card. Some patients do not like the side effects of their medication. They may not be assertive enough to tell the prescriber about their discomfort. The nurse can help patients by rehearsing what to say before the appointment or accompanying them to provide support. Teaching patients to write notes about care providers' instructions and to keep lists of questions for the provider may also increase adherence.

LIVING SKILLS ASSESSMENT. The nursing assessment of a patient who has a serious mental illness should include an analysis of the person's community living skills. Some of the assessment tools presented in Chapter 6 are relevant, particularly those related to cognitive functioning and activities of daily living. Table 14-4 presents a matrix of the skills required for successful functioning in the community. It lists the physical, emotional, and intellectual components of the skills needed for living, learning, and working. The nurse may use these examples in working with the patient to identify strengths, establish goals, and set priorities for skill development. Such a model provides a rational basis for assessing the patient's readiness to function productively in the community. It also provides objective information that can be shared with other mental health care providers.

TABLE **14-4** *Potential Skilled Activities Needed to Achieve the Goal of Psychiatric Rehabilitation*

PHYSICAL	EMOTIONAL	INTELLECTUAL
LIVING SKILLS		
Personal hygiene	Human relations	Money management
Physical fitness	Self-control	Use of community resources
Use of public transportation	Selective reward	Goal setting
Cooking	Stigma reduction	Problem development
Shopping	Problem solving	
Cleaning	Conversational skills	
Sports participation		
Using recreational facilities		
LEARNING SKILLS		
Being quiet	Speech making	Reading
Paying attention	Question asking	Writing
Staying seated	Volunteering answers	Arithmetic
Observing	Following directions	Study skills
Punctuality	Asking for directions	Hobby activities
	Listening	Typing
WORKING SKILLS		
Punctuality	Job interviewing	Job qualifying
Use of job tools	Job decision making	Job seeking
Job strength	Human relations	Specific job tasks
Job transportation	Self-control	
Specific job tasks	Job keeping	
	Specific job tasks	

From Anthony WA: *Principles of psychiatric rehabilitation,* Baltimore, 1980, University Park Press.

The daily "hassles" experienced by people with serious mental illness have also been studied.[28] Daily hassles are concerns, worries, or events that disrupt a person's well-being and daily life. The most common and severe hassles were concerns about money, loneliness, boredom, crime, past, present, and future accomplishments, oral and written communication problems, and physical health.

Specific Populations

YOUNG ADULTS WITH SERIOUS MENTAL ILLNESS. Young patients, generally between the ages of 18 and 35, differ in important ways from older people with serious mental illness. Many of these differences can be traced to deinstitutionalization and an increased emphasis on community-based care. Generally, younger patients have not experienced long psychiatric hospitalizations. For them, short hospital stays at times of crisis or acute exacerbation of symptoms have alternated with care in the community. The personal adaptations necessary for this pattern are different from those needed for long-term hospitalization.

Alternating between hospital and community life, young patients compare themselves with others of their age and expect their lives to be similar to those of their peers. They expect that they should marry, have children, and work. Inability to meet these role expectations and limited ability to cope with community living may lead to abuse of alcohol and drugs or suicidal behavior. Because they do not see themselves as patients, they have little motivation to become involved in treatment or rehabilitation programs or to take medication.

Because their illness interferes with voluntary treatment and ongoing participation in a therapeutic relationship, younger patients are more likely to enter the mental health system through hospital emergency rooms or the legal system. Younger patients may seek help voluntarily or at the insistence of family or friends during times of personal or family crisis. Behavior resulting from poor impulse control is often the precipitating event. Many of these patients enter the mental health system through involvement with the law for offenses such as vandalism and petty assault.

Young patients often become angry in response to their illnesses and may be sarcastic and argumentative. The nurse might represent the success that has been denied to the patient, especially if the nurse and patient are close in age. In this case, anger is related to the situation, not the person. Another factor that often contributes to anger and acting out by these patients is substance abuse. Living in the community offers opportunities to experiment with drugs, which are often appealing to the young person because they facilitate interaction with peers. Unfortunately the interaction of the abused substance, medications, and the biological disorder associated with the illness can have serious consequences. Substance abuse and the problem of dual diagnosis are discussed in Chapter 24.

HOMELESS PEOPLE WITH SERIOUS MENTAL ILLNESS. The process of moving long-term hospital patients to the community is called **deinstitutionalization**. The media have linked deinstitutionalization with homelessness, which leads to the impression that most of the approximately 600,000 homeless people in the United States are mentally ill. Government estimates report that the number of homeless mentally ill is closer to one third, or 200,000 people.[7] This is still a substantial number and represents a particularly challenging population. Homeless people are difficult to reach and less likely to be involved with community resources. They are often, but not always, alienated from their families. They often distrust service systems and providers. Traditional mental health services have been particularly unsuccessful at working with this population because of a lack of flexibility and inability to focus on the patients' priorities. The response of the community is often to demand removal of the homeless, preferably to an institution. This has led to active debate among policymakers and mental health professionals (see Critical Thinking about Contemporary Issues).

The Family

The image of isolated people with serious mental illness who return to a community where they have no connections has been widely publicized. However, most people with mental illness are involved with their families and have frequent contact with family members while they are in the community. It has been reported that approximately 65% of people who have mental illnesses live with their families.[10] Therefore family resources must be assessed when a rehabilitation plan is being developed.

A survey of families of people with mental illness found that professionals did not actively involve caregivers in the treatment of their family member with mental illness, and caregivers ranked more communication with professionals as their greatest need.[4] Although issues of confidentiality and respect for the patient's wishes regarding disclosure of treatment information must always be primary, nurses should strive as much as possible to include family members as partners in the treatment process. Family members can help by identifying potential problem areas and enhancing the patient's compliance with the treatment plan.

COMPONENTS OF FAMILY ASSESSMENT. The nurse who assesses the family as part of a rehabilitation plan should include the following areas:

▼ Family structure, including developmental stage, roles, responsibilities, norms, and values
▼ Family attitudes toward the mentally ill member
▼ The emotional climate of the family (fearful, angry, depressed, anxious, calm)
▼ The social supports that are available to the family, including extended family, friends, financial support, religious involvement, and community contacts
▼ Past family experiences with mental health services
▼ The family's understanding of the patient's problem and the plan of care

---

CRITICAL THINKING *about* Contemporary Issues

What Are the Obligations of Society and the Mental Health Care System to Provide Psychiatric Treatment for Homeless People Who Have Serious Mental Illnesses?

There is an ongoing debate about the provision of mental health services for approximately one third of the homeless population who have a serious mental illness. The primary questions are whether there are resources available to provide the complex array of services needed by this population and, if there are not enough resources, whether the homeless mentally ill should be forced to enter institutional programs.

Homeless mentally ill people tend to cluster in urban areas that have many other disadvantaged groups competing for scarce social and health-care services. Mental health treatment for these patients requires extensive outreach and major changes in traditional patterns of service delivery. Additionally, many service providers do not feel equipped to meet the needs of the homeless mentally ill. When the general public comes into contact with these people, they are often annoyed or embarrassed by their behavior. These factors combine to create pressure to remove homeless mentally ill people from the streets. The proposed solution is usually some form of involuntary reinstitutionalization, perhaps at a lower level of care than the hospital.

Opponents[9,16] of this approach cite civil liberties, including the right to treatment in the least restrictive setting. Consumer advocates have worked long and hard to secure these rights. They fear that a return to acceptance of long-term institutional stays would result in a return to the neglect of mentally ill people. Some suggest that people should have a choice of their living conditions, including homelessness. Others question whether the problem is a lack of resources for services or a refusal to prioritize the needs of a group of people who have little political clout and few who are willing to fight for them.

Proponents of creating involuntary services include some family members and some service providers.[13,37] Families worry about the health and safety of their ill members who are living on the streets. The concept of "asylum" as a place of safety and shelter has been proposed as a way to provide for the needs of these people. Those who would remove the homeless to other settings acknowledge that this is not an ideal solution but believe that it is more humane than leaving people who are often vulnerable to exploitation without assistance. They are pessimistic that resources for community services will be available in the near future. They believe that society is neglecting its responsibility by allowing people who have impaired judgment and decision-making abilities to refuse to be helped. As professionals and citizens, nurses need to consider these issues and form their own opinions.

Some of this information may be obtained from the social worker. However, it is the nurse's responsibility to be available to the family. This includes regular planned contacts with the family and inclusion of the family as part of the treatment team.

TABLE **14-5** *Behaviors Disturbing to Families, by Diagnosis*

BEHAVIORS	SCHIZOPHRENIA	BIPOLAR	DEPRESSION
Lack of motivation	81%	79%	89%
Isolation from others	72	66	72*
Poor eating/sleeping behavior	72	76	88**
Difficulty completing tasks	72	72	77
Poor handling of money	72	75	68
Poor grooming/personal care	64	54	61**
Suspicious of others	64	56	60**
Forgets to do things	64	62	60
Lack of consideration for others	56	65	61**
Excessive arguing	49	62	53**
Talking to self	41	23	25**
Noncompliance with medication	40	45	37
Upsets neighbors and friends	35	46	37**
Breaking or damaging things	29	34	34
Unusual religious beliefs	27	28	14*
Abuse of drugs and alcohol	25	29	22
Inappropriate sexual behavior	17	23	10**
Wandering away	15	14	13
Hitting or hurting others	13	17	15
Suicide attempts	14	23	45**

*Chi square p < .05.
**Chi square p < .01.
From Hatfield A, Coursay R, Slaughter J: Family responses to behavior manifestations of mental illness. *Innovations Res* 3:41, 1994.

FAMILY BURDEN. The mental illness of a family member affects the entire family. This impact is often called **family burden.** Maurin and Boyd[14] reviewed the literature on burden. They differentiate between burden and distress. Distress is the impact of all of the pressures of life on a family member, whereas burden is limited to the impact of the relative who has a mental illness. Table 14-5 lists the kind of behaviors that family members found most disturbing, broken out by diagnosis.[11] The behaviors more often associated with schizophrenia were poor grooming and personal care, suspiciousness, and talking to oneself. The most common behaviors for bipolar illness were lack of consideration of others, excessive arguing, upsetting neighbors and friends, unusual religious beliefs, and inappropriate sexual behavior. Depressed people had more problematic eating and sleeping behaviors and suicide attempts. It is also important to note that on nine other behaviors, such as lack of motivation, poor handling of money, difficulty in completing tasks, and noncompliance with medication, there were no differences between diagnostic groups.

Burden may be objective or subjective. Objective burden is related to the patient's behavior, role performance, adverse effects on the family, need for support, and the financial costs of the illness. Subjective burden is the person's own feeling of being burdened; it is individual and not consistently related to the elements of objective burden. For instance, a patient may lack ambition and remain in a dependent role well into adulthood. Family members who value success and upward mobility would be likely to feel more subjective burden

related to this situation than members who are comfortable with nurturing and supporting someone. By assessing family burden, the nurse can work with the family to identify concerns with which they would like help.

Parker[24] is a nurse who is very active in the National Alliance for the Mentally Ill. She has identified several categories of family response to mental illness. These are useful when assessing subjective burden.

▼ **Grief** is common and is related to the loss of the person they knew before the illness, as well as loss of the future that they expected to share with the ill family member. Because serious mental illness is usually cyclical, grief tends to be recurrent; it subsides during remission and returns during exacerbations. This is especially difficult for families to handle. In addition, social support systems may not recognize or respond to their need because of discomfort with the situation or the related stigma. Family members often feel guilty about the relative's illness. Unfortunately, some theorists of mental illness have reinforced this guilt by blaming family members, especially mothers, for the illness. Although this is becoming less common, guilt still occurs. It is common for those who are close to a person with any serious illness to wonder whether they could have done something to prevent it. For instance, the wife of a heart attack victim may think she could have prevented it if she had not encouraged him to shovel snow. Similarly, parents of a depressed woman may believe that they could have prevented her depression if they had not shared their own worries with her. In neither of these situations did relatives cause the illnesses, but they feel guilt because of their interpretation of the situation. Another source of guilt for relatives of people with mental illness is the need to set limits on the patient's behavior at times. For instance, the family of a patient who is physically abusive may need to arrange involuntary hospitalization if the patient becomes dangerous.

▼ **Anger** may be directed toward the patient, but it is more often felt toward other family members, mental health care providers, or the entire system. Anger within the family relates to differing perceptions of the patient and varied ideas about how to manage the illness. Prolonged stress results in irritability that is often taken out on those to whom one is closest. Anger at the system often is justified because it is related to deficiencies in the accessibility or acceptability of services.

▼ **Powerlessness** and **fear** often result from families' realization that they are dealing with a long-term recurrent illness. Most people believe that the health-care system should cure illnesses. When this is impossible, they feel powerless and frustrated. This understanding can also result in fear about the future of the ill family member and

for themselves. Powerlessness and fear are especially troublesome for parents who are aging and worried about care arrangements for their mentally ill child when they can no longer provide care. Some families also fear ill members who may be dangerous because of the symptoms of the illness.

SOCIAL SUPPORT NEEDS. Norbeck and colleagues[20] have studied families' needs for social support. They identified four categories of support needs. These are presented in Table 14-6 and can be used by the nurse as a guide for assessing family needs.

Nurses can play an important role in offering family members opportunities to discuss their concerns and taking action to meet their needs whenever possible.

> **?** *You are approached by the parent of a hospitalized young adult patient who has a serious mental illness. The family is upset because the discharge plan is to refer the patient to a community program that has not been helpful in the past. What nursing interventions would you suggest in this case?*

TABLE **14-6** *Support Needs Expressed by Family Caregivers*

EMOTIONAL SUPPORT

Acceptance	Absence of stigmatization; acceptance of the caregiver despite his or her relationship to a mentally ill patient
Commitment	Demonstrating to the caregiver a commitment to the well-being of the patient, or sharing the burden of caregiving, if only through contact with the caregiver
Social involvement	Social contacts and companionship for the caregiver
Affective	Showing love and caring for the caregiver, including concern for his or her well-being (with qualities of sympathy, compassion, and occasionally true empathy)
Mutuality	Reciprocity in supportive exchanges

FEEDBACK SUPPORT

Affirmation	Validation of the actions, feelings, and decisions associated with the caregiving role
Listening	Active listening by the support person, provision of a sounding board, and allowing for unburdening by the caregiver
Talking	The opportunity to talk with another person (without the quality of active listening, emotional presence, or the feeling of unburdening)

INFORMATIONAL OR COGNITIVE SUPPORT

Illness information	Information about the patient's illness, care, or supervision
Behavior management	Information about behavior management strategies
Coping	Advice about personal coping strategies for the caregiver
Decision	Help in the decision-making process around caregiving issues and offering solutions
Perspective	Supportive interactions that give the caregiver a new perspective about caregiving or about the caregiving situation

INSTRUMENTAL SUPPORT

Resources	Help in locating resources, negotiating systems, or advocating for needs
Respite	Provision of time off for the caregiver and support for the caregiver's own needs
Care help	Provision of help with the actual tasks of caregiving, including physical care assistance and monitoring activities (watching the patient and setting limits)
Backup	Help is available when needed, including financial help
Household	Help with such home activities as repairs, grocery shopping, and housecleaning

From Norbeck J, Chafetz L, Skodol-Wilson H, Weiss SJ: Social support needs of family caregivers of psychiatric patients from three age groups, *Nurs Res* 40:208, 1991.

The Community

The community greatly influences rehabilitation of its mentally ill members. Mental health professionals have a unique role in the community because they are community members and advocates for people with mental illness and their families at the same time. Care providers, including nurses, should assume a leadership role in assessing the adequacy and effectiveness of community resources and in recommending changes.

Nurses in all settings must be familiar with the community agencies that provide services to people with mental illnesses. Most communities have a social and medical services directory that can be consulted for basic information such as location, type, and cost of the services provided. Most agencies serve people who come from a particular geographical area such as one part of a city or, in a rural area, one or several counties. As nurses gain experience, they will become familiar with other agencies that provide services for the same people. Nurses should pay attention to patients' evaluations of the agencies from which they receive services. This information helps to identify agencies that are responsive and helpful as opposed to those that are difficult for patients to approach.

Personal contact with community agencies can be very useful as part of a community assessment. This may be achieved by making an appointment with an agency staff member. However, a more realistic picture of an agency's services can be obtained by going to the agency with someone who is requesting services. The nurse will see how the agency responds to the patient and how the patient handles personal affairs in the community. The nurse can also provide emotional support if the patient is insecure in a new situation. Nurses should introduce themselves to the staff of the agency and explain that they, as well as the patient, would like to learn more about the services. Collaborative relationships between mental health care providers and community agencies are essential if rehabilitation is to succeed.

A wide range of community services must be available to patients. Those that are directed toward basic needs include provisions for shelter; food, clothing, and household management; income and financial support; meaningful activities; and mobility and transportation. Other services provide for special needs that may differ from one person to the next, such as general medical services, mental health services, habilitation and rehabilitation programs, vocational services, and social services. A third group of services coordinate the system. These include patient identification and outreach, individual assessment and service planning, case management, advocacy and community organization, community information, and education and support.

Planning

Implementation

The Individual

Treatment planning and intervention in rehabilitative psychiatric nursing focus on fostering independence by maximizing the person's strengths. This is directly parallel to the nurse's role in physical rehabilitation. It differs from nursing care that is given to patients when they are acutely ill. During acute illness, people require nurturing. The nurse must provide for all of the basic life functions that the person is unable to manage. However, the relationship becomes less dependent as patients grow stronger and are able to care for themselves. Residual functional deficits may remain. The nurse and patient must work together to find ways for the patient to overcome any remaining impaired areas of functioning.

Three basic interventions are used in psychiatric rehabilitation to help people:
▼ Develop their strengths and potential
▼ Learn living skills
▼ Access environmental supports

Table 14-7 lists the services consumers said they needed, those they were receiving help with, and those with which they wanted more help.[33] The nursing treatment plan should be organized around very specific behavioral goals that are based on a comprehensive assessment of the person's living skills. These goals should build on those that are developed during the acute phase of the illness. This part of the nursing care plan may be called the discharge plan in an inpatient treatment setting. Discharge plans should also be developed in community settings. This will remind the nurse and patient that the expected outcome of nursing care is independent functioning. Even patients who need long-term medication can usually receive maintenance prescriptions from their family physician as part of their general health care program. This helps to put the mental illness into perspective as a chronic health problem that is not so different from other chronic problems the person might have.

The nurse and patient must decide together on the desired level of functioning. If the patient is unwilling to take on activities that the nurse thinks would be helpful, it is important to discover why. Sometimes nurses try to push a patient ahead too rapidly. Behavior that has developed gradually over time cannot be changed quickly. Learning new behavior patterns and giving up old ones is frightening and causes anxiety. The nurse must be sure that the patient's coping skills are adequate to deal with the stress of growth. Feedback must be requested to be sure that the rehabilitation plan continues to address the patient's needs. Sometimes the plan assumes greater importance than the patient. The nurse must prevent this from happening.

DEVELOPING STRENGTHS AND POTENTIALS. The development of the patient's strengths and potentials is im-

TABLE **14-7** *Consumers' Need for Help and Receipt of Help in 15 Areas*

AREA OF NEED	PERCEIVED NEED	RECEIVING HELP	WANT MORE HELP
Keeping busy to avoid getting bored or lonely	51%	25%	37%
Recognizing and controlling symptoms	46	37	35
Finding or getting along with boyfriend, girlfriend, or spouse	53	16	33
Making or getting along with friends	51	19	30
Controlling anger or temper	48	30	27
Getting or keeping a job	61	29	19
Managing money	50	27	19
Housing problems	28	18	19
Maintaining a home	36	18	18
Obtaining Social Security Disability Insurance, Supplemental Security Income, or other benefits	29	20	18
Getting around town	26	14	16
Shopping for groceries, preparing meals	27	14	12
Keeping aftercare appointments	26	15	10
Personal care and grooming	20	7	8
Taking medications	87	88	5

From Uttaro T, Mechanic D: The NAMI consumer survey analysis of unmet needs, *Hosp Community Psychiatry* 45:372, 1994.

portant. Nursing interventions that develop strengths and potentials can help patients develop independent living skills, interpersonal relationships, and coping resources, and thus help meet their special needs. Ultimately, the expected outcome of such interventions is change in the patient's self-concept and an increase in self-esteem. The negative self-concept and low self-esteem that characterize people who have serious mental illnesses interfere with their ability to see themselves as individuals with strengths and potentials. Through experiences of adequacy, self-concept can be altered and self-esteem increased. One intervention that helps patients alter their negative self-perceptions is for nurses to describe their perception of patients' strengths. Nursing interventions in which patients become aware of their strengths fall into two categories: those that occur spontaneously and those that are planned. The following clinical example illustrates a nurse's use of spontaneously occurring situations to increase awareness of strengths.

Clinical Example Theresa, a woman in her fifties, had been in and out of psychiatric hospitals for 30 years and had been living in a supervised apartment in the community for 1 year. Theresa shared the apartment with two roommates. She was a talented musician and had her own baby grand piano. Despite her love for classical music, she played only the "oldies and goodies" her roommates preferred. She said that she didn't want to upset her roommates by practicing classical music. She was afraid that if she brought the issue out in the open she might get so upset she would hurt someone. She offered as evidence the numerous times she'd been placed in seclusion rooms for violent behavior. Clearly, keeping peace was her priority.

The nurse and Theresa discussed her strengths as a peacemaker, as well as ways in which she might calmly ex-

press her own needs to her roommates. The nurse offered to be with Theresa during the discussion. Declining the nurse's offer, Theresa said that even though she was somewhat anxious, she had a clearer understanding of the abilities she had to use in the situation, and she wanted to try to "pick up" for herself in a situation of interpersonal conflict. She carried out her plan and expressed surprise that her roommates accepted her need and quickly arranged 2 hours a day for her to practice. As she told of her success, Theresa smiled, saying she wondered what would have happened if she had tried expressing her needs many months earlier.

Cindy, in her early twenties, had recently moved into the supervised apartment with Theresa and one other roommate. Cindy arrived at the day treatment program crying because she had fainted while at her nursing home job the evening before. She felt that in addition to having been embarrassed, she had failed to live up to the trust invested in her by the director of the nursing home. She had decided to quit her job.

The nurse explored with Cindy the meaning of these events in terms of her many strengths in caring for others. Her sensitivity to anticipated criticism and rejection from the director was related to the same sensitivity that allowed her to respond creatively to others' needs. At this point, Cindy firmly stated that the job was important to her sense of being needed. The nurse encouraged her to call the nursing home, express both her embarrassment and sense of failure, yet state that she wanted to continue working there. Cindy made the phone call with the nurse present for support. Her pleasure at finding out the job was still hers, that she was not viewed unfavorably by the director of nursing, and her sense of personal achievement at having taken a risk and won were so visible and contagious that the other patients staged an impromptu celebration.

Selected Nursing Diagnoses:
▼ *Theresa:* Impaired social interaction related to fear of aggressive impulses, as evidenced by social inhibition
▼ *Cindy:* Chronic low self-esteem related to fear of rejection, as evidenced by feelings of inadequacy

LEARNING LIVING SKILLS. Social skills training uses cognitive and behavioral techniques, as described in Chapter 30, to help people gain the knowledge and skills they need to live in the community. The patient is taught a structured way of examining and modifying his or her own thoughts and behavior that can be continued with decreasing clinician involvement as the patient becomes more skillful at managing difficult situations.[38] These include holding conversations, establishing and maintaining friendships, dating, managing medications, grooming, and the numerous other activities listed in Table 14-4. Social skills training programs typically incorporate videotapes, role-playing, practice, and homework assignments centered around practical problems. They are a most effective psychiatric rehabilitation intervention.[35]

Another important aspect of psychiatric rehabilitation relates to promoting the physical well-being of those with serious mental illness. One nursing study examined the health of people with mental illnesses who rejoined the community following discharge from a psychiatric hospital. It found that the most common physical health problems included high tobacco use, low exercise level, poor oral health, high-risk sexual behavior, and limited contact with physicians and dentists.[17] These findings underscore the need for psychiatric nurses to intervene in a holistic way in all health-care settings with patients who experience serious and long-term psychiatric illness.

Psychoeducation is an approach that supports the rehabilitation process by teaching the patient and family about the mental illness and the coping skills that will help with successful community living. Techniques vary but the information conveyed to the patient and family usually covers all aspects of the illness and its treatment, as shown in Box 14-1. Specific content can be planned to meet the needs of a particular patient or group. Consumers are growing to expect health teaching to be a part of the health-care services they receive. Nurses are well prepared to offer this important service to patients, families, and communities. A more general Patient Education Plan for coping with psychiatric illness is presented on p. 256.

ACCESSING ENVIRONMENTAL SUPPORTS. Supporting people who have serious mental illnesses in community settings requires the development of a wide array of community support programs. Some of these are rehabilitation centers, housing services, employment opportunities, education, crisis intervention and outreach, and case management. When these services are provided, it has been demonstrated that people who would have spent much of their time in the hospital can live successfully in the com-

Box **14-1** *Elements of a Psychoeducation Plan*

Signs and symptoms	Therapeutic strategies
Natural course of the illness	Adaptive coping responses
Possible etiologies	Potential compliance
Diagnostic tests and measures	problems
Indicated lifestyle changes	Early warning signs of
Treatment options	relapse
Expected treatment outcomes	Balancing needs and
Medication effects and side	taking care of oneself
effects	

munity. One longitudinal study found that 75% of a group of former state hospital patients remained in the community 11 years after discharge.[21] Although some required hospital stays during that time, these totaled only 2.6% of the study period. All but one of the patients preferred community life to hospitalization.

Rehabilitation Programs. Psychiatric rehabilitation programs (also called psychosocial rehabilitation) were developed in response to the plight of people who had been discharged from state mental hospitals lacking the skills and resources needed to live independently. Several models are presented here as an overview of some of the psychiatric rehabilitation approaches that have been found to be effective.

Fountain House. Fountain House, in New York City, was established in the late 1940s by a group of former state mental hospital patients. It began as a consumer-operated program, but a decade later employed a professional staff. Many of the current psychiatric rehabilitation programs are built on the Fountain House model.

Fountain House functions as a club in which patients are members. The usual hierarchical distinctions between staff (the healthy) and patients (the ill) do not exist. It is a place where members care about each other and pool their resources and abilities as they work toward increasing independence. Thus Fountain House combats loneliness and isolation while providing a variety of living and work situations that require differing levels of functional ability.

The first month at Fountain House is a residential phase, and members are taught skills necessary for apartment living. Fountain House owns and leases apartments that have staff on call, although not in residence. These supervised apartments allow people to make a gradual transition to independent living in the community.

Fountain House runs several businesses, providing a protected environment in which members can develop self-confidence and job skills. Progressing to a more complex work situation, Fountain House has creatively arranged for transitional employment placements (TEPs). Recognizing that job interviews are tremendously stressful, staff, rather than members, seek out and contract with businesses for jobs. The jobs are assigned to Fountain House rather than

PATIENT EDUCATION PLAN   Coping with Psychiatric Illness

Content	Instructional Activities	Evaluation
Identify and describe common psychiatric diagnoses	Provide handouts outlining behaviors Discuss coping behaviors Assign homework from lay literature Compare mental illness to physical illness	Patient recognizes characteristics of the diagnosis Patient distinguishes between cure and coping
Describe the role of stress in contributing to psychiatric disorders	Sensitize the patient to signs of increased stress Define stress as a test of coping skills Teach relaxation exercises	Patient verbalizes level of stress Patient performs relaxation exercises and describes a reduction in perceived stress
Help to gain a sense of control by recognizing personal pattern of signs and symptoms	Provide feedback when symptomatic behavior occurs Instruct patient to keep a diary of behavior and to identify symptoms	Patient consistently labels symptoms and seeks professional help when necessary
Enhance social and living skills to enable full participation in vocational and recreational activities	Role play social interaction in a variety of situations Review vocational preparation and current level of functioning Assess recreational activities and opportunities for future growth	Patient participates in progressively more rewarding social and work activities
Identify and describe community support systems	Provide a list of community support programs, including self-help groups, mental health-care agencies, and social agencies Invite representatives of programs to speak to patient group Escort to first agency contact	Patient selects community programs that offer needed resources Patient becomes able to access agency independently
Describe and discuss psycho-active medications	Instruct about actions, side effects, and contra-indications to common psychoactive medications Distribute handouts describing the patient's medications Suggest systems to help patient remember when to take medication and how much	Patient describes characteristics of pre-scribed medications Patient reports effects of prescribed medications Patient takes medication as prescribed

Modified from Buckwalter KC, Kerfoot KM: Teaching patients selfcare: a critical aspect of psychiatric discharge planning, *J Psychosoc Nurs Ment Health Serv* 20:15, 1982.

to individuals. Staff assign a member to a transitional employment position for as long as needed. The employer is promised that if members are unable to manage the job or do not show up, Fountain House staff will work in their place. Fountain House members, who share responsibility for a job with staff, can assume increasing responsibility as they are able to handle it. A TEP can easily be transferred from a member who is ready for a more complex work experience to a member who needs a TEP. Furthermore, employers are satisfied because the quality of work is guaranteed.

Ronald Peterson, a veteran of 10 years of residence in a state hospital, speaks poignantly of the loneliness and isolation he felt when he left the state hospital to live alone in a small hotel room. Because he had no job, knew no one, and lived on welfare, it never occurred to him that things could be any different. He said, "You take what you can get. There

is no choice."[25] Eventually becoming a staff member of Fountain House, Peterson spoke for many people trying to adjust to community living when he described the wish for a place where one belongs and is needed.

> I think the greatest need is to have a place to go where you are expected each day, a place where you can be with people like yourself and do things that mean something to yourself and others . . . places to go and be with people who need us to contribute, to take part, to help, and who notice when we're not present and do something about it.[25]

Training in Community Living. The Training in Community Living program attempts to keep patients in their own homes in the community. This program was developed in Madison, Wisconsin, to provide services to former state hospital patients. It has served as a model for community-based programs throughout the United States. In this model, when a person is in crisis and may need hospital admission, a substitute intervention is implemented. Staff are assigned to remain with the person in the community, providing support and assistance. Nurses accompany patients as they perform their usual activities. This real-world experience with the patient enables the nurse to accurately assess the skills that the person needs to learn. The nurse and patient agree on realistic goals. Staff contact is decreased as the patient functions more independently. When patients live with their families, families may also receive counseling and guidance in assisting patients.

Consumer-Run Services. Many of the former mental hospital patients (consumers) who founded Fountain House became dissatisfied with the program after it came under the control of professionals and left. There continues to be a strong feeling among some consumers that psychosocial rehabilitation programs are not truly responsive to their needs unless they are consumer controlled. In recent years there has been slow but steady growth of new consumer-run programs in many communities. Some of these are drop-in centers that provide peer support and a safe place to be, whereas others offer a full range of rehabilitative services.

Successful consumer-run programs include specific elements. They should address needs identified by the members, and participation in all or part of the total program should be voluntary. Help is provided either by members or by others whom the member selects. Consumers are responsible for the administrative direction of the program, and they determine criteria for membership. Finally, the program is mainly accountable to the members and strict confidentiality is maintained.

What is your response to the idea that consumers should run alternative treatment programs? Discuss positive and negative implications.

Residential Services. Housing is consistently identified as a critical element of successful psychiatric rehabilitation services. Appropriate housing must be safe, affordable, and acceptable to the consumer. Early housing programs tended to focus on existing supervised living situations, such as foster care. There was little oversight of these programs, and exploitation of patients was not uncommon. More recently, an array of housing options has been developed under the leadership of consumers and psychiatric rehabilitation professionals. Nonetheless, a recent survey found that people with serious mental illness generally have worse housing and neighborhood circumstances than the overall population. They devote a large share of their monthly income to housing, but the quality of their housing is not high. They are also more likely to live in crime-ridden neighborhoods, which can further reduce their independence and the quality of their life.[19]

Group homes and supervised apartments are the predominant types of housing for people with serious mental illness. Most incorporate some form of rehabilitation program along with housing. Staff supervision ranges from intensive 24-hour awake staffing to telephone consultation, based on the consumer's level of need. Although these programs are a distinct improvement on foster care, there are also drawbacks. Most housing programs focus on providing a "normal" community living experience but fall short of this goal. Supervision needs may lead to organization of housing around levels of care, sometimes requiring consumers to move if their needs become more or less intensive. This can be very disruptive. Consumers rarely have a choice of housemates and they hardly ever lease or own the house in their own names. This type of housing program structure also leads to clustering of group homes or supervised apartments, reinforcing stigmatization and triggering community apprehension.

Some traditional residential programs are now evolving into supported housing programs. This concept was developed by Carling and associates[7] at the Center for Community Change through Housing and Support in Burlington, Vermont. Housing is conceptualized as a basic service that should mirror the housing choices of others in the community. It is permanent and under the control of the resident. Housing program staff help consumers to find affordable housing of their choice. If people decide to live together it is also their choice. Staff may introduce consumers to each other, but they decide whether to establish a household. Mental health and rehabilitative services are flexible and designed to help the person to live successfully in the community. Some supported housing programs are part of comprehensive psychiatric rehabilitation programs and are an element of a broader supportive living approach. In this case staff intervention is directed not only at maintaining the person in housing but also at asserting the consumer to become fully involved in community life. A personal future planning process helps the consumer to identify goals, preferences, and the important people who can help in accomplishing these.

Studies of consumer preference have favored the supportive living approach.[31] In a review of 43 consumer preference surveys, it was consistently found that consumers preferred having their own house or apartment, living alone or with a significant other, and did not want to live with another consumer of mental health services.

Vocational Services. Many psychiatric rehabilitation programs provide vocational rehabilitation services. Prevocational training usually begins within the program itself. Members may be organized into work teams around the activities needed to keep the program running, usually clerical, food service, and maintenance tasks. Aside from the development of marketable work skills, the goal of these programs is to foster good work habits. Some members continue indefinitely in prevocational services. Others may move into temporary employment placements such as those developed at Fountain House. The final stage of vocational rehabilitation is finding competitive employment. Some consumers use vocational services to achieve this goal.

It has been shown that over a short period of time, targeted vocational programs can help people with severe mental illness develop the skills and attitudes necessary to attain employment or entry into the vocational rehabilitation system.[5] In addition, helping people with severe mental illness obtain competitive jobs that correspond with their explicit job preferences increases their job satisfaction and tenure in the job.[2] Box 14-2 lists six principles to be considered in the vocational rehabilitation of people who have serious mental illnesses.

Although mental health service providers support the idea of vocational rehabilitation, they are reluctant and sometimes actively opposed to hiring consumers themselves. If they do, it is often as a janitor, housekeeper, or groundskeeper. Consumers have begun to assert their unique qualifications as counselors and case managers. They have been successfully employed in this role and have achieved good outcomes for themselves and those to whom they provide services.[29]

Besio and Mahler[3] reported the results of a survey about the benefits and problems of employing consumer staff in supported housing services. Benefits to service recipients included more positive staff-recipient relationships, better knowledge of resources and ways to overcome barriers, advocacy, and role modeling. Problems for recipients included concerns about confidentiality and lack of consumer staff training. For the consumer staff, benefits included improved self-esteem, vocational skill development, and increased income. Stress management and the impact of job stress on their mental illness were problems for the consumer staff. The organization benefited from increased sensitivity to consumers and awareness of consumer capabilities by nonconsumer staff, improvement in the relevance of services, and the availability of a pool of good employees.

Box **14-2** *Principles of Vocational Rehabilitation*

Vocational services must be integrated with other rehabilitation services.

There must be an array of vocational options and provision for changes in career goals.

Support and backup services must be provided at the work site.

Job expectations must be realistic, neither too high nor too low.

Compensation should be adequate and should not interfere with ongoing benefits (such as food stamps and medical assistance).

Program development must be based on the realities of the community context related to economic and political considerations.

From Bachrach LL: Psychosocial rehabilitation and psychiatry in the care of long-term patients, *Am J Psychiatry* 149:1455, 1992.

Organizational problems included distrust and stigmatization of consumer staff by their nonconsumer co-workers and the need to accommodate disability-related behaviors. They also reported an improvement in the public image of people with mental illnesses.

Educational Services. Many people with serious mental illnesses have not completed formal education through high school or beyond because of the effects of the illness. Rehabilitation programs often offer remedial education related to vocational services. Education that is offered in a supportive environment can increase self-esteem, improve job qualifications, and encourage some consumers to pursue higher education.

? *Review a book intended for mental health consumers. Critique it in terms of accuracy, practical advice, and emotional tone. Ask a consumer or a family member of a consumer to review the book. Compare your critiques.*

The Family

Family support is very important to the successful rehabilitation of a person with mental illness. The mental illness of a member is often a shock and a source of great stress to the family. Nurses are in a favorable position to help families cope with the stress and adapt to changes in the family structure. Pfeiffer and Mostek[26] have identified three categories of programs for families of people with serious mental illnesses: empowerment, treatment, and education. Empowerment and education programs are discussed here. Family treatment is presented in Chapter 32.

EMPOWERMENT. Walsh,[36] a parent of an adult child who has schizophrenia, has suggested several common trouble spots in family life. Learning ways to handle these troublesome areas empowers the family by giving them a sense of control over their lives. The problem areas include the following:

▼ Disrupted communications
▼ Mechanics of everyday life, including the need for privacy and control over personal space, keeping a regular schedule, television usage, money management, and grooming
▼ Responding to hallucinations, delusions, and odd behavior, particularly coping with violent or suicidal threats
▼ Alcohol and drug use
▼ Need for relatives to remember to take care of themselves

This last area of concern is often ignored by family members and professionals alike. Walsh recommends the following ways to accomplish this:

▼ Accept the fact of a family member with mental illness.
▼ Plan a self-care program.
▼ Continue to pursue personal activities and interests.
▼ Get involved with organizations such as self-help groups or churches.

▼ Avoid the advice and opinions of those who have not lived with a person with mental illness.

▼ Remember that happiness is possible.

▼ Stop blaming yourself.

Reviewing this list gives the nurse some understanding of the pain and stress experienced by the family of a person with mental illness.

Families and mental health care providers sometimes become engaged in power struggles related to the care of the mentally ill family member. This interferes with their ability to work as a team. Nurses should strive to understand the family's fears and concerns and help members to develop effective coping mechanisms. Identifying feelings related to the illness is the first step toward coping. Sharing feelings with each other can be a great relief to people who feel isolated. When feelings are revealed, family members can be supportive of each other, including the ill person. Coping with feelings also allows the person to be receptive to information about the illness and mental health services. The combination of coping and education empowers the family and facilitates their involvement in the recovery process. Because nurses are usually viewed as supportive and helpful, they are in a good position to address the needs of families. Ways that professionals can share power with families are summarized in Box 14-3.

FAMILY EDUCATION. Family education has become a primary nursing intervention in providing rehabilitative services to relatives of people with serious mental illness. Nurses have established workshops for family members that have been well received and have helped families cope with

---

Box **14-3** *Ways Professionals Can Share Power with Families*

Clarify mutual goals.
Do not force families to fit a specific model.
Acknowledge your own limitations.
Work as a team with the family, including co-leading educational groups.
Point out family strengths.
Learn to respond to intense feelings, often directed toward the mental health system.
Encourage family enrichment by spending time on their individual needs.
Provide information about psychiatric illness and medications.
Provide practical advice.
Provide information about community resources.
Encourage involvement in local family support and advocacy groups.
Make a personal commitment.
Acknowledge diverse beliefs.
Develop your own supports.

From Zipple AM, Spaniol L: Current educational and supportive models of family intervention. In Hatfield AB, Lefley HP, editors: *Families of the mentally ill: coping and adaptation,* New York, 1987, The Guilford Press.

---

the challenges presented by the mental illness.[6,15] Programming for these workshops can include information and skill-building exercises. The experiences of the more seasoned family members can be particularly helpful as they can share their successes and failures in using various coping strategies and provide needed social support.

Providing an opportunity for family members to meet one another for mutual support may be especially important. These opportunities may be formal, such as support groups or local chapters of the National Alliance of the Mentally Ill (NAMI), or informal, such as family recreational gatherings.

> **?** *If you were responsible for developing a nursing program for psychiatric rehabilitation, what would it be like? Describe the setting, the program, its goals, and the roles of staff and patients.*

The Community

There are several ways nurses can intervene in the community to encourage the establishment of tertiary prevention programs. Among these are health education, membership in advocacy groups, networking, and political action. It has been noted that stigma decreases with increased formal education. Most nurses have a strong background and a firm belief in health education. Mental health education in the community can have a real impact on the experience of patients in the community. Greater understanding of the behaviors and needs of people with mental illness could increase community acceptance, leading to the development of better services. Thus nurses should take advantage of opportunities to speak to community groups about mental health.

Psychiatric nurses can also perform a valuable service by educating their co-workers and professional colleagues about current research related to serious mental illnesses. Although they are seldom discussed, stigmatizing attitudes toward mental illness exist among health-care workers. These attitudes are transmitted to the general public. Professionals have even taken the lead in opposing the establishment of group homes in their neighborhoods. Well-informed nurses can make health-care workers aware of their prejudices and assist them to change their behavior.

Membership by nurses in community advocacy groups can also be helpful. Nurses can join forces with other professional and lay people who share concerns about the care of the mentally ill. The National Mental Health Association is the largest advocacy group that addresses mental health issues. Members of this organization have been influential in drawing attention to the needs of people with mental illness and in supporting positive legislation at the federal and state levels. They monitor the effectiveness of the mental health care system.

Nurses can also promote working relationships among advocacy groups, professional organizations, self-help groups, and concerned citizens. With limited funding available and health-care costs escalating, the formation of coalitions is essential to lobby for the allocation of resources to mental health care. Psychiatric nurses have taken a leadership role in coalitions to influence reforms in the American health-care system.

The activities of community-wide networks are often directed toward the political system. Aside from allocation of money and other resources, the nature of mental health care in a community is strongly influenced by the political structure of that community. As described in Chapters 8 and 9, environmental and legal issues have a great effect on mental health care delivery. Nurses need to be aware of and involved in the political process. They should communicate directly with legislators at all levels, sharing their interests and concerns. Politicians are well aware of the need to respond to the priorities of their constituents.

Nurses can also become more directly involved in the political system. They can run for office and support other nurses who are legislators. Nurses are often invaluable members of appointed boards and commissions on health care. Their knowledge can be shared with others who are planning community health-care systems. These voluntary activities are time-consuming, but they can have great impact on the health-care system. Community-level policies can either inhibit or facilitate direct care efforts. Active involvement in professional organizations often leads to productive and rewarding community activities. There is a great sense of satisfaction to be derived from selling a community on a new idea and seeing it become a reality.

> **?** *Obtain a copy of a bill considered by your state legislature that is relevant to psychiatric rehabilitation. Explain the effect this legislation would have on the mental health care system, including the potential effect on nursing practice.*

Evaluation

Evaluation of psychiatric rehabilitation services usually covers the impact on the patient and family and the effectiveness of the community service system.

Patient Evaluation

Evaluation of the services provided to patients and family members must focus on the achievement of the expected outcomes of the intervention. Most psychiatric rehabilitation programs rely on both objective and subjective measures of outcome. Objective measures are generally related to the following questions:

▼ Is the person living in housing of personal choice?
▼ Have days of hospitalization in the last year decreased?
▼ How many emergency room visits has the person made?
▼ How many days in the last year have been spent in a transitional employment placement? In competitive employment?
▼ How often does the person have contact with family members? Who are they?
▼ Can the person identify people to provide support in a crisis?
▼ Is the person involved in community activities?
▼ Is the person enrolled in an adult education course? In an academic education program?

The answers to such questions are compared with the individual rehabilitation plans, providing a picture of the success of the services. They should be discussed with program participants and their families as a basis for further planning.

Subjective measures of effectiveness include periodic discussions with patients and families about the progress of rehabilitation. Staff members share their observations about the person's response to the program and invite feedback from the consumers. Many programs also conduct regular consumer satisfaction surveys. More recently, consumers have been employed as advocates to seek information about consumer dissatisfaction and present complaints to program administrators.

COMPETENT CARING A Clinical Exemplar of a Psychiatric Nurse

Iona Bradley, RN, C

Ms. C was one of the first patients in my mobile treatment caseload. She had had multiple admissions to the state hospital. Her psychiatric diagnosis was bipolar disorder. The referral to this new program was made in an attempt to help her to spend more time in the community. We have now been working together for 6 years. Soon after I met her I realized that there were several nursing problems that I would need to address. She had a history of poor compliance with her medications. She was also diabetic and not good about following her prescribed diet. Because of her

diabetes, she had a neurogenic bladder for which an indwelling catheter had been inserted. She was not managing her catheter care very well.

She had been living with an abusive alcoholic boyfriend. Although she knew that this was not a good situation for her, she was unable to break away from him. Her conditional release from the hospital required her to live in supervised housing. This forced her to distance herself from him. A stable living situation also enabled me to observe her behavior over time. I discovered

COMPETENT CARING A Clinical Exemplar of a Psychiatric Nurse—cont'd

that her bipolar cycle involved manic episodes every 21 days. Knowing this, I could work with her to schedule her life to accommodate her cycle. For instance, she is not pressured to attend her daytime psychosocial rehabilitation program during the manic phase. I also observed a relationship between the manic phase of her bipolar disorder and her diabetes. While manic, she craves sweets and is unable to control her carbohydrate intake. I have worked with the residential staff to remove as many sweets as possible from the house when her manic phase is due to happen. If she does eat sweets she becomes irritable and agitated. Because all of her caregivers are aware of this, she is supported until she regains her stable state.

It took a long time to gain Ms. C's trust. I had to demonstrate over and over that I really cared about her. Once she was able to trust me, I was able to focus on some of her physical nursing care needs. Her urinary catheter was a major inconvenience. She didn't always secure the collection bag well and sometimes it would be found around her ankle. In the past, her boyfriend had pulled it out. With a great deal of support, she agreed to the insertion of a suprapubic catheter. This was easier for her to care for and she has even regained some bladder tone. Her diabetes is becoming more fragile. It is expected that she will need to take insulin in the near future. I have found that pharmacy students are available to monitor medication use in the home for patients who are having problems with self-administration or compliance. I have referred Ms. C to that program. I am also teaching the residential staff about meal planning and nutritious diets.

A long-term relationship like this is rewarding but also challenging. Ms. C and I have shared important life experiences. This has led to a closeness that is not a friendship, but is deeper than I have experienced with patients in other settings. I have become a part of her life. I have participated in the realization by her and her boyfriend that they cannot live together. I have had the opportunity to help both of them recognize and deal with their feelings. I feel good that they were able to remain friends while gaining a realistic view of their relationship.

I have learned that working in the community means that the psychiatric nurse has to attend to all of the patient's needs, not just the psychiatric needs. In fact, sometimes the psychiatric needs are not the most important. I have dealt with medical needs, financial needs, needs for housing, and relationship needs. It has been a growth experience for me to be Ms. C's nurse as she has begun to cope with her many problems. It has been very satisfying to be a part of her progress and her road to health.

Program Evaluation

Program evaluation is conducted to inform administrators about the relevance and cost effectiveness of the services they offer. It is often required by funding, regulatory, and licensure agencies to confirm that public mental health dollars are being spent wisely.

Program evaluation is evolving as program funders and the public demand greater accountability from service providers. Community advisory boards, legislators, and consumer advocates are all recognizing the importance of reviewing the effectiveness of individual programs and service systems. As comprehensive community-based service systems for people with serious mental illnesses continue to grow, evaluation approaches will provide direction.

Summary

1. Psychiatric rehabilitation is the tertiary prevention process of helping the person who has a serious mental illness return to the highest possible level of functioning.
2. Assessment related to rehabilitative psychiatric nursing focuses on the individual, the family, and the community. Behaviors that are assessed include activities of daily living, interpersonal relations, self-esteem, motivation, strengths, and compliance. Family assessment focuses on family burden and social support needs.
3. Planning and implementation of rehabilitative psychiatric nursing care consist of developing strengths and potentials, learning living skills, and accessing environmental supports. Family intervention is built on empowerment and education. Nurses intervene at the community level by serving as advocates for mental health services and fighting stigma.
4. Evaluation takes place at the patient and program levels.

your **INTERNET**
connection

Mental Health Education Page: Removing the Stigma of Mental Illness
http://www.metrolink.net/˜jquimby/mh.htm

Alliance for the Mentally Ill/Friends and Advocates of the Mentally Ill
http://www.schizophrenia.com/ami/

Chapter Review Questions

1. Identify whether the following statements are true (T) or false (F).

A. ___ People who have serious mental illnesses and their families experience grief over the loss of potential life achievements.

B. ___ Serious mental illness prevents a person from being successful at work or school.

C. ___ Families of people with mental illness generally want and need to be involved with their ill family member.

D. ___ Consumers of mental health services should not be hired as providers of mental health services.

E. ___ Measures of skills and support, more than psychiatric diagnoses and symptom patterns, determine how well a person with a serious mental illness can function in the community.

2. Fill in the blanks.

A. Tertiary prevention is carried out by the performance of activities identified as _____.

B. The impact on the family of a member's mental illness is often called _____.

C. The process of moving long-term hospital patients to the community is called _____.

D. _____ is the use of cognitive and behavioral techniques to help people gain the knowledge and skills they need to live in the community.

E. The approach that supports the rehabilitation process by teaching the patient and family about the mental illness and the coping skills that will help with successful community living is called _____.

3. Provide short answers for the following questions.

A. Identify four common responses families have to the mental illness of a member.

B. Describe the three basic interventions used in psychiatric rehabilitation.

C. Think about someone you know who has a psychiatric illness. Relate three ways in which you, as a nurse, can help to empower this person and his or her family.

REFERENCES

1. Anthony WA: Psychiatric rehabilitation: key issues and future policy, *Health Aff* 11:164, 1992.
2. Becker D et al: Job preferences of clients with severe psychiatric disorders participating in supported employment programs, *Psychiatr Serv* 47:1223, 1996.
3. Besio SW, Mahler J: Benefits and challenges of using consumer staff in supported housing services, *Hosp Community Psychiatry* 44:490, 1993.
4. Biegel D, Song L, Milligan S: A comparative analysis of family caregivers' perceived relationships with mental health professionals, *Psychiatr Serv* 46:477, 1995.
5. Blankertz L, Robinson S: Adding a vocational focus to mental health rehabilitation, *Psychiatr Serv* 47:1216, 1996.
6. Byre C et al: Wellness education for individuals with chronic mental illness living in the community, *Issues Ment Health Nurs* 15:239, 1994.
7. Carling PJ: Housing and supports for persons with mental illness: emerging approaches to research and practice, *Hosp Community Psychiatry* 44:439, 1993.
8. Deegan PE: Recovering our sense of value after being labeled mentally ill, *J Psychosoc Nurs Ment Health Serv* 31:7, 1993.
9. Federal Task Force on Homelessness and Severe Mental Illness: *Outcasts on Main Street*, Washington, DC, 1992, Interagency Council on the Homeless.
10. Hatfield AB: Families as caregivers: a historical perspective. In Hatfield AB, Lefley HP, editors: *Families of the mentally ill: coping and adaptation*, New York, 1987, The Guilford Press.
11. Hatfield AB, Coursay R, Slaughter, J: Family responses to behavior manifestations of mental illness, *Innovations Res* 3:41, 1994.
12. Hazel KL, Herman SE, Mowbray CT: Characteristics of seriously mentally ill adults in a public mental health system, *Hosp Community Psychiatry* 42:518, 1991.
13. Lamb HR: Will we save the homeless mentally ill? *Am J Psychiatry* 147:649, 1990.
14. Maurin JT, Boyd CB: Burden of mental illness on the family: a critical review, *Arch Psychiatr Nurs* 4:99, 1990.
15. Moller M, Wer J: Simultaneous patient/family education regarding schizophrenia: the Nebraska model, *Arch Psychiatr Nurs* 3:332, 1989.
16. Mossman D, Perlin ML: Psychiatry and the homeless mentally ill: a reply to Dr. Lamb, *Am J Psychiatry* 149:951, 1992.
17. Murphy L, Gass-Sternas K, Knight K: Health of the chronically mentally ill who rejoin the community, *Issues Ment Health Nurs* 16:239, 1995.
18. National Mental Health Advisory Council: *Caring for people with severe mental disorders: a national plan of research to improve services*, Washington, DC, 1991, NIMH.
19. Newman S: The housing and neighborhood conditions of persons with severe mental illness, *Hosp Community Psychiatry* 45:338, 1994.
20. Norbeck J, Chafetz L, Skodol-Wilson H, Weiss SJ: Social support needs of family caregivers of psychiatric patients from three age groups, *Nurs Res* 40:208, 1991.
21. Okin RL, Pearsall D: Patients' perceptions of their quality of life 11 years after discharge from a state hospital, *Hosp Community Psychiatry* 44:236, 1993.
22. Palmer-Erbs V: Psychiatric rehabilitation: a breath of fresh air in a turbulent health-care environment, *J Psychosoc Nurs* 34:16, 1996.

23. Palmer-Erbs V, Anthony W: Incorporating psychiatric rehabilitation principles into mental health nursing, *J Psychosoc Nurs* 33:36, 1995.
24. Parker BA: Living with mental illness: the family as caregiver, *J Psychosoc Nurs Ment Health Serv* 31:19, 1993.
25. Peterson R: What are the needs of chronic mental patients? In Talbott J, editor: *The chronic mental patient: problems, solutions, and recommendations for a public policy,* Washington, DC, 1978, The American Psychiatric Association.
26. Pfeiffer EJ, Mostek M: Services for families of people with mental illness, *Hosp Community Psychiatry* 42:262, 1991.
27. Sartorius N: Rehabilitation and quality of life, *Hosp Community Psychiatry* 43:1180, 1992.
28. Segal SP, VanderVoort DJ: Daily hassles of persons with severe mental illness, *Hosp Community Psychiatry* 44:276, 1993.
29. Sherman PS, Porter R: Mental health consumers as case management aides, *Hosp Community Psychiatry* 42:494, 1991.
30. Steinwachs DM, Kasper JD, Skinner EA: Patterns of use and costs among severely mentally ill people, *Health Aff* 11:178, 1992.
31. Tanzman B: An overview of surveys of mental health consumers' preferences for housing and support services, *Hosp Community Psychiatry* 44:450, 1993.
32. Thompson J, Strand K: Psychiatric nursing in a psychosocial setting, *J Psychosoc Nurs* 32:25, 1994.
33. Uttaro T, Mechanic D: The NAMI consumer survey analysis of unmet needs, *Hosp Community Psychiatry* 45:372, 1994.
34. Vellenga B, Christenson J: Persistent and severely mentally ill clients' perceptions of their mental illness, *Issues Ment Health Nurs* 15:359, 1994.
35. Wallace CJ et al: Effectiveness and replicability of modules for teaching social and instrumental skills to the severely mentally ill, *Am J Psychiatry* 149:654, 1992.
36. Walsh M: *Schizophrenia: straight talk for families and friends,* New York, 1985, William Morrow.
37. Wasow M: The need for asylum revisited, *Hosp Community Psychiatry* 44:207, 1993.
38. Zipple A et al: Cognitive therapy interventions in psychosocial rehabilitation, *Innovations Res* 3:25, 1994.

ANNOTATED SUGGESTED READINGS

Bauer M, McBride L: Psychoeducation: conceptual framework and practical considerations, *J Practical Psychiatry Behav Health* 3:18, 1997.
  Presents two conceptual constructs that can help clinicians achieve more effective psychoeducation with those they treat—host factors and personal cost-benefit analysis—applying these to a case example. Highly recommended.

*Byre C et al: Wellness education for individuals with chronic mental illness living in the community, *Issues Ment Health Nurs* 15:239, 1994.
  Describes a nursing wellness education program for people with chronic mental illness living in the community.

Corrigan P, Garman A: Considerations for research on consumer empowerment and psychosocial interventions, *Psychiatr Serv* 48:347, 1997.
  Challenging discussion of the roles consumers can assume in psychosocial interventions based on a participatory action research framework. Worth reading for the nurse researcher.

*Fishbein S, Manos E, Rotteveel J: A unique colleague support system for mental health professionals-consumers, *J Psychosoc Nurs* 33:41, 1995.
  Describes a support group for "prosumers"—people who both practice in (professionals) and receive services from (consumers) the mental health system.

Fisher D: Health care reform based on an empowerment model of recovery by people with psychiatric disabilities, *Hosp Community Psychiatry* 45:913, 1994.
  Succinct overview and summary of the empowerment model of recovery from psychiatric disabilities.

*Francell E: My role as a consumer-provider: challenges and opportunities, *J Psychosoc Nurs,* 34:29, 1996.
  A first-person account by the author of his history of bipolar and panic disorders and how his experiences help him to help others.

Lamb H: A century and a half of psychiatric rehabilitation in the United States, *Hosp Community Psychiatry* 45:1015, 1994.
  Excellent and thorough historic overview of psychiatric rehabilitation, its theoretical basis, and current concerns about it.

Lefly H: Thinking about recovery: paradigms and pitfalls, *Innovations Res* 3:21, 1994.
  Thought-provoking discussion of the implications of a focus on recovery as a new paradigm of mental health care by a leader in the family advocacy movement.

*Palmer-Erbs V: Psychiatric rehabilitation: a breath of fresh air in a turbulent health care environment, *J Psychosoc Nurs* 34:16, 1996.
  Overview of psychiatric rehabilitation and the opportunity it offers psychiatric nurses to strengthen relationships and create partnerships among consumers of mental health services and their families, nurses, and other providers.

*Palmer-Erbs V et al: Nursing perspectives on disability and rehabilitation. In Anchor K: *Disability analysis Handbook,* Dubuque, Iowa, 1996, Kendall/Hunt.
  Detailed discussion of the perspective nurses bring and the roles they assume in psychosocial rehabilitation.

*Rogers S: National clearinghouse serves mental health consumer movement, *J Psychosoc Nurs* 34:22, 1996.
  Describes this national technical assistance center funded by the federal Center for Mental Health Services.

Salzer M: Consumer empowerment in mental health organizations: concept, benefits and impediments, *Admin Policy Mental Health* 24:425, 1997.
  Proposes a framework for consumer empowerment that involves consumer participation in organizational decision-making, program development and evaluation, access to resources, and opportunities for consumers to develop and run services. Thought-provoking reading.

*Starkey D et al: Inpatient psychiatric rehabilitation in a state hospital setting, *J Psychosoc Nurs* 35:10, 1997.
  Describes an inpatient psychiatric rehabilitation program for patients with serious and persistent mental illness.

Sullivan W: A long and winding road: the process of recovery from mental illness, *Innovations Res* 3:19, 1994.
  Informative report by mental health consumers of those activities, attitudes, and behaviors, initiated by self or others, that were essential to their recovery.

Zipple A et al: Cognitive therapy interventions in psychosocial rehabilitation, *Innovations Res* 3:25, 1994.
  In a practical way, applies cognitive therapy to psychiatric rehabilitation. Good examples of specific interventions.

*Nursing reference.

© 1998 M.C. Escher/Cordon Art, Baarn, Holland.

Chapter 15

The Family's View of the Continuum of Care

Victoria Conn

To multiply the harbors does not reduce the sea. **Emily Dickinson**

LEARNING OBJECTIVES	TOPICAL OUTLINE
After studying this chapter the student should be able to: ▼ **Identify barriers in working with families of persons with mental illness** ▼ **Describe ways to help families in the caregiving of a relative with mental illness** ▼ **Analyze ways to help families across the continuum of psychiatric care**	**Barriers to Care** **Building Bridges** **Anticipating Needs**

Ever since Florence Nightingale, nurses have involved family members in the care of patients with heart disease, cancer, diabetes, and similar disorders. In contrast, the families of patients with mental illnesses were for many years considered to be part of the problem, not part of the solution. Today, new models of working with families and involving family members in the continuum of care are becoming accepted practices. This chapter hopes to sensitize psychiatric nurses to the family's perspective.

BARRIERS TO CARE

An elderly woman was admitted to the hospital from a nursing home because she was having visual hallucinations. The nurse who was assigned to her took time to talk with the patient's son whenever he visited. After a period of treatment limited to vitamin therapy, the patient no longer hallucinated. However, after discharge orders were written, the patient confided that she was again "seeing the little fuzzy animals." The nurse told the son that the doctor had recently prescribed Elavil for the patient's mild depression. With an Eureka expression, he exclaimed, "But Elavil is the medicine she was taking in the nursing home!"

Busy staff may think they have no time to spend with family members. However, as this clinical example shows, making time for contact with families can expedite successful outcomes. When family members are excluded, this opportunity for collaboration is lost. All models of mental illness acknowledge the concept of the interactive family system. According to the vulnerability-stress-coping model, which assumes that symptoms arise at the interface of bio-

264

logical vulnerabilities and environmental stressors, the patient's symptoms can trigger responses in anyone who shares his or her social space, including family members. By the same token, the patient's symptoms can be triggered by interactions with anyone in his or her environment.

Family system theories were used in the 1960s to explain how certain family members, known as identified patients, became and remained symptomatic. Unfortunately, the early researchers made unwarranted assumptions about cause and effect that were pejorative to families. If an ill child relied too much on his or her mother, that was because the mother needed to have someone dependent on her. Parents with unstable marriages were said to need the child's illness in order to hold the marriage together. The unidirectionality of cause and effect was so firmly entrenched that alternative explanations for symptomatology were not explored, families were negatively stereotyped, and the relationship between professionals and families became one of mutual mistrust.

One mother, referring to a past intake interview by a competent and even empathetic social worker, stated, "She was very nice, but I could tell by the questions she asked that she was trying to find out where we had gone wrong." . . . This mother went home and spent a tearful, sleepless night worrying about the things she might have done to cause her son to develop schizophrenia.[1]

My daughter stayed up all night cutting pictures out of magazines to make collages on the outside of manila envelopes. She told me excitedly that she had invented "self-mailing Valentines." I telephoned her doctor, who had recently reduced the dosage of her lithium. Before I could explain, he expressed displeasure that it was I who had made the call and asked to talk to his patient. When she got on the phone, she managed to sound completely normal. Afterwards, she told me, "My doctor thinks you exaggerate because you're a nurse and you need me to be your little patient." He didn't increase the lithium, and a week later she was re-hospitalized.[3]

Another barrier to family-professional collaboration is the fear that establishing an alliance with the family will interfere with the therapeutic alliance with the patient. This is a reasonable assumption under some circumstances, but not always. In the case of a potentially lifetime disorder, the family is likely to be available to the patient longer than any given provider, and allying with the family is a way of ensuring continuity of care. A key issue here is the family's de facto involvement in caregiving. If the patient is receiving caregiving from family members or depends on them for needed services such as housing, failure to involve the family in related decisions is unfair to both the family and the patient.

The discharge plan for a young, single, pregnant woman who was suffering from depression and addiction to cocaine called for her and the future baby to live with her elderly parents. When the parents came in to visit, they were stunned to learn that the discharge date had been changed, and she would be coming home the following day. This was a unilateral decision made by the daughter and her doctor, with no input from the parents.

Perhaps a more controversial issue is confidentiality, which can pose a dilemma to professionals who are seemingly caught between the patient's right to a confidential therapeutic relationship and the family caregiver's right to information. However, there is a distinction between nonconfidential information, which includes diagnostic criteria, treatment modalities, and possible prognosis, and confidential information, which is information that is specific to the particular patient. Professionals should have no problem giving any family nonconfidential information about mental illness because it is public knowledge. If this particular family is providing caregiving services to the patient, they are entitled, like professional caregivers, to all the information they need to support the caregiving role.[9]

Even when a treatment objective involves increasing the patient's autonomy and separation from the family, there are advantages to family involvement. Such a plan is more likely to be carried out if the parents and other relatives understand the goal, agree with it, and contribute their ideas as to how it can be achieved.

Obviously, not all patients with serious mental illness have family members who are willing or able to provide care. The crux of the matter is that for patients requiring long-term treatment and support, family involvement should be the rule, not the exception.

BUILDING BRIDGES

The National Alliance for the Mentally Ill (NAMI) is conducting a national public education campaign to end discrimination against people with mental illness and to educate the public to recognize the prodromal signs so that early detection and prompt, appropriate treatment will become standard practice. Parents, spouses, and other family members are typically the first to recognize that something is wrong, but are unable to determine what that "something" is. Family members in daily contact with their relative notice changes in appetite or sleep patterns, loss of interest in favorite pastimes, slipping performance in school or at work, unexpected religiosity, or social withdrawal. But with the exception of those who already have experienced a psychiatric illness in the family, rarely do they connect these changes with mental illness.

We thought at first he was just having a difficult adolescence. Then we thought he might be into drugs. But mental illness? Not in our family!

When our daughter got religious and started sending hundred dollar bills to Jim and Tammy Baker, we assumed she was just another born again Christian.

But by the time a crisis precipitates the patient's admission into an emergency room or treatment setting, most family members have correctly interpreted these early signs. Their contribution to the patient's history can provide important clues for the appropriate diagnosis and treatment. In the absence of such input, because there are no laboratory tests or other independent measures for these illnesses, important decisions must be based solely on the patient's self-report and presenting behavior. The family's contribution takes on added significance if they have had experience with another ill family member. Close relatives often have similar responses to treatment: If a particular medication has been effective with the patient's relative, it is well worth a trial.

In many cases, however, the family is dealing with this type of crisis for the first time. Nurses and other professionals should be aware that under the circumstances, family members probably are not functioning at their best. They may have been up all night trying to get their relative to agree to come in for evaluation. If the police have been involved, the circumstances have probably been harrowing. Chances are good that the family members will need emotional support, a comfortable place to wait, and perhaps food and drink. The way professionals respond to these needs will make a lasting impression on the family.

> *When I brought my husband to the emergency room for a psychiatric evaluation, I was allowed to accompany him into the cubicle where he was examined. When he shouted that he didn't want me there, the nurse moved me to a nearby spot where he couldn't see me, but I could still hear what was going on. I will always be grateful that they listened to what I had to say, and for how kindly they treated me. If they hadn't done that, I might have needed to be hospitalized myself!*

Later, when things have settled down, family members should be informally assessed for their mental and physical status. Many will need clinical or nonclinical preventive services for themselves, including information about the illness, referral to support groups, and perhaps therapy for individual family members. Some hospitals have established Family Resource Centers that provide educational materials and a place to meet and talk with other families in similar circumstances.

Informed family members who see the patient on a daily basis can provide professionals with information to supplement their own observations, and sometimes they may be more reliable informants than the patient. This was the case when a patient hid his symptoms from his therapist because he wanted her to think that he was profiting from treatment:

> *My brother who lives with us was seeing a therapist once a week, and we couldn't figure out why his only treatment was talking to the therapist and reading books the therapist recommended. He really wasn't even reading the books because he couldn't concentrate. He was hearing voices almost all the time. Finally, I called the therapist and told her what was going on. She was surprised, because my brother hadn't told her he was still hearing voices.*

Confronted with the fragmentation of community resources, and before the widespread use of case managers,

many family caregivers assumed the case manager role by default. Just as families of people with multiple sclerosis help their relatives make necessary adjustments in their lives, families dealing with serious mental illnesses did what they could to help. It is hard to say which is the greater challenge: severe, progressively disabling disorders such as multiple sclerosis, or brain disorders that affect the mental processes without an outward sign of disability. Families who have experienced both situations agree that society treats them differently.

> *I had two sons, one with multiple sclerosis and one with schizophrenia. The one with multiple sclerosis became totally dependent on us for dressing, bathing, and everything else, but he earned a doctoral degree. He was given every kind of assistance: a van to transport his wheelchair, student aides, and a computer. When he was awarded his degree, the whole audience stood up and cheered. Our son with schizophrenia was just as intelligent, but he dropped out of college. No medication helped him, and he began wandering. He got arrested for causing a disturbance in a public place and died under mysterious circumstances in jail.*

The subjective and objective burden of living with a loved one for whom effective treatment has not been found has been called "mourning without end." At the same time, some families say their lives have been tempered in the crucible of experience.

> *We experience this terrible feeling of loss and grieve for the son we knew. We feel cheated out of watching him mature and flower the way adolescents do as they grow into young adults. When I meet his former classmates who are now working, finishing graduate degrees, or married, I am always aware that these things are not possible for him, just the same as someone would feel had their son died. Yet this mourning is strange, because Gary is not dead at all. He is very much still with us, seemingly eternally 13 years old, needing care and attention.[12]*

> *In the dark soul of the night, I grieve for all of us—for the anguish of the past and the present, and the uncertainty of the future. Most of all, I grieve for my son, for his lost hopes and expectations. At the same time, we have emerged from this emotional holocaust as better, stronger, and more tolerant people.*

ANTICIPATING NEEDS

Many family members are candidates for preventive services, but few ever receive them. Parents, children, and siblings are at risk on two counts: heredity and environment. Spouses escape the heredity factor, but are very much affected by living in a stressful environment. Psychoanalysts used to call the intraspousal transfer of symptoms *folie á deux.* Currently, members of support groups for well spouses facetiously refer to their spouses' symptoms as "contagious." A writer who has a son with schizophrenia has compared the ripple effect of mental illness on the family to a large stone skipping across water.[11] The response of members of the family subsystem has been movingly described by Agnes Hatfield, an educator who is a former president of NAMI (Box 15-1).[5]

In the wake of the Oklahoma City bombing, nurses were

Box **15-1** *The Meaning of Mental Illness to the Family*

When a loved one is stricken with mental illness, every member of the family feels pain. Whether the patient is your mother, father, son, daughter, sister, brother, grandchild, or grandparent, you share in his suffering. But you have other feelings that confuse and frighten you.

Before the doctors gave you a diagnosis, you probably went through a long period of uncertainty—trying to make sense of what was happening. You were stunned and bewildered. You hoped that the odd behavior and scary talk would stop, that soon things would be back to normal. Maybe a crisis occurred.

In one way or another, your family member was brought to treatment. Once the diagnosis was made, you began asking questions: "Will my loved one get better and lead a normal life again?" "What have I done wrong?" "Why did this happen to me, to us?"

Your questions and your feelings are quite natural. Your grief, shame, and anger, your sense of helplessness, your hours of anxiety: All are shared by others going through similar experiences. But depending on your relationship to the mentally ill family member, you also have feelings that are not shared by others.

Perhaps it is your child who has fallen ill. Suddenly a promising young person, on the threshold of becoming an adult, takes a sharp turn. Now there is a stranger in your midst. Your once happy and content son or daughter becomes withdrawn, unkempt, and unable to function. He argues, destroys possessions, says and does things that make no sense. You, like other parents, want to protect and nurture your child. When your desire is thwarted, you feel that you have failed. Perhaps you blame him. Such feelings are not unique to parents of mentally ill persons. Parents of children with severe physical illnesses such as cancer or heart disease also tend to blame themselves, to harbor feelings of resentment toward the victim. Because mental illness affects such intensely personal aspects of our being, it is not surprising that parents of mental patients do likewise. Professionals—often unwittingly—may augment your guilt by blaming you for the tragedy

When it is your spouse who becomes mentally ill you have special problems. This is, after all, the person you chose to marry: your mate, companion, and lover. Not only do once-shared responsibilities fall solely on you, but you must try to find help for your spouse. Perhaps help is not welcomed. Without diminishing your partner's status, you must juggle the roles of mother, father, homemaker, and breadwinner all at once.

Other family members may escape the responsibilities that fall to a parent or spouse of the mentally ill person, but they share equally painful feelings. Brothers and sisters are bewildered, hurt, and sometimes ashamed and angry. Grandparents are perplexed and saddened. Adult children find it difficult to assume the role of caretaker when a parent becomes incompetent.

One out of four families has a close relative who is mentally ill. They, like you, typically go through a period of intense searching. Patients, family members, and doctors alike tend to place blame—to identify an event or a person responsible for the breakdown. "Why me?" is an understandable cry.

In time, most families come to accept the illness. Somehow, they find resources to sustain themselves over the rocky period. Many become stronger in the process. When they look back over years of living with chronic mental illness, they almost invariably remember the earliest period as the hardest. They may have been surprised by the amount of energy, resourcefulness, and courage they were able to muster. They come to feel pride in their capacity to face tragedy and conquer defeat.

While no cure is now known for the more severe, chronic mental illnesses, almost everyone can be helped to live worthwhile and meaningful lives. Caring relatives must continue to hope for improvement, set reasonable expectations, and maintain faith in the patient's recuperative and restorative powers. Realities change. What may have been impossible at one time may become quite possible. There will be regressions, plateaus when all anyone can expect to do is "hang on," and forward movement.

A short time ago families who had known mental illness for a long time were asked how it affected them. As might be expected, many reported the negative consequences. But many also saw positive changes in their lives. One mother said she no longer takes life for granted. "I've learned to appreciate the little things in life," she said. "I make it a point to find something to enjoy each day." Other family members reported that they were more compassionate, less judgmental, more understanding of others. Most had made what they considered a more mature reevaluation of their lives, thereby achieving a truer vision of what really counts. They believed that their lives had become more significant, more basic, more meaningful.

Most families, in short, found they had wellsprings of strength they never knew they had until they met the great challenge of mental illness.

From Hatfield A: *Coping with mental illness in the family: a family guide,* Arlington, VA, 1986, The National Alliance for the Mentally Ill.

deployed to care for the victims and to minister to the victims' shocked and grieving families. Serious mental illness can be a comparable catastrophe, and the victims' families suffer a trauma that has been likened to posttraumatic stress syndrome. The reaction differs according to the person's relationship. Aging parents who expected an "empty nest" populated occasionally by visiting grandchildren find themselves in their fifties, sixties, and seventies, sharing the nest with and caring for their adult children. In addition to accepting that their dreams for their child must be dramatically revised, these parents must learn, often by trial and error, to coexist with loved ones whose moods and behaviors

are often baffling and sometimes dangerous. It is not surprising when newsletters of family support groups report heart attacks or strokes suffered in response to a relative's sudden relapse, suicide attempt, or encounter with the law. Less dramatic, but equally unfortunate, are the family members suffering depression, undergoing separation or divorce, or becoming alcoholics or drug users.

Well siblings attracted the attention of early researchers primarily because they had escaped the illness. The question was, "How did the schizophrenogenic mother manage to raise well children?" Some theorized that the siblings were only superficially normal; others surmised that they escaped major pathology by detaching themselves from the family, or because they were neglected by their mothers.

Contemporary researchers have made similar observations, but different interpretations, about the status of siblings. Many surveys have revealed that siblings do suffer problems in living attributable to their family experience, but this has nothing to do with the schizophrenogenic mother hypothesis. The reality is that because the emotional and financial resources of the family are devoted disproportionally to meet the needs of ill siblings, the well siblings' share of the family bounty is decreased. They may resent this, but cannot express their resentment because of survivor's guilt. Consequently, some siblings detach from the family, move thousands of miles away, or become members of helping professions. Others remain involved, often at the expense of career and marriage options.

The 37-year-old sister of a woman diagnosed with schizophrenia graduated from a hospital school of nursing instead of a more expensive college program. She lives in the family home and divides her time between work and being a liaison between her sister's professional caregivers and her parents. Weekends are devoted to her sister, who comes home from the hospital on pass. Of the few men she has dated, none has survived the sister test.

In many ways, the tribulations of well siblings and the offspring of ill parents are similar because in both situations, children and adolescents may be deprived, unintentionally, of needed parental attention. It is ironic that professional caregivers who are very knowledgeable about the effects of childhood trauma in general terms are largely unaware of the specific difficulties faced by children in families preoccupied with mental illness.

The neglect of the children of mothers with serious mental illness begins prenatally. Because of the shift from institutional to community care, there are now significant increases in the number of women with serious mental illness who become pregnant. These women often receive inadequate care because of the lack of coordination between psychiatric services and obstetrical/gynecological services. A women's program at the University of Illinois at Chicago that provides comprehensive prenatal and postpartum psychiatric care for women with severe mental illness received the American Psychiatric Association's 1996 Gold Award because their services were out of the ordinary.

Despite the known risks for the offspring of parents with mental illness, there are very few programs to help them through their developmental stages without problems. The 10% of children who presumably inherit the parent's vulnerability for the illness are often identified when they exhibit emotional problems or conduct disorders in school. However, the remaining 90% seldom come to the attention of mental health professionals unless they seek help as adults, in response to problems in living. Their interpersonal legacy imprints their adult relationships. Possible problems with identity and self-esteem leave them unsure of themselves and uneasily dependent on the approval of others. There may be difficulties with trust and intimacy, an excessive need for perfectionism and control, and a reluctance to make a long-term commitment.

Celebrities such as Marilyn Monroe epitomize both the vulnerabilities and the strengths of offspring. Monroe's ill mother was unable to care for her, and her grandmother, who also had schizophrenia, tried to suffocate her with a pillow when she was 13 months old.[7] Her entire life was haunted by these family ghosts, yet she became one of the most famous actresses of all time.

Box **15-2** *Family Involvement Competencies for Mental Health Professionals*

DEVELOPING A COLLABORATION WITH THE FAMILY
Make a positive first contact
Identify family's needs
Address confidentiality

OFFERING INFORMATION ON MENTAL ILLNESS
Diagnosis, etiology, prognosis, treatments
Long-term course of serious mental illness
Educational sessions

ENHANCING FAMILY COMMUNICATION AND PROBLEM SOLVING
Teach principles of effective communication
Teach problem-solving strategies

HELPING WITH SERVICE SYSTEM USE
Help access entitlements, support, and rehabilitation
Explain the roles of different mental health providers
Establish needed linkages
Translate the language of mental health services
Help access crisis services
Help access housing

HELPING FAMILY MEMBERS MEET OWN NEEDS
Help family members access support services
Understand burden and grief
Assess for stress-related disorders
Offer services or referrals
Encourage self-care
Encourage advocacy

ADDRESSING SPECIAL ISSUES CONCERNING THE PATIENT
Treatment is not working
Illness is of recent onset
Patient has multiple diagnoses
Patient is in jail
Patient refuses treatment

ADDRESSING SPECIAL ISSUES CONCERNING THE FAMILY
The family does not speak English
The family is very important or of high status in the community
The family belongs to an ethnic minority
The family is missing
The family is disinterested

Modified from Glynn S, Liberman R, Backer T: *Involving families in mental health services: competencies for mental health workers,* Los Angeles, 1997, Human Interaction Research Institute.

Six mental health professionals whose mothers or fathers had serious mental illnesses recently contributed their personal accounts to *The Journal of the California Alliance for the Mentally Ill.* Secrecy was their common theme. As children, they were instructed not to talk about the parents' illnesses, and no one talked to them about them. As adults, they were determined to draw attention to the unmet needs of children who face difficult challenges, often with minimal psychological and practical resources at their disposal.

I realize that I had to grow up fast as a child. I recognize that my mother's illness deprived me of having any sort of a carefree, normal childhood. Periodically, I have been angry at one or both of my parents for the atmosphere at home. [2]

As a child it was often difficult to know which of my mother's behaviors were normal and which were due to the illness. [6]

Daddy always had to tell us, "Don't step off the curb!" before we left for school. I was so used to it, it was such a part of my daily routine, that I never realized the absurdity of it. [8]

The professor had just finished a compressed overview on what was known about schizophrenia. "Oh my God!" I gasped, to myself. "That's what my father has." [10]

Diane Marsh, a psychologist and member of NAMI, suggests the following ways for professionals to help young people living in families with mental illness:

▼ Become informed about the family experience of mental illness.

▼ Strengthen and support the family system.

▼ Reach out as early as possible and assure them they are not to blame.

▼ Address the needs of young family members in an age-appropriate manner.

▼ Enlist the help of teachers, principals, guidance counselors, and school psychologists.

▼ Assure them that their needs matter and support their goals.

▼ Offer counseling for those who are experiencing particular difficulty.

Finally, a number of study groups have been commissioned to identify the professional competencies that are required to provide services within this framework. One of these studies, funded by the Center for Mental Health Services and conducted by the Human Interaction Research Institute with the collaboration of the National Alliance for the Mentally Ill, focused specifically on the competencies needed by mental health professionals in order to involve families in treatment. Seven family involvement competencies, listed in Box 15-2, were adapted from the Human Interaction Research Institute report *Involving Families in Mental Health Services: Competencies for Mental Health Workers.* [4] Psychiatric nurses should assess themselves on their ability to reach out to families of those with mental illness in each of these important areas.

Summary

1. Involving the family members of patients with serious mental illnesses in the continuum of care should be standard practice, not only because it benefits the patient, but because it enables the nurse to identify and meet the clinical and nonclinical needs of family members who, because of heredity and environment, are at risk for mental illness and other stress-related disorders. These services to family members should cross the continuum and be preventive, crisis-oriented, and rehabilitative in nature.

2. Patient and family education should be considered a medical necessity because after the treatment has reduced symptoms, the recovering person must reintegrate into appropriate social roles. Family involvement is essential, because families are the natural launching pad for entry or re-entry into the community.

3. This chapter was intended to convey a sense of the continuum of care from the family's perspective. With each new encounter with a patient and family, the psychiatric nurse has a choice: Will it be to fortify the walls, build bridges, or walk with patients and families to new horizons of mental health care?

your **INTERNET**
connection

NAMI: National Alliance for the Mentally Ill
http://www.nami.org

help! A Consumer's Guide to Mental Health Information
http://www.iComm.ca/madmagic/help/help.html

?Chapter Review Questions

1. What preventive strategies from Chapter 12 can you use with the siblings of a patient who is mentally ill?

2. How can families serve as balancing factors, as described in Chapter 13, in helping a person with mental illness who is in crisis?

3. In what ways can the rehabilitative interventions detailed in Chapter 14 be enhanced by including family members?

4. Talk with the family of a psychiatric patient. Listen to their story of how psychiatric illness has affected their lives.

REFERENCES

1. Anderson CM, Reise DJ, Hogarty G: *Schizophrenia and the Family,* New York, 1986, Guilford Press.
2. Bruge D: Thoughts about my mother, *J Calif Alliance Mentally Ill* 7:15, 1996.
3. Francell C, Conn V, Gray P: Families of the chronically mentally ill, *Hosp Community Psychiatry* 39:212, 1988.
4. Glynn S, Liberman R, Backer T: *Involving families in mental health services: competencies for mental health workers,* Los Angeles, 1997, Human Interaction Research Institute.
5. Hatfield A: *Coping with mental illness in the family: a family guide,* Arlington, VA, 1986, The National Alliance for the Mentally Ill.
6. List A: On becoming authentic: a daughter's story, *J Calif Alliance Mentally Ill* 7:37, 1996.
7. Marshall L: Marilyn Monroe: a child of mental illness, *J Calif Alliance Mentally Ill* 7:31, 1996.
8. Poe S: Sailing similar seas, *J Calif Alliance Mentally Ill* 7:16, 1996.
9. Solomon P: Moving from psychoeducation to family education for families of adults with serious mental illness, *Psychiatr Serv* 47:1364, 1996.
10. Steinert P: Why didn't you tell me? *J Calif Alliance Mentally Ill* 7:22, 1996.
11. Wasow M: *The skipping stone: ripple effects of mental illness in the family,* Palo Alto, CA, 1995, Science and Behavior Books.
12. Willick M: Mourning without end. In Andreasen N, editor: *Schizophrenia: mind to molecule,* Washington, DC, 1994, American Psychiatric Press.

ANNOTATED SUGGESTED READINGS

*Doornbos M: The strengths of families coping with serious mental illness, *Arch Psychiatr Nurs* 10:214, 1996.
  Presents research on an important but often forgotten aspect of the clear strengths families possess and their skills related to coping, adaptability, and conflict management.
Jennings A: On being invisible in the mental health system, *J Mental Health Administration* 21:374, 1994.
  This case study, written by a mother about her daughter's sexual abuse as a child and her subsequent experiences as a chronically mentally ill patient, challenges the dominant treatment focus on biology and proposes a new trauma paradigm for the field.
Lefly H: *Family caregiving in mental illness,* Thousand Oaks, Calif, 1996, Sage Publications.

*Nursing reference.

  Superb reference book that should be read by all nurses who need background on how families get blamed, the elements of family burden, the phases of the family cycle, and much more.
Lefly H: *Helping families cope with mental illness,* New York, 1994, Harwood Academic Publishers.
  A "must read" book that covers many perspectives on how professionals can work collaboratively with families.
*Rose L: Families of psychiatric patients: a critical review and future research directions, *Arch Psychiatr Nurs* 10:67, 1996.
  Critical examination of research and identification of gaps in knowledge related to family experience of mental illness. It argues for the need to continue studies of caregiver burden and the resulting stress and suggests future directions for research.
*Saunders J: Walking a mile in their shoes. . . symbolic interactionism for families living with severe mental illness, *J Psychosoc Nurs* 35:8, 1997.
  Excellent article challenging nurses to use the framework of symbolic interactionism to understand how families with mentally ill members define their experiences.
Solomon P: Moving from psychoeducation to family education for families of adults with serious mental illness, *Psychiatr Serv* 47:1364, 1996.
  Good review of psychoeducation and family education in both program structure and effectiveness with suggestions for future policy, program, and research directions for family interventions.
*Tuck I, duMont P, Evans G, Shupe J: The expereince of caring for an adult child with schizophrenia, *Arch Psychiatr Nurs* 11:118, 1997.
  Phenomenological research reporting on how the diagnosis of schizophrenia in a child is experienced by the parent as a destructive force that transforms the family. Implications are discussed and applied to community-based, family-centered mental health care.
Wasow M: *The skipping stone: ripple effects of mental illness on the family,* Palo Alto, Calif, 1995, Science and Behavior Books.
  Content based on findings from the interviews of family members of people with severe mental illness about effects of the illness on members of their immediate and extended family.
Wright E: The impact of organizational factors on mental health professionals' involvement with families, *Psychiatr Serv* 48:921, 1997.
  Identifies the important ways in which attitudinal, occupational, and organizational factors impact on mental health professionals' involvement with patients' families. Thought provoking research.

Applying Principles in Nursing Practice

Have you thought that most people with psychiatric problems were suffering from schizophrenia? Did you ever suspect that one of your friends or family members had an emotional or psychiatric problem but dismissed the idea as impossible? Have you ever worried about the barometer of your own mental health but felt embarrassed to discuss it? If you have answered "yes" to any of these questions, you are in for an awakening. The fact is that almost half of all Americans experience some type of psychiatric problem in their lifetime. Most of these problems are not what nurses commonly think of as a psychiatric illness, but anxiety disorders, mood disorders, and substance use disorders are by far the most common psychiatric disorders, and they are experienced by people more often than many physical illnesses. They are disabling disorders that cause people significant distress, yet they are often underdiagnosed and undertreated. These facts are more than interesting. They suggest that health care professionals need a wide variety of educational and treatment strategies to address these issues.

In this unit you will explore the adaptive and maladaptive coping responses used by people experiencing stress. Some of what you read will surprise you, some of it will concern you, and it is hoped that most of it will intrigue you. It is important that you understand, however, that these psychiatric problems are a common part of the human experience. As such, they merit careful study and consideration by psychiatric nurses like yourself.

Anxiety Responses and Anxiety Disorders

Gail W. Stuart

© 1998 M.C. Escher/Cordon Art, Baarn, Holland.

The fears we know are of not knowing. . . . It is getting late. Shall we ever be asked for? Are we simply not wanted at all? **WH Auden** *The Age of Anxiety*

LEARNING OBJECTIVES

After studying this chapter the student should be able to:

▼ Describe the continuum of adaptive and maladaptive anxiety responses

▼ Identify behaviors associated with anxiety responses

▼ Analyze predisposing factors, precipitating stressors, and appraisal of stressors related to anxiety responses

▼ Describe coping resources and coping mechanisms related to anxiety responses

▼ Formulate nursing diagnoses for patients related to anxiety responses

▼ Assess the relationship between nursing diagnoses and medical diagnoses related to anxiety responses

▼ Identify expected outcomes and short-term nursing goals related to anxiety responses

▼ Develop a patient education plan to promote the relaxation response

▼ Analyze nursing interventions related to anxiety responses

▼ Evaluate nursing care related to anxiety responses

TOPICAL OUTLINE

During the past 20 years, anxiety, a pervasive aspect of contemporary life, has been the subject of more than 600 articles or books. Between 10% and 25% of the population of the United States suffers from an anxiety disorder[17] (Box 16-1). Anxiety has always existed, however, and belongs to no particular era or culture. It derives from the Greek root meaning "to press tight." *Anxious* is related to the Latin word *angere,* which means "to strangle" and "to distress." It resembles the word *anger,* when defined as "grief" or "trouble." It is also related to *anguish,* which is described as "acute pain, suffering, or distress." It involves one's body, perceptions of self, and relationships with others, making it a foundational concept in the study of psychiatric nursing and human behavior.

CONTINUUM OF ANXIETY RESPONSES

In a classic work, May[18] defines anxiety as "diffuse apprehension that is vague in nature and associated with feelings of uncertainty and helplessness." Feelings of isolation, alienation, and insecurity are also present. The person perceives that the core of his or her personality is being threatened. Experiences provoking anxiety begin in infancy and continue throughout life. They end with the fear of the greatest unknown, death.

Defining Characteristics

Anxiety is an emotion and a subjective individual experience. It is an energy and therefore cannot be observed directly. A nurse infers that a patient is anxious based on certain behaviors. The nurse needs to validate this with the patient. Also, anxiety is an emotion without a specific object. It is provoked by the unknown and precedes all new experiences such as entering school, starting a new job, or giving birth to a child.

Box **16-1** *The Prevalence of Anxiety Disorders*

Anxiety disorders are the most common psychiatric disorders in America.
▼ More than 23 million people are afflicted by these debilitating illnesses each year (approximately one out of every four individuals).
▼ Anxiety disorders cost the United States $46.6 billion in 1990 in direct and indirect costs, nearly one third of the nation's total mental health bill of $148 billion.
▼ People with panic disorder spend heavily on health services. One survey found that a patient with panic attacks made an average of 37 medical visits a year, as compared with 5 visits in the general population.
▼ Less than 25% of panic disorder sufferers seek help—mainly because they do not realize their physical symptoms, such as heart palpitations, chest pains, and shortness of breath, are caused by a psychiatric problem.

This characteristic of anxiety differentiates it from fear. **Fear** has a specific source or object that the person can identify and describe. Fear involves the *intellectual appraisal* of a threatening stimulus; anxiety is the *emotional response* to that appraisal. A fear is caused by physical or psychological exposure to a threatening situation. Fear produces anxiety. The two emotions are differentiated in speech; we speak of *having* a fear but of *being* anxious.

Anxiety is communicated interpersonally. If a nurse is talking with a patient who is anxious, within a short time the nurse will also experience feelings of anxiety. Similarly, if a nurse is anxious in a particular situation, this will be readily communicated to the patient. The contagious nature of anxiety can therefore have positive and negative effects on the therapeutic relationship. The nurse must carefully monitor these effects. It is also important to remember that anxiety is part of everyday life. It is basic to the human condition and provides a valuable warning. In fact, the capacity to be anxious is necessary for survival.

The crux of anxiety is self-preservation. Anxiety occurs as a result of a threat to a person's selfhood, self-esteem, or identity. It results from a threat to something central to one's personality and essential to one's existence and security. It may be connected with the fear of punishment, disapproval, withdrawal of love, disruption of a relationship, isolation, or loss of body functioning. Anxiety is experienced when the values a person identifies with existence are threatened. Culture is related to anxiety because culture can influence the values one considers most important. Underlying every fear is the anxiety of losing one's own being. This is the frightening element, but a person can meet the anxiety and grow from it to the extent that the person's values are stronger than the threat.

All people need a balance between courage and anxiety to preserve themselves, fulfill their beings, and affirm their existence. It is only by moving through anxiety-creating experiences that a person achieves self-realization. As May[18] summarizes it, "The positive aspects of selfhood develop as the individual confronts, moves through, and overcomes anxiety-creating experiences."

? *Name two situations that provoke anxiety in you. Compare these to two situations that stimulate fear in you.*

Levels of Anxiety

Peplau[21] identified four levels of anxiety and described their effects:
▼ **Mild anxiety** is associated with the tension of day-to-day living. During this stage the person is alert and the perceptual field is increased. The person sees, hears, and grasps more than before. This kind of anxiety can motivate learning and produce growth and creativity.

▼ **Moderate anxiety,** in which the person focuses only on immediate concerns, involves the narrowing of the perceptual field as the person sees, hears, and grasps less. The person blocks out selected areas but can attend to more if directed to do so.

▼ **Severe anxiety** is marked by a significant reduction in the perceptual field. The person tends to focus on a specific detail and not think about anything else. All behavior is aimed at relieving anxiety, and much direction is needed to focus on another area.

▼ **Panic** is associated with awe, dread, and terror. At this stage details are blown out of proportion. Because of a complete loss of control, the person is unable to do things even with direction. Panic involves the disorganization of the personality. A person can no longer function as an organized human being. There is increased motor activity, decreased ability to relate to others, distorted perceptions, and loss of rational thought. Panic is a frightening and paralyzing experience. The person in panic is unable to communicate or function effectively. This level of anxiety cannot persist indefinitely because it is incompatible with life. A prolonged period of panic would result in exhaustion and death. Little attention has been focused on panic in the nursing literature, yet it is a common and debilitating phenomenon that can be safely and effectively treated.[2,14,25]

The nurse needs to be able to identify which level of anxiety a patient is experiencing by the behaviors observed. Fig. 16-1 shows the range of anxiety responses from the most adaptive response of anticipation to the most maladaptive response of panic. The patient's level of anxiety and its position on the continuum of coping responses is relevant to the nursing diagnosis and influences the type of intervention the nurse implements.

Assessment

Behaviors

Anxiety can be expressed directly through physiological and behavioral changes or indirectly through the formation of symptoms or coping mechanisms developed as a defense against anxiety. The nature of the behaviors displayed depends on the level of anxiety. The intensity of the behaviors increases with increasing anxiety.

In describing anxiety's effects on **physiological responses,** mild and moderate anxiety heighten the person's capacities. Conversely, severe and panic levels paralyze or overwork capacities. The physiological responses associated with anxiety are modulated primarily by the brain through the autonomic nervous system (Fig. 16-2). The body adjusts internally without a conscious or voluntary effort. Two types of autonomic responses exist:

▼ Parasympathetic responses, which conserve body responses

▼ Sympathetic responses, which activate body processes

Studies support the predominance of the sympathetic reaction. This reaction prepares the body to deal with an emergency situation by a fight or flight reaction. It can also trigger the general adaptation syndrome, as described by Selye. When the cortex of the brain perceives a threat, it sends a stimulus down the sympathetic branch of the autonomic nervous system to the adrenal glands. Because of a release of epinephrine, respiration deepens, the heart beats more rapidly, and arterial pressure rises. Blood is shifted away from the stomach and intestines to the heart, central nervous system, and muscle. Glycogenolysis is accelerated and the blood glucose level rises. For some people, however, the parasympathetic reaction may coexist or predominate and produce opposite effects. Other physiological reactions may also be evident. The variety of physiological responses to anxiety that the nurse may observe in patients are summarized in Box 16-2.

Psychomotor manifestations, or **behavioral responses,** are also observed in the anxious patient. Their effects have both personal and interpersonal aspects. High levels of anxiety affect coordination, involuntary movements, and responsiveness and can also disrupt human relationships. In an interpersonal situation anxiety can warn a person to withdraw from a situation where discomfort is anticipated. The anxious patient typically withdraws and decreases interpersonal involvement. The possible behavioral responses the nurse might observe are presented in Box 16-2.

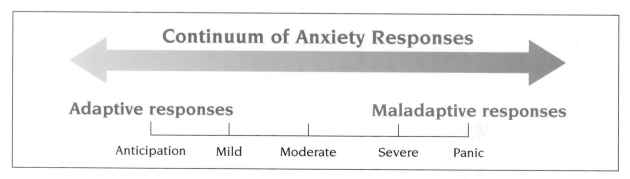

Fig. 16-1 Continuum of anxiety responses.

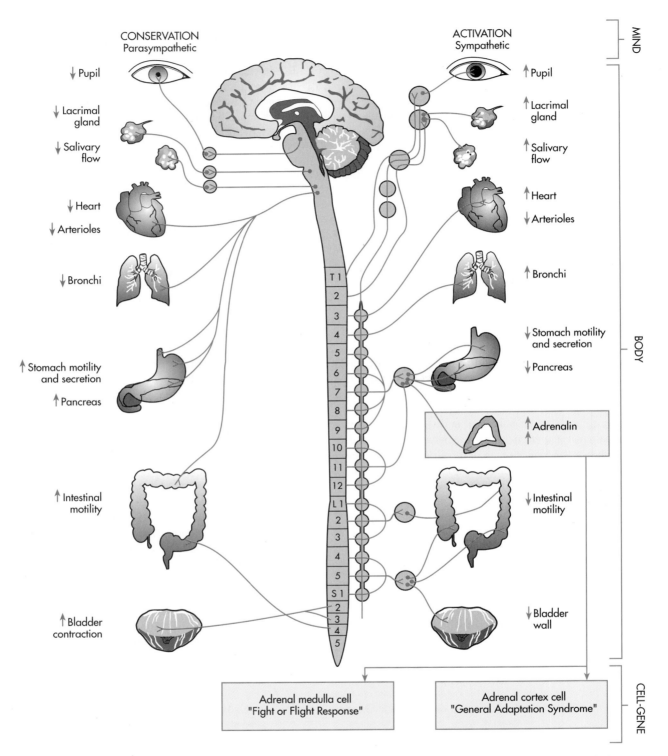

Fig. 16-2 Mind modulation of the autonomic nervous system and its two branches, the parasympathetic (conserving) and the sympathetic (activating), down to the cellular level. (Modified from Rossi EL: *The psychology of mind-body healing*, New York, 1993, WW Norton.)

Box 16-2 *Physiological, Behavioral, Cognitive, and Affective Responses to Anxiety*

PHYSIOLOGICAL		BEHAVIORAL	COGNITIVE	AFFECTIVE
Cardiovascular	**Neuromuscular**	Restlessness	Impaired attention	Edginess
Palpitations	Increased reflexes	Physical tension	Poor concentration	Impatience
Racing heart	Startle reaction	Tremors	Forgetfulness	Uneasiness
Increased blood pressure	Eyelid twitching	Startle reaction	Errors in judgment	Tension
Faintness*	Insomnia	Hypervigilance	Preoccupation	Nervousness
Actual fainting*	Tremors	Rapid speech	Blocking of thoughts	Fear
Decreased blood pressure*	Rigidity	Lack of coordination	Decreased perceptual field	Fright
Decreased pulse rate*	Fidgeting	Accident proneness	Reduced creativity	Alarm
Respiratory	Pacing	Interpersonal withdrawal	Diminished productivity	Terror
Rapid breathing	Strained face	Inhibition	Confusion	Jitteriness
Shortness of breath	Generalized weakness	Flight	Self-consciousness	Jumpiness
Pressure on chest	Wobbly legs	Avoidance	Loss of objectivity	Numbing
Shallow breathing	Clumsy movement	Hyperventilation	Fear of losing control	Guilt
Lump in throat	**Urinary Tract**		Frightening visual images	Shame
Choking sensation	Pressure to urinate*		Fear of injury or death	
Gasping	Frequent urination*		Flashbacks	
Gastrointestinal	**Skin**		Nightmares	
Loss of appetite	Flushed face			
Revulsion toward food	Localized sweating			
Abdominal discomfort	(palms)			
Abdominal pain*	Itching			
Nausea*	Hot and cold spells			
Heartburn*	Pale face			
Diarrhea*	Generalized sweating			

*Parasympathetic response.

Mental or intellectual functioning is also affected by anxiety. Cognitive responses the patient might display when experiencing anxiety are described in Box 16-2.

Finally, the nurse can assess a patient's emotional reactions, or affective responses, to anxiety by the subjective description of the patient's personal experience. Often, patients describe themselves as tense, jittery, on edge, jumpy, worried, or restless. One patient described feelings in the following way: "I'm expecting something terribly bad to happen, but I don't know what. I'm afraid, but I don't know why. I guess you can call it a generalized bad feeling." All these phrases are expressions of apprehension and overalertness. It seems clear that the person interprets his anxiety as a kind of warning sign. Additional affective responses are listed in Box 16-2.

Anxiety is an unpleasant and uncomfortable experience that most people try to avoid. They often try to replace anxiety with a more tolerable feeling. Pure anxiety is rarely seen. Anxiety is usually observed in combination with other emotions. Patients might describe feelings of anger, boredom, contempt, depression, irritation, worthlessness, jealousy, self-depreciation, suspicion, sadness, or helplessness. This makes it difficult for the nurse to discriminate between anxiety and depression, for instance, because the patient's descriptions may be similar.

Close ties exist between anxiety, depression, guilt, and hostility. These emotions often function reciprocally; one

feeling acts to generate and reinforce the others. The relationship between anxiety and hostility is particularly close. The pain experienced with anxiety often causes anger and resentment toward those thought to be responsible. These feelings of hostility in turn increase anxiety.

This cycle was evident in the case of a dependent and insecure wife who was very attached to her husband. She expressed numerous vague fears. In exploring her feelings, she also expressed great hostility toward him and their relationship. This symbolized her helplessness and increased her feelings of weakness. Verbalizing these angry feelings further increased her anxiety and unresolved conflict. Thus anxiety is often expressed through anger, and a tense and anxious person is more likely to become angry.

> **?** *Think of a patient you cared for recently who appeared to be angry or critical. Could this have been the patient's way of dealing with anxiety? If so, how would your nursing interventions have been different?*

Predisposing Factors

Anxiety is a prime factor in the development of the personality and formation of individual character traits. Because of its importance, various theories of the origin of anxiety have been developed.

PSYCHOANALYTIC VIEW. In the beginning of his study of anxiety, Freud regarded it as a purely physiological reaction to a person's chronic inability to reach an orgasm in sexual relations. He believed that unexpressed sexual energy was converted into anxiety. Therefore, alleviation of anxiety merely required improved sexual technique. Not until 30 years later did he see the importance of anxiety for a theory of personality development.[9,10]

His later viewpoint included two types of anxiety: primary and subsequent. Primary anxiety, the traumatic state, begins in the infant as a result of the sudden stimulation and trauma of birth. Anxiety continues with the possibility that hunger and thirst might not be satisfied. Primary anxiety therefore is a state of tension or a drive produced by external causes. The environment is capable of threatening as well as satisfying. This implicit threat predisposes the person to anxiety in later life.

With increased age and ego development, a new kind of anxiety arises. Freud viewed this subsequent anxiety as the emotional conflict between two elements of the personality: the id and the superego. The id represents instinctual drives and primitive impulses. The superego reflects conscience and culturally acquired restrictions. The ego, or I, tries to mediate the demands of these two clashing elements. Freud therefore suggested that one major function of anxiety was to warn the person that the ego was in danger of being overtaken.

INTERPERSONAL VIEW. Sullivan[26] disagreed with Freud. He believed that anxiety could not arise until the organism had some awareness of its environment. He believed that anxiety originated in the early bond between the infant and mother. Through this close emotional bond, anxiety is first conveyed by the mother to the infant. The infant responds as if he and his mother were one unit. As the child grows older, he sees this discomfort as a result of his own actions. He believes that his mother either approves or disapproves of his behavior. In addition, developmental traumas such as separations and losses can lead to specific vulnerabilities.[8,15,23] Sullivan believed that anxiety in later life arises when a person perceives that he or she will be viewed unfavorably or will lose the love of a person he or she values.

Sullivan identified two other aspects of anxiety that are important in the nurse-patient relationship. The first is that a mild or moderate level of anxiety is often expressed as anger. The second is that areas in the personality marked by anxiety often become the areas of significant growth. This can result when the person learns to deal with anxiety constructively, as in a therapeutic relationship.

A person's level of self-esteem is also an important factor related to anxiety. A person who is easily threatened or has a low level of self-esteem is more susceptible to anxiety. This is evident in students with test anxiety. Anxiety is high because they doubt they can succeed. This may have nothing to do with their actual abilities or how much they studied. The anxiety is caused only by their perception of their ability, which reflects their self-concept. They may be well prepared for the examination, but their severe level of anxiety reduces their perceptual field significantly. They may omit, misinterpret, or distort the meaning of the test items. They may even block out all their previous studying. The result will be a poor grade, which reinforces their poor perception of self.

BEHAVIORAL VIEW. Some behavioral theorists propose that anxiety is a product of frustration caused by anything that interferes with attaining a desired goal. An example of an external frustration might be the loss of a job. Many goals may thus be blocked, such as financial security, pride in work, and perception of self as family provider. An internal frustration is evidenced by young college graduates who set unrealistically high career goals and are frustrated by entry-level job offers. In this case their view of self is threatened by their unrealistic goals. They are likely to experience feelings of failure, insignificance, and mounting anxiety.

Other experimental psychologists regard anxiety as a drive that is learned because of an innate desire to avoid pain. They believe that anxiety begins with the attachment of pain to a particular stimulus. If the reaction is strong enough, it may become generalized to similar objects and situations. Learning theorists believe that people who have been exposed in early life to intense fears are more likely to be anxious in later life. In this respect, parental influences are important. Children who see their parents respond with anxiety to every minor stress soon develop a similar pattern. Paradoxically, if parents are completely unmoved by potentially stressful situations, children feel alone and lack emotional support from their families. The appropriate emotional response of parents gives children security and helps them learn constructive coping methods.

Anxiety is also theorized to arise through conflict, which is defined as the clashing of two opposing interests. The person experiences two competing drives and must choose between them. A reciprocal relationship exists between conflict and anxiety. Conflict produces anxiety, and anxiety increases the perception of conflict by producing feelings of helplessness. In this view, conflict derives from two tendencies: approach and avoidance. Approach is the tendency to do something or move toward something. Avoidance is the opposite tendency: not to do something or not to move toward something. There are four kinds of conflict:

▼ **Approach-approach,** in which the person is motivated to pursue two equally desirable but incompatible goals. This type of conflict seldom produces anxiety.

▼ **Approach-avoidance,** in which the person wishes to both pursue and avoid the same goal. The patient who wants to express anger but feels great anxiety and fear in doing so experiences this type of conflict. Another example is the ambitious business executive who must compromise values of honesty and loyalty to be promoted.

▼ **Avoidance-avoidance,** in which the person must choose between two undesirable goals. Because neither alternative seems beneficial, this is a difficult choice usually accompanied by much anxiety.

▼ **Double approach-avoidance,** in which the person can see both desirable and undesirable aspects of both alternatives. This is the kind of conflict experienced by a person living with the pain of one's social and emotional life and destructive coping patterns. The alternative is to seek psychiatric help and expose oneself to the threat and potential pain of the therapy process. Double approach-avoidance conflict feelings are often described as ambivalence.

 Think of an example of each of the four kinds of conflict you have experienced in your life.

FAMILY STUDIES. Epidemiological and family studies show that anxiety disorders clearly run in families and that they are common and of different types.[15,22] Anxiety disorders can overlap, as do anxiety disorders and depression. People with one anxiety disorder are more likely to develop another or to experience a major depression within their lifetime. It has been estimated that only about a quarter of those with anxiety disorders receive treatment. However, these people are high users of health-care facilities, as they seek treatment for the various symptoms caused by anxiety such as chest pain, palpitations, dizziness, and shortness of breath.[19,24]

BIOLOGICAL BASIS. Basic science advances in understanding anxiety have been considerable in recent years.[13]

Some of the most recent developments are described in Chapter 5. For example, investigators have learned that the brain contains specific receptors for benzodiazepines and that these receptors probably help to regulate anxiety. This is related to the activity of the neurotransmitter gamma-aminobutyric acid (GABA), which regulates the activity, or firing rates, of neurons in the parts of the brain responsible for producing anxiety. GABA is the most common inhibitory neurotransmitter in the brain. When it crosses the synapse and attaches or binds to the GABA receptor on the postsynaptic membrane, the receptor channel opens, allowing for the exchange of ions. This results in an inhibition or reduction of cell excitability, and thus a slowing of cell activity. The theory is that people who have an excess of anxiety have a problem with the efficiency of this neurotransmission process.

When a person with anxiety takes a benzodiazepine (BZ) medication, which is from the antianxiety class of drugs, it binds to a place on the GABA receptor next to GABA. This makes the postsynaptic receptor more sensitive to the effects of GABA, enhancing neurotransmission and causing even more inhibition of cell activity (Fig. 16-3). The GABA receptors to which BZs bind are concentrated in two areas of the brain: the limbic system, an area thought to be of central importance for emotional behavior; and the locus ceruleus, the primary manufacturing center of norepinephrine, which is an excitatory neurotransmitter. The effect of GABA and BZ at the GABA receptor in various parts of the brain is a reduced firing rate of cells in areas implicated in anxiety disorders. The clinical result is that the person becomes less anxious.

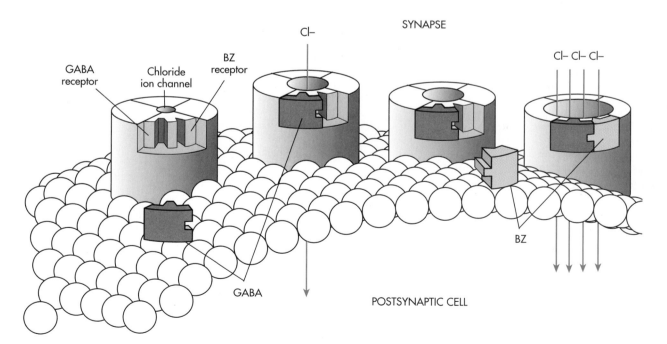

Fig. 16-3   Effects of GABA at the cellular level. *BZ,* Benzodiazepine drug; *Cl−,* chloride ion; *GABA,* gamma-aminobutyric acid.

In the case of a person with panic attacks, both BZs and antidepressant drugs are effective, indicating that panic attacks may involve additional alterations in synaptic functioning in the norepinephrine and serotonin pathways in the brain. Rigorous studies of drugs that relieve or produce anxiety should help provide additional information regarding the biological basis for anxiety disorders.

It has also been shown that a person's general health has a great effect on predisposition to anxiety. Anxiety may accompany some physical disorders such as those listed in Box 16-3. Coping mechanisms may also be impaired by toxic influences, dietary deficiencies, reduced blood supply, hormonal changes, and other physical causes. In addition, symptoms from some physical disorders may mimic or exacerbate anxiety.

Similarly, fatigue increases irritability and feelings of anxiety. It appears that fatigue caused by nervous factors predisposes the person to a greater degree of anxiety than does fatigue caused by purely physical causes. Thus fatigue may actually be an early symptom of anxiety. Patients complaining of nervous fatigue may already be suffering from moderate anxiety and be more susceptible to future stress situations.

Precipitating Stressors

Given these theories about the origin of anxiety, what kinds of events might precipitate feelings of anxiety? Clearly, experiencing or witnessing a source of trauma of any kind has been associated with a variety of anxiety disorders, particularly posttraumatic stress disorder (PTSD).[12,27] Matura-tional, situational, and adventitious crises, as described in Chapter 13, can all precipitate a maladaptive anxiety response. These precipitating stressors can be grouped into two categories: threats to physical integrity and threats to self-system.

THREATS TO PHYSICAL INTEGRITY. These threats suggest impending physiological disability or decreased capacity to perform the activities of daily living. They may include both internal and external sources. External sources may include exposure to viral and bacterial infection, environmental pollutants, safety hazards, lack of adequate housing, food, or clothing, and traumatic injury. Internal sources may include the failure of physiological mechanisms such as the heart, immune system, or temperature regulation. The normal biological changes that can occur with pregnancy and failure to participate in preventive health practices are other internal sources. Pain is often the first indication that physical integrity is being threatened. It creates anxiety that often motivates the person to seek health care.

THREATS TO SELF-SYSTEM. Threats in this second category are pervasive. They imply harm to a person's identity, self-esteem, and integrated social functioning. Both external and internal sources can threaten self-esteem. External sources may include the loss of a valued person through death, divorce, or relocation, a change in job status, an ethical dilemma, and social or cultural group pressures. Internal sources may include interpersonal difficulties at home or at work or assuming a new role, such as parent, student, or employee. In addition, many threats to physical integrity

---

Box **16-3** *Medical Disorders Associated with Anxiety*

CARDIOVASCULAR/RESPIRATORY
Asthma
Cardiac arrhythmias
Chronic obstructive pulmonary disease
Congestive heart failure
Coronary insufficiency
Hyperdynamic beta-adrenergic state
Hypertension
Hyperventilation syndrome
Hypoxia, embolus, infections

ENDOCRINOLOGICAL
Carcinoid
Cushing's syndrome
Hyperthyroidism
Hypoglycemia
Hypoparathyroidism
Hypothyroidism
Menopause
Pheochromocytoma
Premenstrual syndrome

NEUROLOGICAL
Collagen vascular disease
Epilepsy
Huntington's disease
Multiple sclerosis
Organic brain syndrome
Vestibular dysfunction
Wilson's disease

SUBSTANCE RELATED
Intoxications
Anticholinergic drugs
Aspirin
Caffeine
Cocaine
Hallucinogens including phencyclidine ("angel dust")
Steroids
Sympathomimetics
THC

Withdrawal Syndromes
Alcohol
Narcotics
Sedative hypnotics

also threaten self-esteem because the mind-body relationship is an intimate and overlapping one.

This distinction of categories is only theoretical. The person responds to all stressors, whatever their nature and origin, as an integrated whole. No specific event is equally stressful to all people or even to the same person at different times.

Appraisal of Stressors

A true understanding of anxiety requires integration of knowledge from all the various points of view. The Stuart Stress Adaptation Model integrates data from psychoanalytical, interpersonal, behavioral, genetic, and biological perspectives. It is holistic in nature and encourages the assessment of behaviors and the individual's appraisal of stressors in developing appropriate nursing interventions. It also suggests a variety of causative factors and emphasizes the relationship among them in explaining present behavior. It proposes that anxiety disorders can best be understood as an integration of the factors listed in Box 16-4.

Coping Resources

The person can cope with stress and anxiety by mobilizing coping resources in the environment. These may include a variety of intrapersonal, interpersonal, and social factors. Such resources as economic assets, problem-solving abilities, social supports, and cultural beliefs can help the person integrate stressful experiences and adopt successful coping strategies. They can also help the person find meaning in the experience and suggest alternative strategies for mediating stressful events.

> **?** *How might a person's religious or spiritual belief system serve as a resource in coping with a moderate level of anxiety?*

Box **16-4** *Causative Factors in Anxiety Disorders*

- ▼ There is a built-in neurobiological substance that prepares the person to cope with danger.
- ▼ Evolution has affected this substance in such a way that stimuli threatening to survival are selectively avoided.
- ▼ People may be born with a central nervous system that is overly sensitive to stimuli that are generally harmless.
- ▼ Childhood and adult learning experiences may ultimately determine the extent, severity, and nature of the situations that will evoke anxiety.
- ▼ Chronic inability to cope with dangerous situations adaptively could increase the tendency to respond with anxiety.
- ▼ The cognitive functions might permit continual focusing on anxiety reactions, so the mere anticipation of aversive stimuli would provoke anxiety.
- ▼ Such a person might be more vulnerable to insecurities, especially if intelligent and introspective.

Coping Mechanisms

As anxiety increases to the severe and panic levels, the behaviors displayed become more intense and potentially injurious. People seek to avoid anxiety and the circumstances that produce it. When experiencing anxiety, people use various coping mechanisms to try to relieve it (see A Patient Speaks). The inability to cope with anxiety constructively is a primary cause of pathological behavior. To neutralize, deny, or counteract anxiety, the person develops patterns of coping. The pattern used to cope with mild anxiety dominates when anxiety becomes more intense. Anxiety plays a major role in the psychogenesis of emotional illness because many symptoms of illness develop as attempted defenses against anxiety.

The nurse needs to be familiar with the coping mechanisms people use when experiencing the various levels of anxiety. For **mild anxiety,** caused by the tension of day-to-day living, there are several coping mechanisms including crying, sleeping, eating, yawning, laughing, cursing, physical exercise, and daydreaming. Oral behavior, such as smoking

---

 A Patient *Speaks*

It's hard to describe what it feels like. You know something isn't right. Most people don't have to check their doors five or six times before they go to bed. Most people aren't afraid to be near children or feel like they have to count their money over and over again before they can put it back in their wallet. But that's the way my life has been ever since I was a little girl.

Of course I realized I needed help, so I saw a number of different professionals. With one psychologist we discussed every aspect of my childhood and my earliest memories of life. Unfortunately, I finished that therapy still counting everything around me. Next I went to a physician, but he told me that I was just nervous about getting married and things would get better with time. They didn't. Then my mother suggested I go to the university and see someone. That's where I met the psychiatric nurse who did a number of things I'll always remember. First she put me at ease and clearly told me that I wasn't crazy. Then she told me that what I had was obsessive-compulsive disorder and gave me lots of great books and information to read. Finally, she told me that it was a treatable illness and together we devised a treatment plan. It included both medication and behavioral therapy and wow, what a difference! I'm sure glad I was persistent, but I'm even more glad that there are caring professionals out there who can really help. ▼

and drinking, is another means of coping with mild anxiety. When dealing with other people, the individual copes with low levels of anxiety through superficiality, lack of eye contact, use of clichés, and limited self-disclosure. People can also protect themselves from anxiety by assuming comfortable roles and limiting close relationships to those with values similar to their own. Mild levels of anxiety are often handled without conscious thought, and their effects can be easily minimized.

Moderate, severe, and panic levels of anxiety pose greater threats to the ego. They require more energy to cope with the threat. These coping mechanisms can be categorized as task-oriented and ego-oriented reactions.

TASK-ORIENTED REACTIONS. Task-oriented reactions are thoughtful, deliberate attempts to solve problems, resolve conflicts, and gratify needs. They are aimed at realistically meeting the demands of a stress situation that has been objectively appraised. They are consciously directed and action oriented. These reactions can include attack, withdrawal, and compromise.

In attack behavior a person attempts to remove or overcome obstacles to satisfy a need. There are many possible ways of attacking problems, and this type of reaction may be destructive or constructive. Destructive patterns are usually accompanied by great feelings of anger and hostility. These feelings may be expressed by negative or aggressive behavior that violates the rights, property, and well-being of others. Constructive patterns reflect a problem-solving approach. They are evident in self-assertive behaviors that respect the rights of others.

Withdrawal behavior may be expressed physically or psychologically. Physically, withdrawal involves removing oneself from the source of the threat. This can apply to biological stressors, such as smoke-filled rooms, exposure to irradiation, or contact with contagious diseases. A person can also withdraw in various psychological ways, such as by admitting defeat, becoming apathetic, or lowering aspirations. As with attack, this type of reaction may be constructive or destructive. When it isolates the person from others and interferes with the ability to work, the reaction creates additional problems.

Compromise is necessary in situations that cannot be resolved through attack or withdrawal. This involves changing usual ways of operating, substituting goals, or sacrificing aspects of personal needs. Compromise reactions are usually constructive and are often used in approach-approach and avoidance-avoidance situations. Occasionally, however, the person realizes with time that the compromise is not acceptable; a solution must then be renegotiated or a different coping mechanism adopted.

The capacity for task-oriented reactions and effective problem solving is greatly influenced by the person's expectation of at least partial success. This in turn depends on remembering past successes in similar situations. On this basis it is possible to go forward and deal with the current stressful situation. Perseverance in problem solving also depends on the person's expectation of a certain level of pain and discomfort and on the belief in being capable of tolerating the problem. Here lies the balance between courage and anxiety.

> *What coping mechanisms do you use when you are mildly, moderately, and severely anxious? How adaptive or maladaptive are they?*

EGO-ORIENTED REACTIONS. Task-oriented reactions are not always successful in coping with stressful situations. Consequently, ego-oriented reactions are often used to protect the self. These reactions, also called ego defense mechanisms, are the first line of psychic defense. Everyone uses defense mechanisms, and they often help people cope successfully with mild and moderate levels of anxiety. They protect the person from feelings of inadequacy and worthlessness and prevent awareness of anxiety. However, they can be used to such an extreme degree that they distort reality, interfere with interpersonal relationships, and limit the ability to work productively. This results in ego disintegration instead of self-integrity.

As coping mechanisms, they have certain drawbacks. First, ego-oriented reactions operate on unconscious levels. The person has little awareness of what is happening and little control over events. Second, they involve a degree of self-deception and reality distortion. Therefore, they usually do not help the person to cope with the problem realistically. Table 16-1 lists some of the more common ego defense mechanisms with an example of each.

When discussing ego-oriented reactions or defense mechanisms, it is important to note that people often monitor their own levels of emotional tolerance and the need to use ego defenses. Denial may effectively allay anxiety immediately following a stressful event. If denial is gradually eliminated as the stress begins to subside, the person may better adapt to the new situation.

The evaluation of whether the patient's use of certain defense mechanisms is adaptive or maladaptive involves four issues:

▼ The accurate recognition of the patient's use of the defense mechanism by the nurse.
▼ The degree to which the defense mechanism is used. Does it imply a high degree of personality disorganization? Is the person unresponsive to facts about his or her life situation?
▼ The degree to which use of the defense mechanism impedes the patient's progress toward regained health.
▼ The reason the patient used the ego defense mechanism. The nurse will better understand the patient and plan more effective nursing care after considering these areas.

If the ego defense mechanisms fail and the level of anxi-

TABLE **16-1** *Ego Defense Mechanisms*

DEFENSE MECHANISM	EXAMPLE
Compensation: Process by which a person makes up for a perceived deficiency by strongly emphasizing a feature that he or she regards as an asset.	A businessman perceives his small physical stature negatively. He tries to overcome this by being aggressive, forceful, and controlling in business dealings.
Denial: Avoidance of disagreeable realities by ignoring or refusing to recognize them; the simplest and most primitive of all defense mechanisms.	Mrs. P has just been told that her breast biopsy indicates a malignancy. When her husband visits her that evening, she tells him that no one has discussed the laboratory results with her.
Displacement: Shift of emotion from a person or object to another, usually neutral or less dangerous person or object.	A 4-year-old boy is angry because he has just been punished by his mother for drawing on his bedroom walls. He begins to play war with his soldier toys and has them fight with each other.
Dissociation: The separation of a group of mental or behavioral processes from the rest of the person's consciousness or identity.	A man is brought to the emergency room by the police and is unable to explain who he is and where he lives or works.
Identification: Process by which a person tries to become like someone he or she admires by taking on thoughts, mannerisms, or tastes of that person.	Sally, 15 years old, has her hair styled like that of her young English teacher, whom she admires.
Intellectualization: Excessive reasoning or logic is used to avoid experiencing disturbing feelings.	A woman avoids dealing with her anxiety in shopping malls by explaining that shopping is a frivolous waste of time and money.
Introjection: Intense identification in which a person incorporates qualities or values of another person or group into his or her own ego structure. It is one of the earliest mechanisms of the child, important in formation of conscience.	Eight-year-old Jimmy tells his 3-year-old sister, "Don't scribble in your book of nursery rhymes. Just look at the pretty pictures," thus expressing his parents' values.
Isolation: Splitting off of emotional components of a thought, which may be temporary or long term.	A second-year medical student dissects a cadaver for her anatomy course without being disturbed by thoughts of death.
Projection: Attributing one's thoughts or impulses to another person. Through this process one can attribute intolerable wishes, emotional feelings, or motivations to another person.	A young woman who denies she has sexual feelings about a coworker accuses him without basis of trying to seduce her.
Rationalization: Offering a socially acceptable or apparently logical explanation to justify or make acceptable otherwise unacceptable impulses, feelings, behaviors, and motives.	John fails an examination and complains that the lectures were not well organized or clearly presented.
Reaction formation: Development of conscious attitudes and behavior patterns that are opposite to what one really feels or would like to do.	A married woman who feels attracted to one of her husband's friends treats him rudely.
Regression: Retreat to behavior characteristic of an earlier level of development.	Four-year-old Nicole, who has been toilet trained for over a year, begins to wet her pants again when her new baby brother is brought home from the hospital.
Repression: Involuntary exclusion of a painful or conflictual thought, impulse, or memory from awareness. It is the primary ego defense, and other mechanisms tend to reinforce it.	Mr. R does not recall hitting his wife when she was pregnant.
Splitting: Viewing people and situations as either all good or all bad. Failure to integrate the positive and negative qualities of oneself.	A friend tells you that you are the most wonderful person in the world one day, and how much she hates you the next day.
Sublimation: Acceptance of a socially approved substitute goal for a drive whose normal channel of expression is blocked.	Ed has an impulsive and physically aggressive nature. He tries out for the football team and becomes a star tackle.
Suppression: A process often listed as a defense mechanism but really a conscious counterpart of repression. It is intentional exclusion of material from consciousness. At times, it may lead to repression.	A young man at work finds he is thinking so much about his date that evening that it is interfering with his work. He decides to put it out of his mind until he leaves the office for the day.
Undoing: Act or communication that partially negates a previous one; a primitive defense mechanism.	Larry makes a passionate declaration of love to Sue on a date. On their next meeting he treats her formally and distantly.

ety remains high, the person must use exaggerated and inappropriate coping mechanisms. These coping patterns are maladaptive responses that may appear deviant or abnormal. They include the many hidden, unconscious pathways in which the effects of anxiety are converted psychologically.

Obviously, many coping mechanisms are available for minimizing anxiety. Some of these defense mechanisms appear to be essential for maintaining emotional stability. The exact nature and number of the defenses used strongly influence the personality pattern. When these defenses are overused or used unsuccessfully, they cause many physiological and psychological symptoms commonly associated with emotional illness.

Nursing Diagnosis

The nurse who has adequately assessed a patient and uses the Stuart Stress Adaptation Model can formulate a nursing diagnosis based on the patient's position on the continuum of anxiety responses (Fig. 16-4).

Initially the nurse must determine the quality and quantity of the anxiety experienced by the patient. In considering the quality of the anxiety, the nurse might question the appropriateness of the patient's response to the perceived threat. Is it warranted and adaptive or irrational? A problem may exist if the response is out of proportion to the threat. This would indicate that the patient's cognitive appraisal of the threat is unrealistic. The quantity of the reaction is the next consideration in determining the level of anxiety. When anxiety reaches the severe and panic levels, it indicates that the conflict is increasingly problematic for the patient.

The nurse also needs to explore how the patient is coping with the anxiety. Constructive coping mechanisms are protective responses that consciously confront the threat. Destructive coping mechanisms involve repression into the

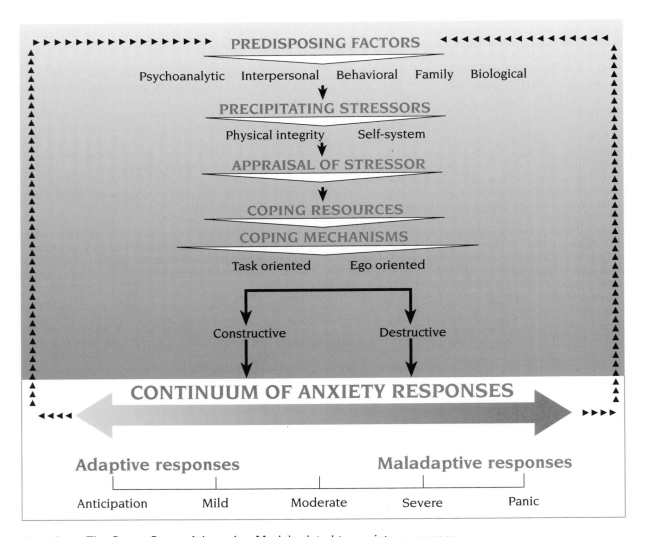

Fig. 16-4 The Stuart Stress Adaptation Model related to anxiety responses.

unconscious. They tend to be ineffective, inadequate, disorganized, inappropriate, and exaggerated. They may be evident in bizarre behavior or symptom formation.

Finally, the nurse needs to determine the overall effect of the anxiety. Is it stimulating growth? Or is it interfering with effective living and life satisfaction? Is it enhancing one's sense of self? Or is it depersonalizing? Whenever possible, the patient should be included in identifying problem areas. This may not always be feasible, however, particularly if the patient's anxiety is at the severe or panic level.

There are three primary NANDA nursing diagnoses concerned with anxiety responses: **anxiety, ineffective coping,** and **fear.** Many additional nursing problems may be identified from the way the patient's anxiety reciprocally influences interpersonal relationships, self-concept, cognitive functioning, physiological status, and other aspects of life.[16] The identification of nursing problems should be as complete as possible to ensure an adequate plan of care. Nursing diagnoses related to the range of possible maladaptive responses and related medical diagnoses are identified in the Medical and Nursing Diagnoses box below. The primary NANDA nursing diagnoses and examples of complete nursing diagnoses are presented in the Detailed Diagnoses box on p. 286.

Related Medical Diagnoses

Many patients with mild or moderate anxiety have no medically diagnosed health problem. However, patients with more severe levels of anxiety usually have neurotic disorders that fall under the category of anxiety disorders in the DSM-IV.[1] A **neurosis** is a mental disorder characterized by anxiety that involves no distortion of reality. Neurotic disorders are maladaptive anxiety responses associated with moderate and severe levels of anxiety.

Psychosis is disintegrative and involves a significant distortion of reality. It can emerge with the panic level of anxiety. Psychotic people feel they are "breaking into pieces." The anxiety of psychosis is not just fear of failure or fear of being unable to cope with the threatening situation. It is the fear that the failure will reveal defeat in the process of living and failure in the process of being.

In addition to differentiating between neurotic and psychotic anxiety responses, the nurse must discriminate between anxiety and other disorders. Anxiety and depression often overlap because anxious patients are often depressed and depressed patients are often anxious. For example, both anxious and depressed patients share the following symptoms: sleep disturbances, appetite changes, nonspecific cardiopulmonary and gastrointestinal complaints, difficulty

---

 ## MEDICAL AND NURSING DIAGNOSES *related to* **Anxiety**

Related Medical Diagnoses (DSM-IV)*	Related Nursing Diagnoses (NANDA)†
Panic disorder without agoraphobia	Adjustment, impaired
Panic disorder with agoraphobia	**Anxiety‡**
Agoraphobia without panic attacks	Breathing pattern, ineffective
Specific phobia	Communication, impaired verbal
Social phobia	Community coping, ineffective
Obsessive-compulsive disorder	Confusion, acute
Posttraumatic stress disorder	**Coping, ineffective individual‡**
Acute stress disorder	Diarrhea
Generalized anxiety disorder	**Fear‡**
	Health maintenance, altered
	Injury, potential for
	Memory, impaired
	Nutrition, altered
	Posttrauma response
	Powerlessness
	Self-esteem disturbance
	Sensory/perceptual alterations
	Sleep pattern disturbance
	Social interaction, impaired
	Thought processes, altered
	Urinary elimination, altered patterns

*From American Psychiatric Association: *Diagnostic and statistical manual of mental disorders,* ed 4, Washington, DC, 1994, The Association.
†From North American Nursing Diagnosis Association: *NANDA nursing diagnoses: definitions and classifications 1997-1998,* Philadelphia, 1997, The Association.
‡Primary nursing diagnosis for anxiety.

DETAILED DIAGNOSES *related to* **Anxiety Responses**

NANDA

Diagnosis Stem	Examples of Complete Diagnoses
Anxiety	Panic level of anxiety related to family rejection, evidenced by confusion and impaired judgment.
	Severe anxiety related to sexual conflict, evidenced by repetitive handwashing and recurrent thoughts of dirt and germs.
	Severe anxiety related to marital conflict, evidenced by inability to leave the house.
	Moderate anxiety related to financial pressures, evidenced by recurring episodes of abdominal pain and heartburn.
	Moderate anxiety related to assumption of motherhood role, evidenced by inhibition and avoidance.
	Moderate anxiety related to poor school performance, evidenced by excessive use of denial and rationalization.
Ineffective individual coping	Ineffective individual coping related to daughter's death, evidenced by inability to recall events pertaining to the car accident.
	Ineffective individual coping related to child's illness, evidenced by limited ability to concentrate and psychomotor agitation.
Fear	Fear related to impending surgery, evidenced by generalized hostility to staff and restlessness.

DSM-IV Diagnoses	Essential Features*
Panic disorder without agoraphobia	Recurrent unexpected panic attacks (Box 16-5), with at least one of the attacks followed by a month (or more) of persistent concern about having additional attacks, worry about the implications of the attack or its consequences, or a significant change in behavior related to the attacks. Also the absence of agoraphobia.
Panic disorder with agoraphobia	Meets the above criteria. In addition, the presence of agoraphobia, which is anxiety about being in places or situations from which escape might be difficult or embarrassing or in which help may not be available in the event of a panic attack. Agoraphobic fears typically involve characteristic clusters of situations that include being outside the home alone, being in a crowd or standing in a line, being on a bridge, and traveling in a bus, train, or car. Agoraphobic situations are avoided, or endured with marked distress or with anxiety about having a panic attack, or require the presence of a companion.
Agoraphobia without history of panic disorder	The presence of agoraphobia without meeting criteria for panic disorder.
Specific phobia	Marked and persistent fear that is excessive or unreasonable, cued by the presence or anticipation of a specific object or situation (such as flying, heights, animals, receiving an injection, or seeing blood). Exposure to the phobic stimulus almost invariably provokes an immediate anxiety response. The person recognizes the fear is excessive, and the distress or avoidance interferes with the person's normal routine.
Social phobia	A marked and persistent fear of social or performance situations in which the person is exposed to unfamiliar people or to possible scrutiny by others. The person fears that he or she will act in a way (or show anxiety symptoms) that will be humiliating or embarrassing. Exposure to the feared situation almost invariably provokes anxiety. The person recognizes the fear is excessive, and the distress or avoidance interferes with the person's normal routine.
Obsessive-compulsive disorder	Either obsessions or compulsions (Box 16-6) are recognized as excessive and interfere with the person's normal routine.
Posttraumatic stress disorder	The person has been exposed to a traumatic event in which both of the following were present:
	The person has experienced, witnessed, or been confronted with an event that involved actual or threatened death or serious injury, or a threat to the physical integrity of oneself or others.
	The person's response involved intense fear, helplessness, or horror.
	The traumatic event is reexperienced, and there is an avoidance of stimuli associated with the trauma and a numbing of general responsiveness.
Acute stress disorder	Meets the criteria for exposure to a traumatic event and experiences three of the following symptoms: sense of detachment, reduced awareness of one's surroundings, derealization, depersonalization, and dissociated amnesia.
Generalized anxiety disorder	Excessive anxiety and worry, occurring more days than not for at least 6 months, about a number of events or activities. The person finds it difficult to control the worry and experiences at least three of the following symptoms: restlessness or feeling keyed up or on edge, fatigue, difficulty concentrating or mind going blank, irritability, muscle tension, sleep disturbance.

*Modified from American Psychiatric Association: *Diagnostic and statistical manual of mental disorders,* ed 4, Washington, DC, 1994, The Association.

Box **16-5** *Panic Attack Criteria*

A panic attack is a discrete period of intense fear or discomfort in which at least four of the following symptoms develop abruptly and reach a peak within 10 minutes:

Palpitations, pounding heart, or accelerated heart rate
Sweating
Trembling or shaking
Sensations of shortness of breath or smothering
Feeling of choking
Chest pain or discomfort
Nausea or abdominal distress
Feeling dizzy, unsteady, lightheaded, or faint
Derealization (feelings of unreality) or depersonalization (being detached from oneself)
Fear of losing control or going crazy
Fear of dying
Paresthesias (numbness or tingling sensations)
Chills or hot flushes

Box **16-6** *Obsession and Compulsion Criteria*

OBSESSION

Recurrent and persistent thoughts, impulses, or images are experienced during the disturbance as intrusive and inappropriate and cause marked anxiety or distress.
The thoughts, impulses, or images are not simply excessive worries about real-life problems.
The person attempts to ignore or suppress such thoughts or impulses or to neutralize them with some other thought or action.
The person recognizes that the obsessional thought, impulses, or images are a product of one's own mind.

COMPULSION

The person feels driven to perform repetitive behaviors (such as handwashing, ordering, checking) or mental acts (such as praying, counting, repeating words silently) in response to an obsession or according to rules that must be applied rigidly.
The behaviors or mental acts are aimed at preventing or reducing distress or preventing some dreaded event or situation; however, these behaviors or mental acts either are not connected in a realistic way with what they are designed to neutralize or prevent or are clearly excessive.

Box **16-7** *Differences between Anxiety and Depression*

ANXIETY

Predominantly fear or apprehension
Difficulty falling asleep (initial insomnia)
Phobic avoidance behavior
Rapid pulse and psychomotor hyperactivity
Breathing disturbances
Tremors and palpitations
Sweating and hot or cold spells
Faintness, lightheadedness, dizziness
Depersonalization (feeling detached from one's body)
Derealization (feeling that one's environment is strange, unreal, or unfamiliar)
Selective and specific negative appraisals that do not include all areas of life
Sees some prospects for the future
Does not regard defects or mistakes as irrevocable
Uncertain in negative evaluations
Predicts that only certain events may go badly

DEPRESSION

Predominantly sad or hopeless with feelings of despair
Early morning awakening (late insomnia) or hypersomnia
Diurnal variation (feels worse in the morning)
Slowed speech and thought processes
Delayed response time
Psychomotor retardation (agitation may also occur)
Loss of interest in usual activities
Inability to experience pleasure
Thoughts of death or suicide
Negative appraisals are pervasive, global, and exclusive
Sees the future as blank and has given up all hope
Regards mistakes as beyond redemption
Absolute in negative evaluations
Global view that nothing will turn out right

concentrating, irritability, and fatigue or lack of energy. Yet there are often discrete (if subtle) differences between the two groups. These are described in Box 16-7.

Also, posttraumatic stress disorder (PTSD) is rarely a patient's only psychiatric diagnosis and it is sometimes difficult to distinguish overlapping independent symptoms from effects of the trauma. Nearly half of all people with PTSD also suffer from major depression, and more than a third from phobias and alcoholism.[12] Behavior that results from child abuse may also take the form of a personality disorder, and the symptoms of PTSD are occasionally mis-

taken for psychotic illness or an organic brain syndrome. This has raised questions regarding the diagnosis of PTSD and how prevalent it is (see Critical Thinking about Contemporary Issues).

Finally, studies show that about 25% of people will experience an anxiety disorder sometime in their life.[17] These are the most common psychiatric disorders in American society. They occur twice as often in women as in men, and obsessive-compulsive disorder is about equally prevalent in women and men. No outstanding differences in the prevalence of anxiety disorders have been found on the basis of race, income, education, or rural versus urban dwelling.[17] The essential features of the medical diagnoses related to anxiety responses are presented in the Detailed Diagnoses box to the left.

Outcome Identification

Goals such as "decrease anxiety" and "minimize anxiety" lack specific behaviors and evaluation criteria. Therefore, these goals are not particularly useful in guiding nursing care and

CRITICAL THINKING *about* Contemporary Issues

Is PTSD in Danger of Becoming Merely a Fashionable Diagnosis That Removes Responsibility for Personal Behavior by Projecting Blame onto Common Traumatic Events?

Epidemiological data show that PTSD is more unusual than usual following exposure to a variety of traumatic events. Research also shows the existence of risk factors other than trauma as predictors of PTSD, and questions have been raised about the differences between people who experience traumatic events and cope adaptively and those who develop PTSD. Other issues have been raised related to the symptoms of PTSD because they may appear immediately after the event or years later. They can remain for less than a month or for many months, or sometimes even years. Other areas of controversy include whether one has to experience the event directly or whether indirect exposure is sufficient, and whether it needs to be an extreme form of trauma and how *extreme* is defined. These questions have led to complaints that PTSD is simply an excuse to obtain disability benefits, win personal injury lawsuits, or evade responsibility for crimes.

The decision to establish PTSD as a diagnosis 15 years ago recognized the rights and needs of victims who were stigmatized, misunderstood, or ignored by the mental health field and it helped to make sense of their suffering. There is considerable evidence that traumatic experiences are associated with PTSD symptoms and that the related symptoms can be very disabling. Current research is revealing interesting findings about the neurobiology of PTSD and the fact that it does not follow the stress response described by Selye, but may be a progressive sensitization of biological systems that leave the person hyperresponsive to a variety of stimuli.[11,28]

Clearly, PTSD is an evolving concept.[27] But the controversy surrounding this diagnosis is likely to continue as long as there are questions about what kinds of events are traumatic, how they are perceived and interpreted, and how personal coping resources and coping responses differ.

evaluating its effectiveness. The expected outcome for patients with maladaptive anxiety responses is as follows:

The patient will demonstrate adaptive ways of coping with stress.

Short-term goals can break this down into readily attainable steps. This allows the patient and nurse to see progress even if the ultimate goal still appears distant.

When the nursing diagnosis describes the patient's anxiety at the severe or panic levels, the highest-priority short-term goals should address lowering the anxiety level. Only after this has been achieved can additional progress be made. The reduced level of anxiety should be evident in a reduction of behaviors associated with severe or panic levels. Following are examples of short-term goals for a particular patient.

After 4 days Mr. Jones will:
▼ Attend and remain seated during all meetings
▼ Participate at least three times during each meeting
▼ Discuss one topic for a minimum of 10 minutes when meeting with his nurse
▼ Attend all occupational therapy sessions
▼ Sleep a minimum of 6 hours a night

When these goals are met, the nurse can assume that the patient's level of anxiety has been reduced. The nurse may then develop new short-term goals directed toward insight or relaxation therapy.

Planning

The main goal of the nurse working with anxious patients is not to free them totally from anxiety. Patients need to develop the capacity to tolerate mild anxiety and to use it consciously and constructively. In this way the self will become stronger and more integrated. As they learn from these experiences, they will move on in their development. Patients must also be convinced that the values to be gained in moving ahead are greater than those to be gained by escape. Anxiety can be considered a war between the threat and the values people identify with their existence. Maladaptive behavior means that the struggle has been lost. The constructive approach to anxiety means that the struggle is won by the person's values. Thus a general nursing goal is to help patients develop sound values. This does not mean that patients assume the nurse's values. Rather, the nurse helps the patient to sort out his or her own values.

Anxiety can also be an important factor in the patient's decision to seek treatment. Because anxiety is undesirable, the patient will seek ways to reduce it. If the patient's coping mechanism or symptom does not minimize anxiety, the motivation for treatment increases. Conversely, anxiety about the therapeutic process can delay or prevent the person from seeking treatment.

The patient should actively participate in planning treatment strategies. If the patient is actively involved in identifying relevant stressors and planning possible solutions, the success of the implementation phase will be maximized. A patient in extreme anxiety initially will not be able to participate in the problem-solving process. However, as soon as anxiety is reduced, the nurse should encourage patient involvement. This participation reinforces that patients are responsible for their own growth and personal development.

Implementation

Severe and Panic Levels of Anxiety

ESTABLISHING A TRUSTING RELATIONSHIP. The patient with severe or panic levels of anxiety may need inpatient treatment or partial hospitalization.[6] To reduce the patient's level of anxiety, most nursing actions are supportive and protective. Initially nurses need to establish an open, trusting relationship. Nurses should actively listen to patients and encourage them to discuss their feelings of anxiety, hostility, guilt, and frustration. Nurses should answer patients' questions directly and offer unconditional acceptance. Their verbal and nonverbal communications should convey awareness and acceptance of patients' feelings. Nurses should remain available and respect the patient's personal space. A 6-foot distance in a small room may create the optimum condition for openness and discussion of fears. The more this distance is increased or decreased, the more anxious the patient may become.[4]

SELF-AWARENESS. Nurses' feelings are particularly important in working with highly anxious patients. They may find themselves being unsympathetic, impatient, and frustrated. These are common feelings of reciprocal anxiety. If nurses are alert to the development of anxiety in themselves, they can learn from it and use it therapeutically. For example, anxiety may indicate some important emotional issue that the patient is unable to identify and verbalize, or it may reflect a conflict within the nurse that is interfering with the ability to be therapeutic. Nurses should be alert to the signs of anxiety in themselves, accept them, and attempt to explore their cause. The nurse may ask the following questions:

▼ What is threatening me?

▼ Have I failed to live up to what I imagine to be the patient's ideal?

▼ Am I comparing myself to a peer or another health professional?

▼ Is the patient's area of conflict one that I have not resolved in myself?

▼ Is my anxiety related to something that will or may happen in the future? Is my patient's conflict really one of my own that I am projecting?

If nurses deny their own anxiety, it can have detrimental effects on the nurse-patient relationship. Because of their own anxiety, nurses may be unable to differentiate between levels of anxiety in others. They may also transfer their fears and frustrations to patients, thus compounding their problem. Finally, nurses who are anxious arouse defenses in patients and other staff that interfere with their therapeutic usefulness. Nurses should strive to accept their patients' anxiety without reciprocal anxiety by continually clarifying their own feelings and role, as indicated in the following clinical example.

Clinical Example Ms. R was a 35-year-old married woman and mother of three children, ages 4, 6, and 9. She was a full-time homemaker and mother. Her husband was a salesperson and spent about 2 nights each week out of town. She came to the clinic complaining of severe headaches that "come upon me very suddenly and are so terrible that I have to go to bed. The only thing that helps is for me to lie down in a dark and absolutely quiet room." She said that these headaches were becoming a real problem for everyone in the family, and her husband told her that she "just had to get over them and get things back to normal."

Mr. W, a psychiatric nurse, offered to see Ms. R in therapy once a week. After 3 weeks, he was asked to present his evaluation, treatment plans, and progress report to the clinic staff at their weekly team conference. Mr. W began his presentation by stating, "This case is really a tough nut to crack. I'll start with the progress report and say that there is none because I can't seem to get past all the complaining this patient does!" He then went on to discuss his evaluation and treatment plan in depth. It became obvious to the other members of the staff that Mr. W saw his patient as a woman who was not living up to her roles and responsibilities. He defended Ms. R's husband even though the husband refused to come to the sessions with his wife. When the psychiatrist asked about the possibility of a medication evaluation for Ms. R, the nurse replied, "Everyone gets headaches. I don't think we should reward or reinforce this woman's complaints."

In reviewing this case the staff noted that Mr. W appeared to have problems relating empathically to his patient because of her particular set of problems and some of his own values and perceptions. Mr. W agreed with this and said he had thought of asking someone else to work with Ms. R. Mr. W's supervisor observed that the nurse had problems with this type of patient in the past, and a more constructive approach would be to increase his supervision on this case, focusing on the dynamics between the patient and nurse that were blocking learning and growth for both of them. Mr. W and his supervisor set a time when they could begin to meet for this purpose.

 What clinical situations or patient problems raise your anxiety?

PROTECTING THE PATIENT. Another major area of intervention is protecting and reassuring the patient of his or her safety. One way to decrease anxiety is by allowing the patient to determine the amount of stress he or she can handle at the time. Nurses should not force severely anxious patients into situations they are not able to handle. They should also not attack their coping mechanisms or try to strip them of these. Rather, nurses should attempt to protect patients' defenses. The coping mechanism or symptom is attempting to deal with an unconscious conflict. Usually patients do not understand why the symptom has developed or what they are gaining from it. They know only that the symptom relieves some of the intolerable anxiety and tension. If they are unable to release this anxiety, their tension mounts to the panic level and they could lose control. It is also important to remember that the severely anxious patient has not worked through the area of conflict and therefore has no alternatives or substitutes for present coping mechanisms.

This principle also applies to severe levels of anxiety, such as obsessive-compulsive reactions and phobias. Nurses should not initially interfere with the repetitive act or force patients to confront the phobic object. They should not ridicule the nature of the defense. Also, nurses should not attempt to argue with patients about it or reason them out of it. Patients need their coping mechanisms to keep anxiety within tolerable limits. Nurses must not reinforce the phobia, ritual, or physical complaint by focusing attention on it and talking about it a great deal. With time, however, nurses can place some limits on patients' behavior and attempt to help them find satisfaction with other aspects of life.

MODIFYING THE ENVIRONMENT. If the patient is hospitalized, the nurse can consult with other members of the health team to identify anxiety-producing situations and attempt to reduce them. The nurse can set limits by assuming a quiet, calm manner and decreasing environmental stimulation. Limiting the patient's interaction with other patients will minimize the contagious aspects of anxiety. Supportive physical measures such as warm baths, massages, or whirlpool baths may also be helpful in decreasing a patient's anxiety.

ENCOURAGING ACTIVITY. The nurse should encourage the patient's interest in activities. This limits the time available for destructive coping mechanisms and increases participation in and enjoyment of other aspects of life. Within the hospital setting the patient may become engaged in simple games, concrete tasks, or occupational or art therapy. The nurse can share some of these activities to provide support and reinforce socially productive behavior. The nurse might also schedule vigorous physical activities such as walking, a sport, or an active hobby. This form of physical exercise helps to relieve anxiety because it provides an emotional release and directs the patient's attention outward.

Similar interventions can be implemented with the severely anxious patient who is not hospitalized. The nurse and patient can plan a daily schedule of activities to be carried out in the community. Family members may be involved in the planning because they can be very supportive in setting limits and stimulating outside activity[7] (see A Family Speaks).

Some nursing interventions can be detrimental and increase anxiety in severely anxious patients. These include pressuring the patient to change prematurely, being judgmental and verbally disapproving of the patient's behaviors, and asking the patient a direct question that brings on defensiveness. Focusing in a critical way on the patient's anxious feelings with other patients present, lacking awareness of one's own behaviors and feelings, and withdrawing from the patient can also be detrimental.

MEDICATION. Nursing intervention may include the administration of medications to the highly anxious patient (Table 16-2). Because anxiety is a pervasive problem, large portions of the population take antianxiety drugs. Americans are now spending more than $500 million each year

A **Family** *Speaks*

My daughter has obsessive-compulsive disorder (OCD). I didn't always know that, and I've spent many years of my life wondering what was wrong with her and if I were to blame. It's not easy living with someone who has an illness like that. At times it is just annoying. At other times it really makes you mad, and still other times you want to burst out laughing, but all that only makes it worse.

I think the one thing the family needs from the mental health care system is for health care professionals to talk with them. The nurse who sees my daughter told me that I can call her with questions, and she explained all about OCD to my husband and me in great detail. Families want to help and support their members who are suffering, but how can we help if we don't know what to do? I used to try to physically stop my daughter from checking things. Then I told her how ridiculous it was. I even tried ignoring it for a while. How was I supposed to know what to do? Things are different now. We've all learned about this illness and how we can best help our daughter. After all, that's all we ever really wanted. ▼

for drugs to relieve anxiety. Among these drugs, the benzodiazepines are often the medication of choice and are the most widely prescribed drugs in the world. They have almost replaced the barbiturates in the treatment of anxiety because of their effectiveness and wide margin of safety. Use of these drugs in combination with alcohol, however, may result in a serious or even fatal sedative reaction. Antidepressants have gained popularity in the treatment of anxiety disorders in light of studies documenting their effectiveness and the low side effect profile of some of them. Antipsychotic drugs are often prescribed for patients experiencing a panic level of anxiety of psychotic proportions.

Although some patients may need to take antianxiety drugs for extended periods, these drugs should always be used in conjunction with nonpharmacological treatments. Potential dangers of benzodiazepines include withdrawal syndrome side effects and addiction. It should be emphasized that psychopharmacology is not a substitute for an ongoing therapeutic relationship. Psychopharmacology can enhance the therapeutic relationship. Chemical control of painful symptoms allows the patient to direct attention to the conflicts underlying the anxiety. More detailed information on medications is presented in Chapter 27.

The Nursing Treatment Plan Summary on p. 292 reviews interventions related to severe and panic levels of anxiety.

TABLE **16-2** *Antianxiety Drugs*

CHEMICAL CLASS GENERIC NAME (TRADE NAME)	USUAL DOSAGE RANGE (MG/DAY)
ANTIANXIETY DRUGS	
Benzodiazepines	
Alprazolam (Xanax)	0.5-4
Chlordiazepoxide (Librium)	20-100
Clorazepate (Tranxene)	7.5-60
Clonazepam (Klonopin)	1.5-2.0
Diazepam (Valium)	10-40
Halazepam (Paxipam)	80-160
Lorazepam (Ativan)	2-6
Oxazepam (Serax)	15-90
Prazepam (Centrax)	10-60
Antihistamines	
Diphenhydramine (Benadryl)	50
Hydroxyzine (Atarax)	100-300
Beta-adrenergic Blocker	
Propranolol (Inderal)	10-40
Anxiolytic	
Buspirone (BuSpar)	10-40
ANTIDEPRESSANT DRUGS	
Clomipramine (Anafranil)	50-200
Fluoxetine (Prozac)	20-80
Sertraline (Zoloft)	50-200
Paroxetine (Paxil)	20-50
Fluvoxamine (Luvox)	50-250
Venlafaxine (Effexor)	150-375
Nefazodone (Serzone)	200-500
Phenelzine (Nardil)	45-90

Moderate Level of Anxiety

The nursing interventions previously mentioned are supportive and directed toward the short-term goal of reducing severe or panic-level anxiety. When the patient's anxiety is reduced to a moderate level, the nurse can begin helping with problem-solving efforts to cope with the stress. Long-term goals focus on helping the patient understand the cause of the anxiety and learn new ways of controlling it.

Education is an important aspect of promoting the patient's adaptive responses to anxiety. The nurse can identify the health teaching needs of each patient and then formulate a teaching plan to meet those needs. Plans should be designed to increase patients' knowledge of their own predisposing and precipitating stressors, coping resources, and adaptive and maladaptive responses.[3] Alternative coping strategies can be identified and explored. Health teaching should also address the beneficial aspects of mild levels of anxiety in motivating learning and producing growth and creativity.

The specific nursing interventions for a moderate level of anxiety were originally described by Peplau[20] and Burd[5]

and reflect the problem-solving process. Short-term goals may be written for each step of this process. Goals include recognition of anxiety, insight into the anxiety, and coping with the threat. They incorporate principles and techniques of cognitive behavioral therapy (see Chapter 30) and can be implemented in any setting: psychiatric, community, home, or general hospital.

RECOGNITION OF ANXIETY. After analyzing the patient's behaviors and determining the level of anxiety, the nurse helps the patient to recognize anxiety by helping him or her explore underlying feelings with such questions as "Are you feeling anxious now?" or "Are you uncomfortable?" It is also helpful for the nurse to identify the patient's behavior and link it to the feeling of anxiety (for example, "I noticed you smoked three cigarettes since we started talking about your sister. Are you feeling anxious?"). In this way the nurse acknowledges the patient's feeling, attempts to label it, encourages the patient to describe it further, and relates it to a specific behavioral pattern. The nurse is also validating inferences and assumptions with the patient.

However, the patient's goal is often to avoid or negate anxiety and he or she may use any of the resistive approaches described in Box 16-8. All these approaches may create feelings of frustration, irritation, or reciprocal anxiety in the nurse, who must recognize personal feelings and identify the patient's behavior pattern that might be causing them.

In attempting to deal with these patient defenses and intervene successfully, the importance of a trusting relationship becomes evident. If nurses establish themselves as warm, responsive listeners, give patients adequate time to respond, and support the patient's self-expression, they will become less threatening. In helping patients recognize their anxiety, nurses should use open questions that move from nonthreatening topics to central issues of conflict. It may be helpful to vary the amount of anxiety to enhance the patient's motivation. In time, supportive confrontation may be used to address the repeated use of a particular resistive pattern. However, if the patient's level of anxiety begins to rise rapidly, the nurse might choose to refocus the discussion to another topic.

INSIGHT INTO THE ANXIETY. Once the patient is able to recognize anxiety, subsequent nursing interventions strive to expand the present context of the patient. The patient may be asked to describe the situations and interactions that immediately precede the increase in anxiety. Together the nurse and patient make inferences about the precipitating causes or biopsychosocial stressors.

The nurse then helps the patient see which values are being threatened by linking the threat with underlying causes, analyzing how the conflict developed, and relating the patient's present experiences to past ones. It is also important to explore how the patient reduced anxiety in the past and what kinds of actions produced relief.

COPING WITH THE THREAT. If previous coping responses have been adaptive and constructive, the patient

NURSING TREATMENT PLAN *Summary* Severe and Panic Anxiety Responses

Nursing Diagnosis Severe/panic level of anxiety
Expected Outcome The patient will reduce anxiety to a moderate or mild level.

Short-term Goals	Interventions	Rationale
The patient will be protected from harm.	Initially accept and support, rather than attack, the patient's defenses. Acknowledge the reality of the pain associated with the patient's present coping mechanisms. Do not focus on the phobia, ritual, or physical complaint itself. Give feedback to the patient about behavior, stressors, appraisal of stressors, and coping resources. Reinforce the idea that physical health is related to emotional health and that this is an area that will need exploration. In time, begin to place limits on the patient's maladaptive behavior in a supportive way.	Severe and panic levels of anxiety can be reduced by initially allowing the patient to determine the amount of stress that can be handled. If the patient is unable to release anxiety, tension may mount to the panic level and the patient may lose control. At this time the patient has no alternative coping mechanisms.
The patient will experience fewer anxiety-provoking situations.	Assume a calm manner with the patient. Decrease environmental stimulation. Limit the patient's interaction with other patients to minimize the contagious aspects of anxiety. Identify and modify anxiety-provoking situations for the patient. Administer supportive physical measures such as warm baths and massages.	The patient's behavior may be modified by altering the environment and the patient's interaction with it.
The patient will engage in a daily schedule of activities.	Initially share an activity with the patient to provide support and reinforce socially productive behavior. Provide for physical exercise of some type. Plan a schedule or list of activities that can be carried out daily. Involve family members and other support systems as much as possible.	By encouraging outside activities, the nurse limits the time the patient has available for destructive coping mechanisms while increasing participation in and enjoyment of other aspects of life.
The patient will experience relief from the symptoms of severe anxiety.	Administer medications that help reduce the patient's discomfort. Observe for medication side effects and initiate relevant health teaching.	The effect of a therapeutic relationship may be enhanced if the chemical control of symptoms allows the patient to direct attention to underlying conflicts.

Box **16-8** *Patient Resistances to Recognizing Anxiety*

Screen symptoms. The patient focuses attention on minor physical ailments to avoid acknowledging anxiety and conflict areas.
Superior status position. The patient attempts to control the interview by questioning the nurse's abilities or asserting the superiority of the patient's knowledge or experiences. The nurse should not respond emotionally to this approach or accept the patient's challenge and compete because this would only further avoid the issue of anxiety.
Emotional seduction. The patient attempts to manipulate the nurse and elicit pity or sympathy.
Superficiality. The patient relates on a surface level and resists the nurse's attempts to explore underlying feelings or analyze issues.
Circumlocution. The patient gives the pretense of answering questions, but actually talks around the topic to avoid it.
Amnesia. This is a type of purposeful forgetting of an incident to avoid confronting and exploring it with the nurse.

Denial. The patient may use this approach only when discussing significant issues with the nurse or may generalize denial to all others, including self. The purpose is often to avoid humiliation.
Intellectualization. Patients who use this technique usually have some knowledge of psychology or medicine. They are able to express appropriate insights and analysis yet lack personal involvement in the problem they describe. They are not actually participating in the problem-solving process.
Hostility. The patient believes that offense is the best defense and therefore relates to others in an aggressive, defiant manner. The greatest danger in this situation is that the nurse will take this behavior personally and respond with anger. This reinforces the patient's avoidance of his or her anxiety.
Withdrawal. The patient may resist the nurse by replying in vague, diffuse, indefinite, and remote ways.

Box **16-9** *Cognitive Behavioral Treatment Strategies for Anxiety Disorders*

ANXIETY REDUCTION	COGNITIVE RESTRUCTURING	LEARNING NEW BEHAVIOR
Relaxation training	Monitoring thoughts and feelings	Modeling
Biofeedback	Questioning the evidence	Shaping
Systematic desensitization	Examining alternatives	Token economy
Interoceptive exposure	Decatastrophizing	Role playing
Flooding	Reframing	Social skills training
Vestibular desensitization training	Thought stopping	Aversion therapy
Response prevention		Contingency contracting
Eye movement desensitization		

should be encouraged to use them. If not, the nurse can point out their maladaptive effects and inform the patient that the present way of life appears unsatisfactory and distressing and that the patient is not attempting to improve the situation. The patient needs to assume responsibility for actions and realize that limitations have been self-imposed. Other people must not be blamed. In this phase of intervention the nurse assumes an active role by interpreting, analyzing, confronting, and correlating cause-and-effect relationships. The nurse should proceed clearly so that the patient can follow while maintaining anxiety within appropriate limits. If the patient's anxiety becomes too severe, the nurse may change topics temporarily.

The nurse can help the patient in problem-solving efforts in various cognitive and behavioral ways. Specifically, cognitive behavioral therapy has been shown to be very effective in treating many anxiety disorders across age groups.[17] These treatments include a number of therapeutic strategies, which can be divided into three groups: anxiety reduction, cognitive restructuring, and learning new behavior. The specific strategies are listed in Box 16-9 and are explained in detail in Chapter 30.

One way of helping the patient cope is to reevaluate the nature of the threat or stressor. Is it as bad as the patient perceives it? Is the cognitive appraisal realistic? Together the nurse and patient might discuss fears and feelings of inadequacy. Does the patient fear that others are as critical, perfectionistic, and rejecting as the patient is of others? Is the conflict based in reality, or is it the result of unvalidated, isolated, and distorted thinking? By sharing fears with family members, peers, and staff, the patient often gains insight into such misperceptions.

Another approach is to help the patient modify behavior and learn new ways of coping with stress.[19] The nurse may act as a role model in this regard or engage the patient in role playing. This can decrease anxiety about new responses to problem situations. One nursing function therefore is to teach the patient how aspects of mild anxiety can be constructive and produce growth. Physical activity should be encouraged as a way to discharge anxiety. Interpersonal resources such as family members or close friends should be incorporated into the nursing plan of care to provide the patient with support.

Often the cause for anxiety arises from an interpersonal conflict. In this case it is constructive to include the people involved when analyzing the situation with the patient. In this way, cause-and-effect relationships are more open to examination. Coping patterns can be examined in light of their effect on others, as well as on the patient.

Working through this problem-solving or reeducative process with the patient takes time because it has to be accepted both intellectually and emotionally. Breaking previous behavioral patterns can be difficult. Nurses need to be patient and consistent and continually reappraise their own anxiety.

PROMOTE THE RELAXATION RESPONSE. In addition to problem solving, one can also cope with stress by regulating the emotional distress associated with it. Long-term goals directed toward helping the patient regulate emotional distress are supportive.

Relaxation can be taught individually, in small groups, or in large-group settings. A Patient Education Plan for teaching the relaxation response is presented on p. 294. It is within the scope of nursing practice, requires no special equipment, and does not need a physician's supervision. As a group of interventions, relaxation can be implemented in various settings. A major benefit for patients is that after several training sessions, they can practice the techniques on their own. This puts the control in their hands and increases their self-reliance. Relaxation training is described in detail in Chapter 30. The Nursing Treatment Plan Summary for patients with moderate anxiety is presented on p. 295.

Evaluation

Evaluation is an ongoing process engaged in by the nurse and patient that is part of each phase of the nursing process. Even before beginning to formulate the nursing diagnosis, the nurse should ask, "Did I critically observe my patient's physiological and psychomotor behaviors? Did I listen to my patient's subjective description of experience? Did I fail to see the relationships between my patient's expressed hostility or guilt and underlying anxiety? Did I assess intellectual and social functioning?" After collecting the data, the nurse should analyze it: "Was I able to identify the precipitating stressor for the patient? What was the patient's perception of the threat?

📖 **PATIENT EDUCATION PLAN** **The Relaxation Response**

Content	Instructional Activities	Evaluation
Describe the characteristics and benefits of relaxation	Discuss physiological changes associated with relaxation and contrast these with the behaviors of anxiety	Patient identifies own responses to anxiety Patient describes elements of a relaxed state
Teach deep muscle relaxation through a sequence of tension-relaxation exercises	Engage the patient in the progressive procedure of tensing and relaxing voluntary muscles until the body as a whole is relaxed	Patient is able to tense and relax all muscle groups Patient identifies muscles that become particularly tense
Discuss the relaxation procedure of meditation and its components	Describe the elements of meditation and help the patient use this technique	Patient selects a word or scene with pleasant connotations and engages in relaxed meditation
Help patient overcome anxiety-provoking situations through systematic desensitization	With patient, construct a hierarchy of anxiety-provoking situations or scenes Through imagination or reality, work through these scenes using relaxation techniques	Patient identifies and ranks anxiety-provoking situations Patient exposes self to these situations while remaining in a relaxed state
Allow the rehearsing and practical use of relaxation in a safe environment	Role play stressful situations with the nurse or other patients	Patient becomes more comfortable with new behavior in a safe, supportive setting
Encourage patient to use relaxation techniques in life	Assign homework of using the relaxation response in everyday experiences Support success of patient	Patient uses relaxation response in life situations Patient is able to regulate anxiety response through use of relaxation techniques

How was this influenced by physical health, past experiences, and present feelings and needs? Did I correctly identify the patient's level of anxiety and validate it?"

When using the criteria of adequacy, effectiveness, appropriateness, efficiency, and flexibility in evaluating the nursing goals and actions, the following questions can be raised:

▼ Were the planning, implementation, and evaluation mutual?
▼ Were goals and actions adequate in number and sufficiently specific to minimize the patient's level of anxiety?
▼ Were maladaptive responses reduced?
▼ Were new adaptive coping responses learned?
▼ Was the care plan reasonable in terms of time, energy, and expense?
▼ Was the nurse accepting of the patient and able to monitor personal anxiety throughout the relationship?

Answering these questions enables the nurse to review the total care provided. The nurse will also identify personal strengths and limitations in working with the anxious patient. Plans may then be made for overcoming the areas of limitation and further improving nursing care.

Summary

1. Anxiety is diffuse apprehension that is vague and associated with feelings of uncertainty and helplessness. It is an emotion without an object that is subjective and communicated interpersonally. Levels of anxiety include mild, moderate, severe, and panic.
2. Patient behaviors related to anxiety include physiological, behavioral, cognitive, and affective responses.
3. Predisposing factors for anxiety responses are described from psychoanalytical, interpersonal, behavioral, family, and biological perspectives. Precipitating stressors include threats to physical integrity and self-system.
4. Coping mechanisms can be categorized as task-oriented reactions such as attack, withdrawal, and compromise, or ego-oriented reactions also known as defense mechanisms.
5. Primary NANDA diagnoses related to anxiety responses are anxiety, ineffective coping, and fear.
6. Primary DSM-IV diagnoses are categorized as anxiety disorders.
7. The expected outcome of nursing care for patients with maladaptive anxiety responses is that the patient will demonstrate adaptive ways of coping with stress.
8. Interventions include establishing a trusting relationship, self-awareness, protecting the patient, modifying the environment, encouraging activity, medication, and learning new ways to cope with stress.
9. The nurse should use the criteria of adequacy, effectiveness, appropriateness, efficiency, and flexibility in evaluating nursing care.

NURSING TREATMENT PLAN *Summary*   Moderate Anxiety Responses

Nursing Diagnosis Moderate level of anxiety
Expected Outcome The patient will demonstrate adaptive ways of coping with stress.

Short-term Goals	Interventions	Rationale
The patient will identify and describe feelings of anxiety	Help the patient identify and describe underlying feelings Link the patient's behavior with such feelings Validate all inferences and assumptions with the patient Use open questions to move from nonthreatening topics to issues of conflict Vary the amount of anxiety to enhance the patient's motivation In time, supportive confrontation may be used judiciously	To adopt new coping responses, the patient first needs to be aware of feelings and to overcome conscious or unconscious denial and resistance
The patient will identify antecedents of anxiety	Help the patient describe the situations and interactions that immediately precede anxiety Review the patient's appraisal of the stressor, values being threatened, and the way in which the conflict developed Relate the patient's present experiences with relevant ones from the past	Once feelings of anxiety are recognized, the patient needs to understand their development, including precipitating stressors, appraisal of the stressor, and available resources
The patient will describe adaptive and maladaptive coping responses	Explore how the patient reduced anxiety in the past and what kinds of actions produced relief Point out the maladaptive and destructive effects of present coping responses Encourage the patient to use adaptive coping responses that were effective in the past Focus responsibility for change on the patient Actively help the patient correlate cause-and-effect relationships while maintaining anxiety within appropriate limits Help the patient reappraise the value, nature, and meaning of the stressor when appropriate	New adaptive coping responses can be learned through analyzing coping mechanisms used in the past, reappraising the stressor, using available resources, and accepting responsibility for change
The patient will implement two adaptive responses for coping with anxiety	Help the patient identify ways to restructure thoughts, modify behavior, use resources, and test new coping responses Encourage physical activity to discharge energy Include significant others as resources and social supports in helping the patient learn new coping responses Teach the patient relaxation exercises to increase control and self-reliance and reduce stress	One can also cope with stress by regulating the emotional distress that accompanies it through the use of stress management techniques

COMPETENT CARING A Clinical Exemplar of a Psychiatric Nurse

Madelyn Myers, BS, RN

As the night shift charge nurse on an adult psychiatric unit, I learned that the graveyard shift was anything but routine. On return to the unit after my days off, I was told that Mr. B's behavior had deteriorated in the last few days. Mr. B was a 68-year-old man with a diagnosis of organic brain syndrome secondary to alcohol abuse. He was unable to stay in bed for more than a few minutes at a time and he was at risk for falls due to his confusion and as a side effect of his tranquilizing medication. The previous nights the staff had found it necessary to contain Mr. B with soft restraints to keep him in bed and reduce the risk of his falling.

After shift report I made my nursing rounds, accounting for all patients and assessing the situation of the unit. Mr. B was obviously distraught and anxious. His first question to me was, "You're not going to rope me, are you?" I sat down to talk with Mr. B to reassure him and explain that it was time for him to get ready for bed. He refused to change his clothing, stating that he just needed to walk around a little longer. I asked the therapeutic assistants if they would walk him around a while longer to try calming him down.

I went to the office to start verifying the day's orders, but found it impossible to get much done as Mr. B was calling me and coming to the nursing office to ask questions very frequently. The staff were also getting frustrated because he seemed very tired but would sit down for only a few minutes before he would jump up again. After I did a few more tasks, I relieved the staff member sitting with Mr. B. I was able to get Mr. B to lie down on his bed only after he saw me take the posey off the bed and out of the room. I watched him as he lay down and he seemed to doze off to sleep almost immediately. Then again just as quickly he awoke and started out of bed. He said, "Something is very wrong with me—I'm afraid I might die." We discussed his anxiety, and I reassured him that one of the staff would sit with him if that would make him feel more secure. He nodded in affirmation. I sat by his bedside. He fell asleep immediately and again repeated his previous pattern of awakening with a start, but this time he just looked over, saw me, and returned to sleep.

A short while later, one of the other staff came to relieve me. I shared with her my concern that Mr. B had been quite anxious and my plan was to sit at his bedside and gradually move the chair back until we were sitting just outside his room but still in his line of sight. This way, he would be reassured that staff were still close by and we could observe him if he tried to get out of bed. That night he actually slept 4 hours with only two brief awakenings. The previous nights he had only dozed for minutes at a time.

The next morning I spoke with the nurse on his team and relayed his fear of dying and of being "roped" with the posey. I shared with her the strategy we used of sitting with him and how he was able to sleep. The new plan of care was placed in his Kardex for all to follow. The next few nights we continued with our plan and each night Mr. B slept a little longer. He would even change into his pajamas before bed. He no longer started to "escalate" at bedtime. As he was sleeping better, Mr. B was also feeling better physically and his anxiety level decreased dramatically. He required less medication for his anxiety; thus he was much more stable on his feet, no longer at risk for falls. Mr. B's ability to perform his ADLs increased over the next week and he was able to return to his previous living situation.

Many of his symptoms seemed to have been from sleep deprivation, high levels of anxiety, and the untoward effects of tranquilizers. This rewarding experience was not an isolated event on the night shift. It seems many people sleep through the night and see only the shadows of the staff making rounds, but there are others for whom the care they receive during these darkened hours makes a critical difference.

 Video **Resources**

Mosby's Psychiatric Nursing Video Series

  Anxiety Disorders (Volume 1)

your **INTERNET**
c o n n e c t i o n

NPAD News: National Panic/Anxiety Disorder News
http://www.npadnews.com

Noodles' Panic-Anxiety Page: The ANXIETY Panic
Internet Resource
http://www.algy.com/anxiety

Chapter Review Questions

1. Match each term in Column A with the correct definition in Column B.

Column A

G. Affective responses

A. Anxiety

C. Cognitive responses

I. Ego-oriented reactions

F. Fear

J. Moderate anxiety

E. Neurosis

D. Panic

H. Psychosis

B. Task-oriented reactions

Column B

A. Diffuse, vague, subjective apprehension with feelings of uncertainty and helplessness

B. Attack behavior, withdrawal behavior, compromise

C. Forgetfulness, confusion, hypervigilance, fear of injury or death, poor concentration and judgment

D. Awe, dread, terror, loss of control, disorganization of the personality

E. A mental disorder characterized by anxiety that involves no distortion of reality

F. An individual ideation with a specific identifiable source

G. Edginess, impatience, uneasiness, tension, nervousness, fright, fear, alarm

H. A mental disorder that involves a disintegration of self, a fear of defeat in the process of being

I. Repression, splitting, denial, dissociation, projection, intellectualization, rationalization

J. Focus is only on immediate concerns, with a narrowing of the perceptual field

2. Fill in the blanks.

A. Difficulty in falling asleep, psychomotor hyperactivity, and selective negative appraisals are characteristic of ___anxiety___. Early morning wakening, psychomotor retardation or agitation, and absolute negative evaluations characterize ___depression___.

B. Recurrent and persistent thoughts, impulses, or images that are intrusive and inappropriate, and cause marked anxiety or distress, are called ___obsessions___.

C. When the patient resists recognizing anxiety and attempts to manipulate the nurse and elicit sympathy or pity, it is called ___emotional seduction___

D. Precipitating stressors that threaten the patient and cause anxiety fall into two categories: threats to ___phys. integrity___ and ___self-esteem___.

E. The two main categories of medications to treat anxiety disorders are the ___benzos.___ and ___antidep.___.

3. Provide short answers for the following questions.

A. Explain the behavioral view that anxiety arises from conflict.

B. Consider the nursing intervention categories for working with the anxious patient. What are some principles you can follow to protect the patient with an anxiety disorder?

C. Describe the criterion of flexibility when evaluating nursing care. How could you have been more flexible last time you worked with an anxious patient?

References

1. American Psychiatric Association: *Diagnostic and statistical manual of mental disorders*, ed 4, Washington, DC, 1994, The Association.
2. Beck CT: A concept analysis of panic, *Arch Psychiatr Nurs* 5:265, 1996.
3. Benham E: Coping strategies: a psychoeducational approach to post-traumatic symptomatology, *J Psychosoc Nurs* 6:30, 1995.
4. Brown P, Yantis J: Personal space intrusion and PTSD, *J Psychosoc Nurs* 24:23, 1996.
5. Burd S: Effects of nursing intervention in anxiety of patients. In Burd SF, Marshall MA, editors: *Some clinical approaches to psychiatric nursing*, New York, 1963, Macmillan.
6. Bystritsky A, Munford PR, Rosen RM, Martin KR, Vapnik T, Gorbis E, Wolson RC: A preliminary study of partial hospital management of severe obsessive-compulsive disorder, *Psychiatr Serv* 47:170, 1996.
7. Calvocoressi L, Lewis B, Harris M, Trufan SJ, Goodman WK, McDougle CJ, Price LH: Family accommodation in obsessive-compulsive disorder, *Am J Psychiatry* 152:441, 1995.
8. Free N, Winget C, Whitman R: Separation anxiety in panic disorder, *Am J Psychiatry* 150:595, 1993.
9. Freud S: *Problem of anxiety*, New York, 1936, WW Norton.
10. Freud S: *A general introduction to psychoanalysis*, New York, 1969, Pocket Books.
11. Glod C, McEnany G: The neurobiology of posttraumatic stress disorder, *J Am Psychiatr Nurses Assoc* 1:196, 1995.
12. Harvard Mental Health Letter, *Post-traumatic stress disorder*, Parts I & II, 12:1, and 13:1, 1996.
13. Hoehn-Saric R, McLeod D: *Biology of anxiety disorders*, Washington, DC, 1993, American Psychiatric Press.
14. Laraia MT: Panic disorder: understanding and education are key to treatment, *Adv Nurse Practitioners* 3:5, 1995.

15. Laraia M, Stuart G, Frye L, Lydiard R, Ballenger J: Childhood environment of women having panic disorder with agoraphobia, *J Anxiety Dis* 8:1, 1994.

16. Massion A, Warshaw M, Keller M: Quality of life and psychiatric morbidity in panic disorder and generalized anxiety disorder, *Am J Psychiatry* 150:600, 1993.

17. Mavissakalian MR, Prien RF: *Long-term treatments of anxiety disorders,* Washington, DC, 1996, American Psychiatric Press.

18. May R: *The meaning of anxiety,* New York, 1950, Ronald Press.

19. Menninger WW: Challenges to providing integrated treatment of anxiety disorders, *Bull Menninger Clin* 58:A86, 1995.

20. Peplau H: Interpersonal techniques: the crux of psychiatric nursing, *Am J Nurs* 62:53, 1962.

21. Peplau H: A working definition of anxiety. In Burd S, Marshall M, editors: *Some clinical approaches to psychiatric nursing,* New York, 1963, Macmillan.

22. Perna G, Bertani A, Caldirola D, Bellodi L: Family history of panic disorder and hypersensitivity to CO_2 in patients with panic disorder, *Am J Psychiatry* 153:1060, 1996.

23. Shear MK: Factors in the etiology and pathogenesis of panic disorder: revisiting the attachment-separation paradigm, *Am J Psychiatry* 153:125, 1996.

24. Shelbourne CD, Wells KB, Judd LL: Functioning and well-being of patients with panic disorder, *Am J Psychiatry* 153:213, 1996.

25. Stuart GW, Laraia MT: Panic disorder with agoraphobia. In McBride AB, Austin JK, editors: *Psychiatric–mental health nursing: integrating the behavioral and biological sciences,* Philadelphia, 1996, WB Saunders.

26. Sullivan HS: *The interpersonal theory of psychiatry,* New York, 1953, WW Norton.

27. Symes L: Posttraumatic stress disorder: an evolving concept, *Arch Psychiatr Nurs* 4:195, 1995.

28. Yehuda R, McFarlane A: Conflict between current knowledge about posttraumatic stress disorder and its original conceptual basis, *Am J Psychiatry,* 152:1705, 1995.

ANNOTATED SUGGESTED READINGS

*Benham E: Coping strategies: a psychoeducational approach to post-traumatic symptomatology, *J Psychosoc Nurs* 6:30, 1995.
Extensive review of the educational approaches the nurse should use in the treatment of patients with PTSD symptomatology.

*Brown P, Yantis J: Personal space intrusion and PTSD, *J Psychosoc Nurs* 24:23, 1996.
Discusses how the direct intrusion of personal space that occurs in much of nursing care adversely affects patients with PTSD and gives suggestions on how to overcome this problem.

Bystritsky A et al: A preliminary study of partial hospital management of severe obsessive-compulsive disorder, *Psychiatr Serv* 47:170, 1996.
This study found efficacy for a program that combined behavioral therapy, medication, and psychosocial intervention for severe and treatment resistant patients with OCD.

Freedy J, Hobfoll S: *Traumatic stress: from theory to practice,* New York, 1995, Plenum Press.
Comprehensively reviews the field of traumatic stress and injury occurring from many sources and the impact on the individual and society. Treatment and research strategies are discussed as well.

Harvard Mental Health Letter, *Post-traumatic stress disorder,* Parts I & II, 12:1, and 13:1, 1996.
This two-part series gives a good overview of PTSD, with case examples, assessment, and treatment. It reviews risk factors, differential diagnoses, and referral sources.

*Laraia M: Biological correlates of panic disorder with agoraphobia: practical perspectives for nurses, *Arch Psychiatr Nurs* 5:373, 1991.
A concise, clear description of the biological theories pertaining to anxiety disorders, with implications for nursing practice and research.

Laraia M et al: Childhood environment of women having panic disorder with agoraphobia, *J Anxiety Disorders* 8:1, 1994.
Research conducted by nurses in an interdisciplinary team on the childhood environment of women with panic disorder.

Mavissakalian M, Prien R: *Long term treatments of anxiety disorders,* Washington, DC, 1996, American Psychiatric Press, Inc.
Comprehensive and easy-to-read review of what is currently known of the long-term outcomes of treating the anxiety disorders.

*Moyers F: Oklahoma City bombing: exacerbation of symptoms in veterans with PTSD, *Arch Psychiatr Nurs* 1:55, 1996
Analyzes the exacerbation of symptoms after the Oklahoma City bombing by veterans from several wars, reviews theories for the etiology of PTSD, and explains the importance of attached meaning to traumatic events.

Roth S: The panic-agoraphobic syndrome: a paradigm of the anxiety group of disorders and its implications for psychiatric practice and theory, *Am J Psychiatry* 153:111, 1996.
Thorough review of panic disorder and agoraphobia combining biological and psychodynamic dimensions that demands a many-sided approach in treating persons with this syndrome.

Smith S, Sherril K, Colenda C: Assessing and treating anxiety in elderly persons, *Psychiatr Serv* 46:36, 1995.
Proposes that treatment of anxiety syndromes in the elderly hinges on a thorough diagnostic evaluation, with attention to the tendency of older adults to prefer somatic descriptors and to view psychiatric illness as stigmatizing.

*Snell F, Padin-Rivera E: Group treatment for older veterans with post-traumatic stress disorder, *J Psychosoc Nurs* 35:10, 1997.
Thorough description of a PTSD treatment program specially designed for older veterans.

*Stuart G, Laraia M: Panic disorder with agoraphobia. In McBride AB, Austin JK, eds: *Psychiatric-mental health nursing: integrating the behavioral and biological sciences,* Philadelphia, 1996, WB Saunders.
A thorough review of panic disorder, including hypothesized etiologies, DSM-IV diagnosis, assessment strategies, and treatment issues.

*Symes L: Post traumatic stress disorder: an evolving concept, *Arch Psychiatr Nurs,* 4:195, 1995.
This inductive inquiry defines the concept of PTSD and highlights unanswered questions in the field.

*Turner D: Panic disorder: a personal and nursing perspective, *J Psychosoc Nurs* 33:5, 1995.
Interesting personal account of a nurse who has panic disorder.

Van Noppen B et al: Learning to live with obsessive-compulsive disorder, *Innovations Res* 2:41, 1993.
Helpful reading for family members trying to cope with the demands of OCD. Information can be generalized to other disorders as well.

*Waddell K, Demi A: Effectiveness of an intensive partial hospitalization program for treatment of anxiety disorders, *Arch Psychiatr Nurs* 7:2, 1993.
Reports on the effectiveness of a 5-week partial hospitalization program based on an integration of biological, cognitive, and behavioral theories.

*Wakefiled M, Pallister R: Cognitive-behavioral approaches to panic disorder, *J Psychosoc Nurs* 35:12, 1997.
Reviews the etiology of panic and cognitive-behavioral approaches to treatment that can be used by nurses.

*Nursing reference.

Psychophysiological Responses and Somatoform and Sleep Disorders

© 1998 M.C. Escher/Cordon Art, Baarn, Holland.

The cure of many diseases is unknown to the physicians of Hellas, because they disregard the whole, which ought to be studied also, for the part can never be well unless the whole is well. **Plato**

Gail W. Stuart

LEARNING OBJECTIVES

After studying this chapter the student should be able to:

▼ Describe the continuum of adaptive and maladaptive psychophysiological responses

▼ Identify behaviors associated with psychophysiological responses

▼ Analyze predisposing factors, precipitating stressors, and appraisal of stressors related to psychophysiological responses

▼ Describe coping resources and mechanisms related to psychophysiological responses

▼ Formulate nursing diagnoses related to psychophysiological responses

▼ Assess the relationship between nursing diagnoses and medical diagnoses related to psychophysiological responses

▼ Identify expected outcomes and short-term nursing goals related to psychophysiological responses

▼ Develop a patient education plan to teach adaptive strategies to cope with stress

▼ Analyze nursing interventions related to psychophysiological responses

▼ Evaluate nursing care related to psychophysiological responses

TOPICAL OUTLINE

Continuum of Psychophysiological Responses
Assessment
  Behaviors
  Predisposing Factors
  Precipitating Stressors
  Appraisal of Stressors
  Coping Resources
  Coping Mechanisms
Nursing Diagnosis
  Related Medical Diagnoses
Outcome Identification
Planning
Implementation
  Psychological Approaches
  Patient Education
  Physiological Support
  Holistic Interventions
Evaluation

Throughout history, philosophers and scientists have debated the nature and extent of the relationship between the mind (*psyche*) and body (*soma*). Recently there has been a renewed interest in holistic health practices, based on the idea that mental processes influence physical well-being and vice versa. Research is attempting to identify the links between thoughts, feelings, and body functioning. Great interest has arisen about the role of the endocrine and immune systems in the development of psychophysiological disorders. Many believe that all illness has a psychophysiological component: Physical disorders have a psychological component and mental disorders a physical one.

CONTINUUM OF PSYCHOPHYSIOLOGICAL RESPONSES

Much of the current thinking about psychophysiological behavior is related to an increased understanding of the role of stress in human life. Stress theory was significantly advanced when Hans Selye[26] published *The Stress of Life* in 1956. Selye described the stress response in detail, creating a greater understanding of the effect of stressful experiences on physical functioning. He identified a three-stage process of response to stress. This generalized response is called the general adaptation syndrome (GAS). These levels of response are

▼ **The alarm reaction.** This is the immediate response to a stressor in a localized area. Adrenocortical mechanisms respond, resulting in behaviors associated with the fight-or-flight response.

▼ **Stage of resistance.** There is some resistance to the stressor. The body adapts and functions at a lower than optimal level. This requires a greater than usual expenditure of energy for survival.

▼ **Stage of exhaustion.** The adaptive mechanisms become worn out and fail. The negative effect of the stressor spreads to the entire organism. If the stressor is not removed or counteracted, death will ultimately result.

Any experience believed by the individual to be stressful may stimulate a psychophysiological response. The stress does not have to be recognized consciously, and often it is not. If people recognize that they are under stress, they are often unable to connect the cognitive understanding of stress with the physical symptoms of the psychophysiological disorder. Fig. 17-1 illustrates the range of possible psychophysiological responses to stress, based on Selye's theory.

Assessment

Behaviors

Many behaviors are associated with psychophysiological disorders. Careful assessment is needed so that organic problems are defined and treated. This type of illness should never be dismissed as "only psychosomatic" or "all in one's head."[10] Serious psychophysiological disorders can be fatal if not treated appropriately.

PHYSIOLOGICAL. The primary behaviors observed with psychophysiological responses are the physical symptoms. These symptoms lead the person to seek health care. Psychological factors affecting the physical condition may involve any body part.[7] The most common organ systems involved are listed in Box 17-1. In addition, longer general hospital stays have been reported to be associated with greater psychological comorbidity, particularly depression, anxiety, and organicity.[25] Such research underscores the importance of linking physiological and psychological assessments.

People are often reluctant to believe that a physical problem may be related to psychological factors. In part, this is because being physically ill is more socially acceptable than having psychological problems. The situation is compounded because the patient has physical symptoms. Denial of the psychological component of the illness may lead to "doctor shopping." The patient searches for someone who will find an organic cause for the illness. This tendency to experience and communicate psychological distress in the form of physical symptoms and to seek help for them in general medical settings is a widespread phenomenon that may involve 30% to 40% of medical patients.[10] The following clinical example illustrates this problem.

Clinical Example Mr. R was a successful 42-year-old executive who had risen quickly to the top of his company. He worked long hours and had difficulty delegating any of his

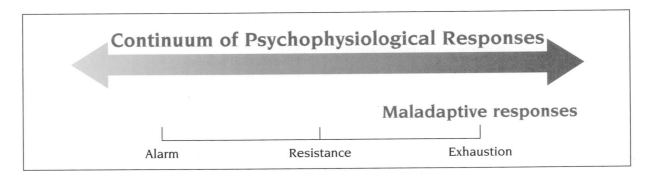

Fig. 17-1 Continuum of psychophysiological responses.

responsibilities. He set high standards for his employees and was believed to be insensitive to human concerns. He viewed himself as tough, but fair. However, he had little sympathy for a worker who requested extra time off for personal business.

Mr. R was married but saw little of his family. He expected his wife and children to do their part to maintain his standing in the community by associating with "the right people." He seldom interacted with his children except to reprimand them if they disturbed him while he was working. His wife reported that their sexual relationship was unsatisfying to her. Mr. R used it for physical release for himself but was not concerned about meeting her needs. She suspected that he was involved in an extramarital affair but did not want to endanger the marriage by confronting him.

Mr. R was expecting to be named to the board of directors of a prestigious philanthropic foundation. He expected that this would add to his social prominence in the community. Shortly before the announcement was to be made, his 14-year-old son was arrested in a drug raid in the lower-middle-class part of town. Mr. R did not get the appointment. He was furious with his son but dealt with his anger by withdrawing still more. One day at work, he experienced an episode of dizziness, followed by a severe headache. He attributed it to tension, took some aspirin, and continued to work. However, after several similar episodes, he decided to consult his family doctor. The physician arrived at a diagnosis of essential hypertension. He tried to discuss work, family, and social behavior with Mr. R but was frustrated by superficial responses. Although concerned about Mr. R's condition and stress level, the doctor gave in to Mr. R's demand for medication to lower his blood pressure. He also advised Mr. R to exercise and to find a relaxing activity.

Box 17-1 *Physical Conditions Affected by Psychological Factors*

CARDIOVASCULAR	SKIN
Migraine	Neurodermatitis
Essential hypertension	Eczema
Angina	Psoriasis
Tension headaches	Pruritus
MUSCULOSKELETAL	
Rheumatoid arthritis	**GENITOURINARY**
Low back pain (idiopathic)	Impotence
RESPIRATORY	Frigidity
Hyperventilation	Premenstrual syndrome
Asthma	**ENDOCRINOLOGICAL**
GASTROINTESTINAL	Hyperthyroidism
Anorexia nervosa	Diabetes
Peptic ulcer	
Irritable bowel syndrome	
Colitis	
Obesity	

Selected Nursing Diagnoses:

▼ Impaired adjustment related to family and work stress, as evidenced by denial and development of physical symptoms
▼ Altered family processes related to rigid role expectations, as evidenced by withdrawal and lack of communication.

Mr. R is typical of many people with stress-related psychophysiological disorders. He is reluctant to admit to a lack of control over his mind and body. He expects a magical cure that will let him follow his usual lifestyle without interruption. He will probably stop taking his medication as soon as he feels better. Distance from the stressor may allow him to function for a while without noticeable symptoms of his hypertension. Sooner or later, however, new stressors will lead to another dizzy spell, headaches, or possibly myocardial infarction or cerebrovascular accident.

PSYCHOLOGICAL. Some people have physical symptoms without any organic impairment, and these are called **somatoform disorders.** They include *somatization disorder,* in which the person has many physical complaints; *conversion disorder,* in which a loss or alteration of physical functioning occurs; *hypochondriasis,* the fear of or belief that one has an illness; *body dysmorphic disorder,* in which a person with a normal appearance is concerned about having a physical defect; and *pain disorder,* in which psychological factors play an important role in the onset, severity, or maintenance of the pain. The next clinical example is a case history of a person with a medical diagnosis of somatization disorder.

Clinical Example Ms. O, a 28-year-old single woman, was admitted to the medical unit of a general hospital for a complete medical work-up. When asked about her main problem during the nursing assessment, she replied, "I've never been very well. Even when I was a child I was sick a lot." Ms. O listed multiple complaints during the physical assessment. These included palpitations, dizzy spells, menstrual irregularity, painful menses, blurred vision, dysphagia, backache, pain in her knees and feet, and a variety of gastrointestinal symptoms including stomach pain, nausea, vomiting, diarrhea, flatulence, and intolerance to seafood, vegetables of the cabbage family, carbonated beverages, and eggs. Except for the food intolerances, none of the symptoms was constant. They occurred at random, making her fearful of going out of her home.

The psychosocial assessment revealed that Ms. O lived with her parents. She was the youngest of three children. Her siblings were living away from the parental home. She had graduated from high school but had poor grades because of her frequent absences. She had tried to work as a clerk in a retail store but was fired because of absenteeism. She did not seem particularly bothered by the loss of her job. She had never tried to find other work, although she had been unemployed for 8 years. When asked how she spent her time, she said that she did some gardening and some housework when she felt well enough. However, she spent most of her time watching television.

Ms. O's parents visited her most of every day. Her mother asked whether she could spend the night in her daughter's room and was displeased when told no. The family had many complaints about the quality of the nursing care, mostly about failures to anticipate the patient's needs, Extensive diagnostic studies failed to reveal any organic basis for Ms. O's physical complaints. When informed that the problem was most likely psychological and advised to obtain psychotherapy, the family protested angrily and refused a referral to a psychiatric clinic. Ms. O was discharged and returned to her parents' home.

Selected Nursing Diagnoses:

▼ Ineffective denial related to physical and emotional health status, as evidenced by repeated medical care visits and refusal to obtain psychiatric treatment

▼ Altered family processes related to mother-daughter dependency issues, as evidenced by excessive caretaking by mother and passivity of daughter

Ms. O shows the dependent behavior that is typical of people with somatization disorder. Her many symptoms allowed her to be taken care of and to avoid the demands of adult responsibility. Her need to be cared for fit with her mother's need to nurture. Therefore, she had little incentive to give up her symptoms. A periodic hospital stay reinforced the seriousness of her problem. Secondary gain related to the gratification of dependency needs is a powerful deterrent to change in many patients. **Secondary gain** is an indirect benefit, usually obtained through an illness or disability. Such benefits may include personal attention, release from unpleasant situations and responsibilities, or monetary and disability benefits.

Another type of somatoform disorder is *conversion disorder.* Symptoms of some physical illnesses appear without any underlying organic cause. The organic symptom reduces the patient's anxiety and usually gives a clue to the conflict. For example, a patient who has an impulse to harm his domineering father may develop paralysis of his arms and hands. The primary gain is that the patient is unable to carry out his impulses. He also may experience secondary gain in the form of attention, manipulation of others, freedom from responsibilities, and economic benefits. Conversion symptoms might include the following:

▼ Sensory symptoms such as numbness, blindness, or deafness

▼ Motor symptoms such as paralysis, tremors, or mutism

▼ Visceral symptoms such as urinary retention, headaches, or difficulty breathing

It is often difficult to diagnose this reaction. Other patient behaviors may be helpful. Patients often display little anxiety or concern about the conversion symptom and its resulting disability. The classic term for this lack of concern

is *la belle indifférence.* The patient also tends to seek attention in ways not limited to the actual symptom.

Hypochondriasis is another type of somatoform disorder. These people have an exaggerated concern with physical health that is not based on any real organic disorders. They fear presumed diseases and are not helped by reassurance. They also tend to seek out and use information about diseases to convince themselves that they are ill or about to become ill. Unlike the conversion reaction, no actual loss or distortion of function occurs. Patients appear worried and anxious about their symptoms. This concern may be based on physical sensations overlooked by most people or on symptoms of a minor physical illness that the patient magnifies. This is often a chronic behavior pattern accompanied by a history of visits to numerous practitioners.

Hypochondriacal behavior is not related to a conscious decision. If a person decides to fake an illness, the behavior is called **malingering**. This is usually done to avoid responsibilities the person views as burdensome. Many otherwise healthy people malinger at one time or another. For instance, a person involved in an automobile accident may feign neck pain to receive insurance money. Often, the person exaggerates symptoms, is evasive, and tells contradictory stories about the illness.

PAIN. Pain is increasingly recognized as more than simply a sensory phenomenon, but as a complex sensory and emotional experience underlying potential disease. Pain is influenced by behavioral, cognitive, and motivational processes requiring sophisticated assessments and multifaceted treatments for its control.[15] Acute pain is a reflex biological response to injury. By definition, chronic pain is pain of a minimum of 6 months' duration. *Somatoform pain disorder* is a preoccupation with pain in the absence of physical disease to account for its intensity. It does not follow a neuroanatomical distribution. There may also be a close correlation between stress and conflict and the initiation or exacerbation of the pain.

The experience, expression, and treatment of pain are subject to cultural norms and biases. For example, in Western cultures, being female is often a predictor of poor pain management because male expressions of pain are typically taken more seriously by health-care practitioners.[30] Also, members of minority groups who seek health care in culturally insensitive settings may have their requests for support in coping with pain misunderstood because support is culturally defined and varies across ethnic and racial groups.[22]

SLEEP. Sleep disorders are common in the general population and among people with psychiatric disorders.[21] Most importantly, sleep disturbances can influence the development and course of mental illnesses and addictive disorders and can also affect treatment and recovery.[4] Insomnia is the most prevalent sleep disorder. Up to 30% of the population have insomnia and seek help for it. Other sleep disturbances include excessive daytime sleepiness, difficulty sleeping during desired sleep time, and unusual nocturnal events such as nightmares and sleepwalking. Sleep disorders are more common in the elderly.[3]

Sleep disorders are classified by the Association of Sleep Disorders Centers (ASDC) into four major groupings with considerable overlap[17]:

▼ Disorders of initiating or maintaining sleep, also known as **insomnia.** Anxiety and depression are major causes of insomnia.

▼ Disorders of excessive somnolence, also known as **hypersomnia.** This category includes narcolepsy, sleep apnea, and nocturnal movement disorders such as restless legs.

▼ Disorders of the sleep-wake schedule, characterized by normal sleep but at the wrong time. These are transient disturbances associated with jet lag and work shift changes. They are usually self-limited and resolve as the body readjusts to a new sleep-wake schedule.[16]

▼ Disorders associated with sleep stages, also known as **parasomnia.** This category includes conditions such as sleepwalking, night terrors, nightmares, and enuresis. These sleep problems are often experienced by children and can have a significant effect on functioning and well-being.[20]

Approximately 40 million Americans suffer from chronic disorders of sleep and wakefulness, such as narcolepsy, sleep apnea, and the insomnias. The majority of those affected are undiagnosed and untreated. An additional 20 to 30 million people experience intermittent sleep-related problems. In addition, millions of other people get inadequate sleep because of demanding work schedules, school, and other lifestyle issues. The consequences of sleep disorders, sleep deprivation, and sleepiness are significant and include reduced productivity, lowered cognitive performance, increased likelihood of accidents, higher morbidity and mortality risk, and decreased quality of life. Furthermore, the consequences span all aspects of modern society, including health care, education, and family and social life.[31]

The assessment of patients with sleep problems is multifaceted, involving a detailed history and medical and psychiatric examinations, extensive questionnaires, the use of sleep diaries or logs, and often psychological testing. Many patients are referred for formal sleep studies, which include all night polysomnography and physiological measures of daytime sleepiness.[6] Many members of the health-care team collaborate within sleep centers to deliver multidisciplinary care.

> **?** *Have you ever had a problem sleeping? Which ASDC grouping would your problem have fit into, and what did you do to relieve it?*

Predisposing Factors

A number of biopsychosocial factors are believed to influence psychophysiological responses to stress. Most of the relationships between physical and psychological processes are still not well described. Thus, it is important for the nurse to consider all possibilities when assessing factors that might predispose the patient to a particular disorder.

BIOLOGICAL.   Some believe that biological factors may predispose a person to psychophysiological illness. Research has linked emotions to arousal of the neuroendocrine system through release of corticosteroids by the hypothalamic-pituitary-adrenal (HPA) axis, as well as to the actions of neurotransmitter systems, particularly norepinephrine and serotonin. More recently, research measuring changes in postsynaptic receptors in response to stress and the effect on neurotransmission (and thus human behavior) is producing interesting results. By understanding the effects of stress and coping strategies at the level of the synapse, clinicians can design effective treatment strategies.[18]

Genetic factors have also been considered. It has been proposed that a biological tendency for particular psychophysiological responses could be inherited. For instance, epidemiological studies have shown that the lifetime prevalence for somatization disorder in the general population is 0.1% to 0.5%, and is more common in women. In the mothers and sisters of affected patients, however, it increases to 10% to 20%. The rate in monozygotic (identical) twins is 29%, and in dizygotic (fraternal) twins it is 10%. Thus, there is clearly an inherited tendency for this disorder. The genetic theory suggests that any prolonged stress can cause physiological changes, which result in a physical disorder. Each person has a "shock organ" that is genetically vulnerable to stress. Thus, some patients may be prone to cardiac illness, whereas others may react with gastrointestinal distress or skin rashes. People who are chronically anxious or depressed are believed to have a greater vulnerability to psychophysiological illness.[14]

Psychoneuroimmunology.   Psychoneuroimmunology is the scientific field that explores the relationship between psychological states and the immune system. Recent research on the ways in which the brain protects itself from cells damaged by trauma, disease, or stress has emerged.[29] This field is based on the mind-body connection that extends to the cellular level (Fig. 17-2).

For example, cells called microglia are found throughout the central nervous system. As numerous as neurons, they form an extensive defensive network in the brain, monitoring and even enhancing normal brain function, and migrating to trouble spots to ingest microbes, dying cells, and other debris. Research has also shown that these cells can lose control and, in some people, exacerbate or even cause several disabling conditions such as stroke, Alzheimer's disease, multiple sclerosis, Parkinson's disease, dementia associated with HIV, and other neurodegenerative disorders.

It has been demonstrated that the immune response can be modified by behavior modification techniques. Researchers are now investigating the possibility of modifying the immune response in the treatment of autoimmune illnesses such as rheumatoid arthritis, systemic lupus erythematosus, myasthenia gravis, and pernicious anemia. Other

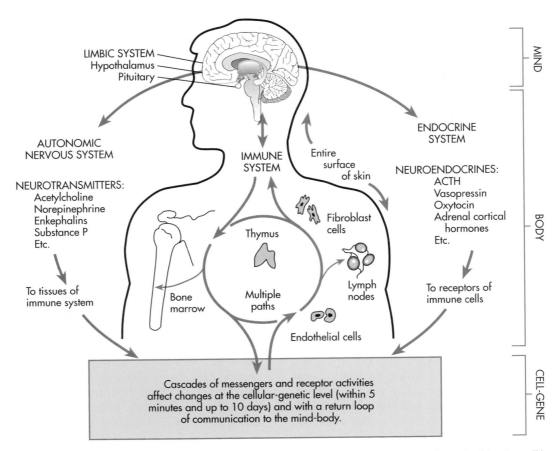

Fig. 17-2 Selye's general adaptation syndrome, updated to emphasize the mind-body-cell/gene communication loop of the immune system. (Modified from Rossi EL: *The psychobiology of mind-body healing*, New York, 1993, WW Norton.)

research is exploring the relationship between the immune system, stress, and cancer. It has been suspected that high stress, especially if prolonged, can decrease the immune system's ability to destroy neoplastic growths.[24,32]

Thus psychoneuroimmunological research has some promising implications. Eventually it may be possible to treat these disabling conditions more effectively and to teach people how to enhance the brain's natural immunity to disease through behavioral changes.

PSYCHOLOGICAL. Philosophers and scientists have long speculated about the roles of personality and stress in the development of illness. In the 1930s and 1940s personality profiles were developed of those prone to several diseases, including hypertension, coronary artery disease (CAD), cancer, ulcers, and rheumatoid arthritis.

Research suggests that a negative affective style marked by depression, anxiety, and hostility may be associated with the development of such chronic diseases as asthma, headaches, ulcers, arthritis, and CAD.[12] The clearest evidence to date relates to the negative effects of chronic hostility on cardiovascular disease. More specifically, Type A behavior, which has been characterized by competitive drive, impa-

tience, hostility, irritability, and aggressiveness, has been shown to predict both the physiological changes that are associated with CAD and the development of CAD itself. Type A people are also more likely to have accidents, to die as a result of accidents or violence, to have migraine headaches, to smoke more, and to have higher levels of serum cholesterol. Thus, Type A behavior appears to be a risk factor not only for cardiovascular disease but also for an array of other disorders. Finally, although such research suggests the possibility of a disease-prone personality, the exact nature of the relationship between personality and susceptibility is unknown. For example, a negative emotional state may

▼ Produce pathological physiological changes
▼ Lead people to practice faulty health behaviors
▼ Produce illness behavior but no underlying pathology
▼ Be associated with illness through other unknown factors

Complementing the research on negative emotional states and disease is the increasing focus on the protective role of positive emotional states. One idea regarding these traits is that of a self-healing personality, which is characterized by enthusiasm.[11] Self-healing, emotionally balanced people are believed to be alert, responsive, and energetic, although they may also be calm and conscientious. They are curious, secure, and constructive. Self-healing personalities also have a sense of continuous growth and resilience and an extra margin of emotional stability that they can call on when their capacities are challenged. Two other positive traits are optimism and perceived control. Optimists appear to have fewer physical symptoms and may show faster recoveries from illness. Belief in personal control, or self-efficacy, appears to affect the likelihood of developing illness by directly influencing the practice of health behaviors and by buffering people against the adverse effects of stress.

> **?** *Think of people you know who always seem to be ill. What personality characteristics do they share? How do they compare with people you know who are hardly ever ill?*

SOCIOCULTURAL. It has been proposed that health, illness, and suffering are patterned by culture and realized as personal worlds of experience.[28] In this view psychophysiological illness derives from the relationships between body, psyche, and society (see Critical Thinking about Contemporary Issues). Illness is not seen as simply the natural unfolding of an exclusively biological process. Rather, its course is also influenced by sociocultural factors. The social course of illness is a concept with at least two meanings.[32]

The first is the idea that the severity of the person's symptoms is influenced by aspects of the social environment. This means that subjectively experienced distress can be increased or decreased by the nature and number of major and minor problems in the person's world, changes in the emotional climate of that world, or in the manner in which the ill person engages in social life.

In the second meaning the symptoms shape and structure the person's social world, as the illness, by its very presence, initiates a series of changes in the person's environment. The resulting chain of illness-related interpersonal events thus becomes a part of the social course of the person's illness. This can be seen in the concept of the *sick role*, first described in the 1950s by Parsons. It proposes that being sick is a social role as well as a condition and that society places certain beliefs and expectations on the person who falls ill.[23] These include the following:

▼ The sick are allowed to be exempt from their usual social responsibilities.

▼ The sick are not seen as being responsible for being ill.

▼ The sick are expected to want to get well.

▼ The sick are expected to seek competent help and cooperate with the helper in trying to get well.

Although the premises of the sick role have been questioned in recent years, they do demonstrate the impact of sociocultural factors on the expression and resolution of psychophysiological responses.

CRITICAL THINKING *about* **Contemporary Issues** **?**

Is Chronic Fatigue Syndrome a Culturally Sanctioned Form of Illness Behavior?

There is much interest in the recently defined chronic fatigue syndrome, which is characterized by exhaustion or fatigue and marked reduction in activity and correlated with a high prevalence of psychiatric disorders and psychophysiological symptoms secondary to stress.[33] This interest results from reports of its growing frequency, substantial morbidity, and unclear pathogenesis. This interest is also fueled by debates about emotional factors related to the illness and questions as to whether it is a discrete disorder.

Currently the diagnosis of chronic fatigue syndrome is more common among women. It has been proposed that it is related to the struggle of American culture with the expanding role of women and the mismatch between women's ambitions and social possibilities.[1] Today, illness and the sick role are the only socially legitimate excuses for abandoning work and the pursuit of achievement. Thus, a diagnosis of chronic fatigue syndrome may provide a legitimate "medical" reason for a variety of psychophysiological responses, allowing the person to withdraw from situations that are intolerable. This example of the cultural shaping of illness and disease underscores society's greater understanding of physical illness and the continued stigmatization of psychiatric illness and emotional distress.

> **?** *Compare this society's beliefs and expectations about the sick role for people with multiple sclerosis, alcoholism, lung cancer, and depression. Do they differ based on each diagnosis and, if so, how and why?*

Precipitating Stressors

Any experience that the person interprets as stressful may lead to a psychophysiological response. Some of these responses are mild and short-lived. Examples include diarrhea before an examination or a dry mouth when speaking before a large group of people. Sometimes the response is more serious and indicates a higher level of anxiety. For instance, a person might feel panicky and experience tachycardia when boarding an airplane. Because the psychophysiological disorder is an attempt to deal with anxiety, information on stressors related to anxiety (Chapter 16) should be reviewed.

One type of stressor that has been shown to cause physical illness and even death is the loss of a significant interpersonal relationship. Siegel[27] has noted that "one of the most common precursors of cancer is a traumatic loss or a feeling of emptiness in one's life." An increased mortality rate has been found among recently widowed people. Similar observations have been made about people admitted to institutions such as nursing homes, who are separated from

PATIENT EDUCATION PLAN **Coping with Stress**

Content	Instructional Activities	Evaluation
Define and describe stress	List feelings that indicate stress Discuss behaviors associated with elevated stress	Patient identifies general behaviors associated with stressful situations
Recognize stressful situations	Ask patient to describe situations personally experienced as stressful Role play the situation (with videotape if possible) Discuss stress-related behaviors observed and feelings experienced	Patient identifies stressful experiences Patient describes own behaviors when stressed
Review common life stressors	Discuss common elements of stressful experiences	Patient identifies stressful aspects of life
Identify adaptive and maladaptive coping mechanisms	Review the role-played stressful situations Discuss alternative ways to cope with the stressors Role play at least one adaptive coping mechanism	Patient identifies and practices adaptive coping mechanisms
Assign use of adaptive strategy to cope with stress	Provide feedback about the effectiveness of the selected coping mechanism	Patient selects an adaptive coping strategy when experiencing stress

significant others. Children who have been separated from their mothers, especially if placed in an impersonal environment, also show a decline in physical health. The effect of a loss may cause both physical and psychological symptoms for an extended period of time. Illnesses and deaths related to loss of a loved person seem to represent the exhaustion phase of the general adaptation syndrome.

Sometimes a psychophysiological problem is a response to an accumulation of rather small stressors. A patient may find it difficult to identify one specific stressor that preceded a particular problem. Careful assessment may reveal a pattern of overwork and overcommitment or a series of seemingly minor events that all required extra effort. Most of the psychophysiological disorders come and go. This may be related to changes in the person's stress level. When the cumulative stress gets too high, the body "calls time out" by developing physical symptoms.

Appraisal of Stressors

The complex interaction between mind and body is perhaps most evident in psychophysiological responses to stress. These responses reinforce the need for an integrated approach to etiology and great sensitivity by the nurse to a person's appraisal of stress and its effects. Social and cultural factors play a particularly important role in the expression of adaptive and maladaptive behaviors. They also must be a prime consideration in planning effective, individualized treatment strategies.

Coping Resources

One of the most important parts of promoting adaptive psychophysiological responses involves changing health habits. People who adopt positive health practices and good health measures can prevent biopsychosocial illnesses. Pa-

A Family *Speaks*

I worry about my husband. He drives himself so hard. I also feel guilty at times because I know he's doing it for me and the children. But I sure would like for him to slow down. Here's a good example of how things go in our house. Every year in the weeks before Christmas he works overtime to give us a little extra money. But then on Christmas Eve, without fail, his ulcer kicks up and we wind up spending part of each holiday in the hospital visiting him.

I know every family has problems and maybe ours aren't so bad. But then again, maybe they are. This last Christmas our doctor recommended that we see a family therapist to discuss the situation. I want to go, but my husband says it's silly. Maybe this year for Christmas I'll ask him to give me that as my present and we'll finally have a really happy New Year. ▼

tient Education Plans that include coping skills training, such as the one above, can increase a person's knowledge about the effect of stress, reduce anxiety, increase a person's feelings of purpose and meaning in life, reduce pain and suffering, and improve coping abilities.

Social support from family, friends, and caregivers is also an important resource for adaptive psychophysiologic responses (see A Family Speaks). It may lower the likelihood of developing maladaptive responses, speed the recovery from illness, and reduce the distress and suffering that accompany illness. Social support groups are another coping resource that can satisfy needs that are unmet by family members and caregivers.

Coping Mechanisms

Psychophysiological disorders may be seen as attempts to cope with the anxiety associated with overwhelming stress. Unconsciously the person links the anxiety to the physical illness. Secondary gain then adds to the psychological relief experienced.

Several of the defense mechanisms described in Chapter 16 may be seen in psychophysiological disorders. *Repression* of feelings, conflicts, and unacceptable impulses often leads to physical symptoms. The maintenance of repression over long periods of time requires a great deal of psychic energy. As the system approaches a state of exhaustion, physical symptoms occur. When a psychological basis for illness is suggested, the patient denies it. This indicates the inability to handle the anxiety that would otherwise be released if the person admitted the psychic conflicts being repressed. The need for this defense should be respected.

Some people respond to psychophysiological illness with *compensation.* They attempt to prove that they are actually healthy by being more active and exerting themselves physically even if told to rest. This coping style is typical of Type A people, who need desperately to prove that they are in control of their bodies, not controlled by them. The opposite of this reaction is the person who uses *regression* as a coping mechanism. This person becomes dependent and embraces the sick role to avoid responsibility and conflict.

Common to each of these coping mechanisms is the need not to confront the basic conflict that is leading to stress and anxiety. This need is so strong that premature attempts to convince the person of psychological conflicts may result in the use of a less adaptive coping mechanism. In extreme cases, if the person is stripped of all efforts to cope and not provided with a substitute, death can result, either from worsening of the organic disorder or from suicide.

Nursing Diagnosis

The nursing diagnosis must reflect the complex biopsychosocial interaction that is the hallmark of psychophysiological disorders. The patient's effort to cope with stress-related anxiety may result in many somatic and emotional disorders. All possible disruptions must be considered when formulating a nursing diagnosis.

The Stuart Stress Adaptation Model (Fig. 17-3) may help in the diagnostic process. A thorough interview will reveal many of the predisposing factors and precipitating stressors present. The nurse must use good communication skills during the interview to enable the patient to share his or her experience as completely as possible. Areas of resistance and gaps in information should be noted as possible indicators of a conflict. These may be explored more completely as trust is established in the nurse-patient relationship.

Questions related to lifestyle and activities may help identify precipitating stressors and coping behaviors. It is particularly important to elicit the patient's view of what is happening. This will provide valuable information about the patient's awareness of the relationship between mind and body. Nonverbal behaviors also give clues about the patient's concerns. Apparent lack of concern may reveal the use of denial suggestive of a conversion disorder.

As the diagnosis is formulated, the nurse must consider the patient's coping in the context of the stress response. Is the patient in a stage of alarm with many coping resources at hand? Or is the patient in the stage of resistance, using coping mechanisms but depleting personal energy resources? Has the patient reached the stage of exhaustion, needing intensive intervention? Determination of the level of stress and coping being used influences the interventions chosen.

There are three primary nursing diagnoses for maladaptive psychophysiological responses. The first is **impaired adjustment,** a state in which the patient is unable to modify his or her lifestyle in order to improve health status. The second is **chronic pain,** a state that continues for more than 6 months. The third is **sleep pattern disturbance,** which is a disruption of sleep time that causes discomfort or interferes with desired lifestyle. Nursing diagnoses related to the range of possible maladaptive responses and related medical diagnoses are identified in the Medical and Nursing Diagnoses box on p. 309. The primary NANDA diagnoses and examples of complete nursing diagnoses are presented in the Detailed Diagnoses box on p. 310.

Related Medical Diagnoses

Medical disorders related to maladaptive psychophysiological responses are classified under the general categories of somatoform disorders, sleep disorders, and psychological factors affecting medical condition.[2] The specific medical diagnoses and essential features in each of these diagnostic classes in the DSM-IV are described in the Detailed Diagnoses box.

Outcome Identification

The expected outcome when working with a patient with maladaptive psychophysiological responses is as follows:

The patient will express feelings verbally rather than through the development of physical symptoms.

This is a long-term goal, and some may never reach it. However, an increased level of self-awareness is beneficial and should be achievable by all patients. An improved ability to deal with conflict will reduce the patient's need to use repression and denial. This in turn will decrease stress and allow the patient to function with fewer episodes of physical illness. In addition, specific goals can be set to address problems related to pain and sleep.

The establishment of goals with these patients is often a

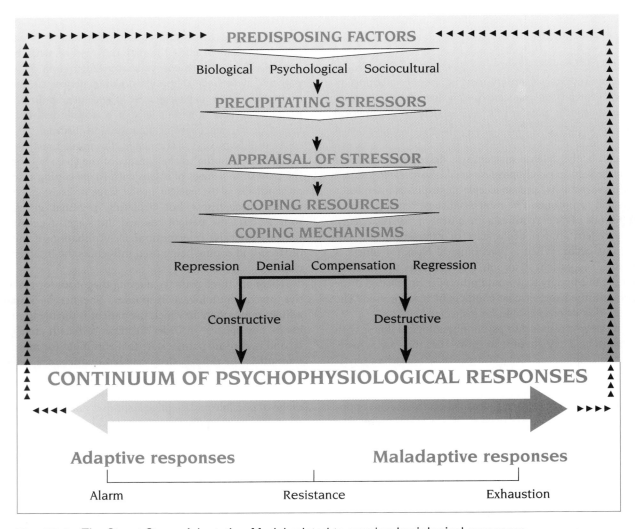

Fig. 17-3 The Stuart Stress Adaptation Model related to psychophysiological responses.

problem. The patient's primary goal is to ease the physical symptoms of the illness, often through medical or surgical treatment. Exploration of psychological conflicts is likely to be seen as unnecessary. This resistance is related to the need to maintain defenses against the extreme anxiety that has led to the illness. The nurse must identify common treatment goals. The nurse also wants the patient to obtain relief from physical symptoms. Many patients undergo medical or surgical treatment and related nursing care. At the same time, the nurse should try to build a trusting relationship so that the patient can feel safe in exploring interpersonal conflicts and feelings.

Significant others must also be considered in developing the plan of care. It is important to explore their understanding of the patient's problem. They can be valuable allies in encouraging the patient to make a lifestyle change, if this is necessary. At the same time, the nurse must recognize that a change in one family member requires a change in all the others. The family may be active participants in the patient's

maladaptive behavioral style. In this case, goals should include addressing the family relationships with the patient.

Planning

Treatment plans for these patients may be lengthy. The nurse must attend to all the patient's biopsychosocial needs. Most patients, while having needs in all areas, have their most urgent needs in a limited area of functioning. Physical disorders are usually disabling and may be life threatening. Psychosocial problems will hinder recovery from the physical illness and must also be given immediate attention.

> **?** *How would you plan care with a patient who denies that problems with his ulcerative colitis are related to work stress and marital conflict, as reported by his wife?*

MEDICAL AND NURSING DIAGNOSES *related to* **Psychophysiological Illness**

Related Medical Diagnoses (DSM-IV)*	Related Nursing Diagnoses (NANDA)†
Somatization disorder	**Adjustment, impaired‡**
Conversion disorder	Anxiety
Hypochondriasis	Body image disturbance
Body dysmorphic disorder	Coping, ineffective individual
Pain disorder	Denial, ineffective
Primary insomnia	Environmental interpretation syndrome, impaired
Primary hypersomnia	Family processes, altered
Narcolepsy	Fear
Breathing-related sleep disorder	Health maintenance, altered
Circadian rhythm sleep disorder	Hopelessness
Psychological factors affecting medical conditions	Mobility, impaired physical
	Nutrition, altered: less than body requirements
	Pain, chronic‡
	Powerlessness
	Self-care deficits
	Self-esteem disturbance
	Skin integrity, impaired
	Sleep pattern disturbance‡
	Social interaction, impaired
	Social isolation
	Spiritual distress

*From American Psychiatric Association: *Diagnostic and statistical manual of mental disorders,* ed 4, Washington, DC, 1994, The Association.
†From North American Nursing Diagnosis Association: *NANDA nursing diagnoses: definitions and classifications 1997-1998,* Philadelphia, 1997, The Association.
‡Primary nursing diagnosis for maladaptive psychophysiological responses.

Implementation

Patients with psychophysiological illnesses are most often seen in general hospital and outpatient settings. They usually seek health care because of symptoms related to physiological functioning. Only after a thorough medical examination can the role of psychosocial stressors in the disorder be evaluated. In some cases a pathophysiological disruption requires physical nursing intervention. If the physical condition is life threatening, this intervention is given highest priority. For instance, a person with a bleeding ulcer needs intensive care to maintain life. However, once the physical crisis is past, the nurse can help the patient avoid similar problems in the future.

Physical illnesses with psychosocial etiologies require psychiatric nursing care. Skilled and compassionate nursing care directed to the patient's physical needs is the first step in establishing the trusting relationship. A person who is in pain, bleeding, or covered with a rash is unable to discuss emotions or interpersonal relationships. The most important principle for patients with psychophysical disorders is to assess the patient's stress level and, whenever possible, act to reduce it. Stress and anxiety are at the root of the patient's problem. The nurse must care for immediate needs before addressing less obvious ones.

Psychological Approaches

The psychophysiological symptom defends the person from overwhelming anxiety. It provides a way to receive help and nurturance without admitting the need for it. Others are protected from expressing frightening aggressive or sexual impulses. Recognizing the defensive nature of the symptom, the nurse should never try to convince the patient that the problem is entirely psychological. Likewise, the attitude that the patient needs only to get his or her life under control to get better is not therapeutic. The patient has not made a conscious choice to be hypertensive or to develop a conversion disorder. The dilemma of these disorders is that the patient consciously would like nothing more than to be cured but is unconsciously unable to give up the symptom. Conscious recognition of the psychological role of the symptom defeats its purpose and is therefore vigorously resisted. An example of this resistance is illustrated in the following clinical example.

Clinical Example Ms. W was a 20-year-old woman admitted to the general hospital after the sudden onset of blindness. There was no evidence of any pathophysiological process affecting her eyes. Assessment revealed that she had witnessed her father's suicide by gunshot at the age of 5, although she claimed to have no memory of this. Her

DETAILED DIAGNOSES *related to* **Psychophysiological Responses**

NANDA Diagnosis Stem	Examples of Complete Diagnosis
Impaired adjustment	Impaired adjustment related to fear of assuming adult responsibilities, evidenced by multiple somatic complaints.
	Impaired adjustment related to inability to express hostile and competitive feelings, evidenced by labile hypertension.
Chronic pain	Chronic pain related to marital conflict, evidenced by back problems and protected gait.
	Chronic pain related to work pressures, evidenced by reports of headaches and facial mask.
Sleep pattern disturbance	Sleep pattern disturbance related to financial and familial concerns, evidenced by difficulty falling asleep and frequent awakening during the night.

DSM-IV Diagnosis	Essential Features*
Somatization disorder	A history of many physical complaints beginning before the age of 30, occurring over a period of several years, and resulting in treatment being sought or significant impairment in social or occupational functioning. The patient must display at least four pain symptoms, two gastrointestinal symptoms, one sexual symptom, and one symptom suggesting a neurological disorder.
Conversion disorder	One or more symptoms or deficits affecting voluntary motor or sensory function, suggesting a neurological or general medical condition. Psychological factors are judged to be associated with the symptom or deficit because the initiation or exacerbation of the symptom or deficit is preceded by conflicts or other stressors. The symptom or deficit cannot be fully explained by a neurological or general medical condition and is not a culturally sanctioned behavior or experience.
Hypochondriasis	Preoccupation with fears of having, or ideas that one has, a serious disease based on the person's misinterpretation of bodily symptoms. The preoccupation persists despite appropriate medical evaluation and reassurance and has existed for at least 6 months. It causes clinically significant distress or impairment in functioning.
Body dysmorphic disorder	Preoccupation with an imagined or exaggerated defect in appearance that causes clinically significant distress or impairment in functioning.
Pain disorder	Pain in one or more anatomical sites is the predominant focus of the clinical presentation. It is of sufficient severity to warrant clinical attention and causes clinically significant distress or impairment in functioning. Psychological factors are judged to have an important role in the onset, severity, exacerbation, or maintenance of the pain.
Primary insomnia	Difficulty initiating or maintaining sleep, or nonrestorative sleep, for at least 1 month that causes clinically significant distress or impairment in functioning.
Primary hypersomnia	Excessive sleepiness for at least 1 month, as evidenced by prolonged sleep episodes or daytime sleep episodes occurring almost daily that cause clinically significant distress or impairment in functioning.
Narcolepsy	Irresistible attacks of refreshing sleep occurring daily over at least 3 months with cataplexy (brief episodes of sudden bilateral loss of muscle tone) and hallucinations or sleep paralysis at the beginning or end of sleep episodes.
Breathing-related sleep disorder	Sleep disruption leading to excessive sleepiness or insomnia judged to be caused by sleep apnea or central alveolar hypoventilation syndrome.
Circadian rhythm sleep disorder	Persistent or recurrent pattern of sleep disruption leading to excessive sleepiness or insomnia that is caused by a mismatch between the sleep-wake schedule required by a person's environment and one's circadian sleep-wake pattern that causes clinically significant distress or impairment in functioning.
Psychological factors affecting medical condition	Presence of a medical condition in which psychological factors influence its cause, interfere with its treatment, constitute additional health risks, or elicit stress-related physiological responses that precipitate or exacerbate its symptoms.

*Modified from American Psychiatric Association: *Diagnostic and statistical manual of mental disorders,* ed 4, Washington, DC, 1994, The Association.

boyfriend had recently been expressing suicidal thoughts to her.

It appeared that the blindness was a conversion reaction. To confirm the diagnosis, the physician decided to interview Ms. W while she was sedated with amobarbital sodium. The interview was videotaped. During the interview, Ms. W was able to see. She read the day's menu and told the time by looking at a clock across the room. She also described her father's suicide. However, when the sedation wore off, Ms. W was again blind. The decision was made to play the videotape for her so that she would recognize the psychogenic nature of her blindness. As the tape was played, she regained the ability to see. However, when it reached the part in which she described her father's suicide, she became deaf.

Selected Nursing Diagnoses:

▼ Ineffective denial related to early life events, as evidenced by symptoms affecting sight and hearing
▼ Impaired social interaction related to boyfriend's depressive thoughts, as evidenced by development of physical symptoms

It is not unusual for a person with a conversion disorder to substitute another symptom if the original one is taken away. This happens because the basic conflict remains. The ego still needs to be defended from experiencing repressed anxiety. The patient really needs assistance in dealing with the conflict. When this is resolved, the symptom will disappear because there is no longer a need for it.

Great skill is needed to intervene therapeutically with patients with maladaptive psychophysiological responses. Psychological approaches include supportive therapy, insight therapy, group therapy, cognitive behavioral strategies, stress reduction, relaxation training, and psychopharmacology. The nurse should be supportive and available to talk with the patient and provide physical care (see A Patient Speaks).

The process of insight-oriented therapy for patients with psychophysiological disorders requires that the patient's underlying feelings be recognized and confronted supportively. As the patient becomes aware of anger, appropriate expression of it may be difficult. The nurse should accept the patient's attempts to express anger and provide feedback. Sometimes patients in this phase of therapy are labeled as hostile or demanding and avoided by nursing staff. This only reinforces their conviction that angry feelings are unacceptable.

The next step in therapy is to identify and explore the patient's defenses. The therapist proceeds very carefully, helping the patient discover and test new, more adaptive coping mechanisms as the dysfunctional ones are given up. The nurse should support the patient in using new behaviors. Spending time with the patient and appreciating the patient's positive qualities will help the patient build self-esteem and confidence. The nurse should be alert to signs of increased anxiety and report these immediately. The physi-

A Patient *Speaks*

All I want to do is to feel better. My husband tells me that I make up all these complaints, but who would want to be sick? It isn't any fun missing out on family and church events because you don't feel good. It isn't fun going to bed with a headache and waking up with back pain day after day after day. On the other hand, my doctors tell me that they can't find anything wrong. Where does that leave me?

Right now I'm working with a nurse who is helping me to learn new habits that may help my physical condition. She has taught me how I can relax myself when I am tense and in pain. She has suggested some activities that I can start doing right now and is also reviewing with me situations and events that seem to trigger my physical problems. Will it help? I don't know, because we're just starting out, but I do know that she is at least one person I can talk to who supports me in my fight to feel like my old self again. ▼

cal disorder may worsen if the therapy moves too rapidly. The therapist may recommend changes in the environment to help the patient function more comfortably. If the patient must consider a job change or another lifestyle change, the nurse can offer time to talk about alternatives.

Patients may also need help in explaining lifestyle change or changes in themselves to significant others. The family is a system, and a change in one component of the system requires adjustment in the other parts. For instance, a man who was very involved in his job and out several nights a week agreed to limit himself to 8-hour work days. This affected the rest of the family. Although his wife had protested for years that he spent too much time away from home, she built her life around his schedule. She spent several evenings a week in other activities. If he were to be at home every evening, she would have to reevaluate her activities and decide whether she should go out or be with him. These are not easy decisions for family members to make.

It is important that any underlying feelings of resentment be revealed and discussed to prevent indirect expression, which would create a new stressor for the patient. Family therapy may be necessary if family members have been supporting the patient's disorder. For instance, families sometimes become adjusted to having a dependent member and unwittingly sabotage efforts to foster independence. Because social support systems may help patients cope with their illnesses, the nurse may need to look for alternatives when the family is not supportive. Self-help groups often provide the needed social support. Group interventions are also helpful in decreasing overuse of health-care services by patients with somatoform disorders.

Nurses must be aware that countertransference often occurs with these patients (see Chapter 2). It is easy to become impatient with a demanding patient who is not acutely ill when sicker patients also need nursing care. Reacting to this behavior by avoidance or anger only adds to the patient's anxiety. Clinical supervision by an experienced psychiatric nurse is highly recommended for nurses who work with these difficult patients. Frequent nursing care conferences are also helpful. If possible, a limited number of staff members should be assigned to the care of these patients. This fosters the development of a trusting relationship.

Patient Education

Health education is important in caring for the patient with a psychophysiological disorder. Such patients usually need instruction about medications, treatments, and lifestyle changes. The patient and family will need information about follow-up care and crisis management (see Chapter 13). In addition, patients should be offered education about ways to cope with anxiety and stress, as described in Chapters 16 and 30. Group classes on stress management may be productive. They may enable patients to share experiences and make suggestions to each other about coping behaviors. Former patients who have made successful life adjustments can also be effective teachers of coping strategies.

> **?** *Do you think that patients with maladaptive psychophysiological responses will be more or less likely to comply with their treatment plans? How might you enhance their adherence?*

Physiological Support

A variety of physiological treatments can also be implemented by the nurse. Relaxation training, described in Chapter 30, can be very helpful in promoting adaptive psychophysiological responses. Encouraging physical activity is also a positive way of promoting stress reduction. Ideally, it should be an activity that the patient enjoys and can share with others. Diet counseling may be helpful in building the person's resistance to stress and illness. Patients under stress should not overuse dietary stimulants such as caffeine. They may need education about the elements of a healthful diet and help in planning balanced meals. A patient who has been relying on alcohol or drugs to cope with stress should be encouraged to find more adaptive coping mechanisms (see Chapter 24).

Finally, the effective treatment of sleep disorders requires that the underlying cause of the sleep problem be identified. Drugs and alcohol often produce fragmented sleep, as does caffeine.[5] Poor sleep hygiene habits may also be a problem,

---

Box 17-2 *Sleep Hygiene Strategies*

Set a regular bedtime and wake-up time 7 days a week.

Exercise daily to aid sleep initiation and maintenance; however, vigorous exercise too close to bedtime may make falling asleep difficult.

Schedule time to wind down and relax before bed.

Avoid worrying when trying to fall asleep.

Guard against nighttime interruptions. Earplugs may help with a noisy partner. Heavy window shades help to screen out light. Create a comfortable bed.

Maintain a cool temperature in the room. A warm bath or warm drink before bed helps some people fall asleep.

Excessive hunger or fullness may interfere with sleep. Avoid large meals before bed. If hungry, a light carbohydrate snack may be helpful.

Avoid caffeine, excessive fluid intake, stimulating drugs, and excessive alcohol in the evening and before bed.

Excessive napping may make it difficult for some people to fall asleep at night.

Do not eat, read, work, or watch television in bed. The bed and bedroom should be used only for sleep and sex.

Maintain a reasonable weight. Excessive weight may result in daytime fatigue and sleep apnea.

Get out of bed and engage in other activities if not able to fall asleep.

TABLE 17-1 *Sedative-Hypnotic Medications and Doses*

SEDATIVE-HYPNOTIC DRUGS	USUAL DOSE (MG/NIGHT)
Flurazepam (Dalmane)	1-2
Temazepam (Restoril)	15-30
Triazolam (Halcion)	0.25-0.5
Zolpidem (Ambien)	10
Secobarbital (Seconal)	100-200
Pentobarbital (Nembutal)	100-200
Chloral hydrate (Noctec)	500-2000

---

and the patient can be encouraged to develop good sleep hygiene habits (Box 17-2). Sedative medications (Table 17-1) can also be used to help induce sleep, but these drugs should be used for only a limited time because of the risk of dependence (see Chapter 27).

Holistic Interventions

A number of interventions practiced by nurses provide a holistic approach to health and illness; research suggests that such approaches are effective in improving immune function and treating the negative effects of stress.[4] Table 17-2 lists proposed uses for the modalities described here.

Therapeutic touch, developed over 20 years ago by nurses Dora Kuntz and Dolores Krieger, proposes that in a healthy person there is an equilibrium between inward and outward energy flow that extends beyond the skin. Illness assumes an imbalance in this energy field or a disruption in

TABLE **17-2** *Proposed Uses for Holistic Interventions*

INTERVENTION	PROPOSED USES
Therapeutic touch	Promote relaxation, reduce anxiety, improve affect, reduce pain (resulting in the need for less pain medication), accelerate healing (in wounds, fractures, and sites of infection), and help terminally ill patients face death.[19]
Acupuncture	Manage pain from dental, facial, low back, musculoskeletal, migraine, surgical, and arthritic sources, postoperative and chemotherapy-related emesis, tennis elbow, depression, cocaine dependence, asthma, and stroke.[13]
Imagery	Envision health; counteract symptoms of stress; regulate blood pressure and heart rate; decrease anxiety about a medical procedure or frightening event; increase internal (strengths, belief systems, and coping strategies) and external (treatments, medicines, surgery, and tests) healing resources; increase empowerment, self-esteem, and independence; reframe negative thoughts.[8,9]

the energy flow. The practitioner of therapeutic touch moves his or her hands approximately 1 to 2 inches above the body of the patient to consciously direct an energy exchange that helps to facilitate healing.

Acupuncture, a modality within the integrated system of traditional Chinese medicine (TCM), is gaining increasing visibility in medical settings in North America and Europe. Theories of cellular communication, patient classification systems, diagnostic categories, and therapeutic approaches with TCM arise from a different model from that of traditional Western medicine. TCM theory is one of energy flow, or chi, through the body along pathways of meridians, or channels. Normal physiologic functioning is experienced when energy moves harmoniously in all directions, and disharmony results if there is too little chi or if the directions of flow are obstructed. The pace and location of the flow of chi can be influenced by the insertion of needles at certain points along the meridians to facilitate harmony.

Imagery, or visualization, is another ancient remedy. It is an internal experience of memories, dreams, fantasies, and visions, which may involve all the senses, and serves as the hypothetical bridge for connecting mind and body, between conscious processing of information and physiologic change. It is a complex phenomenon of mind modulation. Imagery evokes change at the cellular level via activity of the right and left hemispheric brain function and the autonomic, endocrine, immune, and neurotransmitter systems. When used therapeutically, imagery can evoke changes in physiology, perception, and behavioral attitudes that can promote healing.

The Nursing Treatment Plan Summary for patients with maladaptive psychophysiological responses is presented on p. 314.

Evaluation

The evaluation of the nursing care of the patient with psychophysiological illness is based on the identified patient care goals. If goal achievement is not attained, the nurse must ask the following questions:

▼ Was the assessment complete enough to correctly identify the problem?
▼ Did the patient agree with the goal?
▼ Was enough time allowed for goal achievement?
▼ Was I skilled enough to carry out the desired intervention?
▼ Were there environmental constraints that affected goal accomplishment?
▼ Did additional stressors change the patient's ability to cope?
▼ Was the goal achievable for this patient?
▼ What alternative approaches should be tried?

It is very important that neither the patient nor the nurse interpret the lack of goal achievement as a failure. The nurse should look at it as a challenge and convey that attitude to the patient. It is not helpful to add failure to achieve a goal to the patient's collection of stressors. The care of these patients is very complex. The nurse may need to modify the treatment plan several times before finding a successful approach. The most important thing is to keep trying and to encourage the patient to persist in the effort to find health.

Summary

1. The continuum of possible psychophysiological responses to stress based on Selye's theory includes the stages of alarm, resistance, and exhaustion.
2. Patient behaviors related to psychophysiological responses include physical conditions affected by psychological factors, psychological symptoms such as somatization, conversion, body dysmorphic and pain disorders, hypochondriasis, and sleep problems.
3. Predisposing factors are described from biological, psychological, and sociocultural perspectives. Precipitating stressors include any experience the patient interprets as stressful.
4. A variety of coping mechanisms are used in psychophysiological response such as repression, denial, compensation, and regression.
5. Primary NANDA nursing diagnoses for psychophysiological responses are impaired adjustment, chronic pain, and sleep pattern disturbance.

NURSING TREATMENT PLAN *Summary* Maladaptive Psychophysiological Responses

Nursing Diagnosis Impaired adjustment.
Expected Outcome The patient will express feelings verbally rather than through the development of physical symptoms.

Short-term Goals	Interventions	Rationale
The patient will identify areas of stress and conflict and relate feelings, thoughts, and behaviors to them.	Assist patient in identifying stressful situations by reviewing events surrounding the development of physical symptoms. Facilitate the association among cognitions, feelings, and behaviors.	Inability to deal with intrapsychic conflict leads to anxiety and stress, resulting in physiological dysfunction.
The patient will describe present defenses and evaluate whether they are adaptive or maladaptive.	Proceed slowly in analyzing defenses. Explore alternative coping behaviors with the patient. Teach the patient stress management techniques such as relaxation and imagery.	Defenses should not be attacked; rather, the nurse should support positive exploration by the patient and suggest alternative responses.
The patient will adopt two new coping mechanisms to deal with stress.	Give patient positive feedback for new adaptive behaviors. Actively support patient in testing new coping mechanisms. Enlist the support of family and significant others to reinforce change.	Change requires time and positive reinforcement from others. Family members can be important in promoting adaptive responses.
The patient will display a decrease in physical symptoms and greater biological integrity.	Encourage physical activity to reduce stress. Counsel the patient on diet and nutrition needs. Review the patient's sleep habits and promote good sleep hygiene practices.	Wellness requires a balance between biological and psychosocial needs. Interventions focused on the patient's physiological needs can help the patient restore biological integrity.

6. Primary DSM-IV diagnoses are categorized as somatoform disorders, sleep disorders, and psychological factors affecting medical condition.
7. The expected outcome of nursing care is that the patient will express feelings verbally rather than through the development of physical symptoms.

8. Interventions include psychological approaches, patient education, physiological support, and holistic interventions.
9. The care of these patients is complex, and the nurse may need to modify the treatment plan several times before finding a successful approach.

COMPETENT CARING A Clinical Exemplar of a Psychiatric Nurse

Audrey Joseph, MSN, RN

Often it is difficult for healthcare professionals to communicate with their patients about psychosomatic illness. Also, the patient's denial or rejection of this diagnosis does not make the communication process any easier. Psychiatric staff and family members can get caught in the middle when primary care physicians fail to tell their patients that they need a psychiatric evaluation to rule out a psychosomatic illness. I know this from an experience I had that taught me much about psychiatric care.

I was working the evening shift as a staff nurse on an inpatient unit when Mrs. O, an elderly woman, presented herself on the unit for voluntary admission. She was well dressed and quite cheerful. Her medical history revealed that she had visited her family doctor and the emergency room weekly for the last 2 months. She had many diagnostic studies, the results of which were all negative. Mrs. O reported that she was referred by her family doctor for a diagnostic workup. A psychosocial assessment revealed that her husband had recently died and that she lived alone. The patient was allowed to become acclimated to the unit. Then, as the staff explained to her why she was admitted, she became angry and left against medical advice.

About 3 weeks later Mrs. O's son arranged for her to be readmitted because she was constantly going to the emergency room and to her family doctor. She was angry with her son for having her admitted. To keep her in the hospital, he told her that he would have her committed if necessary. On this admission, Mrs. O was neatly dressed but looked tired. Her chief complaint was choking and a general infection throughout her body that was causing a vaginal discharge. Her family doctor still did not tell her that he could not find anything physically wrong with her. She was started on a regimen of antidepressant medication. During the 2 weeks she was in the hospital, she spent most of her time socializing with other patients. She was not interested in psychotherapy and did not develop a therapeutic alliance with the staff.

On her third admission, approximately 2 months later, Mrs. O's family doctor still had not told her that he thought she had a psychosomatic illness. At this time she was disheveled and looked physically ill. Mrs. O spent most of the day in bed. She constantly complained of choking and a vaginal discharge. She admitted that she stopped taking the antidepressant medication right after discharge from the hospital. At this point she was angry with all her children and thought they were all against her. She could not understand why they would not accept the fact that she was physically ill. After 3 weeks of treatment Mrs. O was discharged home. Two years later I met Mrs. O in another psychiatric hospital where she was again admitted for treatment.

Clearly this is not a success story. In fact, it taught me much about the problems of nonintegrated physical and psychiatric systems of care in which patients are treated as parts rather than wholes. I also realized that I shared responsibility for not providing better care for Mrs. O. To this day, she is often in my thoughts, and I now advocate for treating patients broadly within the context of their world view rather than within the narrow realm our society defines as medical care.

Chapter Review Questions

1. Match each term in Column A with the correct definition in Column B.

Column A

___ Body dysmorphic disorder

___ Conversion disorder

___ Hypersomnia

___ Hypochondriasis

___ Insomnia

___ Pain disorder

___ Parasomnia

___ Sleep pattern disturbance

___ Somatization disorder

___ Somatoform disorders

Column B

A. Physical symptoms without organic impairment

B. A history of many physical complaints

C. Loss or alteration of voluntary motor or sensory function that cannot be explained by a medical condition

D. Preoccupation with fears of having a serious disease

E. An imagined or exaggerated defect in appearance

F. A disorder in which psychological factors have an important role in the onset, severity, exacerbation, or maintenance

G. Sleepwalking, night terrors, nightmares, enuresis

H. Narcolepsy, sleep apnea, nocturnal movement disorders

I. Disorders of initiating or maintaining sleep

J. Difficulty falling asleep and frequent awakening during the night

2. Fill in the blanks.

A. The continuum of possible psychophysiological responses to stress, based on Selye's theory, include the stages of _____, _____, _____.

B. A variety of coping mechanisms are used in psychophysiological response such as _____, _____, _____, _____.

C. The expected outcome of nursing care is that the patient will express feelings _____ rather than through the development of _____ symptoms.

D. It is not unusual for a person with _____ _____ to substitute another symptom if the original one is taken away without attention to the underlying stressor.

E. _____ is the scientific field that explores the relationship between psychological states and the immune response.

3. Provide short answers for the following questions.

A. Describe four psychological interventions the nurse might use in the treatment of the patient with a maladaptive psychophysiological response to stress.

B. Define *secondary gain*. Give several examples from your personal experience.

C. Therapeutic touch has gained credibility as a holistic intervention, particularly among nurses, but it continues to be criticized by some health-care providers as unscientific. Support or refute this criticism.

D. Recent research indicates that people with clinical depression who smoke are at higher risk for lung cancer than people without depression who smoke. Based on this information, how would you differ in your educational approach to patients with and without depression who smoke?

REFERENCES

1. Abbey S, Garfinkle P: Neurasthenia and chronic fatigue syndrome: the role of culture in the making of a diagnosis, *Am J Psychiatry* 148:1638, 1991.
2. American Psychiatric Association: *Diagnostic and statistical manual*, ed 4, Washington, DC, 1994, The Association
3. Bachman D: Sleep disorders with aging: evaluation and treatment, *Geriatrics* 47:53, 1992.
4. Bennett C: Expanding the mind-body connection: working women and stress, *Capsules Comments* 2:247, 1996.
5. Blumenthal SJ, Fine T: Sleep abnormalities associated with mental and addictive disorders: implications for research and clinical practice, *J Pract Psychiatry Behav Health* 3:67, 1996.
6. Buysse DJ, Perlis ME: The evaluation and treatment of insomnia, *J Pract Psychiatry Behav Health* 3:80, 1996.
7. Cassileth B, Drossman D: Psychosocial factors in gastrointestinal illness, *Psychother Psychosom* 59:131, 1993.
8. Dossey BM: Using imagery to help your patient heal, *Am J Nurs* 6:41, 1995.
9. Dossey BM, Keegan L, Guzzetta CE, Kolkmeier LG: *Holistic nursing: a handbook for practice*, Gaithersburg, MD, 1995, Aspen.
10. Fava G: The concept of psychosomatic disorder, *Psychother Psychosom* 58:1, 1992.
11. Friedman H: *The self-healing personality: why some people achieve health while others succumb to illness*, New York, 1991, Holt.
12. Friedman H, editor: *Hostility, coping, and health*, Washington, DC, 1992, American Psychological Association.

13. Hammerschlag R, Lewith GT, Bushar H, et al: Discussion of methodological considerations in human trials, *J Alternative Complementary Med* 2:91, 1996.
14. Kaplin HI, Saddock BJ: *Pocket handbook of clinical psychiatry,* ed 2, Baltimore, 1996, Williams & Wilkins.
15. Keefe FJ, Goli V: A practical guide to behavioral assessment and treatment of chronic pain, *J Pract Psychiatry Behav Health* 5:151, 1996.
16. Lamburg L: *Bodyrhythms: chronobiology and peak performance,* New York, 1994, William Morrow.
17. Lilie J, Lahmeyer H: Psychiatric management of sleep disorders, *Psychiatr Med* 9:245, 1991.
18. Lowery BJ, Houldin AD: From stressor to illness: the psychobiological-biological connection, In McBride AB, Austin JK, editors: *Psychiatric–mental health nursing: integrating the behavioral and biological sciences,* Philadelphia, 1996, WB Saunders.
19. Mackey RB: Discover the healing power of therapeutic touch, *Am J Nurs* 4:27, 1995.
20. Mindell J: Sleep disorders in children, *Health Psychol* 12:151, 1993.
21. Moore DP, Jefferson JW: *Handbook of medical psychiatry,* St Louis, 1996, Mosby.
22. Oakley LD, Potter C: *Psychiatric primary care,* St Louis, 1997, Mosby.
23. Parsons T: *The social system,* New York, 1951, The Free Press.
24. Plotnikoff N: *Stress and immunity,* Boca Raton, Fla, 1991, CRC Press.
25. Saravay S et al: Psychological comorbidity and length of stay in the general hospital, *Am J Psychiatry* 148:324, 1991.
26. Selye H: *The stress of life,* New York, 1956, McGraw-Hill.
27. Siegel BS: *Love, medicine, and miracles,* New York, 1986, Harper & Row.
28. Starck P, McGovern J, editors: *The hidden dimension of illness: human suffering,* New York, 1993, National League for Nursing.
29. Streit WJ, Kincaid-Colton CA: The brain's immune system, *Sci Am* 11:54, 1995.
30. Vallerand A: Gender differences in pain, *J Nurs Scholarship* 27:235, 1995.
31. *Wake up America: A national sleep alert,* Report of the National Commission on Sleep Disorders Research, Washington, DC, 1993, US Department of Health and Human Services.
32. Ware N, Kleinman A: Culture and somatic experience: the social course of illness in neurasthenia and chronic fatigue syndrome, *Psychosom Med* 54:546, 1992.
33. Wessely S, Chalder T, Hirsch S, Wallace P, Wright D: Psychological symptoms, somatic symptoms, and psychiatric disorder in chronic fatigue and chronic fatigue syndrome: a prospective study in the primary care setting, *Am J Psychiatry* 153:1050, 1996.

ANNOTATED SUGGESTED READINGS

Birch S, Hammerschlag R, Berman B: Acupuncture in the treatment of pain, *J Alt Comp Med* 2:101, 1996.
A thorough review of this intervention as a treatment for pain in various parts of the body. The research findings in this area are well organized.

Blumenthal S, Fine T: Sleep abnormalities associated with mental and addictive disorders: implications for research and clinical practice, *J Pract Psychiatry Behav Health* 3:67, 1996.
Scientific advances in understanding sleep in chronobiology, sleep physiology, and genetics are reviewed, including specific types of sleep disruptions related to mental illnesses, lifestyle, and gender.

*Dossey B: Using imagery to help your patient heal, *Am J Nurs* 1995:41, 1995.
Clear and concise overview of how nurses can use imagery in their practice.

*Dossey B et al: *Holistic nursing: a handbook for practice,* Gaithersburg, Md, 1995, Aspen Publishers.
Contains concepts important to the practice of contemporary nursing and is intended for students, practitioners, educators, and researchers who desire to expand their knowledge of holism, healing, and spirit.

Holmes E et al: Development of a sleep management program for people with severe mental illness, *Psychiatric Rehab J* 19:9, 1995.
These authors developed a sleep training module, using subject surveys, and evaluated the efficacy of behavioral training of sleep problems for people with severe mental illness.

Keefe F, Goli V: A practical guide to behavioral assessment and treatment of chronic pain, *J Pract Psychiatry Behav Health* 5:151, 1996.
Describes the biobehavioral management of chronic pain. The most useful self-report measures are described, cognitive-behavioral techniques for assessing pain are included, and treatment strategies are reviewed in detail.

*Mackey R: Discover the healing power of therapeutic touch, *Am J Nurs* 1995:27, 1995.
Outline of the basic principles of therapeutic touch and the results of current research on this treatment modality.

*McCain N, Smith J: Stress and coping in the context of psychoneuroimmunology: a holistic framework for nursing practice and research, *Arch Psychiatr Nurs* 8:221, 1994.
Overview of stress and stress management and psychoimmunology with emphasis on behavioral, cognitive, and combination strategies for adaptive coping.

Stoudemire A: *Psychological factors affecting medical conditions,* Washington, DC, 1995, American Psychiatric Press.
Reviews current research on the impact of psychological states on the development and course of particular physical diseases. Excellent resource.

*Nursing reference.

Chapter 18

Self-concept Responses and Dissociative Disorders

Gail W. Stuart

© 1998 M.C. Escher/Cordon Art, Baarn, Holland.

To venture causes anxiety, but not to venture is to lose one's self. And to venture in the highest sense is precisely to be conscious of one's self. **Søren Kierkegaard**

LEARNING OBJECTIVES

After studying this chapter the student should be able to:

▼ Describe the continuum of adaptive and maladaptive self-concept responses

▼ Identify behaviors associated with self-concept responses

▼ Analyze predisposing factors, precipitating stressors, and appraisal of stressors related to self-concept responses

▼ Describe coping resources and coping mechanisms related to self-concept responses

▼ Formulate nursing diagnoses related to self-concept responses

▼ Assess the relationship between nursing diagnoses and medical diagnoses related to self-concept responses

▼ Identify expected outcomes and short-term nursing goals for patients related to self-concept responses

▼ Develop a patient education plan to improve family relationships

▼ Analyze nursing interventions for patients related to their self-concept responses

▼ Evaluate nursing care for patients related to their self-concept responses

TOPICAL OUTLINE

Of all human attributes, the self appears to be the most complex and intangible. The self is the most real aspect of one's experience and it is the frame of reference through which one perceives, conceives, and evaluates one's world. **Self-concept** can be defined as all the notions, beliefs, and convictions that constitute a person's self-knowledge and that influence relationships with others. It includes one's perceptions of personal characteristics and abilities, interactions with other people and the environment, values associated with experiences and objects, and goals and ideals.

Helping professionals of all backgrounds have come to view the self-concept as critical to the understanding of people and their behavior. No two people have identical self-concepts. The self-concept emerges or is learned through each person's internal experiences, relationships with other people, and interactions with the outer world. Because it is the frame of reference through which the person interacts with the world, it has a powerful influence on human behavior. It is impossible to understand a person fully or to predict behavior accurately without understanding the person's internal frame of reference. This involves sharing the person's perceptual world and view of the self. Thus understanding a patient's self-concept is a necessary component of all nursing care.

CONTINUUM OF SELF-CONCEPT RESPONSES

Self-concept

DEVELOPMENTAL INFLUENCES. Most theorists agree that the self-concept does not exist at birth. The self develops gradually as the infant recognizes and distinguishes others and begins to gain a sense of differentiation from others. The boundaries of the self are defined as the result of exploratory activity and experience with one's own body. At first self-differentiation is slow, but with the development of language it accelerates. Use of the child's own name helps with the identification and perception of individuality—of being someone special, unique, and independent. Human language allows clear distinctions to be made between the self and the rest of the world and the ability to symbolize and understand experiences. The continued process of self-concept development is greatly benefited by the following:

▼ Interpersonal and cultural experiences that generate positive feelings and a sense of worth
▼ Perceived competence in areas valued by the individual and society
▼ Self-actualization, or the implementation and realization of a person's true potential

SIGNIFICANT OTHERS. The self-concept is learned in part through accumulated social contacts and experiences with other people. Sullivan[21] called this development "learning about self from the mirror of other people." What a person believes about himself is a function of his interpre-

tation of how others see him, as inferred from their behavior toward him. His concept of self therefore rests partly on what he thinks others think of him. For a young child the most significant others are his parents, who help him grow and react to his experiences. The family provides the person with his earliest experiences of:

▼ Feelings of adequacy or inadequacy
▼ Feelings of acceptance or rejection
▼ Opportunities for identification
▼ Expectations concerning acceptable goals, values, and behaviors

Research indicates that parental influence is strongest during early childhood and continues to have a significant impact through adolescence and young adulthood. Over time, however, the power and influence of friends and other adults increase, and they become significant others to the person.

Culture and socialization practices also affect self-concept and personality development. General cultural patterns and cultural subdivisions, such as social class, have formative influences on one's view of self.

> ? *What sociocultural factors had an impact on your self-concept as you were growing up? Which ones currently influence your self-concept?*

SELF-PERCEPTIONS. Each person can observe one's own behavior the same way that others do and form opinions about oneself. One's perception of reality is selective, however, according to whether the experience is consistent with one's current concept of self. The way a person behaves is a result of how one perceives the situation, and it is not the event itself that elicits a specific response but rather the individual's subjective experience of the event. One's needs, values, and beliefs strongly influence perceptions. People are more likely to perceive what is meaningful and consistent with present needs and personal values. Similarly, people behave in a manner consistent with what they believe to be true. In this case, a fact is not what is but what one believes to be true. Once perceptions are acquired and incorporated into one's self-system, they can be difficult to change. Ways exist to change perceptions, however, including modification of cognitive processes, exposure to drugs, sensory deprivation, and biochemical changes within the body.

As the self-concept develops, it brings a unique perspective of one's relationship with the world. A person with a weak or negative self-concept who is unsure of himself is likely to have narrowed or distorted perceptions. Because he feels easily threatened, his anxiety level will rise quickly and he will become preoccupied with defending himself. In contrast, a person with a strong or positive self-concept can explore his world openly and honestly because he has a background of acceptance and success. Positive self-concepts result from positive experiences leading to perceived competence.

In conclusion, people with positive self-concepts function more effectively. Negative self-concept is correlated with personal and social maladjustment.[11] Fig. 18-1 describes the continuum of self-concept responses from the most adaptive state of self-actualization to the most maladaptive response of depersonalization.

The nurse therefore needs an understanding of various components of the self, including body image, self-ideal, self-esteem, role, and identity, which are briefly discussed here.

Body Image

The concept of one's body is central to the concept of self. The body is the most material and visible part of the self, and, although it does not account for one's entire sense of self, it remains a lifelong anchor for self-awareness. A person's attitude toward one's body may mirror important aspects of one's identity. A person's feelings that one's body is big or small, attractive or unattractive, or weak or strong also reveal something about one's self-concept. Numerous research studies have documented the close positive relationship between self-concept and body image. This association appears to exist in all cultures.

Body image can be defined as the sum of the conscious and unconscious attitudes the person has toward one's body. It includes present and past perceptions as well as feelings about size, function, appearance, and potential. Body image is a dynamic entity because it is continually being modified by new perceptions and experiences. It serves as a target or screen on which the person projects significant personal feelings, anxieties, and values.

As one's body image develops, extensions of the body become important, and anything that extends the effectiveness or control of one's body function can be called one's own. Clothes become identified closely with the body, and in the same way toys, tools, and possessions serve as extensions of the body and help to widen one's sense of self. Position and wealth serve similar functions.

When a person values one's body and acts to preserve and protect it, the body image becomes the basis through which the bodies and possessions of others are also valued. Body image, appearance, and positive self-concept are related. Studies indicate that the more a person accepts and likes one's body, the more secure and free from anxiety one feels. It has also been shown that people who accept their bodies are more likely to manifest high self-esteem than people who dislike their bodies. Problems related to body image are discussed in more detail in Chapter 25.

 What does it mean when one says that "a child lives in his body but an adult lives in his mind"?

Self-ideal

The self-ideal is the person's perception of how one should behave, based on certain personal standards. The standard may be either a carefully constructed image of the type of person one would like to be or merely a number of aspirations, goals, or values that he would like to achieve. The self-ideal creates self-expectations based in part on society's norms, to which the person tries to conform. Formation of the self-ideal begins in childhood and is influenced by significant others, who place certain demands or expectations on the child. With time, the child internalizes these expectations, and they form the basis of the child's own self-ideal. New self-ideals that may persist throughout life are taken on during adolescence, formed from identification with parents, teachers, and peers. In old age additional adjustments must be made that reflect diminishing physical strength and changing roles and responsibilities.

Various factors influence self-ideal. First, a person tends to set goals within a range determined by one's abilities. A person does not ordinarily set a goal that is accomplished without any effort or that is entirely beyond one's abilities. Self-ideals are also influenced by cultural factors as the person compares one's self-standards with those of peers. Other influencing factors include ambitions and the desire

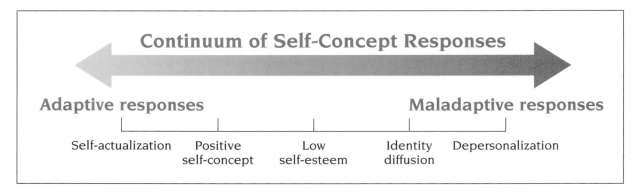

Fig. 18-1 Continuum of self-concept responses.

to excel and succeed, the need to be realistic, the desire to avoid failure, and feelings of anxiety and inferiority. Based on these factors, one's self-ideal may be clear and realistic and thus facilitate personal growth and relations with others, or it may be vague, unrealistic, and demanding. The adequately functioning person demonstrates congruence between one's perception of self and self-ideal. That is, a person sees oneself as being very similar to the person one wants to be.

In summary, self-ideals are important in maintaining mental health and balance. The self-ideal must neither be too high and demanding nor too vague and shadowy, yet it must be high enough to give continuous support to self-respect.

Self-esteem

Self-esteem is a person's personal judgment of one's own worth, based on how well one's behavior conforms to one's self-ideal. The frequency with which a person attains goals directly influences feelings of competency (high self-esteem) or inferiority (low self-esteem) (Fig. 18-2). High self-esteem is a feeling rooted in unconditional acceptance of self despite mistakes, defeats, and failures, as an innately worthy and important being. It involves accepting complete responsibility for one's own life.

Self-esteem is derived from two primary sources: the self and others. It is first a function of being loved and gaining the respect of others. Self-esteem is lowered when love is lost and when one fails to receive approval from others. Conversely, it is raised when love is regained and when one is applauded and praised. The origins of self-esteem can be traced to childhood and are based on acceptance, warmth, involvement, consistency, praise, and respect.[15] Coopersmith[5] described the four best ways to promote a child's self-esteem:

▼ Providing opportunities for success
▼ Instilling ideals
▼ Encouraging aspirations

▼ Helping the child build defenses against attacks to his or her self-perceptions

These should provide the child with a feeling of significance or success in being accepted and approved of by others; a feeling of competence, or an ability to cope effectively with life; and a feeling of power, or control over one's own destiny.

Self-esteem increases with age and is most threatened during adolescence, when concepts of self are being modified and many self-decisions must be made. The adolescent has to choose an occupation and decide whether he is good enough to succeed in a given career. He has to decide whether he is able to participate or is accepted in various social activities.

With adulthood the self-concept stabilizes, and maturity provides a clearer picture of self. The adult tends to be more self-accepting and less idealistic than the adolescent. He has learned to cope with many of his self-deficiencies and to maximize his self-strengths. Not all adults attain maturity; some continue to function as adolescents for many of their adult years.

In later life, self-esteem problems again arise because of the new challenges posed by retirement, loss of spouse, and physical disability. The impact of aging on self-esteem is also affected by the status of older people in American society. Being old in a society that values youth often leads to an assignment of low status and prejudicial attitudes toward the aged. Negative stereotypes of the elderly and the stigmatization that result can decrease self-esteem. Two other potential negative factors are the decreased social interaction of the elderly and their loss of control over their environment, both of which can result in fewer opportunities to validate and confirm one's self-concept.

Research shows a clear relationship between self-reported physical health and self-esteem. The report of a health problem, regardless of its type or severity, is associated with significantly lower self-esteem than is the report of no health problem. In contrast, high self-esteem has been correlated with low anxiety, effective group functioning, and acceptance of others.[3] It is a prerequisite to self-actualization; once self-esteem is achieved, the person is free to concentrate on achieving one's potential.

> **?** *Why do you think low self-esteem is associated with poor interpersonal relations and depressive states?*

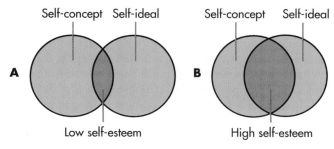

Self-concept   Self-ideal   Self-concept   Self-ideal

A   **B**

Low self-esteem   High self-esteem

Fig. 18-2   A, Person with a low level of self-esteem caused by a large discrepancy between self-concept and self-ideal. **B,** Person with a greater conformity of self-concept and self-ideal and therefore a high level of self-esteem. (From Sundeen SJ et al: *Nurse-client interaction: implementing the nursing process,* ed 6, St Louis, 1998, Mosby.)

Role Performance

Roles are sets of socially expected behavior patterns associated with a person's functioning in various social groups. The person assumes various roles that he tries to integrate into one functional pattern. Because these roles overlap, an understanding of the person requires the nurse to see him in the context of the several roles he occupies. On the basis of his perception of role adequacy in the most ego-involved roles, the person develops a level of self-esteem. High self-esteem results from roles that meet needs and are congruent with one's self-ideal. Many factors, including the following, influence a person's adjustment to the role he or she occupies:

▼ The clarity of the behaviors appropriate to the role and one's knowledge of specific role expectations

▼ The consistency of the response of significant others to one's role

▼ The compatibility and complementarity of various roles

▼ The congruency of cultural norms and one's own expectations for role behavior

▼ The separation of situations that would create incompatible role behaviors

Sex roles affect one's performance in other roles. They are particularly significant to family roles but permeate most others as well and are often the cause of role conflict or disturbance. Another difficult problem faced in growing up is emancipation from one's parents and establishment of an independent life. This primarily occurs during adolescence and early adulthood, when great ambiguity in role definitions occurs. A final crisis is faced during old age, when role behavior must again be changed by aging parents. They rely on their children yet strive to balance their lives with a sense of independence and a high level of self-esteem. Role behavior is intimately related to self-concept and identity, and role disturbances often involve conflicts between independent and dependent functioning.

Personal Identity

The word *identity* is derived from the Latin root *idem,* meaning "the same." It is the organizing principle of the personality. **Identity** is the awareness of being oneself, as derived from self-observation and judgment. It is the synthesis of all self-representations into an organized whole and is not associated with any one accomplishment, object, attribute, or role.

Identity is different from self-concept in that it is a feeling of distinctness from others. It implies consciousness of oneself as an individual with a definite place in the general scheme of things. The person with a sense of identity feels integrated, not diffuse. When a person acts in accordance with his self-concept, his sense of identity is reinforced; when he acts in ways contrary to his self-concept, he experiences anxiety and apprehension. The person with a strong sense of identity sees himself as a unique individual.

DEVELOPMENTAL INFLUENCES. The concept of ego identity was developed by Erikson[7] and built within his formulation of the eight stages of human development. For each stage, Erikson describes a psychosocial crisis that must be resolved for further growth and personality development.

In adolescence the crisis of identity versus identity diffusion occurs. At no other phase of life are the promise of finding oneself and the threat of losing oneself so closely aligned. The adolescent's task is one of self-definition as one strives to integrate previous roles into a unique and reasonably consistent sense of self.

Important in achieving identity is the issue of sexuality, the image of oneself as a male or a female and convictions about what that implies. Society's ideals of masculinity and femininity provide important standards for judging oneself as good, bad, inferior, superior, desirable, or undesirable. These ideals are passed down from generation to generation and become an important part of the culture. If males are defined as superior, this idea becomes part of the self-image of both males and females. If passivity and obedience are feminine ideals in a society, most girls will be taught to be unassertive and obedient.

In addition, much of one's identity is expressed in relationships with others. How a person relates to other people is a central personality characteristic. This presents a paradox in that everyone is a part of humanity yet each person is also separate from all others. Achieving identity is a prerequisite for establishing an intimate relationship.[22] Research has shown that only after a stable sense of identity has been established can one engage in genuinely intimate, mature, and successful relationships.

Healthy Personality

It is possible to describe the healthy personality according to developmental theory and the dynamics of the self. This description may help give perspective to the many aspects of self. A person with a healthy personality would have the characteristics listed in Table 18-1 and be able to perceive oneself and one's world accurately. This insight would create a feeling of harmony and inner peace.

 How do you compare with the qualities of a healthy personality listed in Table 18-1?

Assessment

Behaviors

Assessing the various components of a patient's self-concept is a challenge to the nurse. Because self-concept is the cornerstone of the personality, it is intimately related to anxiety and depression, problems in relationships, acting out, and self-destructive behavior. All behavior is motivated by a desire to enhance, maintain, or defend the self, so the nurse will have extensive information to evaluate. However, the nurse must delve beyond objective and observable behaviors to the patient's subjective and internal world. Only by exploring this area can the nurse understand the patient's actions.

The nurse can begin the assessment by observing the patient's appearance. Posture, cleanliness, makeup, and cloth-

TABLE **18-1** *Qualities of the Healthy Personality*

CHARACTERISTIC	DEFINITION	DESCRIPTION
Positive and accurate body image	Body image is the sum of the conscious and unconscious attitudes one has toward one's body, function, appearance, and potential.	A healthy body awareness is based on self-observation and appropriate concern for one's physical well-being.
Realistic self-ideal	Self-ideal is one's perception of how one should behave or the standard by which behavior is appraised.	A person with a realistic self-ideal has attainable life goals that are valuable and worth striving for.
Positive self-concept	Self-concept consists of all the aspects of the person of which one is aware. It includes all self-perceptions that direct and influence behavior.	A positive self-concept implies that the person expects to be successful in life. It includes acceptance of the negative aspects of the self as part of one's personality. Such a person faces life openly and realistically.
High self-esteem	Self-esteem is one's personal judgment of one's own worth, which is obtained by analyzing how well one matches up to one's own standards and how well one's performance compares with others. It evolves through a comparison of the self-ideal and self-concept.	A person with high self-esteem feels worthy of respect and dignity, believes in his or her own self-worth, and approaches life with assertiveness and zest. The person with a healthy personality feels very similar to the person he or she wants to be.
Satisfying role performance	Roles are sets of socially expected behavior patterns associated with functioning in various social groups.	The healthy person can relate to others intimately, receive gratification from social and personal roles, trust others, and enter into mutual and interdependent relationships.
Clear sense of identity	Identity is the integration of inner and outer demands in one's discovery of who one is and what one can become. It is the realization of personal consistency.	The person with a clear sense of identity experiences a unity of personality and perceives herself or himself to be a unique person. This sense of self gives life direction and purpose.

ing provide data. The nurse might discuss the patient's appearance with him to determine his values related to body image. Observing or inquiring about his eating, sleeping, and hygiene patterns gives clues to his biological habits and self-care.

These initial observations should lead the nurse to ask, "What does my patient think about himself as a person?" The nurse might ask the patient to describe himself or how he feels about himself. What strengths does he think he has? What areas of weakness? What is his self-ideal? Does he conform to it? Does fulfillment of his self-ideal bring him satisfaction? Does he value his strengths? Does he view his weaknesses as important personality deficits, or are they unimportant to his self-concept? What are his priorities? Does he feel unified and self-directed or diffuse and other-directed?

The nurse can then compare the patient's responses to his behavior, looking for inconsistencies or contradictions. How does he relate to other people? How does he respond to compliments and criticisms? The nurse can also examine his or her own affective response to the patient. Is it one of hopelessness, despair, anger, or anxiety? The nurse's own response to the patient is often a good indication of the quality and depth of the patient's pain.

ASSOCIATED WITH LOW SELF-ESTEEM. Low self-esteem is a major problem for many people and can be expressed in moderate and severe levels of anxiety. It involves negative self-evaluations and is associated with feelings of being weak, helpless, hopeless, frightened, vulnerable, fragile, incomplete, worthless, and inadequate. Low self-esteem is a major component of depression, which acts as a form of punishment and anesthesia. Low self-esteem indicates self-rejection and self-hate, which may be a conscious or unconscious process expressed in direct or indirect ways.

Direct expressions of self-hate or low self-esteem may include any of the following:

▼ **Self-criticism.** The patient has negative thinking and believes he is doomed to failure. Although the expressed purpose of the criticism may be self-improvement, there is no constructive value to it and the underlying goal is to demoralize oneself. He might describe himself as "stupid," "no good," or a "born loser." He views the normal stressors of life as impossible barriers and becomes preoccupied with self-pity.

▼ **Self-diminution.** The minimizing of one's ability by avoiding, neglecting, or refusing to recognize one's real assets and strengths.

▼ **Guilt and worrying.** Destructive activities by which the person punishes oneself. They may be expressed through nightmares, phobias, obsessions, or the reliving of painful memories and indiscretions. They indicate self-rejection.

▼ **Physical manifestations.** These might include hypertension, psychosomatic illnesses, and the abuse of various substances, such as alcohol, drugs, tobacco, or food.

▼ **Postponing decisions.** A high level of ambivalence or procrastination produces an increased sense of insecurity.

▼ **Denying oneself pleasure.** The self-rejecting person feels the need to punish himself and expresses this by denying himself the things he finds desirable or pleasurable. This might be a career opportunity, a material object, or a desired relationship.

▼ **Disturbed relationships.** The person may be cruel, demeaning, or exploitive with other people. This may be an overt or a passive-dependent pattern of relating, which indirectly exploits others. Another behavior included in this category is withdrawal or social isolation, which arises from feelings of worthlessness.

▼ **Withdrawal from reality.** When anxiety resulting from self-rejection reaches severe or panic levels, the person may dissociate and experience hallucinations, delusions, and feelings of suspicion, jealousy, or paranoia. Such withdrawal from reality may be a temporary coping mechanism or a long-term pattern indicating a profound problem of identity confusion.

▼ **Self-destructiveness.** Self-hatred can be expressed through accident proneness or attempting dangerous feats. Extremely low levels of self-esteem can lead to suicide.

▼ **Other destructiveness.** People who have overwhelming consciences may choose to act out against society. This activity serves to paralyze their own self-hate and displaces or projects it on victims.

Indirect forms of self-hate complement and supplement the direct forms. They may be chronic patterns and difficult to change in therapy:

▼ **Illusions and unrealistic goals.** Self-deception is the core element; the person refuses to accept a limited here and now. Illusions increase the possibility of disappointment and further self-hate. Examples of illusions are "If I were married, I would be happy" and "Money brings fulfillment." This indirect form of low self-esteem may make the person sensitive to criticism or overresponsive to flattery. It may also be evident in the defense mechanisms of blaming others for one's failures and becoming hypercritical to create the illusion of superiority.

▼ **Exaggerated sense of self.** The person may also attempt to compensate by expressing an exaggerated opinion of his ability. He may continually boast, brag of his exploits, or claim extraordinary talents. An extreme compensatory behavior for low self-esteem is grandiose thinking and related delusions. Another example is evident in the perfectionist. Such people strain toward impossible goals and measure their own worth entirely in terms of productivity and accomplishment.

▼ **Boredom.** This involves the rejection of one's possibilities and capabilities. The person may neglect or reject aspects of himself that have great potential for future growth.

▼ **Polarizing view of life.** In this case the person has a simplistic view of life in which everything is worst or best, wrong or right. He tends to have a closed belief system that acts as a defense against a threatening world. Ultimately this view of life leads to confusion, disappointment, and alienation from others.

The behaviors associated with low self-esteem are described in the clinical example that follows and are summarized in Box 18-1.

Clinical Example Mrs. G was a 66-year-old woman admitted to the psychiatric hospital with a major depressive episode. She told the admitting nurse that "things have been building up for some time now" and she had been seeing a private psychiatrist for the past 6 months who suggested that she enter the hospital. She had been employed in a community college as a librarian until 18 months earlier, when she was forced to retire. Mrs. G said she had been married for 39 years and had two grown children who were married and lived out of state. Her husband had worked as an accountant but had retired a month before. She said that since her retirement she had felt "useless and lost and closed

Box **18-1** *Behaviors Associated with Low Self-esteem*

Criticism of self or others
Decreased productivity
Destructiveness
Disruptions in relatedness
Exaggerated sense of self-importance
Feelings of inadequacy
Guilt
Irritability or excessive anger
Negative feelings about one's body
Perceived role strain
Pessimistic view of life
Physical complaints
Polarizing view of life
Rejection of personal capabilities
Self-destructiveness
Self-diminution
Social withdrawal
Substance abuse
Withdrawal from reality
Worrying

in" by their apartment. She seldom left the apartment, and had lost contact with many of her friends. She said she worried a great deal about their financial situation, especially now that her husband was also retired. He repeatedly reassured her that they had enough money, but she could not stop worrying about it.

Mrs. G said that she liked her job very much and thought she was good at it. A younger woman took her place at the library, and Mrs. G was very bitter when talking about her. She said that, little by little, this woman took over duties Mrs. G was responsible for and one day even cleaned out Mrs. G's desk and took it as her own. Since her retirement, she said, things had been "going downhill steadily." She said she was not a good housewife and disliked cooking. These tasks had become even more difficult since her husband retired because he was "always underfoot and criticizing" what she did. In the past couple of weeks, she had had great difficulty sleeping, a decreased appetite, fatigue, and little interest in her appearance. She said it seemed that all she had to do was "wait around to die."

Selected Nursing Diagnoses:

▼ Self-esteem disturbance related to developmental transition, as evidenced by self-criticism and lack of pleasure in life

▼ Altered role performance related to retirement, as evidenced by feeling useless and failing to complete routine activities

▼ Social isolation related to low self-worth, as evidenced by lack of contact with friends

In this clinical example, Mrs. G's perception of self was closely related to her ability to work. Her retirement created role changes difficult to adapt to. This example points out the close relationship between low self-esteem and role strain. The situation was further compounded by her husband's retirement. Mrs. G's feelings of low self-esteem were evident in her self-criticism, refusal to recognize her own strengths, worrying, physical complaints, and reduced social contacts. The diagnosis of major depressive episode was based on the severity of her feelings of self-depreciation, somatic problems, saddened emotional tone, history of losses, and absence of a manic episode.

Low self-esteem is also a major element of disturbed body image. The following clinical example illustrates the effect of the loss of a body part on a person's self-concept.

Clinical Example Mrs. M was an attractive 32-year-old married woman admitted to the general hospital for a total hysterectomy. Her history was presented in a nursing care conference because she was making many demands and the head nurse noticed that many of the staff were avoiding caring for her. Mrs. M had been married for 2 years and did not have any children. It was observed that Mr. M seldom visited his wife, although she spoke to him over the phone. Mrs. M complained that she was unable to sleep at night and often rang for the nurses with apparently minor re-

quests. She appeared to have established a relationship with one of the evening nurses, who was able to describe some of Mrs. M's concerns.

Mrs. M appeared to have a severe level of anxiety about her hysterectomy. She feared the effect of the surgery on her sexual desires, attractiveness, and ability to have intercourse and respond to her husband. Without her reproductive organs she said she felt "inadequate and no longer like a woman." She said that she and her husband always planned on having children, and she wondered whether her husband might leave her in the future. She also feared that having the hysterectomy would cause her to lose her beauty and youth.

When the nursing staff became aware of Mrs. M's many fears and concerns, they were better able to understand her behavior and plan nursing care. They discussed with her the physiological implications of a hysterectomy and encouraged her to verbalize her feelings. Mr. M was not aware of his wife's concerns, and the nursing staff supported open discussions between them. As the staff were able to identify Mrs. M's concerns, they realized that some of their previous avoidance behavior resulted from their own fears and discomfort. The female nurses had identified with her, and the hysterectomy threatened their own concepts of self, body integrity, and sexual identity.

Selected Nursing Diagnoses:

▼ Body image disturbance related to hysterectomy, as evidenced by expressed fears about her attractiveness and functioning as a woman

▼ Altered family processes related to lack of ability to bear children, as evidenced by limited communication with husband

ASSOCIATED WITH IDENTITY DIFFUSION. Important behaviors that relate to identity diffusion include disruptions in relationships or problems of intimacy. The initial behavior may be withdrawal or distancing. If a person is experiencing an undefined identity, he may wish to ignore or destroy the people who threaten him. The problem is one of gaining intimacy, but it is reflected in isolation, denial, and withdrawal from others. Such patients lack empathy.

A contrasting behavior that may be evident is **personality fusing.** Erikson has pointed out that true intimacy involves a sense of mutuality, which implies a firm self-delineation of the partners, not a diffused merger of two people. If a person is struggling to cope with a weak or undefined identity, however, he may try to establish his sense of self by fusing or belonging to someone else. This may occur in formal relationships, intense friendships, or brief affairs because each can be seen as a desperate attempt to outline one's own identity. However, personality fusion leads to a further loss of identity. Some of these behaviors are evident in this clinical example.

Clinical Example Mrs. P was seen by a psychiatric nurse in the psychiatric outpatient department of a general hospital. She was a well-dressed 24-year-old woman who had numerous somatic complaints, including decreased appetite, frequent headaches, fatigue, and difficulty falling asleep. She reported that she had no energy or interest in doing anything or being with people. She said she dreaded each day and felt abandoned and alone.

She was married at age 17 to the only boy she ever dated in high school. He was 19 at the time and she "looked up to him tremendously." He established a successful career in the insurance business, and she stayed at home to care for the house. She described herself as centering her whole world around him. Three months earlier, he had told her that he wanted a separation and suggested she begin making a new life for herself. He said he intended to move out of the house at the end of the month, but Mrs. P said she hoped he would not do that when he saw how much she loved and needed him.

Mrs. P also described feelings of being unloved and unlovable. She said she felt empty inside and didn't really know who she was. She complained about her appearance and expressed much fear about living alone, finding a job, and getting along with people, especially men.

Selected Nursing Diagnoses:

▼ Personal identity disturbance related to impending separation, as evidenced by feelings of loneliness and abandonment

▼ Self-esteem disturbance related to doubts about self and her abilities, as evidenced by expressed fears of living alone, finding a job, and getting along with people

Many of Mrs. P's behaviors reflect the problem of identity diffusion. She married at an early age before defining her own sense of self as an autonomous individual. Her only experience in a close relationship was with her husband, and she attempted to establish her own identity by living through his. Within the security of the marriage, she managed to avoid any self-analysis, but the impending separation brought forth her fears and self-doubts. She displayed a low level of self-esteem and an unresolved conflict between dependence and independence.

Personality fusion and problems with identity also have serious implications for the larger family system. Dysfunctional families are often characterized by a fusion of ego mass that may be evident in severe symptomatology by one or more family members. This may be expressed in some form of family violence or abuse (see Chapter 39) or in the scapegoating of one family member, who becomes the "diagnosed" or "symptomatic" psychiatric patient (see Chapter 32).

People with identity diffusion may lack a historical-cultural basis of identity and thus display a peculiar lack of ethnicity. This is evident in their sense of history, cultural norms, group affiliations, object choices, lifestyle, and child-rearing practices. A related behavior is the absence of a moral code or any genuine inner value. The behaviors characteristic of identity diffusion are summarized in Box 18-2.

Box **18-2** *Behaviors Associated with Identity Diffusion*

Absence of moral code
Contradictory personality traits
Exploitive interpersonal relationships
Feelings of emptiness
Fluctuating feelings about self
Gender confusion
High degree of anxiety
Inability to empathize with others
Lack of authenticity
Problems of intimacy

ASSOCIATED WITH DEPERSONALIZATION. A more maladaptive response to problems in identity involving withdrawal from reality occurs when the person experiences panic levels of anxiety. This panic state produces a blocking off of awareness, a collapse in reality testing, and feelings of depersonalization and dissociation.[1] **Depersonalization** is a feeling of unreality in which one is unable to distinguish between inner and outer stimuli. In essence, it is a true alienation from oneself. The person has great difficulty distinguishing himself from others, and his body has an unreal or strange quality.

Depersonalization is the subjective experience of the partial or total disruption of one's ego and the disintegration and disorganization of one's self-concept. Because of this, it is the most frightening human experience. It develops as an outcome of uncertainties in human relationships. The person feels unloved and, as a result of his failure to be loved, he fails to love himself. Depersonalization serves as a defense, but it is destructive because it masks and immobilizes anxiety without diminishing its intensity. It can occur in a variety of clinical illnesses, including depression, schizophrenia, manic states, and organic brain syndromes, and it represents the advanced state of ego breakdown associated with multiple personality disorder and psychotic states.

Many behaviors are associated with depersonalization.[18] Primarily, the patient experiences feelings of estrangement as though he were hiding something from himself. He experiences a lack of inner continuity and sameness and feels as if life is happening to him rather than his living by his own initiative. The patient may say that the world appears queer, dreamlike, or frightening. He may experience a loss of identity and express confusion regarding his own sexuality. He may describe related feelings of insecurity, inferiority, frustration, fear, hate, shame, and a loss of self-respect and be unable to derive a sense of accomplishment from any activity.

In depersonalization there may be a loss of impulse control and an absence of feeling and emotion that is shown in impersonality and stiffness in social situations. The person may become lifeless and lack spontaneity and animation. He may plod through each day in a state of numbness and may respond to situations ordinarily eliciting emotion without characteristic love, hate, anxiety, or guilt. A heightened sense of isolation may mark his interpersonal relationships. The person may become increasingly passive, withdrawing from social contacts, failing to assert himself, losing interest in his surroundings, and allowing others to make decisions for him.

Another sign of depersonalization is a disturbance in perception of time, space, and memory. The person may become disoriented and be unable to recognize events as pertaining to yesterday or tomorrow or to plan activities with reference to a schedule. A disturbance of memory may be characterized by aphasia, amnesia, or memory distortion. His thinking and judgment may be impaired and may reflect great confusion and distortion or focus on trivial details. Problems in information processing may be evident in visual hallucinations, and disturbed interpersonal relationships may be reflected in delusions, auditory hallucinations, and incongruent or idiosyncratic communication.

Another behavior associated with depersonalization is a confused or disturbed body image. The person may have a feeling of unreality about parts of his body. He may feel that his limbs are detached or that the size of his body parts is changed, or he is unable to tell where his body leaves off and the rest of the world begins. Some patients describe the feeling that they have stepped outside their bodies and are observing themselves as detached and foreign objects.

Finally, the person may exhibit dissociative behaviors related to **multiple personality disorder**,[6,20] which is the existence of distinct and separate personalities within the same person, each of which dominates the person's attitudes, behaviors, and self-view as though no other personality existed (see A Family Speaks). Because most patients with multiple personality disorder usually conceal their condition, there are only limited periods in their lives when they show overt symptoms that can be easily diagnosed. During these times, patients with multiple personality disorder often show subtle dissociative signs in their affects, thoughts, memories, behaviors, object relations, and transferences. The many behaviors associated with depersonalization and dissociation are summarized in Box 18-3. The following clinical example may further clarify these behaviors.

Clinical Example Mr. S was a 40-year-old man with no history of psychiatric hospitalization. Two months before his present admission, he was severely burned while on the job in a steel-making plant. He sustained second-and-third-degree burns over his face, hands, chest, and back and was treated in the burn center of a large university hospital. Three days before he was to be discharged from the burn unit, he experienced a psychotic episode. He reported hearing voices telling him to kill himself, and he was unable to recall any events surrounding the accident that produced his burns. He said he felt his arms were withering away and

A **Family** *Speaks*

My wife has multiple personality disorder, and it feels like I'm living with several different people. One moment everything is great and the next thing I know she is in a frenzy or a state of rage. There are other problems, too. For example, things keep appearing in our household and no one knows where they came from, or I get calls at work from my wife telling me she is lost and doesn't know how she ended up there. At other times she tells me things and later denies she said them. Sometimes, people come up to my wife and talk like they know her, but she says she's never seen them before. And then there are days when she dresses up and acts just like our teenage daughter.

What is it like to live with someone with this illness? Well, it's unreal and very upsetting. Most of all, it's like living in a world of doubt and uncertainty. Who is this woman I married 12 years ago? What is she all about? What is she capable of doing? These are the questions I ask myself each night as I fall asleep. They are the same ones that go unanswered in the early morning hours. ▼

his eyes were falling into his skull. He was unable to change the dressing on his burns even though he had done this before. When he looked at his arms or chest, his face remained impassive and he showed no emotion. He began to talk continuously about returning to work but was unable to identify how long he had been out on sick leave or the amount of time recommended by his physician for recovery.

With the onset of these symptoms, he was transferred from the burn unit to the psychiatric unit of the hospital. He remained socially isolated on the unit and refused to participate in ward meetings and group activities. At times he wandered into other patients' rooms and took pieces of their clothing. He was later seen wearing this clothing, and the staff intervened to return it to its owners.
Selected Nursing Diagnoses:
▼ Panic level of anxiety related to severe burn injuries, as evidenced by confusion regarding identity, hearing voices, and reported body distortions
▼ Altered thought processes related to psychotic state, as evidenced by confusion and disorientation

This example and the previous discussion show that the various feelings and perceptions associated with depersonalization represent extreme defenses against threats to self that do not alleviate the anxiety and may add to it. The patient views his own behavior as foreign and sees himself as a strong, unknown, and unpredictable being whom he does

Box **18-3** *Behaviors Associated with Depersonalization*

AFFECTIVE
Feelings of loss of identity
Feelings of alienation from self
Feelings of insecurity, inferiority, fear, shame
Feelings of unreality
Heightened sense of isolation
Lack of sense of inner continuity
Inability to derive pleasure or a sense of accomplishment

PERCEPTUAL
Auditory and visual hallucinations
Confusion regarding one's sexuality
Difficulty distinguishing self from others
Disturbed body image
Dreamlike view of the world

COGNITIVE
Confusion
Time disorientation
Distorted thinking
Disturbance of memory
Impaired judgment
Presence of separate personalities within the same person

BEHAVIORAL
Blunted affect
Emotional passivity and nonresponsiveness
Incongruent or idiosyncratic communication
Lack of spontaneity and animation
Loss of impulse control
Loss of initiative and decision-making ability
Social withdrawal

Box **18-4** *Unrealistic Self-expectations: The Tyranny of the Shoulds*

I should have the utmost generosity, consideration, dignity, courage, and unselfishness.
I should be the perfect lover, friend, parent, teacher, student, and spouse. Everyone should love me.
I should be able to find a quick solution to every problem.
I should never feel hurt; I should always be happy and serene.
I should assert myself; I should never hurt anybody else.
I should always be at peak efficiency. I should not be tired, get sick, or make mistakes.

From Horney K: *Neurosis and human growth,* New York, 1950, WW Norton.

not recognize. As both a participant and a spectator, he observes himself with great fear because he is unable to control his own impulses. He cannot completely escape the pain of self-awareness. He therefore disowns his behavior, feelings, thoughts, and body and becomes alienated from his true self.

Predisposing Factors

AFFECTING SELF-ESTEEM. Most research on self-esteem has focused exclusively on its psychosocial determinants. However, a recent study found that self-esteem is partly an inheritable trait and that genetic as well as environmental influences are very important.[19] Specifically, predisposing factors that originate in early childhood can contribute to problems with self-concept. Because the infant initially views himself as an extension of his parents, he is very responsive to both his parents' self-hate and any feelings of hatred toward himself. Parental rejection causes the child to be uncertain of himself and other human relationships. Because of his failure to be loved, the child fails to love himself and is unable to reach out with love to others.

As she grows older, the child may experience lack of recognition and appreciation by parents and significant others. He may learn to feel inadequate because he is not encour-

aged to be independent, to think for himself, and to take responsibility for his own needs and actions. Overpossessiveness, overpermissiveness, or overcontrol, exercised by one or both parents, can nurture a feeling of unimportance and lack of self-esteem in the child. Harsh, demanding parents can set unreasonable standards, often raising them before the child has developed the ability to meet them. Parents may also subject their children to unreasonable, harsh criticism and inconsistent punishment. These actions can cause early frustration, defeatism, and a destructive sense of inadequacy and inferiority. Another factor in creating such feelings may be the rivalry or unsuccessful imitation of an extremely bright sibling or a prominent parent, often creating a sense of hopelessness and inferiority. In addition, repeated defeats and failures can destroy self-worth. In this instance the failure in itself does not produce a sense of helplessness, but internalization of the failure as proof of personal incompetence does.

Unrealistic Self-Ideals. With age, additional factors emerge that can cause and perpetuate feelings of low self-esteem. The person who lacks a sense of meaning and purpose in life also fails to accept responsibility for his own well-being and to develop his capabilities and potential. He denies himself the freedom of full expression, including the right to make mistakes and fail, and becomes impatient, harsh, and demanding with himself. He sets standards that cannot be met. Self-consciousness and observation turn to self-contempt and self-defeat. This results in a further loss of self-trust.

These self-ideals or goals are often silent assumptions, and the person may not be immediately aware of them. They reflect high expectations and are unrealistic. When the person judges his performance by these unreasonable and inflexible standards, he cannot live up to his ideals and, as a result, experiences guilt and low self-esteem. Horney[10] has described these inner dictates as the "tyranny of the shoulds," and some of the common ones are identified in Box 18-4.

The person who overemphasizes these rules or ideals often makes a series of deductions such as the following: "Everyone should love me. If he or she doesn't love me, I have failed. I have lost the only thing that really matters. I am unlovable. There is no point in going on. I am worthless." This inner punishment results in feelings of depression and despair because no human being can fulfill the demands on self. Slavishly striving for these ideals interferes with other activities, such as living a healthy life and having satisfying relationships with other people. These predisposing factors lay the groundwork for feelings of low self-esteem.

AFFECTING ROLE PERFORMANCE

Sex Roles. An important source of strain in contemporary society comes from values, beliefs, and behaviors about sex roles. Research demonstrates that society continues to have clearly defined sex-role stereotypes for men and women. Women are perceived as less competent, less independent, less objective, and less logical than men. Men are perceived as lacking interpersonal sensitivity, warmth, and expressiveness. Moreover, stereotyped masculine traits are more often perceived as desirable than are stereotyped feminine characteristics.

To the extent that these results reflect societal standards of sex-role behavior, both women and men are put in role conflict by the difference in the standards. If a woman adopts behaviors desirable for a man, she risks censure for her failure to be appropriately feminine; if she adopts behaviors seen as feminine, she is deficient in the values associated with masculinity. Likewise, if a man adopts the behaviors seen as desirable for a woman, his masculinity and sexuality may be questioned and his contributions may be devalued or ignored; if he adopts the behaviors associated with masculinity, he risks alienating attributes of his personality associated with warmth, tenderness, and responsiveness. Thus, when a woman steps out of her home, where her sex role has traditionally been defined and confined, and enters the world of work, she may experience heightened role strain. Similarly, the man who arrives home from work in the evening may feel uncertain or in conflict about how he should relate to his school-age son, infant daughter, or working wife.

 Compare the value that two different cultures place on feminine and masculine roles and traits.

Work Roles. Women are still in the minority in most high-status occupations and are clustered near the bottom in terms of professional status and income. In American society, women are socialized to seek an ideal that includes marriage, children, higher education, and satisfying work outside the home. They are increasingly expected to perform in both "feminine" and "masculine" spheres.

This situation has many negative aspects. First, it can be argued that it merely replaces the traditional woman's role with another equally confining one. As the new role is val-

ued, the traditional roles of wife and mother become devalued. Second, although women are expected to assume more "masculine" qualities, a corresponding trend for men to assume more "feminine" behaviors is not apparent. Third, the woman who seeks such an expanded role is faced with reconciling the often conflicting goals of work, marriage, homemaking, and parenting.

Despite social and economic changes, there is often little sharing of tasks when men and women are both gainfully employed. Rather, most industrial societies have witnessed a gradual change in the obligations of women, who now perform a dual role: outside employment and continued responsibility for home and children. The expectation exists that the woman will make the adjustments needed both at home and in her career, including housekeeping and managing; arranging meals, lessons, and appointments; entertaining; caring for the sick; and communicating with the family. There is also the traditional expectation that the wife will be the primary caretaker of the children and will subsume other activities to this end.

One might conclude, therefore, that sex and work roles will continue as a source of stress until care of children, home, and career are viewed as equally valuable and important by both sexes and until gender is regarded as irrelevant to the abilities, personalities, and activities of the people involved. Such a change in attitude should begin with nurses and other mental health clinicians, who indirectly increase role strain by accepting stereotyped views. The cause of mental health might be better served if psychiatric clinicians encourage both men and women to maximize individual potential rather than adjust to existing sex roles.

AFFECTING PERSONAL IDENTITY. Constant parental intervention can interfere with adolescent choices. Parental distrust may lead a child to wonder whether his own choices are correct and to feel guilty if he goes against parental ideas. It may also devalue the child's opinions and lead to indecisiveness, impulsiveness, and acting out in an attempt to achieve some identity. When the parent does not trust the child, the child ultimately loses respect for the parent. It has been found that parents and children do not disagree on significant issues, such as war, peace, race, or religion. Instead, personal and narrow concerns—dating, a party, use of the car, curfews, hairstyles, homework—create the conflict between parents and youth.

Peers may also add to the problem of identity. The adolescent wants to belong, to feel needed and wanted. The peer group, with its rigid standards of behavior, gives him this feeling and provides a bridge between childhood and adulthood. The adolescent loses himself in the fads and the language of the group. However, the group is often a cruel testing ground that can hurt as much as it helps. Taught to be competitive, the young person competes with his friends, putting them down to bring himself up. Membership in the peer group is bought at a high price; the adolescent must surrender much of his identity to belong. Often there is open destruction of self-esteem and insistence on conformity. In sexual relationships adolescents introduce further uncertainty into their lives, which can interfere with developing a stable self-concept.

 Discuss how belonging to a group affects an adolescent's identity.

Precipitating Stressors

TRAUMA. Specific problems with self-concept are initiated by almost any difficult situation to which the person cannot adjust. Specifically, emotional trauma such as sexual and psychological abuse in childhood has been reported by most patients with multiple personality disorder.[13] Abuse, especially ongoing incest and sadistic or ritualistic abuse, is considered to be a major cause of this disorder. A small percentage of patients report no abuse but have experienced a trauma they perceive as life threatening to themselves or to someone else, such as a near drowning or witnessing a violent crime. However, it is believed that the chronic and pervasive dissociation present in multiple personality disorder usually results from prolonged exposure to sexual or physical abuse rather than from an isolated instance of trauma.

ROLE STRAIN. People who experience stress associated with expected roles are said to experience role strain. Role strain is the frustration felt when the person is torn in opposite directions or feels inadequate or unsuited to enact certain roles. In the course of a lifetime a person faces numerous role transitions. These transitions may require the incorporation of new knowledge and alterations in behavior. There are three categories of role transitions:

▼ Developmental
▼ Situational
▼ Health-illness

Developmental transitions are normative changes associated with growth. Situational transitions involve the addition or subtraction of significant others, occurring through birth or death; an example is the birth of one's first child. Health-illness transitions involve moving from a well state to an illness state. Each of these role transitions can precipitate a threat to one's self-concept.

Developmental Transitions. Various developmental stages can precipitate threats to self-identity. Adolescence is perhaps the most critical because it is a time of upheaval, change, anxiety, and insecurity. A serious threat to identity in adulthood is cultural discontinuity. This occurs when a person moves from one cultural setting to another and experiences emotional upheaval. In addition, problems within the social structure, such as political upheavals, economic depression, and high unemployment, can pose threats to identity. In late maturity and old age, identity problems again arise. Menopause, retirement, and increasing physical disability are problems for which people must work out adaptive responses.

Health-Illness Transitions. Some stressors can cause disturbances in body image and related changes in self-concept. One threat is the loss of a major body part, such as an eye, breast, or leg. Disturbances also may result from a surgical procedure in which the relationship of body parts is disturbed. The results of the surgical intervention may be either visible, as with a colostomy or gastrostomy, or invisible, as with a hysterectomy or gallbladder removal. Changes in body size, shape, and appearance can threaten the person's self-perceptions. Threats to body image can result from a pathological process that causes changes in the structure or function of the body, such as arthritis, multiple sclerosis, Parkinson's disease, cancer, pneumonia, and heart disease. The failure of a body part, as in paralysis, is particularly difficult to integrate into one's self-perceptions. The physical changes associated with normal growth and development may pose problems, as may some medical or nursing procedures, such as enemas, catheterizations, suctioning, radiation therapy, dilation and curettage, and organ transplantation.

All these stressors can pose a threat to body image, with resultant changes in self-esteem and role perception. Factors that influence the degree of threat to body image are listed in Table 18-2.

Finally, physiological stressors may also disturb a person's sense of reality, interfere with an accurate perception of the world, and threaten ego boundaries and identity. Such stressors include oxygen deprivation, hyperventilation, biochemical imbalances, severe fatigue, and sensory and emotional isolation. Alcohol, drugs, and other toxic substances may also distort self-concept. Usually these stressors produce only temporary changes.

Appraisal of Stressors

Whether the problem in self-concept is precipitated by psychological, sociological, or physiological stressors, the critical element is the patient's perception of the threat. When

TABLE **18-2** *Factors Influencing Self-concept Based on Health-Illness Transitions*

FACTOR	QUESTION
Meaning of the threat for the patient	Does it threaten the patient's ideal of youth or wholeness and decrease self-esteem?
Degree to which the patient's pattern of adaptation is interrupted	Does it jeopardize the patient's security and self-control?
Coping capacities and resources available	What is the response of significant others, and what help is offered?
Nature of the threat, extent of change, and rate at which it occurs	Is the change that of many small adjustments over time or a great and sudden adjustment?

assessing behaviors and formulating a nursing diagnosis, the nurse must continue to validate observations and inferences to establish a mutual, therapeutic relationship with the patient.

> ? *The incidence of breast cancer is rising in this country. What strategies are women using to promote adaptive self-concept responses?*

Coping Resources

It is important that the nurse and patient review possible coping resources. All people, no matter how disturbing their behavior, have some areas of personal strength,[4] which might include the following:

▼ Sports and outdoor activities
▼ Hobbies and crafts
▼ Expressive arts
▼ Health and self-care
▼ Education or training
▼ Vocation or position
▼ Special aptitudes
▼ Intelligence
▼ Imagination and creativity
▼ Interpersonal relationships

When the patient's positive aspects become evident, the nurse should share them with the patient to expand the patient's self-awareness and suggest possible areas for future intervention.

Coping Mechanisms

SHORT-TERM DEFENSES. An identity crisis may be resolved with either short-term or long-term coping mechanisms. These are used to ward off the anxiety and uncertainty of identity confusion. Logan[14] has described the following four categories of short-term defenses:

▼ Activities that provide temporary escape from the identity crisis
▼ Activities that provide temporary substitute identities
▼ Activities that temporarily strengthen or heighten a diffuse sense of self
▼ Activities that represent short-term attempts to make an identity out of meaninglessness and identity diffusion— that try to assert that the meaning of life is meaningless itself

The first category of temporary escape includes activities that seem to provide intense immediate experiences. These experiences so overwhelm the senses that the issue of identity literally does not exist because the person's entire being is occupied with "right now" sensations. Examples include drug experiences, loud rock concerts, fast car and motorcycle riding, some forms of hard physical labor, exercise or sports, and even obsessive television watching.

The category of temporary substitute identity is derived from being a "joiner"; the identity of a club, group, team, movement, or gang may function as a basis for self-definition. The person temporarily adopts the group definition as his own identity in a type of devotion to the larger entity. Temporary substitute identities can also be obtained by playing a certain role within a group, such as clown, bully, or chauffeur, or by buying objects that are marketed with ready-made identities. Thus, a certain type of cologne, make of car, or article of dress implies built-in personalities the person can adopt as his own.

The third category of defenses involves confronting or challenging something to feel more intensely alive. This is evident in risk taking for its own sake, which creates a feeling of bravado. Competitive activities, such as sports, academic achievement, and popularity contests, also fit into this category. The idea is that competition and comparison with an outsider more sharply define a sense of self. Another example is bigotry and prejudice. By adopting a bigoted stance toward some outgroup or scapegoat, the person can temporarily strengthen self-esteem or ego integrity.

The final category helps to explain the fads that people indulge in with such fervor and that seem so meaningless to others. The sheer force of commitment to fads is an attempt to transform them into something meaningful.

LONG-TERM DEFENSES. Any of these short-term defenses may develop into a long-term one that will be evident in maladaptive behavior. Other resolutions or long-term defenses are also possible. A positive resolution or adaptive response produces an integrated ego identity and unified self. Another type of long-term resolution has been identified as **identity foreclosure**. This occurs when people adopt the "ready made" type of identity desired by others without really coming to terms with their own desires, aspirations, or potential. This is a less desirable long-term resolution, as is adopting a deviant or negative identity.

A **negative identity** is one that is at odds with the values of society. In this case the person tries to define the self in a nonprescribed or antisocial manner. The choice of a negative identity represents an attempt to retain some mastery in a situation in which a positive identity does not seem possible or desirable. The person may be saying, "I would rather be somebody bad than nobody at all." The following clinical example describes the negative identity assumed by an adolescent with a medical diagnosis of conduct disorder—undersocialized, aggressive.

Clinical Example Ken was a 17-year-old boy referred to the local community mental health center by his high school nurse. She made the referral after attending a team conference at school about Ken's repeated behavioral problems. He had a history of aggressive and destructive behavior, poor peer relationships, and low academic performance. The school had suspended him on three occasions, and the result of the team conference was to expel him for the remainder of the school year.

Mr. P, a psychiatric nurse at the mental health center, established a contract to work with Ken and his family. He noted that Ken was an obese young man (112.5 kg) who took little interest in his appearance. His dress was sloppy, his complexion unclean, and his hair oily. He sat slumped in the chair in a disinterested and slightly defiant posture.

As Ken talked about himself, he complained of many pressures he experienced in his part-time job at a local hardware store. He thought the work was too difficult and tiring and that he was qualified for better and more prestigious work. When asked for specifics, he could not identify another job in particular. He also expressed a great deal of harassment from his family. His mother and father had been married for 31 years, and he was the only child of the marriage. His mother worked part-time at a bakery, and his father was recently retired from his job as a supervisor at a local utility company, where he was highly regarded.

Ken said that his father "always had things for me to do." He described how his father signed him up for various team sports—baseball, basketball, football—without acknowledging how much Ken hated sports and how uncoordinated he was. His father also stressed good grades and the necessity of college for success in life. Ken described his mother as passive and polite and said he had little respect for her. He said his aggressive outbursts occurred both at home and at school—whenever he was frustrated. People reacted by staying out of his way. He said he never hurt anyone with his temper. He mostly destroyed property and objects.

Ken avoided the subject of peers but, when asked about friends, said he "hung out" with a couple of boys in the neighborhood. They were older than he was. Most had dropped out of high school and were employed in odd jobs. He denied drug use but said he drank heavily, especially on the weekends. He said he had no girlfriends and wasn't interested in complicating his life "with some broad."

Selected Nursing Diagnoses:

▼ Personal identity disturbance related to fear of failure, as evidenced by aggressive and destructive behavior and poor school performance

▼ Altered family processes related to conflict with parents, as evidenced by avoidance and lack of communication

Ken displays many of the behaviors characteristic of a negative identity. The nurse working with Ken explored his underlying feelings and self-perceptions. Great anger with his father began to surface, and Ken was able to verbalize it. Because he was the only son, he believed he was competing with his father and had to live up to his father's ideals. Ken feared failing in trying to adopt a positive identity and resented the identity his father was trying to impose on him. He thought he had no part in defining it and that it did not represent his real self.

EGO DEFENSE MECHANISMS. Patients with alterations in self-concept may use a variety of ego-oriented mechanisms to protect themselves from confronting their own inadequacies. Typical ego defense mechanisms include fantasy, dissociation, isolation, projection, displacement,

splitting, turning anger against the self, and acting out. These are described in Chapter 16.

Other, more damaging coping mechanisms can also be used to protect self-esteem. These may include the following:

▼ Obesity
▼ Anorexia
▼ Promiscuity
▼ Chronic overworking
▼ Suicide
▼ Delinquency
▼ Crime
▼ Drug use
▼ Family violence
▼ Incest

Nursing Diagnosis

Self-concept is a critical aspect of one's overall personality adjustment. Problems with self-concept are associated with feelings of anxiety, hostility, and guilt. These often create a circular, self-propagating process that ultimately results in maladaptive coping responses (Fig. 18-3).

Most people who express dissatisfaction with life, display deviant behavior, or have difficulty functioning in social or work situations have problems related to self-concept.

The primary NANDA nursing diagnoses related to alterations in self-concept are **body image disturbance, self-esteem disturbance, altered role performance,** and **personal identity disturbance.** Nursing diagnoses related to the range of possible maladaptive responses of the patient are identified in the Medical and Nursing Diagnoses box on p. 334.

Examples of complete nursing diagnoses related to self-concept are presented in the Detailed Diagnoses box on p. 335. However, alterations in self-concept affect all aspects of a person's life. Therefore, many additional problems may be identified by the nurse.

Related Medical Diagnoses

In practice, maladaptive responses indicating alterations in self-concept can be seen in a variety of people experiencing threats to their physical integrity or self-system. These nursing diagnoses are not limited to the psychiatric setting and do not have a discrete category of medical diagnoses associated with them. Because they pertain to basic personality structure and feelings about oneself, they can emerge with many neurotic and psychotic disorders (see A Patient Speaks on p. 336) and may be related to all the diagnostic categories identified in the DSM-IV[2] because all these disorders ultimately reflect on one's view of self. Several specific medical diagnoses deserve particular attention, however, because their dominant features include alterations in self-concept. They are listed in the Medical and Nursing Diagnoses box on p. 334 and include identity problems and

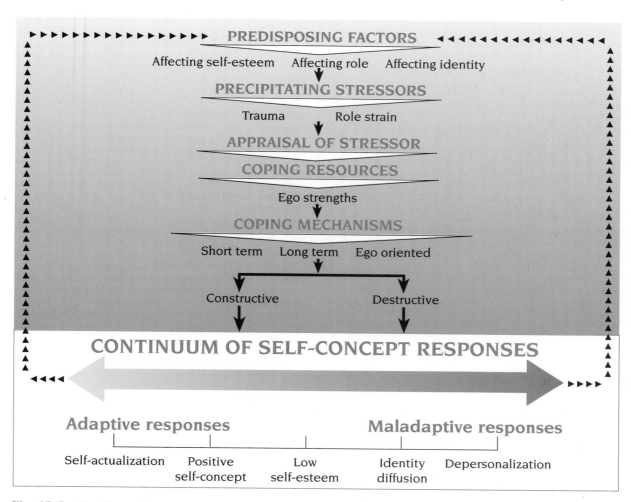

Fig. 18-3   The Stuart Stress Adaptation Model related to self-concept responses.

dissociative identity disorder, also known as multiple personality disorder.

Outcome Identification

The expected outcome when working with a patient with a maladaptive self-concept response is as follows:

The patient will obtain the maximum level of self-actualization to realize his or her potential.

Goals should be as clear and explicit as possible. They should identify realistic steps that the patient can accomplish. In this way the patient's self-confidence will increase, and this will build self-esteem. These goals should emphasize strengths instead of weaknesses. If they are mutually identified, they will motivate the patient and help the patient assume increased responsibility for one's own behavior. Following are examples of goals related to role performance:

Long-term: Mrs. P will resolve role conflict by achieving greater congruency between work and family roles.

Short-term:
After 1 week:
▼ Mrs. P will describe her responsibilities in her work and home roles.
▼ She will identify aspects of these roles that provide her with satisfaction.
▼ She will identify areas of role incompatibility.
After 2 weeks:
▼ She will describe three alternative ways of increasing the complementarity of the roles.
▼ She will discuss the advantages and disadvantages of each alternative.
After 3 weeks:
▼ She will take the necessary measures to implement one of the identified alternatives.

Planning

The nurse's focus is to help the patient understand himself more fully and accurately so that he can direct his own life

MEDICAL AND NURSING DIAGNOSES *related to* **Self-concept Responses**

Related Medical Diagnoses (DSM-IV)*	Related Nursing Diagnoses (NANDA)†
Identity problem	Adjustment, impaired
Dissociative amnesia	Anxiety
Dissociative fugue	**Body image disturbance‡**
Dissociative identity disorder (multiple personality disorder)	Communication, impaired verbal
Depersonalization disorder	Coping, ineffective individual
	Grieving, dysfunctional
	Hopelessness
	Loneliness, risk for
	Personal identity disturbance‡
	Powerlessness
	Role performance, altered‡
	Self-care deficit
	Self-esteem disturbance‡
	Sensory-perceptual alteration
	Sexuality patterns, altered
	Social interaction, impaired
	Social isolation
	Spiritual distress
	Thought processes, altered
	Violence, potential for

*From American Psychiatric Association: *Diagnostic and statistical manual of mental disorders,* ed 4, Washington, DC, 1994, The Association.
†From North American Nursing Diagnosis Association: *NANDA nursing diagnoses: definitions and classifications 1997-1998,* Philadelphia, 1997, The Association.
‡Primary nursing diagnosis for alterations in self-concept.

in a more satisfying way. This means helping him strive toward a clearer, deeper experience of his feelings, wishes, and beliefs; a greater ability to tap his resources and use them for constructive ends; and a clearer perception of his direction in life, assuming responsibility for himself, his decisions, and his actions.

Self-awareness is crucial in bringing about changes in self-concept, but people usually spend little time in introspection. However, certain conditions or events do stimulate self-awareness. This may occur when stimuli from the body are intensified, as in states of pain, fatigue, or anger, or when stimuli from the environment are decreased, as in sensory deprivation or isolation. Self-awareness may be triggered when something unexpected or extraordinary takes place, when the person has succeeded or failed, or when the person is confronted with himself by looking in a mirror, listening to his voice on a tape recorder, or reading an old letter. Special occasions, such as birthdays, anniversaries, New Year's Eve, or a death may stimulate introspection. It may also be initiated when others direct their attention to the person through conversation or touch.

Once the person begins to look at and analyze himself, changes in the self become possible. Often they are the result of feelings of failure, unhappiness, anxiety, inadequacy, doubt, or perceived discrepancies between one's concept of self and the demands of the environment or the expectations of others. Usually changes in the self occur only as a result of experiences and occur gradually. Occasionally, however, a change may take place suddenly. A traumatic experience may force a person to see that something drastic must be done. The nurse should take all these factors into consideration when planning nursing care.

Similarly, the family of origin is a source of many people's self-esteem. Adult contact with parents and siblings can correct misconceptions underlying low self-esteem and allow more positive beliefs. Learning to interact with family members with closeness, but without counterproductive forms of fusion and emotionality, can enable a more mature pattern to develop. Family relationships would therefore be an appropriate focus for patient education. A Patient Education Plan using family systems is presented on p. 337. Chapter 32 has a more detailed discussion of family systems theory and family interventions.

Implementation

The mutually identified goals can be reached by a problem-solving approach that focuses primarily on the present, removes much of the responsibility from the nurse, and actively engages the patient in working on personal difficulties. This approach increases the patient's self-confidence and self-esteem. It requires that the patient first

DETAILED DIAGNOSES *related to* **Self-concept Responses**

NANDA Diagnosis Stem	Examples of Complete Diagnosis
Body image disturbance	Body image disturbance related to fear of becoming obese, as evidenced by refusal to maintain body weight within normal limits
	Body image disturbance related to leukemia chemotherapy, as evidenced by negative feelings about one's body
	Body image disturbance related to cerebrovascular accident, as evidenced by lack of acceptance of body limitations
Self-esteem disturbance	Self-esteem disturbance related to death of spouse, as evidenced by withdrawal from others and feelings of hopelessness
	Self-esteem disturbance related to overly high self-ideals, as evidenced by depressed mood and withdrawal from activities
Role performance, altered	Role performance, altered, related to incompatibility of newly assumed work and family roles, as evidenced by self-criticism and feeling of inadequacy
	Role performance, altered, related to incongruence of cultural and self-role expectations about aging, as evidenced by feelings of frustration and criticism of others
Personal identity disturbance	Personal identity disturbance related to unrealistic parental expectations, as evidenced by running away from home
	Personal identity disturbance related to drug toxicity, as evidenced by confusion and loss of impulse control.

DSM-IV Diagnosis	Essential Features*
Identity problem	Uncertainty about multiple issues relating to identity such as long-term goals, career choice, friendship patterns, sexual orientation and behavior, moral values, and group loyalties
Dissociative amnesia	The predominant disturbance is episodes of inability to recall important personal information, usually of a traumatic or stressful nature, that is too extensive to be explained by ordinary forgetfulness.
Dissociative fugue	The predominant disturbance is sudden, unexpected travel away from home or one's customary place of work, with inability to recall one's past. Confusion about personal identity or assumption of a new identity.
Dissociative identity disorder (multiple personality disorder)	The presence of two or more distinct identities or personality states (each with its own enduring pattern of perceiving, relating to, and thinking about the environment and self). At least two of these identities or personality states recurrently take control of the person's behavior. Inability to recall important personal information that is too extensive to be explained by ordinary forgetfulness.
Depersonalization disorder	Persistent or recurrent experiences of feeling detached from, and as if one is an outside observer of, one's mental processes or body (for example, feeling as if one is in a dream). During the depersonalization experience, reality testing remains intact. The depersonalization causes clinically significant distress or impairment in functioning.

*Modified from The American Psychiatric Association: *Diagnostic and statistical manual of mental disorders,* ed 4, Washington, DC, 1994, The Association.

develop **insight** into her problems and life situation and take **action** to effect lasting behavioral changes. The nurse must thus incorporate both the responsive dimensions (insight oriented) and the action dimensions (action oriented) of the therapeutic relationship described in Chapter 2.

The focus of this approach is on the patient's cognitive appraisal of life, which may contain faulty perceptions, beliefs, and convictions. Awareness of feelings and emotions is also important because they too may be subject to misconceptions. Only after examining the patient's cognitive appraisal of the situation and related feelings can one gain insight into the problem and bring about behavioral change.

Adaptive behavior is based both on insight and on carrying out the solution to the initial problem.

There are principles of nursing care that are applicable to various self-concept problems. These principles are incorporated here within a problem-solving approach and are presented as a progressive sequence. They focus primarily on the level of the patient. However, they may be implemented in conjunction with group or family interventions, and the nurse is expected to include the patient's family, significant others, and community supports whenever possible. Such a mobilization of the patient's coping resources can have both preventive and curative effects.

A Patient *Speaks*   Judy Mays

Thoughts on Mental Illness

It came to me—so clear that I could not deny it,
the pain, the hurt, the anger—I am mentally ill.
I've tried to pretend that I'd get better
putting the hurt away—gutting out the pain
hoping it would eventually pass—yes, eventually pass.
So I did therapy
I talked about what I had experienced,
Perceptual disturbances, they said.
I talked about what unrealness, the flatness—like card-
board.
Depersonalization, they said.
I talked about people making me nervous,
about staying to myself.
You must think rationally, do self-talk, change your
behaviors.
Take these drugs, they said
because I had heard a voice, or felt something
they had not.
I had psychotic symptoms—load her up on Mellaril,
so what if she gets as fat as a pig—keep increasing
the dosage
Too fat? Load her up on Haldol.
But I'm not psychotic—
Oh, but you are schizo-affective, no—let's make
that borderline,
on second thought, maybe major depression
with psychotic features?
No, more like depersonalization disorder
Let's check for temporal lobe epilepsy,
what the hell, it isn't our money—why are you
complaining?
And the therapy goes on—I feel worse
The drugs don't work—
You're resistant to treatment
take some more drugs—they will help you feel better
So I take the damn drugs—is one anti-depressant
any different from another?—how
much of the stuff can you take?
It doesn't do any good
how many times do I have to say that?
Why doesn't my doctor listen?
Why does she keep writing prescriptions for
more of the stuff?
Who is taking this stuff—me, or her? I should
know if it works.

I do therapy with the silicone people,
they who make no mistakes,
who are always clinically correct—always clean
nice people—but inside I am not clean.
I fear that I may be defective,
that some loose part may come undone and all will be
lost.
I'm so scared and I work overtime to find
something positive
something good to come out of all this chaos.
I don't think he understands
when I talk to my therapist I sometimes feel cheap
and shallow because I've bought the time and I know
he would not be talking to me if I hadn't.
I feel frustrated because I've been trapped
in this sickness.
How can they feel the humiliation—the stigma
The ones so well—that they can heal?
Pain, Hurt, and Fear are subjectively private,
but even for me the loneliness is too much.
And so I ask the silicone people,
have you ever been afraid? Yes, they say.
But they don't feel the fear,
and they don't connect with the fear
But I feel it, and—I want the silicone folks to feel it too.
I do not want to hurt by myself
I want someone to also feel the hurt
So all you silicone therapists—hear me:
to hurt when someone IS there but still is NOT,
is the worst kind of hurt of all—listen up. ▼

From South Carolina Self-Help Association Regarding Emotions: *Share the News,* Spring 1993.

Level 1: Expanded Self-awareness

To avoid anxiety, most people resist change. In general, change in the self is easier when threat is absent. Threat forces a person to defend himself, perceptions are narrowed, and the person has difficulty forming new perceptions of himself (see Critical Thinking about Contemporary Issues).

To expand the patient's self-awareness and reduce the element of threat, the nurse should adopt an accepting attitude. Acceptance allows the patient the security and freedom to examine all aspects of oneself as a total human being with positive and negative qualities. The basis of a therapeutic relationship is established by listening to the patient with understanding, responding nonjudgmentally, expressing genuine interest, and conveying a sense of caring and sincerity. Creating a climate of acceptance allows previously denied experiences to be brought into consciousness and explored. This broadens the patient's concept of self

PATIENT EDUCATION PLAN Improving Family Relationships

Content	Instructional Activities	Evaluation
Define the concept of self-differentiation within one's family of origin	Discuss the differences between high and low levels of self-differentiation Ask the patient to identify level of functioning among family members	Patient identifies functioning level in family of origin
Describe the characteristics of emotional fusion, emotional cutoff, and triangulation	Analyze types and patterns of family relationships Diagram family patterns	Patient describes interactional patterns within family Patient identifies own roles and behavior
Discuss the role of symptom formation and symptom bearer in a family	Sensitize the patient to family dynamics and manifestations of stress Encourage communication with family of origin	Patient recognizes family contribution to the stress of individual members Patient contacts family members
Describe a family genogram and show how it is constructed	Use a blackboard to map out a family genogram Assign family genogram as homework	Patient obtains factual information about family Patient constructs family genogram
Analyze need for objectivity and responsibility for changing one's own behavior and not that of others	Role-play interactions with various family members Encourage testing out new ways of interacting with family members	Patient demonstrates a higher level of differentiation in family of origin

CRITICAL THINKING *about* Contemporary Issues

What Is the Recommended Treatment for Multiple Personality Disorder?

Reported cases of multiple personality disorder have increased dramatically in the last decade, yet there are few data on the preferred treatment of this illness. Most recommendations are made based on the experience of individual clinicians rather than on systematic research.

A recent study addressed the efficacy of treatment modalities currently used to treat patients with multiple personality disorder. The findings supported the primacy of psychotherapy and the moderate benefits of psychopharmacology with antidepressant and antianxiety agents.[17] The authors also reported that the length, frequency, and cost of treatment for this illness have major implications for the mental health care system. As a result of inadequate third-party funding and community resources, it is likely that many of these patients will be unable to obtain adequate treatment despite substantial morbidity, social impairment, and risk of continuing a cycle of abuse and violence into future generations.

and helps the patient to accept all aspects of one's personality. It also indicates that the patient is a valued person who is responsible for oneself and is able to help oneself. This is important because the nurse must work with whatever ego strength the patient possesses.

Most patients seen in clinics, the general hospital, and the community setting possess considerable ego strength. However, hospitalized people might have limited ego re-

sources. Psychotic patients experiencing depersonalization and identity confusion often present difficult challenges for the nurse. They tend to isolate themselves and withdraw from reality, so little ego strength is available for problem solving. For this type of patient, expanding self-awareness means first confirming the patient's identity. The nurse should attempt to provide supportive measures to decrease the panic level experienced by this patient. Additional interventions related to anxiety and psychotic states are described in Chapters 16 and 22.

The nurse can spend time with the patient in an undemanding way and approach the patient nonaggressively. Initially the nurse may accept the patient's need to remain nonverbal or attempt to clarify and understand the patient's verbal communication even though it may be distorted or lack apparent logic. Attempts should be made to prevent the patient from being isolated by establishing a simple routine for the patient. If the patient displays bizarre behavior, such as inappropriate laughing or mannerisms, the nurse can set limits on the behavior. It is important to orient the patient frequently to reality and reinforce appropriate behavior.

The patient should be helped to increase the activities that provide positive experiences. This may involve the use of occupational therapy, recreational therapy, or activity groups because success at tasks and increased involvement with objects can increase self-esteem. Movement therapy or body ego technique is a goal-directed way to develop identity, body image, and ego structure. It is predominantly a nonverbal therapy because the emphasis is on movement, not on what the person says.

Depersonalization often leads to poor hygiene and an unkempt personal appearance. Nurses who are aware of their own value systems regarding cleanliness and grooming can help patients unable to care for themselves. They can use patience and repetition to establish health routines and can kindly but firmly encourage patients to care for themselves. Through verbal and nonverbal messages, nurses can encourage patients to take pride in their appearance and reinforce any progress made. Another possible nursing intervention is photographic self-image confrontation. This involves taking photographs of patients and then discussing them. This intervention can provide a means for establishing a nurse-patient relationship and mutually exploring some aspects of the self.

Mutuality is often difficult to establish with a patient experiencing depersonalization. Initially the nurse will deter-mine appropriate activities and incorporate the patient into them without asking for a response. Gradually, however, the nurse can expect greater participation and can involve the patient in decision making. Table 18-3 summarizes the nursing interventions appropriate to level 1.

Sometimes the nurse's attitudes or behaviors can block patients from expanding their self-awareness. These behaviors can take the form of criticism, belittlement, condemnation, condescension, indifference, or insincerity. An impersonal attitude can decrease the patient's self-esteem. Excessive demands or direct challenges to self-concept can result in further withdrawal. Nurses should not allow patients to remain alone or inactive, attempt to shame them into improving their habits, or assume total care for them. If they avoid these behaviors and strive for acceptance, they remove themselves as a source of threat and encourage pa-

TABLE **18-3** *Nursing Interventions in Alterations in Self-concept at Level 1*
GOAL: EXPAND THE PATIENT'S SELF-AWARENESS

PRINCIPLE	RATIONALE	NURSING INTERVENTIONS
Establish an open, trusting relationship.	Reduces the threat that the nurse poses to the patient and helps the patient to broaden and accept all aspects of one's personality	Offer unconditional acceptance. Listen to the patient. Encourage discussion of thoughts and feelings. Respond nonjudgmentally. Convey to the patient that he is a valued person who is responsible for and able to help himself.
Work with whatever ego strength the patient has.	Some degree of ego strength, such as the capacity for reality testing, self-control, or a degree of ego integration, is needed as a foundation for later nursing care.	Identify the patient's ego strength. Guidelines for the patient with limited ego resources are as follows: 1. Begin by confirming his identity. 2. Provide support measures to reduce his level of anxiety. 3. Approach him in an undemanding way. 4. Accept and attempt to clarify any verbal or nonverbal communication. 5. Prevent him from isolating himself. 6. Establish a simple routine for him. 7. Set limits on inappropriate behavior. 8. Orient him to reality. 9. Reinforce appropriate behavior. 10. Gradually increase activities and tasks that provide positive experiences for him. 11. Help him in personal hygiene and grooming. 12. Encourage the patient to care for himself.
Maximize the patient's participation in the therapeutic relationship.	Mutuality is necessary for the patient to assume responsibility for his own behavior and maladaptive coping responses.	Gradually increase the patient's participation in decisions that affect his care. Convey to the patient that he is a responsible person.

tients to lower their defenses. Patients are then prepared to undertake the next step in problem solving.

> ❓ *How do you think that the nurse's level of self-esteem affects nursing interventions in patient's self-concept responses?*

Level 2: Self-exploration

At this level of intervention nurses encourage patients to examine feelings, behavior, beliefs, and thoughts, particularly in relation to the current stressor. The cognitive behavioral strategies described in Chapter 30 are very useful at this time. Patients' feelings may be expressed verbally, nonverbally, symbolically, or directly. For example, self-portrait drawing has been found to facilitate awareness and understanding of sense of self for adult survivors of childhood sexual abuse.[8] Acceptance continues to be important because when nurses accept patients' feelings and thoughts, they are helping them to accept them as well. Nurses should facilitate the expression of strong emotions, such as anger, sadness, and guilt. In a sense, patients' emotions or affects serve as clues to inner thoughts and current behavior.

As the patient focuses his attention on the meaning that experiences have for him, he is clarifying his perceptions and concept of himself and his relationship to the people and events around him. The nurse can elicit his perception of strengths and weaknesses and have him describe his self-ideal. He can be made aware of his self-criticisms.

It is important for nurses to accept and deal with their own feelings before becoming involved in the self-exploration of others. Self-awareness limits the potential negative effects of countertransference in the relationship. It also allows nurses to demonstrate authentic behavior that, in turn, can be elicited and reinforced in the patient. Often patients experience great difficulty in discussing or describing their feelings. This may be because society tends to discourage self-revelation, because some patients are honestly out of touch with their inner self, or because survivors of incest have buried important aspects of the self.[9] In these cases nurses can use themselves therapeutically by sharing feelings, verbalizing how they might feel in the situation, or mirroring their perception of patients' feelings. In this way nurses can help patients explore maladaptive thinking.

The nurse must be careful not to reinforce the patient's self-pity by responding with sympathy. Patients often deny any personal responsibility for their situation and they fail to see how their own behavior precipitates the problem about which they complain. Examples include patients who seek treatment because of things that happened to them (his wife left him, her husband beat her, or his boss fired him, for example) and patients who seek help because of things that have not happened, such as not being happy or not having friends. These patients fail to see that they have

a choice in life and that personal growth and satisfaction involve both risk and responsibility.

The nurse can clarify with the patient that he is not helpless or powerless. He is powerless when he sees himself as such and gives up control and responsibility for his behavior. The patient must accept responsibility for logical consequences of the things he chooses to do or not to do. Only if a patient fully understands the implications of his actions and the scope of his choices can he set goals, explore alternatives, and effect change.

In stressing the importance of behavior, the nurse helps the patient see that he chooses to behave in certain ways. If the patient projects his problems onto the environment, the nurse can discuss with him the difficulty in changing other people and explore the possibilities of changing his own self. This means helping the patient realize that when he says, "I can't," he really means "I don't want to." The nurse should not give the impression that she has the power to change a patient's life. That power lies with the patient alone. However, the nurse can help him to maximize his strengths, use available resources, and see that there is more to life than misery and pain.

Self-exploration need not take place solely within the one-to-one relationship. Family sessions and group meetings can help clarify how the patient appears to others.[12,23] These meetings can supplement the individual sessions with the patient, and similar nursing interventions can be applied within family or group therapy. Regardless of the setting, the nurse collects information on the patient's thinking about himself, logical or illogical reasoning, and reported or observed reactions. Interventions at this level should see the patient progress from denying or attributing contradictory feelings to the external situation, to recognizing a major conflict within himself (Table 18-4).

> ❓ *Do you believe contemporary society encourages or discourages personal responsibility for behavior? Defend your point of view.*

Level 3: Self-evaluation

This level involves hard work for the patient as he critically examines his own behavior, accepts the consequences for it, and judges whether it is the best possible choice. At this point, the problem should be clearly defined and the patient should be helped to understand that his beliefs influence his feelings and behavior. Only by actively and systematically challenging his faulty beliefs and perceptions can he hope for change. Previously identified misperceptions and distortions should be evaluated. Irrational beliefs and unrealistic self-ideals should be identified and analyzed.

The patient's hopelessness should be countered by exploring areas of realistic hope. It is important to point out the mature part of the patient's personality and contrast it

TABLE **18-4** *Nursing Interventions in Alterations in Self-concept at Level 2*

GOAL: ENCOURAGE THE PATIENT'S SELF-EXPLORATION

PRINCIPLE	RATIONALE	NURSING INTERVENTIONS
Help the patient to accept his own feelings and thoughts.	When nurses show interest in and accept the patient's feelings and thoughts, they are helping him to do so as well.	Attend to and encourage the patient's expression of his emotions, beliefs, behavior, and thoughts verbally, non-verbally, symbolically, or directly. Use therapeutic communication skills and empathic responses. Note his use of logical and illogical thinking and his reported and observed emotional responses.
Help the patient to clarify his concept of self and his relationship to others through self-disclosure.	Self-disclosure and understanding one's self-perceptions are prerequisites to bringing about future change; this may, in itself, reduce anxiety.	Elicit his perception of self-strengths and weaknesses. Help him to describe his self-ideal. Identify his self-criticisms. Help him to describe how he believes he relates to other people and events.
Be aware and have control of one's own feelings.	Self-awareness allows the nurse to model authentic behavior and limits the potential negative effects of countertransference in the relationship.	Openness to and acceptance of one's own positive and negative feelings. Therapeutic use of self by sharing one's own feelings with the patient, verbalizing how another might have felt, or mirroring one's perception of the patient's feelings.
Respond empathically, not sympathetically, emphasizing that the power to change lies with the patient.	Sympathy can reinforce self-pity; the nurse should communicate that the patient's life situation is subject to his own control.	Use empathic responses and monitor oneself for feelings of sympathy or pity. Reaffirm to the patient that he is not powerless in the face of his problems. Convey that the patient is responsible for his own behavior, including his choice of maladaptive or adaptive coping responses. Discuss the scope of his choices, his areas of ego strength, and coping resources that are available. Use the support systems of family and groups to facilitate the patient's self-exploration. Help the patient recognize the nature of his conflict and the maladaptive ways in which he tries to cope with it.

to the immature part that causes problems. The behaviors that interfere with effective functioning should be put in perspective so that the patient can see that his maladaptive behavior is only a small part of his total personality.

Success and failure must be placed in perspective. Failures occur every moment of every day and are a natural consequence of human activity. As long as people strive to achieve, they will often not reach their goals. The only way to avoid failure is to do absolutely nothing. Failure may be caused by one's own mistakes, a lack of motivation, or circumstances beyond one's control. Whatever the reason, failure is the unavoidable outcome of human effort. The problem arises when people are labeled or label themselves as

failures. This is illogical and potentially destructive. As an inherent aspect of life, failure should be viewed either as a neutral concept or a positive one for the learning experience it provides.

Unrealistic self-ideals, dependency patterns, and denial are all potential areas that can be analyzed. The patient can be helped to realize that all behavior and coping responses have positive and negative consequences. Contrasts can be drawn between behavior that is destructive, inhibitory, or sabotaging and behavior that is productive, enhancing, or growth producing. The patient must see that he acts in self-defeating ways because some "payoff" or personal gain is in it for him. The patient is probably well aware of the drawbacks of his maladaptive coping responses. The payoffs, or secondary gains, may be more obscure and well repressed. Following are some common payoffs:

▼ Procrastination
▼ Avoiding risks
▼ Retreating from the present
▼ Evading responsibility for one's actions
▼ Avoiding working or having to change

Payoffs specific to the patient's problem should be identified by the nurse and patient together. For example, possible secondary gains from being obese include having people feel sorry for you, having an excuse for not dating or being married, being the focus of dieting attention, or being easily recognized and noticed when with other people. Possible secondary gains for an adult remaining dependent on one's parents might include not having to make one's own decisions, having someone else to blame if things go wrong, being protected from risks and venturing out in the world, not establishing lasting intimate relationships, or not having to establish one's own identity, but rather adopting the values and goals of others.

The nurse becomes more active at this level of intervention by confronting, interpreting, persuading, and challenging. The goal is to increase the patient's objectivity in dealing with stressors. For example, the nurse can show the patient that the same person can nurture and gratify as well as anger and frustrate because both negative and positive qualities coexist in the same person. Supportive confrontation may be particularly effective in pointing out inconsistencies in words and actions. The climate of acceptance established by the nurse in level 1 and the empathic communication developed in level 2 provide a basis for confrontation in level 3. This groundwork is necessary to prevent premature confrontation, which can be destructive.

The nurse may use various aspects of role theory during this level, including helping the patient in role clarification by identifying behaviors, clarifying expectations, and specifying goals related to the role. The nurse can also encourage the patient to participate in any activity in which he can observe his own behavior. Role playing may be particularly effective in providing the patient with feedback and increasing his insight. Through it, he may become more objective about the irrationality and self-destructiveness of his self-criticisms.

Another therapeutic intervention that is particularly useful in promoting the self-esteem and coping mechanisms of the elderly is the use of reminiscence.[16] Reminiscence involves thinking about or relating past experiences, especially those that are personally significant. It has been used to help patients acquire a sense of integrity, enhance self-esteem, and stimulate thinking about oneself. As such, it provides nurses with an opportunity to focus, reflect, and reinforce their patients' uniqueness and enhance their sense of self-worth. Reminiscence is discussed in more detail in Chapter 38.

The nurse-patient relationship is a rich source of infor-

mation for the patient. Within this relationship the patient is enacting and experiencing many of his problem areas, and the nurse can use this as a "study in miniature." The nurse can observe how the patient reacts in the one-to-one situation and share reactions with him to give him feedback on how he affects others. The analysis and use of transference and countertransference reactions constitute the nurse's therapeutic use of self. When a block arises in the relationship or anxiety increases, the nurse should explore its meaning with the patient. The nurse should confront the problem and openly discuss it with him. This can also be done in family or group therapy sessions.

During this level of intervention the patient and nurse critically evaluate the patient's behavior (Table 18-5). Misperceptions, unrealistic goals, and distortions of reality are explored. This provides the patient with sufficient knowledge to progress to the next level of problem solving.

 Think of one of your less desirable habits. What payoff or personal gain does it provide you?

Level 4: Realistic Planning

The nurse and patient are now ready to formulate possible solutions or alternatives. This begins by investigating what solutions were attempted in the past and evaluating their effectiveness. When the patient holds inconsistent perceptions, he is faced with several choices. He can change his perceptions and beliefs to bring them closer to a reality that cannot be changed. Alternatively, he may seek to change his environment to bring it in line with what he believes. When his behavior is inconsistent with his self-concept, he can change his behavior, change the beliefs underlying his self-concept so that they include his behavior, or change his self-ideal while leaving his self-concept intact.

At this time, all possible solutions should be openly discussed with the patient. Nurses must be careful not to use their influence to persuade the patient to do anything that represents their values rather than the patient's. The nurse should help him conceptualize his goals. If they are within his reach, his efforts can be supported. If the patient has conflicting goals, the nurse helps him identify which are more realistic by discussing emotional and practical consequences.

The nurse can work with the patient in various ways. The patient may be encouraged to give up superhuman standards by which he judges his behavior. These standards may set him up for failure. The patient may need to lower his self-ideal and limit his goals. He should be encouraged to renew involvement with life and pursue new experiences for their growth potential.

Role rehearsal, role modeling, and role playing may be used. In role rehearsal the person imagines how a particular situation might take place and how his role might evolve.

TABLE **18-5** *Nursing Interventions in Alterations in Self-concept at Level 3*

GOAL: ASSIST THE PATIENT'S SELF-EVALUATION

PRINCIPLE	RATIONALE	NURSING INTERVENTIONS
Help the patient to define the problem clearly.	Only after the problem is accurately defined can alternative choices be proposed.	Identify relevant stressors with the patient and his appraisal of them. Clarify that the patient's beliefs influence his feelings and behaviors. Mutually identify faulty beliefs, misperceptions, distortions, illusions, and unrealistic goals. Mutually identify areas of strength. Place the concepts of success and failure in proper perspective. Explore the patient's use of coping resources.
Explore the patient's adaptive and maladaptive coping responses to one's problem.	It is then necessary to examine the coping choices the patient has made and evaluate their positive and the negative consequences.	Describe to the patient how all coping responses are freely chosen and have both positive and negative consequences. Contrast adaptive and maladaptive responses. Mutually identify the disadvantages of the patient's maladaptive coping responses. Mutually identify the advantages, or payoffs, of the patient's maladaptive coping responses. Discuss how these payoffs have perpetuated the maladaptive response. Use a variety of therapeutic skills (facilitative communication, supportive confrontation, role clarification, and the transference and countertransference reactions occurring in the one-to-one relationship).

He mentally enacts his role and tries to anticipate the responses of significant others. Role rehearsal is important in anticipating and planning the course of future action. Role modeling occurs when the patient watches someone else playing a certain role so that he is able to understand and emulate those behaviors. The person he observes may be the nurse, a family member, a group member, or a peer. The nurse can help the patient in his role learning by modeling behavior such as expression of feelings, specific socialization skills, or realistic self-expectations. Proceeding one step further, the nurse and patient may role play certain situations to develop alternative solutions.

Visualization can also be used to enhance self-esteem through goal setting. Through the conscious programming of desired change with positive images, expectations are molded. Strong, positive expectations can then become self-fulfilling. To use visualization, the nurse should:

1. Ask the patient to select a positive, specific goal, such as "I will call a friend and suggest we go out together."
2. Help the patient to relax, using a relaxation technique (see Chapter 30).
3. Have the patient repeat the goal phrase several times slowly.
4. Have the patient close his eyes and visualize the goal written on a piece of paper.
5. Have the patient, while relaxed, imagine accomplishing the goal.

The patient should then describe how he feels when the desired goal is reached and how other people respond to him. In this way the patient can gain positive control over his life.

Nursing actions at this level of intervention are summarized in Table 18-6. Ultimately the patient should choose a plan that includes a clear definition of the desired change. Converting a talking decision into an action decision is the final, but most important, step.

Level 5: Commitment to Action

The nurse helps the patient to become committed to his decision and then achieve his goals. The patient's development of self-awareness, self-understanding, and insight is not the ultimate desired outcome of the nursing therapeutic process.

TABLE **18-6** *Nursing Interventions in Alterations in Self-concept at Level 4*
GOAL: HELP THE PATIENT FORMULATE A REALISTIC PLAN OF ACTION

PRINCIPLE	RATIONALE	NURSING INTERVENTIONS
Help the patient identify alternative solutions.	Only when all possible alternatives have been evaluated can change be effected.	Help the patient understand that he can change only himself, not others. If the patient holds inconsistent perceptions, help him to see that he can change his beliefs or ideals to bring them closer to reality, and change his environment to make it consistent with his beliefs. If his self-concept is not consistent with his behavior, he can change his behavior to conform to his self-concept, change the beliefs underlying his self-concept to include his behavior, or change his self-ideal.
Help the patient develop realistic goals.	Goal setting that includes a clear definition of the expected change is necessary	Mutually review how coping resources may be better used by the patient. Encourage the patient to formulate his own (not the nurse's) goals. Mutually discuss the emotional, practical, and reality-based consequences of each goal. Help the patient clearly define the concrete change to be made. Encourage the patient to pursue new experiences for their growth potential. Use role rehearsal, role modeling, role playing, and visualization when appropriate.

Insight alone does not make problems disappear or transform one's world in magical ways. Although a patient may have obtained a high level of insight, he may nevertheless continue to function at a minimum level. Such a patient may be able to discuss with great ease the nature of his problem and the contributing influences, but the problem continues to be unresolved. Some patients actually use their insights to resist moving forward and avoid the hard work involved in making behavioral changes. The value of having the patient gain insight and increase his self-understanding is that he can gain perspective on why he behaves the way he does and what must be done to break maladaptive patterns.

Providing opportunity for the patient to experience success is essential at this time. To help him commit himself to his goal, the nurse can relate to the patient how she sees him, correcting his own poor self-image. In this mirroring technique, the nurse can openly and honestly describe to the patient the healthy parts of his personality and how, by using these parts, he can achieve his goal. The nurse should reinforce his strengths or skills and provide him with opportunities to use them whenever possible.

Sometimes the lack of vocational or social skills may be a causative factor for low self-esteem. If so, nursing intervention can be directed toward gaining vocational assistance for the patient. Group and family involvement may be instrumental in raising self-esteem. The experience of being accepted by others, the sense of belonging and being important to others, and the opportunity to develop interpersonal competence can all enhance self-esteem.

At this point the patient needs much support and positive reinforcement in effecting and maintaining change. For many patients, this means breaking chronic behavior patterns and exposing themselves to real risk. The patient must actively maintain the processes learned to avoid slipping back to the previous behavior. Doing this is difficult and requires that the patient build on the progress he has made in the other levels. Successful change is a continuing process of modifying not only one's behavior but one's environment to help ensure that the change to new ways of behaving is permanent. Otherwise a relapse will occur.

The nurse serves as a transition between the pain of the past and the positive gratification of the future. Both nurse and patient must allow sufficient time for change. A significant period may be required for patterns that developed over months or years to be broken and new ones established. The nurse's role now becomes less active and directive and more confirming of the value, potential, and accomplishments of the patient. A Nursing Treatment Plan

Summary for maladaptive self-concept responses is presented below.

Evaluation

Problems with self-concept are prominent in many psychological disorders. To evaluate the success or failure of the nursing care given in this area, each phase of the nursing process should be reviewed and analyzed by the nurse and patient.

The nurse's assessment should include both the objective and the observable behaviors as well as the subjective perceptions of the patient.

▼ Did the nurse explore the patient's strengths and weaknesses and elicit his self-ideal?

▼ Was information obtained on his body image, feelings of self-esteem, role satisfaction, and sense of identity?

▼ Did the nurse compare responses to his behavior, and were any inconsistencies or contradictions identified?

▼ Was the nurse aware of personal affective response to the patient, and how did this affect the ability to be therapeutic?

The nurse should have adopted a problem-solving approach that placed responsibility for growth on the patient. The most fundamental nursing action should have been to create a climate of acceptance that confirmed the patient's

---

NURSING TREATMENT PLAN *Summary* Maladaptive Self-concept Responses

Nursing Diagnosis Self-esteem disturbance
Expected Outcome The patient will obtain the maximum level of self-actualization to realize his or her potential.

Short-term Goal	Intervention	Rationale
The patient will establish a therapeutic relationship with the nurse.	Confirm the patient's identity. Provide supportive measures to decrease level of anxiety. Set limits on inappropriate behavior. Work with whatever ego strengths the patient has. Reinforce adaptive behavior.	Mutuality is necessary for the patient to assume responsibility for his or her behavior. Some degree of ego integrity is needed for later interventions.
The patient will express feelings, behaviors, and thoughts related to the present stressor.	Help the patient to express and describe feelings and thoughts. Help the patient identify self-strengths and weaknesses, self-ideal, self-criticisms. Respond empathically, emphasizing that the power to change lies within the patient.	Self-disclosure and understanding are necessary to bring about future change. The use of sympathy is not therapeutic because it can reinforce the patient's self-pity. The nurse should communicate that the patient is in control.
The patient will evaluate the positive and negative consequences of his or her self-concept responses.	Identify relevant stressors and the patient's appraisal of them. Clarify faulty beliefs and cognitive distortions. Evaluate advantages and disadvantages of current coping responses.	Only after the problem is defined can alternative choices be examined. It is then necessary to evaluate the positive and negative consequences of current patterns.
The patient will identify one new goal and two adaptive coping responses.	Encourage the patient to formulate a new goal. Help the patient clearly define the change to be made. Use role rehearsal, role modeling, and visualization to practice the new behavior.	Only after alternatives have been explored can change be effected. Goal setting specifies the nature of the change and suggests possible new behavioral strategies.
The patient will implement the new adaptive self-concept responses.	Provide opportunity for the patient to experience success. Reinforce strengths, skills, and adaptive coping responses. Allow the patient sufficient time to change. Promote group and family involvement. Provide the appropriate amount of support and positive reinforcement for the patient to maintain progress and growth.	The ultimate goal in promoting the patient's insight is to have him or her replace the maladaptive coping responses with more adaptive ones.

identity and conveyed a sense of value or worth. In expanding the patient's self-awareness,

▼ How effective was the nurse in promoting full and pertinent self-disclosure?

▼ Was the nurse able to manifest authentic behavior in the relationship and share thoughts and reactions?

▼ What interventions were used, and which ones proved beneficial (validation, reflection, confrontation, suggestion, role clarification, role playing)?

▼ Did the nurse progress on the basis of the patient's readiness and motivation?

▼ Was the patient able to transfer his new perceptions into possible solutions or alternative behavior?

▼ Did they both allow sufficient time for changes to occur?

The degree of overall success achieved through nursing care can be determined by eliciting the patient's perception of his own growth and comparing his behavior to the healthy personality described in this chapter. Not everyone will achieve all these characteristics, but success has been achieved if the patient's potential has been maximized.

Summary

1. The continuum of self-concept responses ranges from the most adaptive state of self-actualization to the most maladaptive response of depersonalization. Components of the self include body image, self-ideal, self-esteem, role, and identity.

2. Patient behaviors related to self-concept responses include low self-esteem, identity diffusion, and depersonalization.

3. Predisposing factors affecting self-concept responses are unrealistic self-ideals, sex and work roles, and challenges to personal identity. Precipitating stressors include role strain and developmental and health-illness transitions.

4. Coping resources focus on the patient's ego strengths, whereas coping mechanisms may be short- or long-term defenses and ego defense mechanisms.

5. Primary nursing diagnoses are body image disturbance, self-esteem disturbance, altered role performance, and personal identity disturbance.

6. Primary DSM-IV diagnoses are categorized as dissociative disorders and identity problem.

7. The expected outcome of nursing care is that the patient will obtain the maximum level of self-actualization to realize his or her potential.

8. Interventions include helping the patient expand self-awareness and engage in self-exploration, self-evaluation, realistic planning, and commitment to action.

9. The degree of success achieved through nursing care can be determined by eliciting the patient's perception of his or her own growth and comparing his or her behavior to characteristics of a healthy personality.

COMPETENT CARING A Clinical Exemplar of a Psychiatric Nurse

Monica Molloy, MSN, RN, CS

Last week one of my patients died.

I have been a nurse for 16 years. I have experienced patients' deaths—many different kinds of deaths, some of them seemingly senseless. I think particularly of young patients with head injuries from motorcycle or automobile accidents. But I understood those deaths. I understood the concept of an accident. What I don't understand is the concept of murder.

In November, a woman was sitting apart from most of the members of a therapy group I lead with a graduate nursing student. I asked her why she didn't join the circle. She replied she was afraid the group didn't want her near them; she thought the odor of her cancer would offend them. When the women in the group responded that they hadn't noticed any odor, she seemed to accept the reassurance offered, but she continued to sit apart.

Last week that woman was murdered.

She was a homeless woman, one of the women that embarrass us as a society. She lived in the Family Center of the homeless

shelter. I'll call her C. I first met her 2 years ago, when the group began. I remember one group session in particular when she and another shelter guest talked about trust issues in the homeless community. Then she moved away. This past fall she returned to the shelter. In addition to neurofibromatosis, she now had cancer. She looked different; she had lost nearly 40 pounds. She had been discharged from a local hospital to the shelter. Despite her willingness to take a risk and to disclose her fears about the odor she thought she had, she essentially remained alone and apart.

C's death has given me one more opportunity to examine what it is to practice psychiatric nursing in the community. When nurses practice in inpatient environments, one of our fundamental responsibilities is to ensure patient safety. Sometimes that safety is interpersonal, sometimes it is environmental. Among the homeless population, environmental safety is tenuous at best. One goal for the group intervention in the shelter community is to enable the women to use themselves and each other as resources to create their own safety zone. Somehow that didn't work with C.

The day after her death, the graduate nursing student and I spent some time with the women in the Family Center community. We went there to be with the women to provide support. We also went there to grieve. And perhaps most of all, we went there

Continued

COMPETENT CARING A Clinical Exemplar of a Psychiatric Nurse—cont'd

to try to answer some questions for ourselves, the same questions all clinicians ask when a patient dies: Did we miss some signs? Could we have done something different?

C's death is mentioned in the group weekly now. New guests use her death to concretize their fears about being homeless, as a metaphor for their own alienation experience. Through her death

C has left a mark on that group and that community. I don't understand the concept of murder any better. I do understand more about the concept of alienation. Acknowledging alienation is a first step to creating a sense of personal safety. It is fundamental to the practice of psychiatric nursing in the community. I learned that from C, and for that I will always be grateful.

your **INTERNET connection**

Guide to Psychotherapy: Self-esteem
http://www.shef.ac.uk/~psysc/psychotherapy/esteem.htm

Multiple Personality & Dissociative Disorders
http://members.tripod.com/~fsvival/index.htm

Chapter Review Questions

1. **Identify whether the following statements are true (T) or false (F).**

   A. ___ People behave in a manner consistent with what they believe to be true.

   B. ___ There is no evidence that genetics plays a role in the inheritance of self-esteem.

   C. ___ Most people who express dissatisfaction with life, display deviant behavior, or have difficulty functioning in social or work situations have problems related to self-concept.

   D. ___ The optimum outcome desired for a patient with alterations in self-concept is enhanced insight into self-concept and its influence on behavior.

   E. ___ Responding with sympathy is an appropriate nursing intervention to help a patient with self-exploration.

2. **Fill in the blanks.**

   A. _____ is a person's perception of how one should behave based on certain personal standards.

   B. A person's judgment of his or her own worth obtained by analyzing how well the person's behavior conforms to his or her self-ideal is called _____.

   C. _____ are sets of socially expected behavior patterns associated with a person's functioning in various social groups.

   D. The organizing principle of the personality is called _____.

   E. _____ is the feeling of unreality in which one is unable to distinguish between inner and outer stimuli.

   F. It is believed that _____ is a precipitating stressor for dissociative disorder and multiple personality disorder.

   G. Thinking about or relating past experiences, especially those that are personally significant, is called _____.

3. **Provide short answers for the following questions.**

   A. Describe the four best ways to promote a child's self-esteem.

   B. Briefly describe the developmental crisis of adolescence.

   C. List six qualities of the healthy personality. Think about someone you admire and evaluate him or her based on each of these qualities.

REFERENCES

1. Allen J: Dissociative processes: theoretical underpinnings of a working model for clinician and patient, *Bull Menninger Clin* 57:287, 1993.
2. American Psychiatric Association: *Diagnostic and statistical manual of mental disorders,* ed 4, Washington, DC, 1994, The Association.
3. Bednar R, Wells M, VandenBos G: Self-esteem: a concept of renewed clinical relevance, *Hosp Community Psychiatry* 42:123, 1991.
4. Burns D: Focusing on ego strengths, *Arch Psychiatr Nurs* 5:202, 1991.
5. Coopersmith S: *The antecedents of self-esteem,* San Francisco, 1967, WH Freeman.
6. Curtin S: Recognizing multiple personality disorder, *J Psychosoc Nurs Ment Health Serv* 31:29, 1993.
7. Erikson E: *Childhood and society,* New York, 1963, WW Norton.
8. Glaister J: Serial self-portrait: a technique to monitor changes in self-concept, *Arch Psychiatr Nurs* 10:311, 1996.
9. Godbey J, Hutchinson S: Healing from incest: resurrecting the buried self, *Arch Psychiatr Nurs* 10:304, 1996.
10. Horney K: *Neurosis and human growth,* New York, 1950, WW Norton.
11. Horowitz M et al: Self-regard: a new measure, *Am J Psychiatry* 153:382, 1996.
12. Klose P, Tinius T: Confidence builders: a self-esteem group at an inpatient psychiatric hospital, *J Psychosoc Nurs Ment Health Serv* 30:5, 1992.
13. Kluft R, Fine C: *Clinical perspectives on multiple personality disorder,* Washington, DC, 1993, American Psychiatric Press.
14. Logan R: Identity diffusion and psychosocial defense mechanisms, *Adolescence* 13:503, 1978.
15. Mruk C: *Self-esteem: research, theory and practice,* New York, 1995, Springer.
16. Nugent E: Reminiscence as a nursing intervention, *J Psychosoc Nurs* 33:7, 1995.
17. Putnam F, Lowenstein R: Treatment of multiple personality disorder: a survey of current practices, *Am J Psychiatry* 150:104, 1993.
18. Ross C, Joshi S, Currie R: Dissociative experiences in the general population: a factor analysis, *Hosp Community Psychiatry* 42:297, 1991.
19. Roy M, Neale M, Kendler K: The genetic epidemiology of self-esteem, *Br J Psychiatry* 166:813, 1995.
20. Stafford L: Dissociation and multiple personality disorder: a challenge for psychosocial nurses, *J Psychosoc Nurs* 31:15, 1993.
21. Sullivan HS: *The interpersonal theory of psychiatry,* New York, 1963, WW Norton.
22. Vaillant G: *The wisdom of the ego,* Cambridge, Mass, 1993, Harvard University Press.
23. Young C, Reed P: Elders' perceptions of the role of group psychotherapy in fostering self-transcendence, *Arch Psychiatr Nurs* 9:338, 1995.

ANNOTATED SUGGESTED READINGS

*Applegate M: Multiphasic short-term therapy for dissociative identity disorder, *J Am Psychiatric Nurses Assoc* 3:1, 1997.
Important and timely article that uses a case study to show how traditional long-term therapy can be redefined in short-term stages when working with patients with dissociative identity disorder.

Bracken B: *Handbook of self-concept,* New York, 1996, Wiley & Sons.
Excellent research-based summary of the developmental, social, and clinical considerations related to self-concept.

Brynat D. Kessler J: *Beyond integration: one multiple's journey,* New York, 1996, WW Norton.
Describes one woman's experiences in reclaiming her life and her achievement of the integration of her psyche.

*Burns D: Focusing on ego strengths, *Arch Psychiat Nurs* 5:202, 1991.
Examines the need for nurses to build on ego strengths of patients and ensure their stable identity.

Cote I: Current perspectives on multiple personality disorder, *Hosp Community Psychiatry* 45:827, 1994.
Concise overview of the incidence, prevalence, and etiology of multiple personality disorder.

*Curtin S: Recognizing multiple personality disorder, *J Psychosoc Nurs* 31:29, 1993
Excellent presentation of the behavioral, clinical, and physiological symptoms associated with MPD.

*Dallam S, Manderino M: Peer group supports patients with MPD/DD, *J Psychosoc Nurs* 35:22, 1997.
Description of the value of group therapy for relatively stable patients with MPD/DD that focuses on the here-and-now and is supportive and psychoeducational in nature.

Grame C: Internal containment in the treatment of patients with dissociative disorders, *Bull Menninger Clinic* 57:355, 1993.
Describes strategies to help patients with dissociative disorders cope with life and work through past traumas. Illustrated with case examples.

*Kerr N: Ego competency: a framework for formulating the nursing care plan, *Perspect Psychiatr Care* 26:30, 1990.
Describes a model of nursing care based on the patient's strengths and deficits. Worthwhile reading.

Kluft R, Fine C: *Clinical perspectives on multiple personality disorder,* Washington, DC, 1993, American Psychiatric Press.
Definitive text on psychotherapeutic approaches and case studies related to MPD.

Mruk C: *Self-esteem: research, theory and practice,* New York, 1995, Springer.
Theoretical constructs, influences on the formation of self-esteem, and programs for self-esteem enhancement are reviewed. Clearly written with practice-oriented sections.

*O'Reilly M: From fragmentation to wholeness: an integrative approach with clients who dissociate, *Perspect Psychiatr Care* 32:5, 1996.
Describes the use of building ego strength, modulating affect, and supporting abreaction to decrease fragmentation in the patient who dissociates.

Phillips J: *The magic daughter: a memoir of living with multiple personality disorder,* New York, 1995, Viking.
Skillfully and sensitively written account that provides insight into what it feels like to have MPD and what the process of therapy is. Highly recommended.

Price B: A model for body-image care, *J Adv Nurs* 15:585, 1990.
Proposes a model of body image care based on five central concepts with practical implications for interventions.

Vaillant G: *The wisdom of the ego,* Cambridge, Mass, 1993, Harvard University Press.
Builds on the work of Erikson in discussing ego development and maturation.

*Nursing reference.

Emotional Responses and Mood Disorders

Gail W. Stuart

© 1998 M.C. Escher/Cordon Art, Baarn, Holland.

Lying awake, calculating the future, Trying to unweave, unwind, unravel And piece together the past and the future, Between midnight and dawn, when the past is all deception, The future futureless . . . **T.S. Eliot**

LEARNING OBJECTIVES

After studying this chapter the student should be able to:

▼ Describe the continuum of adaptive and maladaptive emotional responses

▼ Discuss the epidemiology of mood disorders

▼ Identify behaviors associated with emotional responses

▼ Analyze predisposing factors, precipitating stressors, and appraisal of stressors related to emotional responses

▼ Describe coping resources and coping mechanisms related to emotional responses

▼ Formulate nursing diagnoses related to emotional responses

▼ Assess the relationship between nursing diagnoses and medical diagnoses related to emotional responses

▼ Identify expected outcomes and short-term nursing goals related to emotional responses

▼ Develop a patient education plan to enhance social skills

▼ Analyze nursing interventions related to emotional responses

▼ Evaluate nursing care for patients related to their emotional responses

TOPICAL OUTLINE

Continuum of Emotional Responses
  Grief Reactions
  Depression
  Mania
Assessment
  Behaviors
  Predisposing Factors
  Precipitating Stressors
  Appraisal of Stressors
  Coping Resources
  Coping Mechanisms
Nursing Diagnosis
  Related Medical Diagnoses
Outcome Identification
Planning
  Acute Treatment Phase
  Continuation Treatment Phase
  Maintenance Treatment Phase
Implementation
  Environmental Interventions
  Nurse-Patient Relationship
  Physiological Treatments
  Expressing Feelings
  Cognitive Strategies
  Behavioral Change
  Social Skills
  Mental Health Education
Evaluation

Variations or fluctuations in mood are a natural part of human existence. They indicate that a person is perceiving the world and responding to it. Extremes in mood are also linked with extremes in human experience, such as creativity, madness, despair, ecstasy, romanticism, personal charisma, and interpersonal destructiveness. Moods have fascinated scientists, philosophers, and novelists alike, who romanticize, study, and exaggerate the possible links between mood, deep emotional experience, and talent.[26]

In this text, **mood** is a prolonged emotional state that influences the person's whole personality and life functioning. It pertains to prevailing and pervading emotion and is synonymous with the terms *feeling state* and *emotion*. Like other aspects of the personality, emotions or moods serve an adaptive role. The four adaptive functions of emotions are social communication, physiological arousal, subjective awareness, and psychodynamic defense.

CONTINUUM OF EMOTIONAL RESPONSES

Emotions such as fear, joy, anxiety, love, anger, sadness, and surprise are all normal parts of the human condition. The problem arises in trying to evaluate when a person's mood or emotional state is maladaptive, abnormal, or unhealthy. Grief, for example, is a healthy, adaptive, separative process that attempts to overcome the stress of a loss. Grief work, or mourning, is not a pathological process; it is an adaptive response to a real stressor. The absence of grieving in the face of a loss suggests maladaptation.

The continuum of emotional responses is represented in Fig. 19-1. At the adaptive end is emotional responsiveness. This involves the person being affected by and being an active participant in the internal and external worlds. It implies an openness to and awareness of feelings. If used in such a way, feelings provide us with valuable learning experiences. They are barometers that give us feedback about ourselves and our relationships, and they help us function more effectively. Also adaptive in the face of stress is an uncomplicated grief reaction. Such a reaction implies that the

person is facing the reality of the loss and is immersed in the work of grieving.

A maladaptive response is the suppression of emotions. This may be evident as a denial of one's feelings, a detachment from them, or an internalization of all aspects of one's affective world. A transient suppression of feelings may at times be necessary to cope, as in an initial response to a death or tragedy. However, prolonged suppression of emotion, as in delayed grief reaction, will ultimately interfere with effective functioning.

The most maladaptive emotional responses or severe mood disturbances can be recognized by their intensity, pervasiveness, persistence, and interference with social and physiological functioning. These characteristics apply to the severe clinical states of depression and mania, which complete the maladaptive end of the continuum of emotional responses.

Grief Reactions

Grief is the subjective state that follows loss. It is one of the most powerful emotional states and affects all aspects of a person's life. It forces the person to stop normal activities and focus on present feelings and needs. Most often, it is the response to the loss of a loved person through death or separation, but it also occurs following the loss of something tangible or intangible that is highly regarded. It may be a valued object, a cherished possession, an ideal, a job, or status. As a response to the loss of a loved one, grief is a universal reaction. As a person's dependence on others grows, the chance increases of facing loss, separation, and death, which elicit intense feelings of grief. The capacity to form warm, satisfying relationships with others makes a person vulnerable to sadness, despair, and grief when those relationships are terminated.

As a natural reaction to a life experience, grief is universal. It involves stress, pain, and suffering and an impairment of function that can last for days, weeks, or months. Thus, the understanding of grief is of great importance because of its effect on both physical and emotional health.

The ability to experience grief is gradually formed in the

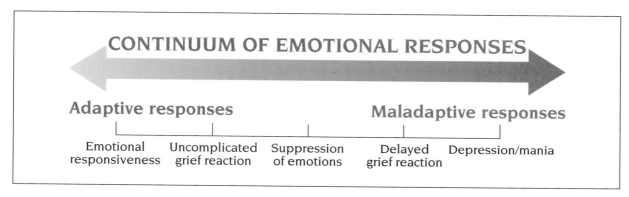

Fig. 19-1 Continuum of emotional responses.

course of normal development and is closely related to the capacity for developing meaningful relationships. Grief responses may be either uncomplicated and adaptive or morbid and pathological. Uncomplicated grief runs a consistent course that is modified by the abruptness of the loss, the person's preparation for the event, and the significance of the lost object. It is a self-limited process of realization; it makes real the fact of the loss.

A maladaptive response to loss implies that something has prevented it from running its normal course. There are two types of pathological grief reactions: the delayed reaction and the distorted reaction. Depression is one type of distorted grief reaction. Persistent absence of any emotion may signal an undue delay in the work of mourning or a delayed grief reaction. The delay may occur in the beginning of the mourning process or slow the process once it has begun, or both. The delay and rejection of grief may occasionally last for many years. The emotions associated with the loss may be triggered by a deliberate recall of circumstances surrounding the loss or by a spontaneous occurrence in the patient's life. A classic example of this is the anniversary reaction, in which the person experiences incomplete or abnormal mourning at the time of the loss, only to have the grieving response recur at anniversaries of the original loss.

Depression

The person who does not mourn can experience a pathological grief reaction known as depression, or melancholia. It is an abnormal extension or overelaboration of sadness and grief. Depression is the oldest and most common psychiatric illness. It has been described as early as 1500 B.C., and it is as familiar as it is mysterious. The word *depression* is used in a variety of ways. It can refer to a sign, symptom, syndrome, emotional state, reaction, disease, or clinical entity. In this chapter it is viewed as a clinical illness that is severe, maladaptive, and incapacitating.

Depression may range from mild and moderate states to severe states with or without psychotic features. Psychotic depression is uncommon, however, accounting for less than 10% of all depressions. Major depression can begin at any age, although it usually begins in the mid-twenties and thirties. Symptoms develop over days to weeks. Approximately one out of eight adults may experience major depression in their lifetime, and it affects 11.5 million people each year, 71% of whom are women. Approximately 15% of severely depressed patients commit suicide. Other complications include marital, parental, social, and vocational difficulties.

The lifetime risk for major depression is 7% to 12% for men and 20% to 30% for women. Among women, rates peak between adolescence and early adulthood.[52] This difference holds true across cultures and continents (see Critical Thinking about Contemporary Issues).[50] Other risk factors include a history of depressive illness in first-degree relatives and a history of major depression.

CRITICAL THINKING *about* **Contemporary Issues**

Is There a Difference in the Experience of Depression Between Black and White Women in America?

It has been suggested that black women's mental health is affected by their double minority status of being black and female in America.[49] Yet the exact incidence of depression in black women is unclear because of controversy regarding misdiagnosis and lack of clinical research. Although it is known that black women report depression more often than black men, little is known about the sociodemographic indicators of risk and depressive symptoms.[27] The assumption that all women share similar experiences does not allow for differences to emerge regarding the diagnostic process, measurement tools, and successful treatment strategies for various cultural groups.[6]

It is clear that depression is an increasing problem for black women. These women are experiencing role changes and additional stressors. Depressed black women may perceive themselves as being devalued by society and may have fewer support systems to buffer stressful events. Depressive symptoms may develop into clinical depression and further decrease the quality of life for black women. Psychiatric nurses can be instrumental in developing protocols and interventions that respond with cultural sensitivity to the psychological and physiological needs of depressed patients and thus improve their overall quality of life.

TABLE **19-1** *Comorbidity of Depression and Other Psychiatric Illness*

	MAJOR DEPRESSIVE DISORDER (%)	DYSTHYMIC DISORDER (%)	DEPRESSION NOS (%)
Alcohol abuse	10	30	67
Drug abuse	19	30	26
Panic disorder	19	7	21
Obsessive-compulsive disorder	35	15	40

Most untreated episodes of major depression last 6 to 24 months. Although some people have only a single episode of major depression and return to presymptomatic functioning, it is estimated that over 50% of those who have such an episode will eventually have another, and 25% of patients will have chronic, recurrent depression.[14]

Depression often occurs along with other psychiatric illnesses (Table 19-1). Up to 43% of patients with major depressive disorders have histories of one or more nonmood psychiatric disorders. These statistics underscore the importance of this health problem and suggest the need for timely diagnosis and treatment. Unfortunately, only one third of all people with depression seek help, are accurately diagnosed, and obtain appropriate treatment.

Research has also revealed the high incidence of depression among patients hospitalized for medical illnesses. These depressions are largely unrecognized and thus are untreated by health care personnel. Depression is found in all severities of medical illness, although its intensity and frequency are higher in more severely ill patients. Available studies suggest that about one third of medical inpatients report mild or moderate symptoms of depression and up to one fourth may have a depressive illness. Certain medical conditions are often associated with depression, especially cancer, stroke, epilepsy, multiple sclerosis, Parkinson's disease, cardiac disease, and a variety of endocrine disorders. Thus depression is a common accompaniment of many major medical illnesses.

Depressive conditions are also highly prevalent in primary care settings. One out of five patients seeing a primary care practitioner has significant symptoms of depression. Yet only about one in 100 patients cites depression as a reason for the most recent visit, and health care providers fail to diagnose major depression in their patients up to 50% of the time.[53] Finally, it has been estimated that depression costs the American economy $43.7 billion in worker absenteeism, lost productivity, and health care.[21]

> **?** *A patient who just underwent cardiac surgery comes for a follow-up visit and tells the physician he is feeling depressed. He is told that depression is a normal response to cardiac illness and he will get over it in time. Do you agree? If not, what nursing actions are indicated?*

Mania

In addition to severe depression, manic episodes may occur.[45] These episodes, like those of depression, can vary in intensity and accompanying level of anxiety from moderate manic states to severe and panic states with psychotic features. Basically, mania is characterized by an elevated, expansive, or irritable mood. **Hypomania** is a clinical syndrome similar to but not as severe as mania.

In the DSM-IV[2] the major affective disorders are separated into two subgroups—bipolar and depressive disorders—based on whether manic and depressive episodes are involved longitudinally. In this classification, major depression may involve a single episode or a recurrent depressive illness but without manic episodes. When there have been one or more manic episodes, with or without a major depressive episode, the category of **bipolar disorder** is used.

Thus a depressive episode with no manic episodes would be classified as a **depressive disorder**. A depressive episode with previous or current manic episodes would be classified as a bipolar disorder or manic depressive illness because the patient experiences both mania and depression. Although bipolar affective disorders are less common than depressive disorders, it is estimated that 0.6% to 0.88% of the adult

MAJOR DEPRESSIVE DISORDER

Major depression is one of the most common clinical problems encountered by primary care practitioners.

Major depression accounts for more bed days (people out of work and in bed) than any other "physical" disorder except cardiovascular disorders, and it is more costly to the economy than chronic respiratory illness, diabetes, arthritis, or hypertension.

Psychotherapy alone helps some depressed patients, especially those with mild to moderate symptoms.

It can be treated successfully by antidepressant medications in 65% of cases.

Success rate of treatment increases to 85% when alternative or adjunctive medications are used or psychotherapy is combined with medications.

BIPOLAR DISORDER

Without modern treatments, patients typically spend one fourth of their adult life in the hospital and fully one half of their life disabled.

Effective medications (lithium and anticonvulsants), often used in combination with psychotherapy, allow 75% to 80% of manic-depressive patients to lead essentially normal lives.

These drugs have saved the U.S. economy more than $40 billion since 1970: $13 billion in direct treatment costs and $27 billion in indirect costs.

population, or approximately 2 million Americans, have bipolar disorder. Risk factors are being female and having a family history of bipolar disorder. The data suggest that people under age 50 are at higher risk of a first attack, whereas those who already have the disorder face increased risk of a recurrent manic or depressive episode as they grow older.[19] Additional facts about depressive and bipolar disorders are presented in Box 19-1.

Assessment

Behaviors

DELAYED GRIEF REACTION. Delayed grief reactions may be expressed by excessive hostility and grief, prolonged feelings of emptiness and numbness, an inability to weep or express emotions, low self-esteem, use of present tense instead of past when speaking of the loss, persistent dreams about the loss, retention of clothing of the deceased, an inability to visit the grave of the deceased, and the projection of living memories onto an object held in place of the lost one. The following clinical example illustrates some of the behaviors associated with a delayed grief reaction.

Clinical Example Mrs. G was a 38-year-old married woman with no history of depression. She came to the local community mental health center complaining of severe throbbing headaches, difficulty falling asleep, fitful and disturbing dreams when asleep, and poor appetite. She said she felt "disgusted" with herself and "useless" to her family. She was living alone with her husband.

Her family history revealed that she had three children: two boys and a girl. Her eldest son, age 20, was attending college out of state, and her daughter, age 19, was living with a girlfriend in the same city. Her youngest son was killed in an automobile accident 2 years before at age 15. She described him as her "baby" and expressed much guilt for contributing to his death. She scolded herself for allowing him to drive to the seashore for the weekend with friends, and said she now worries a great deal about her other two children. She said she was trying to protect them from the dangers of the world, but they resented her advice and concern. On questioning by the nurse, Mrs. G reported that these feelings of sadness and guilt had emerged in the last month and seemed to be triggered by the graduation of her son's high school class.

Selected Nursing Diagnosis:

▼ Dysfunctional grieving related to son's death, as evidenced by somatic complaints and feelings of sadness and guilt

In this example Mrs. G was experiencing a delayed grief reaction precipitated by the event of her deceased son's would-be graduation. She had failed to progress through mourning at her son's death and was just beginning grief work.

DEPRESSION. The behaviors associated with depression vary. Sadness and slowness may predominate, or agitation may occur. The key element of a behavioral assessment is change: Depressed people change their usual patterns and responses. Research indicates that people working through normal mourning respond to their loss with psychological symptoms often indistinguishable from depression, but accepted by them and by their environment as normal. In contrast, patients with depression experience their condition as a change from their usual selves, which often leads them to seek help.

Many behaviors are associated with depression. These can be divided into affective, physiological, cognitive, and behavioral (Table 19-2). Obviously, some are contradictory and incompatible. The lists describe the spectrum of possible behaviors, and not all patients experience all of them.[13]

The most common and central behavior is that of the depressive mood. This is not necessarily described by the patient as depression but as feeling sad, blue, down in the dumps, unhappy, or unable to enjoy life. Crying often occurs. On the other hand, some depressed people do not cry and describe themselves as "beyond tears." The mood disturbance of the depressed patient resembles that of normal unhappiness multiplied in intensity and pervasiveness. Another mood that often accompanies depression is anxiety: a sense of fear and intense worry. Both depression and anxiety may show diurnal variation, that is, a pattern whereby certain times of the day, such as morning or evening, are consistently worse or better.

Some patients may initially deny their anxious or depressed moods but identify a variety of somatic complaints. These might include gastrointestinal distress, chronic or intermittent pain, irritability, palpitations, dizziness, appetite change, lack of energy, change in sex drive, or sleep disturbances. The person often focuses on these symptoms because they are more socially acceptable than the profound feeling of sadness, inability to concentrate, or loss of pleasure in usual activities. In addition, the physical symptoms

TABLE **19-2** *Behaviors Associated with Depression*

AFFECTIVE	PHYSIOLOGICAL	COGNITIVE	BEHAVIORAL
Anger	Abdominal pain	Ambivalence	Aggressiveness
Anxiety	Anorexia	Confusion	Agitation
Apathy	Backache	Inability to concentrate	Alcoholism
Bitterness	Chest pain	Indecisiveness	Altered activity level
Dejection	Constipation	Loss of interest and motivation	Drug addiction
Denial of feelings	Dizziness	Pessimism	Intolerance
Despondency	Fatigue	Self-blame	Irritability
Guilt	Headache	Self-depreciation	Lack of spontaneity
Helplessness	Impotence	Self-destructive thoughts	Overdependency
Hopelessness	Indigestion	Uncertainty	Poor personal hygiene
Loneliness	Insomnia		Psychomotor retardation
Low self-esteem	Lassitude		Social isolation
Sadness	Menstrual changes		Tearfulness
Sense of personal worthlessness	Nausea		Underachievement
	Overeating		Withdrawal
	Sexual nonresponsiveness		
	Sleep disturbances		
	Vomiting		
	Weight change		

may help the person with depression explain why nothing is fun anymore. When patients have a range of somatic symptoms, the nurse should carefully evaluate these complaints but also return to the issues of mood and interest, thus considering the possible diagnosis of depression.

It may also be helpful for the nurse to be familiar with the subgroups of major depressive disorder. The common subgroups and clinical relevance of each are presented in Table 19-3.[14] These subgroups are not all-inclusive and may be varying clinical expressions of the same illness over time, in different age groups, or in relation to specific precipitating stressors. Two of these subgroups merit special attention.

Postpartum Onset. Postpartum mood symptoms are divided into three categories based on severity: blues, psychosis, and depression.[28,48] Postpartum blues are brief episodes lasting 1 to 4 days of labile mood and tearfulness that occur in about 50% to 80% of women within 1 to 5 days of delivery. Treatment consists of reassurance and time to resolve this normal response. Postpartum psychosis can be divided into depressed and manic types. The incidence of postpartum psychosis is low, and the symptoms typically begin 2 to 3 days after delivery. The period of risk for postpartum psychosis is within the first month after delivery. The prognosis is good for acute postpartum psychosis. However, many patients subsequently develop a bipolar disorder. The recurrence rate is 33% to 51%. Postpartum depression may occur from 2 weeks to 12 months after delivery, but usually occurs within 6 months. The risk of postpartum depression is 10% to 15%, but the rate is higher for people with a history of psychiatric disorders.

Seasonal Pattern. Seasonal affective disorder (SAD) is depression that comes with shortened daylight in winter and fall and disappears during spring and summer. It is characterized by hypersomnia, lethargy and fatigue, increased anxiety, irritability, increased appetite with carbohy-

TABLE **19-3** *Major Depressive Disorder Subgroups*

Subgroup	Essential Features	Diagnostic Implications	Treatment Implications	Prognostic Implications
Psychotic	Hallucinations Delusions	More likely to become bipolar than nonpsychotic types May be misdiagnosed as schizophrenia	Antidepressant medication plus a neuroleptic is more effective than are antidepressants alone ECT is very effective	Usually a recurrent illness Subsequent episodes are usually psychotic Psychotic subtypes run in families Mood-incongruent features have a poorer prognosis
Melancholic	Anhedonia Unreactive mood Severe vegetative symptoms	May be misdiagnosed as dementia More likely in older patients	Antidepressant medication is essential ECT is 90% effective	If recurrent, consider maintenance medication
Atypical	Reactive mood Overeating/weight gain Oversleeping Rejection sensitivity Heavy limb sensation Fewer episodes	Common in younger patients May be misdiagnosed as personality disorder	TCAs may be less effective; MAOIs are preferred ?SSRIs preferred	Unclear
Seasonal	Onset, fall Offset, spring Recurrent	More common in nonequatorial latitudes Pattern occurs in major depressive and bipolar disorders	Medications have questionable efficacy Psychotherapy has questionable efficacy Phototherapy is an option	Recurs
Postpartum psychosis/depression	Acute onset (<30 days) in postpartum period Severe, labile mood symptoms 1/1000 is psychotic form	Often heralds a bipolar disorder	Hospitalize Treat medically Antidepressants, ?antipsychotics	50% chance of recurring in the next postpartum period

From Depression Guideline Panel: *Depression in primary care,* vol 1, *Detection and diagnosis, Clinical practice guideline no 5,* Rockville, Md, 1993, US Department of Health and Human Services, Public Health Service, Agency for Health Care Policy and Research, pub no 93-0550.
ECT, Electroconvulsive therapy; *MAOIs,* monoamine oxidase inhibitors; *SSRIs,* selective serotonin reuptake inhibitors, *TCA,* tricyclic antidepressant.

drate craving, and often weight gain.[40] It is believed to be related to abnormal melatonin metabolism. It has also been noted that two to three times as many people are troubled by the winter recurrence of seasonal mood symptoms than exhibit behaviors severe enough to merit clinical diagnosis.

> **?** *Conditions of light and darkness have often been noted to affect mood. Evaluate your environment for exposure to light. Compare it with a hospital environment.*

Suicide. Finally, the potential for suicide should always be assessed in severe mood disturbances. Suicide and other self-destructive behaviors are discussed in detail in Chapter 20. The intensity of anger, guilt, and worthlessness may precipitate suicidal thoughts, feelings, or gestures, as illustrated in the following clinical example.

Clinical Example Mr. W was a 60-year-old man who lived alone. His son and daughter were married and lived in the same state. His wife died 2 years before, and since that time his children had often asked him to move in with either of them. He consistently refused to do this, believing that he and his children needed privacy in their lives. Six months before, he was diagnosed as having advanced prostatic cancer with metastasis. After the diagnosis and because of increasing disability, he left his job and began to receive disability compensation. He visited his children and their families about twice a month and kept his regularly scheduled visits with the medical clinic. The nurses and physicians at the clinic noted that he was "despondent and withdrawn" but viewed this as a normal reaction to his diagnosis and family history. No interventions were implemented based on his emotional needs. A week after attending the clinic for a routine follow-up visit, he went to the cemetery where his wife was buried and at her gravestone shot himself in the head. A groundskeeper of the cemetery heard the shot, discovered what had happened, and called an ambu-

lance. Mr. W was taken to the emergency room of the nearest hospital and, with prompt medical care, survived the suicide attempt.

Selected Nursing Diagnoses:
▼ Potential for self-directed violence related to feelings of depression, as evidenced by gunshot to the head
▼ Hopelessness related to medical diagnosis of metastatic cancer, as evidenced by withdrawal and despondency

This example dramatically makes three important points. First, medical illness often involves a loss of function, body part, or appearance. Therefore, all patients should be assessed for depression. Second, all people experiencing depression and despair have the potential for suicide. Third, nurses can intervene to support the grieving and mourning process, whether it is uncomplicated or pathological. Nursing actions can be preventive, curative, or rehabilitative, based on the nursing assessment and diagnosis.

MANIA. The essential feature of mania is a distinct period of intense psychophysiological activation. Some of the associated behaviors are given in Table 19-4. The predominant mood is elevated or irritable, accompanied by one or more of the following symptoms: hyperactivity, the undertaking of too many activities, lack of judgment in anticipating consequences, pressured speech, flight of ideas, distractibility, inflated self-esteem, and hypersexuality.

If the mood is elevated or euphoric, it is often infectious. Patients report feeling happy, unconcerned, carefree, and devoid of problems. Although such experiences seem enviable, the person has no concern for reality or the feelings of others. The mood is often expansive, and some patients have extraordinary delusions about their power and importance. They characteristically involve themselves in seemingly senseless and risky enterprises.

Alternatively, the mood may be irritable, especially when plans are thwarted. Patients can be contentious and provoked by seemingly harmless remarks. Self-esteem is inflated during a manic episode, and as activity level in-

TABLE **19-4** *Behaviors Associated with Mania*

AFFECTIVE	PHYSIOLOGICAL	COGNITIVE	BEHAVIORAL
Elation or euphoria	Dehydration	Ambitiousness	Aggressiveness
Expansiveness	Inadequate nutrition	Denial of realistic danger	Excessive spending
Humorousness	Needs little sleep	Distractibility	Grandiose acts
Inflated self-esteem	Weight loss	Flight of ideas	Hyperactivity
Intolerance of criticism		Grandiosity	Increased motor activity
Lack of shame or guilt		Illusions	Irresponsibility
		Lack of judgment	Irritability or argumentativeness
		Loose associations	Poor personal grooming
			Provocativeness
			Sexual overactivity
			Social activity
			Verbosity

creases, feelings about the self become increasingly disturbed. Delusional grandiose symptoms are evident, and the patient is willing to undertake any project possible.

In contrast to depressed patients, manic patients are extremely self-confident, with an ego that knows no bounds; they are "on top of the world." Accompanying this magical omnipotence and supreme self-esteem is an equally inordinate lack of guilt and shame. Often they deny realistic danger. The patient's boundless energy, cunning, planning, scheming, and inability to anticipate consequences often lead to irresponsible enterprises and excessive spending, as well as misdemeanors of a sexual, aggressive, or possessive nature. In contrast to depressed patients, manic patients have abundant energy and heightened sexual appetite. Characteristic physical changes are inadequate nutrition, partly because manic patients have no time to eat, and serious weight loss related to their insomnia and overactivity. Extremely manic patients may be dehydrated and require prompt attention.

In addition to mood, speech is often disturbed. As mania intensifies, formal and logical speech is displaced by loud, rapid, and confusing language. As the activated state increases, speech becomes full of plays on words and irrelevancies that can increase to loosened associations and flight of ideas. Some of these behaviors are evident in the next clinical example.

Clinical Example Mr. B was a 30-year-old single man who was admitted to the psychiatric unit of the local community hospital. He had been hospitalized 2 years ago for problems related to alcoholism. He was accompanied to the hospital by a friend who lived with him. His friend said that for the past 2 months Mr. B had been "running on ten cylinders instead of four." He slept and ate little and talked constantly, sometimes so fast that no one could understand what he was trying to say. He had redecorated his bedroom in the apartment twice and had gone into debt buying a new wardrobe. His friend brought him in because his behavior was becoming more erratic and his physical condition was failing.

The nurse who admitted Mr. B asked about his social relationships. He revealed that his girlfriend of 7 years had left him 6 months before for another man. He said that initially he thought she would "see the light," but she had refused to see him since then. Mr. B said this "upset" him a little at the time, but he was sure it was for the best and there were plenty other women waiting for him.

Selected Nursing Diagnosis:
▼ Potential for self-directed violence related to interpersonal rejection, as evidenced by agitated behavior and lack of self-care

Other behaviors found in mania include lability of mood with rapid shifts to brief depression. Such behavior accounts for patients who have loosened associations and alternately laugh and cry. In addition, hallucinations of any type, ideas of reference, and frank delusions may be present with predominant feelings of guilt and thoughts of suicide. Manic episodes are very likely to recur. About 75% of manic patients have more than one episode, and almost all those with manic episodes also have depressive episodes. However, the duration and severity of the manic episodes vary, as do the intervals between relapses and recurrences.

All these clinical examples illustrate the interrelatedness of disturbances of mood with self-esteem and disrupted relationships. Multiple aspects of the patient's life are affected, including physical health. Hypertensive crises, irritable bowel syndromes, coronary occlusions, rheumatoid arthritis, migraine headaches, and various dermatological conditions can occur with severe mood disturbances.

Predisposing Factors

GENETICS. There is wide agreement that heredity and environment play an important role in severe mood disturbances.[11,12] Both bipolar and major depressive disorders run in families, but evidence of heritability is higher for bipolar disorder.
▼ One parent with bipolar disorder: 25% chance in child
▼ Two parents with bipolar disorder: 50% to 75% chance in child
▼ One monozygotic twin with bipolar disorder: 40% to 70% chance in other twin
▼ One dizygotic twin with bipolar disorder: about 20% chance in other twin
▼ One parent with depressive disorder: 10% to 13% chance in child

However, studies using only familial aggregations do not necessarily demonstrate the role of genetics because disturbances may be the result of nutritional, infectious, or psychological factors. Some studies using genetic markers such as color blindness suggest that bipolar affective disorder is transmitted by an X-linked dominant gene. Controversy surrounds the mode of genetic transmission in affective disorders, however, because findings from other studies contradict this hypothesis. Most recent research suggests there are different forms of genetic transmission.

Other evidence includes the following:
▼ A higher frequency of affective disorders in relatives of the patient than in the general population
▼ A higher frequency of psychiatric problems in relatives of the patient with affective disorder than in the general population
▼ Onset of the illness at a characteristic age with no evidence of a precipitating event

Thus, good evidence exists for the role of genetic factors in mood disorders.

AGGRESSION-TURNED-INWARD   THEORY. The aggression-turned-inward theory of Freud views depression as the inward turning of the aggressive instinct, for some reason not directed at the appropriate object and accompanied by feelings of guilt. The process is initiated by the loss of an ambivalently loved object. The person feels angry and loving at the same time and is unable to express anger because it is considered inappropriate or irrational. Also, the person may have developed a pattern throughout life of containing feelings, especially those that are viewed negatively. Angry feelings are then directed inward. Freud believed that if a person went so far as to commit suicide, the act was a strike against the hated and loved object as well as against the self.

Although it is one of the most widely quoted theories of depression, little systematic evidence substantiates it. Some researchers have identified depressed patients who outwardly express anger and hostility. Furthermore, the redirection of hostility at outside objects has not been consistently correlated with clinical improvement. In some instances it may actually have negative effects on the patient's view of self and problem resolution. It should therefore be viewed as one possible theory of causation that is not applicable to all people.

OBJECT LOSS THEORY. The object loss theory of depression refers to traumatic separation of the person from significant objects of attachment. Two issues are important to this theory: loss during childhood as a predisposing factor for adult depressions and separation in adult life as a precipitating stress. The first issue proposes that a child has ordinarily formed a tie to a mother figure by 6 months of age, and once that tie is ruptured, the child experiences separation anxiety, grief, and mourning. Furthermore, this mourning in the early years often affects personality development and predisposes the child to psychiatric illness.

From a research point of view, the connection between early object loss and adult depression is complex. Some cast doubt on the universality of the responses described and suggest that appropriate mothering during the separation period can prevent their occurrence. Other studies indicate that depressed patients seem to experience more parental loss from death, separation, and other causes than do normal and other diagnostic groups. However, that factor alone does not seem sufficiently universal to account for all forms of depression. There is even discussion about the beneficial or immunizing effects of having successfully coped with an early loss in the development of resilience.

A more recent perspective on this theory focuses on the negative impact of maternal depression on infants and children.[16] This is expressed by the infant as flat affect, lower activity, disengagement, and difficulty in being consoled. Among older children it is seen as sadness, submissive helplessness, and social withdrawal. Older children of depressed parents also have a three to four times higher than average rate of adjustment problems, including a range of emotional disorders. These observations lend a different but related view to the object loss theory. They suggest that emotional unavailability may be more stressful to children than physical separation. They also underscore the need for early and aggressive intervention by nurses for parents suffering from depression.

PERSONALITY ORGANIZATION THEORY. Another view of depression focuses on the major psychosocial variable of low self-esteem. The patient's self-concept is an underlying issue, whether expressed as dejection and depression or overcompensated with supreme competence, as displayed in manic and hypomanic episodes. Threats to self-esteem arise from poor role performance, perceived low-level everyday functioning, and the absence of a clear self-identity.

Three forms of personality organization that could lead to depression have been identified.[3] One, based on the "dominant other," occurs because the patient has relied on another for self-esteem. Satisfaction is experienced only through an intermediary. Clinging, passivity, manipulativeness, and avoidance of anger characterize the person with this type of depression. There is a noticeable lack of personal goals and a predominant focus on problems.

Another form of personality disorder results when a person realizes that a desired but unrealistic goal may never be accomplished. This is the "dominant goal" type of depression. This person is usually seclusive, arrogant, and often obsessive. The person sets unrealistic goals and evaluates them with an all-or-nothing standard. An inordinate amount of time is spent in wishful thinking and introverted searches for meaning.

The third type of depression is manifested as a constant mode of feeling. These patients inhibit any form of gratification because of strongly held taboos. They experience emptiness, hypochondriasis, pettiness in interpersonal relationships, and a harsh critical attitude toward themselves and others.

This view of depression looks at patients' belief systems in relation to their experiences. Even in the absence of an apparent precipitating stressor, their depression appears to be preceded by a severe blow to their self-esteem. It emphasizes the crucial position of self-concept in adaptation or maladaptation, and the importance of patients' appraisal of their life situations.

COGNITIVE MODEL. Beck's cognitive model[7] proposes that people experience depression because their thinking is disturbed. He proposes that depression is a cognitive problem dominated by a negative evaluation of self, the world, and the future. This theory is in contrast to others that propose that depressive feelings are primary and negative thinking is secondary. Beck suggests that in the course of development certain experiences sensitize people and make them vulnerable to depression. Such people also acquire a tendency to make extreme, absolute judgments.

The depression-prone person, according to this theory, is likely to explain an adverse event as a personal shortcoming. For example, the deserted husband believes "She left me because I'm unlovable," instead of considering the other possible alternatives, such as personality incompatibility, the wife's own problems, or her change of feelings toward him. As he focuses on his personal deficiencies, they expand to the point where they completely dominate his self-concept. He can think of himself only in a negative way and is unable to acknowledge his other abilities, achievements, and attributes. This negative set is reinforced when he interprets ambiguous or neutral experiences as additional proof of his deficiencies. Comparisons with other people further lower his self-esteem, and thus every encounter with others becomes a negative experience. His self-criticisms increase as he views himself as deserving of blame.

Depressed patients become dominated by pessimism. Their predictions tend to be overgeneralized and extreme. Because they see the future as an extension of the present, they expect their failure to continue permanently. Thus, pessimism dominates their activities, wishes, and expectations.

Depressed people are capable of logical self-evaluation when not in a depressed mood or when only mildly depressed. When depression does occur, after some precipitating life stressors, the negative cognitive set makes its appearance. As depression develops and increases, the negative thinking increasingly replaces objective thinking.

Although the onset of the depression may appear sudden, it develops over weeks, months, or even years as each experience is interpreted as further evidence of failure. As a result of this tunnel vision, depressed people become hypersensitive to experiences of loss and defeat and oblivious to experiences of success and pleasure. They have difficulty acknowledging anger because they think they are responsible for, and deserving of, insults from others and problems in living. Along with low self-esteem, they experience apathy and indifference. They are drawn to a state of inactivity and withdraw from life. They lack all spontaneous desire and wish only to remain passive. Because they expect failure, they lack the ordinary energy to make an effort.

Suicidal wishes can be viewed as an extreme expression of the desire to escape. Suicidal patients see their life as filled with suffering, with no chance of improvement. Given this negative set, suicide seems a rational solution. It promises to end their misery and relieve their families of a burden, and they begin to believe that everyone would be better off if they were dead. The more they consider the alternative of suicide, the more desirable it may seem, and as their life becomes more hopeless and painful, the desire to end it becomes stronger. Naturalistic, clinical, and experimental studies have provided substantial support for this cognitive model of depression.

> **?** *Relate the cognitive model of depression to the adage "mind over matter."*

LEARNED HELPLESSNESS-HOPELESSNESS MODEL. The learned helplessness-hopelessness model was first proposed by Seligman[43] in 1975. He defined helplessness as a "belief that no one will do anything to aid you" and hope-

lessness as a belief that neither "you nor anyone else can do anything." This theory proposes that it is not trauma per se that produces depression, but the belief that one has no control over the important outcomes in life and therefore refrains from adaptive responses. Learned helplessness is both a behavioral state and a personality trait of one who believes that control has been lost over the reinforcers in the environment. These negative expectations lead to hopelessness, passivity, and an inability to assert oneself.

Seligman suggests that people resistant to depression have experienced mastery in life. Their childhood experiences proved that their actions were effective in producing gratification and removing annoyances. In contrast, those susceptible to depression have had lives devoid of mastery. Their experiences proved that they were helpless to influence their sources of suffering and gratification or they controlled too many reinforcers that did not allow for the development of their coping responses against failure.

This model has been revised to include the hopelessness theory of depression.[1] It suggests that inferred negative consequences and negative characteristics about the self contribute to the formation of hopelessness and, in turn, the symptoms of hopelessness depression. Hopelessness theory thus bears a strong similarity to Beck's cognitive model of depression. The hopelessness model is also proposed as a sufficient but not necessary condition for depression. Other physiological and psychological factors can produce symptoms of depression in the absence of an expectation of uncontrollability.

BEHAVIORAL MODEL. The behavioral model views people as capable of exercising considerable control over their own behavior.[32] They do not merely react to external influences. They select, organize, and transform incoming stimuli. Thus people are not viewed as powerless objects controlled by their environments, but neither are they absolutely free to do whatever they choose. Rather, people and their environment affect each other.

The concept of reinforcement is crucial to this view of depression. Person-environment interactions with positive outcomes provide positive reinforcement. Such interactions strengthen the person's behavior. Little or no rewarding interaction with the environment causes the person to feel sad. Thus the key assumption in this model is that a low rate of positive reinforcement is the antecedent of depressive behaviors.

Two particular variables are important. One is that the person may fail to provide appropriate responses to initiate positive reinforcement. The other is that the environment may fail to provide reinforcement and thus worsen the patient's condition. These variables are often apparent because depressed patients have been shown to be deficient in the social skills needed to interact effectively. In turn, other people find the behavior of depressed people distancing, negative, or offensive and often avoid them as much as possible.

Depression is likely to occur if certain positively reinforcing events are absent, particularly those that fall into the following categories:

▼ Positive sexual experiences
▼ Rewarding social interaction
▼ Enjoyable outdoor activities
▼ Solitude
▼ Competence experiences

These may be described as "being sexually attractive," "being with friends," "being relaxed," "doing my job well," and "doing things my own way." Depression also occurs in the presence of certain punishing events, particularly those that fall into three categories:

▼ Marital or interpersonal discord
▼ Work or school hassles
▼ Negative reactions from others

The behavioral model of depression emphasizes an active approach to the person and relies heavily on an interactional view of personality. Treatment is aimed at helping the person to increase the quantity and quality of positively reinforcing interactions and to decrease aversive interactions.

> **?** *How many positive reinforcing events have you experienced this month? How many punishing events? Relate these to your overall mood.*

BIOLOGICAL MODEL. Another major area of research on depression involves a biological model, which explores chemical changes in the body during depressed states. Whether these chemical changes cause depression or are a result of depression is not yet understood. However, significant abnormalities can be demonstrated in many body systems during a depressive illness. These include electrolyte disturbances, especially of sodium and potassium; neurophysiological alterations; dysfunction and faulty regulation of autonomic nervous system activity; adrenocortical, thyroid, and gonadal changes; and neurochemical alterations in the neurotransmitters, especially in the biogenic amines, which act as central nervous system and peripheral neurotransmitters. The biogenic amines include three catecholamines—dopamine, norepinephrine, and epinephrine—as well as serotonin and acetylcholine. Most researchers agree that no single biochemical model adequately explains the affective disorders.

Endocrine System. The possibility of hormonal causes of depression has been considered for many years. Some symptoms of depression that suggest endocrine changes are decreased appetite, weight loss, insomnia, diminished sex drive, gastrointestinal disorders, and variations of mood. New assay techniques have recently detected alterations of hormone activity concurrent with depression. Mood changes have also been observed with a variety of endocrine disorders, including Cushing's disease, hyperthyroidism, and estrogen therapy. Further support for this theory is evi-

dent in the high incidence of depression during the postpartum period, when hormonal levels change.

Current study of neuroendocrine factors in affective disorders emphasizes the disinhibition of the hypothalamic-pituitary-adrenal (HPA) axis and the hypothalamic-pituitary-thyroid (HPT) axis. Two tests based on the neuroendocrine theory and performed clinically may prove to be useful in diagnosing affective illnesses. The first is the corticotropin-releasing factor stimulation test, which evaluates the pituitary's ability to respond to corticotropin-releasing hormone (CRH) and secrete sufficient amounts of adrenal corticotropin hormone (ACTH) to induce normal adrenal activity. The second test is the thyroid-releasing hormone (TRH) infusion test, which differs from the CRH infusion by assessing the pituitary's ability to secrete sufficient amounts of thyroid-stimulating hormones (TSH) to produce normal thyroid activity. These tests may be helpful in differentiating unipolar from bipolar depression and mania from schizophrenic psychosis.

Cortisol. Many depressed patients exhibit hypersecretion of cortisol; this has been used in the dexamethasone suppression test (DST) (dexamethasone is an exogenous steroid that suppresses the blood level of cortisol). The DST is based on the observation that, in patients with biological depression, late afternoon cortisol levels are not suppressed after a single dose of dexamethasone. However, many physical illnesses and some medications can interfere with the test results.

Neurotransmission. One of the dominant theories in the neurobiology of mood disorders is the *dysregulation hypothesis,* which proposes that there is a problem in several of the neurotransmitter systems. Some of them have received more attention than others recently. For example, there is substantial evidence for abnormal regulation of the serotonin (5HT) neurotransmitter system (Fig. 19-2). This dysregulation is in either the amount or the availability of 5HT, in the sensitivity of its receptors in relevant regions of the brain, and in its balance with other neurotransmitters and brain chemicals. Several areas of research support a role for serotonin in depression[33,41,44]:

▼ *Behavior:* 5HT has an important role in brain functions such as aggression, mood, anxiety, psychomotor activity, irritability, appetite, sexual activity, sleep/wakefulness, circadian and seasonal rhythms, neuroendocrine function, body temperature, cognitive function, and pain perception, processes that are abnormal in people with depression.

▼ *Biochemistry:* Research has shown that there is decreased 5HT availability in patients with depression—too little 5HT, its precursor (tryptophan), or its major metabolite (5HIAA) in the cerebrospinal fluid or blood of people with depression and in the postmortem brains of depressed people who died of other causes and in people who committed suicide.

▼ *Neuroimaging:* Multiple brain regions, all rich in 5HT

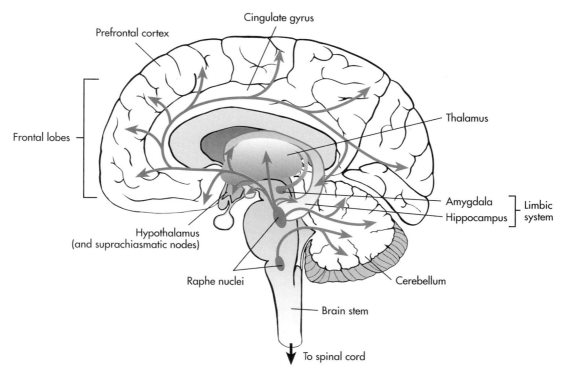

Fig. 19-2   The serotonin neurotransmitter system implicated in depression.

TABLE 19-5 *Prefrontal Cortex and 5HT Interconnections: Implications in Depression*

INTERCONNECTED BRAIN STRUCTURES	HYPOTHESIZED ROLE OF THESE INTERCONNECTIONS IN DEPRESSION
Prefrontal cortex	Covering the frontal lobes, it is unique within the CNS for its strong interconnections with all other areas of the brain; it receives information that has already been processed by other sensory areas and then merges this information with other emotional, historical, or relevant information, thus attending to both feelings and intellect.
Limbic system structures	The prefrontal cortex modulates limbic system activities (emotional and instinctive) by way of these three structures:
	Hippocampus Major importance in cognitive function, including memory.
	Amygdala Major importance in modulating feelings such as aggression, anger, love, and shyness.
	Cingulate gyrus Involved in motivation and interest.
Brainstem	Responsible for regulating the general state of arousal and tone of brain function; also the location of structures that manufacture various neurotransmitters, such as serotonin (5HT), norepinephrine (NE), and dopamine (DA).
Raphe nuclei	Located in the brainstem, they manufacture 5HT; they also modulate excessive stimuli, and the organization and coordination of appropriate responses to these stimuli.
Hypothalamus	This interconnection allows for direct prefrontal input into neuroendocrine function via the hypothalamic-pituitary axes.
Suprachiasmatic nucleus	Located in the hypothalamus, it regulates circadian (24 hour) rhythms and circannual rhythms; thus it is also implicated in seasonal affective disorder.

pathways, show abnormalities in neuroimaging studies in depressed people. An example is the prefrontal cortex, which shows an abnormal slowing of activity (hypometabolism). It covers the frontal lobes, which have an important role in intellectual and emotional activities. Prefrontal cortex hypometabolism affects the function of

many of the brain structures connected with it by way of the 5HT system. It is hypothesized that these interconnections facilitate the varied symptoms of depression (Table 19-5).

▼ *Neuroendocrine:* 5HT has an important role in the secretion of growth hormone, prolactin, and cortisol, all of which are found to be abnormal in people with depression.

▼ *Treatment:* Most clinically effective biological antidepressant agents, such as drugs and ECT, have been found to enhance the neurotransmission of 5HT, although the mechanisms of actions differ from each other.

Finally, there are several important implications of viewing depression as a brain-based illness of the prefrontal cortex[17]:

▼ Cognitive and interpersonal therapies may be viewed as prefrontal rehabilitation because they substitute for, then gradually bring back on line, some of the behaviors and cognitions compromised by prefrontal cortex (PFC) hypoactivity.

▼ Viewing depression as a disease with identified regional brain dysfunction helps to destigmatize depression and reintegrate mood disorders into modern health care.

▼ Changes in brain metabolism identified by neuroimaging studies may help with understanding of how psychosocial stressors such as grief (a hyperactivity in the PFC) may evolve into the clinical syndrome of depression (a hypoactivity in the PFC).

Biological Rhythms. Mood disorders are also typified by periodic variations in physiological and psychological functions.[36] Affective illnesses are usually recurrent, with episodes often occurring and remitting spontaneously. Two subtypes of mood disorders are specifically cyclical in nature: rapid cycling bipolar disorder and depressive disorder with seasonal patterns.[9] In the first, cycles may be days, weeks, months, or years. In seasonal affective disorder, cycles occur annually in the same season each year, as people react to changes in environmental factors such as climate, latitude, or light.

People who are depressed or manic have certain characteristic changes in biological rhythms and related physiology. For instance, body temperature and certain hormones reach their peak earlier than normal; some depressed patients are more sensitive to the absence of sunlight than nondepressed people; and many depressed people experience circadian rhythm disturbances such as diurnal variation and early morning awakening. All-night sleep studies of depressed patients show some basic abnormalities. Sleep problems associated with depression have to do with the timing of rapid eye movement (REM) sleep. The strongest finding is that REM sleep begins too early in the night (Fig. 19-3). It also lasts too long—up to twice as long as the first REM period in nondepressed people. This finding may help to explain why patients report feeling tired even after a night's sleep. There is also decreased total sleep time, an increased percentage of dream time, difficulty in falling asleep, and an increased number of spontaneous awakenings. These and other findings in the area of biological rhythmicity may prove to be valuable diagnostic tools for depression.

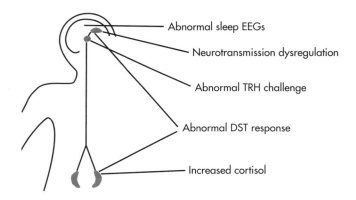

Fig. 19-3 **A**, Normal sleep architecture. **B**, Depressed sleep architecture. Darker areas indicate REM sleep.

Fig. 19-4 Biological factors related to depression.

Research on the biological model has been extensive and of high quality. It has lent support to a biological basis for mood disorders and suggested biological markers of clinical usefulness in diagnosis and treatment. The discovery of neurobiological abnormalities is not surprising and does not preclude psychological causes. Some of the biological bases of depression are shown in Fig. 19-4.

> **?** *A pastor preaches about how depression results from "poor moral character" and "personal weakness." How would you respond?*

Precipitating Stressors

Disturbances of mood are a specific response to stress. Two major types of stress exist. The first is the stress of major life events that is evident to other people. The second type, the minor stress or irritations of daily life, may not be obvious to others. These are the small disappointments, frustrations, criticisms, and arguments that, when accumulated over time and in the absence of compensating positive events, produce a major and chronic negative impact. Stressors that may produce disturbances of mood include loss of attachment, major life events, roles, and physiological changes.

LOSS OF ATTACHMENT. Loss in adult life can precipitate depression. The loss may be real or imagined and may include the loss of love, a person, physical functioning, status, or self-esteem. Many losses take on importance because of their symbolic meaning, which makes the reactions to them appear out of proportion to reality. In this sense, even an apparently pleasurable event, such as moving to a new home, may involve the loss of old friends, warm memories, and neighborhood associations. Loss of hope is another significant stressor often overlooked. Because of the actual and symbolic elements involved in loss, the patient's perception takes on primary importance.

The person is constantly experiencing losses and struggling with integrating them. The intensity of grief becomes meaningful only when the person understands earlier losses and separations. People reacting to a recent loss often behave as they did in previous separations. The intensity of the present reaction therefore becomes more understandable with the realization that the reaction is to earlier losses as well. By definition loss is negative, a deprivation. The ability to sustain, integrate, and recover from loss is a sign of personal maturity and growth.

Uncomplicated grief reactions are the process of normal mourning or simple bereavement. Mourning includes a complex sequence of psychological processes. It is accompanied by anxiety, anger, pain, despair, and hope. The sequence is not a smooth, unvarying course, however; it is filled with turmoil, regressions, and potential problems. Certain factors have been identified that influence the outcome of mourning (Box 19-2).

These factors should be assessed by the nurse for each person experiencing a loss. Two of the factors—the nature of the relationship with the lost person or object and the mourner's perception of the preventability of the loss—have been identified as prime predictors of the intensity and duration of the bereavement. Concurrent crises, the circumstances of the loss, and a pathological relationship with the lost person or object are other factors that contribute to a failure to resolve grief.

Inhibiting Factors. Loss of a loved one is a major stressor for grief reactions. Most people resolve this loss through simple bereavement and do not experience pathological grief or depression. However, various external and internal

---

Box 19-2 *Factors That Influence the Mourning Process*

Childhood experiences, especially the loss of significant others
Losses experienced later in life
History of psychiatric illness, especially depression
Life crises before the loss
Nature of the relationship with the lost person or object, including kinship, strength of attachment, security of attachment, dependency bonds, and intensity of ambivalence
Process of dying (when applicable), including age of deceased, timeliness, previous warnings, preparation for bereavement, expression of feelings, and preventability of the loss
Social support systems
Secondary stresses
Emergent life opportunities

---

factors can inhibit mourning. An external factor may be the immersion of the mourner in practical, necessary tasks that accompany the loss but are not directly connected to the emotional fact of the loss. These tasks may include funeral arrangements, unfinished business of the deceased, or a search for immediate employment. All these tasks foster denial of the loss. Denial also may be encouraged by cultural norms that minimize or negate the finality of the loss. The American norm of "courage in the face of adversity" can prevent an open display of grief.

Mourning may also be inhibited when the bereaved lack support from their social network. Nonsupportiveness suppresses grieving when significant others inhibit mourners' expression of sadness, anger, and guilt, block their review of the lost relationship, and attempt to orient them too quickly to the future. Finally, the widespread use of tranquilizers and antidepressant medications may suppress normal grief and encourage pathological reactions.

Internal factors that inhibit mourning are often fostered by a society that encourages the control and hiding of feelings. Crying, for example, may be seen as weakness, especially in men. Grief and anger are particularly repressed in our society, and this repression may create many emotional problems. Another inhibitor is the belief that the quantity and quality of emotion are unique and cannot be communicated.

In concluding this discussion of loss as a precipitating stressor, it is necessary to place it in proper perspective based on research. Some studies have failed to demonstrate a relationship between loss and depression. Other studies support the relationship but suggest that depression may be the cause of alienation and object loss, and not vice versa. Thus, the following conclusions may be proposed:

▼ Loss and separation events are possible precipitating stressors of depression.

▼ Loss and separation are not present in all depressions.

▼ Not all people who experience loss and separation develop depressions.

▼ Loss and separation are not specific to depression but may act as precipitating events for a variety of psychiatric and medical illnesses.

▼ Loss and separation may result from depression.

LIFE EVENTS. Research conducted on life events and depression reveals that, on average, depressed patients reported almost three times as many important life events during the 6 months before onset of clinical depressive episode as did normal subjects. The events included loss of self-esteem, interpersonal discord, socially undesirable occurrences, and major disruptions of life patterns. Events perceived as undesirable were most often the precipitants of depression. Analysis of the data showed that exit events (separations and losses) more often than entrance events (additions and introductions) were followed by worsening of psychiatric symptoms, physical health changes, impairment of social role performance, and depressive illnesses. The concept of exit events overlaps with the psychiatric concept of loss.

Certain types of events may also prove to be more important than others. For example, childhood physical and sexual abuse has been found to be associated with high depressive symptoms in women.[23] Similarly, Stuart and coworkers[47] researched the early childhood experiences of women with depression in comparison with women who were free of psychiatric diagnosis. They found that the depressed women experienced both parents as rejecting and perceived less warmth from their fathers, described less rational discussion in the resolution of family conflict, experienced significant separation anxiety as children, and grew up in households with more deaths and chronic physical illness.

Most psychiatric clinicians are convinced that a relationship does exist between stressful life events and depression. Some believe that life events play the primary role in depression; others believe that life events simply contribute to the onset and timing of the acute episode. Any definitive conclusions should be made with caution. All people experience stressful life events, but not all people become depressed. This suggests that specific events can contribute only partially to the development of depression.

ROLE STRAIN. In analyzing social role stressors, much of the literature focuses on women. This reflects the predominance of depression among women and the increasing interest in gender socialization processes and women's changing roles.[42] Role strain in marriage emerges as a major stressor related to depression for both men and women. In a classic study Gove[20] examined the rates of mental illness among married men and women. He found higher rates of mental illness for married women, whereas single, divorced, and widowed women have lower rates than men. From this he concluded that being married has a protective effect for males but a detrimental effect for females.

Another role-related risk factor for women is exposure to predictable chronic stressors, many of which occur at the same time. This is particularly problematic given the sociocultural context of contemporary society, which values men's work over that of women and specifically devalues the more traditional forms of women's work. For example, women often experience predictable chronic stressors in their classic role as caregivers. These present specific psychosocial and biological challenges including the following[8]:

▼ The perinatal period, with its subsequent sleep-disrupting infant care demands, which comes immediately after hormonal, biochemical, and social disruptions associated with pregnancy

▼ The predominately female caretaking role for spouses and parents with age-or Alzheimer's-related dementias, which can cause the same sleep disruption experienced by mothers of infants

▼ Achievement-motivated women who take needed time from sleep in order to juggle full-time family and social roles in addition to work and educational commitments

▼ Shift work that does not follow a forward rotation (days to evenings to nights) with adequate adjustment for each shift change

If these special stressors for women are combined with other rhythm-disrupting processes, such as seasonal light changes, and other risk factors for depression, such as family history and inadequate support systems and primary relationships, a woman has a gender-and role-based risk for depression.

> **?** *Describe how the early socialization of young girls in contemporary society might affect their cognitive and emotional coping responses. Compare this to the experiences of young boys.*

PHYSIOLOGICAL CHANGES. Mood may also respond to drugs or a wide variety of physical illnesses (Table 19-6). Drug-induced depressions can follow treatment with antihypertensive drugs, particularly reserpine, and the abuse of addictive substances such as amphetamines, barbiturates, cocaine, and alcohol. Depression may also occur secondary to medical illnesses, such as viral infections, nutritional deficiencies, endocrine disorders, anemias, and central nervous system disorders such as multiple sclerosis, tumors, and cerebrovascular disease. Most chronic debilitating illnesses, whether physical or psychiatric, are accompanied by depression.

The depressions of the elderly are particularly complex because the differential diagnosis often involves organic brain damage and clinical depression.[37] Diagnostic differentiation is complicated. People with early signs of senile brain changes, vascular disease, or other neurological diseases of aging may be more at risk for depression than the

TABLE **19-6** *Physical Illnesses and Drugs Associated with Depressive and Manic States*

	DEPRESSION	MANIA
Infectious	Influenza	Influenza
	Viral hepatitis	St. Louis encephalitis
	Infectious mononucleosis	Q fever
	General paresis (tertiary syphilis)	General paresis (tertiary syphilis)
	Tuberculosis	
Endocrine	Myxedema	Hyperthyroidism?
	Cushing's disease	
	Addison's disease	
	Diabetes mellitus	
Neoplastic	Occult abdominal malignancies (such as carcinoma of head of pancreas)	
	Carcinoid	
	Oat cell carcinoma	
Collagen	Systemic lupus erythematosus	Systemic lupus erythematosus
		Rheumatic chorea
Neurological	Multiple sclerosis	Multiple sclerosis
	Cerebral tumors	Diencephalic and third-ventricular tumors
	Sleep apnea	
	Dementia	
	Parkinson's disease	
	Nondominant temporal lobe lesions	
Cardiovascular	Stroke	
	Coronary artery disease	
Nutritional	Pellagra	
	Pernicious anemia	
Drugs	Steroidal contraceptives	Steroids
	Reserpine	Levodopa
	Alpha-methyldopa	Amphetamines
	Propranolol	Methylphenidate
	Glucocorticoids	Cocaine
	Cycloserine	Monoamine oxidase inhibitors
	Physostigmine	Tricyclic antidepressants
	Alcohol	Thyroid hormones
	Sedative-hypnotics	
	Amphetamine withdrawal	
	Benzodiazepines	
	Neuroleptics	

general population. In the United States there has been a tendency to overdiagnose arteriosclerosis and senility in people over age 65, without recognizing that depression may manifest itself by a slowing of psychomotor activity. Lowered intellectual function and a loss of interest in sex, hobbies, and activities may be taken as signs of brain disease.

Mania can also be secondary to drugs, particularly steroids, amphetamines, and tricyclic antidepressants. It can be triggered by infections, neoplasms, and metabolic disturbances. The evidence that mania can result from pharmacological, structural, and metabolic disturbances suggests that mania, like depression, is a clinical syndrome with multiple causes. The diversity of causes probably involves more than one pathophysiological pathway and challenges any one model of causation, whether biochemical, psychological, genetic, or structural.

Appraisal of Stressors

Debate continues over the nature of depression, that is, whether depression is a single illness with different signs and symptoms or whether several diseases exist. It is clear, however, that there is an interactive effect among predisposing and precipitating factors that are biological and psychosocial in origin.[29] This underscores the importance of one's appraisal of one's life situation and related stressors. Table 19-7 summarizes these major theories of causation.

Coping Resources

Personal resources include one's socioeconomic status (income, occupation, social position, education), family (nuclear, extended), interpersonal networks, and secondary organizations provided by the broader social environment (see A Family Speaks). The far-ranging effects of poverty,

TABLE **19-7** *Summary of Models of Causation of Severe Mood Disturbances*

MODEL	MECHANISM
Genetic	Transmission through hereditary and family history
Aggression turned inward	Turning of angry feelings against oneself
Object loss	Separation from loved one and disruption of attachment bond
Personality organization	Negative self-concept and low self-esteem influence belief system and appraisal of stressors
Cognitive	Hopelessness experienced because of negative cognitive set
Learned helplessness-hopelessness	Belief that responses are ineffectual and that reinforcers in the environment cannot be controlled
Behavioral	Loss of positive reinforcement in life
Biological	Impaired monoaminergic neurotransmission
Life stressors	Response to life stress from four possible sources: loss of attachment, life events, role strain, and physiological changes
Integrative	Interaction of biopsychosocial predisposing and precipitating factors

 A Family *Speaks*

It's hard for me to imagine how life could be so bad that my beautiful and loving 22-year-old daughter couldn't get out of bed in the morning and cried most of the day. It all started when she quit college and returned home and told us about the biggest mistake she had made in her life. While at school, she accidentally got pregnant and then had an abortion. Since that event, she said she felt worthless, immoral, and extremely guilty.

We talked about it, and I suggested that she get help. She saw two different mental health professionals but dropped out of therapy with each one after only a couple of visits. Then one of my friends recommended a nurse who specialized in working with women with depression. My daughter saw her twice a week initially, then once a week, and finally monthly. My daughter was able to open up to this nurse and together they worked at changing my daughter's negative thoughts, feelings, and behaviors. She kept a diary and began to call friends and socialize.

Today, 8 months later, my daughter has a job and is going to college part-time in the evenings. Sometimes when I look at her, she seems like a different person to me—so much more grown up and mature. I'm sorry for her pain, but I know that now she is a stronger and wiser person for having endured it. ▼

discrimination, inadequate housing, and social isolation cannot be ignored or taken lightly.

Research has clearly linked social support to depression. A nursing study among older adults reported that poor physical health and lack of mastery, social resources, and

Box **19-3** *Risk Factors for Depression*

Prior episodes of depression
Family history of depression
Prior suicide attempts
Female gender
Age of onset <40 years
Postpartum period
Medical comorbidity
Lack of social support
Stressful life events
Personal history of sexual abuse
Current substance abuse

economic resources were significant predictors of depression.[4] Such research suggests the importance of nursing interventions that foster the person's ability to develop capacities for coping with life's disruptions. The risk factors for depression are listed in Box 19-3.

Coping Mechanisms

Uncomplicated grief reactions can be normal mourning or simple bereavement. Mourning includes all the psychological processes set in motion by the loss. Mourning begins with the introjection of the lost object. In grieving, the person's feelings are directed to a mental image of the loved one. Thus the mechanism of introjection serves as a buffering mechanism. Through reality testing, the person realizes that the love object no longer exists, and then the emotional investment is withdrawn from it. The ultimate outcome is that reality wins out, but this is accomplished slowly over time. When the mourning work is completed, the ego becomes free to invest in new objects.

A delayed grief reaction uses the defense mechanisms of denial and suppression in an attempt to avoid intense distress. Specific defenses used to block mourning are repression, suppression, denial, and dissociation. Denial of the loss in depression results in profound feelings of guilt, anger, and despair that focus on the person's own unworthi-

Fig. 19-5   The Stuart Stress Adaptation Model related to emotional responses.

ness. Manic and hypomanic episodes are more rare than depressive states. Some believe that mania is a mirror image of depression and that, even though the behaviors are dissimilar, the dynamics and coping mechanisms are related. According to this view, manic behavior is a defense against depression because the person attempts to deny feelings of worthlessness and helplessness.

Nursing Diagnosis

The diagnosis of mood disturbances depends on an understanding of many interrelated concepts, including anxiety and self-concept. One task of the nurse in formulating a diagnosis is to determine whether the patient is experiencing primarily a state of anxiety or depression. It is often difficult to distinguish between the two because they may coexist in one patient and are manifested by similar behaviors. A table distinguishing between anxiety and depression is presented in Chapter 16.

Fig. 19-5 presents the Stuart Stress Adaptation Model with the continuum of emotional responses. The maladaptive responses are a result of anxiety, hostility, self-devaluation, and guilt. This model suggests that nursing care should be centered around increasing self-esteem and encouraging expression of emotions.

The primary NANDA nursing diagnoses related to maladaptive emotional responses are **dysfunctional grieving, hopelessness, powerlessness, spiritual distress,** and **potential for self-directed violence.** Nursing diagnoses related to the range of possible maladaptive responses are identified in the Medical and Nursing Diagnoses box on p. 366. Examples of complete nursing diagnoses are presented in the Detailed Diagnoses box on p. 367.

How do you think "spiritual distress" relates to mood disorders?

MEDICAL AND NURSING DIAGNOSES *related to* **Emotional Responses**

Related Medical Diagnoses (DSM-IV)*	Related Nursing Diagnoses (NANDA)†
Bipolar I disorder	Anxiety
Bipolar II disorder	Communication, impaired verbal
Cyclothymic disorder	Coping, ineffective individual
Major depressive disorder	Grieving, anticipatory
Dysthymic disorder	**Grieving, dysfunctional‡**
	Hopelessness‡
	Injury, potential for
	Loneliness, risk for
	Memory, impaired
	Nutrition, altered
	Powerlessness‡
	Self-care deficit
	Self-esteem disturbance
	Sexual dysfunction
	Sleep pattern disturbance
	Social isolation
	Spiritual distress (distress of the human spirit)‡
	Thought processes, altered
	Violence, potential for self-directed‡

*From American Psychiatric Association: *Diagnostic and statistical manual of mental disorders,* ed 4, Washington, DC, 1994, The Association.
†From North American Nursing Diagnosis Association: *NANDA nursing diagnoses: definitions and classifications 1997-1998,* Philadelphia, 1997, The Association.
‡Primary nursing diagnosis for disturbances in mood.

Related Medical Diagnoses

The psychiatric classification of affective disorders has largely reflected the controversies surrounding the nature, cause, and treatment of these disorders. Although these traditional labels are no longer used in the DSM,[2] nurses know them because they may continue to have some research and clinical value.

One traditional distinction has been to separate patients into those with psychotic versus neurotic affective states. Unfortunately, these terms have acquired multiple meanings and have lost their precision in defining clinical or research practice. Another traditional distinction has been endogenous versus reactive, or exogenous, types of depression. Endogenous depressions were believed to have resulted from early personality development and intrinsic biological processes, whereas exogenous, or reactive types were believed to have occurred in response to external environmental stress, such as recent loss or disappointment. However, research has failed to verify these distinctions. Thus the psychotic-neurotic distinction and the endogenous-reactive dichotomy are better regarded as continuums along which patients may be placed. Most patients are intermediate on the continuum and few are at the extremes. Neither classification is used in the DSM-IV.

Another distinction has been made between primary and secondary affective disorders based on two criteria: chronology and the presence of associated illnesses. Primary affective disorders occur in patients who have been well or whose only previous episodes of psychiatric disease were mania or depression. Secondary affective disorders include feelings of sadness, inadequacy, and hopelessness that occur with another preexisting psychiatric disorder, such as anxiety reactions. They also include symptoms secondary to medical illnesses.

A final distinction is between bipolar and unipolar affective states. It proposes the separation of depressed patients with a history of manic episodes (the bipolar group) from those who have had only recurrent episodes of depression (the unipolar group). Among newer approaches, the bipolar-unipolar distinction has achieved considerable acceptance.[51]

Two major categories of mood or affective disorders are identified in the DSM-IV: bipolar disorders and depressive disorders (see the Medical and Nursing Diagnoses box above. The specific disorders are described in the Detailed Diagnoses box at right. Diagnostic criteria for a major depressive episode and a manic episode are listed in Box 19-4.

Outcome Identification

The expected outcome when working with a patient with a maladaptive emotional response is as follows:

The patient will be emotionally responsive and return to a pre-illness level of functioning.

DETAILED DIAGNOSES *related to* **Emotional Responses**

NANDA Diagnosis Stem	Examples of Complete Diagnosis
Dysfunctional grieving	Dysfunctional grieving related to death of sister, as evidenced by self-devaluation, sleep disturbance, and dejected mood
Hopelessness	Hopelessness related to loss of job, as evidenced by feelings of despair and development of ulcerative colitis
Powerlessness	Powerlessness related to new role as parent, as evidenced by apathy, uncertainty, and overdependency
Spiritual distress	Spiritual distress related to loss of child in utero, as evidenced by self-blame, somatic complaints, and pessimism about the future
Potential for self-directed violence	Potential for self-directed violence related to rejection by boyfriend, as evidenced by self-destructive acts

DSM-IV Diagnosis	Essential Features*
Bipolar I disorder	Current or past experience of a manic episode, lasting at least 1 week, when one's mood was abnormally and persistently elevated, expansive, or irritable. The episode is severe enough to cause extreme impairment in social or occupational functioning. Bipolar disorders may be classified as manic (limited to manic episodes), depressed (a history of manic episodes with a current depressive episode), or mixed (presentation of both manic and depressive episodes).
Bipolar II disorder	Presence or history of one or more major depressive episodes and at least one hypomanic episode. There has never been a manic episode.
Cyclothymic disorder	A history of 2 years of hypomania in which the person experienced numerous periods with abnormally elevated, expansive, or irritable moods. These moods did not meet the criteria for a manic episode, and many periods of depressed mood did not meet the criteria of a major depressive episode.
Major depressive disorder	Presence of at least five symptoms during the same 2-week period, with one being either depressed mood or loss of interest or pleasure. Other symptoms might include weight loss, insomnia, psychomotor agitation or retardation, fatigue, feelings of worthlessness, diminished ability to think, and recurrent thoughts of death. Major depressions may be classified as single episode or recurrent.
Dysthymic disorder	At least 2 years of a usually depressed mood and at least one of the symptoms mentioned for major depression without meeting the criteria for a major depressive episode.

*Modified from the American Psychiatric Association: *Diagnostic and statistical manual of mental disorders,* ed 4, Washington, DC, 1994, The Association.

Box **19-4** *Diagnostic Criteria for Major Depressive and Manic Episodes*

MAJOR DEPRESSIVE EPISODE	MANIC EPISODE
At least five of the following (including one of the first two) must be present most of the day, nearly daily, for at least 2 weeks:	At least three of the following must be present to a significant degree for at least 1 week:
Depressed mood	Grandiosity
Loss of interest or pleasure	Decreased need for sleep
Weight loss or gain	Pressured speech
Insomnia or hypersomnia	Flight of ideas
Psychomotor agitation or retardation	Distractibility
Fatigue or loss of energy	Psychomotor agitation
Feelings of worthlessness	Excessive involvement in pleasurable activities without regard for negative consequences
Impaired concentration	
Thoughts of death or suicide	

Goals of nursing care for patients with severe mood disturbance have the following aims:

▼ To allow recognition and continuous expression of feelings, including denial, hopelessness, anger, guilt, blame, helplessness, regret, hope, and relief, within a supportive therapeutic atmosphere
▼ To allow for gradual analysis of stressors while strengthening the patient's self-esteem
▼ To increase the patient's sense of identity, control, awareness of choices, and responsibility for behavior
▼ To encourage healthy interpersonal ties with others
▼ To promote understanding of maladaptive emotions and to acquire adaptive coping responses to stressors

Specific short-term goals should be generated from behaviors of the patient, present areas of difficulty, and relevant stressors. Goal setting should involve a holistic view of the patient and the patient's world. Goals probably will need to be developed regarding the patient's self-concept, physical status, behavioral performance, expression of emotions, and relationships. All these areas can directly relate to the mood disturbance. The patient's participation in setting these goals can be a significant first step in regaining mastery over his or her life.

Planning

In planning care, the nurse's priorities are the reduction and ultimate removal of the patient's maladaptive emotional responses, restoration of the patient's occupational and psychosocial functioning, improvement in the patient's quality of life, and minimization of the likelihood of relapse and recurrence. Treatment consists of three phases: acute, continuation, and maintenance (Fig 19-6).[31]

Acute Treatment Phase

The goal of acute treatment is to eliminate the symptoms. If patients improve with treatment, they are said to have had a therapeutic response. A successful acute treatment brings patients back to an essentially symptom-free state and to a level of functioning comparable to that before the illness. This phase usually lasts 6 to 12 weeks, and if patients are symptom-free at the end of that time, they are then in **remission**.

Continuation Treatment Phase

The goal of continuation treatment is to prevent **relapse**, which is the return of symptoms, and to promote **recovery**. The risk of relapse is very high in the first 4 to 6 months after remission, and one of the greatest mistakes in the treatment of mood disorders is the failure to continue a successful treatment for a long enough time. This phase usually lasts 4 to 9 months.

Maintenance Treatment Phase

The goal of maintenance treatment is to prevent **recurrence**, or a new episode of illness. This concept is commonly accepted for bipolar illness, but it is new for major depressive disorders. Nonetheless, some research studies point out the effectiveness of maintenance therapy in preventing new episodes or lengthening the interval between them. In the maintenance phase, patients may be on medication indefinitely.

Understanding the phases of treatment for mood disorders is critically important. The nurse should discuss them with the patient and family so that they may join in the therapeutic alliance and have clear expectations about the goals and course of treatment.

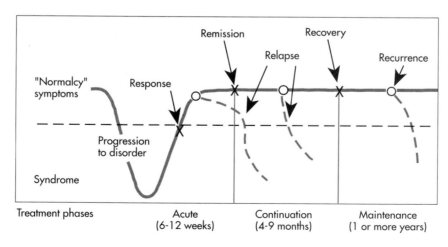

Fig. 19-6 **The phases of treatment for mood disorders.** (From Kupfer DJ: Long-term treatment of depression, *J Clin Psychiatry* 52(suppl):28, 1991.)

> **?** *Your patient tells you she stopped taking her medicine after 2 months because she was feeling better. What would you tell her, based on your understanding of the treatment phases of depression?*

Implementation

Maladaptive emotional responses may emerge at unpredicted moments, can vary in intensity from mild to severe, and can be transitory, recurrent, or stable conditions. Episodes of depression and mania can occur in any setting and can arise in conjunction with existing medical problems. Also, the treatment of mood disturbances can take place in various settings: at home, at an outpatient department, or in a hospital. The best treatment setting for the patient depends on the severity of the illness, available support systems, and resources of the treatment center. In timing intervention, remember that help given when maladaptive patterns are developing is likely to be more acceptable and effective than help given after these patterns have been established. Thus early diagnosis and treatment are associated with more positive outcomes. Recent research has also found that the nature of the therapeutic alliance is an important factor with significant impact on treatment outcome in depression.[30]

The nursing interventions described for severe mood disturbances are based on a multicausal, integrative model of affective disorders. Such a model dismisses the notion of one cause or one cure. Rather, it proposes that affective problems have many determinations and many dimensions that affect all aspects of a person's life. Thus a single approach to nursing care would be inadequate.[25] Nursing interventions must instead reflect the complex nature of the model and address all maladaptive aspects of a person's life.[24] Intervening in as many areas as possible should have the maximum effect in modifying maladaptive responses and alleviating severe mood disturbances. The ultimate aim of these nursing interventions is to teach the patient coping responses and increase the satisfaction gained from interaction with the world. These nursing actions can be implemented in any setting, as seen in the critical pathway for depression on pp. 370-371, which has been developed and is used by one home health agency.

Environmental Interventions

Environmental interventions are useful when the patient's environment is highly dangerous, impoverished, aversive, or lacking in personal resources. In caring for the patient with a severe mood disorder, highest priority should be given to the potential for suicide. Hospitalization is definitely indicated when there is suicidal risk. In the presence of rapidly progressing symptoms and in the absence of support systems, hospitalization is strongly indicated. Nursing care in this case means protecting patients and assuring them that they will not be allowed to harm themselves. Specific interventions for suicidal patients are described in Chapter 20.

Depressed patients must always be assessed for possible suicide. They are at particular risk when they appear to be coming out of their depression, because they may then have the energy and opportunity to kill themselves. Acute manic states are also life threatening. These patients show poor judgment, excessive risk taking, and an inability to evaluate realistic danger and the consequences of their actions. In an acute manic episode, immediate measures must be instituted to prevent death.

Another environmental intervention involves changing the physical or social setting by helping the patient to move to a new environment. Sometimes a change in the general pattern of living is indicated, such as a leave of absence from work, a different job, a new peer group, or leaving a family setting. Changes such as these decrease the immediate stress and mobilize additional support.

Nurse-Patient Relationship

DEPRESSED PATIENTS. Depressed patients resist involvement through withdrawal and nonresponsiveness. Because of their negative views, they tend to remain isolated, verbalize little, think that they are unworthy of help, and form dependent attachments.

In working with depressed patients, the nurse's approach should be quiet, warm, and accepting. The nurse should demonstrate honesty, empathy, and compassion. Admittedly, it is not always easy to give warm, personal care to a person who is unresponsive and detached. The nurse may feel angry, resent the patient's helplessness, or fear rejection. Patience and a belief in the potential of each person to grow and change are needed. If this is calmly communicated, both verbally and nonverbally, in time the patient may begin to respond.

Nurses should avoid assuming an overaggressive or lighthearted approach with the depressed person. Comments such as "You have so much to live for," "Cheer up—things are sure to get better," or "You shouldn't feel so depressed" convey little understanding of and respect for the patient's feelings. They will create more distance and block the formation of a relationship. Also, nurses should not sympathize with the patient. Subjective overidentification by nurses can cause them to experience similar feelings of hopelessness and helplessness and can seriously limit therapy.

Rapport is best established with the depressed patient through shared time, even if the patient talks little, and through supportive companionship. The very presence of the nurse indicates belief that the patient is a valuable person. The nurse should adjust to the depressed patient's pace by speaking more slowly and allowing more time to respond. The patient should be addressed by name, talked with, and listened to. By studying the patient's life and interests, the nurse might select topics that lay the foundation for more meaningful discussions.

CRITICAL PATHWAY — Home Health Care Guide for Depression

Care Elements	Admission	Phase 1 (visits 2-6)	Phase 2 (visits 7-11)	Phase 3 (visits 12-15)	Discharge phase
Disease Process	Complete physical assessment and history. Emergency phone numbers. Instruct on S/S that require immediate attention.	Educate patient/caregiver on depression: definition, treatment for depression, signs and symptoms, causes, predisposing factors.	Instruct patient/caregiver on anxiety.	Reinforce teaching.	Review disease process teaching and S/S or exacerbation to report to health care provider.
Medication	Verify that medications ordered are in the home. Establish basic medication regimen.	Instruct patient/caregiver about medication: purpose, dosage schedule, side effects, action.	Instruct patient/caregiver about medication: purpose, dosage, side effects, action, schedule.	Instruct about medications: purpose, dosage, action, side effects, schedule.	Review medication regimen and instruct on importance of continued compliance.
Nutrition/Hydration	Nutritional assessment.	Teach ways to maintain adequate nutrition and hydration.	Reinforce teaching.	Nutritional assessment.	Review teaching on nutrition/hydration.
Activity	Assess patient's ability to perform ADLs and daily routine.	Help patient to begin developing adequate self-care routine. Instruct on ways to maintain adequate sleep-wake cycle.	Assess self-care routine and sleep/wake patterns.	Instruct on ways to increase social and leisure activities.	Review teaching on activity.
Safety	Assess home environment for risks. Provide emergency phone numbers and instruct on how and when to call for help. Assess for suicidal ideation.	Instruct patient/caregiver on safety measures; assess for suicide risk.	Continue instruction on safety measures; assess for suicide risk.	Continue instruction on safety measures; assess for suicide risk.	Assess for suicide risk.
Interventions	Provide psychotherapeutic counseling. Assess general condition, vital signs, body functions, thought processes, orientation, appearance.	Provide psychotherapeutic counseling. Teach ways to maintain adequate bowel/bladder functioning. Instruct on goal-setting steps, strengths, assets, deficits.	Instruct on behavioral strategies to promote self-worth. Instruct on communication and assertiveness skills. Provide psychotherapeutic counseling. Teach relaxation techniques. Help patient to develop and follow through with goals. Teach thought-stopping techniques.	Instruct on problem-solving and decision-making skills. Continue instruction on communication and assertiveness skills. Provide psychotherapeutic counseling. Continue teaching relaxation techniques. Continue goal setting.	Provide psychotherapeutic counseling.
Tests	Lab/test as ordered. Instruct on frequency/purpose of lab work.	Lab as ordered.	Lab as ordered.	Lab as ordered.	Lab as ordered.

North Mississippi Medical Center Home Health Agency.
D/C, Discharge; *S/S,* signs and symptoms,

Care Elements	Admission	Phase 1 (visits 2-6)	Phase 2 (visits 7-11)	Phase 3 (visits 12-15)	Discharge phase
Psychological/ Sociological	Assess family or other support. Provide information on advance directives, patient rights, responsibilities, plan of care, obtain signatures, set goals, payor criteria, discharge plans.	Assess patient/ caregiver ability to learn. Assess family dynamics. Assess self-esteem and current perception of self.	Assess patient's appraisal of and response to stress. Assess and teach coping skills.	Assess social and leisure activities. Begin D/C teaching.	Complete D/C teaching and D/C patients.
Interteam Services/ Community Referrals	Assess need for other community services. Confirm next physician appointment.	Assist with obtaining needed services (such as social work). Arrange for Meals on Wheels if needed.	Provide information on senior citizens' groups, day programs, and so on.	Evaluate community services.	Plan for future use of community services.
Patient Outcomes	▼ Verbalize S/S that require immediate attention. ▼ Verbalize understanding of emergency number and when to use. ▼ Verbalize understanding of medication schedule and dosage, availability. ▼ Patient/caregiver verbalizes understanding of initial plan of care, services provided, projected length of service. ▼ Agree to plan of care and provide signatures. ▼ Patient verbalizes no thoughts of harming self or others.	▼ Patient verbalizes understanding of disease process of depression. ▼ Verbalizes compliance with and understanding of medications (purpose, dosage, schedule, and side effects) and exhibits therapeutic response to medication. ▼ Verbalizes and demonstrates ways to establish self-care routine. ▼ Verbalizes ways to promote sleep/ wake routine. ▼ Demonstrates improved communication and begins to verbalize feelings. ▼ Verbalizes ways to promote adequate bowel/bladder functioning. ▼ Verbalizes and demonstrates safety measures to prevent injury in the home. ▼ Verbalizes ways to maintain adequate nutrition/hydration.	▼ Verbalizes S/S of anxiety and ways to maintain anxiety at manageable level. ▼ Verbalizes compliance with and understanding of medications (purpose, dosage, schedule, and side effects) and exhibits therapeutic response to medication. ▼ Demonstrates relaxation techniques taught. ▼ Develops one goal for self that is realistic and attainable. ▼ Verbalizes and demonstrates safety measures to prevent injury in the home. ▼ Demonstrates thought-stopping techniques. ▼ Verbalizes adaptive coping strategies for use as alternative to unhealthy responses to stress (such as substance abuse and overeating).	▼ Verbalizes S/S of anxiety and ways to maintain anxiety at manageable level. ▼ Verbalizes compliance with and understanding of medications (purpose, dosage, schedule, and side effects) and exhibits therapeutic response to medication. ▼ Demonstrates relaxation techniques taught. ▼ Develops one goal for self that is realistic and attainable. ▼ Verbalizes and demonstrates safety measures to prevent injury in the home. ▼ Demonstrates thought-stopping techniques. ▼ Verbalizes adaptive coping strategies for use as alternative to unhealthy responses to stress (such as substance abuse and overeating).	▼ Patient/ caregiver verbalizes understanding of teaching on disease process, nutrition/ hydration, active, activity, bowel/bladder functioning, sleep/wake cycle, safety, and medication regimen. ▼ Verbalizes understanding of long-term management of illness and when to notify health care provider of symptoms. ▼ Patient verbalizes no thoughts of harming self or others.

MANIC PATIENTS. In contrast, elated patients may be very talkative and need simple explanations and concise, truthful answers to questions. Although manic patients may appear willing to talk, they resist involvement through manipulation, testing limits, and superficiality. Their hyperactivity, short attention span, flight of ideas, poor judgment, lack of insight, and rapid mood swings all present special problems to the nursing staff.

Manic patients can be very disruptive to a unit and resist engagement in therapy. They may dominate group meetings or therapy sessions by their excessive talking and manipulate staff or patient groups. By identifying a vulnerable area in another person or a group's area of conflict, manic patients are able to exploit others. This provokes defensive and angry responses. Nurses are particularly susceptible to these feelings because they often have the most contact with patients and the responsibility for maintaining the psychiatric unit. When anger is generated, therapeutic care breaks down. Thus the maneuvers of manic patients act as diversionary tactics. By alienating themselves, patients can avoid exploring their own problems.

It is important for nurses to understand how manic patients are able to manipulate others and their reasons for doing so. The treatment plan for these patients should be thorough, well coordinated, and consistently implemented. Constructive limit setting on manic patients' behavior is an essential part of the plan. The entire treatment team must be consistent in their expectations of these patients, and progressive limits must be set as situations arise. Other patients may also be encouraged to carry out the agreed limits. Pressure applied by peers can sometimes be more effective than pressure applied by the staff. Frequent staff meetings are recommended to improve communication, share in understanding the manic patient's behavior, and ensure steady progress.

One goal of nursing care is to increase the patient's self-control, and this should be kept in mind when setting limits. Patients need to see that they can monitor their own behavior and that the staff is there to help them. Also, the nurse should point out that there are many positive aspects to their behavior. The ability to be outgoing, expressive, and energetic is a coping strength that can be maximized.

Physiological Treatments

Physiological treatments include physical care, psychopharmacology, and somatic therapies. They begin with a thorough physical examination and health history to identify health problems and current treatments or medications that may be affecting the patient's mood. The indications for physiological treatment include symptoms that will respond to physiological measures, greater severity of illness, suicidal potential, and need for speed in recovery (Fig. 19-7).

DEPRESSED PATIENTS. In depression, physical well-being may be forgotten or the patient may not be capable of self-care. The more severe the depression, the more impor-

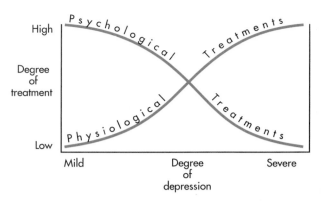

Fig. 19-7 Treatment indications for depression.

tant is the physical care. For example, the nurse may need to monitor the diet of a patient who has no appetite and has lost weight. Staying with the patient during meals, arranging for preferred foods, and encouraging frequent small meals may be helpful. Recording intake and output and weighing the patient daily will help evaluate this need.

Sleep disturbances typically occur. It is best to plan activities according to each patient's energy levels; some feel best in the morning and others in the evening. A scheduled rest period may be helpful, but patients should not be encouraged to take frequent naps or remain in bed all day. Patients with depression experience less stage III and IV sleep, and because these stages depend on the period of wakefulness, napping may worsen sleep disturbances. For many patients, eating regularly, staying active during waking hours, and cutting back on caffeine (especially late in the day) may promote more normal sleep patterns.

The patient's appearance may be neglected and all movements slowed. Nurses may have to help with bathing or dressing. They should do this matter-of-factly, explaining that help is being offered because the patient is unable to do it independently right now. Cleanliness and interest in appearance can be noticed and praised. Nurses must allow patients to help themselves whenever possible. Often nurses might rush the patient or do a task themselves to save time, but this does not facilitate the patient's recovery and should be avoided.

PSYCHOPHARMACOLOGY. Antidepressant medications are often administered to elevate the mood of the depressed patient. They are particularly indicated in severe and recurrent depression. Many antidepressant medications are available on the market (Table 19-8) and new ones can be expected to be released each year.[18,39] The overall success rate of drugs used to treat depression is 60% to 80%.

Despite their success, antidepressant drugs have limitations. Their therapeutic effects begin only after 2 to 6 weeks, and they have side effects that can deter some patients from maintenance. Thus, patient education is essential. Another major problem with some antidepressant medications is their toxicity. Tricyclics are lethal at high doses, which

Table **19-8** *Antidepressant Drugs*

	Usual Adult Dose (mg/day)	Preparations
TRICYCLIC DRUGS		
Tertiary		
Amitriptyline (Elavil)	50-300	PO, IM
Clomipramine (Anafranil)	50-250	PO
Doxepin (Adapin, Sinequan)	50-300	PO, L
Imipramine (Tofranil)	50-300	PO, IM
Trimipramine (Surmontil)	50-300	PO
Secondary		
Desipramine (Norpramin)	50-300	PO
Nortriptyline (Pamelor)	50-100	PO, L
Protriptyline (Vivactil)	15-60	PO
MONOAMINE OXIDASE INHIBITORS		
Isocarboxazid (Marplan)	30-70	PO
Phenelzine (Nardil)	45-90	PO
Tranylcypromine (Parnate)	20-60	PO
SELECTIVE SEROTONIN REUPTAKE INHIBITORS		
Fluoxetine (Prozac)	20-80	PO
Fluvoxamine (Luvox)	50-250	PO
Paroxetine (Paxil)	20-50	PO
Sertraline (Zoloft)	25-200	PO
OTHER ANTIDEPRESSANT DRUGS		
Amoxapine (Asendin)	50-600	PO
Bupropion (Wellbutrin)	50-600*	PO
Maprotiline (Ludiomil)	50-225*	PO
Mirtazapine (Remeron)	15-45	PO
Nefazodone (Serzone)	200-500	PO
Trazodone (Desyrel)	50-600	PO
Venlafaxine (Effexor)	25-375	PO*

*Antidepressants with a ceiling dose because of dose-related seizures.
IM, Intramuscular; *L,* oral liquid; *PO,* oral tablet/capsule.

makes them particularly dangerous for people most in need of them: suicidal patients. In addition, antidepressant medications do not help everyone, and it is difficult to predict who will respond to which drug. Fortunately, those who do not benefit from one drug often do well when switched to another.

Partly in response to patient compliance issues, a number of pharmaceutical companies have established disease management programs for patients being treated for depression with medication. Such programs as *Propartners,* sponsored by Eli Lilly, and *Rhythms,* sponsored by Pfizer, are intended to provide education regarding depression and its treatment, promote a partnership between the patient and the clinician, and encourage the patient to play an active role in getting and staying well. These programs send a variety of educational materials to the patient, such as newsletters and audiotapes, and are designed to support the patient through the acute, continuation, and maintenance phases of treatment. Nurses should ask about these programs from representatives of the pharmaceutical compa-

nies and integrate these learning materials into their own patient education activities.

> **?** *What would you say to a patient who tells you that she doesn't want to take medicines for her depression because they are addictive?*

Somatic Therapies. Electroconvulsive therapy (ECT) is also used with depressed patients, particularly those with recurrent depressions and those resistant to drug therapy. ECT is regarded by many as a specific therapy for patients with severe depressions characterized by somatic delusions and delusional guilt, accompanied by a lack of interest in the world, suicidal ideation, and weight loss.

Sleep deprivation therapy may also be effective in treating depression. Research indicates that depriving some depressed patients of a night's sleep will improve their clinical

TABLE 19-9 *Mood-stabilizing Drugs*

GENERIC (TRADE NAME)	USUAL ADULT DOSE (mg/day)	PREPARATIONS
Lithium (Eskalith, Lithobid, Lithonate)	900-1800	PO, L, SR
Valproate (Depakote)	750 mg/day-60 mg/kg/day	PO, L, SR
Carbamazepine (Tegretol)	200-1600	PO, L, C

C, Chewable tablets; *L,* liquid; *PO,* oral tablet/capsule; *SR,* oral slow-release tablets.

condition. How sleep deprivation works is not known, and the duration of improvement varies.

A final physiological treatment is that of phototherapy, or light therapy, in which patients are exposed to bright artificial light for a specified amount of time each day. Phototherapy appears to be effective in the short-term treatment of patients with mild to moderate seasonal affective disorder (SAD). Electroconvulsive therapy, sleep deprivation, and phototherapy are described in detail in Chapter 28.

MANIC PATIENTS. Manic patients primarily need protection from themselves. They may be too busy to eat or take care of themselves. Eating problems can be handled in the same way as with depressed patients. Manic patients may sleep very little, so rest periods should be encouraged, along with baths, soft music, and whirlpools. These patients may also need help in selecting clothes and maintaining hygiene. Setting limits and using firm actions are effective in physical care.

Psychopharmacology. For many years lithium was considered the drug of choice in the treatment of mania. Care must be taken regarding the narrow therapeutic index of this drug, which requires frequent blood levels and careful patient monitoring. The anticonvulsants valproate and carbamazepine have added to the treatment alternatives (Table 19-9). The overall success rate of these drugs when used to treat bipolar illness is 80%. A more complete discussion of mood-stabilizing medications is presented in Chapter 27.

 Your patient with bipolar disorder tells you that she has stopped taking her medication because she misses the highs that she used to feel and the extra energy she used to have. What would your educational approach be to help her comply with treatment?

Expressing Feelings

Affective interventions are necessary because patients with mood disturbances have difficulty identifying, expressing, and modulating feelings. Feelings that are particularly problematic are hopelessness, sadness, anger, guilt, and anxiety. A range of interventions is available to the nurse in meeting patient needs in this area.

Intervening in emotions requires self-understanding by the nurse. Whether the interventions will be therapeutic de-

A Patient *Speaks*

In depression this faith in deliverance, in ultimate restoration, is absent. The pain is unrelenting, and what makes the condition intolerable is the foreknowledge that no remedy will come—not in a day, an hour, a month, or a minute. If there is mild relief, one knows that it is only temporary; more pain will follow. It is hopelessness even more than pain that crushes the soul. So the decision-making of daily life involves not, as in normal affairs, shifting from one annoying situation to another less annoying—or from discomfort to relative comfort, or from boredom to activity—but moving from pain to pain. One does not abandon, even briefly, one's bed of nails, but is attached to it wherever one goes. And this results in a striking experience—one which I have called, borrowing military terminology, the situation of the walking wounded. For in virtually any other serious sickness, a patient who felt similar devastation would be lying flat in bed, possibly sedated and hooked up to the tubes and wires of life-support systems, but at the very least in a posture of repose and in an isolated setting. His invalidism would be necessary, unquestioned, and honorably attained. However, the sufferer from depression has no such option and therefore finds himself, like a walking casualty of war, thrust into the most intolerable social and family situations. There he must, despite the anguish devouring his brain, present a face approximating the one that is associated with ordinary events and companionship. He must try to utter small talk, and be responsive to questions, and knowingly nod and frown and, God help him, even smile. But it is a fierce trial attempting to speak a few simple words. ▼

William Styron: *Darkness visible,* New York, 1992, Vintage Books.

pends greatly on the nurse's values regarding the various emotions, the nurse's emotional responsiveness, and the ability to offer genuine respect and nonjudgmental acceptance. Nurses must be able to experience feelings and express them if they expect to help patients.

DEPRESSED PATIENTS. Initially the nurse must express hope for depressed patients. They have a genuine need for repeated reassurance. The nurse can reinforce that depression is a self-limiting disorder and that the future will be better. This can be expressed calmly and simply. The intent is not to cheer the patient but to offer hope that, although recovery is a slow process involving weeks or months, the patient will feel progressively better. The nurse may acknowledge the patient's inability to take comfort from this reassurance. For the depressed, only the depression is real; past or future happiness is an illusion (see A Patient Speaks). By affirming belief in recovery, however, the nurse may make the patient's existence more tolerable.

This initial reassurance is a way of acknowledging the patient's pain and despair while also conveying a sense of hope in recovery. It is not the premature reassurance of "Don't worry, everything's going to be just fine." It is an openness to the patient's feelings and acknowledgment of them. This is a very important first step. It lets the patient see that the present state is not permanent. For the depressed patient who lacks time perspective, it directs thoughts beyond the present with genuine hope for tomorrow.

Nursing actions in this area should convey that expressing feelings is normal and necessary. Blocking or repressing emotions is partly responsible for the patient's present pain. Nurses can help patients realize that their overwhelming feelings of dejection and worthlessness are defenses that prevent them from dealing with their problems. Encouraging a patient to express unpleasant or painful emotions can reduce their intensity and make the patient feel more alive and masterful. Thus nursing care should be directed toward helping the patient experience feelings and express them. These actions are a prerequisite to interventions in the cognitive, behavioral, or social areas.

MANIC PATIENTS. Manic patients may have the opposite problem of patients with depression in that they are often too expressive of their feelings. These patients are often hyperverbal and need help from the nurse in pacing and modulating their expression. The nurse must be careful not to criticize or negate the feelings expressed. Rather, helping patients to speak more slowly and to follow one line of thought are important areas for nursing intervention. Manic patients need feedback on the intensity of their self-expressions, as well as the impact of their behavior on other people. Social skills modeling and reinforcement are nursing care activities that can be incorporated into the daily routine. Setting limits, giving simple directions, and keeping focused are other useful nursing interventions.

When the nurse accepts without criticism the anger, despair, or anxiety expressed by the patient, the patient sees that expressing feelings is not destructive or a sign of weakness. Sometimes, however, patients' expression of anger changes their cognitive set from self-blaming to blaming others. It may allow them to see themselves as more effective because it connotes power, superiority, and mastery. How this anger is expressed is important because aggressive behavior can be destructive and can further isolate them. Many patients experiencing both depressive and manic emotional states have problems with expressing anger and need to learn assertive behavior. This important area of nursing intervention is explored in Chapter 29.

Relaxation techniques may also help both manic and depressed patients deal with their anxiety and tension and obtain more pleasure from life. Reducing anxiety to tolerable levels broadens one's perceptual field and allows the nurse to intervene in the cognitive and behavioral areas. Nursing actions to reduce anxiety are described in Chapters 16 and 30.

To successfully implement any of these nursing actions related to the patient's affective needs, the nurse must use a variety of communication skills (see Chapter 2). Particularly important are empathy skills, reflection of feeling, open-ended feeling-oriented questions, validation, self-disclosure, and confrontation. Feelings are the essence of empathy and thus make empathy an essential therapeutic quality. The various other communication skills must also focus on feelings rather than facts. The patient with a severe mood disturbance will challenge the nurse's therapeutic skills and stringently test the nurse's caring and commitment.

Cognitive Strategies

When intervening in the cognitive area, nurses have three major aims, which require that they begin with the patient's conceptualization of the problem:

▼ To increase the patient's sense of control over goals and behavior
▼ To increase the patient's self-esteem
▼ To help the patient modify dysfunctional thinking patterns

DEPRESSED PATIENTS. Depressed patients often see themselves as victims of their moods and environment. They do not see their behavior and their interpretation of events as possible causes of depression. They assume a passive stance and wait for someone or something to lift their mood. One task of the nurse, therefore, is to move patients beyond their limiting preoccupation to other aspects of their world that are related to it. To do this, the nurse must progress gradually. The first step is to help patients explore their feelings. This is followed by eliciting their view of the problem. In so doing, the nurse accepts the patient's perceptions but need not accept the patient's conclusions. Together they define the problem to give the patient a sense of control, a feeling of hope, and a realization that change may indeed be possible.

Nursing actions may then focus on modifying the patient's thinking. Depressed patients are dominated by negative thoughts. Often, despite a successful performance, the patient will view it negatively. Cognitive changes may be brought about in a variety of ways, as described in Chapter 30.

Often, negative thinking is an automatic process of which the patient is not even aware. The nurse can therefore help patients identify their negative thoughts and decrease them through thought stopping or substitution. Concurrently, the patient can be encouraged to increase positive thinking by reviewing personal assets, strengths, accomplishments, and opportunities. Next, the patient can be helped in examining the accuracy of perceptions, logic, and conclusions. Misperceptions, distortions, and irrational beliefs become evident. The patient should be helped to move from unrealistic to realistic goals and to decrease the importance of unattainable goals. All these actions enhance the patient's self-understanding and increase self-esteem. More detailed interventions related to alterations in self-concept, which are inherent in disturbances of mood, are explored in Chapter 18.

Also, because the depressed patient tends to be overwhelmed by despair, it is important to limit the amount of negative evaluation in which he or she engages. One way is to involve the patient in productive tasks or activities; another way is to increase the level of socialization. These benefit the patient in two complementary ways: They limit the time spent on brooding and self-criticism and they provide positive reinforcement.

MANIC PATIENTS. Manic patients also need to gain control over their thoughts and behaviors. Here, however, the challenge is to bring together a patient's scattered thoughts and ideas to help him or her engage in adaptive, goal-directed behavior. The communication skills of focusing, clarifying, and confrontation are useful in redirecting a patient's self-expressions. Once this is accomplished the nurse can begin to help the patient modify dysfunctional thinking. Manic patients often have problems of grandiosity, overestimation of self, and unrealistic pursuits. As in depression, cognitive interventions can help the patient evaluate these thought problems and identify more realistic and ego-supportive goals.

It is also important for the nurse to realize the meaning, nature, and value the manic patient places on behavior and mood change. For example, research has shown that patients with bipolar disorder receive pronounced short- and long-term positive effects from their illness. These include increases in productivity, creativity, sensitivity to surroundings, social outgoingness, and sexual intensity. These effects can provide a great deal of secondary benefit from the illness and can be powerful reinforcers of maladaptive responses, thus making change more difficult. For some patients at some times, the perceived positive consequences of the illness may outweigh their perception of the negative consequences.

Behavioral Change

The ability to accomplish tasks and be productive depends on various factors that apply to both depressed and manic patients. First, expectations and goals should be small enough to ensure successful performance, relevant to their needs, and focused on positive activities. Box 19-5 presents a list of rewarding or potentially rewarding activities.

Next, attention should be focused on the task at hand,

not what has yet to be done or was done incorrectly in the past. Finally, positive reinforcement should be based on actual performance. If such an approach is used consistently over time, the nurse can expect the patient to demonstrate increasingly productive behavior.

Occupational and recreational tasks are usually easily identified by the nurse. These can be most valuable and are well represented in the positive activities list. Another source of accomplishment is movement and physical exercise. Jogging, walking, swimming, bicycling, and aerobics are popular forms of exercise that may be incorporated in a regular program of activity.[22] They are beneficial because they improve the patient's physical condition, release emotions and tensions, and can have an antidepressant effect.

Successful behavior is a powerful reinforcer or antidepressant. However, this idea seldom occurs to depressed patients, who use their despondent mood as a rationalization for inactivity. They instead believe that once their mood lifts, they will be productive again. Such an idea is consistent with a negative cognitive set and a sense of helplessness. However, inactivity prevents satisfaction and social

---

Box **19-5** *List of Possible Positive Activities*

Planning something you will enjoy
Going on an outing (such as a walk, a shopping trip downtown, or a picnic)
Going out for entertainment
Going on a trip
Going to meetings, lectures, or classes
Attending a social gathering
Playing a sport or game
Spending time on a hobby or project
Entertaining yourself at home (for example, reading, listening to music, or watching TV)
Doing something just for yourself (such as buying something, cooking something, or dressing comfortably)
Spending time just relaxing (for example, thinking, sitting, napping, or daydreaming)
Caring for yourself or making yourself attractive
Persisting at a difficult task
Completing a routine task or unpleasant task
Doing a job well
Cooperating with someone else on a common task
Doing something special for someone else, being generous, going out of your way
Seeking out people (for example, calling, stopping by, making a date or appointment, or going to a meeting)
Initiating conversation (for example, at a store, party, or class)
Discussing an interesting or amusing topic
Expressing yourself openly, clearly, or frankly (expressing opinion, criticism, or anger)
Playing with children or animals
Complimenting or praising someone
Physically showing affection or love
Receiving praise, compliments, or attention

recognition. Thus it reinforces a depressive state. Likewise, overactivity or uncompleted activity lowers the self-evaluation of manic patients.

Therefore nursing interventions should focus on activating the patient in a realistic, goal-directed way. Directed activities, strategies, or homework assignments mutually determined by the nurse and patient can reveal alternative coping responses. Many depressed patients benefit from nursing actions that encourage them to redirect their self-preoccupation to interests in the outside world. The timing of these interventions is crucial. Patients should not be forced into activities initially. Also, they will not benefit from coming into contact with too many people too soon. Rather, the nurse should encourage activities gradually and suggest more involvement on the basis of patients' energy.

For severely depressed hospitalized patients, a structured daily program of activities can be beneficial. Because these patients lack motivation and direction, they are slow to initiate actions. The nurse should take into consideration the patient's tolerance to stress and probability of succeeding. The particular task should be neither too difficult nor too time consuming. Success tends to increase expectations of success, and failure tends to increase hopelessness.

Elated patients usually need little encouragement to become involved with others. Because of their short attention span and restless energy, however, they cannot deal with complicated projects. They need tasks that are simple and can be completed quickly. They need room to move about and furnishings that do not overstimulate them.

> **?** *What physiological changes occur as a result of exercise? Relate these to what is currently known about the biology of depression.*

Social Skills

Social factors play a major role in the causation, maintenance, and resolution of affective disorders. Socialization moderates depression by providing an experience incompatible with depressive withdrawal. It also provides increased self-esteem through the social reinforcers of approval, acceptance, recognition, and support.

A major problem is that patients with maladaptive emotional responses are less accomplished in social interaction. In addition, others may avoid them because of their self-absorption, pessimism, or elation. One nursing action to counteract this problem is to help patients improve their social skills. A Patient Education Plan for enhancing social skills is presented below. It applies to patients with either depression or mania.

Involvement with others often is a result of shared activities. The nurse can work with the patient to identify recreational, career, cultural, religious, and personal interests and how to pursue these interests through community groups, organizations, and clubs. Women's groups, single-parent groups, jogging clubs, church groups, and neighborhood associations are all opportunities. Although this may appear to be a simple nursing intervention, it often taxes the nurse's creativity and knowledge of resources.

FAMILY AND GROUP TREATMENT. In addition to a one-to-one relationship, patients with maladaptive emotional responses can benefit from family and group work. Behaviors associated with depression and mania may be contributed to and supported by other family members. The patient's problems in human relationships are examined in light of family patterns, and all members are expected to take responsibility for their share of the continuing pattern. The theory that friends and partners often reinforce and support the patient's maladaptive behavior has been well documented. Much attention and secondary

 PATIENT EDUCATION PLAN **Enhancing Social Skills**

Content	Instructional Activities	Evaluation
Describe behaviors interfering with social interaction.	Instruct the patient on corrective behaviors.	Patient identifies problematic and more facilitative behaviors.
Discuss positive social skills that could be used by the patient.	Model effective interpersonal skills for the patient.	Patient describes specific skills that could be acquired.
Analyze the way in which the patient could incorporate these specific skills.	Use role play and guided practice to allow patient to test these new behaviors.	Patient shows beginning skill in assumed social behaviors.
Encourage patient to test new skills in other situations.	Give the patient homework assignments to do in his or her natural environment.	Patient discusses ability to complete the assigned tasks.
Discuss generalization of new skills to other aspects of the patient's life and functioning.	Give feedback, encouragement, and praise for newly acquired social skills and their generalization.	Patient is able to integrate the new social behaviors in social interactions with others.

gain are usually received from others, who respond by being helpful, nurturing, or annoyed. When the patient acts in a more adaptive way, however, attention given is minimal. Therefore, one goal of family therapy is to have the family reinforce adaptive behavior and ignore maladaptive mood responses. Group therapy can also provide multiple benefits. For example, a format for group treatment of patients with depression or mania can have as its overall aim to increase self-worth and self-esteem through identification with the group and awareness of personal strengths. Specifically, group members can:

▼ Learn more about their own behavior and relationships with others based on feedback from the group
▼ Increase social support through group relatedness
▼ Gain a heightened sense of identity, self-understanding, and control over their own lives
▼ Realize that other people have problems similar to their own, which helps to reduce their sense of loneliness and isolation, thereby also decreasing feelings of hopelessness, helplessness, and powerlessness
▼ Learn new ways to cope with stress from others in the group
▼ More realistically modify their perceptions and expectations of self and others
▼ Allow for the expression of feelings of hopelessness and frustration within the supportive context of the group

Other group interventions have also been described in the literature for patients with bipolar disorder[38] and for depressed women using cognitive behavioral strategies.[34]

Mental Health Education

A final but important aspect of nursing care related to maladaptive emotional responses is mental health education about the nature, extent, and treatments available for mood disorders. Despite its prevalence, most people with depressive illnesses do not seek treatment because many of them do not know that they have a treatable disease. There is a particular need to target outreach to ethnic and racial minority communities.[10]

An important national initiative regarding depression was the publication of clinical practice guidelines on depression by the Agency for Health Care Policy and Research (AHCPR).[14,15] A patient's guide is also available to help consumers. These educational materials are available to professionals and the public and provide the most current information about diagnostic and treatment issues.

Other strategies are also needed. For example, nurses in Arizona have implemented a mental health training program for primary care nurses that addresses primary and secondary prevention issues related to depression.[5] The program emphasizes criteria for assessing depression, presents psychopharmacological and psychotherapeutic content, discusses care coordination among multiple agencies and providers, and addresses referral resources. Cultural and developmental issues for Native Americans, Mexican Americans, the elderly, and adolescents are highlighted. An other innovative strategy is the creation of a slide kit on detecting and treating depression from a nursing perspective.[46] This slide kit is available from Eli Lilly and can be used by nurses to educate students, practitioners, and consumers about this major public health problem.

Nursing care must also address the specific needs of patients and families for education about mood disorders. A psychoeducational approach to depression in women has been found to be effective in increasing their feelings of independence and self-confidence and helping them to manage the stresses associated with being a woman in contemporary society.[35] The psychoeducational model can also be used with families, who are a valuable resource in helping patients deal with their illness. The overall goal of such a program is to improve patient and family functioning and decrease symptomatology by increasing a sense of self-worth and control for both patients and families. Specific information about the reciprocal impact of depression and family life can be outlined (Box 19-6) along with suggestions and strategies designed to help family members cope more effectively with mood disorders.

In summary, the most important ideas that the nurse should try to communicate through mental health education include the following:

▼ Mood disorders are a medical illness, not a character defect or weakness.
▼ Recovery is the rule, not the exception.
▼ Mood disorders are treatable illnesses, and an effective treatment can be found for almost all patients.
▼ The goal of intervention is to not just get better, but to get and stay completely well.

A Nursing Treatment Plan Summary for patients with maladaptive emotional responses is presented on p. 380.

Evaluation

The effectiveness of nursing care is determined by changes in the patient's maladaptive emotional responses and the effect they have on functioning. Problems related to self-concept and interpersonal relationships merge and overlap. Because all people experience life stress and related losses, the nurse can ask a fundamental question related to evaluation: "Did I assess the patient for problems in this area?"

Of particular significance are the many special aspects of transference and countertransference that may occur. The patient's heightened attachment and dependency behaviors and lowered defensiveness can lead to intense transference reactions that should be worked through. Themes of loss and fear of loss, control of emotions and lack of control, and ambivalence predominate. Termination of the nurse-patient relationship may be difficult because the patient experiences it as another loss that requires mourning and integration.

Countertransference can be related to the nurse's own bereavements, attitudes about anger, guilt, sadness, and despair, the ability to confront these emotions openly and objectively, and most importantly, conflicts about death and

Box **19-6** *Outline of Topics for Patient-Family Psychoeducational Sessions on Depression*

I. Defining depression
   A. Definitions and descriptions of depression and mania
   B. How depression differs from "the blues" we all experience (duration, impact on mood, functioning, self-esteem, responsiveness to the environment)
   C. Possible causes: the Stuart Stress Adaptation Model
II. Depression and the interpersonal environment
   A. What depression looks like: interpersonal difficulties
      1. Oversensitivity and self-preoccupation
      2. Unresponsiveness (to reassurance, support, feedback, sympathy)
      3. Behaviors that appear willful
      4. Apparent lack of caring for others, unrealistic expectations
      5. Apparent increased need to control relationships
      6. Inability to function in normal roles, tasks
   B. Negative interactional sequences
      1. Family attempts to coax, reassure, protect (potential for overinvolvement)
      2. Patient is unresponsive, family escalates attempts to help or withdraws
      3. Patient feels alienated, family becomes withdrawn, angry, or both
      4. Family feels guilty and returns to overprotective stance
      5. Patient feels unworthy, hopeless, infantilized
      6. Families burn out over time but remain caught in guilt/anger dilemma
      7. Alienation or overprotection

III. Treatments
   A. Psychotropic medication
   B. Psychotherapies
   C. Other treatments
IV. Coping with depression
   A. What to avoid
      1. Too rapid reassurance
      2. Taking comments literally
      3. Attempting to be constantly available and positive
      4. Allowing the disorder to dominate family life
   B. Creating a balance (neither overresponsive nor underresponsive)
      1. Recognition of multiple realities
      2. Distinguishing between the patient and the disorder
      3. Decreasing expectations temporarily
      4. Providing realistic support and reinforcement
      5. Avoiding unnecessary criticism (but providing feedback when necessary)
      6. Communicating clearly and simply (proverbially)
      7. Providing activity, structure
   C. Taking care of self and family members other than the patient; skills for self-preservation
      1. Time out (away from patient)
      2. Avoiding martyrdom
      3. Accepting own negative feelings
      4. Minimizing the impact of the disorder
   D. Coping with special problems
      1. Suicide threats and attempts
      2. Medication
      3. Hospitalization
      4. Atypical responses

Modified from Keitner G: *Depression and families: impact and treatment,* Washington, DC, 1990, American Psychiatric Press.

loss. Difficulties with any of these issues can be evident in avoidance behavior, preoccupation with fantasies, blocking of feelings, or shortening of sessions. Nursing care will be more appropriate and effective if the nurse is aware of these issues and sensitive to personal feelings and conflicts regarding loss. Supervision and peer support groups can be of great help in this area.

Summary

1. The continuum of emotional responses ranges from the most adaptive state of emotional responsiveness to the more maladaptive states of delayed grief reaction, depression, and mania.
2. Patient behaviors related to emotional responses include delayed grief reaction, depression, and mania.
3. Predisposing factors affecting emotional responses include genetics, aggression turned inward, object loss, personality organization, cognition, learned helplessness-hopelessness, behavioral learning, and biochemistry. Precipitating stressors include loss of attachment, life events, roles, and physiological changes.
4. Coping resources focus on the patient's social and

economic supports and a sense of personal mastery. Coping mechanisms include introjection, denial, and suppression.
5. Primary NANDA nursing diagnoses related to maladaptive emotional responses are dysfunctional grieving, hopelessness, powerlessness, spiritual distress, and potential for self-directed violence.
6. Primary DSM-IV diagnoses include bipolar I and II disorders, cyclothymic disorder, major depressive disorder, and dysthymic disorder.
7. The expected outcome of nursing care is that the patient will be emotionally responsive and return to a preillness level of functioning.
8. Nursing interventions address environmental issues, nurse-patient relationships, physiological treatments, expressing feelings, cognitive strategies, behavioral change, social skills, and mental health education.
9. The effectiveness of nursing care is determined by changes in the patient's maladaptive emotional responses and the effect they have on functioning. Supervision and peer support groups can be helpful to the nurse working with patients with mood disorders.

NURSING TREATMENT PLAN *Summary* **Maladaptive Emotional Responses**

Nursing Diagnosis: Hopelessness
Expected Outcome: The patient will be emotionally responsive and return to preillness level of functioning.

Short-term goal	Intervention	Rationale
The patient's environment will be safe and protective.	Continually evaluate the patient's potential for suicide. Hospitalize the patient when there is a suicidal risk. Help the patient move to a new environment when appropriate (new job, peer group, family setting).	All patients with severe mood disturbances are at risk for suicide; environmental changes can protect the patient, decrease the immediate stress, and mobilize additional resources.

The patient will establish a therapeutic relationship with the nurse.	Use a warm, accepting, empathic approach.
	Be aware of and in control of one's own feelings and reactions (anger, frustration, sympathy).
	With the depressed patient:
	   Establish rapport through shared time and supportive companionship.
	   Give the patient time to respond.
	   Personalize care as a way of indicating the patient's value as a human being.
	With the manic patient:
	   Give simple, truthful responses.
	   Be alert to possible manipulation.
	   Set constructive limits on negative behavior.
	   Use a consistent approach by all health-team members.
	   Maintain open communication and sharing of perceptions among team members.
	   Reinforce the patient's self-control and positive aspects of patient behavior.
		Both depressed and manic patients resist becoming involved in a therapeutic alliance; acceptance, persistence, and limit setting are necessary.

The patient will be physiologically stable and able to meet self-care needs.	Help the patient to meet self-care needs, particularly in the areas of nutrition, sleep, and personal hygiene. Encourage the patient's independence whenever possible. Administer prescribed medications and somatic treatments.	Physiological changes occur in disturbances of mood; physical care and somatic therapies are required to overcome problems in this area.
The patient will be able to recognize and express emotions related to daily events.	Respond empathically, with a focus on feelings rather than facts. Acknowledge the patient's pain and convey a sense of hope in recovery. Help the patient experience feelings and express them appropriately. Help the patient in the adaptive expression of anger.	Patients with severe mood disturbances have difficulty identifying, expressing, and modulating feelings.

NURSING TREATMENT PLAN *Summary*   **Maladaptive Emotional Responses—cont'd**

Nursing Diagnosis: Hopelessness
Expected Outcome: The patient will be emotionally responsive and return to preillness level of functioning.

Short-term goal	Intervention	Rationale
The patient will evaluate thinking and correct faulty or negative thoughts.	Review the patient's conceptualization of the problem but do not necessarily accept conclusions. Identify the patient's negative thoughts and help to decrease them. Help increase positive thinking. Examine the accuracy of perceptions, logic, and conclusions. Identify misperceptions, distortions, and irrational beliefs. Help the patient move from unrealistic to realistic goals. Decrease the importance of unattainable goals. Limit the amount of negative personal evaluations the patient engages in.	This will help to increase sense of control over goals and behaviors, enhance self-esteem, and modify negative expectations.
The patient will implement two new behavioral coping strategies.	Assign appropriate action-oriented therapeutic tasks. Encourage activities gradually, escalating them as the patient's energy is mobilized. Provide a tangible, structured program when appropriate. Set goals that are realistic, relevant to the patient's needs and interests, and focused on positive activities. Focus on present activities, not past or future activities. Positively reinforce successful performance. Incorporate physical exercise in the patient's care plan.	Successful behavioral performance counteracts feelings of helplessness and hopelessness.
The patient will describe rewarding social interactions.	Assess the patient's social skills, supports, and interests. Review existing and potential social resources. Instruct and model effective social skills. Use role playing and rehearsal of social interactions. Give feedback and positive reinforcement of effective interpersonal skills. Intervene with families to have them reinforce the patient's adaptive emotional responses. Support or engage in family and group therapy when appropriate.	Socialization is an experience incompatible with withdrawal and increases self-esteem through the social reinforcers of approval, acceptance, recognition, and support.

COMPETENT CARING A Clinical Exemplar of a Psychiatric Nurse

Virginia A. Reuger, MSN, RN, C

Sure, you read about therapeutic interactions in your nursing textbooks, but every person is not the same, so the only way you learn is by doing, by experiencing. Rarely in school do we have the time to become overinvolved with our patients. We are taught on our psychiatric rotation not to let the boundaries between self and others become blurred. Yet the dynamics of a therapeutic relationship are not real until we come face to face with the situation.

It happened to me, subtly, soon after I started working in a private psychiatric hospital. I was working as a staff nurse on the intensive care unit. I was assigned to the next admission. From the intake sheet, I could see it was another depressed, suicidal patient. But when R and her husband walked onto the unit, I was immediately drawn to her with an empathic feeling. She was tiny, frail looking; her face was thin and drawn. Her long, dark hair partially hid her face. She ignored introductions and stared at the floor. My initial challenge was to establish trust to open channels of communication, assess her suicide potential, and provide a secure environment. Her potential for self-harm was quite high. She was put on strict suicidal precautions. Initially, as I worked with R it required observations of her appearance, gestures, and interests, as well as nonverbal communication. I often had to make inferences, and I shared these with her. I felt like she was testing the waters of trust. R would often wrap herself up in her pink blanket and rock back and forth during our interactions. I found myself wondering what she was thinking.

One day during our time together I asked her about how it felt to be depressed. For her, it was the beginning of self-disclosure. She was able to acknowledge her fear and pain and unmet needs. She talked about what it was like growing up in New York City, living in rat-infested row houses. Her father worked at a bakery and sometimes their only food was the bread he brought home. She had two brothers and two sisters. Eventually she told me her uncle and grandfather lived with them too. As she learned to trust me, she disclosed sexual abuse from her uncle and grandfather. At times the details became so vivid she trembled as she cried. It is hard to express, but there was a sense that we were making contact.

We talked about her present life, her frigidity, her 6-year-old daughter, and the nightmares. She often remarked that her husband and daughter would be better off without her. She believed she could not have a "normal life." R was very bright and talented. She had many hobbies. We started concentrating on these things. I knew her self-esteem was low, and this was the start of some good work.

But being her primary nurse and assigned to her one-to-one daily made me realize I was becoming enmeshed in the situation. I went to my nurse manager for supervision. We discussed several options. I questioned whether I was helping her. I think sometimes nurses want to feel like omnipotent rescuers. I was not sure whether I was fostering independence or dependence. It was important to acknowledge my feelings to someone else openly, to discuss them, and then to move on. Even though I felt a bond, I had to help R find strength on her own. We discussed her upcoming discharge date; we talked about priorities and decisions she had made. We talked about good choices, bad choices, and no choices. She had suffered many setbacks, but she was making plans.

I remember staying late the day of her discharge to say goodbye. R sent me cards at the hospital, dropped gifts off at the admissions office for me, and once tried to reach me at home. It was difficult to not acknowledge these things; I wanted so much to talk to her. But I knew the boundaries of a therapeutic relationship, and I knew she would be fine. I did talk to her outpatient therapist, and he told me she had completed a course in sign language (during her stay R befriended a deaf elderly woman), and she also was attending clown school, something she had always wanted to do—to make people laugh and feel good.

In psychiatric nursing it is important to remember that the art is to offer what you can without dictating the results while recognizing that you are not the only one to contribute to a person's health and happiness. I learned this important lesson from R.

Video **Resources**

Mosby's Psychiatric Nursing Video Series
   Volume 2: Major Depression

Mosby's Chronic Disease Self-management Kits
   Depression Video and Book Kit

your **INTERNET**
connection

Internet Depression Resources List
http://www.execpc.com/-corbeau/

Pendulum's Bipolar Disorder/Manic-Depression Page
http://www.pendulum.org/

Chapter Review Questions

1. **Match each term in Column A with the correct examples in Column B.**

Column A

___Behaviors related to emotional responses

___Coping mechanisms

___DSM-IV diagnoses

___Precipitating stressors

___Predisposing factors

___Seasonal affective disorder

Column B

A. Introjection, denial, suppression

B. Loss, life events, role strain

C. Delayed grief reaction, depression/mania

D. Bipolar, cyclothymia, depression

E. Genetics, early childhood loss, turning anger inward

F. Depression that comes with shortened daylight

2. **Fill in the blanks.**

A. The somatic therapy of _____ is often used for patients with severe depression with somatic delusions and delusional guilt, suicidal ideation, and weight loss.

B. There is substantial evidence for abnormal regulation of the _____ neurotransmitter system in depression.

C. Depressed patients with a history of manic episodes are said to have _____ disorder. Depressed patients who have had only episodes of depression are said to have _____ depression.

D. Prior episodes, family history, prior suicide attempts, female gender, and lack of social support are all _____ factors for depression.

E. The brain structure currently the focus of much research for its role in depression is the _____.

F. Two other psychiatric illnesses that often occur with depression are _____ disorders and _____ disorders.

G. When both medications and psychotherapy are used to treat depression and mania, the success rate of treatment is _____ to _____ %.

H. The goal of the acute phase of treatment for depression is to eliminate symptoms and produce a therapeutic _____. This phase usually lasts _____ to _____ weeks. If patients are symptom free at the end of that time they are said to be in _____.

I. The goal of the continuation phase of treatment for depression is to promote _____ and prevent _____. This phase usually lasts _____ to _____ months.

J. The goal of the maintenance phase of treatment for depression is to prevent _____. This phase may last _____.

3. **Provide short answers for the following questions.**

A. List the responses on the continuum of emotional responses and give a brief definition of each one.

B. What are the three major aims when intervening in the cognitive area with a depressed patient?

C. You are asked to join a peer support group made up of nurses who work with patients with depression. How can such a group be helpful to you? What can you contribute to the group?

D. Design an intervention program for mothers who are depressed and their young children.

REFERENCES

1. Abramson L, Metalsky G, Alloy L: Hopelessness depression: a theory-based subtype of depression, *Psychol Rev* 96:358, 1989.
2. American Psychiatric Association: *Diagnostic and statistical manual of mental disorders,* ed 4, Washington, DC, 1994, The Association.
3. Arieti S, Bemporad J: The psychological organization of depression, *Am J Psychiatry* 137:1360, 1980.
4. Badger T: Physical health impairment and depression among older adults, *Image J Nurs Sch* 25:325, 1993.
5. Badger T, Cardea J, Biocca L, Mishel M: Assessment and management of depression: an imperative for community-based practice, *Arch Psychiatr Nurs* 4:235, 1990.
6. Barbee E: African-American women and depression: a review and critique of the literature, *Arch Psychiatr Nurs* 6:257, 1992.
7. Beck A et al: *Cognitive therapy of depression,* New York, 1979, The Guilford Press.
8. Beeber LS: Depression in women. In McBride AB, Austin JK, editors: *Psychiatric–mental health nursing: integrating the behavioral and biological sciences,* Philadelphia, 1996, WB Saunders.
9. Betrus P, Elmore S: Seasonal affective disorder: Part 1. a review of the neural mechanisms for psychosocial nurses, *Arch Psychiatr Nurs* 5:367, 1991.
10. Brown DR, Ahmed F, Gary LE, Milburn NG: Major depression in a community sample of African Americans, *Am J Psychiatry* 152:373, 1995.
11. Burmeister M: The genetics of bipolar disorder, *J Calif Alliance Mentally Ill* 6:19, 1995.
12. Cadoret RJ et al: Depression spectrum disease, I: the role of gene-environment interaction, *Am J Psychiatry* 153:892, 1996.
13. Costello C: *Symptoms of depression,* New York, 1993, Wiley.

14. Depression Guideline Panel: *Depression in primary care,* vol 1, *Detection and diagnosis, Clinical practice guideline,* no 5, Rockville, Md, 1993, US Department of Health and Human Services, Public Health Service, Agency for Health Care Policy and Research, pub no 93-0550.

15. Depression Guideline Panel: *Depression in primary care,* vol 2, *Treatment of major depression, Clinical practice guideline,* no 5, Rockville, Md, 1993, US Department of Health and Human Services, Public Health Service, Agency for Health Care Policy and Research, pub no 93-0551.

16. Field T: Infants of depressed mothers, *Infant Behav Dev* 18:1, 1995.

17. George MS, Ketter TA, Post RM: Prefrontal cortex dysfunction in clinical depression, *Depression* 2:59, 1994.

18. Glod CA: Recent advances in the pharmacotherapy of depression, *Arch Psychiatr Nurs* 10:355, 1996.

19. Goodwin F, Jamison K: *Manic-depressive illness,* New York, 1990, Oxford University Press.

20. Gove W: The relationship between sex roles, marital status, and mental illness, *Soc Forces* 51:34, 1972.

21. Greenberg P et al: The economic burden of depression in 1990, *J Clin Psychiatry* 54:26, 1993.

22. Gullette ECD, Blumenthal JA: Exercise therapy for the prevention and treatment of depression, *J Pract Psychiatry Behav Health* 9:263, 1996.

23. Hall L, Sachs B, Rayens M, Lutenbacher M: Childhood physical and sexual abuse: their relationship with depressive symptoms in adulthood, *Image J Nurs Sch* 25:317, 1993.

24. Hauenstein EJ: A nursing practice paradigm for depressed rural women: theoretical basis, *Arch Psychiatr Nurs* 10:283, 1996.

25. Heifner CA: Women, depression, and biological psychiatry: implications for psychiatric nursing, *Perspect Psychiatr Care* 32:4, 1996.

26. Jamison K: *Touched with fire: manic-depressive illness and the artistic temperament,* New York, 1993, Free Press.

27. Jones-Webb R, Snowden L: Symptoms of depression among blacks and whites, *Am J Public Health* 83:240, 1993.

28. Kendall-Tackett K, Kantor G: *Postpartum depression: a comprehensive approach for nurses,* Newbury Park, Calif, 1993, Sage.

29. Kendler K et al: The prediction of major depression in women: toward an integrated etiological model, *Am J Psychiatry* 150:1139, 1993.

30. Krupnick JL et al: The role of the therapeutic alliance in psychotherapy and pharmacotherapy outcome: findings in the National Institute of Mental Health Treatment of Depression Collaborative Treatment Program, *J Consult Clin Psychol* 64:532, 1996.

31. Kupfer D: Long-term treatment of depression, *J Clin Psychiatry* 52(suppl):28, 1991.

32. Lewinsohn P, Youngren M, Grosscup S: Reinforcement and depression. In Depue R, editor: *The psychobiology of the depressive disorders,* New York, 1979, Academic Press.

33. Mann JJ, Malone KM, Diehl DJ, Perel J, Cooper TB, Mintun MA: Demonstration in vivo of reduced serotonin responsivity in the brain of untreated depressed patients, *Am J Psychiatry* 153:174, 1996.

34. Maynard C: Comparison of effectiveness of group interventions for depression in women, *Arch Psychiatr Nurs* 7(5):277, 1993.

35. Maynard C: Psychoeducational approach to depression in women, *J Psychosoc Nurs Ment Health Serv* 31:9, 1993.

36. McEnany G: Part I: Rhythm and blues revisited: biological rhythm disturbances in depression, *J Am Psychiatr Nurses Assoc* 2:15, 1996.

37. NIH Consensus Development Conference: *Diagnosis and treatment of depression in late life,* Rockville, Md, 1991, US Department of Health and Human Services, Public Health Service, NIH.

38. Pollack LE: Information-seeking among people with manic-depressive illness, *Image J Nurs Sch* 28:259, 1996.

39. Richelson E: Treatment of acute depression, *Psychiatr Clin North Am* 16:461, 1993.

40. Rosenthal N: *Winter blues: seasonal affective disorder,* New York, 1993, The Guilford Press.

41. Rossen EK, Buschmann MT: Mental illness in late life: the neurobiology of depression, *Arch Psychiatr Nurs* 3:130, 1995.

42. Ruble D, Greulich F, Pomerantz E, Gochberg B: The role of gender-related processes in the development of sex differences in self-evaluation and depression, *J Affect Disord* 29:97, 1993.

43. Seligman M: *Helplessness: on depression, development and death,* San Francisco, 1975, WH Freeman.

44. Shapira B, Newman M, Lerer B: Serotonergic mechanisms in depression: clinical insights and biological correlates, *Isr J Med Sci* 30:162, 1994.

45. Simmons-Alling S: Bipolar mood disorders: brain, behavior, and nursing. In McBride AB, Austin JK, editors: *Psychiatric-mental health nursing: integrating the behavioral and biological sciences,* Philadelphia, 1996, WB Saunders.

46. Stuart G: *Detection and treatment of depression: the nursing perspective, slide kit sponsored by Eli Lilly,* Washington, DC, 1994, American Nurses' Foundation.

47. Stuart G et al: Early family experiences of women with bulimia and depression, *Arch Psychiatr Nurs* 4:43, 1990.

48. Ugarriza D: Postpartum affective disorders: incidence and treatment, *J Psychosoc Nurs Ment Health Serv* 30:29, 1992.

49. Warren B: Depression in African-American women, *J Psychosoc Nurs Ment Health Serv* 32:29, 1994.

50. Weissman M et al: Sex differences in rates of depression: cross-national perspectives, *J Affect Disord* 29:77, 1993.

51. Winokur G, Coryell W, Endicott J, Akiskal H: Further distinctions between manic-depressive illness (bipolar disorder) and primary depressive disorder (unipolar disorder), *Am J Psychiatry* 150:1176, 1993.

52. Work Group on Major Depressive Disorder: Practice guidelines for major depressive disorder in adults, *Am J Psychiatry* 150:1, 1993.

53. Zung W, Broadhead E, Roth M: Prevalence of depressive symptoms in primary care, *J Fam Pract* 37:337, 1993.

ANNOTATED SUGGESTED READINGS

*Shea N et al: The effects of an ambulatory collaborative practice model on process and outcome of care for bipolar disorder, *J Am Psychiatric Nurs Assoc* 3:49, 1997.
Reports important research evaluating the effects of a collaborative outpatient treatment program on patients with bipolar disorder. More research of this type is needed in the field.

Suri R, Burt V: The assessment and treatment of postpartum psychiatric disorders, *J Pract Psychiatry Behav Health* 3:67, 1997.
Complete review of the assessment, clinical characteristics, and psychotherapeutic and psychopharmacologic treatment of the four major types of postpartum depression.

Thase M: Do we really need all these new antidepressants? Weighing the options, *J Pract Psychiatry Behav Health* 3:3, 1997.
Reviews the etiology of depression and the strengths and limitations of the available classes of antidepressants. Highly recommended.

*Webster D, McEnany G: Research and clinical strategies for treatment resistant depression: buyer beware? *J Am Psychiatric Nurs Assoc* 3:17, 1997.
Addresses the clinical aspects of treatment-resistant depression and related research questions.

*Nursing reference.

Self-protective Responses and Suicidal Behavior

Gail W. Stuart

© 1998 M.C. Escher/Cordon Art, Baarn, Holland.

Out, out brief candle! Life's but a walking shadow, a poor player That struts and frets his hour upon the stage And then is heard no more. It is a tale Told by an idiot, full of sound and fury, Signifying nothing. **William Shakespeare** MACBETH, ACT V

LEARNING OBJECTIVES

After studying this chapter the student should be able to:

▼ Describe the continuum of adaptive and maladaptive self-protective responses

▼ Discuss the epidemiology of suicide

▼ Identify behaviors associated with self-protective responses

▼ Analyze predisposing factors, precipitating stressors, and appraisal of stressors related to self-protective responses

▼ Describe coping resources and coping mechanisms related to self-protective responses

▼ Formulate nursing diagnoses related to self-protective responses

▼ Assess the relationship between nursing diagnoses and medical diagnoses related to self-protective responses

▼ Identify expected outcomes and short-term nursing goals related to self-protective responses

▼ Develop a patient education plan to promote compliance with health-care treatment

▼ Analyze nursing interventions related to self-protective responses

▼ Evaluate nursing care related to self-protective responses

TOPICAL OUTLINE

Continuum of Self-protective Responses
  Epidemiology of Suicide
Assessment
  Behaviors
  Predisposing Factors
  Precipitating Stressors
  Appraisal of Stressors
  Coping Resources
  Coping Mechanisms
Nursing Diagnosis
  Related Medical Diagnoses
Outcome Identification
Planning
Implementation
  Protection
  Contracting for Safety
  Increasing Self-esteem
  Regulating Emotions and Behaviors
  Mobilizing Social Support
  Patient Education
  Suicide Prevention
Evaluation

Life is characterized by risk. People must choose the amount of danger to which they are willing to expose themselves. Sometimes these choices are conscious and rational. For instance, the elderly person who decides to stay in the house on an icy day has chosen not to risk falling and possibly fracturing a bone. Other risk-taking behavior is unconsciously determined. Soldiers who volunteer for a suicide mission are probably unaware of their motivation. If asked, they would probably cite patriotism or concern for comrades. Most people go through life accepting some risks as part of their daily routine while carefully avoiding others.

Even though life is risky, most societies have a norm that defines the degree of danger to which people may expose themselves. This norm varies according to age, gender, socioeconomic status, and occupation. In general, the very young, the old, and women are seen as needing to be protected from harm. Great ambivalence is directed at those who engage in potentially self-destructive behavior. Some risk takers are admired, particularly athletes, military personnel, those with dangerous occupations, and those who place themselves in danger to help others. At the same time, feelings of admiration may be accompanied by fear and perplexity about the danger-seeking behavior. The varying attitudes toward cigarette smoking are another example of cultural ambivalence. On one hand, smoking is seen as mature behavior, denoting sophistication and social acceptability. On the other, it is seen as socially alienating, unhealthy, and inconsiderate.

CONTINUUM OF SELF-PROTECTIVE RESPONSES

Protection and survival are fundamental needs of all living things. A continuum of self-protecting responses would have self-enhancement as the most adaptive response, whereas indirect self-destructive behavior, self-injury, and suicide would be maladaptive responses. Self-destructive behavior may thus range from subtle to overt.

Direct self-destructive behavior includes any form of suicidal activity, such as suicide threats, attempts, gestures, and completed suicide. The intent of this behavior is death, and the person is aware of the desired outcome. Indirect self-destructive behavior is any activity detrimental to the person's physical well-being that potentially may result in death. However, the person may be unaware of this potential and deny it if confronted. Examples include eating disorders (see Chapter 25) and abuse of alcohol and other drugs (see Chapter 24). Other examples include cigarette smoking, reckless driving, gambling, criminal activity, socially deviant behavior, stress-seeking behavior, participation in high-risk sports, and noncompliance with medical treatment.

Theories of self-destructive behavior overlap with those of self-concept and disturbances in mood. Careful study of Chapters 18 and 19 will help the reader understand the behaviors discussed in this chapter. To think about or attempt destruction of the self, the person must have low self-regard. Low self-esteem leads to depression, which is always present in self-destructive behavior. The range of self-protective responses is shown in Fig. 20-1.

The levels of behavior in the continuum may overlap. For instance, the girl who learns and excels at gymnastics is building her self-esteem and projecting a positive self-concept. However, if she tries movements she is not prepared for and does not take safety measures, her behavior becomes self-injurious or indirectly self-destructive. Similarly, a diabetic man who has never complied completely with his prescribed diet and medication regimen may become discouraged and intentionally take an overdose of insulin. Thus the nurse must be alert to subtle shifts in the mood and behavior of patients when assessing maladaptive self-protective responses.

Epidemiology of Suicide

About 30,000 people complete the act of suicide each year, making it the eighth leading cause of death in the United States and the third leading killer of young people. The rate of suicide among youth has tripled in the past 30 years. The

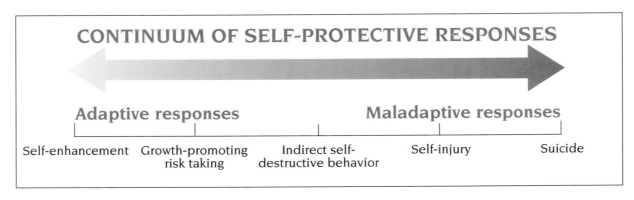

Fig. 20-1 Continuum of self-protective responses.

actual number of suicides may be two to three times higher because of the underreporting that occurs. In addition, many single-car accidents and homicides are, in fact, suicides. Worldwide, at least 1000 suicides occur each day, and 645,680 years of productive life are lost each year in the United States because of deaths by suicide. Of these, 71% occurred among white males, and white females accounted for another 19%. The United States now has one of the highest suicide rates for young men in the world, surpassing Japan and Sweden, countries long identified with high rates of suicide.

Although the base rate of suicide has remained about the same for the past 20 years, the rate has soared for young people ages 15 to 24 and has increased by 25% for the elderly. The highest suicide rate for any group in this country is among people over age 65, especially among those between 75 and 85. Although this group constitutes 26% of the total U.S. population, it accounts for about 40% of suicide deaths. White males over the age of 50 represent the greatest number of these deaths (Fig. 20-2).

Teen suicide in the United States is nearly five times as common among boys as among girls. Suicide is also more common among whites than blacks at all ages. The overwhelming majority of completed suicides are committed by males. Well over half of these males shoot themselves, and the use of guns is increasing rapidly. Women attempt suicide three times as often as men, using potentially less lethal means such as medications and wrist slashing. However, one third of women who complete suicide and over half of those 15 to 29 years of age use guns.

Reports of suicide among young children are rare, but suicidal behavior is not. As many as 12,000 children ages 5 to 14 may be hospitalized in this country every year for deliberate self-destructive acts.

 What factors might contribute to the high rate of suicide among white elderly males?

Assessment

Behaviors

NONCOMPLIANCE. It has been estimated that one half of patients do not comply with their health care treatment plan. People who do not comply with recommended health care activities are generally aware that they have chosen not to care for themselves. They usually have a reason for noncompliance, such as being asymptomatic, not being able to afford the treatment they need, not understanding the treatment, or not having time. Patients may also minimize the seriousness of their problems. Many chronic illnesses are characterized by long periods of stability, during which the person may not be aware of discomfort. This reinforces the noncompliant behavior.

Patients with chronic illnesses often search for healthcare providers who will prescribe less disruptive treatment plans than the ones they are trying to avoid. They are susceptible to questionable practices such as miracle cures and faith healing in their search for the return of complete health. The popular literature is constantly reporting miraculous new treatments for chronic diseases. Most of these lead to more suffering for those who become hopeful and are then disappointed.

The most prominent behavior associated with noncompliance is refusal to admit the seriousness of the health problem. This denial interferes with acceptance of treatment. At the same time, it protects the ego from the anxiety that recognition of impaired health creates. Anxiety may

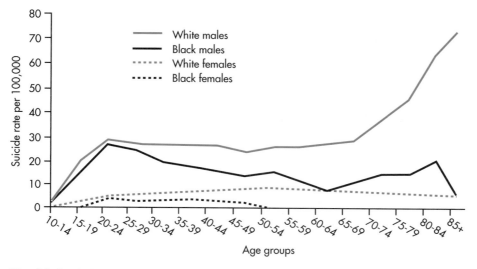

Fig. 20-2 Suicide rates by age group. (From National Center for Health Statistics, National Institute of Mental Health, Washington, DC, 1993.)

also be increased because admission of illness implies recognition of growing older. In a society that values youth, this behavior is not surprising.

An unfortunate aspect of noncompliance is that guilt about not following health care recommendations may also interfere with obtaining regular care. Hypertensive people who have not been taking their medication may be reluctant to have their blood pressure checked because an elevated reading will undermine their defensive system. If the medical system treats these people as children and chastises them for their behavior, they feel even guiltier and are more reluctant to seek health care.

Noncompliant people are also struggling for control. Serious illness is often seen as an attack on the person and a betrayal by the body. Patients need to reassert their control and prove that they are still the master of their fate. The diabetic who cheats on his diet is gambling that he still has control over his body and can resist his problem by will. Most chronically ill people need to test the limits of their control and the validity of the prescribed self-care regimen. The following clinical example illustrates the problem of noncompliance with a prescribed health-care regimen.

Clinical Example Ms. C was a 61-year-old, white married woman who had been in good health most of her life. She had three grown children who had left home and established their own families. She had been a homemaker since her marriage at age 19. She and her husband were both looking forward to his retirement in 6 months. They planned to buy a recreational vehicle and travel around the United States.

Ms. C visited the gynecologist regularly. She was very concerned about having annual Pap smears. Because she was receiving no other regular health care, the nurse practitioner who worked with this physician did a complete physical examination each time Ms. C was seen. On her most recent visit, laboratory studies revealed an elevated blood glucose level. She was then referred to an internist for a more thorough examination. Her diagnosis was diabetes mellitus, adult onset. Ms. C was told that her condition was not serious and could be controlled by diet. She was 20 pounds (9 kg) overweight and was advised that she needed to lose the excess weight. She was instructed about her diet, how to test her urine, and about possible complications of diabetes.

Ms. C was frightened about her condition but did not mention this because no one else seemed very concerned. At first, she was conscientious about following her diet and testing her urine. She felt very well and was proud when she lost 5 pounds. As time went on, Ms. C began to wonder whether she was really so sick. She had never felt ill. On her husband's birthday, she fixed a special dinner and baked a cake. She decided she deserved a reward for "being good" and did not follow her diet. She anxiously tested her urine at bedtime and it was negative. Then her son and his family

visited for a week. She fixed all their favorite foods and ate with them. She still felt fine and decided she did not need to test her urine. When it was time for her next checkup, she postponed calling the physician. She was very busy preparing for retirement travel.

Selected Nursing Diagnosis:

▼ Noncompliance related to fear of the diagnosis of diabetes, as evidenced by lack of adherence to medical treatment plan

 Do you think that noncompliance can ever be an adaptive response? Why or why not?

SELF-INJURY. Society accepts some forms of self-injury as normal. Examples of culturally sanctioned forms include body piercing, cosmetic eyebrow plucking, hair twisting, circumcision, nail biting, and tattoos. Various terms have been used to describe self-injurious behavior: *self-abuse, self-directed aggression, self-harm, self-inflicted injury,* and *self-mutilation.* **Self-injury** can be defined as the act of deliberate harm to one's own body. The injury is done to oneself, without the aid of another person, and the injury is severe enough for tissue damage. Common forms of self-injurious behavior include cutting and burning the skin, banging head and limbs, picking at wounds, and chewing fingers.[26]

Many nurses mistake self-injury for potential suicide. In fact, these are two separate phenomena. Usually the lethality of self-injury is low, and patients who self-injure typically want relief from the tension they feel rather than to kill themselves. Self-injury is also different from other self-destructive behaviors, such as bingeing, drug abuse, smoking, and high-risk activities. Self-injury is a contained event that occurs in a short time span and with an awareness of the consequences of the act.

Self-injurious behavior may be categorized by the type of patient and clinical context in which the behavior occurs:

▼ *People with mental retardation.* Outward-directed aggression among the mentally retarded often coexists with self-injurious behavior.

▼ *Psychotic patients.* Self-injuring acts among psychotic patients tend to be sporadic and often occur in response to command hallucinations or delusions.

▼ *Prison populations.* Self-injury in prisons is difficult to assess because of poor documentation, drug use, and undiagnosed psychiatric disorders. Many self-injurious events among prisoners may be intentionally manipulative, designed to force transfer to a less restrictive facility.

▼ *Character disorders,* particularly borderline personality disorder. This group is often young and female with a poor tolerance of anxiety and anger. They also include patients with eating disorders.

SUICIDAL BEHAVIOR. Suicidal behavior is usually divided into the categories of suicide threats, suicide attempts, and completed suicide. In addition, certain suicide attempts may be called **suicide gestures.** The gesture is a suicide attempt directed toward the goal of receiving attention rather than actual destruction of the self. Use of this term is questionable. It implies that it is only an attention-seeking behavior and should not be taken seriously. This is not true. All suicidal behavior is serious, whatever the intent, and deserves the nurse's serious consideration. Therefore, suicide gestures are included in the general category of suicide attempts.

The **suicide threat** may be veiled but usually occurs before overt suicidal activity takes place. The suicidal person may make a statement such as "Will you remember me when I'm gone?" or "Take care of my family for me." In the context of recent stressors and the person's life situation, statements such as these may be ominous. Nonverbal communication often reveals the suicide threat. The person may give away prized possessions, make a will or funeral arrangements, or systematically withdraw from all friendships and social activities. Sometimes a person may make a direct verbal suicidal threat, but this occurs less often. The threat is an indication of the ambivalence that is usually present in suicidal behavior. It represents the hope that someone will recognize the danger and rescue the person from self-destructive impulses. It may also be an effort to discover whether anyone cares enough to prevent the person from harming him- or herself.

Suicide attempts include any self-directed actions taken by the person that will lead to death if not interrupted. In the assessment of suicidal behavior, much emphasis is placed on the lethality of the method threatened or used. Although all suicide threats and attempts must be taken seriously, more vigorous and vigilant attention is indicated when the person is planning or tries a highly lethal means such as gunshot, hanging, or jumping. Less lethal means include carbon monoxide and drug overdose, which allow time for discovery once the suicidal action has begun.

Assessment of the suicidal person also includes whether the person has made a specific plan and whether the means to carry out the plan are available. The most suicidal person is one who plans a violent death (such as a gunshot to the head), has a specific plan (for example, as soon as his wife goes shopping), and has the means readily available (such as a loaded gun in a desk drawer). This person is exhibiting little ambivalence about a suicide plan. On the other hand, the person who contemplates taking a bottle of aspirin if the situation at work does not improve soon is communicating an element of hope. This person is really asking for help in coping with a poor work situation. The following clinical example illustrates the behavior of a suicidal person.

Clinical Example Mr. Y was a 52-year-old black man employed in the foundry of a large steel mill. He had worked for the company for 20 years. He lived in a rented room in a blue-collar neighborhood near the mill. Most of his neighbors were Appalachian white and southern black families who had moved to the community to work at the mill. There was an undercurrent of racial tension in the neighborhood, but Mr. Y was not involved in conflicts with his neighbors. He had separated from his wife before moving to the community and had no close friends or family. The separation resulted from his violent behavior related to drinking binges.

Mr. Y was seen by the occupational health nurse, Ms. G, when he came to the employee health clinic following a 6-week absence from work. He had been hospitalized for broken ribs and a concussion after he had been beaten and robbed by a gang of adolescents in an alley behind his home. Ms. G was familiar with this patient because he had participated in the company's employee assistance program for alcoholics. When she saw him in the clinic, she immediately noted that he appeared depressed. His face was expressionless, his posture was slumped, and he had lost weight. He appeared disheveled, which was a change from his usual neat appearance. He said he did not feel ready to return to work, but he had received a letter from the personnel office requesting that his condition be evaluated by the company's physician. His speech was slow and halting and so soft that he could barely be heard. He told Ms. G that he had a request to make of her. He knew from past conversations that she was an animal lover. He wanted her to take his pet dog because he did not feel able to care for it adequately, and the neighbors who kept it while he was in the hospital had neglected it.

Ms. G was very concerned about Mr. Y and asked him how he was spending his time. He said he kept the television on and he thought a lot. When asked, he said he felt "too shaky" to go outside unless he absolutely had to. He thought the boys who attacked him were still in the neighborhood. Ms. G asked if he had thought about harming himself. Mr. Y looked startled, then admitted that he saw no other solution to his problem. "It makes sense. I don't have anybody. If you take Rover, I can go." With further questioning, he admitted that he had a loaded revolver at home and planned to use it after he left the clinic. Ms. G realized that Mr. Y needed help immediately and initiated plans for hospitalization.

Selected Nursing Diagnoses:

▼ Potential for self-directed violence related to impoverished social environment, as evidenced by intent to kill self with a gun

▼ Powerlessness related to recent neighborhood attack, as evidenced by expressed feelings of despair and hopelessness

Completed suicide may take place after warning signs have been missed or ignored. Some people do not give any easily recognizable warning signs. Research done on completed suicide has of necessity been retrospective. However, it can be informative to interview survivors. This procedure is known as the *psychological autopsy*.[12] It is a retrospective review of the person's behavior before the suicide. The information obtained can be used to better understand suicidal behavior and to enhance the effectiveness of primary prevention activities.

Significant others of suicidal people, including survivors, have many feelings about this behavior. An element of hostility exists in suicidal behavior. Often the message to significant others, stated or implied, is "You should have cared more." At times, when the person survives the attempt, this message may be transmitted in a manipulative way. An example is the adolescent girl who discovers that her boyfriend is dating someone else and takes an overdose of over-the-counter sleeping pills. If she sets the scene so that she will almost inevitably be discovered and makes sure that her boyfriend hears of her behavior, she is behaving in a hostile, manipulative way. A remorseful response by the boyfriend would be reinforcing and increase the likelihood that she will repeat the behavior. It is important to treat these attempts seriously and help the patient develop healthier communication patterns. People who do not really intend to die may do so if they are not discovered in time.

When suicide is successful, the survivors are left with many feelings that they cannot communicate to the involved object, the dead person (see A Family Speaks). This may lead to an unresolved grief reaction and depression. Some suicide prevention centers have become involved in *postvention*.

Survivors are helped, either individually or in groups, to express their feelings and work through their grief.

In summary, the suicidal patient may have many different clinical behaviors. Mood disturbances are often present, as are somatic complaints. It has been noted that hopelessness may be more important than depression in explaining suicidal ideation.[3] Nurses should take a careful medical and psychiatric history, paying specific attention to the mental status examination described in Chapter 6 and the psychosocial history, and evaluate the patient for recent losses, life stresses, and substance use and abuse (see Critical Thinking about Contemporary Issues).

Contrary to common opinion, directly questioning the patient about suicidal thought and plans will not cause the patient to take suicidal action. Rather, most people want to be prevented from carrying out their self-destruction. Most patients are relieved to be asked about these feelings. One of the most important questions to ask of suicidal patients is whether they think they can control their behavior and refrain from acting on their impulses. If patients cannot do this, immediate psychiatric hospitalization is indicated.

Finally, the nurse may find it helpful to use an assessment tool to explore self-protective responses. Fig. 20-3 presents a nursing assessment tool developed for this purpose by the Division of Psychiatric Nursing at the Medical University of South Carolina. Factors the nurse must consider in the assessment of the self-destructive patient are listed in Box 20-1.[8]

 A Family *Speaks*

My husband died last year. He didn't commit suicide, but he took his own life just as surely as if he had pulled the trigger of a gun. Only his weapon was a cigarette. You see, 2 years ago his doctor discovered a cancer lesion on his lung. At that time my husband was told he needed to lose weight, cut down on his drinking, and most of all, stop smoking. But my husband wasn't a very good patient.

Sometimes I blame myself for not doing more. I nagged for a while, but that only seemed to make our marriage worse. My husband said that what he did with his life was his own choice and that his father had smoked all of his life and lived until he was 84. My husband died at age 62.

One good thing has come out of this tragedy, however. My son has stopped smoking and has vowed he will never touch another cigarette for as long as he lives. That small goodness gives me comfort and some sense of hope. ▼

CRITICAL THINKING *about* *Contemporary Issues*

Are Health Care Professionals Missing Suicidal Behavior in Their Patients?

It has been reported that 8 out of 10 patients who commit suicide talked about it with someone before completing the act. Often the person they talk with is a health care professional. The problem is that care providers often miss the signs and symptoms of depression and the subtle indicators of self-destructive intentions.

There is evidence, for example, that 30% of all people who complete and attempt suicide visit primary care physicians within 1 month before their attempt. Among the elderly, more than 80% give clues of their intent. Of the elderly who commit suicide, 75% are known to have visited their personal physician in the month before they took their life. In one study, health-care professionals reported a surprisingly small amount of probing for depressive or suicidal symptoms, even when they were mentioned by the patient. Most interesting, patients 55 and older, who were possibly at the highest risk, reported no health professional inquiries about suicidal thinking and perceived the least amount of attention or interest in their mental state.[11] It thus appears that much work needs to be done to alert health-care providers to the severity and extent of this problem and to help them to better evaluate patients for potential self-destructive responses.[25]

SUICIDE/SELF-HARM ASSESSMENT

Complete on admission if indicated by Risk Factor Assessment or any time when suicidal risk is suspected.

Directions:
1. Answer Question I.
2. Complete Section II by circling one of the three descriptors for each Key Factor that BEST describes the patient.
3. Complete Section III.
4. Add the points for each circled item in Sections I, II, and III to obtain the total score.

I. Is the current admission precipitated by suicide attempt?		Yes 2 No 1	
II. Key Factors	**High Risk (1:1)**	**Moderate Risk (q15min observation)**	**No Precautions**
Contract for safety	Unwilling to contract OR Unable to contract because of impaired reality testing (hallucinations, delusions, dementia, delirium, dissociation) 2	Contracts but is ambivalent or guarded 1	Reliably contracts for safety 0
Suicide plan	Has plan with actual or potential access to planned method 2	Has plan without access to planned method 1	No plan 0
Plan lethality	Highly lethal plan (gun, hanging, jumping, carbon monoxide) 2	Low lethality of plan 1	Low lethality of plan (superficial scratching, head banging, pillow over face, biting, holding breath) 0
Elopement risk	High elopement risk 2	Low elopement risk 1	No elopement risk 0
Suicidal ideation	Constant suicidal thoughts 2	Intermittent or fleeting suicidal thoughts 1	No current suicidal thoughts 0
Attempt history	Past attempts of high lethality 2	Past attempts of low lethality 1	No previous attempts 0
Symptoms (circle those that apply) hopelessness helplessness anhedonia guilt/shame anger/rage impulsivity	5-6 symptoms present 2	3-4 symptoms present 1	0-2 symptoms present 0
Current morbid thoughts (reunion fantasies, preoccupation with death)	Constantly 2	Frequently 1	Rarely 0
III. RN's Subjective Appraisal of Patient's Reliability:	Pt. replies not trustworthy; several nonverbal cues Pt. replies questionably, trustworthy, at least one nonverbal cue Pt. replies trustworthy		4 3 0

Scoring Key:
High Risk Precautions (1:1) = 10 or more

Moderate Risk Precautions (q15min observation) = 4-9

Moderate Risk Precautions = 4-9

No Precautions = 0-3

Total Score _____

Assessed by (RN): _____

Date: _____

Time: _____

Fig. 20-3 **Suicide/self-harm assessment.** (Courtesy of Psychiatric Nursing, Institute of Psychiatry, Medical University of South Carolina.)

Box *20-1* *Factors in the Assessment of the Self-destructive Patient*

ASSESSING CIRCUMSTANCES OF AN ATTEMPT
Precipitating humiliating life event
Preparatory actions: acquiring a method, putting affairs in order, suicide talk, giving away prized possessions, suicide note
Use of violent method or more lethal drugs/poisons
Understanding of lethality of chosen method
Precautions taken against discovery

PRESENTING SYMPTOMS
Hopelessness
Self-reproach, feelings of failure and unworthiness
Depressed mood
Agitation and restlessness
Persistent insomnia
Weight loss
Slowed speech, fatigue, social withdrawal
Suicidal thoughts and plans

PSYCHIATRIC ILLNESS
Previous suicide attempt
Mood disorders
Alcoholism or other substance abuse
Conduct disorders and depression in adolescents
Early dementia and confusional states in the elderly
Combinations of the above

PSYCHOSOCIAL HISTORY
Recently separated, divorced, or bereaved
Lives alone
Unemployed, recent job change or loss
Multiple life stresses (move, early loss, breakup of important relationship, school problems, threat of disciplinary crisis)
Chronic medical illness
Excessive drinking or substance abuse

PERSONALITY FACTORS
Impulsivity, aggressivity, hostility
Cognitive rigidity and negativity
Hopelessness
Low self-esteem
Borderline or antisocial personality disorder

FAMILY HISTORY
Family history of suicidal behavior
Family history of mood disorder, alcoholism, or both

Predisposing Factors

No one theory adequately explains self-destructive responses or guides therapeutic intervention. Behavior theory suggests that self-injury is learned and reinforced in childhood or adolescence. In contrast, psychological theory focuses on significant defects in early stages of ego development. It suggests that self-destructive behavior may have its roots in early interpersonal trauma and that unmanaged anxiety may provoke continued episodes of self-injury. Interpersonal theories propose that self-injury may result from interactions that leave the child feeling guilty and worthless. A history of abuse or incest may then precipitate self-destructiveness if negative perceptions have been internalized and acted upon and there is a lack of secure attachments. Other predisposing factors related to self-destructive behavior include the inability to communicate needs and feelings verbally, feelings of guilt, depression, and depersonalization, and fluctuating emotions.

Five domains of predisposing factors—psychiatric diagnosis, personality traits and disorders, psychosocial and environmental factors, genetic and familial variables, and biochemical factors—contribute to a theoretical biopsychosocial model for understanding self-destructive behavior over the life cycle.[7,8]

PSYCHIATRIC DIAGNOSIS. More than 90% of adults who end their lives by suicide have an associated psychiatric illness.[2] There are three broad psychiatric disorders that put people at particular risk for suicide:
▼ Mood disorders
▼ Substance abuse
▼ Schizophrenia

Recent studies suggest that patients with panic disorder also have increased risk of suicide, and adolescents who kill themselves tend to have depression and conduct disorders. In addition, a high percentage of these youth abused alcohol or drugs.[4]

Suicide is the most serious complication of mood disorders, with 15% of those with these illnesses ending their lives by suicide. Suicide is particularly common in depressed elderly men.[10] Patients with bipolar disorder and psychotic depression are at greatest risk. Alcohol use is associated with 25% to 50% of suicides. In patients with alcohol dependence, suicide often occurs late in the disease and is often related to some interpersonal loss or the onset of medical complications. Schizophrenia, a disease that affects 1% of the population, carries a high incidence of suicide; 10% to 13% of patients with schizophrenia commit suicide. The risk is greatest for patients under age 40 who feel hopeless, are suicidal, fear mental disintegration, have made previous suicidal attempts, have a chronic or relapsing course to their illness, and do not comply with treatment.[6]

PERSONALITY TRAITS. The three aspects of personality that are most closely associated with increased risk of suicide are hostility, impulsivity, and depression. These traits are important because they cross diagnostic groups. In addition, borderline personality disorder and antisocial personality disorder are more highly correlated with suicidal behavior (see Chapter 22). The coexistence of antisocial and depressive symptoms appears to be a particularly lethal combination in both adults and young people. The association between hostility and suicide stems from the notion proposed by Freud that the suicidal person turns rage inward against the self. Other studies have found that suicidal people are more socially withdrawn, have lower self-esteem, are less trusting of others, expect bad things to happen to them, feel powerless over their lives, and have a rigid and inflexible way of thinking.

> ? *How might the personality traits of hostility, impulsivity, and depression contribute to the development of substance abuse?*

PSYCHOSOCIAL MILIEU. This domain is concerned with social supports, life events, and chronic medical illnesses. Recent bereavement, separation or divorce, early loss, and decreased social supports are all important factors related to potential suicide.[22] Precipitants of suicidal behavior are often humiliating life events such as interpersonal problems, public embarrassment, loss of a job, or the threat of incarceration. In addition, evidence shows that knowing someone who attempted or committed suicide or exposure to suicide through the media may make one more vulnerable to self-destructive behavior. This appears to be a particularly important factor in cluster suicides.

The strength of social supports is also important. It has been well documented that the strength and quality of these supports are important to the etiology of psychiatric problems, compliance with treatment, and response to therapeutic interventions. Finally, diseases with chronic and debilitating courses often precipitate self-destructive behavior. The prevalence of physical illness varies from 25% to 70% of suicides and appears to be an important factor in 11% to 51%. Among the disorders most often associated with suicide are cancer, Huntington's chorea, epilepsy, musculoskeletal disorders, peptic ulcer disease, and HIV/AIDS.

FAMILY HISTORY. A family history of suicide is a significant risk factor for self-destructive behavior. Explanations for this association include identification with and imitation of a family member who has committed suicide, family stress, and transmission of genetic factors. Families of suicide victims have a significantly higher rate of suicide than do families with members who are nonsuicidal but mentally ill. In addition, monozygotic twins have a higher concordance rate for suicide than dizygotic twins. It will be important to distinguish the contribution of a family history of suicide from a family history of affective disorder to better identify high-risk groups for clinical intervention.

BIOCHEMICAL FACTORS. There is growing evidence of an association between suicide or suicidal tendencies and a low level of the brain neurotransmitter serotonin (5HT). Recent interest in the role of 5HT levels and activity in suicide stems from two main areas of study: an increase in the understanding of abnormal serotonin transmission in the etiology of mental illness, particularly depression and schizophrenia; and a better appreciation that antidepressant drugs enhance the efficacy of serotonin. This suggests that 5HT must be in balance for adaptive emotional responses. This balance can be assessed by measuring the amounts of

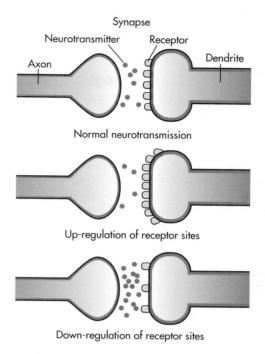

Fig. 20-4 Levels of postsynaptic serotonin (5HT) receptors. There are more receptors when there is too little serotonin (up-regulation) and fewer receptors when there is too much serotonin (down-regulation).

neurotransmitter produced, and the amount of its metabolites (the leftover products of neurotransmitter breakdown, or turnover). Thus, the amount of the metabolite for serotonin, 5HIAA, that can be measured in the blood and spinal fluid is an indication of the amount of serotonin originally available in the brain.

The brain also attempts to regulate or balance neurotransmitter levels in another way. The number of postsynaptic 5HT receptors in the brain is affected by the available levels of 5HT. There are more of these receptors if there is too little 5HT (up-regulation) and fewer of them if there is too much 5HT (down-regulation) (Fig. 20-4). Mood disorders are hypothesized to be the result of an imbalance or deficiency of neurotransmitters, particularly 5HT. Antidepressant drugs generally increase the amount or efficiency of 5HT, thus increasing the amount of metabolites and affecting the numbers of 5HT receptors.

Recently, several research studies have found that a deficiency in serotonin and its metabolite, 5HIAA, and an increase in one of the 5HT postsynaptic receptors ($5HT_{2A}$) are implicated in suicidal behavior.[17] For example, depressed patients with low serotonin levels have stronger suicidal tendencies than those with normal levels. Among people hospitalized for violent suicide attempts, those with low levels of 5HIAA in their spinal fluid are 10 times more likely to kill themselves within a year. Similarly, schizophrenic patients who have attempted suicide have significantly lower 5-HIAA concentrations than those who do not. In postmortem studies of the brains of suicide victims, researchers have discovered an excess of nerve receptors for serotonin, indicating a compensation in the brain for low levels of serotonin.[20] Finally, a combination of impulsive aggressiveness and feelings of hopelessness, associated with serotonin deficiency, is more common in men than in women. This may explain why men kill themselves much more often even though women have a higher rate of depression.

Because of the increased rate of suicide globally and the high suicide risk in psychiatric patients, it would be beneficial to be able to identify high-risk people for suicide prevention and treatment. Thus, in addition to demographic, psychosocial, personality, and behavioral indicators for suicide risk, a simple blood test that could provide an additional method for identifying those at greatest risk for suicide would be a significant advantage for the mental health field. Although there is currently no biological test that shows a differentiation between people who commit suicide and those who do not, there is a great deal of interest in finding such a biological marker for suicide.

 Do you believe suicide is a fundamental human right and should be allowed by society? Why or why not?

Precipitating Stressors

Self-destructive behavior may result from almost any stress the person feels as overwhelming. Stressors are somewhat individualized, as is the person's ability to tolerate stress. All self-destructive behaviors may be seen as attempts to escape from uncomfortable or intolerable life situations. Anxiety is therefore central to self-destructive behavior.

The anxiety associated with a deliberate attempt at self-destruction is overwhelming. It is difficult to imagine if it has not been experienced. Most people cringe from contemplating their own deaths, much less initiating self-destruction. Self-death is experienced differently from the death of another because self-death literally cannot be experienced. In a sense, those who destroy themselves actually destroy everything else but themselves.

In contrast, people engaged in gradual self-destructive behavior tend to deny their eventual deaths, usually believing that they can assume control at any time. This fantasy of control, although it alleviates anxiety, also helps to perpetuate the behavior. When the sense of self-worth is extremely low, self-destructive behavior reaches its peak. At this point, suicidal behavior is likely. Suicide implies a loss of the ability to value the self at all.

Appraisal of Stressors

Given the review of predisposing and precipitating factors in this chapter, it is evident that suicide prediction is not

Box **20-2** *Suicide Risk Factors*

PSYCHOSOCIAL
Hopelessness
Caucasian race
Male gender
Advanced age
Living alone
HISTORY
Prior suicide attempts
Family history of suicide attempts
Family history of substance abuse
DIAGNOSTIC
General medical illnesses
Psychosis
Substance abuse
Mood disorder

possible to any meaningful degree.[16] What is possible and essential is for the nurse to assess each patient for known suicidal risk factors (Box 20-2) and determine the meaning of each of these elements for potential suicidal behavior.[14]

Coping Resources

Patients with chronic, painful, or life-threatening illnesses may engage in self-destructive behavior. Often these people consciously choose to kill themselves. Quality of life becomes an issue that overrides quantity of life. An ethical dilemma may arise for nurses who become aware of the patient's choice to engage in this behavior. There are no easy answers to the question of how to resolve this conflict.[23] Nurses must do so according to their own belief system.

Self-destructive behavior may be related to many social and cultural factors. Durkheim,[15] in his pioneering study of suicidal behavior, identified three subcategories of suicide, based on the person's motivation:

▼ *Egoistic suicide* results from the person being poorly integrated into society.
▼ *Altruistic suicide* results from obedience to customs and habit.
▼ *Anomic suicide* results when society is unable to regulate the individual.

Durkheim believed the structure of society has a great influence on the individual. Society may either help or sustain individuals or lead them to self-destruction (see A Patient Speaks).

Social isolation may lead to loneliness and increase the person's vulnerability to suicide. People who are actively involved with others in their communities are more able to tolerate stress. Those who lose the ability to participate in social activities are more likely to turn to self-destructive behavior. Religious involvement is particularly supportive to many people during difficult times.

A Patient *Speaks*

The following are notes left by patients who committed suicide.

▼ *Please forgive me and please forget me. I'll always love you. All I have was yours. No one ever did more for me than you; oh please pray for me, please.*

▼ *To Whom It May Concern,*

I, Mary Smith, being of sound mind, do this day make my last will as follows: I bequeath my rings, diamond and black opal to my daughter-in-law, Doris Jones, and any other of my personal belongings she might wish. What money I have in my savings account and my checking account goes to my dear father, as he won't have me to help him. To my husband, Ed Smith, I leave my furniture and car.

▼ *I hate you and all of your family and I hope you never have peace of mind. I hope I haunt this house as long as you live here and I wish you all the bad luck in the world.*

▼ *Dear Daddy:*

Please don't grieve for me or feel that you did something wrong, you didn't. I'll leave this life loving you and remembering the world's greatest father.

I'm sorry to cause you more heartache, but the reason I can't live anymore is because I'm afraid. Afraid of facing my life alone without love. No one ever knew how alone I am. No one ever stood by me when I needed help. No one brushed away the tears I cried for "help" and no one heard. I love you Daddy, Jeannie. ▼

Are you surprised to learn that in North America more people die by suicide than by homicide? Do you think this fact requires a reallocation of social resources? If so, in what way?

Coping Mechanisms

A patient may use a variety of coping mechanisms to deal with self-destructive feelings, including denial, rationalization, and regression. In addition, the patient might display magical thinking. These coping mechanisms may stand between the person and self-destruction. They defend the person from strong emotional responses to life events that are a serious threat to the ego. If they are removed, underlying depression will become overt and may lead to suicidal behavior.

Suicidal behavior indicates the imminent failure of the coping mechanisms. A suicidal threat may be a last-ditch effort to get enough help to be able to cope. Completed suicide represents the total failure of adaptive coping mechanisms.

Nursing Diagnosis

When considering the nursing diagnosis of self-destructive behavior, the nurse must incorporate information about the seriousness and immediacy of the patient's harmful activity. The nurse must consider the information obtained in the assessment to identify accurately the patient's need for nursing intervention (Fig. 20-5). Validation of the nursing diagnosis with the patient is essential. However, denial is a prominent defense with most self-destructive disorders. The patient may not be able to agree with a statement that confronts this behavior. The primary concern is to communicate, through the diagnosis, the level of protection the patient needs. In the case of self-destructive behavior, caution is recommended in determining the level of risk. It is better to overestimate the patient's level of risk than to allow serious injury to occur.

Primary NANDA nursing diagnoses related to maladaptive self-protective responses are **risk for self-mutilation, noncompliance,** and **potential for self-directed violence.** Because of the nature of the disorders associated with self-destructive behavior, other nursing diagnoses are often applied in the care of these patients. Nursing diagnoses related to the range of possible maladaptive responses are listed in the Medical and Nursing Diagnoses box on p. 397. Examples of complete nursing diagnoses related to self-protective responses are presented in the Detailed Diagnoses box on p. 397.

Related Medical Diagnoses

Suicidal behavior is not identified as a separate diagnostic category in DSM-IV.[1] Several medical diagnostic classifications of the DSM-IV include actual or potential self-destructive behavior among their defining criteria. The medical diagnoses in which this behavior is listed as possible include bipolar disorder, major depression, noncompliance with treatment, schizophrenia, and substance use disorders. Their essential features are described in the Detailed Diagnoses box on p. 397.

Outcome Identification

The expected outcome when working with a patient with maladaptive self-protection responses is as follows:

The patient will not physically harm oneself.

Careful setting of priorities is necessary with the self-destructive patient. Highest priority should be given to preservation of life. The nurse must identify goals related to immediately life-threatening behavior. For example, the actively suicidal person must first be prevented from acting on impulses.

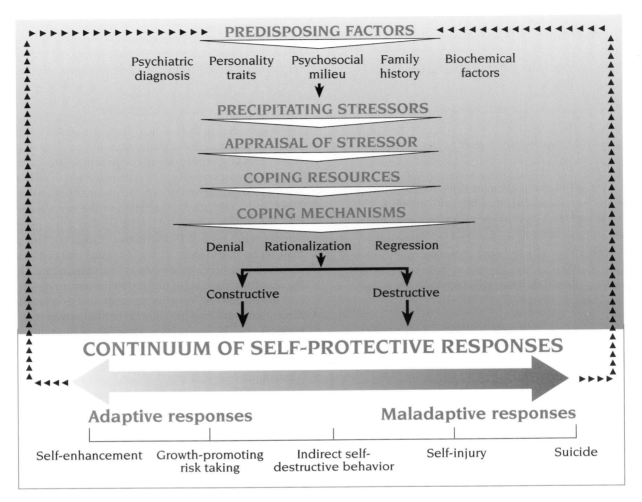

Fig. 20-5 The Stuart Stress Adaptation Model related to self-protective responses.

In dealing with self-destructive behavior, the nurse and the patient may appear to have incompatible goals. Suicidal patients may resist attempts to protect them and may actively try to evade their observers. However, most of these patients have some ambivalence. The nurse, in setting positive, life-preserving goals, is appealing to the healthy part of the person's self that wants to survive and be better able to cope with life. The very act of seeking help is an expression of this healthy aspect of the personality. The positive attitude of the nurse in setting constructive goals conveys a sense of hope to a patient who may be feeling hopeless. Communicating hope is often the most therapeutic element in any nursing intervention with a suicidal patient.

Planning

The nursing care plan for the person with self-destructive behavior must focus first on protecting the patient from harm. In addition, the plan must address the factors that contributed to the patient's dangerous behavior. Later, the nurse can

attend to the development of insight into the suicidal behavior and substitution of healthy coping mechanisms.

Suicidal patients can be treated in a variety of settings. The decision about which setting is most appropriate for a given patient is based on the assessment of risk (Fig. 20-6).[19] The first issue is how ambivalent or resolute the patient is. People who seem very intent and have a specific plan for action should be admitted to an inpatient setting where they can be monitored closely. Another important factor in determining the treatment setting is the patient's judgment. Anything that impairs a patient's judgment and rational decision-making capacity greatly increases the risk of a suicide attempt and is a good indication for inpatient treatment. A final issue is the availability of a responsible family member or close friend willing to stay with the patient through the immediate crisis until the suicidal ideation abates. Sometimes this may require several family members taking shifts and watching the patient around the clock. In the final analysis, however, the safety of the patient is the top priority.

MEDICAL AND NURSING DIAGNOSES *related to* **Self-protective Responses**

Related Medical Diagnoses (DSM-IV)*	Related Nursing Diagnoses (NANDA)†
Bipolar disorder	Adjustment, impaired
Major depressive disorder	Anxiety
Noncompliance with treatment	Body image disturbance
Schizophrenia	Coping, family, ineffective: compromised
Substance use disorders	Coping, ineffective individual
	Denial, ineffective
	Risk for self-mutilation‡
	Noncompliance‡
	Self-esteem disturbance
	Spiritual distress
	Violence, potential for‡

*From American Psychiatric Association: *Diagnostic and statistical manual of mental disorders,* ed 4, Washington, DC, 1994, The Association.
†From North American Nursing Diagnosis Association: *NANDA nursing diagnoses: definitions and classifications 1997-1998,* Philadelphia, 1997, The Association.
‡Primary nursing diagnosis for self-destructive behavior.

 DETAILED DIAGNOSES *related to* **Self-protective Responses**

NANDA

Diagnosis Stem	Examples of Complete Diagnosis
Risk for self-mutilation	Risk for self-mutilation related to feelings of tension and worthlessness, as evidenced by cutting of arms and legs
	Risk for self-mutilation related to command hallucinations, as evidenced by dissection of calf
Noncompliance	Noncompliance with taking antihypertensive medication related to asymptomatic behavior, as evidenced by unchanged elevation of blood pressure
	Noncompliance with 1800-calorie-per-day diabetic diet related to denial of illness, as evidenced by gain of 10 pounds since last clinic visit
Potential for self-directed violence	Potential for self-directed violence related to loss of spouse, as evidenced by purchase of a gun and discussions of death
	Potential for self-directed violence related to phencyclidine (PCP) abuse, as evidenced by extreme psychotic disorganization and lack of body boundaries

DSM-IV Diagnosis	Essential Features*
Bipolar disorder	Presence of a manic episode and no past depressive episodes (see Chapter 19 for details)
Major depressive disorder	The presence of at least five symptoms nearly every day during the same 2-week period, with one being either depressed mood or loss of interest or pleasure (see Chapter 19 for details)
Noncompliance with treatment	Noncompliance with an important aspect of the treatment for a mental disorder or a general medical condition
Schizophrenia	Presence of two or more of the following symptoms for a 1-month period: delusions, hallucinations, disorganized speech, disorganized behavior, negative symptoms (see Chapter 21 for details)
Substance use disorders	Presence of substance dependence or substance abuse (see Chapter 24 for details)

*Modified from the American Psychiatric Association: *Diagnostic and statistical manual of mental disorders,* ed 4, Washington, DC, 1994, The Association.

Implementation

Common elements exist in nursing intervention with all patients who exhibit self-destructive behavior. First, nurses must consider their own responses to people who are trying to harm themselves. It can be difficult for a person who is happy and involved in life to imagine the depth of despair that leads to suicidal impulses or the lack of caring for the self that results in physically, psychologically, and socially damaging behavior, even if not immediately lethal. On the other hand, nurses who are depressed and dissatisfied with their own life may be threatened by interacting with patients who are more upset because they may fear similar consequences for themselves. These nurses may also overidentify

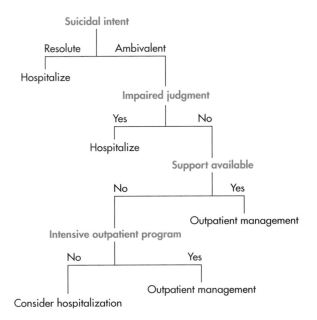

Fig. 20-6 Decision tree to determine treatment setting.

with the patient, which limits their ability to help. A therapeutic approach is empathic and nonjudgmental, with subjective responses limited by awareness of one's own attitudes.

All possible efforts must be made to protect patients and to motivate them to choose life. Nurses should align themselves with the patients' wish to live and then help them to be responsible for their own behavior. However, nurses must also understand that some patients will choose death despite their best efforts to intervene. Nurses must therefore develop a realistic understanding of the patient's responsibility for his or her own life and accept the possibility of losing a suicidal patient even with the best nursing care.

> *A friend tells you that suicidal patients are intent on dying and will ultimately succeed despite all intervention. How would you respond?*

Protection

The highest priority nursing activity with self-destructive patients is to protect them from inflicting further harm on themselves and, if suicidal, from killing themselves. The message of protection is conveyed to patients verbally and nonverbally.

Verbally, patients are informed of the nurse's intention not to allow harm to come to them. The nurse might say, "I understand that you are feeling impulses to harm yourself. I will be here with you to help you control those impulses. I will do whatever is necessary to protect you. I'd like to talk with you about how you are feeling whenever you are able to share that with me."

The nonverbal communication should reinforce and agree with the verbal. Obviously, dangerous objects such as belts, sharp implements, glass, and matches should be taken from the suicidal patient. It is impossible to make an environment perfectly safe. Even walls and floors can cause injury if patients throw themselves against them. However, the removal of dangerous objects gives a message of concern. One-to-one observation of the suicidal patient also communicates caring. This observation should be carried out sensitively, with the nurse neither hovering over nor remaining aloof from the patient. The patient's nonverbal cues can guide the one-to-one interaction. It is important to remain alert until the mental health team and the patient agree that the self-destructive crisis is over. Suicidal patients may appear to be feeling much better immediately before making an attempt. This is attributed to the feeling of relief experienced when the decision has been made and the plans finalized. Nurses have been fooled by this behavior pattern, relaxing their vigilance, only to have patients kill themselves when they are allowed to be alone for a moment.

Contracting for Safety

An important aspect of protecting the patient involves coming to an agreement about the nature of the therapeutic relationship. This can involve the use of contracts in which the patient agrees not to inflict self-harm for a specified period of time. The patient further agrees to contact the clinician if he or she is tempted to act on self-destructive impulses. The patient also agrees to give away any possibly lethal articles such as guns or pills. Hospitalization is indicated if the patient is not willing to agree to these terms. Outpatients and clinicians need names and telephone numbers to cover any emergencies. Finally, supportive others should be involved in the contracting process. Families and friends are important allies in caring for a suicidal patient.

After a trustworthy contract has been made, the nurse can take some additional steps to ensure the patient's safety. First, the patient should be supervised at all times. The patient should never be left alone. Second, the nurse can monitor any medications the patient receives. For example, many antidepressants are fatal in overdose. This suggests that the patient should have only a few days' supply if treated as an outpatient. The nurse should note that tricyclic antidepressants are associated with a higher rate of death in the event of overdose than the newer SSRI antidepressants, and that the benzodiazepines may disinhibit a patient, resulting in less control over self-destructive impulses (see Chapter 27).

> *Your depressed patient has been prescribed a tricyclic antidepressant because it is less expensive than other antidepressants. However, she lives in a rural area and cannot have the prescription filled every few days. You are worried about potential overdose. What alternatives can you identify?*

Increasing Self-esteem

Self-destructive people have low self-esteem. The nurse may intervene by treating the patient as someone deserving attention and concern. Positive attributes of the patient should be recognized with genuine praise. An attempt to make up reasons to praise the patient is usually recognized as artificial and lowers the patient's self-esteem. The message is that the patient is so bad that one has to search for positive characteristics. When getting to know the patient, the nurse should be alert to strengths that can be built on to provide the patient with positive experiences. It is also important to reinforce reasons for living and promote the patient's realistic expectations. Chapter 18 describes interventions the nurse can use to enhance a patient's self-esteem.

Regulating Emotions and Behaviors

Nursing care should also be directed toward helping patients become aware of their feelings, label them, and express them appropriately. Anger is often a difficult feeling for these patients. The angry patient must be helped to deal constructively with anger through anger management skills. These are described in Chapter 29. Anxiety can also be overwhelming. Chapter 16 discusses anxiety-reducing interventions.

It may be helpful to assist patients with self-destructive responses to explore the predisposing and precipitating factors influencing their behavior. Once the acute crisis is over, the nurse can help the patient understand high-risk times and triggers, the feelings that are stimulated, dysfunctional thinking patterns, and resultant maladaptive coping responses. Plans can then be made to test out new coping mechanisms. For instance, during times of stress, the patient can[21]:

▼ Increase involvement with others
▼ Initiate a physical activity
▼ Engage in relaxation and tension-reducing activities
▼ Process feelings by talking with someone or writing in a journal

These and other examples of cognitive behavioral strategies are described in Chapter 30.

Mobilizing Social Support

Self-destructive behavior often reflects a lack of internal and external resources. Mobilization of social support systems is an important aspect of nursing intervention. Significant others probably have many feelings about the patient's self-destructive behavior. They need an opportunity to express their feelings and make realistic plans for the future. Family members must be made aware of control issues and helped to encourage self-control by the patient. Both the patient and the family may need help to see that caring can be expressed by fostering self-care, as well as by providing care. Families of suicidal patients may be frightened of future suicidal activity. They need to be aware of behavioral clues to suicide and of community resources that can help with crises. Suicidal behavior often recurs. False reassurance should be avoided. A better approach is to foster improved

communication and an ability to cope in the family. The nurse may help people sort out their feelings and may want to refer significant others for individual intervention or family therapy.

If a patient commits suicide, it is important to intervene with the survivors, who may be at risk for suicidal behavior.[9] They need someone who can listen to them and let them know that their feelings are not abnormal. They need to be able to discuss their beliefs about why the death occurred and helped to find some meaning in the experience. Family members should be encouraged to support one another. Survivors are often stigmatized and may need assistance in dealing with this.

Community resources may also be important for the long-term care of the self-destructive person. Self-help groups may provide the recovering patient with needed peer support. Family therapy may help in the reintegration of a family group that has been disrupted by the patient's recent experiences. Public health nurses, clergy, and other community-based helping people can provide the patient and family with day-to-day support. The nurse may be active in explaining resources to the patient and initiating referrals to other agencies.

Patient Education

Patient education is another important aspect of nursing intervention. Education must be timed carefully. Patient readiness is essential if behavior change is to result. Patients who are noncompliant with prescribed health-care regimens may not understand the nature of their problem. The nurse should assess the patient's knowledge and initiate appropriate teaching. A Patient Education Plan for a patient who is noncompliant with medical treatment is presented on p. 400. Many patients are willing to participate in self-care if it makes sense to them. Teaching ways to monitor health status may also be helpful. For example, if hypertensive patients learn to check their blood pressure, they can learn to associate their health care activities with their physiological response.

Patients following medication regimens, such as psychotropic medication for the previously suicidal patient, should know the prescribed dosage, frequency, and side effects. Information about how to handle any future crises should be provided to the patient. If the nurse has explained the possible reason for the patient's behavior, this may be reinforced at termination of the relationship to help the patient integrate the experience into his or her self-concept. Helping a patient to work through self-destructive behavior can be an extremely rewarding aspect of psychiatric nursing.

Suicide Prevention

Finally, nurses need to be aware of several important strategies that may help to prevent suicide. These are listed in Box 20-3. Educational measures and suicide curricula in schools are other helpful interventions. These programs try to break down taboos about suicide and describe the symp-

PATIENT EDUCATION PLAN   Compliance Counseling

Content	Instructional Activities	Evaluation
Assess patient's knowledge of self-care activities.	Ask patient to describe usual diet, exercise, and medication patterns.	Patient describes usual behavior.
	Validate whether described behaviors match self-care instruction received in the past.	Patient repeats directions.
Identify areas in which patient behavior differs from healthy self-care practices.	Describe healthy self-care behavior to patient, provide written patient education materials, encourage patient to describe reasons for not performing recommended self-care.	Patient discusses compliance problems.
Discuss alternative approaches to self-care	Help patient to identify alternative self-care behaviors that would be more acceptable. Enable patient to talk about feelings related to illness and treatment regimen.	Patient decides on different approach and shares feelings related to illness.
Agree on a reward for compliant behavior	Ask patient what reward he or she would choose for taking good care of him- or herself.	Patient identifies reward.
Reinforcement.	Praise patient for making a commitment to a healthier lifestyle.	Patient recognizes renewed commitment to self-care.

Box **20-3** *Suicide Prevention Strategies*

> Gun control and decreased availability of lethal weapons
> Limitations on the sale and availability of alcohol and drugs
> Increased public and professional awareness about depression and suicide
> Less attention and reinforcement of suicidal behavior in the media
> Establishment of community-based crisis intervention clinics
> Campaigns to decrease the stigma associated with psychiatric care
> Increased insurance benefits for psychiatric and substance abuse disorders

toms of depression to students, teachers, and parents.[18,24] The development of prevention clinics in communities may be helpful. Such clinics might offer expert clinical assessment and treatment combined with strong community links, increased social supports, family education, and hotlines staffed with mental health professionals. Another effective suicide prevention strategy is telephone services to the elderly that provide home assistance, need assessment, and emotional support.[13] In addition, education of the public and health-care providers is needed to increase knowledge about the early warning signs of self-destructive behavior and implement effective treatment strategies. A Nursing Treatment Plan Summary for patients with maladaptive self-protective responses is presented at right.

Evaluation

Evaluation of the nursing care of the self-destructive patient requires careful daily monitoring of the patient's behavior.

Patient involvement in evaluation of their progress can provide reinforcement and an incentive to work toward a goal. Modifications of the care plan are often necessary as patients reveal more of themselves and their needs to the nurse. As soon as possible, patients should participate in the planning, evaluation, and modification process.

Unfortunately, self-destructive behavior tends to recur. Nurses sometimes become discouraged and angry with patients who return again and again with the same behavior. When this occurs, nurses may be caught in the trap of feeling responsible for patient behavior. Nurses who have given the best nursing care possible have done as much as they can for the patient. It is impossible to change the total life situation for the patient. The nurse can only help to identify alternative behaviors and provide encouragement for change. If the patient returns, the nursing process must begin again with an attitude of hope that this time the patient will learn and grow more and be better able to live a satisfying life.

A final issue related to suicidal behavior is the impact of a completed suicide on the clinical staff. Psychiatric nurses will inevitably experience a patient suicide. When a patient commits suicide, staff response can split the interdisciplinary treatment team. Thus interventions must be aimed not only at helping the individual clinician heal, but also at preserving the integrity of the treatment team. The following activities can help this process[5]:

▼ Have an immediate review of the event by the treatment team to acknowledge feelings, and plan care for the other patients.

▼ Hold a patient community meeting to help patients accept the reality of the loss.

▼ Call an additional meeting of the treatment team 2-3 days after the suicide to further process the suicide.

NURSING TREATMENT PLAN *Summary*   Maladaptive Self-protective Responses

Nursing Diagnosis: Potential for self-directed violence
Expected Outcome: The patient will not physically harm him- or herself.

Short-term Goal	Intervention	Rationale
The patient will not engage in self-injury activities.	Observe closely. Remove harmful objects. Provide a safe environment. Provide for basic physiological needs. Contract for safety if appropriate. Monitor medications.	Highest priority is given to life-saving patient care activities. The patient's behavior must be supervised until self-control is adequate for safety.
The patient will identify positive aspects of oneself.	Identify patient's strengths. Encourage the patient to participate in activities that he or she likes and does well. Encourage good hygiene and grooming. Foster healthy interpersonal relationships.	Self-destructive behavior reflects underlying depression related to low self-esteem and anger directed inward.
The patient will implement two adaptive self-protective responses.	Facilitate the awareness, labeling, and expression of feelings. Help the patient to recognize unhealthy coping mechanisms. Identify alternative means of coping. Reward healthy coping behaviors.	Maladaptive coping mechanisms must be replaced with healthy ones to manage stress and anxiety.
The patient will identify two social support resources that can be helpful.	Help significant others to communicate constructively with the patient. Promote healthy family relationships. Identify relevant community resources. Initiate referrals to community resources.	Social isolation leads to low self-esteem and depression, perpetuating self-destructive behavior.
The patient will be able to describe the treatment plan and its rationale.	Involve patient and significant others in care planning. Explain characteristics of identified health-care needs, nursing care needs, medical diagnosis, and recommended treatment and medications. Elicit response to nursing care plan. Modify plan based on patient feedback.	Understanding of and participation in health-care planning enhance compliance.

▼ Conduct an in-house memorial service to facilitate grieving.

▼ Participate in a continuous quality improvement critical incident review to help staff understand the suicide and objectively review the treatment.

▼ Identify opportunities for continuous process improvement.

▼ Acknowledge anniversary reactions.

If a variety of these activities are provided for the healing of other patients and the treatment team, recovery can occur and growth result.

Summary

1. The continuum of self-protective responses ranges from the most adaptive state of self-enhancement to the maladaptive responses of indirect self-destructive behavior, self-injury, and suicide.

2. Self-destructive behaviors may range from subtle to overt and include noncompliance with medical treatment plan, self-injury, and suicidal behavior.

3. Predisposing factors affecting self-protective responses include psychiatric diagnosis, personality traits, psychosocial milieu, family history, and biochemical factors. Precipitating stressors may be any stress the person perceives as overwhelming.

4. Coping resources focus on social support systems, and coping mechanisms may include denial, rationalization, and regression.

5. Primary nursing diagnoses are high risk for self-mutilation, noncompliance, and potential for self-directed violence.

6. Suicide is not identified as a separate diagnostic category in the DSM-IV. Medical diagnostic classifications of the DSM-IV that include actual or potential self-destructive behavior are bipolar disorder, major depression, schizophrenia, and substance use disorder.

7. The expected outcome of nursing care is that the patient will not physically harm him- or herself.

8. Nursing interventions include protecting the patient, contracting for safety, increasing self-esteem, regulating emotions and behaviors, mobilizing social support, educating the patient, and preventing suicide.

9. Evaluating nursing care requires daily monitoring of the patient's behavior. The nurse must not become discouraged if self-destructive behavior recurs, but approach the patient with the hope that this time the patient will grow and be better able to live a satisfying life.

COMPETENT CARING Clinical Exemplar of a Psychiatric Nurse

Philip Macaione, BS, RN

After 18 years of acute care nursing practice with a specialty in ICU, ER, and trauma nursing, I sought a new challenge and began psychiatric nursing practice. Having had the opportunity to associate professionally with hundreds of patients over the years who were experiencing critical and life-threatening situations, I felt well equipped to deal with psychiatric emergencies, until that seemingly routine day shift on an inpatient adult unit.

Ms. W had been committed to our unit as a dual-diagnosis patient. She was referred from our county emergency room. She had been found near-stuporous, wandering the city streets, and was thought to be homeless. She was addicted to heroin, cocaine, and alcohol. She also suffered from multiple personality disorder, anxiety disorder, major depression, and schizotypical disorder. She was 6′2″ and weighed more than 300 pounds. Her hospital course over the previous 2 weeks was highlighted by her continued acting-out behaviors. These included disrupting the milieu, verbal, physical, and sexual threats to others, seeking the medication of other patients, noncompliance with her treatment plan, and defiance of unit rules and policies. Needless to say, she was a nursing challenge and required a firm, consistent approach by the staff and a constant vigil over her behavior.

One morning her behavior deteriorated to the point where staff intervened by placing her in scrubs and escorting her to the seclusion room to maintain her safety and that of the other patients. I explained to her that during this time out I would help her to begin processing her behavior and identify more effective coping strategies. I gave her a PRN medication for her agitation and anxiety and suggested that she begin writing her thoughts and feelings down in her journal. After about a half hour, she verbally contracted for safety, seemed aware of her actions, and was resting quietly on her mattress. She also said that she was "feeling much better now" and thanked me for my help. I decided to put her on 15-minute checks but leave her in open-door seclusion until we agreed that she was ready to return to the milieu. I remember thinking, "Wow, I did a good job with this patient, and she is really making progress."

After years of nursing practice I notice that I have developed a sixth sense when I feel that something is just not right. On the surface Ms. W seemed to be in control, but my sixth sense drew me back to the seclusion room only minutes after I had left her. As I walked into the room I did a double take and thought to myself, "This can't be happening." Unfortunately, it was. Ms. W had managed, in the moments that had elapsed since I had left her side, to tear up her journal into small pieces, place the scraps between her legs, and ignite them with a cigarette lighter we later discovered she had hidden in her vagina. She was madly waving the fire between her legs to produce more flames. Her scrub pants and mattress were now on fire.

At this point I just reacted. I ran to her, pulled away the mattress, patted down the flames on her pants, and yelled for help. The smoke alarm had gone off, and within seconds other staff arrived. I instructed them to remove the patient to the corridor and give her first aid. This was no easy task given the patient's size and level of agitation. I then activated the fire procedure, grabbed the fire extinguisher, and returned to the seclusion room. By now the smoke was thick, but I pulled the pin of the fire extinguisher, aimed, and released the foam. Within seconds, the fire was extinguished. The fire department had now arrived and moved in to deal with the smoldering mattress. Ms. W suffered no injuries and was discharged to a boarding house about 1 week later.

I learned a great deal from this incident and think I am a better nurse because of it. The staff response and teamwork in reacting to this crisis were extraordinary. I also think that the many years of critical decision-making opportunities afforded me throughout my nursing practice made me well equipped to handle this seemingly routine shift on our unit. Most of all, I have a greater appreciation and respect for the sixth sense of nurses, which may be the mark of truly competent nursing care.

Chapter Review Questions

1. Identify whether the following statements are true (T) or false (F).

A. _F._ Suicide rates are highest for adolescent males.

B. _T._ The most prominent behavior associated with noncompliance is refusal to admit the seriousness of the health problem.

C. _F._ A suicide gesture is an attention-seeking behavior and should not be reinforced by focusing on it.

D. _T._ Physical diseases with chronic and debilitating courses often precipitate self-destructive behavior.

E. _T._ There is currently no biological test that is an accurate predictor of suicide.

F. _F._ The newer SSRI antidepressant medications have a higher rate of death by overdose than the older tricyclics.

2. Fill in the blanks.

A. The retrospective review of a person's behavior in the time preceding the suicide is called the _psych. autopsy_

B. The psychiatric disorders that put people at particular risk for suicide are _mood disorders_, _substance abuse_, and _schizophrenia_

C. Mood disorders are hypothesized to be the result of an imbalance or deficiency of neurotransmitters, particularly _serotonin_.

D. _communicating hope_ is often the most therapeutic element in any nursing intervention with a suicidal patient.

E. The three personality traits most closely associated with increased risk of suicide are _hostility_, _impulsivity_, and _depression_.

F. When a patient agrees not to inflict self-harm for a specified period of time it is called _contracting for safety_

3. Provide short answers for the following questions.

A. It has been observed that patients often act less depressed and seem to be in better spirits immediately before attempting suicide. Explain the reason for this behavior.

B. Identify the five factors to assess in the self-destructive patient.

C. Describe how you would determine the best treatment setting for a patient expressing suicidal thoughts.

D. There is currently much discussion about the wisdom and the ethics of assisted suicide. Discuss your position on this subject, first as a consumer of health care and then as a nurse.

References

1. American Psychiatric Association: *Diagnostic and statistic manual of mental disorders,* ed 4, Washington, DC, 1994, The Association.
2. Beautrais A et al: Prevalence and comorbidity of mental disorders in persons making serious suicide attempts: a case-control study, *Am J Psychiatry* 153:1009, 1996.
3. Beck A, Steer R, Beck J, Newman C: Hopelessness, depression, suicidal ideation, and clinical diagnosis of depression, *Suicide Life Threat Behav* 23:139, 1993.
4. Brent D et al: Psychiatric risk factors for adolescent suicide: a case-control study, *J Am Acad Child Adolesc Psychiatry* 32:521, 1993.
5. Bultema J: Healing process for the multidisciplinary team: recovering post-inpatient suicide, *J Psychosoc Nurs* 32:19, 1994.
6. Caldwell C, Gottesman I: Schizophrenia—a high-risk factor for suicide: clues to risk reduction, *Suicide Life Threat Behav* 22:479, 1992.
7. Cardell R, Horton-Deutsch S: A model for assessment of inpatient suicide potential, *Arch Psychiatr Nurs* 8:366, 1994.
8. Chiles J, Strohsall K: *The suicidal patient: principles of assessment, treatment, and case management,* Washington, DC, 1995, American Psychiatric Press.
9. Constantino R, Bricker P: Nursing postvention for spousal survivors of suicide, *Issues Ment Health Nurs* 17:131, 1996.

10. Conwell Y et al: Relationships of age and axis I diagnoses in victims of completed suicide: a psychological autopsy study, *Am J Psychiatry* 153:1001, 1996.

11. Coombs D et al: Presuicide attempt communications between parasuicides and consulted caregivers, *Suicide Life Threat Behav* 22:289, 1992.

12. Cooper C: Psychiatric stress debriefing, *J Psychosoc Nurs* 33:21, 1995.

13. DeLeo D, Carollo G, Dello Buono M: Lower rates associated with a tele-help/tele-check service for the elderly at home, *Am J Psychiatry* 152:632, 1995.

14. Depression Guideline Panel: *Depression in primary care: detection, diagnosis, and treatment: quick reference guide for clinicians,* no 5, Rockville, Md, 1993, US Department of Health and Human Services, Public Health Service, Agency for Health Care Policy and Research.

15. Durkheim E: *Suicide,* New York, 1951, The Free Press.

16. Hughes D: Can the clinician predict suicide? *Psychiatr Serv* 46:449, 1995.

17. Mann J, Arango V: Integration of neurobiology and psychopathology in a unified model of suicidal behavior, *J Clin Psychopharmacol* 12:2S, 1992.

18. Orbach I, Bar-Joseph H: The impact of a suicide prevention program for adolescents on suicidal tendencies, hopelessness, ego identity, and coping, *Suicide Life Threat Behav* 23:120, 1993.

19. Oxley S, Meter S: The assessment and management of the suicidal patient, *J Pract Psych Behav Health* 1:327, 1996.

20. Pandy G, Pandy S, Dwivedi Y: Platelet serotonin-2A receptors: a potential biological marker for suicidal behavior, *Am J Psychiatry* 152:850, 1995.

21. Pawlicki C, Gaumer C: Nursing care of the self-mutilating patient, *Bull Menninger Clin* 57:380, 1993.

22. Rich C et al: Suicide, stressors, and the life cycle, *Am J Psychiatry* 148:524, 1991.

23. Rosenbluth M, Kleinman I, Lowy F: Suicide: the interaction of clinical and ethical issues, *Psychiatr Serv* 46:919, 1995.

24. Shaffer D: Preventing suicide in young people, *Innovations Res* 2:3, 1993.

25. Skoog I et al: Suicidal feelings in a population sample of nondemented 85-year-olds, *Am J Psychiatry* 153:1015, 1996.

26. Winchel R, Stanley M: Self-injurious behavior: a review of the behavior and biology of self-mutilation, *Am J Psychiatry* 148:306, 1991.

ANNOTATED SUGGESTED READINGS

*Barstow D: Self-injury and self-mutilation, *J Psychosoc Nurs* 33:19, 1995.
    Describes behaviors, functions, staff responses, and treatment approaches to this difficult patient population.

*Bultema J: Healing process for the multidisciplinary team: recovering post-inpatient suicide, *J Psychosoc Nurs* 32:19, 1994.
    Excellent discussion of ways to help the staff heal after a completed suicide in an inpatient unit.

Canetto S: Gender and suicide in the elderly, *Suicide Life Threat Behav* 22:80, 1992.
    Thought-provoking discussion of why elderly women are less likely to be suicidal than men. Integrates sociocultural aspects of suicidal behavior and suggestions for prevention.

*Cardell R, Horton-Deutsch S: A model for assessment of inpatient suicide potential, *Arch Psychiatr Nurs* 8:366, 1994.
    Describes a comprehensive nursing model for exploring factors that play a role in inpatient suicide.

Chiles J, Strohsall K: *The suicidal patient: principles of assessment, treatment, and case management,* Washington, DC, 1995, American Psychiatric Press.
    One of the most comprehensive texts on the many aspects of suicide.

*Cugino A et al: Searching for a pattern: repeat suicide attempts, *J Psychosoc Nurs* 30:23, 1992.
    Reports on nursing research examining repeat suicide attempters.

*Egan M et al: The "no suicide contract": helpful or harmful? *J Psychosoc Nurs* 35:31, 1997.
    Challenging article that explores the theoretical underpinnings of patient contracting to determine its usefulness to psychiatric nursing practice. Concludes that more research is needed in this area.

*Faye P: Addictive characteristics of the behavior of self-mutilation, *J Psychosoc Nurs* 33:36, 1995.
    Presents explanations of addictive behavior related to self-mutilation and considerations for successful nursing interventions.

*Green J, Grindel C: Supervision of suicidal patients in adult inpatient psychiatric units in general hospitals, *Psychiatr Serv* 47:859, 1996.
    Excellent example of nursing research examining the use of various levels of supervision for suicidal patients, the advantages and disadvantages of these interventions and the issues of cost and reimbursement for the services.

*Loughrey L et al: Patient self-mutilation: when nursing becomes a nightmare, *J Psychosocial Nurs* 35:30, 1997.
    Makes a case that staff members who manage the patient who wounds himself have a need for administrative support, education, and counseling to relieve guilt, conflict, and stress.

*Neville D, Barnes S: The suicidal phone call, *J Psychosoc Nurs* 23:14, 1985.
    Classic article that discusses issues related to interacting with a suicidal person on the telephone, recommending information that should be collected and helpful and unhelpful responses.

*Pawlicki C, Gaumer C: Nursing care of the self-mutilating patient, *Bull Menninger Clinic* 57:380, 1993.
    Excellent summary of nursing interventions for working with patients who self-mutilate. Clear and practical.

*Rickelman B, Houfek J: Toward an interactional model of suicidal behaviors: cognitive rigidity, attributional style, stress, hopelessness and depression, *Arch Psychiatr Nurs* 9:158, 1995.
    Explores major theoretical and research findings for model development. Includes nursing interventions and implications for nursing research.

Werth J: *Rational suicide? Implications for mental health professionals,* New York, 1996, Taylor & Francis.
    Assumes the point of view that it is possible to make a rational decision to commit suicide. Controversial and stimulating reading.

*Nursing reference.

© 1998 M.C. Escher/Cordon Art, Baarn, Holland.

Neurobiological Responses and Schizophrenia and Psychotic Disorders

Mary D. Moller and Millene F. Murphy

How do I get away Away from you—voices? How do I leave you behind me forever? You who echo my feelings haunt my thoughts and ravage my nights . . . How do I get away from you? I sing at the top of my voice and still I hear you. I talk loud and listen to people and still I hear you. Is there a me without you? No, the answer comes loud and clear, there is no me without you. As long as I have feelings you will be my echo. As long as I have thoughts you will be the ghost. As long as there is night you will be in the darkness. **Sharon LeClaire**

LEARNING OBJECTIVES

After studying this chapter the student should be able to:

▼ Describe the continuum of adaptive and maladaptive neurobiological responses

▼ Discuss the prevalence of schizophrenia and other psychotic disorders

▼ Identify behaviors associated with maladaptive neurobiological responses

▼ Analyze predisposing factors, precipitating stressors, and appraisal of stressors related to maladaptive neurobiological responses

▼ Describe coping resources and coping mechanisms related to maladaptive neurobiological responses

▼ Formulate nursing diagnoses related to maladaptive neurobiological responses

▼ Assess the relationship between nursing diagnoses and medical diagnoses related to maladaptive neurobiological responses

▼ Identify expected outcomes and short-term nursing goals related to maladaptive neurobiological responses

▼ Develop a family education plan to promote adaptive neurobiological responses

▼ Analyze nursing interventions related to maladaptive neurobiological responses

▼ Evaluate nursing care related to maladaptive neurobiological responses

TOPICAL OUTLINE

Continuum of Neurobiological Responses
Assessment
  Behaviors
  Predisposing Factors
  Precipitating Stressors
  Appraisal of Stressors
  Coping Resources
  Coping Mechanisms
Nursing Diagnosis
  Related Medical Diagnoses
Outcome Identification
Planning
Implementation
  Interventions in the Crisis and Acute Phases
  Interventions in the Maintenance Phase
  Interventions in the Health Promotion Phase
Evaluation

Psychiatric nurses are often challenged when providing nursing care to patients with schizophrenia and other psychotic disorders. These are complex disorders and probably involve a number of syndromes. The behaviors associated with these disruptions in brain function are difficult to understand and sometimes frightening. Patients who experience psychoses are frightened by their experiences. They have difficulty forming close relationships because of the demands of the illness for their attention and energy. They tend to be alienated from society.[8] Caring nurses must strive to make contact with patients who are psychotic and help them toward wellness and rehabilitation. A Patient Speaks describes one person's experience with psychosis.

> **?** *Read the patient's description of psychosis a second time. Focus on identifying the feelings that might be associated with these experiences.*

CONTINUUM OF NEUROBIOLOGICAL RESPONSES

The symptoms of psychosis are clustered within five major categories of brain function: cognition, perception, emotion, behavior, and socialization, which is also called relational. Fig. 21-1 presents the continuum of responses related to neurobiological functioning.

Assessment

Schizophrenia is a serious and persistent brain disease. It is an illness that results in psychotic behavior, concrete thinking, and difficulties in processing information, interpersonal relationships, and problem solving.[2] Table 21-1 presents information on the impact of schizophrenia.

Behaviors

Attempts at defining psychosis are varied and often related to the theoretical orientation of the person who is making the definition. Typically, psychosis is defined within the context of a patient's perception of reality and the resulting behavior. This has led to a bias toward treatment focused on reorienting the person to the "correct" reality.

Schizophrenia is an illness that results in psychotic behavior. It is actually one of a group of related disorders that are heterogeneous in pathophysiology, predisposing factors, precipitating stressors, and related behaviors. Other psychotic disorders include schizophreniform disorder, schizoaffective disorder, delusional disorder, brief psychotic disorder, shared psychotic disorder (folie à deux), psychotic disorder due to a general medical condition, and substance-induced psychotic disorder.[1] In addition, psychosis is sometimes present in other disorders such as depression with psychotic features and manic episodes of bipolar disorder.

 A Patient *Speaks*

Psychosis is real. Its main feature is a loss of consciousness of the self in such a way that I can no longer discern my relationship to the reality that my body is in. This would not be destructive, except that I have done it inadvertently; I have done it without consciousness and have not provided for my body. My body, then, goes on without me. It wanders aimlessly and does not know to keep warm in the cold. It does not know how to avoid attack by violence. It does not know to protect itself from fire and deep water and the traffic that races down the highway.

My brain comes up with fantastical ideas about who I might be, since I am not there to tell it. Perhaps I am the Queen of Hearts, or a messenger from another planet, or even Jesus Christ himself. And why not? My brain distorts the reality of the senses: Is this burner hot, or cold? Is this coat wet or dry? Is this chair a chair, or, what exactly is this anyway, and for that matter, what in the world are you?

Maybe bugs are jumping out of my mind and onto that wall over there. Maybe there's a current coming up from the earth and into my feet and trying to pull me in. My brain can think of every kind of combination and definition, every kind of idea that it can put together, for it has a nearly infinite number of choices. It has all it has ever experienced, all the sounds, all the sights, all the sensations, all the dreams, all the fantasies, all the nightmares.

My brain chooses its manifestation according to what emotions were available to it when I was in charge. Only I am not there to add my discernment, my wisdom, and my awareness according to what I have learned. My brain goes haywire then. It has no person to guide it, no captain, no helm, and no rudder. It has no fingers at the keyboard. It wanders through its innerspace like the steel ball that is thrown into nothing and bounces at random from arbitrarily placed spots in the pinball machine.

What is this I, then, that is gone, and where did it go? It is consciousness. It is awareness. It is the presence of the I in me. It is ego. It is my separation. It is the part in me that tells me the difference between me and the world. It is the I-ness of me that holds me upright like a spine and says, "You will not fall into this tree, or this song, or this ocean of water or air, and it will not fall into you. The I that is gone is the intelligence that says I am me, and you are you." ▼

From Corday R: *Psychosis, the inner experience*, Boulder, Colo, 1991, Common Loon Productions.

CONTINUUM OF NEUROBIOLOGICAL RESPONSES

Adaptive responses		Maladaptive responses
Logical thought	Occasional distorted thought	Thought disorder/delusions
Accurate perceptions	Illusions	Hallucinations
Emotions consistent with experience	Emotional overreaction or underreaction	Difficulty processing emotions
Appropriate behavior	Odd or unusual behavior	Disorganized behavior
Social relatedness	Withdrawal	Social isolation

Fig. 21-1   Continuum of neurobiological responses.

TABLE **21-1** *Impact of Schizophrenia on the Individual and Society*

▼ About one in every 100 people suffers from schizophrenia, or 2.5 million Americans, regardless of race, ethnic group, or gender.

▼ In three out of four cases it begins between the ages of 17 and 25.

▼ 95% of people with schizophrenia have it for their lifetime.

▼ The annual cost of family caregiving and crime- and welfare-related expenditures due to schizophrenia is $33 billion in the United States.

▼ More than 75% of taxpayer dollars spent on treatment of mental illness are used for people with schizophrenia.

▼ People with schizophrenia occupy 25% of all inpatient hospital beds.

▼ An estimated one third to one half of homeless people in the United States have schizophrenia.

▼ Schizophrenia is ranked fourth worldwide in terms of burden of illness. The top three are unipolar depression, alcohol use, and bipolar disorder.

▼ Schizophrenia is a chronic illness, 5 times more common than multiple sclerosis, 6 times more common than insulin-dependent diabetes, 60 times more common than muscular dystrophy, and 80 times more common than Huntington's disease.

▼ Of patients with schizophrenia, 25% do not respond adequately to traditional antipsychotic medication.

▼ 20% to 50% of patients with schizophrenia attempt suicide; 10% succeed.

The word *schizophrenia* was introduced in 1911 by the Swiss psychiatrist Bleuler. He believed that the schizophrenias were multidimensional and organic in nature. He also believed that these illnesses were strongly influenced and could be shaped by psychological factors. The word *schizophrenia* is a combination of two Greek words, *schizein*, "to split," and *phren*, "mind." Bleuler's reference was not to a "split personality," which refers to separate identities, but to his belief that a split occurred between the cognitive and emotional aspects of the personality. Confusion about the meaning of the word *schizophrenia* continues to exist today.

COGNITION. **Cognition** is the act or process of knowing. It involves activities of awareness and judgment that enable the brain to process information in a way that ensures accuracy, storage, and retrieval. People with schizophrenia are sometimes unable to produce complex logical thoughts and express coherent sentences because the neurotransmissions traveling through the brain's malfunctioning information processing system are accelerated, delayed, or blocked. Behaviors related to problems in information processing associated with schizophrenia are often called cognitive deficits. They include problems with all aspects of memory, attention, form and organization of speech (formal thought disorder), decision making, and thought content (delusions) (Box 21-1).

Information processing depends on anatomical and neurophysiological brain processes as well as prior learning. It involves organizing sensory input into behavioral responses. Sensory input is screened according to the focus of the person's attention and ability to remember, learn, discriminate, interpret, and organize information (Fig. 21-2).

> **?** *Describe how your cognitive processing differs from that of a person of the opposite sex, an older generation, another race, and another socioeconomic class. What are the results of these differences?*

The information processing of people with schizophrenia may be altered by brain deficits. However, interferences with cognitive function often keep people with schizophrenia from realizing that their ideas and behavior are different

Box **21-1** *Problems in Cognitive Functioning*

MEMORY

Difficulty retrieving and using stored memory
Impaired short-term/long-term memory

ATTENTION

Difficulty maintaining attention
Poor concentration
Distractibility
Inability to use selective attention

FORM AND ORGANIZATION OF SPEECH (FORMAL THOUGHT DISORDER)

Loose associations
Tangentiality
Incoherence/word salad/neologism
Illogicality
Circumstantiality
Pressured/distractible speech
Poverty of speech

DECISION MAKING

Failure to abstract
Indecisiveness
Lack of insight
Impaired concept formation
Impaired judgment
Illogical thinking
Lack of planning and problem-solving skills
Difficulty initiating tasks

THOUGHT CONTENT

Delusions
    Paranoid
    Grandiose
    Religious
    Somatic
    Nihilistic
    Thought broadcasting
    Thought insertion
    Thought control

Fig. 21-2 Brain information processing model.

ferentiate symptoms from manipulative behavior, staff place restrictions on patients. When people with schizophrenia repeatedly ask the same question, such as what time it is or how to get somewhere, it is important for the nurse to provide the requested information in a kind and matter-of-fact manner that does not cause embarrassment or decrease the person's self-worth.

Attention is the ability to focus on one activity in a sustained, concentrated manner. Disrupted attention is an impairment in the ability to attend, observe, and concentrate on external reality. Disturbances in attention are common in schizophrenia and include difficulty completing tasks, difficulty concentrating on work, and easy distractibility. Easy distractibility refers to a patient's attention being drawn easily to irrelevant external stimuli such as noises, books out of order on a bookshelf, or people passing by. In addition, the patient who is experiencing auditory hallucinations often has problems with attention.

These impairments are not constant and often shift depending on the brain activity required. This generates much frustration for all involved, especially the patient, who often expresses frustration about inability to complete tasks because "my mind is always wandering." The nurse needs to be prepared to redirect the patient back to the task at hand. The nurse will also need to repeat directions often in short, simple phrases.

> **?** *The parents of a young man who has schizophrenia tell you that they are frustrated by their son's unwillingness to return to work. Based on your understanding of the cognitive disorders related to schizophrenia, how would you respond?*

Malfunctions in information processing produce other disturbances in thinking that interfere with coherent com-

from others. This is particularly evident in their self-perception of worth and abilities. They tend to dramatically overestimate or underestimate their own capability. Hospitalization is often viewed as a sign that others are trying to get rid of the person with schizophrenia. The increased brain dysfunction during an acute episode makes it difficult for the patient to realize his or her need for help.

Memory is the retention or storage of knowledge about the world. Additional information about memory and its assessment can be found in Chapters 5, 6, and 23. Memory problems associated with schizophrenia include forgetfulness, disinterest, and lack of compliance. It is critical for the nurse to understand the frustration this symptom causes for patients. They commonly seek validation of the correctness of task accomplishment, ask whether it is time to attend a group function or an appointment, and ask permission to make a telephone call just to verify whether they remember phone numbers. Often, because they fail to dif-

Box **21-2** *Form and Content of Speech Related to Psychotic Disorders*

LOOSE ASSOCIATIONS

Nurse: "Do you have enough money to buy that candy bar?"

Patient: "I have a real yen for chocolate. The Japanese have all the yen and have taken all our money and marked it. You know, you have to be careful of the Marxists because they are friends with the Swiss and they have all the cheese and all the watches and that means they have taken all the time. The worst thing about Swiss cheese is all the holes. People have to be careful about falling into holes."

Nurse: "It sounds like you are worried about your money."

Patient: "Yes, I have it all here in my wallet and you can't have it and the bank can't have it either."

INCOHERENCE

Nurse: "What does your family like to do at Christmas?"

Patient: "I believe they took Christmas from the Russians to get all the cars into the ocean and make jello. You could go and get the Christmas but you couldn't do it because the keylars have the fan."

TANGENTIALITY

Nurse: "I'm interested in learning more about your landscape paintings."

Patient: "My interest in art goes back to my parents who lived on a farm in Indiana. They had lots of haystacks, kind of like they do in Ohio, but you know, the hay is different colors in different states so that gave me the ability to paint so many different colors of yellow. Some people don't really like bright yellow hay, but I do. If I make the hay really bright yellow, then I make the barns a dull red, because barns really shouldn't be painted with bright red paint. Bright red should be saved for fire engines and fire hydrants and stop signs."

ILLOGICAL SPEECH

Nurse: "Do you think your medicine is helping you think more clearly?"

Patient: "I used to think my medicine helped me think. But I realized that it was me who took the medicine, so it wasn't the medicine that helped me think. Medicine can't think, don't you realize that? Maybe you should take some medicine to help you think better. But if you do, I would have to give it to you because it is the fact I took it myself that my thinking is better, so, no, I don't think the medicine is helping me think better."

DISTRACTIBLE SPEECH

Nurse: "I would like to talk with you about your understanding of schizophrenia."

Patient: "I know it's got something to do with my brain. What perfume are you wearing? It must be from France. Is that where that picture was taken? Your hair is different than when that picture was taken. Was that about 4 years ago?"

CLANG ASSOCIATIONS

Patient: "I got a new shirt but the buttons become loose. Do you suppose Lucifer's buttons become lucent or are they lucid like Lucy's lucky ducky?"

"I want to sing ping pong that song wong kong long today hey way."

POVERTY OF CONTENT OF SPEECH

Nurse: "Do you want to go to the grocery store?"

Patient: "Yeah, uh huh, well what would I do with the, uh, the stuff that is over there on top of it? Do they, uh, have the, the, you know, the thing to do it with the wheels on the floor. I, uh, guess they should let me."

---

munication. **Form and organization of speech** problems may include loose associations, word salad, tangentiality, illogicality, circumstantiality, pressure of speech, poverty of speech, distractible speech, and clanging. These behaviors are described in Chapter 6. Box 21-2 presents nurse-patient dialogues that reflect problems in the form and organization of speech related to psychotic disorders.

Recognizing that speech is a reflection of cognitive processing helps the nurse appreciate the considerable difficulties a person with schizophrenia has in communicating needs clearly. The nurse will need to focus attention and use active listening to understand the patient. The nurse who is making an honest attempt to identify and clarify what a patient wants does not need to be afraid of offending the patient by seeking to understand. It is essential to remember that the patient is sincerely trying to answer, no matter how difficult or bizarre the answer is. The nurse's responsibility is to identify one or two key verbal or nonverbal responses and seek validation. This is usually achieved through simple trial and error.

Decision making means arriving at a solution or making a choice. Components of decision making include insight, judgment, logic, decisiveness, planning, ability to carry out decisions, and abstract thought. Lack of insight is

probably one of the greatest problems in schizophrenia because patients generally do not believe that they are ill or different in any way. Unfortunately, many clinicians confuse lack of insight with denial and treat people who have schizophrenia as if their symptoms were willful and within conscious control.

Faulty logic is often identified through the speech of people with schizophrenia who display the behaviors of thought disorder. When there are cognitive deficits in decision making, the patient makes decisions based on erroneous inferences, yet cannot understand that the judgment was faulty. Other people with schizophrenia are simply unable to reach a decision. For them, life is difficult at best. They wrestle with even simple decisions such as which coffee cup to use. Plans based on faulty decision making do not serve the intended purpose. This symptom creates much of the frustration related to schizophrenia. Following through on decisions is also a problem for people who have schizophrenia. Often this is mistaken as loss of motivation. Motivation involves having a desire, not having the ability to follow through. People with schizophrenia typically have difficulty initiating tasks of any kind because of other problems related to components of decision making.

Concrete thinking typically replaces abstract thought in

schizophrenia, particularly during acute episodes. It is indicated by the absence of abstracting abilities and by several key indicators. Patients often have difficulty with multiple-stage commands. In other words, if the nurse approaches the patient and presents the daily schedule and gives directions about the time and place of group and occupational therapies, the information is not all processed and the brain perceives an overload. The patient will probably miss one or more of the directions.

Another example of concrete thinking is difficulty with time management. People with schizophrenia describe this behavior as "trying to tell time with clocks that have no minute or second hands." This is why patients often are late or miss events and appointments altogether. This may create fear in patients who have to be alone for long periods of time or are required to be places at specific times. Some patients have developed clever ways to determine time, such as getting watches with built-in alarms and monitoring certain television programs.

Difficulty managing money is another result of concrete thinking. People with schizophrenia often lose their ability to understand the concept of dollars and cents and are exploited by other people. A patient may agree to buy items without having enough money just because he sees some money in his wallet. He may not remember to pay for items he gets in a store or leave a restaurant without paying for the meal. Unfortunately, many nonhospitalized patients get into legal trouble because of this cognitive problem.

Literal interpretation of words and symbols is one of the most problematic behaviors related to concrete thinking. People with schizophrenia have difficulty abstracting the English language. Patients' descriptions of literal interpretation are presented in the following clinical examples.

"I was standing in the medication line and the nurse asked me to take my pills. So I took the medicine cup and held it in my hand. The nurse asked me again to take my pills and I didn't know what to do. She began to lose her patience as I stood there holding the medicine cup. She then told me to put the pills in my mouth and to swallow them with the water she handed me. I could follow each of the instructions and eventually 'took my pills.'"

An example of literal interpretation of symbols is described by this patient: "It took me at least 15 minutes to walk down the street because I stopped every time the light changed from green to red. I didn't understand that the traffic signal was only for cars."

Sometimes this problem advances to the point where the patient interprets a metaphor literally, as described in this example: "I remembered the expression 'step on a crack and break your mother's back.' One day I was walking down the street and stepped on a crack in the sidewalk. That same day my mother had fallen off a step stool after getting a can of soup from the kitchen cupboard and fractured two vertebrae in her back. For 9 months I believed that I had caused

this accident to happen." This is also called *magical thinking.*

Nursing implications regarding patient teaching for the person experiencing concrete thinking are profound. Consider this example: A nurse was instructed to collect a sterile urine specimen from a newly admitted male patient. The patient exhibited terror and strongly resisted. When the nurse gently asked him why he was so frightened, he replied, "I don't want to become sterile."

The role of the nurse is to help with decision making in a nonpunitive, supportive manner, recognizing that these symptoms represent neurological disabilities over which the patient has little control. The nurse functions in a rehabilitative role and needs to provide information as clearly and concretely as possible. The language used should involve simple words in short phrases that are easy to understand. The nurse also needs to seek validation regarding how instructions were heard to clarify confusion and misunderstanding.

> **?** *It is important to involve the patient in planning nursing care. Describe how you would accomplish this if the patient has cognitive problems that interfere with decision-making ability.*

Content of thought is the last problem in cognitive functioning and includes the presence of delusions. A delusion is a personal belief based on an incorrect inference of external reality. One of the mind's primary functions is to produce thoughts. Thoughts provide a sense of identity. They rarely begin as the logical product we consider a thought. Thoughts are produced as a result of intricate processes that involve screening and filtering internal and external stimuli and use multiple feedback loops in the brain. Recognizing the complexity of this process helps the nurse appreciate the unyielding way in which a person defends personal beliefs.

Recalling the cognitive deficits already described helps the nurse understand why people with schizophrenia sometimes have different beliefs from others. It is also important to realize that a delusion does not always last. It is common for a belief to be fixed for only a few weeks or few months, particularly in the less severe forms of schizophrenia. Many patients have reported the relief they experienced when they realized the belief was actually a delusion, just a symptom, not the actual truth.

The inability of the brain to process data accurately can result in paranoid, grandiose, religious, nihilistic, and somatic delusions. The delusions can be complicated further by thought withdrawal, thought insertion, thought control, or thought broadcasting. Types of delusions are described in Chapter 6.

Delusions represent an elaborate interplay between brain physiology, current environmental stimuli, and the person's frame of reference regarding the world. Delusions have several characteristics that must be identified before effective interventions can be planned. Delusions can become intertwined with hallucinations. They may be a single thought or pervade the person's entire cognitive process. They can represent a complete thought or only a portion of an idea. Delusions may be systematized, which means they are restricted to a specific area of belief such as family or religion, or nonsystematized, meaning they extend into many areas of a person's life, so new people and new information are incorporated into the delusion.

PERCEPTION. Perception is identification and initial interpretation of a stimulus based on information received through sight, sound, taste, touch, and smell. Remembering the complex interplay of brain functions among brain stem, diencephalon, and cortex for each of the five senses, it is important to recognize that perceptual problems are often the first symptoms in many brain illnesses. Hallucinations and illusions are perceptual distortions that occur in maladaptive neurobiological responses. Although hallucinations are most commonly associated with schizophrenia, only 70% of people with this illness experience them. They can also occur in a manic or depressive illness, as well as in delirium. It is essential to stress that hallucinations and delusions can occur in any illness that disrupts brain function. Hallucinations arise from any of the five senses. They are described in Table 21-2.

> **?** *A young woman is hospitalized in a forensic psychiatric unit because she attempted to kill her preschool children. She says her dead mother's voice told her to do this because the devil would get them unless they were in heaven with her. Is this a delusion, a hallucination, or both? Would knowing the woman's sociocultural background influence your response? Why or why not?*

Another category of perceptual behaviors involves **sensory integration** and includes pain recognition, stereogenesis, graphesthesia, right/left recognition, and recognition and perception of faces. Symptoms related to these are common in schizophrenia yet often are assessed inaccurately within a behavioral instead of a perceptual context. Sensory integration disruptions often lead to deliberate acts of self-harm, as described in this clinical example.

Clinical Example During an initial physical assessment a nurse noted many superficial scars on the left arm of a young woman who had just completed an 8-week education program on symptom management in schizophrenia. The nurse said, "Tell me about those scars," to which the patient replied: "Before I knew it was okay to talk about my symptoms I often lost sensation in my left arm and hand and thought my arm was poisoned or dead. I tried to determine if I was alive or not. I could see myself walking and see

TABLE 21-2 *Sensory Modalities Involved in Hallucinations*

SENSE	CHARACTERISTICS
Auditory	Hearing noises or sounds, most commonly in the form of voices.
	Sounds that range from a simple noise or voice, to a voice talking about the patient, to complete conversations between two or more people about the person who is hallucinating.
	Audible thoughts in which the patient hears voices that are speaking what the patient is thinking and commands that tell the patient to do something, sometimes harmful or dangerous.
Visual	Visual stimuli in the form of flashes of light, geometric figures, cartoon figures, or elaborate and complex scenes or visions.
	Visions can be pleasant or terrifying, as in seeing monsters.
Olfactory	Putrid, foul, and rancid smells such as blood, urine, or feces; occasionally the odors can be pleasant.
	Olfactory hallucinations are typically associated with stroke, tumor, seizures, and the dementias.
Gustatory	Putrid, foul, and rancid tastes such as blood, urine, or feces.
Tactile	Experiencing pain or discomfort with no apparent stimuli.
	Feeling electrical sensations coming from the ground, inanimate objects, or other people.
Cenesthetic	Feeling body functions such as blood pulsing through veins and arteries, food digesting, or urine forming.
Kinesthetic	Sensation of movement while standing motionless.

and feel my right arm, so I thought I was probably alive but I didn't know for sure, so I used to take a knife and poke tiny holes in my skin. I couldn't feel the knife yet I saw blood. It was when I saw the blood that I knew I was still alive."

Selected Nursing Diagnoses:

▼ Altered sensory perception, tactile, related to disrupted sensory integration, as evidenced by explanation of scars on right arm

▼ Risk for self-mutilation related to perceptual disturbance, as evidenced by scars from past episodes of cutting left arm

The concept of pain and pain recognition has been well studied. Knowing that the parietal lobe is the major site of pain recognition helps the nurse to see this as a neurobiologically based symptom. Visceral pain recognition involves integration of stimuli from the spinal cord through the brainstem, diencephalon, and cortex using intricate feedback circuits. People with schizophrenia generally have poor visceral pain recognition and need to have an in-depth assessment of physical complaints, as described by the patient in the next clinical example.

Clinical Example "I told my case manager that I had a stomach ache, some diarrhea, and vomiting and felt like I had the flu. I had a fever, so she took me to the doctor, who said I probably had the flu and should just go home and rest. After a few days I got real sick and had to be taken to the emergency room, where they discovered my appendix had ruptured, and I had to have a very long and complicated surgery."

It is not uncommon for people with schizophrenia to think they have a bad cold and have it diagnosed as pneumonia. Unfortunately, the physical needs of psychiatric patients are often disregarded.

Sensory integration perceptions are included in standard neurological examinations under the category *soft signs*, meaning that they represent a neurological deficit in an undetermined location but are consistent with brain injury to the frontal or parietal lobes. These terms refer to the ability to identify objects by touch. Stereogenesis is the ability to recognize an object only by touch, such as reaching into a paper bag filled with objects and identifying a key. Astereogenesis is the inability to do this. Graphesthesia is the recognition of letters "drawn" on the skin, such as recognizing the letters C-A-T "drawn" on one's back. Agraphesthesia is the inability to do this. Table 21-3 lists several neurological soft signs common in schizophrenia that should be assessed carefully during a baseline evaluation of each patient. Problems in these functions contribute to difficulty with fine motor actions of the hand, and the patient may appear clumsy. Problems with right/left discrimination also contribute to lack of coordination and ability to carry out directions involving right and left.

TABLE **21-3** *Neurological Soft Signs: Prefrontal Cortical Dysfunction in Schizophrenia*

Astereognosis: inability to recognize objects by the sense of touch (such as differentiating a nickel from a dime)
Agraphesthesia: inability to recognize numbers or letters traced on the skin
Dysdiadochokinesia: impairment of the ability to perform smooth, alternating movements (such as turning the hand face up and face down rapidly)
Mild muscle twitches, choreiform and ticlike movements, grimacing
Impaired fine motor skills and abnormal motor tone
Increased rate of eye blinking
Abnormal smooth pursuit eye movements (SPEM): difficulty following movement of objects

Hard signs: loss of function, weakness, diminished reflexes, paralysis caused by a CVA or tumor

Misidentification and perception of faces can contribute to fear, aggressiveness, withdrawal from interactions, and hostility. This symptom involves self-recognition as well and often is present when patients refuse to look in a mirror or avoid eye contact.

When perceptions are altered, concurrent symptoms in cognitive functions are common. Studies have shown that 90% of people who experience hallucinations also have delusions, whereas only 35% who experience delusions also have hallucinations. Approximately 20% of patients have mixed sensory hallucinations, usually auditory and visual.

Environmental factors can stimulate hallucinations. In general, objects that are reflective, such as television screens, photo frames, and fluorescent lights can contribute to visual hallucinations. Auditory hallucinations can be caused by excessive noise and by sensory deprivation. The nurse needs to be acutely aware of environmental stimuli and the patient's response or lack of response. Patients may withdraw from sensory stimuli in an attempt to decrease sensory responses.

Emotion. In psychiatry emotions are described in terms of mood and affect (see Chapter 6). Mood is defined as an extensive and sustained feeling tone that can be experienced for a few hours or for years and can noticeably affect the person's world view. (Chapter 19 includes a complete description of mood and mood disorders.) Affect refers to behaviors such as hand and body movements, facial expression, and pitch of voice that can be observed when a person is expressing and experiencing feelings and emotions. Terms related to affect include *broad, restricted, blunted, flat,* and *inappropriate.* What is considered normal varies greatly among cultures. *Broad* and *restricted* are usually considered within the range of normal, whereas *blunted, flat,* and *inappropriate* represent symptoms. Disorders of affect refer to expression of emotion, not the experience of emotion. Patients describe affective symptoms in the following examples:

▼ "I remember trying to smile for 3 years, but my face didn't work."
▼ "My face was as stiff as your fingers would be if you tied them to popsicle sticks for 3 months and then tried to use them to thread a needle."

Patients describe tremendous frustration with these affective symptoms because others assume that they do not experience any emotion. These descriptions demonstrate why patients are commonly misjudged as appearing bored, disinterested, and unmotivated.

Emotion refers to moods and affects that are connected to specific ideas. Emotions are generated from an interplay of neural activity among the hypothalamus, amygdala, hippocampus, and higher cortex centers such as the association cortices. The hypothalamus, in addition to its hormonal functions, is the emotional coordinating center. Emotions can be hyperexpressed or hypoexpressed. People with schizophrenia commonly have symptoms of hypoexpression. Some patients perceive that they no longer have any feelings. Problems of emotion usually seen in schizophrenia include alexithymia, apathy, anhedonia, and a decreased ability to feel intimacy and closeness:

▼ **Alexithymia:** difficulty naming and describing emotions
▼ **Apathy:** lack of feelings, emotions, interests, or concern
▼ **Anhedonia:** inability or decreased ability to experience pleasure, joy, intimacy, and closeness

In addition to problems with emotions and affect, people with schizophrenia can also have mood disorders. A full-blown depression may develop in up to 60% of people with schizophrenia. A diagnosis of schizoaffective disorder is given to the patient who meets the diagnostic criteria for schizophrenia as well as bipolar disorder or major depression.

Understanding the effect of brain malfunctions on the emotions and affect of the person with schizophrenia is important for promoting constructive communication and problem solving. It is important to recognize that people with brain illnesses often have an uncanny ability to sense the emotions of others, yet they may have difficulty identifying the emotion they have perceived. This creates special problems in caring for the patient.

Caregivers often confuse feelings that are a direct result of brain malfunction and those that are an indirect product of social difficulties resulting from illness. Examples of feelings that are a direct result of brain malfunction include paranoid hostility and emotional flattening. An example of feelings that are an indirect product of social difficulties caused by illness is frustration over not being able to achieve one's potential. When patients and caregivers have difficulty identifying feelings and emotions, barriers in communication usually result.

BEHAVIOR AND MOVEMENT. Definition of "normal" behavior is based on culture, age appropriateness, and social acceptability. Maladaptive neurobiological responses cause behaviors that are odd, unsightly, confusing, difficult to manage, and puzzling to others. With exploration, many behaviors can be explained. Some make perfect sense in the context of information provided by the patient.

> **?** *Describe unusual behaviors that you have observed in patients with maladaptive neurobiological responses. Were you able to discover the reason for the behavior? Can you think of possible explanations for wearing several layers of clothing in very hot weather? Refusing to bathe? Hugging oneself and rocking?*

Maladaptive movements associated with schizophrenia include catatonia, extrapyramidal side effects of psychotropic medications, abnormal eye movements, grimacing, apraxia/echopraxia, abnormal gait, and mannerisms. Catatonia is a stuporous state in which the patient may require complete physical nursing care, similar to that for a comatose patient, sometimes interspersed with unpredictable

outbursts of aggressive behavior. (Extrapyramidal side effects of psychotropic medication are described in Chapter 27.) Grimacing refers to abnormal facial movements that are beyond the patient's control and are not caused by psychotropic medications. Abnormal eye movements include difficulty following a moving target, absence or avoidance of eye contact, decreased or rapid eye blinking, and frequent staring. These are common ocular motor symptoms found in 40% to 80% of people with schizophrenia.

Apraxia is difficulty carrying out a purposeful, organized task that is somewhat complex, such as dressing. Echopraxia is defined as purposeless imitation of movements by other people. This symptom may not always be purposeless but can illustrate a delusion, as described by the patient in the following clinical example.

Clinical Example "I thought the nurse was my mirror and I had to do what the mirror showed me, so I copied everything she did. As long as I could see her I could feel connected to myself and my surroundings, but she didn't understand how important it was for me to be around her and watch what she did. Of course I couldn't explain what was happening to me at the time because I was psychotic, so she put me in seclusion and restraints."
Selected Nursing Diagnosis:

▼ Altered thought processes related to maladaptive information processing, as evidenced by belief that the nurse was a mirror

Staggering, intentional stepping, and walking with the toes touching the ground first are abnormal gaits common in people with schizophrenia. Mannerisms involve gestures that seem contrived and are not appropriate to the situation, such as stopping in the middle of a sentence to whirl two fingers around.

Maladaptive behaviors in schizophrenia include deteriorated appearance, lack of persistence at work or school, avolition, repetitive or stereotyped behavior, aggression and agitation, and negativism. Deterioration in appearance includes disheveled and dirty clothes, sloppy and unkempt appearance, poor or absent personal grooming, and lack of personal hygiene. This is often the first set of symptoms to occur and is a signal to the family that something is happening to their loved one. Accompanying deterioration in appearance is lack of persistence at work or school. As problems in brain function begin to appear, the cognitive skills seem to "short circuit" and the person can no longer perform routine tasks. As deterioration continues the person begins to experience avolition, which means lack of energy and drive. This is a result of the brain changes (which may be occurring rapidly) and frustration with the inability to accomplish tasks that required little effort in the past. Unfortunately, at this point most people with schizophrenia are mislabeled as lazy, disinterested, and unmotivated.

As deterioration continues, patients often engage in repetitive or stereotyped behaviors. These appear similar to obsessive-compulsive behavior but are related to a private meaning rather than to thoughts. Examples include having to eat foods in a certain way, wearing only certain clothes, walking four steps forward and one step back, or being able to drink only half a glass of water at a time.

Aggression, agitation, and the potential for violence unfortunately are often used to describe the typical person with schizophrenia. The person with schizophrenia generally is the victim rather than the aggressor. However, people experiencing psychoses are sometimes violent, especially when their illness is out of control. Agitation is common for anyone who is living with a chronic illness for which there is no cure. It is important to identify and document situations that seem to be triggers for agitated behavior (see Chapter 29). People who have schizophrenia tend to become agitated when there is performance anxiety, particularly related to carrying out tasks that previously posed no difficulty. Abnormal movements and behaviors in schizophrenia are summarized in Box 21-3.

SOCIALIZATION. Socialization is the ability to form cooperative and interdependent relationships with others. This was placed last among the five major brain functions because problems with the others must be understood to appreciate the relational consequences of maladaptive neurobiological responses. Social problems are often the major source of concern to families and health-care providers because these tangible effects of illness are often more prominent than the symptoms related to cognition and perception.

Social problems may result from the illness directly or indirectly. Direct effects occur when symptoms prevent the person from socializing within accepted sociocultural norms or when motivation deteriorates. Regardless, the result is social withdrawal and isolation from life's activities. Behaviors directly causing these problems include inability to communicate coherently, loss of drive and interest, deterioration of social skills and personal hygiene, and paranoia.

Indirect effects on socialization are secondary consequences of the illness. An example is low self-esteem related to poor academic and social achievement. Significant social discomfort and further social isolation may result. Specific problems in the development of relationships include social inappropriateness, disinterest in recreational activities, gender identity confusion, and stigma-related withdrawal by friends, families, and peers.

Social inappropriateness relates directly to cognitive deficits and results in behaviors such as suddenly beginning loud, evangelistic prayer in public, toileting in public, standing in the middle of a street trying to direct traffic, dressing bizarrely, and engaging in intimate conversation with total strangers. Social inappropriateness often involves bizarre sexual behavior such as public masturbation, running nude in the street, or making inappropriate sexual advances. Sometimes bizarre sexual behavior is related to gender identity confusion. It is not uncommon, particularly with temporal lobe involvement, for people with schizophrenia to be unable to recognize their genitalia as their own. This often is the reason for sudden undressing and what appears to be public masturbation, when it actually may be a patient's futile attempt at reality testing.

Stigma also presents major obstacles to developing relationships and adversely affects quality of life.[31] Stigma, which literally means mark of shame, is a major cause of the social isolation of people with schizophrenia. Stigma often spreads to the whole family, who may be having their own schizophrenia-related social problems stemming from embarrassment about having the illness in the family. They may avoid talking about it, or if they do want to talk they may not know how. Stigma and rejection may discourage them from talking. Family members may feel like social outcasts for having this illness in the family. One family member explained, "For the rest of my life I will be dealing not only with the heartbreak of my brother's illness, but with negative response, stigma, and ignorance in my home town that will affect me deeply. I know, because the last 10 years of it already has been sheer hell."

> **?** *Describe your own attitudes and behaviors and those of your peers toward people who have maladaptive neurobiological responses and their families.*

POSITIVE AND NEGATIVE SYMPTOMS OF SCHIZOPHRENIA. The symptoms of schizophrenia have been organized in various ways over time, depending on the evolving understanding of brain function in this disorder, as well as efficacy of antipsychotic drugs. A prominent system for categorizing the symptoms of schizophrenia lists them as

---

Box **21-3** *Abnormal Movements and Behaviors in Schizophrenia*

MOVEMENTS	BEHAVIORS
Catatonia, waxy flexibility, posturing	Appearance
Extrapyramidal side effects of psychotropic medications	Aggression/agitation/violence
Abnormal eye movements	Repetitive or stereotyped behavior
Grimacing	Avolition
Apraxia/echopraxia	Impersistence at work or school
Abnormal gait	
Mannerisms	

"positive" (additional behaviors) and "negative" (deficit of behaviors) symptoms[24a] (Table 21-4). Five core symptom clusters are presented in Fig. 21-3. With minimum overlap, this model incorporates the positive and negative symptom clusters with cognitive deficits, mood disturbances, and some of the social and occupational dysfunction common in schizophrenia.

Predisposing Factors

BIOLOGICAL. Behaviors related to maladaptive neurobiological responses have been described in writing and art since biblical times. Causes proposed for these strange behaviors ranged from demon possession, bad blood, and witchcraft to the full moon. Fortunately, modern science is now identifying many clues to the actual causes of these disorders. (Biological factors related to schizophrenia are discussed in detail in Chapter 5.)

Schizophrenia is a heterogeneous neurodevelopmental brain disorder.[29] It is not known what accounts for the disruptions in brain function causing the diverse symptoms of schizophrenia, but there are interesting results from research that have implications for a multifactorial etiology of schizophrenia.

Genetics. The specific genetic defects that cause schizophrenia have not yet been identified, but family studies have shown increased risk for the disease and other psychiatric illnesses in people with a first-degree relative with schizophrenia. Whereas there is a 1% lifetime risk of developing schizophrenia in the general population, the monozygotic (identical) twin of a person with schizophrenia has a 50% risk for the disorder, and a dizygotic (fraternal) twin has a 15% risk for the disorder. In some monozygotic twin pairs, the schizophrenic twin was noted to become permanently different from the unaffected identical twin by the age of 5, although symptoms of schizophrenia did not appear until young adulthood. These early childhood differences included excessive shyness, hyperactivity, bed wetting, aggressiveness, poor concentration and coordination, tantrums, hand-washing compulsions, reversion to baby talk, and delays in learning to walk and speak.[36] Children with a biological parent with schizophrenia have a 15% risk for it, and if both parents have schizophrenia the risk goes up to 35%. Children with a biological parent with schizophrenia who were adopted at birth by a family with no incidence of the disorder have the same risk as if they had been raised by their biological parents.[13] Thus there is compelling evidence for both a genetic predisposition for the disorder and additional environmental or random factors, as evidenced by the fact that identical twins share 100% of genes, but only 50% of the risk for schizophrenia.

Neurobiology. Multiple studies show anatomical, functional, and neurochemical abnormalities in the living and postmortem brains of people with schizophrenia. Research suggests that the prefrontal cortex and the limbic cortex may never fully develop in the brains of patients with schizophrenia. The two most consistent neurobiological re-

TABLE **21-4** *Positive and Negative Symptoms of Schizophrenia*

POSITIVE SYMPTOMS
An excess or distortion of normal function, usually responsive to traditional antipsychotic drugs
Psychotic Disorders of Thinking
Delusions (paranoid, somatic, grandiose, religious, nihilistic, or persecutory themes, and thought broadcasting, insertion, or control)
Hallucinations (auditory, visual, tactile, gustatory, olfactory)
Disorganization of Speech and Behavior
Positive formal thought disorder (incoherence/word salad, derailment, illogicality, loose associations, tangentiality, circumstantiality, pressured speech, distractible speech, or poverty of speech)
Bizarre behavior (catatonia, movement disorders, deterioration of social behavior)

NEGATIVE SYMPTOMS
A diminution or loss of normal function, usually unresponsive to traditional antipsychotics and more responsive to atypical antipsychotics
Affective flattening: limited range and intensity of emotional expression
Alogia: restricted thought and speech
Avolition/apathy: lack of initiation of goal-directed behavior
Anhedonia/asociality: inability to experience pleasure or maintain social contacts
Attentional impairment: inability to mentally focus

search findings in schizophrenia are imaging studies showing decreased brain volume and abnormal function,[18] and neurochemical studies showing alterations of numerous neurotransmitter systems. Particular focus has been on the frontal cortex, implicated in the negative symptoms of schizophrenia; the limbic system (in the temporal lobes), implicated in the positive symptoms of schizophrenia; and the neurotransmitter systems connecting these regions, particularly dopamine and, more recently, serotonin. Therefore, psychotic behaviors are probably related to lesions in the frontal, temporal, and limbic regions of the brain and dysregulation of the dopamine and serotonin neurotransmitter systems.[7,18,33]

Imaging Studies. CT and MRI studies of brain structure show decreased brain volume in people with schizophrenia: There are larger lateral and third ventricles; atrophy in the frontal lobe, cerebellum, and limbic structures (particularly the hippocampus and amygdala); and increased size of sulci (fissures) on the surface of the brain. These findings all suggest loss or underdevelopment of brain tissue. There is a trend for enlarged ventricles to be associated with two indicators of poor prognosis: early age of onset and poor premorbid functioning (functioning before the first diagnosis).[21]

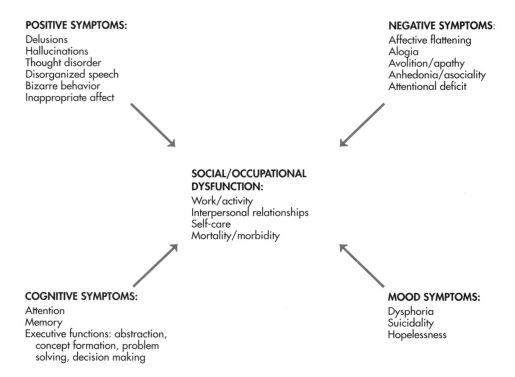

POSITIVE SYMPTOMS:
Delusions
Hallucinations
Thought disorder
Disorganized speech
Bizarre behavior
Inappropriate affect

NEGATIVE SYMPTOMS:
Affective flattening
Alogia
Avolition/apathy
Anhedonia/asociality
Attentional deficit

SOCIAL/OCCUPATIONAL DYSFUNCTION:
Work/activity
Interpersonal relationships
Self-care
Mortality/morbidity

COGNITIVE SYMPTOMS:
Attention
Memory
Executive functions: abstraction,
 concept formation, problem
 solving, decision making

MOOD SYMPTOMS:
Dysphoria
Suicidality
Hopelessness

Fig. 21-3 **Core symptom clusters in schizophrenia.** (Modified from Eli Lilly: *Schizophrenia and related disorders: a comprehensive review and bibliography slide kit,* Indianapolis, 1996, Lilly Neuroscience.)

PET scans usually demonstrate decreased cerebral blood flow to the frontal lobes during specific cognitive tasks in people with schizophrenia. This frontal hypometabolism is thought to account for some problems with attention, planning, and decision making. Recently, the thalamus (which lies in the center of the brain, near the temporal lobes and hippocampus, and regulates sensory input, serving as a filter or relay station between the cerebral cortex and the rest of the brain) was found to be smaller than average and to have reduced activity in some schizophrenic patients. This may explain some of the problems in sensory filtering and information processing in many people with schizophrenia.[7] The basal ganglia, part of the extrapyramidal system, are responsible for various aspects of movement, such as the inhibition of unwanted movement and the promotion of motor learning and planning, and may also play a role in cognitive function with their rich connectivity to the frontal lobes. The basal ganglia are overactive in people with schizophrenia, perhaps accounting for movement and speech abnormalities.[21]

Neurotransmitter Studies. Research in the area of neurotransmission has led to the **dysregulation hypothesis** of schizophrenia: A persistent impairment in one or more neurotransmitter or neuromodulator homeostatic regulatory mechanisms causes unstable or erratic neurotransmission. This theory postulates that there are overactive dopamine pathways in the mesolimbic area while prefrontal mesocortical dopaminergic pathways are hypoactive, and

that there is an imbalance between dopamine and serotonin neurotransmitter systems (and probably others as well).[14]

Dopamine has been implicated the longest in neurotransmitter studies of schizophrenia. This is because it has long been known that mind-altering drugs such as amphetamines and cocaine increase brain levels of dopamine and produce psychosis[14] and because early on it was understood that the conventional antipsychotic drugs exerted their therapeutic effects by blocking dopamine receptors. Dopamine is important in responses to stress, and has many connections to the limbic system. The prefrontal cortex has few dopamine receptors of its own, but it may regulate dopamine in other circuits in the brain. Also, dopamine is present in high levels in the brain during late adolescence, when schizophrenia usually first appears. Dopamine is found in three parts of the brain:

▼ Substantia nigra motor center, affecting movement and coordination
▼ Midbrain, involving emotion and memory
▼ Hypothalamic-pituitary connection, involving emotional responses and stress-coping patterns

Dopamine has four major pathways in the brain (see Fig. 21-4):

▼ Mesocortical: innervates the frontal lobes. Function: insight, judgment, social consciousness, inhibition, and highest level of cognitive activities (reasoning, motivation, planning, decision-making). Negative symptoms: affective flattening or blunting, poverty of speech or

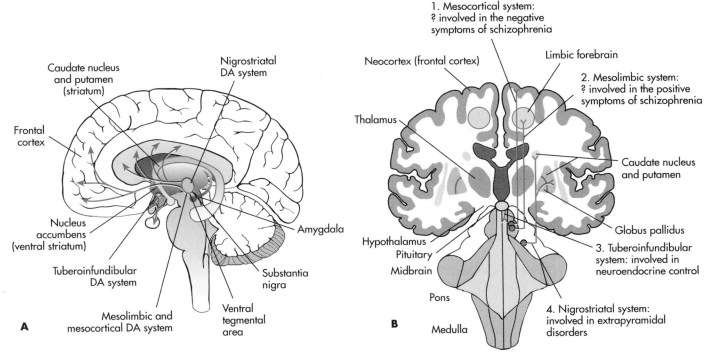

Fig. 21-4 **A,** A midsagittal section shows the approximate anatomical routes of the four dopamine tracts. **B,** A coronal section shows the sites of origin and the targets of all four tracts.
(Modified from Kandel E, Schwartz J, Jessell T: *Principles of neural science,* ed 3, New York, 1991, Elsevier.)

speech content, blocking, poor grooming, lack of motivation, anhedonia, social withdrawal, cognitive defects, and attention deficits(see Table 21-4)

▼ Mesolimbic: innervates the limbic system. Function: associated with memory, smell, automatic visceral effects, and emotional behavior. Positive symptoms: hallucinations, delusions, disorganized speech, and bizarre behavior (see Table 21-4)

▼ Tuberoinfundibular: originates in the hypothalamus and projects to the pituitary. Function: endocrine function, hunger, thirst, metabolism, temperature control, digestion, sexual arousal, and circadian rhythms (implicated in some of the endocrine abnormalities seen in schizophrenia and some of the side effects of antipsychotic drugs)

▼ Nigrostriatal: originates in the substantia nigra and terminates in the caudate nucleus–putamen complex (neostriatum). Function: innervates the motor and extrapyramidal systems (implicated in some of the movement side effects of antipsychotic drugs)

Serotonin, in addition to mediating many brain functions (see Chapter 19), has recently been implicated in schizophrenia. It has a modulating effect on dopamine, and some atypical antipsychotic drugs (Clozaril, Risperdal, and Zyprexa) are combination serotonin/dopamine blocking agents, accounting for their improved efficacy in the treatment of the negative symptoms of schizophrenia.[30,35]

Neurodevelopment. It is now clear that the multiple structural, functional, and chemical brain deviations seen in schizophrenia are usually present long before the symptoms appear, probably from the earliest years of life, and perhaps before birth. It is not clear yet whether these changes are caused by genetic programming defects or environmental injury, or both, creating a vulnerability that remains dormant until later developmental events occur.

There is not agreement that the intrauterine environment or early infant events are linked to the development of schizophrenia. Some research has found a greater frequency of prenatal and perinatal complications among schizophrenics, such as poor nutrition, stress, tobacco, alcohol, street drugs, caffeine, maternal viral infection, and some pharmacological agents common in childhood neurological dysfunction. This research suggests that some disruption in fetal neural development may change the way the brain matures throughout childhood and adolescence, affecting the myelination, migration, and interconnections of young neurons, and thus may contribute to brain abnormalities common in schizophrenia. Research has shown that some preschizophrenic children show subtle abnormalities involving attention, coordination, and emotional responses long before they exhibit overt symptoms of schizophrenia.[29,37]

Viral Theories. There is mixed evidence that prenatal exposure to the influenza virus, particularly during the second trimester, may be one of the factors in the etiology of schizophrenia in some people but not in others. This theory is supported by research findings that more people with schizophrenia are born in the winter. This finding suggests a seasonal cause, such as viral infections, which are more common in winter and may occur in utero or in early childhood in some vulnerable people.[14]

Multifactorial Hypothesis. Finally, it can be proposed that societal demands for increased behavioral independence and future planning, along with effects of normal maturational changes, may contribute to the increase in susceptibility for schizophrenia for the genetically and developmentally vulnerable adolescent and young adult. Research that identifies young people at risk for schizophrenia so that early interventions can prevent the illness from occurring, or modify the impact and severity of the disorder, is just beginning to evolve[38] and holds much promise for the future. It is essential that nurses adapt neurobiological knowledge to social and behavioral interventions and caring, taking an active role in acquiring and applying this knowledge.[9]

PSYCHOLOGICAL. In the past, in the absence of identified biological causes for schizophrenia, psychological, sociological, and environmental influences became the focus. For most of the twentieth century schizophrenia has been seen as an illness caused partly by the family and partly by some individual character flaw. The mother was believed to be anxious, overprotective, or cold and unfeeling; the father was distant or overbearing. Marital conflict and families that stayed together for the sake of the children were blamed. There were theories describing a "schizophrenogenic" mother and theories that described how communicating in double messages could "double bind" a person into developing schizophrenia.

Schizophrenia was also seen by some as failure to accomplish an early stage of psychosocial development. For example, an infant's inability to form a trusting relationship could lead to a lifetime of intrapsychic conflict. Schizophrenia was seen as the most severe example of inability to cope with stress. Disturbances in identity, inability to attach to a love object, and inability to control basic drives also served as key theories.

It is critically important for psychiatric nurses to realize that with the psychobiological discoveries of recent years, most of these psychodynamic theories have found little scientific support. In addition, they can have a very negative impact on patient and family alliances with mental health care professionals.

? *The "schizophrenogenic" mother was described as one who gave her child conflicting and confusing messages about their relationship, resulting in schizophrenia. How would this theory affect the mothers of people with schizophrenia, their relationships with their ill children, and their relationships with care providers?*

SOCIOCULTURAL AND ENVIRONMENTAL. Some theorists proposed that poverty, society, and cultural disharmony could cause schizophrenia or that people chose to become schizophrenic to cope with the insanity of the modern world. Others proposed that schizophrenia was caused by living in the city or living in isolation in the country. Although accumulated stress related to environmental factors is likely to contribute to the onset of schizophrenia and to relapses, neurobiological findings point to other causes for the primary development of psychotic disorders.

Precipitating Stressors

BIOLOGICAL. Interference in a brain feedback loop that regulates the amount of information that can be processed at a given time has been identified as one possible biological stressor. Normal information processing occurs in a predetermined series of neural activities. Visual and auditory stimuli are initially screened and filtered by the thalamus and sent for processing by the frontal lobe. If too much information is sent at once, or if the information is faulty, the frontal lobe sends an overload message to the basal ganglia. The basal ganglia in turn send a message to the thalamus to slow down transmissions to the frontal lobe.[14] The decreased function of the frontal lobe impairs the ability of this feedback loop to perform. There is less ability to regulate the basal ganglia, and ultimately, the message to slow down transmissions to the frontal lobe never occurs. The result is information-processing overload and the neurobiological responses described in the beginning of this chapter.

Another possible biological stressor is the abnormal gating mechanisms that may occur in schizophrenia. Gating is an electrical process involving electrolytes. It refers to inhibitory and excitatory nerve action potentials and the feedback occurring within the nervous system related to completed nerve transmissions. Decreased gating is demonstrated by a person's inability to selectively attend to stimuli. For example, at a baseball game the person with schizophrenia would be unable to differentiate the noise from the crowd, the organ, the team, or the public address system. Normally, when people hear a loud noise they become startled; however, when the noise is repeated, there is a decreased startle response. For example, if you hear a neighbor setting off firecrackers on the Fourth of July you become startled. When you hear a second explosion, you are generally less startled. The person with schizophrenia is just as startled the second time, and maybe even more than the first. This inability to gate a noise stimulus causes people to become frightened in crowds or wherever there is increased noise.[4]

Symptom Triggers. Precursors and stimuli often precede a new episode of the illness. The word *trigger* is used to describe these stressors. Common triggers of neurobiological responses related to health, environment, attitudes, and behaviors are listed in Table 21-5. Patients with schizophrenia can learn to recognize triggers that they are particularly reactive to, and they can be taught to avoid them if possible,

TABLE **21-5** *Neurobiological Response Symptom Triggers*

HEALTH
Poor nutrition
Lack of sleep
Out-of-balance circadian rhythms
Fatigue
Infection
Central nervous system drugs
Lack of exercise
Barriers to accessing health care

ENVIRONMENT
Hostile/critical environment
Housing difficulties (unsatisfactory housing)
Pressure to perform (loss of independent living)
Changes in life events, daily patterns of activity
Interpersonal difficulties, disruptions in interpersonal
  relationships
Social isolation
Lack of social support
Job pressures (poor occupational skills)
Stigmatization
Poverty
Lack of transportation (resources)
Inability to get/keep a job

ATTITUDES/BEHAVIORS
"Poor me" (low self-concept)
"Hopeless" (lack of self-confidence)
"I'm a failure" (loss of motivation to use skills)
"Lack of control" (demoralization)
Feeling overpowered by symptoms
"No one likes me" (unable to meet spiritual needs)
Looks/acts different from others who are of the same age,
  culture
Poor social skills
Aggressive behavior
Violent behavior
Poor medication management
Poor symptom management

and to contact their mental health care provider for help if they cannot.

Appraisal of Stressors

   STRESS DIATHESIS. There is no scientific research indicating that stress causes schizophrenia. However, studies of relapse and symptom exacerbation provide evidence that stress, one's appraisal of the stressor, and problems with coping may predict the return of symptoms.[8,31] The **stress diathesis model** described in a classic work by Liberman and colleagues[16] states that schizophrenic symptoms develop based on the relationship between the amount of stress that a person experiences and an internal stress tolerance threshold. This is an important model because it integrates biological, psychological, and sociocultural factors. In this way it is similar to the Stuart Stress Adaptation Model, which is used as the organizing conceptual framework of this text.

Coping Resources

Coping skills tend to be learned from parents. Children and young adults with schizophrenia need to be actively taught these skills because they have difficulty internalizing them from observation. Family resources such as parental understanding of the illness, finances, availability of time and energy, and ability to provide ongoing support influence the course of illness.

   It is important to remember that the mix of disabilities and resources of a particular patient is related to the type and location of the brain dysfunction. Thus it is essential to assess mental status carefully to identify the person's strengths. For instance, some people with maladaptive neurobiological responses are highly intelligent but unable to express themselves well. Others may be artistically talented but not skilled at verbal communication. Exploring these areas of strength helps the nurse in planning individualized nursing interventions.

Coping Mechanisms

Patients attempt to protect themselves from the frightening experiences caused by their illnesses. Regression is related to information-processing problems and expenditure of large amounts of energy in efforts to manage anxiety, leaving little for activities of daily living. Projection is an effort to explain confusing perceptions by assigning responsibility to someone or something. Withdrawal is related to problems establishing trust and preoccupation with internal experiences. Families often express denial when they first learn of their relative's diagnosis. This is the same as the denial that occurs whenever one receives information that causes fear and anxiety. It allows the person to gather internal and external resources and adapt to the stressor gradually.

Nursing Diagnosis

In formulating the nursing diagnosis the nurse should review the complete nursing assessment as illustrated in the Stuart Stress Adaptation Model (Fig. 21-5). Nursing diagnoses take into account the functional level, stressors, and support systems of the patient and should be prioritized according to the patient's stage of illness (crisis, acute, maintenance, or health promotion). Nursing diagnoses associated with maladaptive neurobiological responses are presented in the Medical and Nursing Diagnoses box on p. 421. Primary NANDA nursing diagnoses include **impaired verbal communication, sensory/perceptual alterations, impaired social interaction, social isolation,** and **altered thought processes.** Examples of complete nursing diagnoses are presented in the Detailed Diagnoses box on p. 422.

Related Medical Diagnoses

The medical diagnoses associated with maladaptive neurobiological responses include the schizophrenias, schizophreniform disorder, schizoaffective disorder, delusional

Fig. 21-5 The Stuart Stress Adaptation Model related to neurobiological responses.

disorder, brief psychotic disorder, and shared psychotic disorder. These diagnoses and related essential features are presented in the Detailed Diagnoses box.

Outcome Identification

The expected outcome of patient care is as follows:

The patient will live, learn, and work at a maximum possible level of success, as defined by the individual.

Prevention of relapse and early intervention are key components of a successful outcome. Relapse is defined as the return of symptoms severe enough to interfere with activities of daily living.[27] It can be prevented only by thorough, ongoing symptom monitoring.[3,27] Planning therapeutic interventions depends on goals related to diagnosis and level of wellness.

Short-term goals identify the steps that will lead the patient to successfully accomplish the expected outcome. Examples include the following:

▼ The patient will initiate conversation with at least one person daily.

▼ The patient will participate in medication education group.

▼ The patient will identify medications and describe the prescribed dose, expected effects, possible side effects, and actions to take if questions arise.

MEDICAL AND NURSING DIAGNOSES *related to* **Maladaptive Neurobiological Responses**

Related Medical Diagnoses (DSM-IV)*	Related Nursing Diagnoses, NANDA†
Schizophrenia	Adjustment, impaired
Paranoid type	Anxiety
Disorganized type	**Communication, Impaired Verbal‡**
Catatonic type	Coping, family: potential for growth
Undifferentiated type	Coping, ineffective family: compromised
Residual type	Coping, ineffective individual
Schizophreniform disorder	Management of therapeutic regimen, individual or family:
Schizoaffective disorder	effective or ineffective
Delusional disorder	Personal identity disturbance
Brief psychotic disorder	Role performance, altered
Shared psychotic disorder	Self-care deficit (bathing/hygiene, dressing/grooming)
	Self-esteem disturbance
	Sensory/Perceptual Alterations (specify)‡
	Social Interaction, Impaired‡
	Social Isolation‡
	Thought Processes, Altered‡
	Caregiver role strain, risk for

*From American Psychiatric Association: *Diagnostic and statistical manual of mental disorders,* ed 4, Washington, DC, 1994, The Association.
†From North American Nursing Diagnosis Association: *NANDA nursing diagnoses: definitions and classifications 1997-1998,* Philadelphia, 1997, The Association.
‡Primary nursing diagnosis for maladaptive neurobiological responses.

▼ The patient will describe preferred living situation following hospital discharge.
▼ The patient will practice community living skills such as food preparation, housekeeping, care of clothing, money management, and use of public transportation.

Planning

When a person is in the crisis or acute stage of illness, care is often given in a hospital. The overall goal is to help the patient to reach stability while establishing a foundation for habilitation. Because of the complex psychosocial needs of patients with maladaptive neurobiological responses, planning for discharge begins with admission. All patient resources must be studied. The family resources are particularly important because families are the providers of care for at least 65% of patients with schizophrenia.[12] Federal law requires that patients and, with patients' permission, family members be present at treatment planning meetings. This facilitates a smooth transition from the hospital to home. Recognizing the burden of caring for loved ones with schizophrenia,[12,15] families must decide what resources they are able to use to assist the patient. These resources may include time, energy, knowledge, and money. The discharge plan must be based on the reality of available resources.

Care of the patient in the maintenance phase occurs at home or in another community setting. The focus of this phase is to assist with habilitation. The process of habilitation begins with learning to identify symptom triggers and prodromal symptoms. Prodromal symptoms are the first to occur at the beginning of an illness. Successful habilitation involves the identification of symptom management techniques that reduce the potential for relapse and maintain stability. Additional information about the rehabilitation of people with maladaptive neurobiological responses is included in Chapter 14.

When stability has been attained, the health promotion phase begins. The goal is to collaboratively develop and implement symptom management techniques that prevent relapse. When patients and families recognize that relapse prevention is possible, they become empowered and can enjoy a quality of life that places the patient rather than the illness in control.

Implementation

Intervention modalities encompass the full range of psychosocial and psychobiological treatments and must include the patient, family, and caretaker if possible.[2] The modality chosen should be based on predisposing factors, precipitating stressors, coping resources, coping mechanisms, and the patient's responses.

The core problems related to cognition, perception, emotion, behavior, and socialization create significant difficulties for people with schizophrenia. These problems affect the implementation of the nursing treatment plan. Table 21-6 outlines areas of difficulty and related nursing interventions in working with a patient who is psychotic. These issues must be addressed in order to maximize the patient's recovery and enhance compliance with the treatment plan.

DETAILED DIAGNOSES *related to* **Maladaptive Neurobiological Responses**

NANDA Diagnosis Stem	Examples of Complete Diagnosis
Impaired verbal communication	Impaired verbal communication related to formal thought disorder, as evidenced by loose associations.
Sensory/perceptual alteration (specify)	Sensory/perceptual alteration (auditory) related to physiological brain dysfunction, as evidenced by verbal reports of "hearing voices that say bad things about me."
Social isolation	Social isolation related to inadequate social skills, as evidenced by inappropriate sexual advances toward members of both sexes.
Altered thought processes	Altered thought processes as related to physiological brain dysfunction, as evidenced by stated belief that staff members are really actors who were hired by parents to watch him.

DSM-IV Diagnosis	Essential Features*

Schizophrenia	At least two of the following, each present for a significant portion of time during a 1-month period:
	  Delusions
	  Hallucinations
	  Disorganized speech
	  Grossly disorganized or catatonic behavior
	  Negative symptoms
	For a significant portion of the time since the onset of the disturbance, one or more major areas of functioning such as work, interpersonal relations, or self-care is markedly below the level achieved before the onset. Continuous signs of the disturbance persist for at least 6 months.

Paranoid type	Preoccupation with one or more delusions or frequent auditory hallucinations.
Disorganized type	All of the following are prominent: disorganized speech, disorganized behavior, flat or inappropriate affect; does not meet the criteria for catatonic type.
Catatonic type	At least two of the following dominate the clinical picture: motor immobility as evidenced by catalepsy or stupor; excessive motor activity; extreme negativism or mutism; peculiarities of voluntary movement, as evidenced by posturing, stereotyped movements, prominent mannerisms, or prominent grimacing; echolalia or echopraxia.
Undifferentiated type	Symptoms meeting the first general criteria for schizophrenia are present, but criteria for other types are not met.
Residual type	Criteria for schizophrenia are not met, nor are those for any other subtype. There is continuing evidence of the disturbance, indicated by negative symptoms or attenuated presence of two or more symptoms included in the general criteria.
Schizophreniform disorder	Meets criteria for schizophrenia and an episode lasts at least 1 month but less than 6 months. Specify with or without good prognostic features based on at least two of the following: onset of prominent psychotic symptoms within 4 weeks of first noticeable change in behavior or functioning, confusion or perplexity at the height of the psychosis, good premorbid social and occupational functioning, and absence of blunted or flat affect.
Schizoaffective disorder	An interrupted period of illness including a major depressive episode or manic episode concurrent with symptoms of schizophrenia. During the same period of illness, there have been delusions or hallucinations for at least 2 weeks in the absence of prominent mood symptoms. Symptoms of a mood episode are present during a substantial part of the illness.
Delusional disorder	Nonbizarre delusions (situations that could occur, such as being followed, poisoned, or having a disease) lasting at least a month. Has never met criteria for schizophrenia. Apart from the impact of the delusion, functioning and behavior are not markedly affected.
Brief psychotic disorder	Presence of at least one of the following: delusions, hallucinations, disorganized speech, or grossly disorganized or catatonic behavior. (Behaviors are not culturally sanctioned.) Duration between 1 day and 1 month, with eventual return to premorbid functioning. The presence (brief reactive) or absence of marked stressors should be noted, as should onset within 4 weeks postpartum.
Shared psychotic disorder (folie à deux)	A delusion develops in a patient in the context of a close relationship with someone who already has a delusion. The delusions of the people involved are similar in content.

*Modified from the American Psychiatric Association: *Diagnostic and statistical manual of mental disorders,* ed 4, Washington, DC, 1994, The Association.

TABLE **21-6** *Behavioral Strategies for People with Psychosis*

CORE PROBLEMS	NURSING INTERVENTIONS
Anxiety	Teach patient the symptoms related to anxiety.
	Help patient to identify what triggers anxiety.
	Help patient use symptom management techniques to cope with anxiety.
	Assess whether anxiety is a relapse trigger and, if so, make a plan to reduce anxiety while still in the moderate stage.
Depression	Teach patient the symptoms related to depression.
	Help patient use symptom management techniques to cope with depression.
	Assess whether depression is a relapse trigger and, if so, make a plan to reduce depression while still in a mild stage because there is a high correlation between depression and being able to perform activities of daily living.
Inability to learn from experience	Review both positive and negative experiences.
	Identify what was successful in helping the patient achieve the desired goal and what was not successful.
Problems with cause-and-effect reasoning	Analyze each experience to see what went well and what did not.
	Help patient sequence events leading to the outcome in each experience.
	Rehearsal may be helpful in enacting an event before it occurs.
Difficulty assessing passage of time	Teach patient how to use clocks to tell time.
	Teach patient to use environmental cues such as the sun going down or a certain radio program to orient oneself to time of day.
	Help patient create and maintain a calendar of scheduled activities.
Concrete thinking	Realize that the patient sees every problem as having one solution.
	Teach patient to look at other possible solutions to problems.
	Realize that the patient often thinks there is only one way to do a task.
	Create alternative ways to approach situations.
Difficulty telling background from foreground information	Teach patient to distinguish between important and unimportant information.
	Teach patient to focus on only the important information.
	Help patient learn to avoid or minimize confusion caused by excess stimulation from noise and large crowds.
Slowed information processing	Give patients time to process and respond to information.
	Minimize anxiety because this increases information processing difficulties.
	Demonstrate genuine interest in trying to understand what the patient is saying.
	Be clear and simple when communicating with patient.
Difficulty screening information to share	Teach patient to identify people who are safe to talk to about one's illness.
	Teach patient to go to these people when the symptoms are creating problems.
	Let patient know that you understand the illness and are a safe person to talk with.
Communication difficulties	Use active listening to understand the patient.
	Clarify what the patient is trying to tell you.
	Listen for the theme.
	Seek validation from patient on what is communicated.
	Help patient with vocabulary as needed.
	Use the literal meaning of words.
	Have patient repeat back what was heard.
	Help patient understand the words and phrases used.
Problems expressing needs	Help patient to identify and prioritize needs.
	Help patient to express needs in ways that others will understand.
	Role play conversations and practice negotiating with others.
Low self-concept	Help patient identify and maximize his or her strengths and positive characteristics.
	Use role play to handle common situations patients face.
	Give positive feedback when patient handles a situation well.
	Analyze a problem to determine how it could have been better handled.
Forced isolation due to stigma	Maximize patient's understanding of his or her illness.
	Teach patient to minimize stigmatizing behaviors when possible.
	Identify comments that are difficult to handle.
	Teach ways to handle stigma and rude comments.
	Develop concrete humorous comebacks.
	Role play various situations with the nurse being the patient.

Continued

TABLE **21-6** *Behavioral Strategies for People with Psychosis—cont'd*

CORE PROBLEMS	NURSING INTERVENTIONS
Difficulty with perception and interpretation of sensory stimuli	Review problematic situations with the patient. List and assess the thought processes in interpreting events. Help patient reality test and reframe problematic interpretations. Reinforce positive and productive processes.
Poor attention span and difficulty completing tasks	Help patient break tasks into small sequential steps. Help the patient keep focused on a single task, a step at a time. Do not emphasize completing the task. Give directions to patient one step at a time.
Inappropriate social behaviors	Identify the patient's thought processes that lead to the behavior. Ask patient about the behavior. Help correct inaccurate perceptions. Help patient identify undesirable outcomes of the behavior. Teach appropriate social skills.
Difficulty with decision making	Help patient to determine desired outcomes. Help patient to prioritize goals and categorize them into short and long term. Help patient establish a timeline for attainment of each goal. Help establish small, concrete steps to achieve desired goals. Ensure that these small steps are achievable by the patient and are culturally and value congruent.

Interventions in the Crisis and Acute Phases

Unstable neurobiological responses require constant observation and monitoring of health, behavior, and attitudes. Nursing interventions in this phase should focus on restoring adaptive neurobiological responses while providing for the safety and well-being of the patient.

PATIENT SAFETY. Patient safety is a critical issue during the crisis and acute phases, particularly in light of the fact that 10% of patients with schizophrenia commit suicide (see Chapter 20). Environmental safety factors should be attended to, including the availability of sharp and dangerous objects, as well as the placement of furniture, art objects, and pictures. It is important to maintain constant vigilance with the patient and carefully explain all actions involving the patient. Patients may accidently harm themselves because of impaired judgment or responding to hallucinations or delusions. For example, a patient with a badly abscessed tooth refused to go to the dentist. He was afraid the dentist would plant a radio in his tooth that would broadcast his thoughts to those who were trying to harm him. The concern of the health care providers was that the infection was interfering with the patient's health and making the psychosis worse. Unfortunately, patients often have difficulty distinguishing between people who are trying to help them and those who they believe seek to harm them.

Staff can create safety issues for patients when they fail to respond to patient needs in a caring and appropriate manner. Patients should not feel threatened, belittled, anxious, ignored, rejected, boxed in, or controlled by staff. Helping the patient to reduce anxiety and feel safe and accepted decreases the incidence of harmful behaviors toward self and others.

MANAGING DELUSIONS. Patients cope with delusions in several ways. Some adapt by learning to live with them.

Others deny the presence of these troublesome symptoms. Still others seek to understand the symptom and become empowered to manage delusions when they occur. The art of communicating with people who have delusions requires the development of trust. Patients with cognitive disorders have difficulty processing language; therefore, the beginning of trust is more readily accomplished through nonverbal communication. Patients with delusions perceive the environment as much more stimulating than others do. It is essential for the nurse to approach the patient with calmness, empathy, and gentle eye contact. Patients report they can literally "feel the vibrations" of others and can "sense if the nurse is with me or against me." Once trust is established, the use of clear, direct, and simple statements becomes significant in communicating with people who have delusions.

> **?** *Describe nonverbal nursing approaches that would foster the development of trust between a nurse and a delusional patient.*

These patients are keenly sensitive to rejection. When they sense anxiety and avoidance in the nurse they often feel annoyed, inadequate, and hopeless. Sensing rejection by health-care professionals can also lead to anger on the part of the patient.

If patients perceive that the nurse is going along with the delusion, they become confused, particularly if they sense that the nurse is trying to get their cooperation. The nurse should not attempt a logical explanation of the delusion because it will not be possible to identify one. Only the patient understands the logic behind the delusion and is not able to express it until after the delusion has reached conscious

Box **21-4** *Strategies for Working with Patients with Delusions*

PLACE THE DELUSION IN A TIME FRAME AND IDENTIFY TRIGGERS.

Identify all of the components of the delusion by placing it in time and sequence.

Identify triggers that may be related to stress or anxiety.

If delusions are linked to anxiety, teach anxiety management skills.

Develop a symptom management program.

ASSESS THE INTENSITY, FREQUENCY, AND DURATION OF THE DELUSION.

Fleeting delusions can be worked out in a short time frame.

Fixed delusions, endured over time, may have to be temporarily avoided to prevent them from becoming stumbling blocks in the relationship.

Listen quietly until there is no need to discuss the delusion.

IDENTIFY EMOTIONAL COMPONENTS OF THE DELUSION.

Respond to the underlying feelings rather than the illogical nature of the delusions.

Encourage discussion of fears, anxiety, and anger without assuming that the delusion is right or wrong.

OBSERVE FOR EVIDENCE OF CONCRETE THINKING.

Determine whether the patient takes you literally.

Determine whether you and the patient are using language in the same way.

OBSERVE SPEECH FOR SYMPTOMS OF A THOUGHT DISORDER.

Determine whether the patient exhibits a thought disorder (is talking in circles, going off in tangents, easily changing subjects, and unable to respond to your attempts to redirect).

It may not be the appropriate time to point out discrepancy between fact and delusion.

OBSERVE FOR THE ABILITY TO ACCURATELY USE CAUSE-AND-EFFECT REASONING.

Determine whether the patient can make logical predictions based on past experiences.

Determine whether the patient can conceptualize time.

Determine whether the patient can access and use meaningfully his or her recent and long-term memory.

DISTINGUISH BETWEEN THE DESCRIPTION OF THE EXPERIENCE AND THE FACTS OF THE SITUATION.

Identify false beliefs about real situations.

Promote the patient's ability to reality test.

Determine whether the patient is hallucinating, as this will strengthen the delusion.

CAREFULLY QUESTION THE FACTS AS THEY ARE PRESENTED AND THEIR MEANING.

Sometimes talking with the patient about the delusion will help him or her see that it is not true.

If you take this step before the previous steps are completed it may reinforce the delusion.

DISCUSS CONSEQUENCES OF THE DELUSION WHEN THE PERSON IS READY.

When the intensity of the delusion lessens, discuss the delusion when the patient is ready.

Discuss the consequences of the delusion.

Allow the patient to take responsibility for his or her behavior, daily activities, and decision making.

Encourage the patient's personal responsibility for and participation in wellness and recovery.

PROMOTE DISTRACTION AS A WAY TO STOP FOCUSING ON THE DELUSION.

Promote activities that require attention to physical skills and will help the patient use time constructively.

Recognize and reinforce healthy and positive aspects of the personality.

---

awareness. On gaining insight into the illness and symptoms, the patient can differentiate experiences with delusions from those that are reality based. In the meantime, the nurse should not underestimate the power of a delusion and the patient's inability to differentiate the delusion from reality.

It is normal for the nurse to feel confused by a delusion. The nurse must carefully assess the content of the delusion without appearing to probe. It is also important to assess the context and environmental triggers for the delusional experience. The nurse must avoid becoming incorporated into the delusion. However, this is difficult if the nurse has achieved a trusting relationship with the patient because people who are significant to the patient in reality may also become part of the delusional world.

Box 21-4 identifies strategies helpful in working with the patient who is delusional, and Box 21-5 identifies barriers to intervening. The intervention plan must be followed exactly by the entire treatment team. If the nurse resorts to "trying anything" to gain compliance, care will be inconsistent and will create an even more chaotic environment for the patient, who already has great difficulty identifying reality.

MANAGING HALLUCINATIONS. Approximately 70% of hallucinations are auditory, 20% are visual, and the remaining 10% are gustatory, tactile, olfactory, kinesthetic, or cenesthetic. Therapeutic nursing interventions for hallucinations involve understanding the characteristics of the hallucination and identifying the related anxiety level. Table 21-7 describes intensity levels, characteristics, and observable behaviors commonly associated with hallucinations.

The goal of intervention with patients who are hallucinating is to help them to increase awareness of these symptoms so that they can distinguish between the world of psychosis and the world experienced by others. The first step toward achieving this goal is facilitative communication. Unfortunately, patients experiencing these symptoms are often laughed at, belittled, and ignored when these symptoms emerge.

Learning about a person's hallucinations helps avoid the roadblocks to communication these symptoms can create

Box *21-5* *Barriers to Successful Intervention for Delusions*

BECOMING ANXIOUS AND AVOIDING THE PERSON

Anxiety leads to annoyance, anger, a sense of hopelessness and failure, feelings of inadequacy, and potential laughing at or discounting the patient.

REINFORCING THE DELUSION

Do not go along with the delusion, especially to get the cooperation of the patient.

ATTEMPTING TO PROVE THE PERSON IS WRONG

Do not attempt a logical explanation.

SETTING UNREALISTIC GOALS

Do not underestimate the power of a delusion and the patient's need for it.

BECOMING INCORPORATED INTO THE DELUSIONAL SYSTEM

This will cause great confusion for the patient and make it impossible to establish boundaries of the therapeutic relationship.

FAILING TO CLARIFY CONFUSION SURROUNDING THE DELUSION

If the complexity and many intricacies of the delusion are not clearly understood, the delusion will become more elaborate.

BEING INCONSISTENT IN INTERVENTION

The intervention plan must be firmly adhered to; if you resort to "trying anything," approaches will become inconsistent and the patient less able to identify reality.

SEEING THE DELUSION FIRST AND THE PERSON SECOND

Avoid saying "the person who thinks he's being poisoned."

when unrecognized. Left unattended, hallucinations will continue and may escalate. Nurses may become so involved in planning what to say that they forget about the importance of listening. Listening and observing are the keys to successful intervention with the person who is hallucinating.

Hallucinations are very real to the person having them, just as dreams during sleep are very real. The hallucinating person may have no way to determine whether these perceptions are real.[33] It usually does not even occur to the person to verify the experience. An analogy might be hearing an ordinary weather report on the radio and not thinking to question whether the voice is from a real person. Inability to perceive reality accurately can make life difficult. Therefore, hallucinations can be considered problems needing a solution. This is best accomplished when the person can talk freely about the hallucinations. Nurses also need to be able to talk about hallucinations because they are useful indicators of the current level of symptoms in ongoing monitoring of a psychotic illness. To facilitate monitoring, the patient needs to be comfortable telling the nurse about symptoms.

Patients often learn not to discuss their unusual experiences with anyone because they have received negative responses from people who think their ideas are strange. The experience of hallucinations can be especially troublesome for the patient who does not have anyone to talk to about them. Being able to talk about one's hallucinations is a greatly reassuring and self-validating experience. This discussion can take place only in an atmosphere of genuine interest and concern.

For those who have never experienced a hallucination, it can be difficult to understand that the person has no control over it. People with true psychosis have no direct voluntary control over the brain malfunction that causes hallucinations. This means that they cannot just will them away. Ignoring hallucinations may increase the confusion of the already chaotic brain filled with delusional ideas and disjointed thoughts. If the person is left alone to sort out reality without the input of trusted health-care providers, the symptoms may overwhelm available coping resources. Interactive discussion of hallucinations is a vital element in the development of reality-testing skills. Communicating right at the time of the hallucination is particularly helpful. Honesty, genuineness, and openness are the foundation for effective communication during hallucinations.

Modulation of sensory stimulation to an optimal level is another useful technique for helping the patient minimize the perceptual confusion. Some patients do well with minimal environmental stimulation, whereas others find that noise and distraction help to drown out the hallucinations. It is essential to find out how the patient has previously managed hallucinations.

Command hallucinations are a special type of hallucination that are potentially dangerous. They may lead a person to perform harmful acts such as cutting off a body part or striking out at someone at the instruction of voices. Fear caused by these often frightening hallucinations can also lead to dangerous behaviors such as jumping out a window. Because of the potential seriousness of this symptom, intervention is crucial.

Intervening during the acute phase of hallucinations requires patience and the ability to spend time with the patient. Box 21-6 outlines strategies useful in working with patients who experience hallucinations. Four basic principles are helpful during this phase: maintain eye contact, speak simply in a slightly louder voice than usual, call the patient by name, and use touch. The patient needs sensory validation to override the abnormal sensory processes that are occurring in the brain. Unfortunately, traditional interventions focus on isolating the patient. Isolating a person during this time of intense sensory confusion often reinforces the psychosis. As with delusions, consistency is the essential ingredient to a successful intervention plan.

PSYCHOPHARMACOLOGY. The new wave of psychopharmacology described in Chapter 27 promises to improve patient response to antipsychotic medications. Drugs that are more site and symptom specific and provide a better re-

TABLE **21-7** *Levels of Intensity of Hallucinations*

LEVEL	CHARACTERISTICS	OBSERVABLE PATIENT BEHAVIORS
Stage I: Comforting **Moderate level of anxiety** Hallucination is generally pleasant.	The hallucinator experiences intense emotions such as anxiety, loneliness, guilt, and fear and tries to focus on comforting thoughts to relieve anxiety. The person recognizes that thoughts and sensory experiences are within conscious control if the anxiety is managed. **Nonpsychotic**	Grinning or laughter that seems inappropriate. Moving lips without making any sounds. Rapid eye movements. Slowed verbal responses as if preoccupied. Silent and preoccupied.
Stage II: Condemning **Severe level of anxiety** Hallucination generally becomes repulsive.	Sensory experience is repulsive and frightening. The hallucinator begins to feel a loss of control and may attempt to distance self from the perceived source. Person may feel embarrassed by the sensory experience and withdraw from others. **Mild psychotic**	Increased autonomic nervous system signs of anxiety such as increased heart rate, respiration, and blood pressure. Attention span begins to narrow. Preoccupied with sensory experience and may lose ability to differentiate hallucination from reality.
Stage III: Controlling **Severe level of anxiety** Sensory experiences become omnipotent.	Hallucinator gives up trying to combat the experience and gives in to it. Content of hallucination may become appealing. Person may experience loneliness if sensory experience ends. **Psychotic**	Directions given by the hallucination will be followed rather than objected to. Difficulty relating to others. Attention span of only a few seconds or minutes. Physical symptoms of severe anxiety such as perspiring, tremors, inability to follow directions.
Stage IV: Conquering **Panic level of anxiety** Generally becomes elaborate and interwoven with delusions.	Sensory experiences may become threatening if person doesn't follow commands. Hallucinations may last for hours or days if there is no therapeutic intervention. **Severe psychotic**	Terror-stricken behaviors such as panic. Strong potential for suicide or homicide. Physical activity that reflects content of hallucination such as violence, agitation, withdrawal, or catatonia. Unable to respond to complex directions. Unable to respond to more than one person.

sponse with fewer side effects will ultimately improve patient adherence. Traditional antipsychotics currently provide some measure of symptom relief for 80% of patients.[22] The atypical clozapine helps approximately 30% of the 20% not responding to the traditional antipsychotics.[2,20] Risperidone and olanzapine, examples of atypical antipsychotic drugs, do not have the life-threatening side effects associated with clozapine. Table 21-8 summarizes the medications most often prescribed for maladaptive neurobiological responses.

Interventions in the Maintenance Phase

Nursing interventions that focus on teaching self-management of symptoms and identifying symptoms indicative of relapse are most useful in the maintenance phase. Patient teaching should involve caregivers whenever possible (see A Family Speaks).[10,32] A Family Education Plan for understanding the world of psychosis[25] is presented on p. 430. Behavioral interventions that teach patients skills for coping with psychotic symptoms include cognitive reframing regarding the cause of symptoms, gaining control over

symptoms, and behavioral coping strategies.[5] In addition, patients and families should be taught the stages of relapse.

STAGES OF RELAPSE. Five stages of relapse have been identified. It is important to recognize that the first two do not involve symptoms that indicate psychosis. This is relevant because this is the crucial time to intervene. In the first two stages the patient can seek and use feedback constructively.

Stage one is **overextension**. In this stage the patient complains of feeling overwhelmed. Symptoms of anxiety are intensified and great energy is used to overcome them. Patients describe feeling overloaded, being unable to concentrate on or complete tasks, and tend to forget words in the middle of sentences. Other symptoms of overextension include increasing mental efforts to perform usual activities, decreasing performance efficiency, and easy distractibility.

Stage two is **restricted consciousness**. The previous symptoms of anxiety are joined by symptoms of depression. The depression is more intense than usual daily mood variations. There are added dimensions of appearing bored, apathetic, obsessional, and phobic. Somatization may occur. The patient seems to withdraw from everyday events and

Box **21-6** *Strategies for Working with Patients with Hallucinations*

ESTABLISH A TRUSTING, INTERPERSONAL RELATIONSHIP.

If the nurse is anxious or frightened, the patient will be anxious or frightened.

Be patient, show acceptance, and use active listening skills.

ASSESS FOR SYMPTOMS OF HALLUCINATIONS INCLUDING DURATION, INTENSITY, AND FREQUENCY.

Observe for behavioral clues that indicate the presence of hallucinations.

Observe for clues that identify the level of intensity and duration of the hallucination.

Help the patient to record the number of hallucinations that are experienced each day.

FOCUS ON THE SYMPTOM AND ASK THE PATIENT TO DESCRIBE WHAT IS HAPPENING.

Empower the patient by helping him or her to understand the symptoms experienced or demonstrated.

Help the patient gain control of the hallucinations, seek helpful distractions, and minimize intensity.

IDENTIFY WHETHER DRUGS OR ALCOHOL HAVE BEEN USED.

Determine whether the person is using alcohol or drugs (over-the-counter, prescription, or street drugs).

Determine whether these may be responsible for or exacerbate the hallucinations.

IF ASKED, POINT OUT SIMPLY THAT YOU ARE NOT EXPERIENCING THE SAME STIMULI.

Respond by letting the patient know what is actually happening in the environment.

Do not argue with the patient about differences in perceptions.

When a hallucination occurs, do not leave the person alone.

SUGGEST AND REINFORCE THE USE OF INTERPERSONAL RELATIONSHIPS AS A SYMPTOM MANAGEMENT TECHNIQUE.

Encourage the patient to talk to someone trusted who will give supportive and corrective feedback.

Help the patient in mobilizing social supports.

HELP THE PATIENT DESCRIBE AND COMPARE CURRENT AND PAST HALLUCINATIONS.

Determine whether there is a pattern to the patient's hallucinations.

Encourage the patient to remember when hallucinations first began.

Pay attention to the content of the hallucination; it may provide clues for predicting behavior.

Be especially alert for command hallucinations that may compel the patient to act in certain way.

Encourage the patient to describe past and present thoughts, feelings, and actions as they relate to hallucinations.

HELP THE PATIENT IDENTIFY NEEDS THAT MAY BE REFLECTED IN THE CONTENT OF THE HALLUCINATION.

Identify needs that may trigger hallucinations.

Focus on the patient's unmet needs and discuss the relationship between them and the presence of hallucinations.

DETERMINE THE IMPACT OF THE PATIENT'S SYMPTOMS ON ACTIVITIES OF DAILY LIVING.

Provide feedback regarding the patient's general coping responses and activities of daily living.

Help the patient recognize symptoms, symptom triggers, and symptom management strategies.

TABLE **21-8** *Antipsychotic Drugs*

GENERIC NAME (TRADE NAME)	DRUG DOSAGE EQUIVALENCE (MG)	USUAL MAINTENANCE DOSAGE RANGE (MG/DAY)
TYPICAL DRUGS		
Chlorpromazine (Thorazine)	100	300-1400
Thioridazine (Mellaril)	100	300-800*
Mesoridazine (Serentil)	50	100-500
Perphenazine (Trilafon)	10	8-64
Trifluoperazine (Stelazine)	5	10-80
Fluphenazine (Prolixin)	2	5-40
Thiothixene (Navane)	4-5	10-60
Haloperidol (Haldol)	2	5-50
Loxapine (Loxitane)	15	50-250
Molindone (Moban)	10-15	25-250
ATYPICAL DRUGS		
Clozapine (Clozaril)	100	300-600
Risperidone (Risperdal)	—	4-6
Olanzapine (Zyprexa)	10	5-20

*Upper limit to avoid retinopathy.

limit external stimulation as a way to protect against the upcoming loss of control.

The first appearance of psychotic features occurs in stage three, **disinhibition.** Symptoms may resemble those of hypomania and usually include the emergence of hallucinations and delusions that the patient no longer is able to control. Previously successful defense mechanisms tend to break down.

In stage four, **psychotic disorganization,** clearly psychotic symptoms occur. Hallucinations and delusions intensify and the patient ultimately loses control. This stage is characterized by three distinct phases:

▼ The patient no longer recognizes familiar environments or people and may accuse family members of being impostors. Extreme agitation is possible. This phase is called *destructuring of the external world.*

▼ The patient loses personal identity and may refer to the self in the third person. This subphase is called *destructuring of the self.*

▼ Total fragmentation is the total loss of the ability to differentiate reality from psychosis and may be called *loudly psychotic.* The patient experiences complete loss of control. Hospitalization is usually required at this point, and

A Family *Speaks*

When our daughter, Sue, was in college, she began to change quite suddenly. She had been almost a perfect child. She got good grades all the way through high school, and we never worried that she would get into trouble. In fact, we used to feel sorry for our friends who suspected that their children were experimenting with drugs and sex, hanging out with wild friends, and failing at school.

What a shock it was when we visited Sue and she had completely changed. Her room was a mess. She was wearing sloppy clothes and obviously needed a bath. When we asked what was wrong, she denied there was a problem and then became angry and refused to say anything more to us at all. When we got home, we called a counselor at the college, who told us that Sue was about to flunk out. She had not been attending classes, and other students had been reporting that she was "living in her own world."

We returned to the college to take our daughter home. We immediately took her to a psychiatrist who said that she was schizophrenic and referred her to a hospital. We were frightened, confused, and depressed. We had little understanding of schizophrenia, except that it is a terrible disease that people never recover from and they usually end up in a hospital forever. We also felt guilty that we had perhaps failed Sue in some way. What a relief it was to talk with her primary nurse. She immediately scheduled us for a family education group that met at the hospital. Every time that she was working when we visited, she made sure to spend time so that we could ask questions, and we had a million of them. Most important, she told us about the Alliance for the Mentally Ill. It was so reassuring to meet and talk with other family members who knew what we were going through. We know now that our daughter may never achieve the potential that we thought she once had, but she can lead a productive life. We continue to learn with her about how that will happen for her. ▼

family members may have to enlist law enforcement officers to take the patient to the hospital. When this happens it is extremely devastating and embarrassing to both the patient and the family.

Stage five, **psychotic resolution,** usually occurs in the hospital. The patient is generally medicated and still experiencing psychosis, but the symptoms are "quiet." The person may appear to follow instructions in a robotic manner and often looks dazed. Unfortunately, many patients are discharged in this stage because they are compliant or they no longer have insurance benefits.

> **?** *Identify how you would approach a patient and family regarding the need for a change in the treatment plan at each stage of the relapse process. Why is it important to identify relapse as soon as possible?*

An example of how well patients can recognize their symptoms compared with staff and families is described in the following clinical example.

Clinical Example During a class on relapse and symptom management, a patient was asked what symptoms caused a return to the hospital. The patient responded, "It was my red dots." When asked to explain, he said, "I see red dots all the time, but when they change in a way that I can no longer tell the difference between my red dots, brake lights of the car in front of me, or stop lights, I know it's time to go back to the hospital for a medication check." A staff member said, "So that's why you are always staring at the exit sign, because it's red?" The patient nodded, and the staff member continued with, "So why didn't you tell us?" The patient simply said, "You didn't ask."

This example clearly demonstrates the need not only to teach patients about symptoms indicative of relapse, but also to ask what they already know about their own symptoms.

MANAGING RELAPSE. The key to managing relapse is awareness of the onset of behaviors indicating relapse. About 70% of patients and 90% of families are able to notice symptoms of illness recurrence. Almost all patients know when symptoms are intensifying.[29] These and other studies also identify a prodromal phase before relapse. A prodromal phase is the time between the onset of symptoms and the need for treatment. With the majority of patients and families indicating a prodromal period longer than 1 week, it is essential that nurses collaborate with the patient, family, and residential staff regarding the onset of relapse. Box 21-7 presents a guide for patients on how to best handle a potential relapse.

Identifying and managing symptoms help to decrease the number and severity of relapses. Teaching this to patients and families is a cost-effective intervention that can provide control over one's life and decrease the number or length of hospitalizations.

Tools such as the Moller-Murphy symptom management assessment tool (MM-SMAT)[24,26] can help the patient to self-report symptoms, difficulties in activities of daily living, problems with medications, and ways of managing symptoms. Once patients can validate their experiences they are empowered to manage symptoms rather than have the symptoms rule their lives.

> ? *In what ways is self-assessment of symptoms an empowering experience for patients? How might it positively affect the nurse-patient relationship?*

When assessing symptom stability of any chronic illness, it is important to evaluate whether daily symptoms are better, about the same, or worse than usual. Some patients with schizophrenia have psychotic symptoms daily yet are able to maintain adaptive responses and carry out activities of daily living. Relapse for these patients is usually indicated by an increase in symptom intensity.

The nurse conducting discharge teaching or working in an outpatient or residential setting must stress the lengthy recuperation process, with special emphasis on the sedative qualities of the medication used to prevent relapse. When families and residential supervisors who do not understand the length of time needed for recuperation complain that the patient just wants to sit around, smoke, and watch tele-

FAMILY EDUCATION PLAN Understanding Psychosis

Content	Instructional Activities	Evaluation
Describe psychosis.	Introduce participants and leaders. State purpose of group. Define terminology associated with psychosis.	The participant will describe the characteristics of psychosis.
Identify the causes of psychotic disorders.	Present theories of psychotic disorders. Use audiovisual aids to explain brain anatomy, brain biochemistry, and major neurotransmitters.	The participant will discuss the relationship between brain anatomy, brain biochemistry, and major neurotransmitters and the development of psychosis.
Define schizophrenia according to symptoms and diagnostic criteria.	Lead a discussion of the diagnostic criteria for schizophrenia. Show a film on schizophrenia.	The participant will describe the symptoms and diagnostic criteria for schizophrenia.
Describe the relationship between anxiety and psychotic disorders.	Present types and stages of anxiety. Discuss steps in reducing and resolving anxiety.	The participant will identify and describe the stages of anxiety and ways to reduce or resolve it.
Analyze the impact of living with hallucinations.	Describe the characteristics of hallucinations. Demonstrate ways to communicate with someone who is hallucinating.	The participant will demonstrate effective ways to communicate with a person who has hallucinations.
Analyze the impact of living with delusions.	Describe types of delusions. Demonstrate ways to communicate with someone who has delusions. Discuss interventions for delusions.	The participant will demonstrate effective ways to communicate with a person who has delusions.
Discuss the use of psychotropic medications.	Provide and explain handouts describing the characteristics of psychotropic medications that are prescribed for schizophrenia.	The participant will identify and describe the characteristics of medications prescribed for self/family member.
Describe the characteristics of relapse and the role of compliance with the therapeutic regimen.	Help the participants to describe their own experiences with relapse. Discuss symptom management techniques and the importance of complying with the therapeutic regimen.	The participant will describe behaviors that indicate an impending relapse and discuss the importance of symptom management and compliance with the therapeutic regimen.
Analyze behaviors that promote wellness.	Discuss the components of wellness. Relate wellness to the elements of symptom management.	The participant will analyze the effect of maintaining wellness on the occurrence of symptoms.
Discuss ways to cope adaptively with psychosis.	Lead a group discussion focused on coping behaviors and the daily problems of living with psychosis. Propose ways to create a low-stress environment.	The participant will describe ways to modify lifestyle to create a low-stress environment.

vision, the nurse is encouraged to provide information. This clinical example illustrates this behavior.

Clinical Example A 26-year-old man with a medical diagnosis of schizophrenia who experienced a lengthy relapse was discharged from the acute care setting and admitted to a residential group home affiliated with a local mental health center. He was later asked to leave both community-based treatment programs because he was not able to actively engage in the required therapies. He was discharged to the care of his parents, who were to motivate him to take his medications and engage him in some type of therapy eventually leading to a job. The parents were active in the Alliance for the Mentally Ill. After months of frustration the parents attended a program on relapse and learned about the lengthy rehabilitation period required. They were encouraged to make sure their son ate well and kept up daily hygienic practices, to stop trying to force him to go out, and

to support his basic needs based on the wellness model. After 6 months he said one day that he wanted to play a sport at which he had previously excelled. He was encouraged to practice and entered competition. After that positive experience he was able to reenter life within the limits of his neurobiological responses.

Selected Nursing Diagnoses:

▼ Social isolation related to low energy during recovery, as evidenced by resistance to involvement in activities

▼ Caregiver role strain related to parents' unrealistic expectations for rapid recovery, as evidenced by positive response to education about relapse and recovery

Anxiety and depression are often overlooked as major contributors to poor health-related practices of people with schizophrenia. Common observable behaviors related to anxiety include pacing, restlessness, irritability, quickness to anger, or withdrawal. The high incidence of suicide in people with schizophrenia mandates the importance of assessing lethality, potential dangerousness toward self, and risk of leaving treatment against medical advice. Because of impaired information processing, patients should also be assessed for potential dangerousness to others.

Finally, a variety of symptom management techniques have been found useful by patients. Box 21-8 categorizes these techniques. Patients who have found other symptom management techniques should be encouraged to use them as long as the technique is not harmful to self or others. The following six steps can serve as a guide to the teaching of effective symptom management techniques:

1. Identify problem symptoms.
2. Identify current symptom management techniques.
3. Identify specific support systems.
4. Discuss additional symptom management techniques.
5. Eliminate nonproductive symptom management.
6. Develop new symptom management plan.

RELAPSE AND MEDICATIONS. The most common causes of relapse relate in some way to medications. Unfor-

---

Box **21-7** *A Patient Guide for Handling Potential Relapse*

Go to a safe environment with someone who can help you if help is needed. This person should be able to monitor behavior that indicates the relapse is getting worse.

Reduce the stress and demands on you. This includes reducing stimuli. Some people find a quiet room where they can be alone, perhaps with soft music. Relaxation techniques or distraction techniques may work for you. A quiet place where you can talk with one person you trust is often helpful.

Take medications if this is part of your program. Work with your prescriber to determine whether medications may be useful to reduce relapse. Medications are most helpful when used with a safe, quiet environment and stress reduction.

Talk to a trusted person about what the voices are saying to you or about the thoughts you are having. The person needs to know ahead of time that you will call them if you need help.

Avoid negative people who say such things as, "You are thinking crazy" or "Stop that negative talk."

Box **21-8** *Symptom Management Categories and Techniques*

CATEGORY I: DISTRACTION
Talking with friends
Listening to music or dancing
Prayer/meditation
Watching television
Working
Writing
Going for a walk or a ride

CATEGORY II: FIGHTING BACK
Positive self-talk
Positive thinking
Yelling at the voices
Not paying attention to the thoughts
Avoiding situations that increase symptoms

CATEGORY III: HELP SEEKING
Going to a mental health treatment center
Talking with a health-care professional
Seeking the support of a family member

CATEGORY IV: ATTEMPTS TO FEEL BETTER
Eating
Taking a bath or shower
Hugging a pillow or stuffed animal
Taking medication
Relaxation exercises

CATEGORY V: ISOLATION
Going to bed
Staying home

Should Inpatient and Residential Mental Health Care Facilities Be Caffeine and Nicotine Free?

Many patients are faithful to their treatment regimens but, because of a daily intake of over 250 mg of caffeine, experience a decrease in effectiveness of most antipsychotic and antianxiety drugs as well as lithium. In addition, a nicotine intake of more than 10 to 20 cigarettes daily dramatically decreases the effectiveness of antipsychotic drugs.[11] Because of the effects of nicotine and caffeine on maladaptive neurobiological responses and the effectiveness of medications, many inpatient psychiatric units have eliminated use of these substances. Smoking has also been banned because of the direct and indirect impact on health.

This is a major change in psychiatric settings. Until recently, coffee and cigarettes were an important part of the inpatient culture. Cigarettes, in particular, were used as rewards in token economy behavioral management plans. Patients often measured the course of the day from one cigarette break to the next. Given this history of reinforcement of these habits, some believe that it is cruel to deprive chronically hospitalized people of one of their few pleasures. Others believe that these restrictions are not in keeping with the philosophy of individual choice and the value that adults should make their own health-related decisions.

Limits on smoking and caffeine are based on the obligation of a health-care program to promote healthful behavior. Careful attention should be paid to patient education and programs that help with withdrawal. An issue that needs more attention is the impact on a newly admitted person of sudden withdrawal from these highly addictive substances. Nurses need to assess preadmission use of caffeine and nicotine carefully. The impact of withdrawal must be considered when evaluating response to medications. In addition, the nurse should be aware of the possibility of withdrawal symptoms, help the patient understand them, and design alternatives to sudden withdrawal from these substances if the patient is addicted to them.

tunately, one of the first things nurses often do in assessing relapse is blame the patient for not taking medications. The nurse should realize that relapse is likely to occur whether the patient is taking medications or not, particularly if the patient has poor health practices. However, there will be a distinct difference in the onset, quality, and length of relapse based on compliance with the treatment regimen.[2,30]

Caffeine and nicotine can affect the action of psychotropic medications (see Critical Thinking about Contemporary Issues). Predicting the success of any medication is impossible if the patient consumes alcohol or other drugs. Research on a variety of ethnic groups has also determined that enzyme variations among population groups cause medications to act and metabolize differently in people of different backgrounds.[19]

Studies consistently show that without medication, people with schizophrenia relapse at a rate of 60% to 70% within the first years of diagnosis. For those who are faithful to the medication regimen, the relapse rate is approximately 40%, but drops to 15.7% with a combination of medications, group education, and support.[22] This statistic has tremendous implications for the role of patient education.

Patients who are compliant yet still relapse tend to have rapid onset of mood-related symptoms and recover quickly with minimal or no change in their antipsychotic medications. These patients usually volunteer for treatment and are generally able to trace the onset of their relapse to an identifiable stressor. Nonadherent patients tend to have gradual onset of relapse with prominent psychotic features and generally enter treatment through an involuntary hospital commitment. They usually require a longer hospitalization and a change in medication. Typically they cannot trace the onset of the relapse to any specific trigger.

Even with support, education, and adherence to the treatment regimen relapse still occurs. This emphasizes the need for ongoing symptom monitoring and identification of factors leading to nonadherence. Cooperative medication management can be fostered if the patient is included as an equal partner in treatment.[34] This only occurs when the patient is taught about the effects and side effects of the medication and staff and family are sensitive to feedback from the patient about how the medication makes him or her feel.

Even with education, medication nonadherence still occurs. In a study of 253 psychiatric inpatients interviewed on the day of discharge from a short hospital stay, more than half did not know the name and dosage of the psychiatric medications prescribed for them or why they were supposed to take them; 68% of the patients knew the names of all their psychiatric medications, but only 53% knew when to take them.[6] These results are surprising because all patients had attended both group and individual medication instruction classes during the hospitalization. Considering the cognitive symptoms of an acute episode of schizophrenia, the results are less surprising and implications for ongoing postdischarge medication instruction become clear.

Interventions in the Health Promotion Phase

Teaching in the health promotion phase focuses on prevention of relapse and symptom management. Patient teaching methods that involve simple, clear, and concrete instructions including repetition and return demonstrations are the most helpful.[28] One of the keys to preventing relapse includes identifying symptom triggers and strategies for managing them. Box 21-9 summarizes nursing interventions to prevent relapse.

Relatives often do not know how to react to more autonomous functioning and need as much teaching and support as the patient.[15,32] Studies have shown that psychotherapy may be helpful in the rehabilitative phase of recovery as pa-

Box **21-9** *Nursing Interventions to Prevent Relapse*

Identify symptoms that signal relapse.
Identify symptom triggers.
Select symptom management techniques.
Identify coping strategies for symptom triggers.
Identify support system for future relapse.
Document action plan in writing and file with key support people.
Facilitate integration into family and community.

tients deal with the neurobiological deficits that often become apparent to them only then.[28] The focus of the psychotherapy is usually supportive and nonconfrontational.

Many families make comments such as, "When we learned our son's diagnosis was schizophrenia, it was like he had died." Thus, it is understandable that schizophrenia remains a closely held secret in many households. These attitudes often prevent families from effectively coping with schizophrenia.

The situation may be complicated by incorrect advice from health professionals who tell or imply to families that they caused or perpetuated the illness. Parental guilt stemming from self-blame further blocks communication within the family. Parents often do not know how to talk with their ill child, and perhaps even fear him or her. Clearly this situation does not help parents face the many problems they encounter in their additional roles of case manager, residential supervisor, and legal guardian.

Parents must also act as negotiators between the assigned case manager, guardian, and an adult child. No one knows a person better than the family, but it can be emotionally painful and draining to be a loving, nurturing, advocating parent in one situation, a treatment-enforcing case manager in another, and residential supervisor to an outside case manager in yet another.

Simultaneous patient/family teaching about symptom management and medication compliance is useful at this stage. Patient and family education may also dispel myths and provide suggestions for improving communication with the treatment team.

Research shows that structured rehabilitation programs provide significant improvement in function and coping skills (see Chapter 13). There are four programs with structured curricula and participant manuals that have as their main goal either to rehabilitate the patient or to help the family cope more effectively with chronic mental illness.

▼ The **Three Rs Psychiatric Rehabilitation Program** is for patients with chronic mental illness and their families.[28] The three Rs are relapse, recovery, and rehabilitation. The aim of the program is to teach patients to use a wellness model to manage their illness and integrate back into the community. Developed by advanced practice psychiatric rehabilitation nurses, this program has shown a significant decrease in hospitalization of its participants.[24]

▼ **Liberman's Skill Training Program** has as its aim the rehabilitation of patients by teaching life skills.[17] The patient is taken through a structured set of modules that teach coping strategies in order to effect life changes.

▼ **McFarlane's Family Education Program** is aimed at teaching families about schizophrenia and helping them to cope with the illness.[23] This is the only program that is exclusively for families and uses professionals specifically trained to conduct the program.

▼ **Journey of Hope** is a self-help program developed by the National Alliance for the Mentally Ill (NAMI) for families of people with chronic mental illness. It is a scripted program that uses family members trained to facilitate the program.

A Nursing Treatment Plan Summary for the patient with maladaptive neurobiological responses is presented on pp. 434-435.

Evaluation

Evaluation of the nursing care provided to patients who have maladaptive neurobiological responses is based on input from the patient and family. Because these are serious, long-term illnesses, care is often episodic. Relapse should not be interpreted as a failure of the nursing intervention but should be considered in the context of the patient's life situation.

To evaluate the nursing intervention, the following questions may be asked:

▼ Is the patient able to describe the behaviors that characterize the onset of a relapse?

▼ Is the patient able to identify and describe the medications prescribed, reason for taking them, frequency of taking them, and possible side effects?

▼ Does the patient participate in relationships with other people at a comfortable level?

▼ Is the patient's family aware of the characteristics of the illness and able to participate in a supportive relationship with the patient?

▼ Are the patient and family informed about available community resources such as rehabilitation programs, mental health care providers, educational programs, and support groups, and do they use them?

Summary

1. Maladaptive neurobiological responses are related to disruptions in brain functioning and affect cognition, perception, emotion, behavior, and relatedness. Adaptive neurobiological responses include logical thought, accurate perceptions, emotions consistent with experiences, behavior consistent with cultural norms, and re-

NURSING TREATMENT PLAN *Summary* Maladaptive Neurobiological Responses

Nursing Diagnosis: Altered thought processes
Expected Outcome: The patient will live, learn, and work at a maximum possible level of success, as defined by the individual.

Short-term Goals	Interventions	Rationale
The patient will participate in brief, regularly scheduled meetings with the nurse	Initiate a nurse-patient relationship contract mutually agreed on by nurse and patient. Schedule brief (5- to 10-minute), frequent contacts with the patient. Consistently approach the patient at the scheduled time. Extend length of sessions gradually based on patient's agreement.	The establishment of a trusting relationship is fundamental to developing open communication. A patient with altered thought processes cannot tolerate extended, intrusive interactions and functions best in a structured environment.
The patient will describe delusions and other altered thought processes.	Demonstrate attitude of caring and concern. Validate the meaning of communications with the patient. Help the patient to identify the difference between reality and internal thought processes.	Patients are very sensitive to others' responses to their symptoms. A respectful, interested approach will enable the patient to discuss unusual and frightening thoughts. Identification of reality by a trusted person is helpful.
The patient will identify and describe the effect of brain disease on thought processes.	Provide information about causes of psychoses. Discuss the relationship between the patient's behaviors and brain function. Involve significant others in educational sessions.	Understanding of the physiological basis for altered thought processes helps the patient to recognize symptoms and feel in control of the illness. Significant others can provide support and experience less stigma if they are informed about the illness.
The patient will identify signs of impending relapse and describe actions to take to prevent relapse.	Help patient and significant others to identify behaviors related to altered thought processes that indicate threatened relapse. Identify community resources and mutually plan actions directed toward prevention of relapse.	Relapse can be predicted if the patient and family are alert to warning signs. Early intervention allows the patient to control the course of the illness. Family members can help the patient to identify symptoms and provide support for seeking assistance.
The patient will describe symptom management techniques that are helpful in living with altered thought processes.	Describe symptom management techniques that other patients have used. Ask the patient to describe techniques used to manage symptoms. Encourage the patient to take control of the illness by using symptom management techniques.	Many patients with psychoses continue to have delusions after the acute phase of the illness has passed. Patients can function better if they learn ways to manage the symptom.

latedness. Maladaptive neurobiological responses include thought disorder (delusions), misperceptions (hallucinations), inability to experience emotions, bizarre behavior, and social isolation.

2. The behaviors associated with maladaptive neurobiological responses include cognitive, perceptual, emotional, behavioral, and relational responses.

3. Predisposing factors for maladaptive neurobiological responses are described from biological, psychological, and sociocultural perspectives. Precipitating stressors

include biological characteristics, environmental stress, and symptom triggers.

4. Coping resources are individualized and depend on the nature and extent of the neurobiological disruption. Family resources are very important. Coping mechanisms may include regression, projection, and withdrawal and represent the person's attempt to control the illness.

5. Primary NANDA nursing diagnoses are impaired verbal communication, sensory/perceptual alterations, im-

NURSING TREATMENT PLAN *Summary*   Maladaptive Neurobiological Responses—cont'd

Nursing Diagnosis: Altered thought processes

Expected Outcome: The patient will live, learn, and work at a maximum possible level of success, as defined by the individual.

Short-term Goals	Interventions	Rationale
The patient will engage in a trusting relationship with the nurse.	Initiate a nurse-patient relationship contract mutually agreed on by nurse and patient. Establish mutual goals related to social interaction. Establish trust by consistently meeting the elements of the plan and engaging in open and honest communication.	Patients who have maladaptive neurobiological responses often have difficulty trusting others. Difficulty with information processing causes problems interpreting the communication of others.
The patient will discuss personal goals related to social interaction.	Encourage the patient to describe current relationship patterns. Discuss past relationship experiences. Identify problems associated with social interaction. Explore goals.	The patient may be unaware of the characteristics of mutually satisfying interpersonal relationships. Honest feedback from the nurse can help the patient to identify the reasons for past problems. Knowledge of the patient's relationship goals leads to the development of realistic behavioral change.
The patient will identify behaviors that interfere with social relationships.	Share observations about the patient's behavior in social situations.	Identification of problematic behavior helps the patient and nurse target changes.
The patient will practice alternative social behaviors with the nurse.	Discuss possible behavioral changes that will facilitate the establishment of social relationships. Role play alternative behaviors. Provide feedback.	Practice will help the patient to gain comfort with new behaviors. Feedback provides reinforcement for successful behavioral change.
The patient will select one person and practice social interaction skills.	Discuss experience of practicing new behavior with another person. Discuss ways of maintaining a relationship.	The patient will need ongoing feedback and support related to maintaining behavioral change.

paired social interaction, social isolation, and altered thought processes.

6. Primary DSM-IV diagnoses are schizophrenia, schizophreniform disorder, schizoaffective disorder, delusional disorder, brief psychotic disorder, and shared psychotic disorder.

7. The expected outcome of nursing care is that the patient will live, learn, and work at a maximum possible level of success as defined by the individual.

8. The nursing care plan must be based on an understanding of the patient's disabilities, strengths, and preferences. Patient and family education about symptom management and relapse prevention is a critical element of the plan.

9. Primary nursing interventions for patients with maladaptive neurobiological responses include intervention in delusions, intervention with hallucinations, medication management, and patient and family education about symptom management and relapse.

10. Evaluation is based on the patient's satisfaction with the level of functioning and on the ability to communicate improvement or impending relapse.

COMPETENT CARING A Clinical Exemplar of a Psychiatric Nurse

Melody Sewell, MSN, RN

I had the unique opportunity to broaden my skills as a psychiatric nurse by working with J, a psychotic patient. I learned invaluable lessons in patience and acceptance as I watched the thought processes of this young man unfold. He also taught me important lessons in caring as we built our therapeutic relationship.

J was a well-groomed, handsome 26-year-old white man with a 9-year history of paranoid schizophrenia. He displayed an intense facial expression. He was admitted to our 22-bed adult psychiatric unit for a second time within the year. Although he had a high level of functioning, he neglected to acknowledge his limits. This was evidenced by his working more than 60 hours per week in landscaping for the previous 6 months. The patient had been followed up on an outpatient basis monthly since his discharge last year. The psychiatrist working with him noted increasing symptoms of paranoia exacerbated by job-related stress.

J was admitted to the unit with a marked weight loss, guarded affect, and minimal interaction. Reiterating that, "I need to get back to my job—the bills must be paid," he expressed the importance of maintaining his independence from his parents and retaining his employment and apartment. He was on the unit 1 week. A pending discharge date was set for 2 days hence despite his minimal disclosure and apparent lack of progress. I was concerned he would return to the same environmental demands and deteriorate further if our treatment was not effective. This might also increase his risk for rehospitalization, which would further threaten his self-esteem and feelings of independence.

When I arrived at work, another patient reported to me that J was tearful, expressing feelings of helplessness and worthlessness. From my perspective he clearly was not ready for discharge without prompt constructive intervention. I realized that this would be difficult, however, because he withdrew from almost all interaction.

I approached J, providing a quiet, comfortable area free from distractions and allowing for privacy. When I expressed my observation of his red and swollen eyes, he immediately responded, "I wear contacts." I provided an atmosphere of trust, building on my rapport with him that dated back to his previous hospitalization, and continued to offer myself in a nonjudgmental manner, encouraging him to explore issues that were perpetuating internal conflicts. This time my intervention worked. His once-guarded affect softened as tears filled his eyes.

He spoke of job-related stressors, his need to maintain independence from his parents, and his desire to provide for himself without government financial assistance. He elaborated on his feelings of failure as a son. When further explored, issues of his father's difficulty accepting the limitations associated with the mental illness of his only son became apparent. J explored this and realized that he had to accept responsibility for his own actions and provide boundaries for himself to maintain his sense of independence. To do so, he could no longer overextend himself and be able to maintain good functioning.

When encouraged to continue talking, he expressed concerns about his sexuality. He greatly desired companionship but realized the chronicity of his illness. Painfully exploring the insight of his diminished ability to provide financially for a family, he cried. I empathized with his pain but also confirmed that he was a sexual being with options. At the end of our discussion, we established concrete steps to implement upon discharge. One of these included finding a job with fewer physical and time demands. He also expressed his gratitude to me, since he could now see that his symptoms had prevented any constructive interactions or positive outcomes previously.

Throughout the discussion with J, I maintained an atmosphere of mutual interaction. He vacillated between tearfulness and guarded behavior, expressing that our interaction was uncomfortable for him at times. I also observed occasional twitching of his thumbs, which I assessed for possible extrapyramidal symptoms.

J was discharged with plans to implement the changes we had discussed. He expressed hope, admitting that he had previously thought of leaving the hospital and "traveling around the country to get away from everything and just see where I might end up." Now, with some pertinent education coupled with concrete steps to guide him, he was leaving the hospital with a sense of direction and hopeful intentions for his life.

Through a comprehensive care approach and expressed respect for my patient, J and I were able to set attainable goals for his discharge, allowing him to leave the hospital with a sense of control and hope. I think about him often, especially on my hectic and sometimes discouraging days in psychiatric nursing, and quietly smile, knowing the difference one nurse can make.

your **INTERNET**
connection

NARSAD: National Alliance for Research on Schizophrenia and Depression
http://www.mhsource.com/narsad.html

The Schizophrenia Home Page
http://www.schizophrenia.com

? Chapter Review Questions

1. Match each term in Column A with the correct definition in Column B.

Column A

___Attention

___Perception

___Hallucinations

___Mood

___Cognition

___Anhedonia

___Affect

___Decision making

___Memory

___Soft signs

Column B

A. The act or process of knowing

B. The retention and storage of knowledge learned

C. The ability to focus on one activity in a sustained, concentrated manner

D. Insight, judgment, logic, decisiveness, planning, and abstract thought

E. Identification and initial interpretation of a stimulus based on information from the senses

F. Perceptual distortions

G. Neurological deficits consistent with frontal or parietal lobe damage

H. An extensive and sustained feeling tone affecting the person's world view

I. Inability to experience pleasure, joy, intimacy, and closeness

J. Behaviors and expressions that show during experiences of feelings

2. Fill in the blanks.

A. The five areas affected by maladaptive neurobiological responses related to disruptions in brain functioning are _____, _____, _____, _____, and _____.

B. Difficulty carrying out a purposeful, organized, complex task is called _____.

C. One of the current dominant biological theories of schizophrenia that proposes abnormal neurotransmission is the _____.

D. _____ are precursors and stimuli that often precede a new episode of schizophrenia and can serve as warnings to the patient and mental health care provider.

E. The five stages of relapse in schizophrenia are _____, _____, _____, _____, and _____.

3. Identify whether the following statements are true (T) or false (F).

A. ___ Studies show multiple abnormalities in the brains and behaviors of many people with schizophrenia before they become symptomatic.

B. ___ The majority of hallucinations experienced by people with schizophrenia are visual.

C. ___ Atypical antipsychotic drugs should be used only when the patient does not respond to conventional treatments.

D. ___ Teaching during the health promotion phase focuses on relapse prevention and symptom management.

E. ___ The self-help program developed by the National Alliance for the Mentally Ill is called the Three Rs.

4. Provide short answers for the following questions.

A. Review the positive and negative symptoms of schizophrenia. How would their presence or absence affect the treatment plan you design for your patient?

B. One of your patients with schizophrenia and her husband tell you they would like to have children. They ask you to explain the risk factors for having children with the disorder. How would you respond?

C. Spend some time in a crowded place and make a detailed list of the things you notice about people that make them stand out or blend into the crowd. How can you use this knowledge to help your socially isolated patients?

REFERENCES

1. American Psychiatric Association: *Diagnostic and statistical manual*, ed 4, Washington, DC, 1994, American Psychiatric Press.

2. American Psychiatric Association: Practice guideline for the treatment of patients with schizophrenia, *Am J Psychiatry* 154:4, Supplement, 1997.

3. Baker KP: The development of the self-care ability to detect early signs of relapse among individuals who have schizophrenia, *Arch Psychiatr Nurs* 9:261, 1995.

4. Braff D: Information processing and attention dysfunctions in schizophrenia, *Schizophr Bull* 19:233, 1993.

5. Bruun CV: Cognitive remediation in schizophrenia: a review of the literature, *Continuum* 3:221, 1996.

6. Clary C, Dever A, Schweizer E: Psychiatric inpatients' knowledge of medication at hospital discharge, *Hosp Community Psychiatry* 43:140, 1992.

7. Cohen BM, Wan W: The thalamus as a site of antipsychotic drugs, *Am J Psychiatry* 153:104, 1995.

8. DiNiro DA: Perceived alienation in individuals with residual-type schizophrenia, *Issues Ment Health Nurs* 16:185, 1995.

9. Fox JC, Kane CF: Information processing deficits in schizophrenia. In McBride AB, Austin JK. editors: *Psychiatric–mental health nursing: integrating the behavioral and biological sciences*, Philadelphia, 1996, WB Saunders.

10. George RD, Howell CC: Clients with schizophrenia and their caregivers' perceptions of frequent psychiatric rehospitalizations, *Issues Ment Health Nurs* 17:573, 1996.

11. Goff D, Henderson D, Amico E: Cigarette smoking in schizophrenia: relationship to psychopathology and medication side effects, *Am J Psychiatry* 149:1189, 1992.

12. Hatfield AB, Gearon JS, Coursey RD: Family members' ratings of the use and value of mental health services: results of a national NAMI survey, *Psychiatr Serv* 47:825, 1996.

13. Karno M, Norquist GS: Schizophrenia: epidemiology. In Kaplan HI, Saddock BJ, editors: *Comprehensive textbook of psychiatry*, ed 6, Philadelphia, 1995, Williams & Wilkins.

14. Knable MB, Kleinman JE, Weinberger DR: Neurobiology of schizophrenia. In Schatzberg AF, Nemeroff CB, editors: *Textbook of psychopharmacology*, Washington, DC, 1995, American Psychiatric Press.

15. Kopelowicz A, Liberman RP: Self-management approaches for seriously mentally ill persons, *Directions Psychiatr Nurs* 1:7, 1995.

16. Liberman RP et al: The nature and problem of schizophrenia. In Bellack AS, editor: *Schizophrenia: treatment, management, and rehabilitation*, New York, 1984, Grune & Stratton.

17. Liberman RP, Kopelowicz A, Young AS: Biobehavioral treatment and rehabilitation of schizophrenia, *Behav Ther* 25:89, 1994.

18. Lim KO, et al: Cortical grey matter volume deficit in patients with first-episode schizophrenia, *Am J Psychiatry* 153:1548, 1996.

19. Lin K, Poland R, Nakasaki G: *Psychopharmacology and psychobiology of ethnicity*, Washington, DC, 1993, American Psychiatric Press.

20. Littrell KH, Littrell SH: Choosing an antipsychotic in the treatment of schizophrenia: conversions to olanzapine, *J Am Psychiatr Nurs Assoc* 3:S18, 1997.

21. McCarely RW et al: Neuroimaging and the cognitive neuroscience of schizophrenia, *Schizophr Bull* 22:703, 1996.

22. McFarlane WR et al: From research to clinical practice: dissemination of New York State's family psychoeducation project, *Hosp Community Psychiatry*, 44:265, 1993.

23. McFarlane WR: Families in the treatment of psychotic disorders, *Harvard Ment Health Lett* 10:4, 1995.

24. Moller MD, Murphy MF: The three r's rehabilitation program: a prevention approach for the management of relapse symptoms associated with psychiatric diagnoses, *Psychiatr Rehab J* 20(3):42, Winter 1997.

24a. Moller MD, Rasmussen NA: Coping with negative symptoms of schizophrenia, *Primary Care Psychiatry* 2(suppl 1):5, 1996.

25. Moller MD, Wer J, Murphy MF: *Recovering from psychosis: a wellness approach*, Nine Mile Falls, Wash, 1997, Psychiatric Rehabilitation Nurses, Inc.

26. Murphy MF, Moller MD: Relapse management in neurobiological disorders: the Moller-Murphy symptom management assessment tool, *Arch Psychiatr Nurs* 7:226, 1993.

27. Murphy MF, Moller MD: Symptom management and relapse prevention: a wellness approach, *Directions Psychiatr Nurs* Fall 1997.

28. Murphy MF, Moller MD: The three r's rehabilitation program: a wellness approach to the rehabilitation of psychiatric disorders, *Int J Psychiatr Res* Fall 1997.

29. Parnas J: New views on the psychopathology of schizophrenia. In *Current approaches to psychosis, diagnosis and management*, Excerpta Medica, Belle Mead, NJ, 1997, Reed Elsevier Company.

30. Patel JK et al: Chronic schizophrenia: response to clozapine, risperidone, and paroxetine, *Am J Psychiatry* 154:543, 1997.

31. Perese EF: Unmet needs of persons with chronic mental illness: relationship to their adaptation to community living, *Issues Ment Health Nurs* 18:19, 1997.

32. Rose LE: Caring for caregivers: perceptions of social support, *J Psychosoc Nurs* 35:18, 1997.

33. Ruppin E, Reggia JA, Horn D: Pathogenesis of schizophrenic delusions and hallucinations: a neural model, *Schizophr Bull* 22:105, 1996.

34. Ruscher SM, de Wit R, Mazmanian D: Psychiatric patients' attitudes about medication and factors affecting noncompliance, *Psychiatr Serv* 48:82, 1997.

35. Smith GS et al: Serotonergic modulation of dopamine measured with $[^{11}C]$ raclopride and PET in normal human subjects, *Am J Psychiatry* 154:490, 1997.

36. Torrey EF et al: Prenatal origin of schizophrenia in a subgroup of discordant monozygotic twins, *Schizophr Bull* 20:423, 1994.

37. Wright P, Takei N, Rifkin L, Murray RM: Maternal influenza, obstetric complications, and schizophrenia, *Am J Psychiatry* 152:1714, 1995.

38. Yung AR et al: Monitoring and care of young people at incipient risk of psychosis, *Schizophr Bull* 22:283, 1996.

Annotated Suggested Readings

American Psychiatric Association: Practice guideline for the treatment of patients with schizophrenia, *Am J Psychiatry* 154(suppl):4, 1997.
A state-of-the-art review of research that is translated into practice guidelines for the health care practitioner treating patients with schizophrenia.

*Landeen J et al: Factors influencing staff hopefulness in working with people with schizophrenia, *Issues Ment Health Nurs* 17:457, 1996.
This study of staff in various health care settings found that knowing clients as people, sharing client success, and receiving recognition for their accomplishments significantly influenced their sense of hopefulness when working with patients with schizophrenia.

*McCay E, Ryan K, Amey S: Mitigating engulfment: recovery from a first episode of psychosis, *J Psychosoc Nurs* 34:40, 1996.
Describes an outpatient coping group with young adults in the first phases of psychotic illness. Working through and making sense of the illness experience, stigma, and a wish to be disassociated from the formal mental health system were themes of the group.

*Nihart M: Atypical antipsychotics and the pharmacology of olanzapine, *J Am Psychiatric Nurses Assoc* 3(S):2, 1997.
A good review of the neurobiology of schizophrenia and the importance of the atypical antipsychotic drugs in the treatment of this illness.

Weiden P, Zygmunt: Medication noncompliance in schizophrenia, *J Pract Psychiatry Behav Health* 3:106, 1997.
Reviews issues related to assessing compliance and identifying noncompliance. Practical and highly recommended.

Yung A et al: Monitoring and care of young people at incipient risk of psychosis, *Schizophr Bull* 22:283, 1996.
The preliminary report of a schizophrenia prevention program case that finds young people at risk, follows them prospectively, and intervenes early when indicated. An interesting concept and a worthwhile program model.

*Nursing reference.

© 1998 M.C. Escher/Cordon Art, Baarn, Holland.

Social Responses and Personality Disorders

Carol K. Perlin

The emptiness caused by dissatisfaction with mere achievement and the helplessness that results when the channels of relation break down have brought forth a loneliness of soul such as never existed before. **Karl Jaspers** EXISTENZPHILOSOPHIE

LEARNING OBJECTIVES

After studying this chapter the student should be able to:

▼ Describe the continuum of adaptive and maladaptive social responses

▼ Identify behaviors associated with social responses

▼ Analyze predisposing factors, precipitating stressors, and appraisal of stressors related to social responses

▼ Describe coping resources and coping mechanisms related to social responses

▼ Formulate nursing diagnoses related to social responses

▼ Assess the relationship between nursing diagnoses and medical diagnoses related to social responses

▼ Identify expected outcomes and short-term nursing goals related to social responses

▼ Develop a patient education plan to promote patients' adaptive social responses

▼ Analyze nursing interventions related to social responses

▼ Evaluate nursing care related to social responses

TOPICAL OUTLINE

Continuum of Social Responses
  Adaptive and Maladaptive Responses
  Development Through the Life Cycle
Assessment
  Behaviors
  Predisposing Factors
  Precipitating Stressors
  Appraisal of Stressors
  Coping Resources
  Coping Mechanisms
Nursing Diagnosis
  Related Medical Diagnoses
Outcome Identification
Planning
Implementation
  Establishing a Therapeutic Relationship
  Family Involvement
  Milieu Therapy
  Limit Setting and Structure
  Protection from Self-Harm
  Focusing on Strengths
  Behavioral Strategies
Evaluation

To find satisfaction in life, people must be able to establish positive interpersonal relationships. People who are involved in such relationships experience closeness with each other while keeping their separate identities. This type of closeness is called *intimacy* and is characterized by sensitivity to the other person's needs.[36] There is also mutual validation of personal worth in these relationships. Rogers[31] has described other characteristics of healthy relatedness, including open communication of feelings, acceptance of the other person as valued and separate, and empathic understanding. In a similar way, friendships are "voluntary, primary, enduring, possible across the life span, . . . with no fixed legal or social norms, with limits, and with a reciprocal quality of exchange that includes intimacy and love."[5]

To become deeply involved with another person, an individual must be willing to risk revealing private thoughts and feelings. This can be frightening, especially if one has had past difficulty sharing feelings with other people. Fear of exposing private feelings often makes people reluctant to become involved in intimate relationships. People who have extreme difficulty in relating closely to others may have behaviors that are characteristic of the medical diagnostic category of personality disorders.

Personality disorders are usually recognizable by adolescence or earlier and continue throughout most of adulthood. They are deeply ingrained, enduring, inflexible, and maladaptive patterns of response that are severe enough to cause dysfunctional behavior or profound distress.[7,21] Personality disorders are common. It has been estimated that about 6% to 13% of the general population suffer from these illnesses. However, only one fifth of these people are receiving treatment.[32] At least some of these disorders are associated with greater mortality due to suicide. A recent study of suicide victims with personality disorders found that they almost always had a depressive syndrome, psychoactive substance abuse disorder, or both.[19]

> **?** *Based on your experiences, compare family, friends, and nurse-patient relationships. Describe how they are alike and different.*

CONTINUUM OF SOCIAL RESPONSES

Every person has the potential to be involved in many levels of relationships, from intimacy to casual contacts. Intimate and interdependent relationships provide security and instill the self-confidence necessary to cope with the demands of daily life. A lack of intimacy with family members and friends leaves only superficial encounters, taking away many of life's most meaningful experiences. The support of significant others frees energy for involvement with social groups, work groups, and the community. Mature adults can be involved at all these levels and feel satisfied with the quality of their relationships.[17]

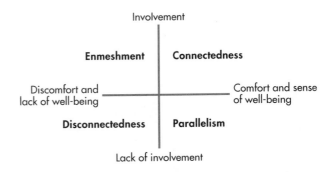

Fig. 22-1 States of relatedness. (From Hagerty BMK, Lynch-Sauer J, Patusky KL, Bouwsema M: An emerging theory of human relatedness, *Image* 25:291, 1993.)

The concept of relatedness has been analyzed and described. Hagerty and associates[18] have identified four states of relatedness depending on the dimensions of involvement or lack of involvement and comfort and sense of well-being or discomfort and lack of well-being (Fig. 22-1). The state of connectedness indicates that the person is actively involved in satisfying relationships. Disconnectedness relates to a lack of involvement that is not satisfactory to the person. Parallelism is a lack of involvement that is comfortable for the person. Enmeshment occurs when the person is involved in relationships but is unable to maintain clear boundaries. Connectedness involves high levels of belonging, mutuality, reciprocity, and synchrony; the reverse is true for disconnectedness.

Adaptive and Maladaptive Responses

Within a relationship the participants usually develop a continuum of dependent and independent behavior. Ideally, these behaviors are balanced, which is described as interdependence. The interdependent person can decide when to rely on others and when it is appropriate to be independent. An interdependent person can let another be dependent or independent without needing to control that person's behavior. All people are responsible for controlling their own behavior while receiving support and help from significant others as needed. Adaptive social responses therefore include the ability to tolerate solitude and the expression of autonomy, mutuality, and interdependence.

Interpersonal relationship behaviors may be represented on a continuum that ranges from healthy interdependent interactions to those involving no real contact with other people (Fig. 22-2). At the midpoint of the continuum, a person experiences loneliness, withdrawal, and dependence. The maladaptive end of the continuum reflects the dominance of manipulation, impulsiveness, and narcissism. People with these responses often have a history of problematic relationships in the family, on the job, and in the social arena.

Development Through the Life Cycle

INFANCY. From birth until 3 months the infant does not perceive physical separation between self and mother. Al-

Fig. 22-2   Continuum of social responses.

though physical differentiation occurs at about 3 months, psychological differentiation does not begin until 18 months. This period between 3 and 18 months is the symbiotic stage of development.[24] The infant is completely dependent on others. Trust develops as needs are met consistently and predictably. The infant experiences the environment as unconditionally loving, nurturing, and accepting. Feelings of positive self-worth result from the infant's complete dependence on an environment that is good and loving. This creates a capacity for empathic understanding in future relationships.

PRESCHOOL YEARS. Masterson[24] calls the period between 18 months and 3 years of age the separation-individuation stage. Separation includes all the experiences, events, and developmental achievements that promote self-differentiation and a sense of being separate and unique. Individuation is the evolution of the child's internal psychological structure and growing sense of separateness, wholeness, and capability. The toddler ventures away from the mother to explore the environment. During this phase, a sense of object constancy develops.[2] This means that the child knows that a valued person or object continues to exist when it cannot be directly perceived. Games such as peek-a-boo teach object constancy. At the beginning of the separation-individuation process, the child seeks the parents' reassurance, support, and encouragement. If the response to autonomous behavior is positive and reinforcing, there is a foundation for building a solid sense of self and future relationships characterized by interdependence, commitment, and a capacity for interpersonal growth.

CHILDHOOD. The internal development of morality and empathic feelings occurs between the ages of 6 and 10 years. During this period a supportive environment that encourages the budding sense of self fosters development of a positive, adaptive self-concept. Conflict occurs as adults set limits on behavior, often frustrating the child's efforts toward independence. However, loving, consistent limit setting communicates caring and helps the child develop interdependence. The older child adopts the parents' guidelines for behavior and a value system begins to appear. In school the child begins to learn cooperation, competition, and

compromise. Peer relationships and approval of adults from outside the family, such as teachers, scout leaders, and friends' parents become important.

PREADOLESCENCE AND ADOLESCENCE. By preadolescence the person becomes involved in an intimate relationship with a friend of the same sex, a best friend. This relationship involves sharing. It offers another chance to clarify values and recognize differences in people. This is usually a very dependent relationship. There are often active efforts to exclude others. However, as adolescence develops, the dependence on a close friend of the same sex usually yields to a dependent heterosexual relationship. While young people are involved in these dependent relationships with peers, they are asserting independence from their parents. Friends support each other in this struggle, which often includes rebellious behavior. Parents can help the adolescent grow by providing consistent limits and a caring tolerance of rebellious outbursts. Another step toward mature interdependence is taken as the person learns to balance parental demands and peer group pressures.

YOUNG ADULTHOOD. Adolescence ends when the person is self-sufficient and maintains interdependent relationships with parents and peers. Decision making is independent, taking the advice and opinions of others into account. The person may marry and begin a new family. Occupational plans are made and a career begun. The mature person demonstrates self-awareness by balancing dependent and independent behavior. Others are allowed to be dependent or independent as appropriate. Being sensitive to and accepting the feelings and needs of oneself and others is critical to this level of mature functioning. Interpersonal relationships are characterized by mutuality.

MIDDLE ADULTHOOD. Parenting and adult friendships test the person's ability to foster independence in others. Children gradually separate from parents, and friends may move away or drift apart. The mature person must be self-reliant and find new supports. Pleasure can be found in the development of an interdependent relationship with children as they grow. Decreased dependent demands by children creates freedom that can be used for new activities.

LATE ADULTHOOD. Change continues during late adulthood. Losses occur, such as the physical changes of aging, the death of parents, loss of occupation through retirement, and later the deaths of friends and one's spouse. The need for relatedness must still be satisfied. The mature person grieves over these losses and recognizes that the support of others can help resolve the grief. However, new possibilities arise, even with a loss. Old friends and relatives cannot be replaced, but new relationships can develop. Grandchildren may become important to the grandparent, who may delight in spending time with them. The aging person may also find a sense of relatedness to the culture as a whole. Life has deeper meaning in relation to one's perception of personal accomplishments and contributions to the welfare of society. The mature older person can accept whatever increase in dependence is necessary but also retain as much independence as possible. Even loss of physical health does not necessarily force the person to give up all independence. The ability to maintain mature relatedness throughout life enhances one's self-esteem.

Assessment

Behaviors

The behaviors observed in people with personality disorders are characterized by chronic, maladaptive social responses. The DSM-IV has grouped the personality disorders into three clusters based on descriptive similarities: Cluster A includes personality disorders of an odd or eccentric nature (paranoid, schizoid, and schizotypal personality disorders). Cluster B are of an erratic, dramatic, or emotional nature (antisocial, borderline, histrionic, and narcissistic personality disorders). Cluster C includes disorders of an anxious or fearful nature (avoidant, dependent, and obsessive-compulsive personality disorders).[1]

The patient may report or exhibit one or more of the following findings in the course of the nursing assessment.[20]

▼ Cluster A personality disorders: aloofness, anger, anxiety in social situations, eccentric behavior, suspicion of others, isolation, hypersensitivity
▼ Cluster B personality disorders: chronic irritability, frequent suicidal thoughts, poor frustration tolerance, alternating social withdrawal and overinvolvement, manipulativeness, impulsiveness, detachment from loved ones, anxiety, history of multiple jobs, controlling behavior, hypersensitivity to criticism
▼ Cluster C personality disorders: isolation, withdrawal, compulsive work habits, preoccupation with work, inability to engage in leisure activities, extreme criticism of others, anxiety, inability to assume responsibility for behavior

A specific classification of interpersonal and behavioral characteristics associated with each of the personality disorders is presented in Box 22-1.

People with Cluster B personality disorders have unique character features that can make the provision of nursing care complicated and difficult.[15] For example, borderline patients who often mutilate themselves appear to represent a subgroup of especially high users of psychiatric treatment who are at particularly high risk for suicidal behavior, comorbid major depression, and eating disorders.[9] For this reason, the nursing assessment and implementation of care for people with borderline, antisocial, and narcissistic personality disorders are emphasized in this chapter. Common maladaptive responses of people with Cluster B personality disorders include manipulation, narcissism, and impulsivity.

MANIPULATION. People who use manipulative behaviors present a particularly difficult nursing problem. They treat others as objects, as illustrated in the following clinical example.

Clinical Example Mr. Y was a 20-year-old single man who was committed to an inpatient psychiatric unit by a judge for a psychiatric evaluation. He had been charged with sale of illicit drugs, statutory rape of his 15-year-old pregnant girlfriend, and contributing to the delinquency of a minor. He had been arrested on the grounds of a junior high school, where he was selling PCP and barbiturates to a group of young teenagers.

In jail Mr. Y had been observed to be "crazy" by the guards. He paced his cell, chanted, and threw his food on the floor. Because of this behavior, the judge agreed to order a psychiatric evaluation. On arrival at the psychiatric unit Mr. Y continued to behave in the same manner. However, his behavior did not seem typical of psychosis. There was no evidence of hallucinations or disorders of thought or affect. When unaware that he was observed, Mr. Y seemed relaxed and was noted at one time to be talking with another patient. By the day after admission he seemed to be free of his symptoms. At this point the staff began to describe him as a "nice guy." He complimented female staff members and behaved toward them in a pleasantly seductive manner. He was respectful to the physicians and agreed to abide by all the rules. He was helpful with other patients. In group meetings he admitted that he had behaved badly in the past and described how he had been led astray by his friends. He said he became involved in drugs because he wanted to be "one of the gang" and he needed money so he "had to" start selling drugs. By the end of his first week in the hospital he had received the sympathy of all the other patients and the staff.

Nine days after admission, after visiting hours, it was noted that Mr. Y and two other patients looked lethargic. Their speech was slurred, and their gaits ataxic. The nursing staff immediately collected urine and blood specimens for toxicological analysis. The unit was searched for hidden drugs, but none were found. The results of the toxicology screening tests were positive for barbiturates. Suspicion was immediately focused on Mr. Y because the other patients involved were young adolescents with no history of drug

Box **22-1** *Classification of Personality Disorders*

Type and Disorder	Characteristics
CLUSTER A: ODD, ECCENTRIC	
Paranoid	Pervasive unwarranted mistrust of others, manifested by jealousy, envy, and guardedness
	Hypersensitivity, frequent feelings of being mistreated and misunderstood
	Restricted affect, evidenced by lack of tenderness and poor sense of humor
Schizoid	Inability to form social relationships, absence of warm and tender feelings for others
	Indifference to praise, criticism, and feelings of others
	Apparently little or no desire for social involvement, few if any close friends
	Generally reserved, withdrawn, and seclusive, preference for solitary interests or hobbies
	Dull or flat affect, appears cold or aloof
Schizotypal	Various oddities of thought, perception, speech, and behavior
	Possible magical thinking, ideas of reference, paranoid ideation, illusions, depersonalization, peculiarities in word choice, social isolation, and inappropriate affect
CLUSTER B: DRAMATIC, EMOTIONAL, ERRATIC, IMPULSIVE	
Antisocial	General disregard for others' rights and feelings
	History of persistent antisocial behavior
	Poor school or job performance
	Inability to maintain close relationships, especially a sexually intimate one
	Superficial charm, often with manipulative and seductive behavior
Borderline	Instability in interpersonal behavior, marked by intense and unstable relationships
	Impulsive and unpredictable behavior
	Profound, inappropriate shifts in mood and affect
	Poor identity with uncertainty in such areas as self-image, sexual preference, and values
Histrionic	Lively, dramatic, attention-seeking behavior
	Tantrums and angry outbursts
	Demanding, egocentric, inconsiderate behavior
	Manipulation and divisiveness
	Seductive or charming behavior, superficial personal attachments
Narcissistic	Exaggerated sense of self-importance, manifested by extreme self-centeredness
	Preoccupation with fantasies involving power, success, wealth, beauty, or love
	No capacity for empathy
	Need for constant admiration and attention
	Manipulative behavior
CLUSTER C: ANXIOUS, FEARFUL	
Avoidant	Anxiety and fearfulness
	Low self-esteem, hypersensitivity to potential humiliation, rejection, or shame
	Social withdrawal accompanied by longing for close relationships
Dependent	Extreme self-consciousness accompanied by feelings of inadequacy and helplessness
	Dependency in relationships, subordinating own needs and leaving major decisions to others
	Overly passive and compliant
Obsessive-compulsive	Inability to express affection
	Overly cold and rigid demeanor
	Preoccupation with rules, trivial details, and other expressions of conformity
	Superior attitude, need to control
	Tendency toward perfection, valuing work more than pleasure or relationships

From *Psychiatric nurse review,* Springhouse, Pa, 1990, Springhouse Corp.

abuse. When confronted, Mr. Y seemed amazed that he could be suspected and pointed out his past behavior as a model patient. He admitted that he had behaved strangely and wondered whether someone had "slipped" him some drugs. He was convincing but was warned that if he was involved in any way with drugs, he would be sent directly back to jail.

Mr. Y began to pressure the physicians for their decision on his ability to be held responsible for his actions. He seemed to be actively engaged in therapy and promised to continue with outpatient treatment if recommended for probation. He also convinced his family of his good intentions, and they agreed to allow him to move into their house. On the basis of these indications of positive behavioral change, Mr. Y received a recommendation for probation, which was carried out by the judge.

Three months after discharge from the hospital, Mr. Y and a friend were arrested for operating a PCP-manufacturing laboratory in a friend's garage.

Selected Nursing Diagnoses:

▼ Impaired social interaction related to need for control, as evidenced by illegal behavior and treating people like objects

▼ Defensive coping related to inability to identify relationship problems, as evidenced by manipulation of others

There is usually little motivation to change because manipulative behavior often has rewards for the person, facilitating the accomplishment of a desired goal. The manipulator is goal-oriented or self-oriented, not other-oriented. However, the person is skilled at giving the impression of involvement with others. In this clinical example Mr. Y was able to gain the confidence of the staff in order to have support in court. This is typical of a person with an antisocial personality disorder.

The manipulative person is unaware of a lack of relatedness and assumes that all interpersonal relationships are formed to take advantage of others. This person cannot imagine an intimate, sharing relationship. The manipulator believes in maintaining control at all times to avoid being controlled. Patients with borderline personality disorder are often manipulative. This results in their inability to participate in mature interpersonal relationships, as illustrated in the next clinical example.

Clinical Example Ms. S is a 23-year-old woman who was admitted to a general hospital psychiatric unit. She had lacerated her wrists superficially three times during the week before admission. Each time she cut herself, she had telephoned her therapist, a psychiatric clinical nurse specialist. Because her therapist was about to leave for vacation and she was concerned about the safety of Ms. S, the nurse decided to hospitalize her.

On admission Ms. S appeared mildly depressed. She gave the impression of a guilty child who had been punished. She denied any current self-destructive thoughts. During the physical assessment, the nurse noted that there were many scars on the patient's body. When asked about these, she claimed she was abused as a child. Her therapist's records described the scars as the result of much self-mutilation since the age of 16. This had been her main reason for seeking therapy. There was also a history of sexual promiscuity.

Ms. S described herself as a failure, stating that she had "the best parents in the world, but they did not get the daughter they deserve." She said she was a drifter who had never been able to settle on a career, a lifestyle, or any consistent friends. She didn't know who or what she was. When asked how she felt, she responded, "Most of the time, I don't feel anything, just empty." She had no signs of psychosis.

Ms. S was placed on constant observation to prevent further cutting. All sharp objects were removed from her room. At first she was very cooperative and superficially friendly to other patients. Because of her smooth adjust-

ment, constant observation was discontinued after 3 days. She was also given a schedule of activities and informed that she was responsible for following it. The next day, an X-Acto knife was missing from the activities therapy room. Ms. S was found in the bathroom, bleeding from several small cuts on her ankles. This sequence was repeated several times. Each time the constant observation was discontinued, she found a sharp object and cut herself.

She was also very labile emotionally. She had unpredictable outbursts of anger, similar to temper tantrums. However, these outbursts passed as quickly as they came, never lasting more than a few minutes. She also began to categorize the staff as "good guys and bad guys." When she was with staff members she liked, she was pleasant, complimenting them on their kind and understanding attitudes toward her. With staff she disliked, she was sullen and uncooperative, comparing them unfavorably to the others. Eventually the staff began to bicker about her care, some believing she was spoiled and others that she was neglected.

Ms. S remained in the hospital during her therapist's absence. When the therapist returned, Ms. S refused to see her. The frequency of angry outbursts increased dramatically. However, following frequent visits from her therapist, Ms. S began to request discharge. Behavioral criteria for discharge were set, including no self-mutilation and no temper tantrums. She met the criteria and was discharged back to outpatient treatment.

Selected Nursing Diagnoses:

▼ Risk for self-mutilation related to anxiety about her therapist's vacation, as evidenced by lacerating her wrists

▼ Self-esteem disturbance related to unclear goals and expectations, as evidenced by describing herself as a failure

▼ Impaired social interaction related to inability to tolerate close relationships, as evidenced by splitting staff into "good guys" and "bad guys"

The diagnosis of borderline personality disorder is more often given to female patients. Some have questioned whether this is evidence of sex role stereotyping.[34] Masterson[24] notes the borderline person's failure to achieve object constancy during the separation-individuation stage of psychosocial development. Because of this, the person relates to another as a series of disconnected parts rather than as a whole. The borderline person cannot recall the image of someone who is absent. He or she is not able to mourn the loss of another person. When someone fails to meet the borderline person's needs, the relationship is likely to end.

People who fail to complete separation from the mother and develop autonomy in childhood often repeat this developmental crisis at adolescence. Behaviors characteristic of this phase include the following:

▼ Clinging

▼ Depression accompanied by rage and defended by acting out or neurotic behavior

▼ Detachment and withdrawal

Many of these behaviors can be seen in the preceding clinical example. Because of their inability to become involved in reciprocal interpersonal relationships and the related manipulativeness, these patients are frustrating for nursing staff. It must be remembered that their behavior is not consciously planned but is a defense against a fear of loneliness.

NARCISSISM. The term *narcissism* comes from the Greek myth of Narcissus, who fell in love with his own reflection in the waters of a spring and died. The flower that bears his name sprang up at the site of his death.

Many successful people are narcissistic. Acting, modeling, professional sports, and politics are usually attractive occupations to people with this personality trait. In these contexts self-centeredness is usually expected. However, problems occur when the person does not gain the status they think they deserve or loses status. The frustration caused by lack or loss of recognition may be expressed as anger, depression, substance abuse, or other maladaptive behaviors.

People with narcissistic personality disorders have persistently fragile self-esteem, driving them to search constantly for praise, appreciation, and admiration. The clinical example that follows demonstrates narcissistic entitlement, which describes an egocentric attitude, envy, and rage when others are seen as critical or not supportive.

Clinical Example Ms. T, the psychiatric clinical nurse specialist, was called to the emergency room to see Mr. F. He was accompanied by his wife. The nurse knew from the intake form that Mr. F was a 44-year-old man with no psychiatric history. His chief complaint was that he had gone into a "blind rage" when he had an argument with his wife earlier in the evening and he had punched her in the arm. He was frightened by his loss of control and said that he felt like a failure. Both Mr. and Ms. F denied any history of violence, although Mr. F said that his first marriage ended "because of my anger."

Mr. F appeared quite anxious; he was tapping his foot and wringing his hands, and he avoided eye contact with Ms. T. After a short time, however, he became more verbal, and he willingly explained what had led to the "blow up." He had been self-employed for the past 10 years and had been "highly successful," expanding his company nationally. He told Ms. T that his father was a "multimillionaire" and that he had been on his way to exceeding his father's wealth. It seemed important to impress Ms. T by dropping the names of well-known people, whom he described as his friends.

Ms. F angrily interrupted him, saying "that's important to you—who you know and how it looks." Ms. F then explained that business began slipping 2 years ago. Despite several profitable years, he had never invested or saved money. When sales fell, instead of cutting expenses and downsizing the company, he continued to live lavishly, making extravagant purchases. It was this situation that led to their argument. When Ms. F accused her husband of taking them to the brink of financial collapse, he went into a rage and punched her.

Ms. F began sobbing, and Mr. F seemed not to notice. He said he felt like his life was falling apart and that he must be the failure his father always said he was. He angrily referred to his "rich brother," who, in his father's eyes, was the perfect son. He became tearful, and Ms. F then turned to her husband, attempting to provide support and reassurance.

Selected Nursing Diagnoses:
▼ Impaired social interaction related to need for approval by others, as evidenced by attempts to impress others and inability to respond to wife's distress
▼ Risk for violence directed at others related to impulsivity, as evidenced by acts engaged in during "blind rage"
▼ Altered family processes related to inconsistency between goals of husband and wife, as evidenced by wife's reaction to patient's description of his problem
▼ Defensive coping related to fear of failure, as evidenced by bragging and name-dropping
▼ Chronic low self-esteem related to perceived lack of caring and approval from father, as evidenced by stated need to exceed his father's success and description of himself as "a failure" in his father's eyes

Narcissism and impulsivity often go together.[13] This was demonstrated in the previous clinical example, in which Mr. F's impulsiveness was shown by his extravagance, inability to establish and follow a life plan, failure to learn by experience, poor judgment, and unreliability.

The behaviors related to maladaptive social responses are summarized in Table 22-1. Patients often exhibit combinations of these behaviors. The nurse must be able to identify the complex behavior associated with high levels of stress and anxiety. In some cases a usual mode of behavior, such as manipulation, may be exaggerated or combined with a change in behavior. For instance, manipulative people may withdraw when confronted by their manipulations and may be rejected by those they have been trying to manipulate. In other instances the behavior resulting from stress may be different from the person's usual style of relatedness. A per-

TABLE **22-1** *Behaviors Related to Maladaptive Social Responses*

BEHAVIOR	CHARACTERISTICS
Manipulation	Others are treated as objects
	Relationships center around control issues
	Person is self-oriented or goal-oriented, not other-oriented
Narcissism	Fragile self-esteem
	Constant seeking of praise and admiration
	Egocentric attitude
	Envy
	Rage when others are not supportive
Impulsivity	Inability to plan
	Inability to learn from experience
	Poor judgment
	Unreliability

son who is usually outgoing may withdraw when under great stress. It is helpful to include a description of the patient's usual relationships in the nursing assessment. This provides a baseline of behavior for that person against which the nurse measures the patient's progress.

Predisposing Factors

A variety of factors—within the individual, between the individual and significant others, and environmental—may lead to maladaptive social responses. Although much research has been done on disorders that affect interpersonal relationships, there are no specific conclusions about their causes. A combination of factors probably is involved. The nurse must explore all relevant areas during the nursing assessment.

DEVELOPMENTAL FACTORS. The capacity for relatedness results from a developmental process. Anything that interferes with that process decreases the person's ability to develop healthy relationships. Parents who were deprived of caring as children may not know how to meet this need in their own children. Lack of attention or stimulation by the parent deprives an infant of a sense of security. This results in failure to establish basic trust. The person may develop a suspicious attitude toward others continuing throughout life. The quality of parenting is also important. A child may be well fed and receive perfect physical care but without any communication of parental caring. A child who is treated as an object may become an adult who treats others as objects.

> **?** *Describe aspects of contemporary American culture that are likely to negatively affect child-raising practices. What are the implications for mental health services? What preventive activities would be helpful?*

A longitudinal study of the childhood antecedents of personality disorders that are diagnosed in adolescence was recently conducted. The four childhood conditions examined in the study were conduct problems, depressive symptoms, anxiety or fear, and immaturity. Findings indicated that predictive relationships with specific personality disorders were found for all four antecedents. Thus antecedents of adolescent personality disorder can be identified 10 years earlier through an accurate assessment of emotional and behavioral problems.[4] So too, childhood sexual abuse and other early traumatic events have been found to be risk factors for the later development of personality disorders.[21]

Many people with maladaptive social responses are enmeshed in a family system that obstructs further development and makes change difficult and hazardous. Families of borderline and narcissistic people often operate with the unspoken ground rule that independence and separation from the family imply rejection of family values. The parents often reenact their own developmental conflicts through their children, and role reversals (for example, parent as child) are common. Features of these families include various degrees of restrictiveness from the extrafamilial world, absence of clear-cut lines of authority, confusion of parental executive and nurturing roles, blurred generational boundaries, generations of family patterns in which people are labeled as good and bad, and the generational transmission of irrational forms of thinking and relating.

Current thinking suggests two factors that may promote the development of antisocial behavior: having an alcoholic parent and being abused as a child. Children of alcoholic parents are more likely to be aggressive as a result of dysfunctional family dynamics characterized by a predominance of anger and other negative affects.[30] The nurse needs to assess the nature of family interactions and gather information related to possible child abuse and alcohol abuse as part of comprehensive data collection. Child abuse is discussed in Chapter 39 and alcoholism in Chapter 24.

BIOLOGICAL FACTORS. Growing evidence suggests that the development of major personality disorders is determined by environmental factors that interact with biological factors such as lack of anxiety tolerance, aggressiveness, and genetic vulnerability to certain affects.[23] Twin studies of the effects of heredity and environment on the development of personality disorders conclude that these disorders occur on a continuum with normal personality traits.[22] Abnormal behaviors, except those related to attachment and dependency, showed a strong genetic component. There is also support for the theory that behavioral disorders occur when a person with a strong genetic predisposition experiences unusual life stress.

Growing evidence supports the premise that biological factors influence the development of antisocial personality. Low levels of serotonin have been reported in people prone to aggressive and impulsive behaviors. Recent studies have also found that low thresholds for limbic system stimulation are likely to occur in people with antisocial behavior. Finally, a study of monozygotic twins presents convincing evidence that antisocial behavior is inheritable.[16] Thus, biological predisposing factors appear to interact with environmental factors such as parental hostility, deficient parental role modeling, and reinforcement of vindictive behavior in the genesis of antisocial personality disorder.[35]

Finally, there is some evidence that a subgroup of patients with borderline personality disorder have biological abnormalities similar to those found in mood disorders.[6] This is as yet inconclusive. There is a possibility that dopaminergic function may contribute to the transient psychotic symptoms experienced by some borderline patients. Some studies have found an inverse relationship between serotonin and aggressive or suicidal behavior. These findings are suggestive of multiple biochemical disruptions related to maladaptive social responses. Further research is needed to clarify the role of neurotransmitters in the development of personality disorders.

SOCIOCULTURAL FACTORS. Sociocultural factors can also influence the person's ability to establish and maintain relatedness. Many forces in American culture make people feel isolated and lonely. Friendships are often short term because of the mobility involved in many occupations. Family relationships are more distant as adult children move away and see their parents only occasionally. Friends are often closer than siblings.

Warren[37] has developed the following criteria for social isolation:

▼ *Stigmatized environment.* The person is labeled as different, is aware of this, and is hesitant, unwilling, or does not know how to participate in social interactions.

▼ *Societal indifference.* The person experiences loneliness or lacks close relationships.

▼ *Personal-societal disconnection.* Society reacts to the stigmatized person by denying access to close relationships.

▼ *Personal powerlessness.* Society's rejection causes people to believe they are powerless to control their lives.

Involuntary social isolation also affects the disabled and chronically ill of any age. People with terminal illnesses or disfiguring disorders are often stigmatized and avoided by others. This is also true for people with long-term psychiatric problems. Although an effort has been made to decrease chronic institutionalization, many strongly resist integrating disabled people into the community. This involuntary isolation may result in a variety of maladaptive social responses as the person tries to cope with loneliness.

Immigration continues to be a reality in the United States and many other parts of the world. As people move into entirely different cultures, they may feel alienated and frightened about customs they do not understand. Sometimes immigrants form separate communities to preserve their traditions. These close-knit communities help to meet relationship needs but create barriers to broader community participation. Unfortunately, they also focus attention on the group, often attracting discriminatory behavior.

Closeness is the ideal in American culture. At the same time, people are given the message that they need to be careful in deciding whom to trust. This can cause confusion and a feeling of insecurity. Rising crime rates cause fear and reluctance to risk closeness or contact with strangers. Some urban residents, particularly the elderly, become lonely prisoners in their homes.

Precipitating Stressors

Maladaptive social responses are the result of experiences that influence the person's emotional growth. In most instances a series of life events predisposes a person to have relationship problems. Many people cope with their interpersonal problems and say they are reasonably satisfied with their relationships. However, additional stress can cause a somewhat satisfying interpersonal life to become disrupted. Response to stressors is highly individual, and the nurse should remember that the person experiences an increase in

anxiety as a result of the stressor. This is at the root of the behavioral disruption.

SOCIOCULTURAL STRESSORS. Stressors leading to relationship difficulties may be sociocultural. For instance, there can be instability in the family. Divorces are common. Mobility has broken up the extended family, depriving people of all ages of an important support system. Less contact occurs between the generations. Tradition, which provides a powerful link with the past and a sense of identity, is less observable when the family is fragmented. Interest in ethnicity and "roots" may reflect the efforts of isolated people to associate themselves with a specific identity. The many stresses on the family have made it more difficult for family members to accomplish the developmental tasks related to intimacy.

Nurses who work in general hospitals often encounter patients with maladaptive social responses. Even a reasonably well-adjusted person may have difficulty maintaining a satisfying level of intimacy while hospitalized. The patient's feeling of isolation is enhanced by the impersonal hospital environment. Sometimes patients need to be isolated because of infection, or in the psychiatric setting to control behavior. They are then susceptible to the effects of sensory deprivation. Creative nursing care is needed to lessen this problem. For instance, a patient who is in isolation for infection control could be given a schedule of times when staff will be present. This should include time to talk. Family members should be encouraged to visit, telephone, and share current activities. On the other hand, sensory overload may be a problem for patients in critical care units. This can also lead to loneliness and separation from others.

PSYCHOLOGICAL STRESSORS. Many psychological theories have been proposed to explain problems in establishing and maintaining satisfying relationships. It is known that high anxiety levels result in impaired ability to relate to others. A combination of prolonged or intense anxiety with limited coping ability is believed to cause severe relationship problems.

It has been suggested that the person with borderline personality disorder is likely to experience an incapacitating level of anxiety in response to life events that represent increased autonomy and separation, (such as high school or college graduation, going away to camp, marriage, birth of a child, employment, job promotion). The person who has narcissistic personality disorder tends to experience high anxiety, causing relationship difficulties, when the significant other no longer adequately nourishes the person's fragile self-esteem. These relationships often move through predictable stages:

1. Idealization and overvaluation
2. Disappointment when unrealistic needs for maintaining self-esteem are not met
3. Rationalization and devaluation
4. Rejection of the other person based on "narcissistic injury"

Typically, these people go through life repeating this pattern on the job, in marriages, and in friendships.

Appraisal of Stressors

The mature person who can participate in healthy relationships is still vulnerable to the effects of psychological stress. A person's appraisal of the stressor is critically important in this regard. A series of losses or a single significant loss may lead to problems in establishing future intimate relationships. The pain of a loss can be so great that the person avoids future involvements rather than risk more pain. This response is more likely if the person had difficulty with developmental tasks pertinent to relatedness. Losses of significant others may cause difficulty with future relationships, but other types of losses may do the same. For example, the loss of a job decreases a person's self-esteem. This can also result in future withdrawal and problems unless the person has a well-established support system.

Coping Resources

When a person is having problems with relationships, it is important for the nurse to assess the person's coping resources. For many people, when one relationship is troublesome or lost, others are available to offer support and reassurance. Those who have broad networks of family and friends have many resources to draw upon. Sometimes they need encouragement to reach out for help.

Some people do not have readily available human supports but have other ways of managing interpersonal problems. Pets can be an important way of expressing relatedness. Isolated elderly people often focus their need to give and receive affection on a dog or cat. Sometimes a person who is troubled about a relationship will use creative ways to express feelings. Use of expressive media such as art, music, or writing allows the person to explore and resolve an upsetting experience. Others are helped by reading, exercise, looking at art, dancing, or listening to music.

> **?** *Identify a novel, a popular song, or a work of art that would have meaning for a person who is trying to cope with an interpersonal loss.*

Coping Mechanisms

Behaviors associated with maladaptive social responses are attempts to cope with anxiety related to threatened or actual loneliness. However, they are not healthy and sometimes have the unintended effect of driving people away. Thus the person is always caught in the approach-avoidance conflict of the need-fear dilemma, searching for some degree of human contact on one hand and pushing people away on the other.

Manipulative people view other people as objects. Their defenses protect them from potential psychological pain related to the loss of a significant other. People with antisocial

personality disorder often use the defenses of projection and splitting. **Projection** places responsibility for antisocial behavior outside oneself. For instance, a patient may rationalize using drugs by saying, "Everybody I know uses cocaine. Why shouldn't I?" **Splitting** is characteristic of people with borderline and narcissistic personality disorders as well. It is the inability to integrate the good and bad aspects of oneself and objects. An object is anything outside of the self, animate or inanimate, to which the person has an attachment. An object could be a parent, a friend, or a teddy bear. Characteristics of splitting include the following:

▼ Alternately expressing opposite sides of a conflict while appearing unconcerned about the contradiction
▼ Inconsistent lack of impulse control with periodic expression of primitive impulses and no concurrent anxiety
▼ Dividing perceptions of objects (people and things) into "all good" and "all bad"
▼ Fluctuation between "all good" and "all bad" perceptions
  Defense mechanisms characteristic of people with borderline personality disorder include
▼ Denial of responsibility for acting out behavior and denial of painful or threatening feelings
▼ Devaluation of another, which makes the borderline person appear good by contrast
▼ Idealization of positive traits of others
▼ Projective identification, in which the borderline person projects various parts of oneself onto different people
▼ Dissociation to block out feelings
▼ Isolation and avoidance of self-discolsure[28]

Projective identification is a complex defense mechanism. When the borderline patient projects parts of himself or herself onto others, these people are often not consciously aware of this. However, they may begin to behave like the projected parts.[14] For example, a patient projects onto a nurse cruel, punishing parts of oneself. The projection reverberates with something in the nurse that had been submerged, and the nurse will tend to react to the patient in a cruel, punishing manner. Likewise, staff who have received idealized projected parts of the patient will tend to respond in an overly involved, protective, indulgent manner. An example of projective identification is demonstrated by Ms. T in the following clinical example.

Clinical Example A nurse, Ms. M, was describing her relationship with a borderline patient, Ms. T, who had been on the unit for approximately 2 weeks. She explained that Ms. T had become negativistic and increasingly demanding to the point that her demands had no bounds. For the past week Ms. T had been calling Ms. M "Nurse Ratched." If that was not difficult enough, Ms. T was also telling new patients on the unit about what a tyrant Ms. M was. Further inquiry made it clear that soon after Ms. T had cast Ms. M into "Nurse Ratched's" role, she started to react to the patient far more rigidly than was typical for her. Indeed, most of her interactions with Ms. T were now focused on policy adherence and strict limit setting. Without knowing it, Ms. M was on her way to repeating a script straight out of the movie *One Flew Over the Cuckoo's Nest.*

Selected Nursing Diagnosis:

▼ Self-esteem disturbance related to use of the defense mechanism of splitting, as evidenced by need to belittle the nurse

Finally, the defense mechanisms of splitting and projective identification help explain why different staff members often see the same patient in very different ways, as illustrated in Fig. 22-3.

 Compare the processes of empathic understanding and projective identification.

Nursing Diagnosis

When diagnosing maladaptive social responses, the nurse should consider the extent and nature of maladaptive behaviors, coping mechanisms, and the predisposing factors and precipitating stressors leading to the behaviors. The nurse may formulate a nursing diagnosis by using the Stuart Stress Adaptation Model (Fig. 22-4) as a guide. Nursing diagnoses associated with maladaptive social responses and related medical diagnoses are presented in the Medical and Nursing Diagnoses box on p. 451. Primary NANDA diagnoses include **personal identity disturbance, self-esteem disturbance, risk for self-mutilation, impaired social interaction,** and **risk for violence.** Examples of complete nursing diagnoses are presented in the Detailed Diagnoses box on p. 452.

Related Medical Diagnoses

Medical diagnoses related to maladaptive social responses are categorized as personality disorders. Personality is composed of temperament, which is inherited, and character, which is learned.[3]

In general the distinguishing characteristics of the personality disorders are that they are:

▼ Chronic and long-standing
▼ Not based on a sound personality structure
▼ Difficult to change

Personality disorders are described in the Detailed Diagnoses box.

 Describe one of your own personality traits that is due to temperament and one that is due to character.

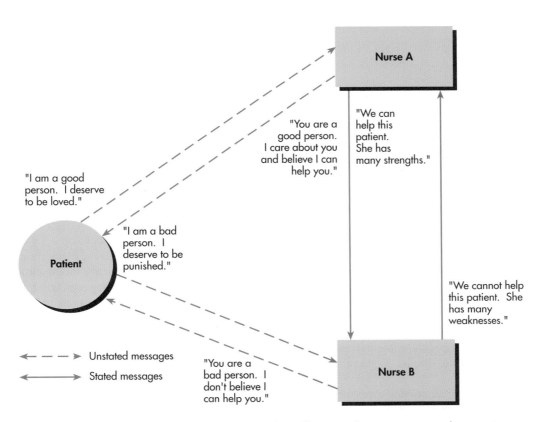

Fig. 22-3 Projective identification and splitting affects patient-to-nurse and nurse-to-nurse communication.

Fig. 22-4   The Stuart Stress Adaptation Model related to social responses.

Outcome Identification

The expected outcome for nursing care of the patient with maladaptive social responses is the following:

The patient will obtain maximum interpersonal satisfaction by establishing and maintaining self-enhancing relationships with others.

Short-term goals are more specific to the patient's problems. They may progress from simpler to more complex changes in behavior.

It can be difficult to set mutual nursing care goals with a patient who has problems with relatedness. This is partly because mutuality must be based on a strong nurse-patient relationship. It is difficult to develop a strong relationship with a patient who fears intimacy. In addition, setting a goal implies a commitment to change. Many patients who have maladaptive social responses are reluctant to commit themselves to change. Because most of these behavioral problems also serve as coping mechanisms, there is additional resistance to change.

For these reasons, even though it is desirable to have the patient's full participation, it may be necessary for the nurse to set initial goals. To overcome a problem with relatedness, the person must be involved with others. At first, the other person may be the nurse, but eventually others will take the nurse's place.

MEDICAL AND NURSING DIAGNOSES *related to* **Maladaptive Social Responses**

Related Medical Diagnoses (DSM-IV)*	Related Nursing Diagnoses (NANDA)†
Paranoid personality disorder	Adjustment, impaired
Schizoid personality disorder	Anxiety
Schizotypal personality disorder	Coping, ineffective family
Antisocial personality disorder	Coping, ineffective individual
Borderline personality disorder	Family processes, altered
Histrionic personality disorder	Management of therapeutic regimen, individual or family:
Narcissistic personality disorder	effective or ineffective
Avoidant personality disorder	**Personal Identity Disturbance‡**
Dependent personality disorder	Role performance, altered
Obsessive-compulsive personality disorder	**Self-esteem Disturbance‡**
	Self-mutilation, Risk for‡
	Social Interaction, Impaired‡
	Social isolation
	Thought processes, altered
	Violence, Risk for‡
	Self-directed
	Directed at others

*From American Psychiatric Association: *Diagnostic and statistical manual of mental disorders,* ed 4, 1994, The Association.
†From North American Nursing Diagnosis Association: *NANDA nursing diagnoses: definitions and classifications 1997-1998,* Philadelphia, 1997, The Association.
‡Primary nursing diagnosis for maladaptive social responses.

Short-term goals with these patients may focus on reducing acting-out behaviors and modifying specific communication patterns. Examples include the following:

▼ The patient will use verbal communication as an alternative to acting out.
▼ The patient will verbally identify angry feelings when they occur during a one-to-one interaction.

These goals must be developed with the patient's active participation.

Learning to relate more directly and openly causes anxiety. Therefore, the patient's ability to tolerate anxiety must be considered when setting goals. Increasing the anxiety level before the patient has increased coping ability and environmental supports may reinforce use of maladaptive coping behaviors.

Planning

The nursing care plan provides a guide for intervention and promotes consistency among the nursing staff members who provide care to the patient. This is particularly important when working with patients with maladaptive social responses.[8] Planning also includes attending to the patient's educational needs. A Patient Education Plan for modifying impulsive behavior is presented on p. 453. However, it is the nurse's responsibility to help patients and their families to understand the nature and treatment of any of the disorders that cause maladaptive social responses.

Implementation

Establishing a Therapeutic Relationship

No matter what type of maladaptive social response the patient is experiencing, nursing care is based on accessibility. The nurse must be physically present with the patient regularly so that there is an opportunity for interaction. There must also be psychological accessibility. This means that the nurse shows interest in the patient. The nurse tries to understand the patient by clarifying meanings and validating perceptions. The nurse is also empathic. If the nurse-patient relationship is a healthy one, the patient can learn how to find satisfaction in other human relationships (see A Patient Speaks on p. 453).

Family Involvement

Because intimate relationships are always affected by maladaptive social responses, significant others must be involved in the plan of care (see A Family Speaks). This is especially important for manipulative patients, who often shift attention away from themselves by creating conflict between the family and the staff. For instance, the patient may complain to family members about poor nursing care. At the same time the patient may tell the staff about mistreatment by the family. Staff and family are then in conflict. Attention is distracted from the patient, who avoids the discomfort of self-examination. When the staff finally realizes what is happening, the result is usually anger at the patient. Nurses should be aware of this tendency and avoid a puni-

DETAILED DIAGNOSES *related to* **Maladaptive Social Responses**

NANDA Diagnosis Stem	Examples of Complete Diagnosis
Personal identity disturbance	Personal identity disturbance related to early developmental arrest, as evidenced by difficulty defining self boundaries
Self-esteem disturbance	Self-esteem disturbance related to physical abuse during childhood, as evidenced by verbalized unhappiness with personal accomplishments
Risk for self-mutilation	Risk for self-mutilation related to fear of rejection, as evidenced by cutting self after visits from parents
Impaired social interaction	Impaired social interaction related to rejection of sociocultural values, as evidenced by stated belief that rules do not pertain to self
Risk for violence: self-directed	Risk for self-directed violence related to need to punish self, as evidenced by repeated burning of hands and feet when criticized
Risk for violence: directed at others	Risk for violence directed at others related to use of projection as evidenced by blaming, argumentativeness, and recent purchase of a handgun

DSM-IV Diagnosis	Essential Features*
Paranoid personality disorder	A pervasive distrust and suspiciousness of others such that their motives are interpreted as malevolent, beginning in early adulthood and present in a variety of contexts
Schizoid personality disorder	A pervasive pattern of detachment from social relationships and a restricted range of expression of emotions in interpersonal settings, beginning in early adulthood and present in a variety of contexts
Schizotypal personality disorder	A pervasive pattern of social and interpersonal deficits marked by acute discomfort with and reduced capacity for close relationships and by cognitive and perceptual distortions and eccentricities of behavior, beginning in early adulthood and present in a variety of contexts
Antisocial personality disorder	A pervasive pattern of disregard for and violation of the rights of others occurring since age 15
Borderline personality disorder	A pervasive pattern of instability of interpersonal relationships, self-image, and affects, and marked impulsivity beginning by early adulthood and present in a variety of contexts
Histrionic personality disorder	A pervasive pattern of excessive emotionality and attention seeking, beginning by early adulthood and present in a variety of contexts
Narcissistic personality disorder	A pervasive pattern of grandiosity (in fantasy or behavior), need for admiration, and lack of empathy beginning by early adulthood and present in a variety of contexts
Avoidant personality disorder	A pervasive pattern of social inhibition, feelings of inadequacy, and hypersensitivity to negative evaluation, beginning by early adulthood and present in a variety of contexts
Dependent personality disorder	A pervasive and excessive need to be taken care of that leads to submissive and clinging behavior and fears of separation, beginning by early adulthood and present in a variety of contexts
Obsessive-compulsive personality disorder	A pervasive pattern of preoccupation with orderliness, perfectionism, and mental and interpersonal control, at the expense of flexibility, openness, and efficiency, beginning by early adulthood and present in a variety of contexts

*Modified from the American Psychiatric Association: *Diagnostic and statistical manual of mental disorders,* ed 4, Washington, DC, 1994, The Association.

tive response. When manipulative patients are hospitalized, this behavior occurs many times. The patient returns home, still relating to others as objects. Family involvement is also important to promote and maintain positive change for the patient and family.

> **?** *How would you help family members to participate in the treatment of a person with a personality disorder?*

Milieu Therapy

Because it is difficult and takes a long time to change maladaptive social responses, most patients are treated in the community. However, sometimes hospitalization is needed. For instance, the person with a borderline personality disorder may be self-destructive, or the antisocial person may require a structured environment with limit setting. Day treatment or partial hospitalization programs have been found to have unique advantages for the treatment of patients with borderline personality disorder.[25] Such treatment can offer patients the optimal level of intensiveness

PATIENT EDUCATION PLAN Modifying Impulsive Behavior

Content	Instructional Activities	Evaluation
Describe characteristics and consequences of impulsive behavior.	Select a situation in which impulsive behavior occurred. Ask the patient to describe what happened. Provide the patient with paper and a pen. Instruct the patient to keep a diary of impulsive actions, including a description of events before and after the incident.	The patient will identify and describe an impulsive incident. The patient will maintain a diary of impulsive behaviors. The patient will explore the causes and consequences of impulsive behavior.
Describe behaviors characteristic of interpersonal anxiety and relate anxiety to impulsive behavior.	Discuss the diary with the patient. Help the patient to identify interpersonal anxiety related to impulsive behavior.	The patient will connect feelings of interpersonal anxiety with impulsive behavior.
Explain stress-reduction techniques.	Describe the stress response (see Chapters 16 and 17). Demonstrate relaxation exercises (see Chapter 30). Help the patient to return the demonstration.	The patient will perform relaxation exercises when signs of anxiety appear.
Identify alternative responses to anxiety-producing situations.	Using situations from the diary and knowledge of relaxation exercises, help the patient to list possible alternative responses.	The patient will identify at least two alternative responses to each anxiety-producing situation.
Practice using alternative responses to anxiety-producing situations.	Role-play each of the identified alternative behaviors. Discuss the feelings associated with impulsive behavior and the alternatives.	The patient will describe the relationship between behavior and feelings. The patient will select and perform anxiety-reducing behaviors.

and containment, resulting in less regressive dependency and acting-out behavior.

The milieu, as found in hospitals, residential treatment, or outpatient programs, can effectively provide patients with an opportunity to gain insight into their behavior.[11] Aside from staff limit setting, patients with maladaptive social responses learn from other patients about how much acting out will be tolerated. The patient responds well to a therapeutic milieu in which mature, responsible behavior is expected. Milieu work with these patients is most effective if it focuses on the following:

▼ Realistic expectations
▼ The process of decision making
▼ The process of interactional behaviors in the here and now

Nursing roles in milieu therapy include:

▼ Provide a structured environment
▼ Serve as an emotional sounding board
▼ Clarify and diagnose conflicts

Consistent clinical supervision is also very important because countertransference is usually an issue when caring for these patients (see Chapter 2). Positive countertransference by some staff members, and negative by others, leads to splitting and staff conflict. Whenever these behavioral patterns emerge while there is a manipulative patient on the

A Patient *Speaks*

When I was hospitalized, the nurses were my link with the outside world. They were with me more than anyone else. They were also my link to the treatment that was prescribed by my psychiatrist. The doctor left PRN orders because he thought I was a mature woman who could decide when I needed medication. I often felt a loss of dignity when the nurse questioned my need for the PRN medication. Because the medicine decreased my anxiety, I think I was the best judge of when I needed it. Because the doctor made me responsible for requesting the medication, it was not the nurse's job to question my need for it unless I asked for more than was prescribed. Even if someone is in the hospital, they need to be treated with dignity and respect. They are sick, not children and not stupid. Nothing hurts more than being treated like a second-class citizen by people who are in a more powerful position. It is much easier to work with a nurse who is kind and supportive. ▼

A Family *Speaks*

It seems like my brother was always a problem. When we were growing up, he got us both into trouble all the time. Finally I learned to ignore his schemes and stay away from him. As he got older, the situation got worse. Our parents kicked him out of the house, but he would come back and promise to change and they would let him back in. Then it would start all over again. He began to get into trouble with the law. First there was vandalism for spray-painting graffiti on a building; then he was with a gang of kids who stole a car. He said he was just along for the ride, but I didn't really believe him.

The rest of the family was pretty embarrassed about his behavior. I thought about telling people I was adopted so they wouldn't think I was like him. I didn't do that because I knew it would hurt my parents and they had enough trouble already. I'll never forget the night when the phone rang at 4:00 AM and it was my brother saying he was in jail. He had been caught with drugs in a stolen car and had also resisted arrest. My parents refused to bail him out and he didn't have any money. The next day he called again to say that he was at the local psychiatric hospital. He had threatened to kill himself in jail, so they sent him to the hospital to see whether he was really mentally ill.

My parents were really upset about this development. I think it was actually a good thing, though, because the doctors and nurses at the hospital explained to us that he has a personality disorder. It did help to know that there might be a reason for his behavior, although he hasn't really changed much. I think my parents are beginning to accept this, but I know it's really hard for them. ▼

psychiatric unit, the staff must examine their level of involvement with the patient.[29]

Dyckoff addresses countertransference issues related to the borderline patient.[10] Countertransference feelings may include impulses to rescue, support, hurt, admire, identify with, or accept compliments from the patient. The principles of milieu treatment for patients with Cluster B personality disorders include the following:

▼ Establish control with no option to escape involvement

▼ Provide an experienced, consistent staff

▼ Implement a strict hierarchical structure with rules that are firm and consistently enforced

▼ Provide support while the patient learns to experience painful feelings

Limit Setting and Structure

The way the nurse approaches limit setting can make the difference between a productive hospital experience and one that is nonproductive or counterproductive. Angry, punitive limit setting confirms the patient's expectations. Suppressive and rigid limits create obstacles to self-exploration and therapeutic change. This approach also confirms the patient's belief of having little or no control over life situations. It is essential that the nurse not view limits as a way of controlling the patient.

For example, a patient with antisocial personality structure engages in physically aggressive acting-out behavior. One way of dealing with this might be to emphasize the need for medications and to tighten up restrictions. The treatment team might also issue an ultimatum, such as "One more similar episode, and we're going to have to transfer you to another hospital." A more positive way of approaching the situation could be: "I can't understand why you're putting the team in the position of having to reassess continuation of your stay in this hospital. Has there been some change about wanting to help yourself?" The difference in the latter approach is emphasis on the idea that the patient has responsibility for life situations; the control and the decisions are the patient's. It also communicates an attitude of respect, which could boost the patient's self-esteem. The more the nurse is able to align with the nonregressed aspects of the patient's ego, the better are the chances for improved functioning.

Manipulative patients must also be held responsible for their behavior. They are skilled at placing responsibility on others. Staff members must communicate with each other so that consistent messages are given. These patients recognize any inconsistency and use it to focus attention on others. They usually resist rules. Staff and family members must collaborate in enforcing clear limits. Manipulative patients sometimes lie. It is important to confront the patient who consciously lies.

Masterson[24] describes guidelines for treating borderline patients that incorporate several of these principles. He emphasizes the need for availability of staff attention combined with structured discipline. There must be an expectation that the patient will meet standards of healthy behavior. Failure to meet the standard is identified, and acting out is confronted. Loss of control may be dealt with by room restriction, with the patient instructed to think about the episode so that it may be discussed in therapy. The length of the restriction should be based on the seriousness of the behavior. These approaches may lead to depression. The depressed feelings should be directed into formal psychotherapy sessions, but the staff can act as role models for appropriate behavior. A school program, occupational therapy, and the milieu may be used to teach age-appropriate social and achievement skills. Reality orientation may also be necessary.

Should Constant Close Observation Be the Primary Nursing Approach for Borderline Patients with Impulsive Self-harming Behavior?

Patients with borderline personality disorder are most often hospitalized because of impulsive attempts at self-mutilation or suicide. The nursing intervention of constant close observation is usually initiated to protect the patient from impulsive behavior. This intervention activates the patient's conflicts about close relationships. Splitting may become evident as the patient establishes preferences for the staff assigned to observation. The patient is challenged to outwit the staff and find opportunities to act out. When efforts are made to decrease the level of observation, the patient's attachment conflicts become evident. There is often an effort to maintain the undivided attention of staff by renewed self-harming behavior.

Gallop[12] suggests that nurses can help these patients to assume responsibility for their behavior and find ways to change it. The nurse should enlist the patient's help in defining and describing the harmful behavior. Identification of behavioral cues and triggers allows the patient to request assistance, thereby becoming an active participant in the therapeutic process. Nurses are less judgmental about the patient because they understand the source of the behavior and can be sensitive to the patient's feelings. The challenge to nurses is to maintain the patient's safety while facilitating behavioral change.

> **?** *You believe that a manipulative adolescent patient is exploiting another patient by "borrowing" money, clothing, and snacks. When confronted, the first patient claims that the items were gifts, "because we're friends." Do you think that limit setting is needed? If so, how would you set appropriate limits?*

Protection from Self-Harm

The deliberate self-destructive or self-mutilating behavior of the borderline patient is very difficult to treat (see Chapter 20). Often the nursing staff must observe the patient constantly to prevent serious physical harm. At the same time, these patients have intense dependency needs related to an unresolved separation-individuation developmental phase. This makes it extremely difficult to wean them from constant staff attention, and contact must be decreased very gradually. Observation may need to be increased again if the patient seems out of control. Patient involvement in planning for decreased observation may be helpful. The patient must be reassured that less contact does not equal no contact. Consistent, scheduled time with a staff member is recommended. Primary nursing is particularly effective with a patient who needs to work

through these separation issues (see Critical Thinking about Contemporary Issues).

Focusing on Strengths

Patients with maladaptive social responses often are effective leaders within the patient group. A useful nursing approach is to encourage them to identify and use their strengths. They may be given responsibilities within the patient care unit and can be helpful to other patients. They are often intelligent and can participate actively in planning their own care. However, they are extremely resistant to recognizing or dealing with feelings and need consistent encouragement to verbalize these emotions.

Nurses become frustrated with these patients because they seem to be so aware of what is happening and in control of most situations, yet so unaware of others' needs. Nurses must remember that these patients have little tolerance for intimacy. Their maneuvering of others is a way to keep them at a safe distance. These patients are often charming, and it is easy to become involved with them. However, as soon as other people make demands or show signs of emotional closeness, the patients dilute the relationship by withdrawing, frustrating others, or distracting attention from themselves.

Journal writing is a nursing intervention that can be helpful to patients who have difficulty with close relationships. Keeping a diary of their thoughts and feelings helps them identify the various aspects of their interpersonal experiences and review them over time. Sebastian[33] has found that keeping a journal helps patients develop object constancy. It gives them an opportunity to see continuity of people and relationships. The nurse can review the journal with the patient to help in making connections among experiences. Interpersonal strengths can be identified and reinforced. The nurse can also note behavioral strengths that the patient has not yet identified and help the patient in recognizing these as well.

Behavioral Strategies

Various behavioral strategies can help decrease antisocial behavior (see Chapter 30). The patient is usually impatient with delays in gratification. Material rather than emotional rewards are preferred. Thus, reinforcers used in a behavior modification program should be concrete and readily available. For example, points may be accumulated to qualify for privileges, such as a trip to the canteen. Other reinforcers might be a visit or a favorite food. Ignoring undesirable behavior is the least reinforcing but is not always possible. If behavior is disruptive and there must be a response, it should be matter of fact and one not desired by the patient. For instance, removal from contact with others for a specific period of time may discourage undesirable behavior, whereas a lecture that attracts attention may be a reinforcer.

Behavioral contracting has been tried with borderline patients. Miller[27] describes the contract as a mutually negotiated agreement that is explicit and specifies the responsibilities of both parties. She describes the advantages of behavioral contracting as:

▼ Emphasizing the need for the patient's active collaboration in treatment
▼ Decreasing vulnerability to regression
▼ Reducing anxiety about medicolegal issues
▼ Helping the treatment team identify countertransference feelings and splitting more quickly
▼ Countering an unrealistic sense of timeliness by establishing a prearranged discharge date

When a contract is negotiated, control is shared between the nurse and the patient. The nurse-patient contract is based on patient-identified strengths, learning needs, and goals. However, the patient must agree to basic expectations. These usually include agreement to refrain from harmful behavior, as well as defining the length of time that the contract will be in effect.

Finally, cognitive-behavioral therapy (see Chapter 30) has been shown to be effective in working with patients with borderline personality disorder. A group format used by nurses focuses treatment modules on deficits in emotional control and regulation, interpersonal effectiveness, and distress tolerance.[26] Reinforcement of the patient's new coping skills outside of the group setting was also seen as an important aspect of successful treatment.

A Nursing Treatment Plan Summary for the patient with maladaptive social responses is presented at right.

Evaluation

Evaluating the success of nursing intervention is difficult when the focus is on the quality of the therapeutic relationship. Because the relationship is central to effective nursing care, it is threatening for many nurses to examine their ability to relate to others. This type of evaluation must take place on two levels. One level focuses on the nurse and the nurse's participation in the relationship. Self-examination may be useful in accomplishing this, especially if the nurse reviews an interaction immediately. Blind spots about one's own feelings that may be present while involved with the patient may become clearer in retrospect. However, self-evaluation is colored by self-perceptions. Supervision from an experienced nurse therapist can be very helpful in identifying aspects of the relationship that may be less obvious to the nurse. Constructive supervision can help nurses identify the dynamics of the relationship. It can also help them deal with patients' resistance to change. No matter how experienced, nurses' perceptions of their participation in a relationship are affected by their self-concept. The need for supervision continues throughout their career.

The second level of evaluation focuses on the patient's behavior and the behavioral changes that the nurse works to facilitate. The patient is the primary source of input about these changes. Perceived changes in behavior should be validated with the patient to see whether the patient is also aware of change. Sharing feelings and intimate thoughts denotes increased trust and a willingness to risk self-revelation. Nonverbally the patient also reveals responses to the therapeutic relationship. Accessibility to the nurse for scheduled meetings indicates trust and involvement in the relationship. Eye contact usually occurs more often when one person is comfortable with another. Initiation of activities with others indicates more openness to relatedness. Increased decision making and assumption of leadership roles imply improved self-esteem and increasing self-confidence. Such behaviors can be observed, documented, and validated with other staff members. Therefore, these are useful evaluation criteria.

Significant others may also contribute to the evaluation. They have known the patient before the occurrence of any behavioral problem and can provide information about the patient's behavioral norms. They are particularly helpful in providing information about changes that continue when the patient is in the community. Some patients have difficulty transferring new behavior to their usual life settings. Involving families in this type of assessment helps to teach the family the behaviors learned by the patient. It gives them an idea of what is reasonable to expect from the patient.

Several questions may help the nurse to evaluate the outcomes of intervention with the patient who has maladaptive social responses:

▼ Has the patient become less impulsive, manipulative, or narcissistic?
▼ Does the patient express satisfaction with the quality of his or her relationships?
▼ Can the patient participate in close relationships?
▼ Does the patient express recognition of positive behavioral change?

Summary

1. In a healthy relationship, the people involved experience intimacy with each other while maintaining separate identities. Adaptive social responses include the capacity for solitude, autonomy, mutuality, and interdependence.

2. The behaviors associated with disruptions in relatedness include manipulation, impulsivity, and narcissism.

3. Predisposing factors for maladaptive social responses are described from developmental, biological, and sociocultural perspectives. Precipitating stressors that affect social responses include sociocultural values and norms and psychological pressures.

4. A wide array of relationships and interests provide coping resources. Coping mechanisms related to social responses may include idealization of others, devaluation of others, projection, acting out, splitting, and projective identification.

5. Primary NANDA nursing diagnoses are personal iden-

NURSING TREATMENT PLAN *Summary*   Maladaptive Social Responses

Nursing Diagnosis: Impaired social interaction
Expected Outcome: The patient will obtain maximum interpersonal satisfaction by establishing and maintaining self-enhancing relationships with others.

Short-term Goals	Interventions	Rationale
The patient will participate in a therapeutic nurse-patient relationship.	Initiate a nurse-patient relationship contract mutually agreed on by patient and nurse. Develop mutual behavioral goals. Maintain consistent behavior by all nursing staff. Communicate honest responses to the patient's behavior. Provide honest, immediate feedback about behavioral change. Maintain confidentiality. Demonstrate accessibility.	An atmosphere of trust facilitates open expression of thoughts and feelings. A trusting relationship enables the patient to risk sharing feelings. Honest responses reinforce openness. Staff consistency creates a predictable environment that creates trust.
The patient will describe interpersonal strengths and weaknesses.	Provide opportunities to demonstrate strengths, such as helping other patients, assuming leadership roles. Help to analyze experiences that are perceived as failures. Communicate acceptance of the patient as a person while not accepting maladaptive social behavior.	Patients with maladaptive social responses are unable to identify accurately their interpersonal strengths and weaknesses, leading to fear of closeness and fear of failure. It is important to help the patient to separate behavioral incidents from total self-worth and recognize that one can be liked even if imperfect.
The patient will establish or reestablish one interpersonal relationship that is mutually satisfying and adaptive.	Provide consistent feedback about adaptive and maladaptive social behavior. Encourage patient to describe successful and unsuccessful relationship experiences orally or in a written journal. Help patient in initiating or resuming a relationship with one other person. Review aspects of this relationship with the patient. Reinforce the patient's adaptive social responses. Evaluate with the patient alternatives to maladaptive social responses.	Describing and evaluating one's behavior requires taking responsibility for the behavior and its consequences. Patients need to go beyond understanding or insight to engaging in actual behavioral change. It is important for the nurse to help the patient evaluate whether one's responses are adaptive or maladaptive. Alternatives can then be identified to further the patient's goal achievement.

Nursing Diagnosis: Risk for self-mutilation
Expected Outcome: The patient will select constructive rather than self-destructive ways of coping with interpersonal anxiety.

Short-term Goals	Interventions	Rationale
The patient will not engage in self-mutilation.	Develop a contract with the patient to notify staff when anxiety is increasing. Provide close 1:1 observation of the patient when necessary to maintain safety. Remove all potentially dangerous objects from the patient and the environment. Provide prescribed medications.	When the patient is unable to cope with anxiety, safety is the nurse's highest priority. A contract helps the patient assume responsibility and explore healthier coping responses.

Continued

tity disturbance, self-esteem disturbance, risk for self-mutilation, social isolation, and risk for violence (self-directed or directed at others).

6. Primary DSM-IV diagnoses are paranoid, schizoid, schizotypal, histrionic, antisocial, narcissistic, obsessive-compulsive, dependent, avoidant, and passive-aggressive personality disorders.

7. The expected outcome of nursing care is that the patient will obtain maximum satisfaction by establishing and maintaining self-enhancing relationships with others.

NURSING TREATMENT PLAN *Summary* Maladaptive Social Responses—cont'd

Nursing Diagnosis: Risk for self-mutilation
Expected Outcome: The patient will select constructive rather than self-destructive ways of coping with interpersonal anxiety.

Short-term Goals	Interventions	Rationale
The patient will describe self-mutilating episodes.	Help the patient review these events. Identify cues and triggers that precede self-mutilating behavior. Help the patient explore feelings related to these episodes.	Self-mutilation is often a way of relieving extreme anxiety. Structured interpersonal support can help the patient review these events.
The patient will describe alternatives to self-mutilation.	Suggest alternative behaviors such as seeking interpersonal support or engaging in an adaptive anxiety-reducing activity.	The nurse can help the patient review the full range of adaptive responses. Supportive but critical evaluation is necessary for behavioral change.
The patient will implement one new adaptive response when experiencing high interpersonal anxiety.	Help the patient select new adaptive responses. Reinforce the patient's adaptive behavior. Identify positive consequences of the adaptive responses. Discuss ways these may be generalized to other situations.	The nurses should take an active role in setting limits, examining patient behaviors, and reinforcing adaptive actions. These new learned responses can also be reviewed for their applicability to other life events.

8. The plan of nursing care must be realistic, considering the patient's ability to tolerate anxiety, and promote consistency of interventions.

9. Primary nursing interventions for patients with maladaptive social responses include establishing a therapeutic relationship, family involvement, milieu therapy, limit setting and structure, protection from self-harm, focusing on strengths, and behavior modification.

10. Evaluation is based on the patient's recognition of improvement of the quality and quantity of interpersonal relationships.

COMPETENT CARING A Clinical Exemplar of a Psychiatric Nurse

Ernestine Cosby, BSN, RN, C

I met Ms. X when she was admitted to my unit. She was 35 years old with a diagnosis of borderline personality disorder and a history of five hospitalizations. Her previous hospitalizations were characterized by being in restraints for destructive behavior to herself and others, intense negative relationships with staff, and depression with a history of four suicide attempts. Ms. X had been a nun for 8 years until her self-destructive behavior became unmanageable at the convent, necessitating her first psychiatric admission. The order of nuns continued their involvement with her even when she was unable to return to the convent. They helped find a teaching position for her in one of their schools.

Ms. X was the oldest of four siblings, all girls, with parents who provided "things" but not affection. She had hoped to fill the emptiness she felt all the time in the convent. She discovered that being a nun didn't make it "all better." On this admission she was depressed and had made a suicide attempt by overdosing on pills. She was distrustful, unable to express anger, impulsive, and demanding. By the second day with us she was actively engaged in staff splitting, making requests that could not be met no matter how we tried and cutting herself following conflict with staff.

Predictably, the staff engaged in conflict with each other over how to deal with the patient. Because I often talked with her, my peers elected me to coordinate a plan to focus on the splitting, angry outbursts, and self-destructive behaviors. I was aware of two things I liked about Ms. X: her sense of humor and her ability to write. I spent the next few days meeting with her at planned times. My goals were to establish rapport, attempt to engage her involvement, and establish some level of trust. I was anxious about the potential for creating dependency on me. But with her involvement I planned to help her branch out from me to others.

This patient's strengths included an ability to express herself through writing. I offered several options of times when the staff had agreed that they could be with her one-on-one for 20 minutes. She selected her preferred times. We agreed that she would keep a journal of the issues, feelings, needs, or concerns to discuss with staff at the designated times. She would also write how she felt after each meeting with staff. Another nurse and I met with the patient to make a list of emergencies that would require an immediate response from the staff.

Ms. X and I met to review her contacts with the other staff.

COMPETENT CARING A Clinical Exemplar of a Psychiatric Nurse—cont'd

Initially this involved only complaints about the staff or how they talked to her. Eventually, she was able to explore her involvement in the interaction. Then she was able to listen to my feedback and later to ask other staff for their feedback. This process continued to provide stepping stones to engage her involvement in contracting to work on her self-destructive behavior, trying other coping skills to deal with anger, branching out to interact with patients, and recognizing her own manipulative behavior.

This process had peaks and valleys throughout. She would greet me in the morning (my worst time) at the door with a hostile and provoking interaction. She later explained the fear she experienced each day when it neared time for me to leave. She feared that I would not return, and at other times she would wish harm to me. This was reflected in her early morning behavior. The rewarding part of working with this patient was her continued attempt to carry out what she contracted to do, even though under protest most of the time. The staff and I were able to recognize her progress in the milieu, with staff and patients. This took longer for her to acknowledge, but one day she was able to write and share an interaction with staff that did not end in her losing control or cutting. She was ecstatic that she used options that she had worked out and that had resulted in a positive outcome. Since her discharge Ms. X has not required inpatient hospitalization. In outpatient therapy she has continued to be actively involved in her treatment.

your INTERNET connection

BPD Central: Borderline Personality Disorder
http://members.aol.com/BPDCentral/index.html

Borderline Personality Disorder Page
http://www.cmhc.com/disorders/sx10t.htm

Chapter Review Questions

1. For each personality disorder listed in Column A, select the cluster from Column B to which it belongs.

Column A

A. ___ Antisocial personality disorder
B. ___ Avoidant personality disorder
C. ___ Borderline personality disorder
D. ___ Dependent personality disorder
E. ___ Histrionic personality disorder
F. ___ Narcissistic personality disorder
G. ___ Obsessive-compulsive personality disorder
H. ___ Paranoid personality disorder
I. ___ Schizoid personality disorder
J. ___ Schizotypal personality disorder

Column B

Cluster A
Cluster B
Cluster C

2. Fill in the blanks.

A. Personality disorders are usually recognizable by _____ and continue throughout much of _____.

B. Patients with _____ are high users of psychiatric treatment and are particularly at risk for suicidal behavior, depression, and eating disorders.

C. Low levels of the neurotransmitter _____ have been reported in people prone to aggressive and impulsive behaviors.

D. The inability to integrate the good and bad aspects of oneself and of objects is called _____.

E. _____ occurs when one projects part of oneself onto different people.

F. Clinical supervision is important for the psychiatric nurse working with patients with personality disorders because _____ is often an issue when working with these patients.

G. A _____ is a mutually negotiated agreement that is explicit and specifies the responsibilities of both the patient and the clinician.

3. Provide short answers for the following questions.

A. Identify the three distinguishing characteristics of personality disorders.

B. Describe the two levels of evaluation necessary when working with patients with personality disorders.

C. In the United States, the diagnosis of borderline personality is most often given to females; males most often are given the diagnosis of antisocial personality disorder. Discuss the impact of American culture on this issue. Explore how these diagnoses are made in other cultures.

D. Analyze yourself and members of your family in relation to their states of relatedness: connectedness, disconnectedness, parallelism, and enmeshment.

REFERENCES

1. American Psychiatric Association: *Diagnostic and statistical manual of mental disorders,* ed 4, revised Washington, DC, 1994, The Association.
2. Amey S: Transitional objects, phenomena, and relatedness: understanding and working with individuals with borderline personality disorder, *J Am Psychiatr Nurses Assoc* 2:143, 1996.
3. Bates J, Wachs T, VandenBos G: Trends in research on temperament, *Psychiatr Serv* 46:661, 1995.
4. Bernstein D et al: Childhood antecedents of adolescent personality disorders, *Am J Psychiatry* 153:7, 1996.
5. Caroline HA: Explorations of close friendship: a concept analysis, *Arch Psychiatr Nurs* 7:236, 1993.
6. Coccaro EF, Kavoussi RJ: Biological and pharmacological aspects of borderline personality disorder, *Hosp Community Psychiatry* 42:1029, 1991.
7. Derksen J: *Personality disorders: clinical and social perspectives,* New York, 1995, Wiley.
8. Doenges ME et al: *Psychiatric care plans: guidelines for planning and documenting care,* Philadelphia, 1995, FA Davis.
9. Dulit R et al: Clinical correlates of self-mutilation in borderline personality disorder, *Am J Psychiatry* 151:1305, 1994.
10. Dychoff D et al: The investigation of behavioral contracting in patients with borderline personality disorder, *J Am Psychiatr Nurses Assoc* 2:71, 1996.
11. Field S: Milieu-based treatment of the borderline patient: a self psychology perspective, *Continuum* 1:133, 1994.
12. Gallop R: Self-destructive and impulsive behavior in the patient with a borderline personality disorder: rethinking hospital treatment and management, *Arch Psychiatr Nurs* 6:178, 1992.
13. Gallop R, McCay E, Esplen MJ: The conceptualization of impulsivity for psychiatric nursing practice, *Arch Psychiatr Nurs* 6:366, 1992.
14. Goldstein W: Clarification of projective identification, *Am J Psychiatr* 148:2, 1991.
15. Greene H, Ugarriza D: Borderline personality disorder: history, theory and nursing intervention, *J Psychosoc Nurs* 33:26, 1995.
16. Grove W et al: Heritability of substance abuse and antisocial behavior: a study of monozygotic twins reared apart, *Biol Psychiatry* 27:1293, 1990.
17. Hagerty BMK et al: Sense of belonging: a vital mental health concept, *Arch Psychiatr Nurs* 6:172, 1992.
18. Hagerty BMK, Lynch-Sauer J, Patusky KL, Bouwsema M: An emerging theory of human relatedness, *Image* 25:291, 1993.
19. Isometsa E et al: Suicide among subjects with personality disorders, *Am J Psychiatry* 153:667, 1996.
20. Keopnick S, Wade A: *Psychiatric care planning,* Springhouse, Pa, 1993, Springhouse Corp.
21. Link P: *Clinical assessment and management of severe personality disorders,* Washington, DC, 1996, American Psychiatric Press.
22. Livesley WJ, Jang KL, Jackson DN, Vernon PA: Genetic and environmental contributions to dimensions of personality disorder, *Am J Psychiatr* 150:1826, 1993.
23. Livesley WJ, Schroeder ML: Dimensions of personality disorder, *J Nerv Ment Dis* 179:320, 1991.
24. Masterson JF: *Treatment of the borderline adolescent,* New York, 1985, Brunner/Mazel.
25. Miller B: Characteristics of effective day treatment programming for persons with borderline personality disorder, *Psychiatr Serv* 46:605, 1995.
26. Miller C, Eisner W, Allport C: Creative coping: a cognitive-behavioral group for borderline personality disorder, *Arch Psychiatr Nurs* 8:280, 1994.
27. Miller LJ: The formal treatment contract in the inpatient management of borderline personality disorder, *Hosp Community Psychiatry* 41:985, 1990.
28. Miller S: Borderline personality disorder from the patient's perspective, *Hosp Community Psychiatry* 12:1215, 1994.
29. Piccinino S: The nursing care challenge: borderline patients, *J Psychosoc Nurs Ment Health Serv* 28:22, 1990.
30. Pollock VE et al: Childhood antecedents of antisocial behavior: parental alcoholism and physical abusiveness, *Am J Psychiatry* 147:1290, 1990.
31. Rogers C: *On becoming a person,* Boston, 1961, Houghton Mifflin.
32. Samuels J et al: DSM-III personality disorders in the community, *Am J Psychiatry* 151:1055, 1994.
33. Sebastian L: Promoting object constancy: writing as a nursing intervention, *J Psychosoc Nurs Ment Health Serv* 29:21, 1991.
34. Simmons D: Gender issues and borderline personality disorder: why do females dominate the diagnosis? *Arch Psychiatr Nurs* 6:219, 1992.
35. Sperry L: *Handbook of diagnosis and treatment of the DSM-IV personality disorders,* New York, 1995, Brunner/Mazel.
36. Sullivan H: *The interpersonal theory of psychiatry,* New York, 1953, WW Norton.
37. Warren BJ: Explaining social isolation through concept analysis, *Arch Psychiatr Nurs* 7:270, 1993.

ANNOTATED SUGGESTED READINGS

*Hampton M: Dialectical behavior therapy in the treatment of persons with borderline personality disorder, *Arch Psychiatr Nurs* 11:96, 1997.
Describes the use of dialectical behavior therapy, which is a form of cognitive-behavioral therapy, and its effectiveness in reducing inpatient hospital days, suicide attempts, and therapy attrition.
*Henson R: Analysis of the concept of mutuality, *Image* 29:77, 1997.
Excellent exploration of the concept of mutuality and the impact it can have on balancing power and respect and promoting productive provider-patient communication.

*Nursing reference.

Cognitive Responses and Organic Mental Disorders

Sandra J. Sundeen

© 1998 M.C. Escher/Cordon Art, Baarn, Holland.

Cogito, ergo sum. I think, therefore I am. **Descartes**

LEARNING OBJECTIVES

After studying this chapter the student should be able to:

▼ Describe the continuum of adaptive and maladaptive cognitive responses

▼ Identify behaviors associated with cognitive responses

▼ Analyze predisposing factors, precipitating stressors, and appraisal of stressors related to cognitive responses

▼ Describe coping resources and coping mechanisms related to cognitive responses

▼ Formulate nursing diagnoses related to cognitive responses

▼ Assess the relationship between nursing diagnosis and medical diagnosis related to cognitive responses

▼ Identify expected outcome and short-term nursing goals related to cognitive responses

▼ Develop a family education plan to help caregivers to cope with maladaptive cognitive responses

▼ Analyze nursing interventions related to cognitive responses

▼ Evaluate nursing care related to cognitive responses

TOPICAL OUTLINE

The ability to think and reason is a distinguishing feature of the human being. This ability created civilization and allowed progress from the Stone Age to the Space Age. Knowledge is growing at such a rapid rate that there is an overwhelming demand for a person to assimilate new information. Society has moved from the time when power meant physical strength, to the use of money to acquire power, to an era in which power lies in information.

Intellectual functioning is highly valued. Most people fear the possibility of losing their cognitive abilities (reasoning, memory, judgment, orientation, perception, and attention). These functions allow the person to make sense of experience and interact productively with the environment. Maladaptive cognitive responses leave the affected person in a state of confusion, unable to understand experience and unable to relate current to past events. Memory is a key cognitive ability because to exercise judgment, make decisions, or even to be oriented to time and place, the person must remember past experiences. Therefore, memory loss is a particularly frightening experience.

CONTINUUM OF COGNITIVE RESPONSES

Learning Model of Cognition

Psychology is the discipline that has historically been most involved in studying cognition. Experimental psychologists have been interested in defining the process of learning and developing models to explain learned behavior. Learning is a persistent change in the person's behavior related to a particular situation. It results from experience rather than instinct, reflex, or maturation. The behavioral model of learning relates behavioral change to reinforcement. When a person experiences a **stimulus,** several behavioral **responses** are available. The person is most likely to select the response that has been **reinforced** in the past. In other words, the person has learned a particular response to a given stimulus or set of stimuli. If the response is not reinforced, an alternative behavior may be substituted. If the new behavior is reinforced, the person is more likely to continue to behave in that way. The following clinical example illustrates this process.

Clinical Example Johnny M, age 3, asked his mother for a cookie. Ms. M told Johnny that he could have a cookie after he picked up his toys. Johnny began to kick and scream. Ms. M cuddled Johnny, gave him a cookie, and picked up the toys. When she discussed this experience with her neighbor, Ms. P, the mother of four children, Johnny's mother learned that he had a temper tantrum and that the behavior was likely to continue if she gave in to Johnny's demands. The next time Johnny demanded a cookie, Ms. M again requested that he pick up his toys first. Johnny began his temper tantrum. His mother placed him in another room and told him again that when he picked up his toys, he could have a cookie. After a few minutes, Johnny quieted, then came out and put away his toys. His mother responded with cuddling and a cookie. Over time the temper tantrums disappeared.

By reinforcing Johnny's tantrums with cookies and cuddling, Ms. M had taught him that his behavior was effective. When she stopped reinforcing Johnny's negative behavior, he learned that another behavior was more effective in meeting his needs. Gradually, with continued reinforcement, the potential for effective behavior increased. Learning theorists believe that this sequence is responsible for the development of many human behaviors. They also believe that behavior can be changed, or learning can take place, by altering the reinforcement.

This process is depicted in Fig. 23-1. Because response number 1 is not reinforced, it tends not to recur. Instead, the person tries response number 2. It is reinforced and thus will tend to recur the next time the stimulus is produced. Reinforcement need not be a reward, although rewards are certainly powerful reinforcers. Punishment can also be a reinforcer of behavior. In the preceding example, spanking Johnny would probably have been less effective than leaving him alone because he would still be receiving his mother's attention. Also, a reinforcer need not be a material object. The cuddling may have been as effective in reinforcing Johnny's behavior as the cookie.

Social-Cognitive Model

Another major group of learning theorists proposes a social-cognitive model.[28] While recognizing that reinforcement of behavior is important, they believe that behavior is based on additional information about the environment. In this case, the stimulus is perceived as a **sign** that a desired resource may be available from the environment (for example, a cookie). This perception creates a **demand** that, when combined with knowledge about the environment, leads the person to seek gratification. The person's perception of the

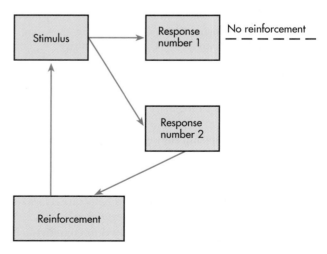

Fig. 23-1 The associationist, or behavioral, model of learning.

environment is called a **cognitive map.** Cognitive learning theorists would say that the change in Johnny's cookie-seeking behavior resulted from a change in his perception of his mother's behavior as a part of his environment. Her changed behavior blocked the pathway that had previously led him to a cookie, so he had to find a new route.

Observational learning is another example of the social-cognitive model. It has been shown that people learn from watching others in similar situations. If Johnny had an older brother who stole cookies when his mother was not looking, he might have tried this as an alternative path to his reward. Role modeling is a form of observational learning that is often used by nurses to teach health-related behavior. Application of the behavioral and cognitive theories of learning in psychiatric nursing practice is presented in Chapter 30.

Piaget's Developmental Model of Cognition

Human cognitive development has been described by Piaget[19] and is summarized in Table 23-1. His research revealed three stages in the development of thought processes. The first developmental stage is the period of sensorimotor intelligence. This phase lasts from birth until the development of language, usually about 2 years of age. This stage is action oriented, with the actions first directed toward the self and then gradually incorporating more space and the ability to locate the self in space. Also, memory begins for objects that are out of sight. This is a necessary condition for the development of language using words to describe objects that are not present. The baby who plays peek-a-boo is practicing this ability.

The second stage is the period of preparation and organization of concrete operations (categories, relations, and numbers). This period lasts from 2 to 12 years of age and is divided into two substages.

The first substage of preoperational behavior lasts from about 2 to 5 years of age. The child then enters the substage of concrete operations. At this point, the child is "capable of relatability, i.e., combinations, associations, negations and reversibility."[7] They learn to solve problems of conservation. For instance, if an object changes in shape, its weight remains the same. During this period, children develop the capacity for syllogistic reasoning, which means that an action leads to a reaction or consequence. This enables them to make and follow rules. They also develop the ability to quantify experience.

The third stage is the period of formal operations. This develops between ages 12 and 14 years, resulting in the ability to conceptualize at an adult level. The period of formal operations enables people to explore idealistic concepts and to measure reality against possibilities. This pertains to observations of significant others, such as parents, and of cultural institutions, such as government and religions. The same process is applied to the self in the form of self-criticism. This developmental process provides the foundation for continued cognitive growth as life experiences enrich and modify the person's perceptions of the world.

In some people, cognitive responses do not develop fully or, once developed, deteriorate. When maladaptive cognitive responses occur during childhood, they are generally called developmental disabilities or mental retardation. The reader is referred to a textbook of pediatric nursing for a discussion of these disorders. This chapter considers maladaptive cognitive responses in the adult. In most cases the person has developed to the level of formal operations. Although they may occur at any age, maladaptive cognitive responses are most common in the elderly. It is highly recommended that this chapter be read in conjunction with Chapter 38 because the content of the two chapters is complementary.

Maladaptive cognitive responses include inability to make decisions, impaired memory and judgment, disorientation, misperceptions, decreased attention span, and difficulties with logical reasoning. They may occur episodically or be present continuously. Depending on the stressor, the condition may be reversible or characterized by progressive deterioration in functioning. Fig. 23-2 illustrates the continuum of cognitive responses.

TABLE **23-1** *Piaget's Levels of Cognitive Development*

STAGE	AGE (YEARS)	CHARACTERISTICS
Sensorimotor	Birth to 2	Action oriented No language Develops awareness of body in space Develops memory for missing objects
Preparation and organization of concrete operations		
Preoperational phase	2 to 5	Symbolism appears Objects defined by function Magical thinking Imaginative play
Concrete operations	5 to 12	Capable of relatability Syllogistic reasoning Makes and follows rules Quantifies experience Understands conservation
Formal operations	12 to 14 and older	Abstraction Development of ideals Criticism of others Self-criticism

? *Cognitive functioning is affected by the person's level of anxiety. Compare the cognitive functioning of a person experiencing a mild level of anxiety with that of one in a state of panic.*

CONTINUUM OF COGNITIVE RESPONSES

Adaptive responses		Maladaptive responses
Decisiveness	Periodic indecisiveness	Inability to make decisions
Intact memory	Forgetfulness	Impaired memory and
Complete orientation	Mild transient confusion	judgment
Accurate perception	Occasional misperceptions	Disorientation
Focused attention	Distractibility	Serious misperceptions
Coherent, logical	Occasional unclear	Inability to focus attention
thought	thinking	Difficulties with logical
		reasoning

Fig. 23-2 Continuum of cognitive responses.

Assessment

Behaviors

Maladaptive cognitive responses are most apparent in people who have a medical diagnosis of delirium, dementia, and amnestic and other cognitive disorders (DSM-IV).[1] Discussions in this chapter focus primarily on delirium and dementia because these are the medical diagnostic categories that nurses encounter most often. Assessment relies heavily on both biological findings (see Chapter 5) and results of the mental status examination (see Chapter 6).

ASSOCIATED WITH DELIRIUM. Delirium is characterized by clouded awareness involving sensory misperceptions and disordered thought. Disordered thought processes include disturbed attention, memory, thinking, and orientation. There are also disturbances of activity patterns and the sleep-wake cycle. Generally there is a rapid onset and brief course of illness. The degree of impairment usually fluctuates. The delirious person may have occasional periods of mental clarity, but the condition is usually worse at night. This clinical example illustrates behavior that is typical of a patient who is delirious.

Clinical Example Ms. S was brought to the emergency room of a general hospital by her parents. She was a 22-year-old single woman who was described as having been in good health until 2 days before admission, when she complained of malaise and a sore throat and stayed home from work. She worked as a typist in a small office and had a stable employment record. According to her parents, she had an active social life and there were no significant conflicts at home.

On admission, Ms. S was extremely restless and had a frightened facial expression. Her speech was garbled and incoherent. When she was approached by an unfamiliar person, she would become agitated, trying to climb out of bed and striking out aimlessly. Occasionally she would slip into a restless sleep. Her temperature on admission was 104° F (40° C) rectally, pulse was 108 per minute, and respirations were 28 per minute. Her skin was hot, dry, and flushed. Her mother said she had had only a few sips of water in the last 24 hours and had not urinated at all, although she had had several episodes of profuse diaphoresis.

Her ability to cooperate with a mental status examination was limited. She would respond to her own name by turning her head. When her mother asked her where she was, she said "home," but could not say where her home was. She would give only the month when asked for the date and said it was January, when the actual date was February 19. She also refused to give the day of the week. A neurological examination was negative for signs of increased intracranial pressure or for localizing signs of CNS disease.

The tentative medical diagnosis was delirium secondary to fever of unknown origin. Symptomatic treatment of the fever, including intravenous fluids, an aspirin suppository, and cool water mattress, was begun immediately while further diagnostic studies were carried out. Nurses caring for the patient noticed continued restlessness and disorientation. Her speech was still incoherent. In addition, they noticed that she was picking at the bedclothing. Suddenly she became extremely agitated, trying to get out of bed and crying out, "Bugs, get away, get bugs away." She was brushing and slapping at herself and the bed. As her mother and the nurse talked with her and held her, she gradually became calmer but periodically would continue to slap at "the bugs" and need reassurance and reorientation.

Later in the day additional laboratory results became available. A lumbar puncture was normal, as were skull x-ray films. Results of toxicological screening of blood were also negative. The electroencephalogram revealed diffuse slowing. There was an elevated white blood count and electrolyte imbalance consistent with severe dehydration. Cultures of her throat and blood were both positive for beta-hemolytic streptococci, so intravenous antibiotic therapy was begun at once while other supportive measures were continued.

As the infection gradually came under control and the fever decreased, Ms. S's mental state improved. A week later, when she was discharged from the hospital, her cognitive functioning was completely normal, with the exception of amnesia for the time during which she was delirious.

Selected Nursing Diagnoses:

▼ Hyperthermia related to infection, as evidenced by elevated temperature; hot, dry, flushed skin; and diaphoresis

▼ Fluid volume deficit related to decreased fluid intake, as evidenced by anuria for 24 hours and hot, dry, flushed skin

▼ Risk for injury related to fear and disorientation, as evidenced by agitated behavior

▼ Impaired verbal communication related to altered brain chemistry, as evidenced by garbled and incoherent speech

▼ Sensory/perceptual alteration (visual) related to altered brain chemistry, as evidenced by hallucination of bugs

▼ Altered thought process related to altered brain chemistry, as evidenced by disorientation

Ms. S demonstrates many behaviors often seen in patients who have delirium. The behaviors have a sudden onset and are related to alterations in neurochemical and electrical responses in the brain as a result of the stressor that causes the maladaptive response. Disorientation is generally present, sometimes in all three spheres of time, place, and person. Thought processes are usually disorganized. Judgment is poor, and little decision-making ability exists. Stimuli may be misinterpreted, resulting in illusions or distortions of reality. An example of an illusion is the perception that a polka-dot drape is actually covered with cockroaches. Delirious patients may hallucinate. These hallucinations are usually visual and often take the form of animals, reptiles, or insects. They are real to the person and very frightening. Assaultive or destructive behavior may be the patient's attempt to strike back at a hallucinated image. At times, patients with delirium also exhibit a labile affect, changing abruptly from laughter to tearfulness, and vice versa, for no apparent reason. There may also be loss of usual social behavior, resulting in such acts as undressing, playing with food, and grabbing at others. Delirious patients tend to act on impulse.

Other behaviors may be specifically related to the cause of the behavioral syndrome. For example, the fever and dehydration experienced by Ms. S were a result of her systemic streptococcal infection, as was her brain syndrome. It is very important to describe observations of behavior carefully. This helps identify the stressor. Treatment is usually conservative until a specific stressor has been isolated. Although

most patients recover, it is possible for the person to develop long-term disabilities or die as a result of the stressor's severity. If adequate intervention does not take place, delirium may become dementia.

ASSOCIATED WITH DEMENTIA. Dementia is a maladaptive cognitive response that features a loss of intellectual abilities and interferes with usual social or occupational activities. The loss of intellectual ability includes impairment of memory, judgment, and abstract thought. The patient with dementia does not have the clouding of awareness that is seen with delirium. Changes in personality often occur. The personality change may appear as either alteration or accentuation of the person's usual character traits. The onset of dementia is usually gradual. It may result in progressive deterioration or the condition may become stable. In some cases the process of dementia can be reversed, and the person's intellectual functioning improves if the underlying stressors are identified and treated.

Dementia may occur at any age but most often affects the elderly. Alzheimer's disease is the most common type of dementia, accounting for about 65% of cases.[15] It is estimated that 4 million people in the United States have Alzheimer's disease at an annual cost of $80 billion.[21,23] After 75 years of age, Alzheimer's is the fourth leading cause of death. Dementia results from structural and neurochemical brain changes. These changes may be related to accidental or surgical trauma, a chronic infection such as tertiary syphilis, cerebrovascular disruptions such as arteriosclerosis or chronic hypertension, or an unknown cause. *Senility* is a nonspecific term and usually applies to those who have degenerative brain disease of unknown cause. Because of the negative connotation, use of the terms *senility* or *senile* is discouraged. The following clinical example demonstrates behaviors associated with dementia.

Clinical Example Mr. B is a 73-year-old widower who has resided in a retirement home for 3 years. He chose to move to the retirement home after the death of his wife, although his son encouraged him to live with him and his family. Mr. B stated that he did not want to burden his family and would be happier with others of the same age. He did well for the first 18 months. He was an active participant in social groups both in the home and in his church, which he continued to attend regularly. He also visited his son once a week and enjoyed seeing his grandchildren and puttering around his son's house.

About 18 months ago Mr. B began to seem forgetful. He would ask the same question several times and on occasion prepared for church on a Friday or Saturday. He also became irritable and accused his son of not caring about him and abandoning him in "that place." Mr. B spent many hours taking papers from his desk and studying them. When asked what he was doing, he would say, "Attending to my business." He began to withdraw from activities and make flimsy excuses to avoid playing his favorite card game, gin rummy. When he was persuaded to play, he usually quit in frustration because he could not remember which cards had been played. At times Mr. B was quite anxious. He periodically seemed well oriented and expressed great concern about the changes he was experiencing, wondering if he was "going crazy."

Because of the concern of the retirement home staff, Mr. B was scheduled for a complete physical examination by his family physician and for a psychiatric evaluation by the geriatric psychiatric nurse consultant who came to the retirement home weekly. The physical examination revealed generally good health for a man of Mr. B's age. He suffered from a mild hearing loss and slight prostatic hypertrophy. Hypertension had been diagnosed 10 years before this examination but was well controlled by diuretics. Neurological examination revealed normal reflexes, normal muscle strength, a slight intention tremor, normal response to sensation, normal cranial nerves, and no disturbance of gait. An electroencephalogram was normal, as were a skull x-ray film and the results of laboratory studies of blood and urine. Computed tomography studies of the brain revealed some atrophy of the cerebral cortex.

The mental status examination confirmed the deficits in cognitive functioning that had been observed by the nursing home staff and Mr. B's son. He was oriented to person and place but stated that the date was April 6, 1958. The real date was March 11, 1997. He also thought the day of the week was Friday, when it was actually Tuesday. He correctly identified the season of the year as spring. Mr. B was able to give correctly his birth date, the date of his son's birth, and the year he began to work at his first job. He spoke at length and with great detail about his exploits as a young man. However, he could not repeat the names of three objects after 5 minutes and could not remember what he had eaten for lunch or the last name of the man who shared his room. He became distressed when he was trying to answer these questions. His vocabulary was excellent, as was his fund of general information. However, he was unable to remember the names of the two most recent presidents. However, he could recite the names of the eight presidents preceding them.

Mr. B's judgment was somewhat impaired. When asked what he would do if he found a stamped, addressed, sealed envelope, he said he would "read it, then mail it." His ability for abstract thinking was slightly concretized. His attention span and ability to concentrate were normal. His eye-hand coordination was disrupted, as demonstrated by his difficulty in copying simple figures. A hand tremor was evident both when he was drawing and when he signed his name.

His affect was appropriate in quality and quantity to the content of the discussion. He appeared depressed when talking about his memory loss but cheerful and proud when describing his grandchildren. No abrupt mood swings were noted. The flow of speech was of a normal rate and volume. Content of speech was logical and coherent, except when Mr. B was trying to remember and describe recent events, when it became somewhat disjointed.

As a result of the data gathered in the physical and mental status examinations, he was diagnosed as having dementia not otherwise specified.

Over the next several months Mr. B's condition continued to deteriorate gradually. He became increasingly forgetful and began to confabulate or fabricate stories. He was less conforming to social norms and needed reminding about hygiene and appropriate dress. He also became seductive with female residents and staff, making suggestive remarks and occasionally fondling someone. Visits to his son's home became impossible as his behavior deteriorated. His memory of the identity of family members sometimes was confused. He would misidentify his daughter-in-law as his wife and his grandson as his son. More and more, his conversation consisted of rambling reminiscences of his life in his youth. His son and health-care providers began to discuss plans to move Mr. B to the Assisted Living Program associated with his retirement home. Because he is surrounded with caring people, Mr. B continues to live with dignity and respect despite his progressively limited ability to communicate.

Selected Nursing Diagnoses:

▼ Impaired verbal communication related to cognitive impairment, as evidenced by recent memory loss and confabulation
▼ Impaired social interaction related to altered thought processes, as evidenced by loss of conformity to social norms
▼ Bathing/hygiene self-care deficit related to cognitive impairment, as evidenced by failure to perform personal hygiene activities without reminders
▼ Dressing/grooming self-care deficit related to cognitive impairment, as evidenced by need for assistance in selecting appropriate clothing
▼ Altered thought processes related to cognitive impairment, as evidenced by disorientation and memory loss

The behaviors associated with dementia reflect the brain tissue alterations that are taking place. In Alzheimer's disease behavioral change occurs slowly in the early and late stages and rapidly in the middle stage.[24] The cognitive changes are related to the actions of stressors that interfere with the functioning of the cerebral cortex. Other areas of the brain may be affected as well, which is one reason for performing a complete medical and neurological examination. Another reason is that although the condition may be irreversible, progression may be stopped by identifying the stressor and treating the underlying dysfunction. For instance, treatment of hypertension may prevent further occurrence of small hemorrhages, which are a possible cause of dementia. Recent research has shown that many cases of dementia may be reversible. It has also been found that depression in the elderly is often misinterpreted as dementia and therefore not treated appropriately. This happens so often that the condition has been labeled **pseudodementia.** Behaviors related to delirium, dementia, and depression are compared in Table 23-2. One study found that people who have vascular dementia are more likely to have depression at any stage of their illness than are people with severe Alzheimer's disease.[9] Another study identified more severe behavioral retardation, depression, and anxiety in patients with vascular dementia than in those with Alzheimer's disease.[25]

? *Depressed elderly people are often misdiagnosed as demented. What nursing observations will help in determining whether a patient's mental disorder is primarily affective or cognitive?*

A common behavior related to dementia is disorientation. Usually, time orientation is affected first, then place, and finally person. This behavior can be distressing to the patient, who may be aware of this difficulty and embarrassed or frightened by it. This is particularly true if the person's mental acuity is fluctuating. In these instances the person is aware, during periods of lucidity, of the confusion and disorientation experienced at other times.

Memory loss is another prominent characteristic of dementia. Immediate recall and recent memory are most seriously affected. Remote memory may be intact, although it will deteriorate as the condition progresses. In the last clinical example, Mr. B had trouble remembering what he had eaten for lunch but gave accurate dates for significant events earlier in his life. Most aging people dwell on the past, but people with recent memory loss have difficulty shifting to the present and at advanced stages may seem to live in the past. This is exemplified by Mr. B's misidentification of his grandson and his daughter-in-law.

Another behavior related to memory loss is confabulation. This is a confused person's tendency to make up a response to a question when he or she cannot remember the answer. For instance, when Mr. B was asked whether he knew one of the female residents of the home, he replied, "Of course I know her. I used to play gin with her husband." Actually, the woman's husband had been dead for many

TABLE **23-2** *Comparison of Delirium, Depression, and Dementia*

	DELIRIUM	DEPRESSION	DEMENTIA
Onset	Rapid (hours to days).	Rapid (weeks to months).	Gradual (years).
Course	Wide fluctuations; may continue for weeks if cause not found.	May be self-limited or may become chronic without treatment.	Chronic; slow but continuous decline.
Level of consciousness	Fluctuates from hyperalert to difficult to arouse.	Normal.	Normal.
Orientation	Patient is disoriented, confused.	Patient may seem disoriented.	Patient is disoriented, confused.
Affect	Fluctuating.	Sad, depressed, worried, guilty.	Labile; apathy in later stages.
Attention	Always impaired.	Difficulty concentrating; patient may check and recheck all actions.	May be intact; patient may focus on one thing for long periods.
Sleep	Always disturbed.	Disturbed; excess sleeping or insomnia, especially early-morning waking.	Usually normal.
Behavior	Agitated, restless.	Patient may be fatigued, apathetic; may occasionally be agitated.	Patient may be agitated or apathetic; may wander.
Speech	Sparse or rapid; patient may be incoherent.	Flat, sparse, may have outbursts; understandable.	Sparse or rapid; repetitive; patient may be incoherent.
Memory	Impaired, especially for recent events.	Varies day to day; slow recall; often short-term deficit.	Impaired, especially for recent events.
Cognition	Disordered reasoning.	May seem impaired.	Disordered reasoning and calculation.
Thought content	Incoherent, confused, delusions, stereotyped.	Negative, hypochondriac, thoughts of death, paranoid.	Disorganized, rich content, delusional, paranoid.
Perception	Misinterpretations, illusions, hallucinations.	Distorted; patient may have auditory hallucinations; negative interpretation of people and events.	No change.
Judgment	Poor.	Poor.	Poor; socially inappropriate behavior.
Insight	May be present in lucid moments.	May be impaired.	Absent.
Performance on mental status exams	Poor but variable; improves during lucid moments and with recovery.	Memory impaired; calculation, drawing, following directions usually not impaired; frequent "I don't know" answers.	Consistently poor; progressively worsens; patient attempts to answer all questions.

From Holt J: *Am J Nurs* 93:32, 1993.

years and Mr. B had never met him. This behavior should not be viewed as lying or an attempt to deceive. Rather, it is the person's way of trying to save face in an embarrassing situation. He is aware that he should know the answer to the question and gives an answer that seems reasonable, not entirely disbelieving it himself. It is not unlike the situation in which a person meets an acquaintance and cannot recall the other's name or where they met. The person acts as if these facts are remembered, hoping that the other will offer clues about his or her identity. Denial of memory loss may also be related to the dementia's effect on the cognitive abilities needed for awareness of the problem.[22]

As Alzheimer's disease progresses, patients often develop **aphasia, apraxia,** and **agnosia.** Aphasia is difficulty finding the right word, apraxia is inability to perform familiar skilled activities, and agnosia is difficulty recognizing well-known objects, including people.[29] These behaviors are related to the effect of the illness on the temporal-parietal-occipital association cortex.

Vocabulary and general information may be less affected by dementia, at least until its very late stages. This depends on when the information was learned. Facts learned early in life may be recalled well, whereas those learned recently may be quickly forgotten, as demonstrated by Mr. B's performance in listing the last 10 presidents.

These patients may have labile affective behavior, particularly if the limbic system has been affected by the disease process. There may also be some deterioration in social skills. Impulsive sexual advances may occur. These reflect decreased inhibition and impaired judgment. Often this behavior is also an attempt to establish interpersonal contact and is a way of asking for caring from others. It is also a way of reinforcing an important part of the person's identity, which is becoming less secure as mental functioning declines. Alteration in sexual functioning associated with Alzheimer's disease causes great concern for patients and their partners. Loss of erection ability is a common problem among men who have Alzheimer's.[5] It is uncertain whether this is physiological or psychological in origin. However, both the patient and the sexual partner can benefit from continued sexual intimacy.

Restlessness and agitation are other behaviors that occur with dementia. Extreme agitation may occur at night; this is sometimes called the **sundown syndrome.** It probably results from tiredness at the end of the day combined with fewer orienting stimuli, such as planned activities, meals, and contact with people.

> **?** *Based on your understanding of sundown syndrome, describe nursing interventions that would decrease the severity of this problem.*

Disorientation can result in fear and agitation. When behavior becomes extremely agitated, it is called a **cata-**strophic reaction. Swanson and colleagues[26] have described the following precipitating factors related to catastrophic reactions:

▼ A change in cognitive status, resulting in difficulty organizing and interpreting information; sensory or cognitive overload or misinterpretation of sensory stimuli may be contributing factors.
▼ Side effects of medications.
▼ Psychosocial factors resulting in increased demands to remember, such as fatigue, changes in routines or care-givers, and disorienting stimuli.
▼ Environmental factors, including changes in the environment, noise, and decreased light.

The term *confusion* is often used when referring to the person with cognitive impairment. Although widely accepted as nursing and medical jargon, this term has not been specifically defined. It is better to use specific terms when describing a patient's behavior.

Kolanowski[16] synthesized the concepts that resulted from several studies of disturbing behaviors in people with dementia. She identified five types of behaviors. These are summarized in Table 23-3.

Some people who have maladaptive cognitive responses function at a level that is lower than would be expected based on objective measurements of their impairment. This type of functional deficit is called **excess disability.**[2] This problem adds to the frustration of the patient and to the burden placed on caregivers. Paradoxically, caregivers may contribute to the development of excess disability by performing activities for the person rather than coaching and assisting when needed. Functional abilities are then lost more rapidly.

Often patients who have a cognitive impairment are referred to a clinical psychologist for testing. This referral should be made for a specific purpose because the testing is time consuming, expensive, and tiring for the patient. Some reasons for psychological testing include measuring the extent of the disability, identifying the stressors causing the disruption, understanding the dynamics of the problem, developing guidelines for therapeutic intervention, and obtaining a prognosis for recovery.

Predisposing Factors

Maladaptive cognitive responses are usually caused by a biological disruption in the functioning of the central nervous system (CNS). The CNS requires a continuous supply of nutrients to function. Any interference with the provision of supplies to the brain will cause functional disruptions. For instance, the difficulties in cognition experienced by some elderly people result from arteriosclerotic changes in cerebral blood vessels. These changes deprive the brain of needed oxygen, glucose, and other essential chemicals. Other vascular abnormalities, such as transient ischemic attacks (small strokes), cerebral hemorrhage, and multiple small infarcts in brain tissue caused by chronic hypertension can also result in cognitive impairments.

TABLE **23-3** *Disturbing Behaviors Characteristic of Dementia*

BEHAVIOR	DESCRIPTION	EXAMPLES
Aggressive psychomotor behavior	An increase in gross motor movement that has the effect of harming or repelling another	Hitting, kicking, pushing, scratching, assaultiveness
Nonaggressive psychomotor behavior	An increase in gross motor movement without an apparent negative effect on others, but draws attention because of its repetitive nature	Restlessness, pacing, wandering
Verbally aggressive behavior	Vocalizations that have the effect of repelling others	Demanding, disruptive, manipulative, screaming, complaining, negativism
Passive behavior	A diminution of behavior, that is, a decrease in gross motor movement accompanied by apathy and a lack of interaction with the environment	Decreased activity, loss of interest, apathy, withdrawal
Functionally impaired behavior	Loss of ability to perform self-care, the expression of which may be aversive and burdensome	Vegetative behaviors, incontinence, poor personal hygiene

Modified from Kolanowski AM, Disturbing behaviors in demented elders: a concept synthesis, *Arch Psychiatr Nurs* 9:188, 1995.

AGING. Aging itself predisposes the person to maladaptive cognitive responses. It is now accepted that loss of mental abilities is not automatically associated with aging. A cumulative degeneration of brain tissue is associated with aging, but it is not extensive enough to be particularly noticeable in most people. If other stressors are added, however, the person may experience difficulty. Some toxins collect in brain tissue, and a lifetime of exposure to a toxic chemical or heavy metal may result in maladaptive cognitive responses.

NEUROBIOLOGICAL. Alzheimer's disease is the most prevalent cause of maladaptive cognitive responses. Intensive research has focused on identifying the causes, characteristics, and treatment for Alzheimer's disease. Investigators have found that characteristic alterations occur in brain tissue[11]:

▼ Neuritic plaques, which consist of beta-amyloid, a starchlike protein and remains of dying nerve cells. Plaques also contain altered glial cells.
▼ Neurofibrillary tangles, which are twisted clumps of protein fibers. Tangles contain a substance called tau protein, which seems to interfere with internal transport in neurons.

These phenomena are found in the cortex (affecting cognition), the amygdala, and the hippocampus, the center for short-term memory. This is consistent with the emotional changes and short-term memory loss characteristic of Alzheimer's disease. In addition, there is atrophy of the associational areas of the cortex. Alterations have also been noted in the neurotransmitter systems. In particular, there is a serious deficiency of acetylcholine. Additional information regarding the biological aspects of Alzheimer's disease is included in Chapter 5.

Vascular dementia is much less common than dementia of the Alzheimer's type. This was previously called multi-infarct dementia because of the underlying cause. It results from disruptions in the cerebral blood supply. Patients with hypertensive vascular disease may experience this type of dementia as the result of the sudden closure of the lumen of arterioles related to pressure changes. Atherosclerosis may lead to the formation of thrombi or emboli. In either case, the outcome is infarction of the brain tissue in the area supplied by the affected blood vessels. The resulting cognitive problems are related to the area of the brain involved. Another brain disorder that results in dementia is associated with HIV. AIDS dementia complex is discussed in Chapter 40.

Some metabolic disorders, such as chronic liver disease, chronic renal disease, and vitamin deficiencies, can result in maladaptive cognitive responses. Vitamin B–complex deficiency, particularly thiamine, is believed to cause the Wernicke-Korsakoff syndrome found in some chronic alcoholics. A prominent feature of this syndrome is a severe deficit in cognitive functioning. Malnutrition increases the person's risk of organic brain disease. This is often a problem in the elderly, who may lack the physical or financial resources needed for an adequate diet. However, young people with anorexia nervosa or bulimia nervosa are also at risk for cognitive impairment.

GENETIC. Genetic abnormalities may also be a cause. An example of a hereditary degenerative brain disease is Huntington's chorea, which is inherited as an autosomal dominant trait. Progress has been made in identifying genetic markers that indicate a potential for developing Alzheimer's disease. Recent studies have also indicated that risk for development of Alzheimer's disease is greater for relatives of people with the illness than it is for those with no family history.[3,18] The risk is greatest for relatives of people who developed Alzheimer's disease before age 55. It also occurs more often in people with Down's syndrome, another hereditary brain disorder. For additional discussion of genetic factors related to Alzheimer's disease, see Chapter 5.

A degree of cognitive impairment may be found along with other maladaptive psychiatric responses. For instance, a delusional person may seem disoriented because he misidentifies his location. People who have affective disorders may have short attention spans. Depression may also result in memory disorders, although it is often difficult to determine whether the problem is related to memory loss or lack of motivation. The predisposing factors related to these maladaptive cognitive responses are also related to the primary problem.

Precipitating Stressors

Any major assault on the brain is likely to disrupt cognitive functioning. Three major systemic problems may contribute to maladaptive cognitive responses: hypoxia, metabolic disorders, and toxicity, including infection. There are four types of hypoxia: anemia, histotoxicity (conditions that prevent cells from metabolizing oxygen), hypoxemia (problems with ventilation), and ischemia.

HYPOXIA. Anemic hypoxia may be insidious in onset. Possible stressors include aspirin ingestion, resulting in occult bleeding; other occult blood loss; or deficiencies of iron, folic acid, or vitamin B$_{12}$. Histotoxic hypoxia may be related to such stressors as dehydration, hyperthermia, or hypothermia. A possible stressor related to hypoxemic hypoxia is chronic obstructive lung disease. Others might include asthma or an acute respiratory tract infection. Ischemic hypoxia can result from congestive heart failure, atherosclerosis, hypotension, hypertension, or increased intracranial pressure resulting from a tumor, subdural hematoma, or normal pressure hydrocephalus.

METABOLIC DISORDERS. Metabolic disorders often affect mental functioning, especially when severe or of long duration. Endocrine malfunctioning, whether it involves underproduction or overproduction of hormones, can adversely affect cognition. For example, the thyroid hormone greatly influences mental alertness. People with hypothyroidism are sluggish and retarded in their thinking. Those with severe hypothyroidism (myxedema) may develop psychotic behavior characterized by delusional thinking. People with hyperthyroidism, on the other hand, are often hyperalert and agitated. Other endocrine disorders that may cause cognitive disruptions include hypoglycemia, hypopituitarism, and adrenal disease.

> **?** *Based on a review of neurophysiology, compare the effects of hypoxia, hypothyroidism, and hypoglycemia on cerebral functioning.*

TOXICITY AND INFECTION. Toxic and infectious agents may also result in behavior typical of maladaptive cognitive responses. Toxins may originate within the patient or in the external environment. An example of an internally generated toxin is the elevated blood level of urea found in a patient with renal failure. Environmental toxins include various poisonous substances, such as toxic wastes and animal venoms. Acute viral and bacterial infections occur in the CNS, resulting in inflammation and impaired functioning.

Infections in other body systems may also impair the CNS if temperature is extremely elevated. Chronic infections also affect the brain. One such condition is the neural manifestation of tertiary syphilis, general paresis. This is seldom seen because of the early treatment of syphilis. It has also been determined that people who are infected with human immunodeficiency virus type 1 (HIV-1) often develop an organic brain syndrome called AIDS dementia complex.

Prescription and over-the-counter drugs are also potential toxic stressors. Thorough assessment of drug use is critical with elderly patients because of their increased sensitivity to drugs and because confusion could lead to difficulty in following directions for taking drugs. Interactions between drugs or between drugs and other substances, particularly alcohol, may also lead to disruptions in cognitive functioning.

STRUCTURAL CHANGES. Conditions that alter the structure of brain tissue are also reflected in impaired cognitive functioning. Tumors may cause proliferation or displacement of tissue, thus altering its function. Trauma, whether accidental or surgical, may result in a change in ability to process information. The specific effect depends on the location of the lesion.

SENSORY STIMULATION. Sensory underload or overload can result in cognitive dysfunction. People who are placed in environments with minimal stimuli seem to develop internally produced stimuli in the form of hallucinations. In contrast, the constant light and activity in intensive care units (ICUs) have led to confusion, delusions, and hallucinations, sometimes called ICU psychosis. However, it is difficult to determine how much of the cognitive impairment results from the sensory experience as opposed to other concurrent stressors, such as the introduction of multiple drugs into the system and the result of massive assaults on physical integrity.

> **?** *Sensory overload or sensory deprivation may lead to maladaptive cognitive responses. In what way is this information significant in planning the nursing care of a patient who is confined to a seclusion room?*

Appraisal of Stressors

Unfortunately, many times the specific stressor related to cognitive impairment cannot be identified. Understanding of the biochemical process of the brain and the response of brain and nervous tissue to stressors is still limited. As knowledge grows, specific biological components may be identified in the etiology of all psychiatric disorders. The fields of psychiatry and neurology may merge at some time as knowledge grows more sophisticated. For example, deficiency in the neurotransmitter acetylcholine has been observed in patients with Alzheimer's disease. It is not known whether this is a cause or effect of the illness.

In general, in assessing maladaptive cognitive responses, physiological causes are ruled out first, then psychosocial stressors are considered. Even when physiological factors are present, psychosocial stress may further compromise the person's thought process. Thus, a person's appraisal of the stressor is critically important. Each patient must receive a complete assessment so that nursing care can be planned in a holistic manner.

Coping Resources

Individual and interpersonal resources are important to the person who is attempting to cope with maladaptive cognitive responses. The person who has a varied repertoire of skills may be able to substitute for functional losses. For instance, it has been noted that people with Alzheimer's disease who have higher levels of educational attainment deteriorate less rapidly than those who have less education.

Interpersonal resources are extremely important to the person with a cognitive impairment. Family members and friends often have a calming influence on the agitated person. They can provide the nurse with information about the person's usual lifestyle and ensure that the environment contains familiar objects. Caregivers also need coping resources. These can often be found by attending self-help groups such as the Alzheimer's Disease and Related Disorders Association. The importance of family involvement is illustrated in A Family Speaks.

Coping Mechanisms

How a person copes with maladaptive cognitive responses is greatly influenced by past experience. A person who has developed a reservoir of effective coping mechanisms is better able to handle the onset of a cognitive problem than one who has not.

Because the basic behavioral disruption in delirium is altered awareness, which reflects the severe biological disturbance in the brain, psychological coping mechanisms are not generally used. Therefore, the nurse must protect the patient from harm and provide a substitute for the patient's coping mechanisms by constantly reorienting the patient and reinforcing reality.

The patient's response to the onset of dementia often mirrors that person's basic personality. For instance, a person who has usually reacted to stress with anger directed toward other people and the environment will probably react similarly when limitations in intellectual abilities occur. A person who is more apt to direct anger inward and become depressed will be more likely to respond with depressive behaviors. A person who has relied on a mechanism such as intellectualization will be more threatened by loss of intellectual ability than a person who has used a mechanism such as reaction formation.

A characteristic of early dementia is the mechanism of denial. Those with dementia attempt to pursue their usual daily routine and make light of memory lapses. They may

A Family *Speaks*

My mother, Margaret, is 78 years old and has been in a nursing home for the past 3 years. She is diagnosed with dementia. There are days when she does not recognize me and there are some days when she does, but her mood may not be very pleasant. Many days she only sits in her chair and responds to nothing. Often she cannot feed herself or express her needs. I visit her nearly every day.

The nurses in the home are my only link to my mother. The doctor visits weekly but rarely communicates with me unless there is an emergency. The nurse gives me information about my mother's condition and listens to me when I have concerns about her. In the beginning the nurses were indifferent to me, and I worried that they were the same with my mother. I brought pictures of the family to the nursing home and shared them with the nurses. They began to see that her life had been very different. It allowed them to see a person instead of a patient. This helped them treat her with more respect and dignity. Now I really depend on the nurses to let me know how my mother is doing from day to day. ▼

be able to use some environmental resources to help them cope. For instance, a businessman who is experiencing difficulty with recent memory might ask his secretary to remind him of all his appointments and provide him with the names of the people with whom he is meeting and the meeting's purpose. As the impairment progresses, the person may become very resistant to any limitations on his independence. For instance, the family of a patient with Alzheimer's disease might become very concerned about her ability to continue to drive a car safely. The patient probably would be very reluctant to give up her driver's license and would deny that she was having any problem.

Regression is often used to cope with advanced dementia. It may be caused in part by deterioration in mental function. It probably also results from the problem's behavioral manifestations, which cause the patient to become more dependent on others for the fulfillment of basic needs such as nutrition and hygiene. Encouraging patients to perform self-care also supports their use of healthier coping mechanisms.

As cognitive ability decreases, efforts to cope become more obvious. For instance, a family member may complain that a relative has "always been irritable, but is now belligerent when he doesn't get his way." In other cases the patient's behavior may be perceived as a personality change.

Some behaviors that are probably attempts to cope with loss of cognitive ability include suspiciousness, hostility, joking, depression, seductiveness, and withdrawal. Because it is threatening to admit that a close relative has dementia, family members may focus on the coping mechanism instead of the real problem, thus participating in the denial of the underlying cognitive impairment.

Nursing Diagnosis

The nursing diagnosis of the person with cognitive impairment must consider both the possible underlying stressors and the patient behaviors. Fig. 23-3 summarizes the Stuart Stress Adaptation Model related to maladaptive cognitive responses.

Most cognitive impairment disorders are physiological in origin. Therefore, the nurse must consider the patient's physical needs, as well as the psychosocial behavioral problems. For instance, the delirious patient may be reacting to an infection or a drug overdose. The identified problem and all its effects must be reflected in a complete nursing diagnosis. Many people who are demented are also elderly. They experience many effects of the aging process in addition to impaired cognitive functioning. A thorough nursing diag-

Fig. 23-3 The Stuart Stress Adaptation Model related to cognitive responses.

nosis reflects all these influences on the patient's behavior. In addition, the nature of a cognitive impairment may inhibit the patient's ability to participate in the care planning process. The nurse must rely on observational skills and on the input of significant others to arrive at an accurate, relevant diagnosis. If the nursing diagnosis cannot be validated with the patient, a family member familiar with the person's behavioral patterns should be involved. The primary NANDA nursing diagnosis related to maladaptive cognitive response is **altered thought processes.** The range of common NANDA nursing diagnoses and the DSM-IV medical diagnoses are included in the Medical and Nursing Diagnoses box below. The primary NANDA diagnoses and examples of complete nursing diagnoses are presented in the Detailed Diagnoses box on p. 474.

Outcome Identification

The expected outcome related to the patient who has maladaptive cognitive responses is the following:

The patient will achieve optimum cognitive functioning.

Goals may be directed toward an improved ability to process information, if this is realistic, or toward optimum use of the abilities the patient retains if the impairment is irreversible. For example, a goal for a patient who is disoriented because of drug withdrawal might be that the patient will verbalize the complete date within 3 days.

In contrast, a goal for a patient who is disoriented because of chronic alcoholism and who is not in withdrawal might be that within 1 month the patient will find his own bed every night without assistance.

This patient may never be able to remember the exact date but may not need that information if he is to function in a protected setting. The first patient, however, will need that information. In addition, the nurse can use the assessment of the patient's orientation to time to assess the current status of mental functioning. Goals should be realistic to avoid discouragement. If the second patient had been required to learn the date, frequent confrontation with deteriorated cognitive skills might result, leading to frustration, higher anxiety, and possibly less effective coping.

If an identified stressor is causing the patient's behavioral disruption, goals that focus on the stressor should also be developed. For instance, if a person is delirious because of a fever, a goal might state that the patient's temperature will be maintained below 100° F (37.8° C).

When the cause of the elevated temperature is identified, appropriate goals will be written to address that problem. For example, dehydration may be a stressor contributing to an elevated temperature. A related nursing goal would then be that the patient's fluid intake will be at least 3000 ml in each 24-hour period.

As the various elements of the person's behavior are explored and documented, nursing goals must be updated and modified; new goals must be added; and accomplished goals must be deleted.

 MEDICAL AND NURSING DIAGNOSES *related to* **Maladaptive Cognitive Responses**

Related Medical Diagnoses (DSM-IV)*	Related Nursing Diagnoses (NANDA)†
Delirium due to a general medical condition	Anxiety
Substance-induced delirium	Communication, impaired verbal
Delirium due to multiple etiologies	Coping, ineffective family: compromised
Dementia of the Alzheimer's type	Coping, ineffective individual
Vascular dementia	Health maintenance, altered
Dementia due to other general medical conditions	Home maintenance management, impaired
Substance-induced persisting dementia	Injury, potential for
Dementia due to multiple etiologies	Mobility, impaired physical
Amnestic disorder due to a general medical condition	Role performance, altered
Substance-induced persisting amnestic disorder	Self-care deficit (specify)
	Bathing/hygiene, feeding, dressing/grooming, toileting
	Sensory/perceptual alterations (specify)
	Visual, auditory, kinesthetic, gustatory, tactile, olfactory
	Sleep pattern disturbance
	Social interaction, impaired
	Social isolation
	Thought Processes, Altered‡
	Trauma, potential for

*American Psychiatric Association: *Diagnostic and statistical manual of mental disorders,* ed 4, Washington, DC, 1994, The Association.
†From North American Nursing Diagnosis Association: *NANDA nursing diagnoses: definitions and classifications 1997-1998,* Philadelphia, 1997, The Association.
‡Primary nursing diagnosis for maladaptive cognitive responses.

DETAILED DIAGNOSES *related to* **Maladaptive Cognitive Responses**

NANDA Diagnosis Stem	Examples of Complete Diagnoses
Altered thought processes	Altered thought processes related to severe dehydration, as evidenced by hypervigilance, distractibility, visual hallucinations, and disorientation to time, place, and person
	Altered thought processes related to barbiturate ingestion as evidenced by altered sleep patterns, delusions, disorientation to time and place, and decreased ability to grasp ideas
	Altered thought processes related to brain disorder as evidenced by inaccurate interpretation of environment, deficit in recent memory, impaired ability to reason, and confabulation

DSM-IV Diagnosis	Essential Features*
Delirium (general criteria) (to be applied to all other categories of delirium)	Disturbed consciousness accompanied by a cognitive change that cannot be accounted for by a dementia.
	Impaired ability to focus, sustain or shift attention.
	Cognitive changes including impaired recent memory, disorientation to time or place, language disturbance or perceptual disturbance.
	Develops over a short time; tends to fluctuate during the course of a day.
Delirium due to a general medical condition	Evidence that the cognitive disturbance is the direct result of a general medical condition.
Substance-induced delirium	Evidence of substance intoxication or withdrawal, medication side effects, or toxin exposure judged to be related to the delirium.
Delirium due to multiple etiologies	Evidence of multiple causes for the delirium.
Dementia (general criteria) (to be applied to all other categories of dementia)	Development of multiple cognitive deficits including memory impairment and at least one of the following: aphasia, apraxia, agnosia, or disturbed executive functioning (ability to think abstractly and plan, initiate, sequence, monitor, and stop complex behavior).
	Must cause severe impairment in social or occupational functioning.
Dementia of the Alzheimer's type	Gradual onset with continuing cognitive decline. All other causes of dementia must be ruled out.
Vascular dementia	Focal neurological signs and symptoms or laboratory evidence of cerebrovascular disease that are judged to be related to the dementia.
Dementia due to other general medical conditions	Evidence that the general medical condition (such as HIV, traumatic brain injury, Parkinson's disease, Huntington's disease, Pick's disease, Creutzfeldt-Jakob disease, normal-pressure hydrocephalus, hypothyroidism, brain tumor, vitamin B_{12} deficiency) is etiologically related to the dementia.
Substance-induced persisting dementia	Deficits do not occur exclusively during a delirium and persist beyond the usual duration of substance intoxication or withdrawal.
	Evidence that the deficits are related to persisting effects of substance use (such as drug of abuse, medication).
Dementia due to multiple etiologies	Evidence that the dementia has more than one etiology.
Amnestic disorder (general criteria)	Development of memory disorder, as evidenced by impaired ability to learn new information or to recall previously learned information.
	Disturbance causes significant impairment in social or occupational functioning and represents a significant decline from a previous level of functioning.
	Does not occur exclusively during the course of delirium or dementia.
Amnestic disorder due to a general medical condition	Evidence that the disturbance is directly related to a general medical condition (including physical trauma).
Substance-induced persisting amnestic disorder	Evidence that the memory disturbance is etiologically related to the persisting effects of substance use (such as drug of abuse, medication).

*Modified from the American Psychiatric Association: *Diagnostic and statistical manual of mental disorders,* ed 4, Washington, DC, 1994, The Association.

FAMILY EDUCATION PLAN   **Helping a Family with a Cognitively Impaired Member**

Content	Instructional Activities	Evaluation
Explain possible causes of maladaptive cognitive responses.	Describe predisposing factors and precipitating stressors that may lead to impaired cognition, provide printed reference materials.	The family identifies possible causes of the patient's disorder.
Define and describe orientation to time, place, and person.	Define the three spheres of orientation, role play interpersonal responses to disorientation	The family identifies disorientation and provides reorientation.
Relate level of cognitive functioning to ability to communicate.	Describe the impact of maladaptive cognitive responses on communication, demonstrate effective communication techniques, videotape and discuss return demonstration.	The family adjusts communication approaches to the patient's ability to interact.
Describe effect of maladaptive cognitive responses on self-care behaviors.	Describe the usual progression of gain or loss of self-care ability related to nature of disorder, encourage the family to help in providing care to patient, provide written instructional materials.	The family helps with activities of daily living as required by the patient's level of biopsychosocial functioning.
Refer to community resources.	Provide a list of community resources, arrange to meet with staff members of selected community programs, visit meetings of selected programs and self-help groups.	The family describes various programs that provide services relevant to the patient and family's needs and contacts appropriate programs or self-help groups when needed.

Planning

The nursing care plan for a patient with maladaptive cognitive responses must address all of the person's biopsychosocial needs. In most cases, the person either has or is at risk for physiological problems in addition to the psychosocial disruption. Life-threatening problems always receive the highest priority for nursing intervention. Protection of the person's safety is almost always a concern with these patients.

Mental health education related to patients with impaired cognition is often directed toward the family. They are often the caregivers for these patients. The nurse can help them cope with this difficult and demanding responsibility by providing them with information. Harvis and Rabins[12] found that educational approaches were helpful for caregivers of patients with dementia. One useful topic was information about problematic behaviors and problem solving for the caregiver. Another was providing information on stress reduction, including individual ways to decrease stress, the use of respite care, and participation in a peer support group. A Family Education Plan for families of cognitively impaired people is presented above.

Implementation

Intervening in Delirium

PHYSIOLOGICAL NEEDS. Highest priority is given to nursing interventions that will maintain life. If the person is too disoriented or agitated to attend to basic physiological needs, nursing care must be planned to meet these needs. Nutrition and fluid balance may be maintained by intravenous therapy. If the patient is very agitated or restless, restraint may be necessary to keep the intravenous line open. However, restraints can increase agitation and anxiety and thus should be used only when absolutely necessary. A disoriented patient should never be restrained and left alone.

Sleep deprivation may be another problem. Intervention is important because lack of sleep can add to already existing cognitive dysfunction. Because sedative medication may complicate attempts to identify the original stressor, the physician may be reluctant to prescribe sedation. Nursing measures such as a back rub, a glass of warm milk, and soothing conversation may help a less agitated patient relax and fall asleep. The presence of a family member is also reassuring to the patient. Disoriented patients need to be in a lighted room. Shadows may be misinterpreted and add to the patient's fear. Also, environmental objects help the patient orient to place and person.

> ? *Do you think it is safer to use physical (mechanical) restraints than to use chemical restraints (medication) with an agitated delirious patient?*

HALLUCINATIONS. Disoriented patients may need to be protected from hurting themselves or others, particularly during hallucinations. Visual hallucinations of delirium are often very frightening. Patients may try to run away or even jump out a window. Patients' rooms must be safe, with security screens and a minimum of extra furniture or other objects placed where they might hurt themselves. These patients often require one-to-one nursing observation and repetitive verbal reorientation.

It is tempting to help a frightened patient eliminate the hallucinated object. For instance, the patient might request help in brushing the bugs off the sheets. Agreeing to do this is not usually therapeutic. By participating in this activity, the nurse is nonverbally communicating to the patient that the hallucinated objects are real. This can make the patient even more frightened. In reality the hallucinations will continue until the underlying stressor is eliminated. A more appropriate response is to orient the patient continually to the reality of being sick and hospitalized. In addition, the patient can be assured that the nursing staff and physician are there to help and to keep the patient safe. Family members should also be helped to respond in a supportive way.

COMMUNICATION. Patients with maladaptive cognitive responses need clear messages and instructions. Choices should be kept to a minimum. Independent decision making can be introduced into the plan of nursing care as the patient improves. Decisions related to orientation may be especially difficult for the patient. To respond appropriately to the question "What time would you like to take your bath?" requires knowledge of the present time and some idea of the usual routine.

Simple, direct statements are reassuring and most likely to result in an appropriate response. Orienting phrases such as "here at the hospital" or "now that it's June" can be woven into a conversation. Patients who have difficulty dressing or feeding themselves need matter-of-fact, specific directions. Confused patients need to be fed or dressed in a manner that allows them to maintain their dignity. Families can often help with this. Helping the patient can lessen the family's anxiety, and the patient may be reassured by the family's physical closeness and concern.

PATIENT EDUCATION. While recovering, patients may be concerned about what happened to them. The health care team needs to discuss this issue and arrive at a conclusion about the disruption in functioning that occurred. This should then be explained to patients and their families. The nurse should assess the patient's understanding of the nature of the problem, the stressors that were involved, any ongoing therapy that will be required, and preventive measures that will decrease the probability of a recurrence. Teaching may have to be repeated several times before the patient copes with personal feelings and understands the information. Written materials can be helpful to patients who are having residual problems processing information. The teaching should include at least one responsible family member so that the information will be reinforced when the patient goes home.

If the patient is discharged from the hospital with a residual deficit in cognitive functioning, a community health nursing referral may be helpful. The community health nurse can then continue to implement the nursing care plan and validate the patient's compliance with the treatment plan. See the critical pathway for a geropsychiatric unit.

Intervening in Dementia

Nursing care of the patient with dementia is similar in some respects to that of the patient with delirium. Usually the stressors involved do not present an immediate threat to life; thus highest priority is given to nursing care that will help the patient maintain an optimum level of functioning. This will differ for each patient. Often an attitude of hopelessness evolves in those who work with chronically ill people. This can lead to stereotyping and decreased ability to see and appreciate the uniqueness of each person. It is challenging to search for this uniqueness and rewarding to find it. Individualized nursing care is probably most important for those who will be institutionalized for a long time.

Nursing approaches must address the patient's need for social interaction. Some interventions that have been helpful include discussion groups with structured agendas, exercise groups to promote physical activity, reality orientation groups, sensory stimulation, and parties appropriate to the time of the year or to recognize important events such as birthdays. Arranging for visits from community volunteer groups provides stimulation as well as an opportunity to socialize. Referral to other members of the treatment team, especially the occupational, recreational, art, music, and dance therapists, may be indicated.

PHARMACOLOGICAL APPROACHES. Pharmacological approaches to the treatment of dementia are related to theories about the cause of the disorder. Much of the research seeks a treatment for Alzheimer's disease. Tacrine (Cognex) was the first drug to receive approval as a specific treatment for this disorder. In doses up to 160 mg per day, it has been found to delay the progression of Alzheimer's. It maximizes the function of cholinergic neurons by inhibiting the enzyme acetylcholinesterase, preventing the degradation of acetylcholine.

Much current research is focused on identifying pharmacological agents that can protect neurons from progressive death that is caused by Alzheimer's disease. Brain functions involving glutamate, calcium, and free radicals are being targeted in this research. Other brain research related to cognitive disorders is investigating the role of phospholipid metabolism and the usefulness of antiinflammatory drugs, nerve growth factor, and estrogen.[17] Table 23-4 lists some of the drugs being investigated for the treatment of Alzheimer's disease.

Donepezil (Aricept) is another new acetylcholinesterase inhibitor (the enzyme that breaks down acetylcholine) for the treatment of mild to moderate Alzheimer's disease. Like tacrine, donepezil allows a greater concentration of acetyl-

Hospital Guide for Elderly Patients with Cognitive Impairment

	PREADMISSION	DAY 1	DAY 2	DAY 3	DAY 4	DAYS 5-7/ DISCHARGE
CONSULTS	Neurology Neuropsychiatric testing	Neurological, Medical, Neuropsychiatry, VNA/Home Health				
TESTS	SMA 7-12, CBC, VDRL, Sed rate, B$_{12}$ Folate, T$_{3-4}$, TSH; MRI or CT w/n 6 mo; Obtain CXR & ECG	Anything not done preadmission	Evaluate labs, ECG for medication monitoring		TB Test	
ASSESSMENTS*	Preadmission criteria met Medical records Family/patient interview Patient's support systems ADLs & related activities MMSE, CMAI, CDS, Blessed, ADAS, AIMS	Initial psychiatric eval, CDS, MMSE, Behav-AD, WPS; Nursing assessment; CMAI sleep agitation; monitor progress	Complete/repeat scales, Monitor tx, AIMS, CDS, MMSE, WPS	Repeat	Repeat	Repeat
ANXIETY/ SAFETY LEVEL	Assess for falls, violence, suicidality, fears about hospitalization	Order groups: Environment, Awareness, ADLs, Reminiscing, Exercise, OT/RT	Engage in groups	Repeat	Repeat	Repeat
MEDICATIONS	Obtain list of Rx & OTCs, Doses, Purpose, S/E	Eval need for PRNs for agitation/sleep	Pharmacologic tx for identified behavioral/ emotional sx	Eval for changes in sx & med needs	Repeat	Repeat
TEACHING	Provide family informational sheets and GeroPsychiatry Program info sheets	Eval educational needs of patient, family, caregiver, & select a program	Plan family mtg; include inter-disciplin team members	Repeat	Family mtg: health teaching/ after care issues	Family mtg: Review recall of teaching & reinforce
SPECIAL NEEDS	Potential patient needs: diet, mobility, vision, hearing, etc Discuss partial hospitalization potential with family	Eval for partial hospitalization placement needs at D/C; implement fall risk protocol	Determine partial hospitalization needs; discuss placement	Repeat	Decide on partial hospitalization, notify adm, arrange transportation	Refer for other special needs
DISCHARGE PLAN	Preliminary D/C needs & date; Disposition Contract	Discuss w/family: finances, community resources; D/C plans	Maintain family contact/ involvement	Repeat	Repeat; Arrange D/C	Repeat; Confirm D/C plans with agencies; pack pt.

Modified from Behavioral Intensive Care Unit, Institute of Psychiatry and Behavioral Sciences, Medical University of South Carolina, Charleston, SC, 1997.

*Assessments: MMSE = Mini Mental State Exam, GPHP = Geriatric Partial Hospitalization Program, CMAI = Cohen Mansfield Agitation Inventory, CDS = Cornell Depression Scale, AIMS = Abnormal Involuntary Movement Scale, WPS = Washington Paranoia Scale, Blessed = Blessed Dementia Scale, ADAS = Alzheimer's Disease Assessment Scale, Behav-AD = Behavioral Pathology in Alzheimer's Disease Rating Scale, VNA = Visiting Nurses Association.

TABLE **23-4** *Psychopharmacologic Agents in Development for the Treatment of Alzheimer's Disease*

AGENT	DEVELOPER
CHOLINESTERASE INHIBITORS	
ENA 317	Sandoz
Metrofinate	Miles/Bayer
CHOLINOMIMETICS	
Physostigmine FKS 508	Forest Labs
Xanomeline	Eli Lilly
GABA AND BENZODIAZEPINE AGENTS	
Sarmazenil	Roche
CGP 35348	Ciba-Geigy
N-METHYL D-ASPARTATE ANTAGONISTS	
Dizocilpine	Merck
MAO-B INHIBITORS	
Lazabemide	Roche
OTHER AGENTS	
Nerve growth factor agonists	Genentech
Lipid peroxidase inhibitors	Otsuka
Adenosine A1 receptor agonists	Marion Merrell Dow
Histamine H3 receptor agonists	Gliatech
Transdermal nicotine	
Nonsteroidal antiinflammatory agents	
Vitamin E	

Modified from Kumar V et al: Advances in pharmacotherapy for decline of memory and cognition in patients with Alzheimer's Disease, *Psychiatr Serv* 47:249, 1996.

choline in the brain, thereby improving cholinergic function. Acetylcholine, associated with memory and learning, is in short supply in patients with Alzheimer's disease.

Medications must be used with care when treating persons with dementia. Elderly people are very sensitive to medications and combinations of medications. Drugs with anticholinergic effects and benzodiazepines (which interfere with learning) should be avoided.

ORIENTATION. Disorientation is a common problem of people with cognitive impairment. Nursing interventions should help the patient function in the environment. In an institution it is helpful to mark patient rooms with large, clearly printed signs indicating the occupant's name. This also reminds forgetful people of others' names. Personal possessions can also be orienting devices. A favorite rocking chair, a hand-made afghan, or a family picture gives the person a sense of identity and helps to identify a personal area of the institution. Everyone needs a personal space. A light in the room at night helps the person remain oriented and decreases nighttime agitation. Some authorities recommend the use of small amounts of antipsychotic medications, such as phenothiazines and butyrophenones, to help patients rest because barbiturate sedatives may cause paradoxical agitation in patients with organic brain syndromes.

Clocks with large faces aid in orientation to time. A digital clock is not recommended because the confused person may not identify it as a clock. Calendars with a separate page for each day and large writing also help with time orientation. Newspapers provide other orienting stimuli and help to stimulate interest in current events. An institutional newspaper provides a creative outlet that focuses on patient strengths and helps patients maintain awareness of the environment.

Reality orientation is generally helpful to patients with cognitive impairments. Orientation includes the dimensions of time, place, and person. Systematic reality orientation includes attention to each of these dimensions. This approach often takes place in a group. It is most effective if the group meets daily, if possible, and at a consistent time. A pattern of group activity should be established. For instance, the group might begin with each person introducing himself or herself, followed by informing the group of the date and time. A review of the schedule for the day is often helpful. A brief time is allowed for questions. In general, this type of group should last only 15 to 20 minutes. If the members become fatigued, their cognitive ability will deteriorate.

COMMUNICATION. Recent memory loss is another common behavior. Patients may be frustrated when constantly confronted with evidence of failing memory. Conversational focus can be directed toward topics that the patient initiates. Most patients feel more comfortable talking about remote memories and may derive pleasure from discussing past experiences. Misperceptions of the present can be dealt with gently and diplomatically. For example, if an elderly woman who has been widowed for 10 years says that she expects her husband to come home soon, the nurse might reply, "You must have loved your husband very much. Sometimes it seems to you that he's still here." Explicitly or implicitly agreeing that her husband will "come home" is fostering false hope, perhaps leading to a disappointment. Abrupt confrontation with the reality of her husband's death is cruel and will increase her anxiety. Considerations about reality orientation are discussed in Critical Thinking about Contemporary Issues.

Farran and Keane-Hagerty[8] have recommended communication techniques for nurses who provide care for patients with dementia. The nurse should introduce himself or herself at each interaction with the patient. There should be an attitude of unconditional positive regard. Empathy, warmth, and caring are important. Verbal communication should be clear, concise, and unhurried. The voice should be modulated in relationship to the patient's ability to hear. Shouting may be interpreted as anger by a person who hears well. The use of pronouns should be avoided. Questions that require "yes" and "no" answers are best. Behavior should be requested one step at a time and if repetition is required, it should be stated in exactly the same way as originally. Nonverbal communication skills are also important. A pleasant,

Is Reality Orientation Always the Best Nursing Intervention for Patients Who Are Experiencing Progressive Memory Loss?

Reality orientation is often recommended as a nursing intervention for patients who are disoriented. The rationale for this is that patients are reassured by being in touch with where they are in time and place. For the same reason, clocks and calendars are placed where patients can see them. Reality orientation is appropriate for patients who can process the information that is given to them. However, in the case of progressive memory loss related to dementia the question arises as to whether repeated efforts at reality orientation serve patients' needs.

Jones[13] describes a situation in which a patient was distressed at the nursing staff's attempts to convince him that he was in a hospital. When a nurse participated in his life situation as he was experiencing it and responded as if she were in his workplace with him, he was much happier. The nurse's rationale for this intervention was that she was helping him to reminisce, which is an important developmental task for the elderly. Richards[20] refers to the delicate balance nurses must maintain between providing the patient with needed information about the environment and denying the patient's inability to process that information in a meaningful way. This means that nurses must question the automatic use of reality orientation as the best intervention for every disoriented patient.

calm, supportive tone of voice should be used. Verbal and nonverbal communication must be congruent. Sometimes nonverbal techniques, especially touch, may be reassuring to the patient. The nurse should try to understand who the patient was in the past. This can be accomplished by encouraging reminiscence and talking with family members. Pictures or music may help the patient to remember past experiences.

Farran and Keane-Hagerty[8] further suggest providing an environment of "sheltered freedom." This includes a predictable, unhurried schedule and the assignment of a primary nurse. Distraction or diversion along with decreased stimulation should be used if a patient appears to become agitated. Appropriate use of humor and flexibility on the part of the nurse help the patient to function in the environment.

REINFORCEMENT OF COPING MECHANISMS. Previously helpful coping mechanisms are often used by the patient with maladaptive cognitive responses. Sometimes these attempts to cope may be hard to understand unless placed in the appropriate context. An older man who pats and pinches nurses and makes lewd remarks may have had past success dealing with his anxiety by behaving seductively. An elderly woman who hoards food in her room may equate food with security. An aging person who has been suspicious of others in the past may become more suspicious

over time. Because of the protective nature of these behaviors, they should not be actively confronted. Rather, the nurse should try to discover the source of the person's anxiety and attempt to alleviate it, thus allowing the person to behave less defensively.

WANDERING. Wandering is a behavior that causes great concern to caregivers. In fact, it often leads to institutionalization or to the use of restraints. Fopma-Loy[10] recommends that nurses observe patients carefully to identify situations that contribute to wandering behavior. She suggests that mapping of the behavior may be useful when attempting to understand it and plan appropriate interventions. In some cases, medications may cause agitation and restlessness. Some patients are extremely sensitive to stress and tension in the environment. Their wandering may be an attempt to get away. Similarly, if patients are aware that an activity they dislike is about to occur, such as bathing or medication administration, they may try to avoid it. If wandering meets needs for attention, efforts to control the behavior may actually reinforce it.

Fopma-Loy suggests decreasing stress in the environment, especially at night, when many people have decreased stress tolerance. Eliminating distracting background noise or shadows may help. Safe areas should be provided where patients can move about freely. If possible, this should include an outside area with adequate staff supervision to ensure safety. Environmental design can be used to camouflage doorways or to incorporate distractions. Any method of increasing orientation can also decrease the need to wander. However, it is important to base nursing intervention on observation and analysis of the motivation for the patient's behavior.

DECREASING AGITATION. Patients may also become agitated when pushed to do something unfamiliar or unclear. Expectations should be explained simply and completely. If the patient can make choices, they should be offered. An individual daily schedule of activities can help the person prepare for and plan his or her day. If a patient refuses to participate in an activity, continued insistence usually leads to increased agitation and sometimes loss of behavioral control, resulting in a catastrophic response. The best approach may be to wait a few minutes and then return to see whether the patient will agree to the request. In the interim the approach to the patient can be examined to see whether the nurse might have contributed to the problem. Perhaps the patient thought the nurse was too controlling and a power struggle developed, or perhaps the nurse initiated the request abruptly, not allowing the patient a time for transition.

FAMILY AND COMMUNITY INTERVENTIONS. Many people with dementia live in the community with their families. It is important to support these caregivers because the patient usually derives great benefit from being with them. When hospitalization occurs, careful discharge planning is needed.[6]

Teusink and Mahler[27] have identified a family reaction process in relatives of patients with Alzheimer's disease. The

TABLE **23-5** *Pattern of Family Members' Responses to Alzheimer's Disease*

STAGE	FAMILY BEHAVIOR	INTERVENTION
Denial	May ignore severe memory loss; may use intact remote memory as evidence of no problem; may interfere with treatment planning.	Education. Supportive confrontation.
Overinvolvement	Sacrifice of usual family activities; reluctance to seek help, often related to ethnicity.	Determine cultural norms; help to see problems related to overinvolvement.
Anger	Reaction to burden of care and feeling of abandonment by patient; often projected or displaced onto care provider.	Help to recognize and express feelings; be aware of countertransference.
Guilt	Reaction to recognition of anger and wish that patient would die; may also be caused by past interpersonal experiences with the patient.	Educate about the illness and what the family can and cannot control; help to make decisions about care, even if patient objects.
Acceptance	Resolution of other stages; realistic understanding of what to expect and what can be done.	Provide support and knowledge as required.

Modified from Teusink JP, Mahler S: Helping families cope with Alzheimer's disease, *Hosp Community Psychiatry* 35:152, 1984.

same sequence of responses is probably characteristic of families of people with other dementing illnesses. This five-stage process closely parallels the grieving process identified in the significant others of dying people.[14] The stages are presented in Table 23-5.

Families may need assistance in providing 24-hour care for the patient. Home care agencies may provide nursing and homemaking services to enable patients to remain in their own homes. If family members are not available during the day, adult day-care centers are available in some communities. These programs provide help with activities of daily living, recreation, health supervision, rehabilitation, exercise, and nutrition. Families also receive support and assistance, particularly during the first few weeks of attendance, when the patient may be resistant because of difficulty adapting to a new experience. However, one study found that although caregivers recognized that supportive services were available, they tended not to use them.[4] A Nursing Treatment Plan Summary for patients who have maladaptive cognitive responses is presented at right.

Evaluation

Expectations of the patient who has cognitive difficulty must be realistic but not pessimistic. One evaluation criterion is the appropriateness of the nursing goal to the patient. The nurse should assess whether the expectation is too high or too low. Levels of expectation can be increased until the patient is clearly unable to function and then lowered to the realistic level.

The evaluation of the nursing care of the patient who has maladaptive cognitive responses is based on achievement of the identified nursing care goals. If goals are not achieved, the nurse should ask the following questions:

▼ Was the assessment complete enough to correctly identify the problem?
▼ Were the goals individualized for the patient?

▼ Was enough time allowed for goal achievement?
▼ Did I have the skills needed to carry out the identified interventions?
▼ Were there environmental factors that affected goal achievement?
▼ Did additional stressors affect the patient's ability to cope?
▼ Was the goal achievable for this patient?
▼ What alternative approaches could be tried?

Colleagues are helpful in evaluating the nursing care plan. They may suggest alternative interventions or provide feedback about transference-countertransference issues. For instance, nurses who work with aging patients with dementia may respond to concerns about their own aging or that of their parents and have difficulty seeing patients as unique persons. Hallucinating patients often arouse anxiety in nurses, who may then respond with their own defense mechanisms. Regular supervision can help nurses to develop enhanced self-awareness and to determine when a particularly anxiety-provoking situation has bothered them and why.

Summary

1. The continuum of cognitive responses is related to the learning, social-cognitive, and developmental models.
2. Behaviors related to cognitive responses vary depending on whether the maladaptive response is acute and likely to resolve, as in delirium, or progressive and chronic, as in dementia. Behaviors are related to disturbances in thought, memory, reasoning, judgment, orientation, perception, and attention.
3. Predisposing factors are related to aging, neurobiological functioning, and genetic factors. Precipitating stressors are categorized as hypoxic, metabolic, toxic and infectious, structural, and related to sensory stimulation.
4. Coping resources are based on individual and interpersonal supports. Coping mechanisms include intellectualization, rationalization, denial, and regression.

| NURSING TREATMENT PLAN *Summary* | Maladaptive Cognitive Responses |

Nursing Diagnosis: Altered thought processes
Expected Outcome: The patient will achieve optimum cognitive functioning.

Short-term Goals	Interventions	Rationale
The patient will meet basic biological needs.	Maintain adequate nutrition, monitor fluid intake and output, monitor vital signs. Provide opportunities for rest and stimulation. Help with ambulation if necessary. Help with hygiene activities as needed.	Basic biological integrity is necessary for survival. Interventions related to survival are given high priority for nursing intervention.
The patient will be safe from injury.	Assess sensory and perceptual functioning. Provide access to eyeglasses, hearing aids, canes, walkers, and so on. Observe and remove safety hazards (such as obstacles, slippery floors, open flames, and inadequate lighting). Supervise medications if necessary. Protect from injury during periods of agitation with one-to-one nursing care; use restraints only if absolutely necessary.	Maladaptive cognitive responses usually involve sensory and perceptual disorders that can endanger the patient's safety.
The patient will experience an optimum level of self-esteem.	Provide reality orientation. Establish a trusting relationship. Encourage independence. Identify interests and skills; provide opportunities to use them. Give honest praise for accomplishments. Use therapeutic communication techniques to help patient communicate thoughts and feelings.	Cognitive impairment is a threat to self-esteem. A positive nurse-patient relationship can help the patient to express fears and feel secure in the environment. Recognition of accomplishments also raises self-esteem.
The patient will maintain positive interpersonal relationships.	Initiate contact with significant others. Encourage patient to interact with others; involve in group activities. Teach family and patient about the nature of the problem and the recommended health-care plan. Allow significant others to help in patient care if they wish. Meet with significant others regularly and provide them with an opportunity to talk. Involve patient and family in discharge planning.	Caring relationships with others promote a positive self-concept. Communication by significant others can often be understood more easily than that of strangers. Family and friends can provide help in knowing the patient's habits and preferences. Involvement of significant others in caregiving often helps them cope with the stress of the patient's health problem.

5. The primary NANDA nursing diagnosis is altered thought processes.
6. Primary DSM-IV diagnoses are categorized as dementia, delirium, and amnestic disorder.
7. The expected outcome of nursing care is that the patient will achieve the optimum level of cognitive functioning.
8. Interventions related to delirium include caring for physiological needs, responding to hallucinations, therapeutic communication, and patient education. Interventions related to dementia include pharmacological approaches, orientation, therapeutic communication, reinforcement of coping mechanisms, responding to wandering, decreasing agitation, and family and community approaches.
9. Evaluation of nursing care is based on goal accomplishment and involves feedback from the patient, significant others, peers, and supervisors.

COMPETENT CARING A Clinical Exemplar of a Psychiatric Nurse

Alison Meeks, RN, MS

I worked on a unit that was set up to care for patients with behavioral problems as a result of their dementia. I vividly remember one call we received about a patient who was described as violent, explosive, confused, and in need of total care in activities of daily living. When the patient arrived on the unit I discovered that Ms. S weighed 90 pounds, had long beautiful hair up in a bun, and was ambulatory. She thought she was going to a hotel, so we took her bags and served her lunch while we interviewed her husband, who was her primary caregiver.

His was a very sad story. Tearfully he reported that his wife no longer loved him, that she was very malicious, and that she became physically violent at least once a day. He wanted to go on vacation while she was in the hospital, which some of the staff felt was probably the reason for this admission. However, he has been caring for his wife for 5 years with little or no help from the community or family members and it was clear that he needed a break. It would be hard, however, because this would be the first time they had been apart from each other in their 58 years of marriage.

Ms. S had a mini-mental exam score of 12, and had great difficulty visually interpreting her environment. For example, she thought a comb was a knife and the garbage can was her purse. She was also very sensitive to her environment. If the unit was loud and a lot of people were walking around, she became more active and often had the potential for getting hurt or hurting someone else. During periods of activity on the unit, such as shift change, we escorted Ms. S to her room, where she would fold clothes or go through one of four pocketbooks we put together for her. The reason we needed four pocketbooks was that she would misplace one and we would not be able to find it. This symptom presented great problems at home for the caregiver because anything left out would be moved and often never be found. Our solution was to set up several baskets of safe items for Ms. S to rummage through.

She became physically violent three times during her 10-day hospitalization. Each incident occurred when staff entered her room and she accused staff of breaking into her home. We started to knock on her door before entering and would have something for her such as a pocketbook, a book, or her stockings in our hands. That seemed to solve that problem. Another intervention that worked for Ms. S was music. She always liked ballet and now thought she was a retired dancer. We never challenged this and listened to her wonderful stories about dance and other dancers.

When her husband came back from vacation Ms. S did not recognize him. He was hurt and said we had done nothing to help her. We worked extensively with her husband by having him come and observe our interventions with Ms. S. Our goal was to help him realize the level of her impairment. He soon realized that her actions were not malicious. We diagnosed a urinary tract infection during her admission, which we treated and prescribed .5 milligrams of Haldol each morning, which helped to decrease her explosive episodes. We also enlisted the help of family members, friends, and a home health provider to care for Ms. S. I made one home visit after discharge and gave suggestions on how to make the home safe for Ms. S.

Four weeks after discharge Mr. S mailed the nurses a letter thanking us for giving him his life back. He explained that he felt he should have been better able to care for his wife on his own before her hospitalization, and that he had even contemplated suicide because of the overwhelming burden of caring for his wife. It seemed to us that in this case, we touched the lives of two rather than one.

your **INTERNET connection**

Alzheimer's Association
http://www.alz.org/

Family Caregiver Alliance
http://www.caregiver.org/

Chapter Review Questions

1. Match each term in Column A with the correct definition in Column B.

Column A

___Delirium
___Denial
___Piaget
___Dementia
___Agnosia
___Pseudodementia
___Sundown syndrome
___Aphasia
___Apraxia
___Excess disability

Column B

A. Creator of the developmental model of cognition

B. Difficulty recognizing well-known objects

C. Disturbed consciousness and cognitions developing over a short time

D. May ignore memory loss, interfering with treatment planning

E. Depressed, missed in the elderly, is not treated appropriately

F. Gradual onset with continuing cognitive decline

G. Difficulty finding the right word

H. Extreme agitation, occurring at night

I. Cognitive responses functioning at a lower level than one would expect

J. Inability to perform familiar skilled activities

2. Fill in the blanks.

A. The brain lesions that are characteristic of Alzheimer's disease are _____ and _____.

B. The person's perception of the environment is called a _____.

C. The term _____ refers to extreme agitation related to dementia.

3. Provide short answers for the following questions.

A. Select one of Piaget's levels of cognitive development, identify the age range during which it normally occurs, and list its characteristics.

B. List three coping strategies that you would suggest to the caregiver of a person who has a moderate level of cognitive impairment due to dementia.

C. Describe a discharge plan for a person who has been hospitalized for treatment of delirium related to combining prescription medicine and alcohol.

References

1. American Psychiatric Association: *Diagnostic and statistical manual of mental disorders,* ed 4, Washington, DC, 1994, The Association.
2. Beck C et al: Dressing for success: promoting independence among cognitively impaired elderly, *J Psychosoc Nurs Ment Health Serv* 29:30, 1991.
3. Cohen GE: Alzheimer's disease: clinical update, *Hosp Community Psychiatry* 41:496, 1990.
4. Collins C, Stommel M, Given CW, King S: Knowledge and use of community services among family caregivers of Alzheimer's disease patients, *Arch Psychiatr Nurs* 5:84, 1991.
5. Davies HD, Zeiss A, Tinklenberg JR: 'Til death do us part: intimacy and sexuality in the marriages of Alzheimer's patients, *J Psychosoc Nurs Ment Health Serv* 30:5, 1992.
6. Dellasega C, Shellenbarger T: Discharge planning for cognitively impaired elderly adults, *Nurs Health Care* 13:526, 1992.
7. Engelhardt K: Piaget: a prescriptive theory for parents, *Matern Child Nurs J* 3:1, 1974.
8. Farran CJ, Keane-Hagerty E: Communicating effectively with dementia patients, *J Psychosoc Nurs Ment Health Serv* 27:13, 1989.
9. Fischer P, Simanyi M, Danielczyk W: Depression in dementia of the Alzheimer type and in multiinfarct dementia, *Am J Psychiatry* 147:1484, 1990.
10. Fopma-Loy J: Wandering: causes, consequences, and care, *J Psychosoc Nurs Ment Health Serv* 26:8, 1988.
11. Grinspoon L, editor: Update on Alzheimer's disease, Part I, *Harvard Ment Health Lett* 11(8):1, Feb 1995.
12. Harvis KA, Rabins PV: Dementia: helping family caregivers cope, *J Psychosoc Nurs Ment Health Serv* 27:7, 1989.
13. Jones CP: In Sam's shop, *Am J Nurs* 94:51, 1994.
14. Jones PS, Martinson IM: The experience of bereavement in caregivers of family members with Alzheimer's disease, *Image J Nurse Sch* 24:172, 1992.
15. Kaplan HI, Sadock BJ: *Synopsis of psychiatry,* ed 6, Baltimore, 1991, Williams & Wilkins.
16. Kolanowski AM: Disturbing behaviors in demented elders: a concept synthesis, *Arch Psychiatr Nurs* 9:188, 1995.
17. Kumar V, Goldstein MZ, Doraiswamy PM: Advances in pharmacotherapy for decline of memory and cognition in patients with Alzheimer's disease, *Psychiatr Serv* 47:249, 1996.
18. Li G et al: Age at onset and familial risk in Alzheimer's disease, *Am J Psychiatry* 152:424, 1995.

19. Piaget J: *The child and reality: problems of genetic psychology,* New York, 1973, Grossman Publishers.
20. Richards BS: Alzheimer's disease: a disabling neurophysiological disorder with complex nursing implications, *Arch Psychiatr Nurs* 4:39, 1990.
21. Selkoe DJ: Amyloid protein and Alzheimer's disease, *Sci Am* special issue, 1993.
22. Sevush S, Leve N: Denial of memory deficit in Alzheimer's disease, *Am J Psychiatry* 150:748, 1993.
23. Skelton WP, Skelton NK: Alzheimer's disease: recognizing and treating a frustrating condition, *Postgrad Med* 90:33, 1991.
24. Stern RG et al: A longitudinal study of Alzheimer's disease: measurement, rate, and predictors of cognitive deterioration, *Am J Psychiatry* 151:391, 1994.
25. Sultzer DL et al: A comparison of psychiatric symptoms in vascular dementia and Alzheimer's disease, *Am J Psychiatry* 150:1806, 1993.
26. Swanson EA, Maas ML, Buckwalter KC: Catastrophic reactions and other behaviors of Alzheimer's residents: special unit compared with traditional units, *Arch Psychiatr Nurs* 7:292, 1993.
27. Teusink JP, Mahler S: Helping families cope with Alzheimer's disease, *Hosp Community Psychiatry* 35:152, 1984.
28. Tolman EC: *Purposive behavior in animals and man,* New York, 1932, Century.
29. Ugarriza DN, Gray T: Alzheimer's disease: nursing interventions for clients and caretakers, *J Psychosoc Nurs Ment Health Serv* 31:7, 1993.

ANNOTATED SUGGESTED READINGS

*Abraham I et al: Multidisciplinary assessment of patients with Alzheimer's disease, *Nurs Clin North Am* 29:113, 1994.
  Compares and contrasts the clinical assessment of a patient who has Alzheimer's disease when performed by the various members of the multidisciplinary team, demonstrating the important contribution of each team member.
American Psychiatric Association: Practice guidelines for the treatment of patients with Alzheimer's disease and other dementias of late life, *Am J Psychiatry* 154:5, 1997.
  A state-of-the-art review of research that is translated into practice guidelines for the health care provider treating patients with Alzheimer's disease.
Breitner J, Walsh K: Diagnosis and management of memory loss and cognitive disorders among elderly persons, *Psychiatr Serv* 46:29, 1995.
  Discusses the key differences among delirium, dementia, and psychiatric disorders as causes of cognitive impairment in the elderly. Particularly useful for advanced practice nurses or those who work in geriatric settings.

*Nursing reference.

Colenda C: Managing agitated dementia patients: a decision analysis approach, *J Pract Psychiatry Behav Health* 3:156, 1997.
  Uses agitated behaviors in dementia patients as an example of applying decision trees to clinical decision making. Highly recommended.
*Fopma-Loy J, Austin J: An attributional analysis of formal caregivers' perceptions of agitated behavior of a resident with Alzheimer's disease, *Arch Psychiatr Nurs* 7:217, 1993.
  This nursing study applied attributional theory to the expectations of nursing home staff regarding the behavior of patients.
*Hall G: This hospital patient has Alzheimer's, *Am J Nurs* 91:45, 1991.
  Contains a good overview of the nursing care of a patient who has Alzheimer's disease.
*Hamdy R et al: *Alzheimer's disease: a handbook for caregivers,* ed 2, St Louis, 1994, Mosby.
  Provides a wealth of information about Alzheimer's disease. It is designed to be used by caregivers of people who have this illness but is very useful for nurses as well. Highly recommended.
Kumar V, Goldstein M, Doraiswamy P: Advances in pharmacotherapy for decline of memory and cognition in patients with Alzheimer's disease, *Psychiatr Serv* 47:249, 1996.
  Excellent reference for medication information related to cognitive problems.
*Liken M, Collins C: Grieving: facilitating the process for dementia caregivers, *J Psychosoc Nurs* 31:21, 1993.
  Addresses the nursing interventions that assist caregivers to cope with both predeath and postdeath when a loved one has a dementia.
Patkar A, Kunkel E: Treating delirium among elderly patients, *Psychiatr Serv* 48:46, 1997.
  Contains practical information presented in a concise manner with specific treatment recommendations.
Powell L, Courtice K: *Alzheimer's disease: a guide for families,* Reading, Mass, 1993, Addison-Wesley.
  Recommended as a reference for families with practical information that can be applied to everyday caregiving.
*Rentz C: Reminiscence: a supporting intervention for the person with Alzheimer's disease, *J Psychosoc Nurs* 33:15, 1995.
  Describes a creative nursing approach using photograph albums to help elderly patients who have Alzheimer's disease to reminisce.
*Rossby L, Beck C, Heacock P: Disruptive behaviors of a cognitively impaired nursing home resident, *Arch Psychiatr Nurs* 6:98, 1992.
  Good example of the use of research to analyze a nursing care problem and identify interventions.

Chemically Mediated Responses and Substance-Related Disorders

Linda V. Jefferson

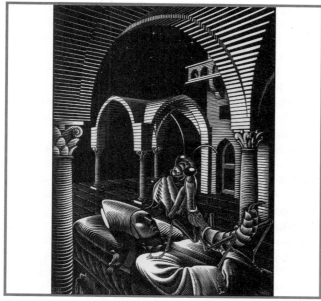

© 1998 M.C. Escher/Cordon Art, Baarn, Holland.

*Sleepmonger, deathmonger, with capsules in my palms each night, eight at a time
from sweet pharmaceutical bottles I make arrangements for a pint-sized journey.
I'm the queen of this condition. I'm an expert on making the trip and now they say
I'm an addict. Now they ask why. Why!* **Anne Sexton** The Addict*

LEARNING OBJECTIVES

After studying this chapter the student should be able to:

▼ Describe the continuum of adaptive and maladaptive chemically mediated responses

▼ Discuss trends in the use of alcohol and drugs

▼ Identify behaviors associated with chemically mediated responses

▼ Analyze predisposing factors, precipitating stressors, and appraisal of stressors related to chemically mediated responses

▼ Describe coping resources and coping mechanisms related to chemically mediated responses

▼ Formulate nursing diagnoses related to chemically mediated responses

▼ Assess the relationship between nursing diagnoses and medical diagnoses related to chemically mediated responses

▼ Identify expected outcomes and short-term nursing goals related to chemically mediated responses

▼ Develop a patient education plan to promote patients' adaptive chemically mediated responses

▼ Analyze nursing interventions related to chemically mediated responses

▼ Evaluate nursing care related to chemically mediated responses

TOPICAL OUTLINE

Continuum of Chemically Mediated Responses
Definition of Terms
Attitudes Toward Substance Abuse
Prevalence
Assessment
Screening for Substance Abuse
Behaviors of Abuse and Dependence
Dual Diagnosis
Predisposing Factors
Precipitating Stressors
Appraisal of Stressors
Coping Resources
Coping Mechanisms
Nursing Diagnosis
Related Medical Diagnoses
Outcome Identification
Planning
Implementation
Biological Interventions
Intervening to Maintain Abstinence
Psychological Interventions
Social Interventions
Working with Dually Diagnosed Patients
Intervening with Impaired Colleagues
Preventive Interventions
Evaluation

*From Anne Sexton: *Live or die,* © 1966 by Anne Sexton. Reprinted by permission of Houghton Mifflin Co.

Psychoactive substances have been used by people in almost all cultures since prehistoric times. These substances have been seen as enhancers of individual and social functioning. People continue to use them for relief of negative emotional states, such as depression, fear, and anxiety; relief from fatigue or boredom; and as a break from daily routines through altered states of consciousness. Alcohol and drugs also continue to be used in various religious ceremonies. Ethical and legal considerations aside, moderate use for any of these purposes would probably not result in major social or individual harm. However, all cultures have recognized the negative effects of alcohol and drug use. Excessive use of these substances has contributed to profound individual and social problems.

Any drug that can produce pleasurable changes in mental or emotional states has potential for abuse. Drugs that cause the most marked and immediate desirable effects have the greatest abuse potential. Alcohol and cocaine are very popular because they produce effects on the brain within minutes. Drugs of abuse include legal drugs, such as alcohol and prescription drugs, illegal drugs, such as heroin, cocaine, and marijuana, and household products such as inhalants.

CONTINUUM OF CHEMICALLY MEDIATED RESPONSES

Definition of Terms

A person may achieve a state of relaxation, euphoria, stimulation, or altered awareness in several ways. The range of these chemically mediated coping responses is illustrated in Fig. 24-1. Although there is a continuum from occasional drug use to frequent drug use to abuse and dependence, not everyone who uses drugs becomes an abuser, nor does every abuser become dependent. The definitions of the terms *use, abuse,* and *dependence* have changed through the years and vary greatly in the addiction literature. The nurse must realize that what one person or health-care professional means by addiction is not necessarily meant by another.

Reading and discussion should start with agreement about the meanings of terms.

Substance abuse, as described in the *Diagnostic and Statistical Manual of Mental Disorders,* fourth edition (DSM-IV),[2] refers to continued use despite related problems. The term **substance dependence,** related to either drugs or alcohol, indicates a severe condition, usually considered a disease. There may be physical problems as well as serious disruptions in the person's work, family, and social life. The psychosocial behaviors related to substance dependence are often called **addiction.** For most purposes, the terms *dependence* and *addiction* are used interchangeably. **Dual diagnosis** is the coexistence of substance abuse and psychiatric disorders within the same person.

Withdrawal symptoms and tolerance are signs that the person is **physically dependent** on the drug. **Withdrawal symptoms** result from a biological need that develops when the body becomes adapted to having the drug in the system. Characteristic symptoms occur when the level of the substance in the system decreases appreciably. **Tolerance** means that with continued use, more of the substance is needed to produce the same effect. Physical dependence can occur independently from the symptoms of substance dependence. For example, a patient who receives narcotics for chronic pain may develop both tolerance and withdrawal, yet not have any of the other problems related to substance dependence such as preoccupation with getting the drug, loss of control, or use despite problems. This person would be described as physically dependent on the narcotic but would not be called a drug addict.

Many people progress from use to abuse at some time in their lives. However, only about 1 in 10 people progress from use to abuse to dependence. Once use has begun, the risk of becoming dependent is influenced by many biological, psychological, and sociocultural factors. Whether substance abuse is a disease is controversial. Nonetheless, use of the disease model can aid in the acceptance and treatment of substance-related disorders.

Fig. 24-1   Continuum of chemically mediated coping responses.

Attitudes Toward Substance Abuse

Substance abuse is viewed differently, depending on the substance used, the person using it, and the setting in which it is used. Nurses should be aware of these social and cultural attitudes and recognize their impact on individual users and people close to them. For instance, a businessman who starts arguments after a few drinks with his associates would not usually be considered an alcohol abuser. If the same person was caught nipping from a bottle in his desk, he would probably be considered to have a drinking problem. Despite convincing evidence of medical problems related to smoking and the effects of secondary smoke inhalation and the fact that practice guidelines for the treatment of patients with nicotine dependence have been released,[3] tobacco abuse is still widely accepted in the United States (Box 24-1). On the other hand, a person who smokes opium would be considered deviant even if the behavior took place in private.

> *Can you describe other examples of sociocultural mixed messages about the use of tobacco, alcohol, and marijuana? How would you as a health professional go about changing these attitudes?*

Changing laws related to consumption, sale, and serving of alcohol and drugs may reflect changing attitudes toward their use (see Critical Thinking about Contemporary Issues). Driving while intoxicated (DWI) laws are becoming tougher. When groups of friends go out, it is common for one to be the designated driver and not drink. Places that serve alcoholic beverages can be held liable if a customer overindulges and then causes an accident. Mandatory sentencing for certain drug offenses is intended to show an unaccepting attitude toward drug abuse.

Many nurses have negative attitudes toward alcoholics and other drug abusers. Some have had negative experiences with family members or friends who have had substance-related problems. This may influence the nurse's ability to assess and care for these patients. Nurses often see substance abusers at their worst, during a medical or psychiatric crisis. They see these patients returning repeatedly for alcohol or drug-related health problems. Nurses rarely have contact with alcoholics and drug addicts who have recovered from their addiction because they are ill less often. When they do seek health care, these patients may try to hide their substance abuse history. The best way for nurses to change negative attitudes is to attend open meetings of self-help groups. There they will meet recovering alcoholics and addicts who have overcome tremendous odds to remain sober and lead healthy, productive lives.

Prevalence

The United States still has one of the highest levels of substance abuse in the industrialized world. Substance abuse is involved in numerous chronic illnesses, hospitalizations, emergency room visits, and deaths. Recent data from the National Household Survey on Drug Abuse revealed that in 1992 approximately 83% of people in the United States age 12 and older had used alcohol sometime in their lives.[27] About 10 million people (5%) reported heavy alcohol use in the past month. In contrast, 36% had used illicit drugs and 12% had used prescription drugs for nonmedical reasons sometime in their lives. Overall, use of alcohol and illicit drugs appears to increase into the mid-twenties, level off, and then decrease with age. Both the lifetime prevalence

Box **24-1** *Nicotine as a Substance of Abuse*

Cigarette smoking among teenagers rose in 1995 for the fourth year in a row. Although approximately one-fourth of the U.S. population smokes, 90% of all new smokers are under the age of 18. The federal government aims to reduce smoking among children and adolescents by 50%. It began this initiative in August 1996 when President Clinton signed an executive order that subjects tobacco to regulation by the Food and Drug Administration. The FDA claims authority over cigarettes by defining them as the delivery system for the addictive drug nicotine. The legislative changes are directed at reducing access (for example, by eliminating mail order, vending machine, and self-service sales) and limiting the appeal (for example, eliminating cartoons and other child-directed advertisements) to children. This initiative marks the first major successful attack on the cigarette industry in the United States.

CRITICAL THINKING *about* Contemporary Issues

Should All Drugs Be Legalized?

In 1993 Joycelyn Elders, then–surgeon general of the United States, stated that she was in favor of legalizing drugs. Those who agree with her position argue that substance abuse is a public health problem and that criminalization of drug abusers creates a barrier to treatment. In addition, they point to the criminal activity that results from illegal sale of abused substances and the use of tax dollars to combat crime rather than support treatment programs.

Opponents say that they doubt legalization will decrease the crime associated with drug use. They worry about the enormous health-care costs that could be associated with providing treatment for chronic drug users. They believe that ready availability of drugs would encourage experimentation and result in increased rates of addiction. They are also strongly opposed to government sanction of what they view as an immoral behavior.

and the intensity of alcohol use were greater among males. In addition, whites reported higher levels of alcohol use than blacks or Hispanics. Those with more education were more likely to use alcohol, but heavy use was more common among the less educated and unemployed.

Adolescence is a critical time for the first experience with drugs. Although teenagers tend to progress from nicotine, alcohol, and marijuana (also known as the "gateway" drugs) to drugs that are perceived to be more dangerous, drug use patterns seem to be most related to availability. The percentage of high school seniors who had ever used an illicit drug reached a high of 65% in the United States in 1981, then steadily decreased to 41% by 1992. However, by 1995 the rate had again risen to 48%.[28] Nearly 1 in 20 high school seniors in 1995 reported daily marijuana use. Lifetime use of LSD (5% to 10%), stimulants (15%), and inhalants (20%) continued an upward trend for all high school students in 1995. Lifetime prevalence rates for heroin were low (2%) compared to other drugs, but were still two to three times higher than they had been years before. Information about substance abuse by adolescents is provided in Chapter 37.

MULTIPLE SUBSTANCE USE. Simultaneous or sequential use of more than one substance is very common. People do this to enhance, lessen, or otherwise change the nature of their intoxication or to relieve withdrawal symptoms. Use of alcohol with cocaine, or alcohol with heroin ("speedballing") is especially common. Heroin users often combine alcohol, marijuana, and benzodiazepines with heroin. Multiple drug use is particularly dangerous if synergistic drugs, such as barbiturates and alcohol, are used. It also complicates substance abuse assessment and intervention because the patient may be demonstrating effects of or withdrawal from several drugs at the same time.

DUAL DIAGNOSIS. In the addicted population, there is no greater prevalence of psychiatric illness than in the general population. However epidemiologic surveys have found that people with psychiatric disorders were more prone to substance disorders than the general population. Those with severe mental illness were especially vulnerable, with lifetime prevalence of approximately 50%.[16] For example, people with schizophrenia were more than four times as likely to have a substance use disorder during their lifetimes, and those with bipolar disorder were more than five times as likely to have such a diagnosis than people in the general population.

Many studies show that despite their prevalence, substance disorders are underdetected and underdiagnosed in acute care psychiatric settings.[24] Failure to detect substance abuse disorder results in misdiagnosis of the psychiatric disorder, suboptimal pharmacological treatment, neglect of appropriate interventions for substance abuse, and inappropriate treatment planning and referral. This underdetection can be caused by a combination of factors including clinicians' lack of awareness of the high rates of substance disor-

ders in psychiatric populations; the inadequacy of standardized assessment tools in this population; patients' denial, minimization, and failure to acknowledge their substance-related problems; and patients' cognitive, psychotic, and other impairments related to their psychiatric illness.[23]

SUBSTANCE-RELATED DISORDERS IN NURSES. Despite claims that health care professionals have a higher rate of substance abuse than the general public, there is little information to support this. In fact, at least one major epidemiological study contradicts these claims. Trinkoff found that nurses were no more likely to have used illicit drugs and were less likely to have had alcohol abuse problems than nonnurses.[35] The Epidemiologic Catchment Area Study[16] surveyed the mental health status of 20,000 people in five locations across the United States. Based on prevalence figures from this study, about 10% of registered nurses probably have problems with alcohol or drug abuse/dependence. Because there are 2.2 million registered nurses in the United States, the number of RNs with drug- or alcohol-related problems would be estimated at 220,000.

State board of nursing disciplinary records provide additional information. According to statistics from the data bank of the National Council of State Boards of Nursing, 53% of all disciplinary actions taken against registered nurses in 1995 were drug related, down from 94.4% in 1987 and 68% in 1991. These figures could reflect a decrease in the problem, a decrease in reporting of the problem, or earlier and more effective treatment. Unfortunately, it is still a common practice to deal with a nurse who has a drug problem by ignoring the problem, firing the nurse, or asking for the nurse's resignation rather than reporting it to the state licensing board. Therefore, these data may only reflect a small segment of the problem.

Alcohol is the drug of choice for nurses, as in the general population. Also, as in the general population, the nurse's choice of substance is influenced by availability and exposure.[26] Of all health-care professionals, physicians and nurses use parenteral narcotics the most in their practices. Therefore, they are more likely to choose these drugs for their own use. Among narcotics the drug of choice for nurses is Demerol. Anesthesiologists and nurse anesthetists tend to favor fentanyl, a potent, short-acting narcotic. In general, health-care professionals tend to abuse prescription drugs rather than "street" drugs, whether they acquire them by prescription or diversion.

Assessment

Although accurate assessment of a patient's patterns of drug and alcohol use is important, it is sometimes very difficult to accomplish. Alcohol and drug addicts may use many defense mechanisms when discussing their chemical use. They tend to deny how much they use and its relationship to problems in their lives. They often rationalize their substance use. Patients should not be criticized for these unconscious mechanisms. They are often not aware of the extent or effects of their use. It is also true that some patients purposely distort the truth about drug use to avoid feared consequences. The nurse must be aware of these behaviors and take them into account. On the other hand, the nurse should be aware that only about 1 in 10 people who drink develop substance dependence at some point in their lives. Thus, one should not jump to the conclusion that a person is in denial if he or she relates no alcohol-related problems.

Screening for Substance Abuse

Fortunately, there are ways to increase the accuracy of assessment. One must first be asking the right questions. People who drink, take drugs, or do both tend to be around others who drink and use drugs as they do. They do not have a good idea of what "normal" use patterns are. Therefore, even people who deny drug and drinking problems are apt to answer certain questions truthfully. These questions are included in screening tools, which are the first level of assessment for alcohol and drug dependence.

Simple screening tools are available that are very useful in identifying people who are probably addicted to drugs. One of these, the Brief Drug Abuse Screening Test (B-DAST), is presented in Box 24-2. It is a true/false self-administered questionnaire. Each item has a one-point value. Scores of 6 or above suggest significant drug abuse problems. Patients who score above established cutoff

scores are considered to be addicted. Because the tools can be incorrect, all people screened positive for addiction should be further assessed according to diagnostic criteria.

CAGE. The CAGE questionnaire is one of the simplest and most reliable screening tools for alcohol abuse. CAGE is an acronym for the four questions it contains (Box 24-3). Answering "yes" to one or more questions indicates that alcohol abuse is likely. Further assessment would be needed to make a diagnosis. The CAGE questionnaire is recommended as an initial screening tool in a variety of settings because its questions and scoring can be remembered easily and included in any interview. The wording should be adapted to fit the general conversation, being sure to focus on Cutting down, Annoyance by criticism, Guilty feelings, and Eye-openers. Other tools for screening for substance abuse are found in Chapter 6.

> **?** *Given that CAGE is such a simple screening tool, why do you think it is not used more often in routine nursing assessments?*

BREATHALYZER. The simplest biological measure to obtain is blood alcohol content (BAC) by use of a breathalyzer. Alcohol in any amount has an effect on the central nervous system. The behaviors that can be expected from a nontolerant person at different concentrations of alcohol in

---

Box **24-2** *Brief Drug Abuse Screening Test (B-DAST)*

Instructions: The following questions concern information about your involvement and abuse of drugs. Drug abuse refers to (1) the use of prescribed or over-the-counter drugs in excess of the directions and (2) any nonmedical use of drugs. Carefully read each statement and decide whether your answer is yes or no. Then circle the appropriate response.

YES NO   1. Have you used drugs other than those required for medical reasons?
YES NO   2. Have you abused prescription drugs?
YES NO   3. Do you abuse more than one drug at a time?
YES NO   4. Can you get through the week without using drugs (other than those required for medical reasons)?
YES NO   5. Are you always able to stop using drugs when you want to?
YES NO   6. Have you had "blackouts" or "flashbacks" as a result of drug use?
YES NO   7. Do you ever feel bad about your drug abuse?
YES NO   8. Does your spouse (or parents) ever complain about your involvement with drugs?
YES NO   9. Has drug abuse ever created problems between you and your spouse?
YES NO   10. Have you ever lost friends because of your use of drugs?
YES NO   11. Have you ever neglected your family or missed work because of your use of drugs?
YES NO   12. Have you ever been in trouble at work because of drug abuse?
YES NO   13. Have you ever lost a job because of drug abuse?
YES NO   14. Have you gotten into fights when under the influence of drugs?
YES NO   15. Have you engaged in illegal activities in order to obtain drugs?
YES NO   16. Have you ever been arrested for possession of illegal drugs?
YES NO   17. Have you ever experienced withdrawal symptoms as a result of heavy drug intake?
YES NO   18. Have you had medical problems as a result of your drug use (e.g., memory loss, hepatitis, convulsions, bleeding, etc.)?
YES NO   19. Have you ever gone to anyone for help for a drug problem?
YES NO   20. Have you ever been involved in a treatment program specifically related to drug use?

From Skinner HA: *Addict Behav* 7:363, 1982.
(Items 4 and 5 are scored in the "no," or false, direction.)

Box **24-3** *The CAGE Questionnaire*

Have you ever felt you ought to *C*ut down on your drinking?
Have people *A*nnoyed you by criticizing your drinking?
Have you ever felt bad or *G*uilty about your drinking?
Have you ever had a drink first thing in the morning to
   steady your nerves or get rid of a hangover (*E*ye-opener)?
Scoring: One "yes" answer calls for further inquiry.

From Ewing JA: *JAMA* 252:1905, 1984.

TABLE **24-1** *Comparison of Blood Alcohol Concentrations with Behavioral Manifestations of Intoxication*

BLOOD ALCOHOL LEVEL	BEHAVIORS
0.05 to 0.15 g/dl	Euphoria, labile mood, cognitive disturbances (decreased concentration, impaired judgment, loss of sexual inhibitions)
0.15 to 0.25 g/dl	Slurred speech, staggering gait, diplopia, drowsiness, labile mood with outbursts
0.3 g/dl	Stupor, aggressive behavior, incoherent speech, labored breathing, vomiting
0.4 g/dl	Coma
0.5 g/dl	Severe respiratory depression, death

From Antai-Otong D: Helping the alcoholic patient recover, *Am J Nurs,* August 1995.

the blood are shown in Table 24-1. Remember that a person who has developed tolerance to alcohol would not demonstrate these behaviors and could have a high BAC without showing any signs of impairment. A level above 0.10% without associated behavioral symptoms indicates the presence of tolerance. The higher the level without symptoms, the more severe the tolerance. High tolerance is a sign of physical dependence.

BLOOD AND URINE SCREENING. Blood and urine are the body fluids most often tested for drug content, although saliva, hair, breath, and sweat analysis methods have been developed and are being refined. Identification and measurement of drug levels in the blood are useful for treating drug overdoses or complications in emergency room and other medical settings. Otherwise, urine drug screening is the method of choice because it is noninvasive. Urine drug screening is sometimes used to test prospective employees and athletes for evidence of drug use. It is also used by drug treatment personnel to determine whether patients have used drugs while in treatment. Urine drug screening is often used in court to validate a person's drug use related to criminal activity.

The person being tested may try to alter the sample to hide drug use. The most common ways to do this are diluting the specimen with water from the toilet or substituting a "clean" specimen donated by a friend for the "dirty" specimen. To help prevent these practices, the specimen is often collected on random days under direct observation of a same-sex staff member. Another way is to have the person leave jackets, sweaters, purses, and so forth outside the stall, place drops of dye in the toilet water to alter its color, and test the specimen for temperature. Fresh, undiluted urine should feel warm through the cup and should be approximately 37° C.

The length of time that drugs can be found in blood and urine varies according to dosage and the metabolic properties of the drug. All traces of the drug may disappear within 24 hours or may still be detectable 30 days later.

Random urine testing for drugs is required for members of some occupations, including some nurses. This practice has been challenged as an invasion of privacy and an intrusion on professional integrity. What is your opinion about random urine testing for nurses?

Behaviors of Abuse and Dependence

There are many biopsychosocial consequences of using alcohol and drugs. Some are very serious and have led to great social concern. Lifestyles associated with drug abuse carry risks. Accidents are frequent and violence is common. Self-neglect is the norm, contributing to physical and mental disease. The drugs and lifestyle also lead to complications of pregnancy and the risk of fetal abnormalities and fetal drug dependence.

Users of intravenous drugs and their sexual partners are at high risk for infection with bloodborne pathogens, particularly hepatitis B (HBV) and the human immunodeficiency virus (HIV), which causes the acquired immunodeficiency syndrome (AIDS). It is common for addicts to share needles when they are using drugs in a group. Because the needles are not cleaned, blood is transferred from one person to the others. This is an ideal situation for the transmission of HIV or HBV.

Additional information regarding the consequences of substance abuse is included in Table 24-2.

CNS DEPRESSANTS. This term is used for any drug that depresses excitable tissues at all levels of the brain. These drugs are also called sedative-hypnotics. Their primary effects are to reduce anxiety (the calming, antianxiety, or sedative effect), induce sleep (the hypnotic effect), or both. Included in this class are alcohol, barbiturates, and benzodiazepines. The signs and symptoms of the use of, overdose by, and withdrawal from CNS depressants are listed in Table 24-2. It should be noted that cross-tolerance develops among all drugs in this category. This means that as tolerance develops to one drug, it develops to all other drugs in this category as well. For example, a chronic alcoholic will need very high doses of benzodiazepines to control signs of withdrawal.

Alcohol. Although alcohol is a sedative, it creates an initial feeling of euphoria. This is probably related to decreased inhibitions. Symptoms of sedation of different central nervous system structures increase as the amount drunk increases.

Approximately 15% of drinkers progress to alcoholism. Fig. 24-2 demonstrates characteristic elements of this process. The behaviors are categorized into phases according to severity. A person's drinking may begin like everyone else's, or a person may be able to drink more alcohol than others before feeling intoxicated. In either case, the person likes the feeling, and continues to drink whenever possible. Gradually, drinking occurs more often and in larger quantities. As this happens, drinking begins to cause problems in the person's life, which are quickly explained away. The problems increase, the drinking increases, physical and psychological dependence develops, and the person begins to drink to avoid withdrawal symptoms. Or, the person drinks in binges. Not everyone progresses in the same way or displays all of these characteristics, and the time period over which the progression occurs varies widely. The following clinical example illustrates many of the behaviors described. Mr. H has the medical diagnoses of alcohol dependence and alcohol withdrawal delirium.

Clinical Example Mr. H was admitted to the detoxification center of a large metropolitan hospital in acute alcohol withdrawal. He was delirious and having visual hallucinations of bugs in his bed. He was extremely frightened, thrashing around in bed and mumbling incoherently. Because he had a long and well-documented history of alcohol abuse, family members were contacted and confirmed that he had recently stopped drinking after a 2-week binge.

The patient had been a successful lawyer with a large practice. He specialized in corporate law and conducted much business over lunch or dinner. He also kept a well-stocked bar in his office to offer clients a drink. Without his really being aware of it, Mr. H's drinking gradually increased. After a few years he was drinking almost nonstop from lunchtime to bedtime. He then began to have a Bloody Mary with breakfast "just to get myself going."

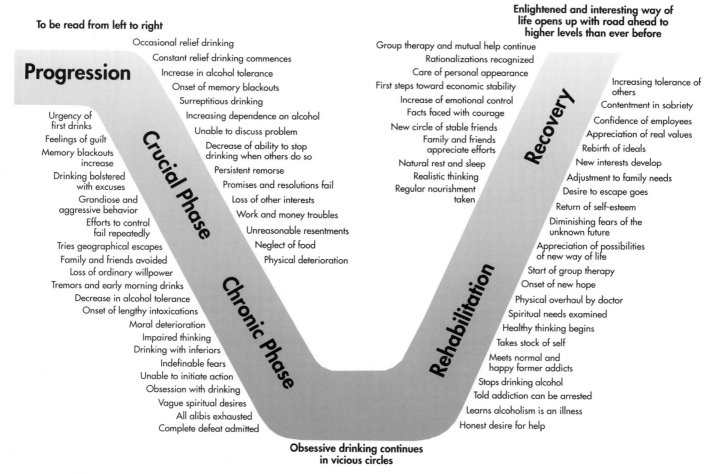

Fig. 24-2   The progression and recovery of the alcoholic. (From Jellinek EM: *QJ Stud Alcohol* 13:672, 1952.)

TABLE 24-2 *Characteristics of Substances of Abuse*

Substance	Route (most common first)	Common Street Names	Dependence: physical/psychological	Use Signs and Symptoms	Overdose Signs and Symptoms	Withdrawal Signs and Symptoms	Special Considerations/Consequences of Use
DEPRESSANTS							
Alcohol	Ingestion	Booze, brew, juice, spirits	Yes/Yes	Depression of major brain functions such as mood, cognition, attention, concentration, insight, judgment, memory, affect, and emotional rapport in interpersonal relationships. Extent of depression is dose dependent and ranges from lethargy through anesthesia and death.	Unconsciousness, coma, respiratory depression, death	*General depressant withdrawal syndrome:* Tremors; agitation, anxiety, diaphoresis, increased pulse and blood pressure, sleep disturbance, hallucinosis, seizures, delusions, DTs *Postacute withdrawal:* Mood swings, difficulty sleeping, impaired cognitive functioning, increased emotionality, overreaction to stress.	Chronic alcohol use leads to serious disruptions in most organ systems: malnutrition and dehydration; vitamin deficiency leading to Wernicke's encephalopathy and alcoholic amnestic syndrome; impaired liver function, including hepatitis and cirrhosis; esophagitis, gastritis, pancreatitis; osteoporosis; anemia; peripheral neuropathy; impaired pulmonary function; cardiomyopathy; myopathy; disrupted immune system; and brain damage. High susceptibility to other dependencies.
Barbiturates	Ingestion, injection	Barbs, beans, black beauties, blue angels, candy, downers, goof balls, G.B., nebbies, reds, sleepers, yellow jackets, yellows	Yes/Yes	Psychomotor impairment, increased reaction time, interruption of hand-eye coordination, motor ataxia, nystagmus. Decreased REM sleep leading to more dreams and sometimes nightmares.		*Low-dose benzodiazepine withdrawal:* Therapeutic doses for no more than 6 months; subtle symptoms, peak in about 12 days; wax and wane for 6-12 months; several symptom-free days, followed by acute anxiety, dilated pupils, elevated pulse, and blood pressure.	Dependence on barbiturates and benzodiazepines may develop insidiously; users may underreport the actual amount taken because of guilt about multiple prescriptions and abuse.
Benzodiazepines	Ingestion, injection	Downers	Yes/Yes			*High-dose benzodiazepine withdrawal:* Peaks in 2 to 3 days for short-acting drugs and 5 to 8 days for longer-acting; symptoms usually gone in 2 weeks.	
STIMULANTS							
Amphetamines	Ingestion, injection	A, AMT, bam, bennies, crystal, diet pills, dolls, eye-openers, lid poppers, pep pills, purple hearts, speed, uppers, wake-ups	Yes/Yes	Sudden rush of euphoria, abrupt awakening, increased energy, talkativeness, elation. Agitation, hyperactivity, irritability, grandiosity, pressured speech. Diaphoresis, anorexia, weight loss, insomnia. Increased temperature, blood pressure, and pulse. Tachycardia, ectopic heartbeats, chest pain. Urinary retention, constipation, dry mouth. *High dose:* Slurred, rapid, incoherent speech. Stereotypic movements, ataxic gait, teeth grinding, illogical thought processes, headache, nausea, vomiting. *Toxic psychosis:* Paranoid delusions in clear sensorium; auditory, visual, or tactile hallucinations. Very labile mood. Unprovoked violence.	Seizures. Cardiac arrhythmias, coronary artery spasms, myocardial infarctions, marked increase in blood pressure and temperature that can lead to cardiovascular shock and death	*Crash:* Depression, agitation, anxiety, and intense drug craving followed by fatigue, depression, loss of drug desire, insomnia, desire for sleep followed by prolonged sleep then extreme hunger, renewed drug cravings, anergia, and anhedonia, which may increase for 1 to 4 days.[20]	Certain amphetamines prescribed for attention deficit hyperactivity disorder in children because of a paradoxical depressant action. Sometimes these medications are stolen and abused. May be used alternately with depressants.
Cocaine	Inhalation, smoking, injection, topical	Bernice, bernies, big C, blow, C, charlie, coke, dust, girl, heaven, jay, lady, nose candy, nose powder, snow, sugar, white lady. Crack = conan, freebase, rock, toke, white cloud, white tornado	Yes/Yes			Pattern varies widely among patients; anxiety, depression, irritability, fatigue may last several weeks[15]; craving may return; relapse is a risk. Sometimes a user stops stimulants purposely to decrease tolerance, decreasing the amount needed to get high.	Cocaine use may lead to multiple physical problems: destruction of the nasal septum related to snorting, coronary artery vasoconstriction, seizures, cerebrovascular accidents; transient ischemic episodes, sudden death related to respiratory arrest, and myocardial infarction. Intravenous use of stimulants may lead to the serious physical consequences described under Opiates
OPIATES							
Heroin	Injection, ingestion, inhalation	H, horse, harry, boy, scag, shit, smack, stuff, white junk, white stuff	Yes/Yes	Euphoria, relaxation, relief from pain, "nodding out" (apathy, detachment from reality, impaired judgment, and drowsiness); constricted pupils, nausea, constipation, slurred speech, respiratory depression.	Unconsciousness, coma, respiratory depression, circulatory depression, respiratory arrest, cardiac arrest, death. Anoxia can lead to brain abscess	*Initially:* Drug craving lacrimation, rhinorrhea, yawning, diaphoresis. *In 12-72 hr:* Sleep disturbance, mydriasis, anorexia, piloerection, irritability, tremor, weakness, nausea, vomiting, diarrhea, chills, fever, muscle spasms, flushing, spontaneous ejaculation, abdominal pain, hypertension, increased rate and depth of respirations.	Intravenous use leads to risk for infection with bloodborne pathogens, such as HIV or hepatitis B. Other infections (skin abscesses, phlebitis, cellulitis, and septic emboli causing pneumonia, pulmonary abscess, or subacute bacterial endocarditis) may occur as a result of lack of asepsis or contaminated substances.
Morphine	Injection						
Meperidine	Injection, ingestion						

Drug	Routes of Administration	Common Names	Dependence (Physical/Psychological)	Effects	Overdose	Withdrawal	Long-Term Effects
Codeine	Ingestion, injection					*Protracted withdrawal:* Changes in respirations and temperature, decreased self-esteem, anxiety, depression, drug hunger, and abnormal responses to stressful situations. Lasts up to 6 months.[18]	Chronic use leads to lack of concern about physical well-being, resulting in malnutrition and dehydration. Criminal behavior may occur to acquire money for drugs.
Opium	Smoking, ingestion						
Methadone	Ingestion						
MARIJUANA	Smoking, ingestion	Acapulco gold, aunt mary, broccoli, dope, grass, grunt, hay, hemp, herb, J, joint, joy stick, killer weed, maryjane, pot, ragweed, reefer, smoke, weed	No/Yes	Altered state of awareness, relaxation, mild euphoria, reduced inhibition, red eyes, dry mouth, increased appetite, increased pulse, decreased reflexes, panic reaction.	Toxic psychosis	None	Pulmonary problems. Interference with reproductive hormones. May cause fetal abnormalities.
HALLUCINOGENS	Ingestion, smoking	Acid, big D, blotter, blue heaven, cap, D, deeda, flash, L, mellow yellows, microdots, paper acid, sugar, ticket, yello	No/No	Distorted perceptions and hallucinations in the presence of a clear sensorium. Distortions of time and space, illusions, depersonalization, mystical experiences, heightened sense of awareness. Extreme mood lability. Tremor, dizziness, piloerection, paresthesias, synesthesia, nausea, and vomiting. Increased temperature, pulse, blood pressure, and salivation. Panic reaction, "bad trip."	Rare with LSD: convulsions, hyperthermia, death	None	Flashbacks may last for several months. Permanent psychosis may occur.
PHENCYCLIDINE (PCP)	Smoking, ingestion	Angel dust, DOA, dust, elephant, hog, peace pill, supergrass, tic tac	No/No	Intensely psychotic experience characterized by bizarre perceptions, confusion, disorientation, euphoria, hallucinations, paranoia, grandiosity, agitation. Anesthesia. Apparent enhancement of strength and endurance. Rage reactions. May be agitated and hyperactive with tendency toward violence or catatonic and withdrawn or vacillate between the two conditions. Red, dry skin; dilated pupils, nystagmus, ataxia, hypertension, rigidity, and seizures.	Seizures, coma, and death	None	If flashbacks occur, they are mild and usually not disturbing.
INHALANTS	Inhalation	Spray, rush, bolt, huffing, bagging, sniffing	Yes/Yes	*Psychological:* Belligerence, assaultiveness, apathy, impaired judgment. *Physical:* Dizziness, nystagmus, incoordination, slurred speech, unsteady gait, depressed reflexes, tremor, blurred vision, euphoria, anorexia.	Lethargy, stupor/coma, respiratory arrest, cardiac arrhythmia	Headaches, chills, abdominal cramps, delirium, tremors (not common)	Death from inhalants can occur in different ways: Sudden death is caused by cardiac arrhythmia—sometimes this happens the first time the child uses inhalants. Suicide may be a result of impaired judgment. Injury: Under the influence of inhalants, youth feel invulnerable. Burns and frostbite can also be caused by these chemicals. Permanent cognitive impairment may require an individual to reside in a structured setting.

His wife reported that he had become irritable, particularly if she questioned his drinking. On two occasions he had hit her during their arguments. She was seriously considering divorce. He had also become alienated from his children, who appeared frightened of him. Infrequently he would feel guilty about his neglect of his family and plan a special outing. Most of the time he was too drunk to carry out his plans. The family had also become less involved in activities with friends. Mrs. H and the children felt embarrassed about his behavior and did not invite anyone to their home. On two occasions, Mr. H had tried to stop drinking. The first time he went to a private hospital, where he was detoxified. He abstained from drinking for about a month after discharge.

He then lost an important case and decided to have "just one drink" to carry him through the crisis. Soon his drinking was again out of control. His second hospitalization was at a general hospital with an active alcoholism rehabilitation program. He was introduced to Alcoholics Anonymous and started taking disulfiram (Antabuse). This program worked until he decided that he could manage without medication. A couple of weeks later his co-workers persuaded him to "help celebrate" at an office party. This was the start of a binge that ended when he had an automobile accident on the way home from a bar. A passenger in the other car was killed, and Mr. H was charged with vehicular homicide and driving under the influence of alcohol. He stopped drinking abruptly, which resulted in his current hospital admission 3 days later.

Selected Nursing Diagnoses:

▼ Sensory-perceptual alteration, visual, related to neurobiological changes induced by acute alcohol withdrawal, as evidenced by hallucinations of bugs in the bed
▼ Ineffective individual coping related to repeated drinking, as evidenced by work and family problems and denial of drinking problems
▼ Risk for injury related to drinking and driving, as evidenced by recent automobile accident
▼ Risk for violence directed at others related to lack of control of behavior when drunk, as evidenced by past pattern of violent behavior

Barbiturates. Barbiturates include barbital, amobarbital (Amytal), phenobarbital, pentobarbital (Nembutal), secobarbital (Seconal), and butabarbital. These drugs were once widely prescribed for their sedative and hypnotic effects. However, many problems were associated with their use, and they have been the major cause of overdose death from accidental poisonings and suicide. They produce excessive drowsiness, even at therapeutic doses. Also, tolerance to them develops rapidly. Like alcohol, barbiturates are depressants that cause an initial response of euphoria. Thus they are popular street drugs. Barbiturate use leads to both physical and psychological dependence. There is a synergistic effect between alcohol and barbiturates, meaning that either drug potentiates the effects of the other. For this reason, combinations of these drugs are particularly dangerous and can lead to accidental overdose and death. Despite these drawbacks, barbiturates are very useful for the treatment of epilepsy and general depressant withdrawal syndromes.

Benzodiazepines. In the 1960s benzodiazepines replaced barbiturates as the preferred treatment for anxiety and related disorders. This was based on three beliefs about these drugs:

▼ They would relieve anxiety without drowsiness.
▼ They had a wide therapeutic index (the difference between the therapeutic dose and the lethal dose).
▼ They were nonaddicting.

It is now known that benzodiazepines do cause drowsiness, although less than barbiturates. They are also addicting, causing both physical and psychological dependence. They lead to the same withdrawal symptoms as alcohol. Because benzodiazepines are longer acting, the symptoms are less intense and continue over a longer period of time. They are safer in terms of overdoses. Despite their drawbacks, they are still widely prescribed in the United States. The clinical uses of benzodiazepines are described in Chapter 27.

STIMULANTS. The stimulants have the ability to stimulate the central nervous system at many levels. The most common of these are the amphetamines and cocaine. People use these drugs for the feelings of euphoria, relief from fatigue, added energy, and alertness they provide. The signs and symptoms of use, overdose, and withdrawal are basically the same for all drugs in this class (see Table 24-2).

Amphetamines. The amphetamine drugs include amphetamine, methamphetamine, dextroamphetamine, and benzphetamine. Amphetamines are thought to act by crowding norepinephrine and dopamine out of storage vesicles and into the synapse. The increase of these catecholamines at the receptors causes increased stimulation. It was once believed that amphetamines did not cause physical dependence, but clear patterns of tolerance and withdrawal have been described. Tolerance develops to the euphoria and the pleasant effects of these drugs but not to the wakefulness effects. Prolonged or excessive use of amphetamines can lead to psychosis, which is almost identical to paranoid schizophrenia.

In the 1950s and 1960s amphetamines were widely prescribed for weight loss and relief of fatigue and depression. Their effectiveness for both conditions was only temporary and often led to dependency. In 1970 the Food and Drug Administration (FDA) restricted the legal use of amphetamines to three types of conditions: narcolepsy, hyperkinetic behavior in children, and short-term weight reduction programs. Today it is clear that the abuse potential of amphetamines outweighs the benefit of their medical use for almost any reason. Safer treatments for these conditions have been found and are generally preferred.

Cocaine. Cocaine may be a drug of recent popularity, but it has been around for thousands of years. Cocaine is usually inhaled as a powder, injected intravenously, or smoked.

The smokable form of cocaine is produced by a process called freebasing. The "crack" form of freebase cocaine is produced by "cooking" street-grade cocaine in a baking soda solution. Its name is derived from the cracking sound it makes when it is smoked.

The euphoria caused by cocaine is short acting, starting with a 10-to 20-second rush and followed by 15 to 20 minutes of less intense euphoria. A person who is high on cocaine feels euphoric, energetic, self-confident, and sociable. Although cocaine was not initially thought to produce physical dependence, a pattern of withdrawal symptoms very similar to that seen in amphetamine users has been observed, beginning with intense craving and drug-seeking behavior. The relapse rate for patients who try to discontinue cocaine use is very high. Cocaine use has been known to result in sudden death.

Biochemically, cocaine blocks the reuptake of norepinephrine and dopamine. Because more neurotransmitter is present at the synapse, the receptors are continuously activated. It is believed that this causes the euphoria. At the same time, presynaptic supplies of dopamine and norepinephrine are depleted. This causes the "crash" that happens when the effect of the drug wears off.

Cocaine use has been glamorized by the publicity given to it by movie stars, sports figures, and other well-known people. This makes it particularly inviting to adolescents who regard famous people as role models.

Addiction to barbiturates ("downers") and stimulants ("uppers"), particularly the amphetamines, often occurs simultaneously. Sometimes a patient who has been using downers develops a need for uppers to provide enough energy to function. The next clinical example illustrates this pattern. Ms. W's pattern is not uncommon. Aside from street use, many people slip into drug abuse without being aware of the consequences of their behavior.

Clinical Example Ms. W was a 34-year-old woman who was moderately overweight. She had tried various diets on her own with little success. A friend told her about a "diet doctor" who had a reputation for helping his patients lose weight with minimum deprivation. Ms. W decided to see the physician and was accepted for treatment. She was given a diuretic and appetite depressant medication. The latter contained amphetamines. She began to lose weight as soon as she started the prescribed regimen and was delighted. She also liked the additional burst of energy she felt every time she took her medication. She completed projects that she had been planning to work on for months. However, her family began to complain because she was irritable and very restless. In addition, she developed insomnia and roamed about the house at night.

On the urging of her husband, she went to her family physician. She felt guilty about seeing another physician for her weight problem, so did not tell her regular physician about this. With the history of insomnia, irritability, and recent weight loss, her physician thought she might be depressed. He ordered an antidepressant medication and a barbiturate sedative. Ms. W soon found that she was able to sleep well with her sedative. However, she felt slightly hung over in the morning and still wanted to lose more weight, so she continued with her diet pills as well. For a while she was able to function well. Gradually, however, she found that she needed two sedatives and then she also began to use extra stimulants. Her husband questioned her drug use. Ms. W had read about drug abuse and with her husband's help identified that she had a problem. She decided to see her family physician again and this time told him the whole story. He then advised a brief hospitalization so she could be withdrawn from both drugs under medical supervision. Ms. W was very embarrassed by her addiction. While in the hospital, she needed a great deal of nursing support to integrate this experience.

Selected Nursing Diagnoses:
▼ Ineffective individual coping related to dependence on stimulants and depressants, as evidenced by inability to function without the drugs and the development of tolerance
▼ Altered role performance related to drug dependence, as evidenced by family concern over her behavior
▼ Altered nutrition, more than body requirements, related to repeated dieting failures, as evidenced by seeking out a doctor who would help her lose weight with minimal deprivation

OPIATES. The opiates include opium, heroin, meperidine, morphine, codeine, and methadone. Meperidine, morphine, and codeine are frequently used analgesics. Methadone is used to treat addiction to other opiates. It can be used either to aid withdrawal or to provide maintenance at a stable dose. It is useful because it does not interfere with the ability to function productively, as other narcotics do. Patients taking a maintenance dose of methadone may work and live normally, although still addicted to narcotics.

Opiate use is less widespread than depressant or stimulant use but is still a serious social problem. Although some people use opiates for years with few problems, people with opiate addiction often deteriorate mentally and physically until they are unable to function productively. Illegal behavior such as stealing or prostitution to acquire money for drugs may result from addiction. Obtaining and using drugs becomes an all-consuming passion.

One characteristic of narcotic addiction is the development of tolerance, which also increases the expense of the habit. Physiological effects of narcotics are included in Table 24-2.

The most important psychological response to opiate use is euphoria, or feeling high. This powerful, pleasurable response causes the person to use the drug repeatedly, leading to addiction. Other psychological effects of narcotics include apathy, detachment from reality, and impaired judgment. The phrase "nodding out" describes this group of behaviors combined with drowsiness. The next clinical example demonstrates the behaviors associated with opiate abuse.

Clinical Example Mr. C was a 35-year-old man who had been jailed for auto theft. He was believed to be a member of a large ring of automobile thieves in a major metropolitan area. His previous arrest record included several episodes of armed robbery and breaking and entering. A few hours after he had been jailed, Mr. C complained of abdominal cramps and appeared very anxious. His nose and eyes were running, there were beads of perspiration on his brow, and he was rocking back and forth on his bunk. The guard called Ms. V, the correctional health nurse.

Ms. V observed Mr. C and performed a brief physical assessment. She noted that his pupils were dilated, his blood pressure was elevated, and he had gooseflesh. In addition, there were multiple needle tracks on his arms. She asked him directly about drug use, and he admitted that he had been addicted to heroin. He stated that his addiction began in 1967 while he was stationed with the army in Vietnam. When he returned to the United States, he remained in the army for 18 months and was able to stop using drugs altogether. He planned to get a job and attend school after leaving the service. He related that he was disturbed by the attitude of people toward Vietnam veterans. While he was still in the service, he was able to use peer support to cope with his feelings. However, after his discharge, he was reluctant to talk about his military experience. Others seemed disinterested, embarrassed, or hostile when he talked about it.

Mr. C had difficulty finding a civilian job. He was an artillery specialist in the army and found that it was difficult to apply this experience. He began to have nightmares and flashbacks of his combat experiences. Because of the anxiety associated with this, he finally returned to drugs. Without a job, he used illegal means to finance his habit and therefore repeatedly went to jail.

Ms. V discussed Mr. C's problem with the physician in the prison health department. They decided to assess Mr. C's eligibility for a methadone drug treatment program and to request consultation from a counselor at the local veterans counseling center.

Selected Nursing Diagnoses:
▼ Ineffective individual coping related to inability to obey the law, as evidenced by repeated arrests
▼ Altered role performance related to difficulty adjusting to civilian life, as evidenced by inability to find a job or seek out peer support
▼ Social isolation related to unresolved stressful military experiences, as evidenced by reliance on drugs rather than people
▼ Risk for violence directed at others, related to compelling need for drugs, as evidenced by history of armed robbery

Withdrawal from narcotics is extremely uncomfortable but not usually life threatening. Overdosage of narcotics, on the other hand, is very dangerous. It can lead rapidly to coma, respiratory depression, and death. Accidental overdoses among narcotic addicts sometimes occur, particularly because the user is uncertain of the drug's strength. Drugs are usually cut with inert (and sometimes toxic) substances before they are sold, resulting in the availability of varied strengths on the streets.

Natural Opiates. In 1975 natural substances that acted very much like morphine were isolated in the brain. It was later learned that these biochemicals, known as endorphins or enkephalins, were neurotransmitters that bond with opiate receptors in the brain and pituitary gland. Release of these "natural opiates" results in a feeling of euphoria. This understanding has led to a theory of drug cravings: When large amounts of artificial opiates are taken over a long period of time, the brain responds by cutting off production of endorphins in an attempt to restore homeostasis. As the artificial opiates leave the system, there are no natural opiates to take their place. This deprivation is experienced as craving. Details of these mechanisms continue to be studied.

MARIJUANA. Marijuana is sometimes classified as a hallucinogenic drug, but it rarely causes hallucinations. It causes sedation, but is not primarily a CNS depressant. The active ingredients in marijuana are the tetrahydrocannabinoids (THC). The marijuana cigarette can be smoked as it is, or through a water-pipe, or "bong," to cool the hot vapors. Marijuana generally produces an altered state of awareness accompanied by a feeling of relaxation and mild euphoria. Effects depend on the potency of the drug, as well as the setting and the experience of the user. Strength can vary widely from 1% to 30% THC, with the average for 1995 being 6%.[12]

Prolonged use may lead to apathy, lack of energy, loss of desire to work or be productive, diminished concentration, poor personal hygiene, and preoccupation with marijuana. This cluster of symptoms is known as the **amotivational syndrome.** Although study findings are controversial, there seems to be general support for the existence of such a syndrome. Use of very large doses can lead to a toxic psychosis that clears as the substance is eliminated from the body. Marijuana may also precipitate psychosis when used by schizophrenics whose symptoms are otherwise controlled with antipsychotic drugs. It does not appear to lead to psychosis in nonschizophrenic people.

The main physiological effects of marijuana are mild (see Table 24-2). Tolerance develops in heavy users, but there is no withdrawal pattern. Marijuana has been reported to have medicinal benefits in alleviating glaucoma as well as the nausea and vomiting associated with chemotherapy used in cancer treatment. However, its effectiveness for these purposes is controversial. It appears at best to have no greater efficacy than drugs already on the market. Thus its use for medicinal purposes has been limited legally in the United States.

> **?** *Supporters of legalization of marijuana say that the penalties are too severe for the behavior and that marijuana is no more harmful than legal substances such as alcohol and nicotine. What is your position on the legalization of marijuana?*

HALLUCINOGENS. Drugs that create experiences very similar to those typical of a psychotic state have been called *hallucinogens*, although they generally produce perceptual distortions, not true hallucinations. They have also been called psychedelic or mind-revealing drugs. LSD, peyote, mescaline, and psilocybin are commonly used hallucinogens, with LSD being the most commonly used.

LSD is generally swallowed. It is colorless and tasteless and is often added to a drink or food, such as a sugar cube. It may be given to a person without that person knowing. Pleasurable effects of hallucinogen use include intensification of sensory experiences. Colors are described as more brilliant, and sounds, smells, and tastes are heightened. Sometimes users of these drugs report synesthesia, or a crossover of sensory experiences during which music may be seen or colors may be heard. Space and time are distorted.

The hallucinogens do not appear to cause physical dependence, but tolerance develops if they are used regularly. Hallucinogens also lead to self-destructive behavior because they cause impaired judgment. Vulnerable people who take these drugs may experience "bad trips," sometimes resulting in psychotic episodes. They may experience paranoid, grandiose, or somatic delusions, usually accompanied by vivid hallucinations. The hallucinatory experience may be pleasant or frightening. Patients who are psychotic are not in contact with reality and often misinterpret environmental events. They may be unable to attend to any of their biological needs and may inadvertently hurt themselves or others in response to hallucinations or while trying to escape from the frightening experience. Because there is no physical dependence, withdrawal symptoms do not occur. Usually there is a gradual decrease in psychotic behavior, although the patient may have flashbacks for several months. These brief recurrences of the hallucinogenic experience can be frightening. Patients often express the fear that they are crazy and will never be free of the after effects of the drug.

> **?** *A college classmate who is not a nursing major tells you that she overheard her 12-year-old brother talking with a friend about "doing microdots." You suspect that he was talking about LSD. What would you advise her to do?*

PCP. PCP use was very popular in the 1970s but today is much less common than LSD in all age groups.[27,28] As a street drug it may be ingested, but it is often smoked in a mixture with another substance, such as marijuana. Severity of symptoms are dose dependent. At low doses (less than 5 mg) the user experiences a euphoric, floating feeling, along with heightened emotionality and incoordination. Distorted perceptions such as objects floating or growing in size, inability to judge distance, or feelings of being outside one's body are common. At higher doses PCP use may precipitate an intensely psychotic experience characterized by extreme agitation. Patients may become violent toward themselves or others. Because the drug is an anesthetic, PCP-intoxicated people feel little or no pain and may pound their heads into a wall or strike out violently, causing serious injury to themselves or others. Physical manifestations of PCP intoxication are noted in Table 24-2.

PCP may cause or exacerbate a previously controlled psychosis. The unpredictability of the reaction to PCP makes it an extremely dangerous drug.

INHALANTS. The use of inhalants by youth to obtain a high is becoming more prevalent. There are approximately 1,400 products that can be inhaled. The most common inhalants include butane (lighter fluid), gas, air fresheners, rubber cement, correction fluid, and nitrous oxide (whippets). It is estimated that approximately 21% of eighth graders in the United States have used inhalants at least once in their lives. Children and adolescents choose inhalants as a means of obtaining a high because of the quality of the high, the rapid onset of the effect, the low cost, and the ease of availability.

The nurse must be alert to the physical indicators of inhalant abuse when completing an assessment. These signs include residue from paint, glue, or substances noted on the clothes, hands, or face, especially around the nose. Youth may also have symptoms of a cold, such as a runny nose, or pimples or sores around the mouth. These are caused by the abrasive effect of the chemicals on the skin. Finally, it is essential that nurses take a leadership role in educating children and adults about the nature of inhalant abuse.

> **?** *You are working as a nurse in a local high school in which a 15-year-old student recently died while inhaling butane. The principal approaches you requesting that students not be told that inhalants were involved in the death because it might "give other students ideas." How would you respond?*

CODEPENDENCY. When the term *codependency* was first coined in 1979, it referred to people who had become dysfunctional as a result of living in a committed relationship with an alcoholic. It was said that the alcoholic was addicted to the bottle, and the codependent was addicted to the alcoholic. The major focus was initially on the spouse of the alcoholic.

The concept is really not a new one. Al-Anon was created in the 1930s specifically to help family members of alcoholics cope with their own problems, which stem from living with an alcoholic. However, the codependency movement stresses the lasting effects of growing up in an alcoholic home. Adult children of alcoholics (ACOA) are believed to share certain characteristics as adults because they all struggled to survive the chaos of growing up with an alcoholic parent. The major aspects of the condition are

▼ Overinvolvement with a dysfunctional person
▼ Obsessive attempts to control the dysfunctional person's behavior
▼ A strong need for approval from others
▼ Constantly making personal sacrifices to help the dysfunctional person be "cured" of the problem behavior.[10]

As the movement has grown, however, the definition has broadened to include almost anyone who has had anything to do with a dysfunctional person, either while growing up or as an adult. Anyone who can identify with the laundry list of symptoms associated with codependency (most notably low self-esteem, need to please others, and overresponsibility for others) can identify with the term.

The positive aspect of this movement is that it may allow many people who are unhappy with themselves to reframe their life situation and improve their functioning in very significant ways, with or without formal counseling. In fact, many people who otherwise would never have recognized their own dysfunction identify with the characteristics of codependency and are motivated to seek specific counseling and self-help groups. ACOA and codependency self-help groups, based on the 12-step recovery program of AA, have sprung up all over the country. Dozens of self-help books have been published by people who self-identify with the concept and who offer recommendations about how to recover from it and also by mental health professionals, who write based on case reports and clinical impressions. Counselors and other clinicians have developed specific recovery programs for codependents. Theories have evolved to explain the development of various symptoms and the legitimacy of some recommended approaches. The negative side of the movement is that some people use the label to blame problems on current or past relationships without taking responsibility for their own part in the process.

Despite the popularity of this movement, there is no sound research basis for the existence of a clinical syndrome distinct for ACOA.[38] The issue is that symptoms generally accepted to be part of the syndrome, such as low self-esteem and difficulty forming close personal relationships, are not unique to children of alcoholics. One major problem is the post hoc nature of identification of the syndrome. The nature of codependency calls for people to look back in time and create a causal link between present psychological distress and parental alcoholism. In addition, this type of analysis deemphasizes more current individual and environmental causal factors and stresses the primary effect of the parent's alcoholism. For example, there may be several complex, interrelated factors outside the home environment that contribute to psychological problems. Identifying the parent's behavior as the cause of current problems tends to minimize individual capacity and responsibility for adjustment and positive change. However, some research indicates that most children who grow up in alcoholic homes escape without serious psychological or emotional problems.

Whether a clearly identifiable and unique syndrome exists or not, it is easy to understand how children who grow up in alcoholic homes can develop low self-esteem. As an adult this is often manifest in a preoccupation with the lives, feelings, and problems of others. Although codependents want their loved ones to stop drinking or using drugs, their behavior may have the opposite effect and enable the person to continue drug or alcohol use.

The nurse may observe some of these behaviors in family members of substance-dependent patients, in the patients themselves, or in nurses and other professionals. Simple questions to family members about efforts they have made to try to control the addict's use may uncover the pattern. Questions to the patient about relationships with others may indicate that growing up in an alcoholic home may have contributed to his or her own substance abuse problem. Listening to colleagues talk about their family and friends may reveal similar patterns in their relationships. Nurses tend to find great satisfaction in caring for others. When this behavior is the person's only source of self-esteem, it is done at the expense of personal health and welfare. It takes on a compulsive quality that is evidence of codependence.

Dual Diagnosis

A patient may have a substance use disorder, a psychiatric disorder, or both concurrently. The types of relationships between substance use and psychiatric disorders are listed in Box 24-4. One can precede and cause the other, such as when the alcoholic becomes severely depressed or when the depressed person uses alcohol to treat the depression. It is often impossible to distinguish the two disorders, especially early in the assessment process. To complicate matters further, substance abuse may cause psychiatric symptoms such as hallucinations or paranoia, even though the person has no separate psychiatric diagnosis. Therefore, assessment of people with potential coexisting conditions is best accomplished in three stages:

1. Detection
2. Diagnostic assessment
3. Specialized assessment[11]

Because substance use problems are so common among psychiatric patients, mental health clinicians should routinely assess all patients for these problems.

Detection of substance abuse in patients with psychiatric illness is most effective when multiple instruments or types of assessment are used. A combination of interview, screen-

Box **24-4** *Relationships between Substance Use and Psychiatric Disorders*

Substance use may be causing the psychopathology (a substance-induced mental disorder). This is the most common situation. Some of the more common substance-induced disorders are alcohol-induced depressive disorders, cocaine-induced psychotic disorders, and stimulant-induced anxiety disorders.

Substance use may be secondary to the psychopathology in various ways:

Patients may use substances to self-medicate the symptoms of their mental disorder (for example, alcohol may be used to try to alleviate the symptoms of an anxiety disorder, such as social phobia).

Patients may use substances to enhance symptoms of the mental disorder (as in the use of stimulants by manic patients).

Patients may use substances in an attempt to counter side effects of medications they are taking for a mental disorder (for example, a patient with schizophrenia may use cocaine in an attempt to counter neuroleptic side effects).

The mental disorder and the substance-use problems may be coincidental and not related to each other.

From Miele G, Trautman K, Hasin D: Assessing comorbid mental and substance-use disorders: a guide for clinical practice, *J Pract Psychiatry Behav Health* 2:272, 1996.

ing tools, information from collateral sources, and laboratory tests including urine drug screens should be used. *Diagnostic assessment* is done according to DSM-IV criteria. However, the nurse should be aware that psychiatric patients may be especially vulnerable to small amounts of substances. For example, even small amounts of cocaine may precipitate a psychotic episode in a patient with schizophrenia. *Specialized assessment* can follow the more general diagnostic assessment to obtain more detailed information necessary for treatment planning. The special problems posed by patients who are dually diagnosed can be seen in the following clinical example.

Clinical Example Robbie is a 25-year-old, single, white male who began using alcohol and drugs at age 16, around the time he dropped out of school. He continued to live with his mother and spent most of his time in his room, although there were long periods of time when she did not know where he was. His mother reported that he increasingly isolated himself and acted so strangely that others did not feel comfortable around him.

Over the next couple of years Robbie's behavior became increasingly bizarre until one day his mother observed him pacing, talking to himself, saying strange and threatening things aloud, and pounding his fists together. She obtained an emergency petition and the police took him to the emergency room for an evaluation. He was diagnosed as schizophrenic, stabilized on medication, and returned to his

mother's home with an appointment for outpatient follow-up. However, he did not return to the clinic, stopped taking his medication, and was rehospitalized a month later. This time he was placed on Prolixin and promised to return to the clinic as scheduled in 2 weeks. He seemed to do well for a few days until he resumed drinking and smoking marijuana. He disappeared for several weeks, and was found by his mother wandering the city streets, dirty, unkempt, reeking of alcohol, and talking to himself again. During the subsequent rehospitalization, he admitted also using cocaine and heroin occasionally. He was referred to AA and assigned to a social worker, who helped him to obtain social services.

Soon he was getting a disability check every month, which exacerbated his problems. Every month he cashed his check as soon as he got it and went on a binge of drug and alcohol use until his money was gone, usually in about a week. Unable to afford such heavy use for the remainder of the month, Robbie approached people on the streets and demanded money. Eventually, he was picked up by the police for aggressive panhandling. By the time he was 24, Robbie was well known by the police and emergency rooms in town. He'd been hospitalized at least a dozen times and arrested for numerous petty crimes. His mother, doctor, and social worker were totally exasperated by his failure to comply. When the new Dual Diagnosis Clinic opened in the Mental Health Center, Robbie was one of the first referrals.

Predisposing Factors

Several models or etiologies have been proposed for substance abuse. Belief in a particular model influences the assessment and intervention. Awareness of the differences between these models helps the nurse understand why patients, as well as other professionals, hold many different views about substance abuse treatment. Much research has been conducted concerning the factors that predispose a person to becoming chemically dependent. These factors may be biological, psychological, or sociocultural.

BIOLOGICAL. A key biological factor is the tendency of substance abuse to run in families. Most genetic research has focused on alcoholism; very little is known about other drugs of abuse. There is much evidence from adoption, twin, and animal studies that heredity is significant in the development of alcoholism. Some research has identified subtypes of alcoholism that differ in inheritability. One type of alcoholism is associated with an early onset, inability to abstain, and an antisocial personality. This type appears to be limited to males and primarily genetic in origin. Another type tends to be associated with onset after age 25, inability to stop drinking once started, and a passive-dependent personality. This type seems to be influenced much more by the environment.[9]

Although still controversial, some researchers believe that they have identified a gene associated with transmission of alcoholism. There is now compelling evidence that variants of the DRD2 gene are associated with alcoholism and some other drug problems.[29] It is theorized that this genetic abnormality blocks feelings of well-being. This results in a tendency toward anxiety, anger, low self-esteem, and other negative feelings. There is a craving for a substance that will take the bad feelings away. People with such a disorder need alcohol or some other psychoactive drug just to feel "normal." This genetic finding is only one of many predisposing factors in the etiology of substance abuse. It is important to understand that the larger etiological role appears to be played by environmental factors and still unidentified genes.

> **?** *If genetic factors are clearly identified as major influences on the development of alcoholism in some people, what ethical issues are likely to be debated?*

Biological differences in the response to alcohol may influence susceptibility. For example, many Asian people experience a physiological response to alcohol including flushing, tachycardia, and an intense feeling of discomfort. This appears to be related to the tendency for Asians to have a genetically inactive form of the enzyme aldehyde dehydrogenase. This leads to a buildup of the toxic substance acetaldehyde, an alcohol metabolite, which causes the symptoms. This response may help explain why Asian-Americans have the lowest level of alcohol consumption and alcohol-related problems of the major racial and ethnic groups in the United States.

PSYCHOLOGICAL. Many psychological theories have attempted to explain the factors that predispose people to developing substance abuse. Psychoanalytic theories see alcoholics as fixated at the oral stage of development, thus seeking need satisfaction through oral behaviors such as drinking. Behavior or learning theories view addictive behaviors as overlearned, maladaptive habits that can be examined and changed in the same way as other habits. Family system theory emphasizes the pattern of relationships between family members through the generations as an explanation for substance abuse. It is easy to see how belief in any particular theory would influence assessment and treatment.

Clinicians have observed a link between substance abuse and several psychological traits such as depression, anxiety, antisocial personality, and dependent personality. There is little evidence that these psychological problems existed before or caused substance abuse. It is just as likely that they resulted from drug and alcohol use and dependence.

Many studies have tried to find common personality traits among people addicted to alcohol or drugs. No addictive personality has been identified. Studies show a wide variety of personality types among alcoholics. Observed personality patterns result from the effects of the alcohol or drug on previously normal psychological functions, combined with ineffective responses to these effects.

Another theory of substance abuse focuses on the human tendency to seek pleasure and avoid pain or stress. Drugs create pleasure and reduce physical or psychological pain. Because pain returns when the effect of the drug wears off, the person is powerfully attracted to repeated drug use. It has been suggested that some people are more sensitive to the euphoric effects of drugs and are more likely to repeat their use. This repeated drug use leads to more problems and initiates the downhill spiral of substance use.

Some substance abusers have psychological problems related to childhood experiences. Many have histories of childhood physical or sexual abuse. Most have low self-esteem and difficulty expressing emotions. These problems may have influenced the initial use of drugs and progression into dependence. The nursing care of survivors of abuse is discussed in Chapter 39.

SOCIOCULTURAL. Several sociocultural factors influence a person's choice whether to use drugs, which drugs to use, and how much to use. Attitudes, values, norms, and sanctions differ according to nationality, religion, gender, family background, and social environment. Assessment of these factors is necessary to understand the whole person. Combinations of factors may make a person more susceptible to drug abuse and interfere with recovery.

Nationality and ethnicity influence alcohol use patterns. For example, it has been found that northern Europeans have higher alcoholism rates than southern Europeans. Values may influence the way in which addiction is viewed. Some believe that addiction results from moral weakness or lack of willpower. Unfortunately, a moralistic approach may cause the person to feel guilty, often resulting in drinking to alleviate the guilt.

Formal religious belief can also affect drinking behavior. Members of religions that discourage the use of alcohol have much lower rates of alcohol use and alcoholism than members of those that accept or encourage its use. Of the major religious groups in the United States, Roman Catholics have the highest rate of alcoholism and Jews the lowest. During assessment, however, the nurse should not assume certain use or nonuse patterns related to ethnic or religious factors.

Gender differences also have been noted in the prevalence of substance abuse.[31] Research is needed to determine the influence of biological as opposed to sociocultural reasons for this. However, powerful gender-related cultural factors help to shape substance-using behaviors. There is much less acceptance of female alcoholism, which is often hidden. Women tend to deny having a drinking problem even longer than men do. In the United States more women than men abuse prescription drugs such as diazepam. This is more socially acceptable and sometimes even encouraged. In contrast, use of antianxiety drugs is viewed as weak and unmasculine, whereas the ability to drink large amounts of alcohol is considered manly.

Finally, broad, sociocultural factors have influenced drug use, abuse, and treatment since the 1960s. Multiple social crises have contributed to the risk for drug abuse in poor neighborhoods. Affordable and decent housing and shelter are difficult to find. Job opportunities are limited, and many jobs are low paying. Social programs often inadvertently foster development of single-parent families. The dropout rate in inner-city schools is high, and advanced education is difficult to obtain. Living in neighborhoods dominated by these problems, along with poor health-care access, crime, and violence creates vulnerability to the escape some people find in drugs and alcohol. However, it is important to recognize that the majority of people living in these circumstances are not addicted to drugs, which supports the belief that many factors influence the development of drug use patterns.

 What sociocultural factors have you observed that encourage the use of drugs and alcohol?

Precipitating Stressors

WITHDRAWAL. If a person becomes physically dependent on a substance, substance abuse may continue simply to avoid withdrawal symptoms. The person may no longer get much effect from the substance other than its ability to prevent withdrawal.

Symptoms of withdrawal from particular drugs of abuse are listed in Table 24-2. Medically, withdrawal from CNS depressants is the most dangerous. It is important for the nurse to understand the expected symptoms of withdrawal and the associated medical dangers. With appropriate medical and nursing management, excessive discomfort and risk of serious complications can be minimized.

It is possible to predict the severity and duration of withdrawal symptoms by following three general guidelines:

▼ The longer the period of time between last use and appearance of withdrawal symptoms and the longer these symptoms last, the less intense they will be.

▼ The longer the half-life of the drug, the longer withdrawal symptoms will last.

▼ The longer the half-life of the drug, the less intense the withdrawal symptoms will be.

For example, if a person has alcohol withdrawal symptoms within 2 hours after the last drink, the withdrawal syndrome will probably be more intense than if the symptoms appear after 18 hours. As another example, the withdrawal symptoms from methadone, which has a long half-life, are less severe than from heroin. Alcohol is the model for the withdrawal syndrome and is presented in more detail.

When a large amount of alcohol is ingested, unpleasant symptoms usually occur. If overindulgence is short-lived, symptoms are caused by the direct effect of alcohol on body cells. This results in headache and stomach and intestinal distress—the typical hangover. However, if heavy drinking occurs over a long time, a decrease in blood alcohol level may cause symptoms of withdrawal.

Alcohol sedates the central nervous system. When alcohol is withdrawn, the symptoms resemble a rebound reaction in the CNS. The first symptoms usually occur 4 to 6 hours after the last drink and include agitation, anxiety, tremors, diaphoresis, insomnia, nausea, vomiting, mild tachycardia, and hypertension. The severity of symptoms depends on the quantity, frequency, and duration of consumption and how quickly the blood level drops. Symptoms usually disappear in hours or days but could last as long as 2 weeks. A person who drinks large amounts over long periods of time may develop more severe symptoms, sometimes progressing to delirium tremens (DTs), which may be fatal.

Grand mal seizures, sometimes called "rum fits," may occur, usually 6 to 48 hours after the last drink. A history of seizures or photophobia may predispose a person in withdrawal to seizures. Conditions such as hypomagnesemia, hypoglycemia, and respiratory alkalosis have also been associated with seizures. Other causes of seizures should be explored, including trauma and use of other drugs. Seizures occurring after 10 to 14 days of abstinence generally indicate dependence on a long-acting CNS depressant.

Alcoholic hallucinosis is characterized by auditory, visual, or tactile hallucinations in the absence of other psychotic behavior. It usually occurs about 48 hours after the last drink. The person is usually oriented and rational, and may not even admit to hallucinations unless reassured that they are not caused by mental illness. One way to obtain this information is to ask the patient about nightmares and vivid daydreams. This condition generally lasts for a few hours or a day, although it may last 1 to 2 weeks and in rare instances becomes chronic. The person experiencing alcoholic hallucinosis is not disoriented. Disorientation should be reported immediately because it may herald the onset of alcohol withdrawal delirium.

Alcohol withdrawal delirium (DTs) is a medical emergency because it can be fatal even with appropriate medical intervention. It is characterized by an exaggeration of earlier symptoms plus paranoia, disorientation, delusions, visual hallucinations, elevated vital signs, vomiting, diarrhea, and diaphoresis. Alcohol withdrawal delirium usually occurs 3 to 5 days after the last drink and lasts 2 to 3 days.

The Clinical Institute Withdrawal Assessment–Alcohol, Revised (CIWA-AR)[33] was developed for use in monitoring the symptoms of alcohol withdrawal to determine appropriate intervention. An opioid withdrawal assessment (CINA) has also been developed. Nurses may find these tools helpful in monitoring patient responses to medication and other aspects of nursing care. Table 24-2 summarizes the important aspects of withdrawal from the opioids and other abused substances.

Appraisal of Stressors

The reasons why a person initiates use of substances vary widely. Curiosity, desire to be grown up, desire to rebel against authority, peer pressure, desire to ease the pains of living, desire to feel good—all of these are stressors and may apply. If use of the substance brings about the desired effects, then use is likely to continue. As the amount and frequency of substance use increase, so do the perceived stressors, which lead to more use. If substance use becomes associated with relief from emotional and social pain in the person's mind, then these stressors will lead to more substance use. Perceiving the substance as the answer to these problems, the person fails to develop healthier coping mechanisms. Gradually it takes more and more of the substance to get the same effect.

Coping Resources

Coping resources vary tremendously from person to person. Comprehensive assessment of a patient with a substance abuse problem must include assessment of the personal, social, and material assets available to the person. Assessment of motivation and social supports is particularly important. What is the patient's motivation to change the substance use pattern? It could be that the patient is sick and tired of being sick and tired, or may have been ordered to complete a treatment program after receiving a driving while intoxicated (DWI) charge. What social supports does the patient have? Family, friends, and co-workers may be available for support, or the patient may be homeless and have no family or friends. What is the status of the patient's health? The health status may be perfect, or the patient may have hepatitis, AIDS, or other complications of abuse. What social skills does the patient have? Some patients are very adept in social interactions, and some are withdrawn, quiet, and isolated. Patients may or may not have developed problem-solving skills in other areas of their lives. They may or may not have other social, material, and economic assets to support recovery. They may or may not have intellectual skills and personality traits that contribute to positive change.

Coping Mechanisms

Mechanisms used by the patient to cope with stress depend partly on how the patient appraises stress on a cognitive, emotional, and psychological level. Although the patient may have used substances in response to certain stressors, the substance use may have escalated to the point where it has become an additional stressor. Patients who use problem-focused coping mechanisms will take responsibility for the substance use problem and either find ways to

change or seek help in doing so. These are constructive coping mechanisms. Patients may also use destructive cognitive or emotion-focused coping mechanisms. Patients who use cognitive coping mechanisms change the meaning of the substance abuse problem so that it becomes a nonproblem, saying that there is no problem ("It's just the thing to do") or devaluing a desired object ("I didn't want that job anyway"). Patients who use emotion-focused coping mechanisms try to decrease emotional stress by minimization of the extent of use ("I only had a couple of beers") or the consequences of use ("We don't fight about it too much"), denial ("I don't have a problem. I can quit anytime I want"), and rationalization ("If you had the problems I have you'd drink too"). It is impossible in the initial assessment to sort out the facts from the distortions caused by these coping mechanisms. This is one reason why assessment is an ongoing process. Information from collateral sources and continued observation of behavior over time are essential.

Nursing Diagnosis

After completion of the nursing assessment the nurse synthesizes the data regarding the patient's drinking or drug use behavior. Using the Stuart Stress Adaptation Model (Fig. 24-3) and the NANDA classification system, appropriate nursing diagnoses are identified.

Addiction problems are very complex. They affect nearly every aspect of the patient's functioning.[32] The nurse should be sure that the nursing diagnoses selected reflect the whole person. At least 27 nursing diagnoses are common in addiction nursing practice,[1] which can be grouped into four categories: biological, cognitive, psychosocial, and spiritual. Nursing diagnoses related to chemically mediated responses and medical diagnoses for substance-related disorders are listed in the Medical and Nursing Diagnoses box on p. 504. The primary NANDA diagnoses include **sensory-perceptual alteration, altered thought processes, ineffective individual coping,** and **altered family processes.** Examples of complete nursing diagnoses are presented in the Detailed Diagnoses box on p. 505.

Related Medical Diagnoses

Disorders that are related to substance abuse are included in DSM-IV[2] in two ways. First, diagnoses that are primarily related to alcohol or drug use are categorized as substance-related disorders. The essential features of these are presented in the Detailed Diagnoses box. A patient with a substance-related disorder who is also diagnosed with another Axis I psychiatric disorder is considered to be **dually diagnosed.**

Second, if substance-induced intoxication or withdrawal is associated with another type of mental disorder, the diagnosis is located in that category. For example, if a person is depressed related to alcohol withdrawal, the medical diag-

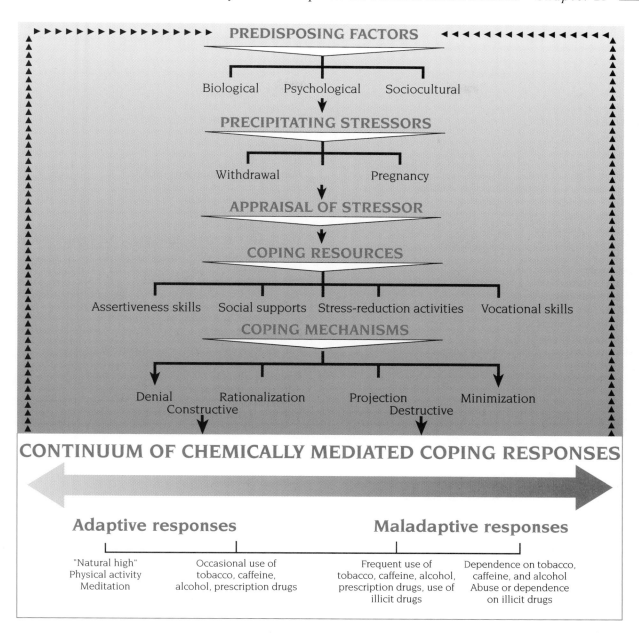

Fig. 24-3   The Stuart Stress Adaptation Model related to substance abuse.

nosis would be substance-induced (withdrawal) mood disorder. The categories that include substance-induced diagnoses are delirium, dementia, amnestic, psychotic, mood, anxiety, sex, and sleep.

> ? *How would you respond to a patient who prefers street drugs over prescribed medication because of the side effects of the medication?*

Outcome Identification

The expected outcome related to withdrawal is as follows:
The patient will overcome addiction safely and with a minimum of discomfort.

Short-term goals related to this phase of recovery may include the following:

▼ The patient will withdraw from dependence on the abused substance.

MEDICAL AND NURSING DIAGNOSES *related to* **Chemically Mediated Responses**

Related Medical Diagnoses (DSM-IV)*	Related Nursing Diagnoses (NANDA)†
Alcohol abuse	**Biological Responses**
Alcohol dependence	Growth and development, altered
Alcohol intoxication	Infection, potential for
Alcohol withdrawal	Injury, potential for
Amphetamine (or related substance) abuse	Nutrition, altered
Amphetamine (or related substance) dependence	Self-care deficit
Amphetamine (or related substance) intoxication	**Sensory-perceptual Alteration‡**
Amphetamine (or related substance) withdrawal	Sexual dysfunction
Caffeine intoxication	Sleep pattern disturbance
Cannabis abuse	**Cognitive Responses**
Cannabis dependence	Knowledge deficit
Cannabis intoxication	Management of therapeutic regimen, individual or family:
Cocaine abuse	effective or ineffective
Cocaine dependence	Noncompliance
Cocaine intoxication	**Thought Processes, Altered‡**
Cocaine withdrawal	**Psychosocial Responses**
Hallucinogen abuse	Anxiety
Hallucinogen dependence	Communication, impaired verbal
Hallucinogen intoxication	**Coping, Ineffective Individual‡**
Hallucinogen persisting perception disorder (flashbacks)	**Family Processes, Altered: Alcoholism‡**
Inhalant abuse	Growth and development, altered
Inhalant dependence	Parenting, altered
Inhalant intoxication	Self-esteem disturbance
Nicotine dependence	Social isolation
Nicotine withdrawal	Violence, potential for
Opioid abuse	**Spiritual Responses**
Opioid dependence	Grieving, dysfunctional
Opioid intoxication	Hopelessness (also psychological)
Opioid withdrawal	Powerlessness
Phencyclidine (or related substance) abuse	Spiritual distress
Phencyclidine (or related substance) dependence	
Phencyclidine (or related substance) intoxication	
Sedative, hypnotic, or anxiolytic abuse	
Sedative, hypnotic, or anxiolytic dependence	
Sedative, hypnotic, or anxiolytic intoxication	
Sedative, hypnotic, or anxiolytic withdrawal	
Polysubstance dependence	
Other (or unknown) substance abuse	
Other (or unknown) substance dependence	
Other (or unknown) substance intoxication	
Other (or unknown) substance withdrawal	

*From American Psychiatric Association: *Diagnostic and statistical manual of mental disorders,* ed 4, Washington, DC, 1994, The Association.
†From North American Nursing Diagnosis Association: *NANDA nursing diagnoses: definitions and classifications 1997-1998,* Philadelphia, 1997, The Association.
‡Primary nursing diagnosis for chemically mediated response.

▼ The patient will be oriented to time, place, person, and situation.
▼ The patient will report symptoms of withdrawal.
▼ The patient will correctly interpret environmental stimuli.
▼ The patient will recognize and talk about hallucinations or delusions.

For people dependent on drugs or alcohol, the expected outcome is the following:

The patient will abstain from all mood-altering chemicals.

Studies have shown that most people who are dependent on a drug or alcohol cannot safely return to any level of use of any addicting drug. If they do, eventually the vast majority return to their old addictive patterns. However, patients

DETAILED DIAGNOSES *related to* **Chemically Mediated Responses**

NANDA Diagnosis Stem	Examples of Complete Diagnosis
Sensory-perceptual alteration	Sensory-perceptual alteration related to hallucinogen ingestion, as evidenced by visual hallucination of snakes in the bed
Altered thought processes	Altered thought processes related to alcohol withdrawal, as evidenced by disorientation to time, person, and place
Ineffective individual coping	Ineffective individual coping related to cocaine abuse of 6 months' duration, as evidenced by loss of job and lack of personal goals
Altered family processes: alcoholism	Altered family processes related to alcoholism, as evidenced by marital conflict and avoidance of the family and home by the children

DSM-IV Diagnosis	Essential Features*
Substance dependence	Maladaptive pattern of substance use characterized by any three of the following within 12 months: tolerance; withdrawal; using more of the substance or using for longer than planned; persistent desire or unsuccessful efforts to cut down or control use; much time spent in efforts to obtain, use, or recover from use; interference with social, occupational, or recreational activities; continued use despite knowledge of use-related recurrent physical or psychological problems
Substance abuse	Maladaptive pattern of substance use characterized by one or more of the following within 12 months: recurrent use resulting in failure to meet role obligations, recurrent use in physically hazardous situations, recurrent use-related legal problems, continued use despite persistent or recurrent use-related social or interpersonal problems, has never met the criteria for dependence for this class of substance

*Modified from the American Psychiatric Association: *Diagnostic and statistical manual of mental disorders,* ed 4, Washington, DC, 1994, The Association. A single set of essential features has been developed for substance dependence and substance abuse. The essential features of intoxication and withdrawal vary according to the substance and are listed in Table 24-2.

often become very anxious at the thought of never again using the substance to which they are addicted. Therefore, it may be helpful to focus on short-term goals. Short-term goals related to abstinence may include the following:

▼ The patient will agree to remain drug and alcohol free for 1 week, with the agreement to be renewed weekly.
▼ The patient will make a daily commitment to abstain.
▼ The patient will attend at least two support group meetings weekly.
▼ The patient will contact a supportive person if he or she experiences an urge to use an addictive substance.

Development of some kind of support system is an essential expected outcome for drug-dependent patients. Once abstinence and support system goals are established, attention can turn to learning about dependence and recovery and developing alternative coping skills. Goals related to the person's job, relationships, or education should be deferred until later, unless any are a roadblock to recovery. For instance, a person is usually encouraged to focus on self and not on a relationship. However, if the person's spouse is an alcoholic and violence in the home is common, then the priority shifts to finding a safe place to live.

Goals should be worded so that it is clear that the patient is responsible for behavior. Addicted patients often want others to do the work for them. Nurses sometimes comply because they want to be helpful. However, such behavior does not help in the long run. Writing the goals and a specific plan of action into a contract and providing the patient with a copy of the contract will reinforce the patient's responsibility. The contract should be signed by both the nurse and the patient.

Planning

The nursing care plan should be developed by considering the expected long-and short-term outcomes of intervention. Priority must be given to the most immediate needs. For patients who are experiencing drug withdrawal, the highest priority is given to stabilization of the patient's physiological status until the crisis of withdrawal is over.

Once safety needs are met, abstinence and support system issues must be addressed. Plans related to these needs must be made in collaboration with the patient, considering the overall assessment and taking into account the patient's current life situation and desires. Family members and supportive friends should be included in the planning process. This will help them to understand the problems the patient may encounter as recovery continues.

The nurse must be aware that it is rare for an addicted person suddenly to stop substance use forever. Most addicts try at least once and usually several times to use the substance in a controlled way. It is important for addicts to know that they should return to treatment after these relapses. They can learn from what they did and try to prevent further relapses. These issues should be addressed openly in the planning process.

Implementation

The nurse encounters patients with substance abuse problems in all health-care settings. The types of interventions recommended depend largely on the setting in which the nurse works. When encountering these patients outside addiction treatment programs, the nurse may be able to refer the person to treatment. If a patient has a history of seizures or serious withdrawal symptoms or is at risk for developing symptoms because of a heavy, chronic use pattern, the first referral should be to a detoxification program. Otherwise, referral should be to the program that appears to match the patient's level of severity. Research is being conducted to determine the relationship between patient variables and treatment variables to ensure the best treatment outcome. This treatment-matching approach holds promise for improving effectiveness and efficiency of care.

Biological Interventions

Substance abusers often come into contact with the health-care system because of a physiological crisis. It may be related to overdose, withdrawal, allergy, or toxicity. There may be physical deterioration caused by the damaging effects of drugs, including such conditions as malnutrition, dehydration, and various infections, including HIV. When an acute physical condition is present, it takes priority over the other health needs of the patient. It is particularly important to attend to the condition that the patient has identified as the problem. The nurse is then seen as potentially helpful and will have more credibility when other aspects of the addiction are addressed.

INTERVENING IN WITHDRAWAL. Substances with potentially life-threatening courses of withdrawal include alcohol, barbiturates, and benzodiazepines. Withdrawal from opiates and stimulants can be extremely uncomfortable but is generally not dangerous, although a patient may become suicidal during the acute phase of cocaine withdrawal. Withdrawal from the general depressants, opiates, and stimulants is treated by gradual tapering of a drug in the same classification as well as by treatment with symptom-specific medications. There is no identified acute withdrawal pattern associated with marijuana, hallucinogens, or PCP.

Withdrawal symptoms may occur despite efforts to prevent them. Substance abusers do not always give accurate drug use histories, although it is extremely important to obtain as specific an assessment as possible. If the amount of substance used has been understated or if multiple abuse is undetected, withdrawal symptoms may occur. The possibility of seizures should always be anticipated. Emergency equipment should be at hand. Drug abuse should always be considered possible when unexpected seizures occur. If drug abuse is suspected, the physician should be informed so that blood and urine specimens can be collected for laboratory analysis and an appropriate treatment plan initiated.

Depressant Drug Withdrawal. Withdrawal from all depressant drugs (alcohol and benzodiazepines) is similar and is called the **general depressant withdrawal syndrome.**[37] If the patient is physically dependent on a depressant drug, withdrawal symptoms may occur when the blood level of the drug drops. Symptoms appear and peak at various times according to the half-life of the drug involved. These symptoms are generally the opposite of the symptoms of use. Because some of these symptoms are at best uncomfortable and at worst life threatening, medical and nursing interventions are planned to prevent severe withdrawal symptoms.

The process of helping an addict safely through withdrawal is called **detoxification.** Actually, the liver detoxifies the substance. Medications and nursing actions only help to relieve the symptoms. Gradual weaning from the substance may be instituted, especially if the person is addicted to prescription drugs such as barbiturates or benzodiazepines. Another approach is the use of a longer-acting, cross-tolerant drug with a similar action to prevent the occurrence of withdrawal symptoms. The dose of the substituted drug is then tapered down and eventually discontinued. A recommended dosing schedule is as follows: Librium 200-400 mg given as the loading dose, followed by 50 mg given every 2-4 hours as needed to lightly sedate the patient. The total dose given in the first 24 hours (called stabilization dose) is then given in four divided doses the following day. The dose is then tapered over the next 3 to 5 days, with continued monitoring for the potential reemergence of symptoms.[4]

Some programs measure withdrawal symptoms every 2 to 4 hours using the CIWA-AR and then establish medication doses based on these scores. It is prudent to base dosages on objective measures so that the patient is not overmedicated because of overreporting of symptoms or undermedicated because of staff reluctance to treat. Fewer than 5% of patients with alcohol withdrawal develop severe symptoms. Treatment programs are also using critical pathways to plan, implement, and document care during detoxification. Excerpts from one such tool is presented in Fig. 24-4.

Detoxification is best accomplished in a setting in which there can be close monitoring of the patient. This can be an inpatient unit, a crisis stabilization unit, or an outpatient setting.

A quiet, calm environment is helpful for patients experiencing the general depressant withdrawal syndrome. This helps the patient relax and decreases nervous system irritability. Reassurance in a calm, quiet tone of voice is also helpful. To help maintain the patient's orientation, the nurse should place a clock within sight and give frequent, low-key reminders about who they are, where they are, the

CRITICAL PATHWAY	Excerpts from Alcohol Detoxification

INTERDISCIPLINARY ACTION	DATE: PREADMISSION	INITIALS AND TIME	DATE _____ DAY 1	INITIALS D	INITIALS N	DATE: _____ DAY 2	INITIALS D	INITIALS N
ASSESSMENT	▼ Confirm I.D. ▼ Screening tool ▼ Assess for other drug dependency ▼ Verify insurance		▼ Physical/psychological assessment, PRN ▼ Withdrawal scale q4h and PRN ▼ H&P ▼ VS q4h while awake ▼ Assess seizure history			▼ Physical/psychological assessment, PRN ▼ Withdrawal scale q4h and PRN ▼ VS BID ▼ Observe for seizure activity ▼ Screen for malnutrition and contributing factors		
TREATMENTS/ INTERVENTIONS			▼ If history of seizures, pad bed rails, place airway at bedside			▼ If seizure history, initiate insert		
TESTS			▼ Labs ▼ CXR for + PPD ▼ Urine tox screen ▼ Urine U/A			▼ Labs ▼ Urine screen		
CONSULTS/REFERRALS	▼ Consider comorbidities list		▼ Nutrition consults as needed			▼ Other consults PRN		
MEDICATIONS			▼ Diazepam ▼ Vitamin ▼ Thiamine ▼ Tetanus			▼ Diazepam ▼ Vitamin ▼ Thiamine		
NUTRITION/ELIMINATION			▼ Double portions ▼ Special concerns			▼ Double portions ▼ Special concerns		
ACTIVITY/SAFETY			▼ Up ad lib on unit ▼ Off unit with escort			▼ Up ad lib on unit ▼ Off unit with escort		
PATIENT TEACHING/DISCHARGE PLANNING			▼ Unit rules ▼ Assess home meds ▼ 12-step group			▼ Community group ▼ HIV info group ▼ Nurse 1:1 ▼ FU arrangements		

D = 7 AM-7 PM
N = 7 PM-7 AM

Continued

Fig. 24-4 Excerpts from alcohol detoxification critical pathway.

nurse's name, and the day of the week. If possible, another patient who is further along in detoxification may be assigned as a buddy so that the patient is not left alone. A family member may also help.

The patient in withdrawal should be treated symptomatically. Fluids should be encouraged only if the person is dehydrated. Eating should be encouraged, and vitamins are usually ordered. Tylenol or Kaopectate, if ordered, may be given for discomfort or diarrhea. A small amount of milk may be offered frequently to help manage epigastric distress. Seizure precautions should be taken. A cool washcloth can be offered for use on the forehead if the patient is feeling warm or diaphoretic. Position changes, assistance with ambulation, and changing damp clothing are also indicated. Evidence suggests that offering this type of intense, supportive care can reduce withdrawal symptoms rapidly and often dramatically without medications. If the patient is receiving large doses of benzodiazepines, the nurse should monitor

CRITICAL PATHWAY	**Excerpts from Alcohol Detoxification Goals and Outcomes Sheet—cont'd**					

| | | **GOAL ACHIEVED** | | | **OUTCOMES ACHIEVED** | |
PROBLEMS	**INTERMEDIATE GOALS***	**DATE**	**INITIALS**	**OUTCOME(S)**	**DATE**	**INITIALS**
1. ALCOHOL WITHDRAWAL	1. Absence of hallucinations, seizures, or DTs 2. VS stable 3. Medical/psychological problems treated if present	1. 2. 3.		1. Rating on withdrawal scale of 0-5 2. Withdrawal medication discontinued. 3. Stabilization of comorbid medical and psychiatric illness	1. 2. 3.	
2. NUTRITIONAL DEFICITS	Adequate oral intake			Eating 90% of meals without n/v		
3. KNOWLEDGE DEFICITS	Verbalizes alcoholism's effect on physical, psychosocial, and spiritual life			Verbalizes knowledge of disease process of alcoholism		
4. LACK OF SUPPORT SYSTEMS	Verbalizes willingness to involve various support systems.			1. Selects desired support systems. 2. Makes plan for involvement.	1. 2.	
5. LIVING CONDITIONS	Need for changes in living situation will be determined to support alcohol-free lifestyle			Verbalizes resources available for drug-free living situations Develops plan for changes in living situation to support alcohol-free lifestyle		

*Each goal may be keyed to specific modalities of intervention such as "12-step group," "staff 1:1."

Fig. 24-4, cont'd Excerpts from alcohol detoxification critical pathway.

for signs of toxicity, such as ataxia and nystagmus. The patient always should be treated with respect and dignity.

Opiate Withdrawal. Opiate detoxification follows the same principles as detoxification from general depressants. The substitution drug usually used is methadone, an opiate agonist. The maximum initial dose is 30 mg, with supplementation possible if symptoms of withdrawal persist after several hours of observation.[4] The dosages may be increased by as much as 10 mg every 2 to 3 days until stabilization of symptoms, based primarily on objective criteria. Most patients are stabilized on a dose of 60 to 100 mg.[36]

INTERVENING IN TOXIC PSYCHOSIS. Users of LSD, PCP, and stimulants often come to the emergency room in acute toxic psychosis. The behavior may be quite similar to that of the schizophrenic patient. However, there may be no history of abnormal behavior. Careful assessment of an acute psychotic reaction, particularly in an adolescent or young adult, should include exploration of drug use. It may be necessary to interview friends of the patient to obtain this information. An attempt should be made to identify the specific drug used, although LSD and PCP may be taken without the knowledge of the person involved.

There is an important difference in the nursing approach to users of PCP and amphetamine as opposed to those who have an adverse reaction to LSD. Unless the psychiatric symptomatology is severe, LSD users experiencing a "bad trip" often respond to reassurance and may be "talked down." Patients should be oriented frequently and discouraged from closing their eyes because this may make the symptoms worse.

However, victims of PCP-induced psychosis do not respond well to attempts at interaction. Agitated PCP and amphetamine users are more likely to strike out in response to their misperceptions and panic. They are potentially more harmful to themselves and others. This aggression may be totally unprovoked. In addition, because PCP is also an anesthetic, these patients feel little or no pain. For this reason, they seem to have enormous strength. They do not feel pain when they exceed the limits of their muscular capability and may continue pushing, pulling, or hitting until they seriously injure themselves or others.

Other elements of treatment are basically the same for acutely agitated LSD and PCP users. Both require a safe environment that has minimum stimulation. Staff should not perform any procedures without a thorough explanation, should not touch the patient without permission, and should avoid rapid movements in the patient's presence. Adequate staff should be present to control impulsive behavior. Vital signs should be monitored and other physiological needs met. Although restraints may exacerbate muscle damage and agitation, they may be necessary, especially if a seclusion room is not available. Benzodiazepines are the treatment of choice, followed by high-potency antipsychotic medications if benzodiazepines are ineffective. Gastric lavage may be necessary for persistent symptoms or if an overdose has been taken, although this is not recommended for PCP users because it increases agitation.

Intervening to Maintain Abstinence

Maintaining abstinence from the abused substances is one of the most difficult issues in working with patients who have substance-related disorders. In addiction treatment, mild levels of anxiety and depression can generate motivation for change. Therefore, these symptoms should not be treated with medication unless they significantly interfere with the patient's functioning and participation in the treatment plan. However, a number of pharmacological therapies can help patients decrease cravings and maintain abstinence.

ANTABUSE THERAPY. A long-term biological approach to substance abuse is the prescription of **disulfiram (Antabuse)** for alcoholics. This drug interrupts the metabolism of alcohol, causing a buildup of a toxic substance in the body if the person uses alcohol in any form. The physiological response may include a severe headache, nausea and vomiting, flushing, hypotension, tachycardia, dyspnea, diaphoresis, chest pain, palpitations, dizziness, and confusion. Rarely, it can lead to respiratory and cardiac collapse, unconsciousness, convulsions, and death. Antabuse should never be given without the patient's stated willingness to comply. It is also important that the patient agree to take Antabuse only after careful instruction about the potential consequences of drinking while taking the drug. This instruction should include a written list of alcohol-containing preparations to be avoided, including cough medicines, rubbing compounds, vinegar, aftershave lotions, and some mouthwashes. Drinking must be avoided for 14 days after Antabuse has been discontinued. This medication cannot prevent someone who is determined to drink from drinking. This person can simply wait until the Antabuse has been excreted. However, it helps to prevent impulsive drinking because the person has to wait to be able to drink safely. This treatment should be used in conjunction with other supportive therapies, not by itself.

> **?** *Describe the information that should be provided to a patient who is to be treated with Antabuse. What issues related to informed consent should be considered in the use of this drug?*

NALTREXONE. Naltrexone, an opiate antagonist, has demonstrated effectiveness in reducing the amount of drinking, severity of craving, and relapse among alcoholics in treatment. It is believed to act in the following way: Alcohol intake increases the number of endorphins (naturally occurring opioids) in the brain. Naltrexone, in doses of approximately 50 mg/day, appears to block the effects of these endorphins, thus reducing the reinforcing effects of alcohol.[13,30] Naltrexone is the first drug approved by the FDA for the treatment of alcohol dependence since the approval of Antabuse more than 40 years ago.

OPIATE AGONISTS. Long-term opiate addicts who meet federal criteria for opiate dependence may be eligible for maintenance with methadone or LAAM. LAAM is a longer-acting opiate agonist. Patients in maintenance programs remain on stable doses of one of these substitute drugs for years—even for the rest of their lives. They must report to the clinic daily (for methadone) or every other day (for LAAM) or may be given take-home doses for certain days if they qualify. This treatment approach is controversial because these substitution drugs are narcotics. However, addiction to methadone does not cause impaired functioning; thus the person can be productive while addicted. Those in favor of methadone maintenance point out the benefits of avoiding the debilitating effects of heroin addiction and the lifestyle associated with obtaining illegal drugs on the streets.

> **?** *Methadone maintenance is essentially substituting a legal narcotic for an illegal one. Do you believe that this is a responsible practice? State the reasons for your position.*

ACAMPROSATE. Recently, researchers have found that a new drug, acamprosate, helps to prevent relapse in alcoholism.[17] This new drug has no sedative, antianxiety, muscle relaxant, or antidepressant properties and produces no withdrawal symptoms. It appears to work by lowering the activity of receptors for the excitatory neurotransmitter glutamate. Chronic alcohol abuse increases the number of these receptors and their resultant latent excitability may account for the high rate of relapse in the first few months after withdrawal.

COCAINE VACCINE IN DEVELOPMENT. One of the most exciting breakthroughs in the field is the development of a cocaine vaccine that is designed to be part of a comprehensive approach to treating cocaine addiction. A therapeutic vaccine that induces anticocaine antibodies and prevents the drug from crossing the blood/brain barrier will be used on an experimental basis beginning in 1998. It may prove to be a powerful tool to inhibit the reinforcing activity of the drug.

PREGNANCY. Because most of the drugs that are abused cross the placental barrier, women should be counseled about the possible effects of substance use during pregnancy.

Congenital abnormalities have occurred in infants of mothers who have taken drugs. A fetal alcohol syndrome has been identified, which involves a pattern of physical growth and mental deficiencies. In addition, use during pregnancy of drugs that cause physical dependence can result in the birth of an addicted baby who must be withdrawn from the drug. The safest pregnancy is one in which the mother is totally drug and alcohol free with one exception: For pregnant women addicted to heroin, methadone maintenance is safer for the fetus than acute opiate detoxification.

> **?** *Some policymakers have proposed that pregnant women who abuse substances should be jailed, placed under house arrest, or committed to a mental hospital until the baby is born. Do you agree with this? Support your position. Do you have the same opinion related to all abused substances, including alcohol and nicotine?*

Psychological Interventions

Before initiating nursing intervention with a substance-abusing patient, the nurse must develop self-awareness of feelings and attitudes about the problem (see A Patient Speaks). It is recommended that a value clarification approach be used, as described in Chapter 2. Most people have had personal contact with substance abuse by family, friends, or colleagues. This problem creates many negative feelings. It is important that the nurse be able to differentiate feelings associated with past situations from those aroused by contacts with patients and their families. A supervisor, teacher, or senior clinical nurse can be of assistance when a nurse is having difficulty sorting out these feelings.

Traditional addiction treatment is based on the concepts of addiction as a disease, total abstinence from all substances, immersion in 12-step recovery programs, direct confrontation of denial and other defense mechanisms (generally in group sessions), and a lifelong recovery process. Groups are usually led by recovering alcoholic/addict counselors. Ambivalence, resistance, and denial are viewed as characteristics of the disease of addiction. Confrontation is viewed as necessary to break through these defenses. Through the years, a practice of using very harsh and confrontational counseling techniques has evolved. Although some people respond well to these approaches, others do not. Despite their popularity, clinical outcome studies do not support such confrontational strategies, and some of the traditional programs have adopted gentler approaches.

While traditional addiction treatment was being offered in specialized addiction treatment programs, psychiatric patients with substance abuse problems continued to be treated in psychiatric and mental health programs. Many psychiatric professionals viewed alcoholism and other drug addictions as secondary to psychiatric disorders. They believed that the substance abuse would cease when the person's primary psychiatric disorder was resolved. Patients often were given tranquilizers to treat what was believed to be their underlying pathology. However, instead of abstaining from their substance of choice, many patients became addicted to the tranquilizers as well. Psychiatric treatment models operated from a different philosophical base, which was effective in dealing with psychiatric problems but less effective in dealing with addiction. Differences in treatment philosophies and backgrounds of providers contributed to a developing rift between psychiatric clinicians and addiction counselors. Dually diagnosed patients were often caught in the middle of this rift.

Over the years, approaches for the treatment of addictions developed that incorporated knowledge of both addictions and mental health strategies. These have been slow to gain acceptance in the separatist treatment communities. However, in the 1980s, because of the interaction of many forces in the mental health and substance abuse fields, the division lessened. More and more addiction counselors began to incorporate family counseling and cognitive behavioral techniques into their repertoires. Psychiatric clinicians began to better understand addiction as a separate disorder. Dual diagnosis programs evolved and mental health approaches were adapted for the primary treatment of addiction.

Although these newer approaches vary, they generally involve creation of an alliance between the therapist and the patient, inclusion of the patient in the setting of treatment goals (even if the patient's goal is not total abstinence), avoidance of confrontation, brevity of treatment, and use of professional therapists. More than just a series of techniques, they offer a completely new way of being with the

A Patient *Speaks*

I have abused drugs and alcohol for many years. One thing that has been important is for nurses to spend time with me so I can learn to trust them. It helps when they make sure I schedule treatment appointments and keep them. Substance abuse education is very important, and it has to be repeated over and over.

I've been through detoxification many times. Some of the nurses in those programs have coddled me. This makes it easy for me to dance around issues of sobriety. I've had the best success with the nurse who will get in my face and cut me no slack. The nurses who have high expectations leave me enough room to help myself, but not enough to be dishonest. There needs to be a balance of empathy and toughness. It's not easy, but that's the role for the nurse to establish. ▼

patient. Even more importantly, they have demonstrated efficacy in the treatment of patients with substance abuse disorders. Some of these newer approaches are described here.

MOTIVATIONAL INTERVIEWING. Motivational interviewing[25] is a way of preparing people to change addictive behavior. It is based on the concept that lack of motivation is a challenge for the therapist's skills, not a fault of the patient's. There are specific strategies designed to elicit self-motivating statements and build on them. Examination of past behaviors is aimed at identifying the positive aspects of it and reframing failures as successes. For example, instead of focusing on the fact that the patient returned to drinking after only 1 month, the focus is on how the patient managed to stay sober during that 1 month. Although many techniques can be used, the most important element of treatment is the attitude of the therapist. There must be high regard for the patient and genuine efforts to develop a facilitative relationship.

Five basic principles are used with this approach:

▼ Express empathy, particularly in the first session, because it sets the tone for everything to follow. Following through with a telephone contact after the initial visit and a personalized letter after missed sessions helps motivate the patient to stay in treatment.

▼ Explore discrepancies, particularly between the patient's present behavior and broader goals. A comprehensive assessment should be done and findings and their interpretation should be shared with the patient.

▼ Avoid argumentation, particularly because this sets up a power struggle and initiates the confrontation-denial trap. Ambivalence is normal and it is more therapeutic for the clinician to engage the patient in evaluating the costs of maintaining behaviors versus the costs of change.

▼ Roll with resistance, particularly when it is viewed as the therapist's problem rather than the patient's. The therapist's job is to ask questions in a way that helps the patient to understand and work through resistances.

▼ Support self-efficacy, particularly emphasizing that no one but the patient can change his or her behavior.

SOLUTION-FOCUSED THERAPY. Solution-focused therapy shares some of the patient-centered underpinnings of motivational interviewing. The main assumption of solution-focused therapy is that people have the skills and resources necessary to solve their own problems.[5] They need help in uncovering these strengths and finding the answers within themselves. This belief leads to an entirely different way of relating with patients. There is little direct resistance and denial because the nurse is not trying to sell a professional answer to the problem. The nurse accepts and works within the patient's frame of reference. In the traditional model, patients are expected to learn and adapt to the frame of reference of the treatment model; those who do not are considered difficult, resistant, or in denial. In solution-focused therapy, the nurse is expected to adapt to the frame of reference of the patient. Rather than wearing the hat of an expert and trying to fit the patient's problem into some kind of category, the nurse wears the hat of a student and tries to learn—to totally understand—the patient's unique way of conceptualizing the problem. Only then can the nurse help the patient.

Other principles are as follows:

▼ The simplest interventions are best. Start with these.

▼ Change is inevitable. Change is such a part of everyday life that the patient cannot prevent it from occurring. Help the patient to examine times, as short as they may be, when the problem did not exist, or when it was handled well.

▼ The present and future hold the key to success. Help orient the patient away from the past and toward the future and a solution.

▼ Cooperation with the patient is paramount.

Two kinds of questions used in this type of therapy are particularly useful.

▼ *Miracle questions* serve the purpose of orienting the patient to a future when the problem is solved. The question can be worded as follows: "Suppose that one night, while you are asleep, there is a miracle and the problem that brought you into therapy is solved. However, because you are asleep you don't know that the miracle has already happened. When you wake up in the morning, what will be different that will tell you that this miracle has taken place?"

▼ *Scaling questions* help patients to put their problems, priorities, successes, emotional investments in relationships, and level of self-esteem on a numerical scale. An example is, "On a scale from 1 to 10, with 1 meaning you have no confidence at all in your ability not to drink today and 10 meaning you are absolutely positive you will not take a drink today, how confident are you that you will not take a drink?" Solution-focused therapy is well-suited to pursing the goal of maximizing a patient's potential. It empowers patients by helping them to direct their own treatment and take responsibility for its outcomes.[8]

COGNITIVE-BEHAVIORAL STRATEGIES. Cognitive-behavioral approaches have been specifically designed for the treatment of patients with substance abuse disorders. Cognitive strategies are based on the belief that by identifying and modifying dysfunctional thinking patterns, patients can reduce or eliminate negative feelings and maladaptive responses such as substance use. Contingency management is one behavioral approach that has been successfully applied in many substance abuse treatment programs. In this strategy, rewards (often in the form of vouchers that can be exchanged for desired items) are given for adaptive behavior (such as compliance with treatment or clean urine). Behavioral contracting is also a useful approach. It involves creating a written agreement with the patient that specifies targeted patient behavior and consequences. These cognitive-behavioral treatment strategies are discussed in more detail in Chapter 30.

> ? *Discuss the significance of the substance abuser's level of self-esteem to the recovery process. Describe nursing interventions designed to enhance self-esteem.*

WORKING WITH CODEPENDENCY. Whether or not codependency exists as an independent phenomenon is not important in treatment planning. However, it is important not to discount the patient's identification with the codependency movement or the syndrome. Having a label for problems makes them more legitimate and easier to accept for some people. The codependency label has popular appeal. It is nonstigmatizing because the cause does not lie within the self, but with another person. The nurse should accept the patient's view of the problem as a legitimate starting point for a therapeutic alliance. Then the patient can be helped to understand how behavior that once allowed survival in a dysfunctional family no longer serves this purpose. The nurse can help the patient to move gradually away from anger and fear and toward responsibility for self-fulfillment.

Interventions center around the patient's primary identified problems, and may include assertiveness training, challenging cognitive distortions, teaching self-affirmations, and relaxation training. Because physical and sexual abuse are common in alcoholic families, specific assessment and intervention strategies must be implemented to identify and help patients with these types of problems. Referral to specialized programs may be useful. Additional information about appropriate interventions for survivors of abuse and violence is in Chapter 39. ACOA self-help groups may be useful. The nurse should suggest that the patient try several self-help groups before deciding to be actively involved in any one group. The nurse should also monitor how the patient responds to participation in these groups. Some groups are more positive and forward-focused than others.

Alcoholism is known to run in families. People who grew up in an alcoholic home often develop alcohol problems themselves or may marry alcoholics. It is clear that both biological and environmental factors contribute to generational transmission of this disorder. Thus it is common for a patient to be alcoholic and have an alcoholic parent. Intervention is most effective if it addresses intergenerational patterns.

INTERVENING IN RELAPSE. Although it is great when a person is able to quit drinking alcohol or using drugs forever on the first attempt, this does not usually happen. Most people in recovery have one or more slips in their attempt to stay sober. Continued use leads to a full-scale relapse, and many addicts return to their previous lifestyle. Without condoning substance use, it is important for the nurse to teach the patient ways of minimizing the possibility of slips and ways of preventing a slip from turning into a relapse.

The nurse should help the patient identify the environmental triggers that led to previous use or relapse. Some examples are driving down a street where the patient used to buy drugs, getting into an argument with a loved one, going to parties, or the sights and sounds associated with the drug-using environment. The patient is asked to avoid these environmental triggers as much as possible, especially early in recovery. Eventually the patient is taught to cope with many of them. Sometimes it is helpful to bring triggers into the treatment setting and teach the patient how to cope with the support of the nurse. This behavioral technique is called cue exposure. Paraphernalia associated with use, substances simulating the appearance of the drug, or movie clips with use on the screen can all be used as cues. Nurses teach patients to recognize their physical and psychological responses to cues and to cope with them when they occur. When cues are repeatedly not followed by drug use, they lose their potency. Avoidance of triggers (cues), coping with them, and development of new cognitive behavioral skills become part of the patient's relapse prevention plan (see Chapter 30).

Another key element of the relapse prevention plan includes what to do if the person actually uses drugs or alcohol. It must be taught that a slip does not make the patient a failure or a bad person. It must be learned that there are many decision points between first thinking of using drugs or alcohol, actual use, and relapse. It should be clear that the patient will be welcomed back into treatment if a slip occurs. Otherwise, guilt will cause a loss of perspective and feelings of hopelessness. There is a sense of failure in abstinence that gives a reason for continuing to use drugs. This kind of thinking is called the abstinence violation effect.[22] It can be one of the causes of a full-blown relapse.

Social Interventions

FAMILY COUNSELING. Reliable support from caring people is crucial to the recovery of substance abusers. However, the family is often frustrated with the patient's behavior and finds it difficult to be supportive. The family seldom understands the nature of addiction and generally does all the wrong things in its attempt to help the substance abuser. The family often tries to protect the patient from consequences. Many times, family members cover up by making excuses to employers and other family members for the person's erratic behavior. They also tend to blame themselves for the behavior and go to great lengths to avoid confrontation with the user. All of these behaviors are called enabling behaviors. By shielding the person from the consequences of drug use, the family enables the person's continued use of the drug.

Addiction is a family problem (see A Family Speaks). Everyone in the family suffers, not just the alcoholic or drug addict. Some problems families experience include guilt, shame, resentment, insecurity, delinquency, financial

A Family *Speaks*

When I met Jim in 1983, I knew he dabbled in drugs but I still married him. I had no idea how his growing drug abuse problem would affect my life over the next decade. In 1986 Jim entered treatment for his heroin addiction for the first time. I was impressed with the nurses in that program. They were compassionate, understanding, and knowledgeable about addiction. They taught Jim the first steps in the recovery process and supported him through the difficult changes that he had to make to maintain a drug-free lifestyle.

One nurse was particularly helpful to me as a family member of a newly recovering addict. She stood out because she consistently showed genuine concern for Jim and me. She always asked about Jim by name. She talked like he was an individual, not just one of the patients in the program. This allowed me to open up to her. I was finally able to ask if some of the things he was going through were normal, and I was very relieved to find out that they were! In contrast, another nurse on the staff talked down to all the patients. Neither the patients nor the family members felt they could talk to her.

Despite all the help he received, Jim relapsed after a few months of being clean. I was disappointed, but I had learned about relapse and I refused to give up on him. After 5 more years, Jim entered a methadone maintenance program. By then our marriage was falling apart. A nurse in the program had special training in working with families. We saw her together. With her help, Jim was able to recognize that he, not I, was responsible for his addiction. He became more responsible for himself. I learned about how I had enabled his addiction and how I would have to change for our drug-free marriage to succeed. It seemed like each of us could hear what the nurse said better than we could hear each other. Now, 4 years later, Jim is still taking methadone, and we are still together. I want nurses to know that little kindnesses as well as bigger interventions can make a positive difference in the lives of drug addicts and their families. ▼

troubles, isolation, fear, and violence. Families think their problems would be solved if their loved one simply stopped using drugs or alcohol. However, they can get help even if the user refuses. They should also realize that without help, many of the negative patterns of behavior developed over years of dysfunctional family life will continue after sobriety.

The nurse should encourage family members to seek counseling from a professional experienced in addiction treatment. Referral to AlAnon, a support group for friends and family of alcoholics, or NarAnon, for friends and family of narcotic addicts, is also helpful. These groups are based on the same 12 steps as AA and NA except that they are powerless over their alcoholic/addict instead of the substance itself. These families need to learn to pay attention to their own needs. They need to stop covering up for the addict. They need to be direct in their communication. They also need to know that they are not alone. These issues are evident in the following clinical example.

Clinical Example Mr. B was a 45-year-old man who was admitted to the medical unit of a general hospital with a diagnosis of gastritis. He complained of abdominal pain, nausea, and vomiting. He had a slightly elevated temperature of 37.5° C (100° F). When the admitting nurse who was completing the nursing assessment asked Mr. B about alcohol use, he said he had "a couple of beers" after work every day. He also reported that his wife had left him the day before admission. He said he was not sure why she left, but he was sure she would be back. Mrs. B did come to the hospital to visit her husband. His primary nurse met with them together and asked Mrs. B why she left. She said she was tired of putting Mr. B to bed every night after he passed out from drinking and did not want to continue to call his employer saying he was sick when he was really hung over. She had threatened to leave before, but Mr. B had always begged her to stay and she had relented. She had married him because she felt sorry for him. He had been living alone and was not taking good care of himself. She revealed that her first husband was also an alcoholic and her father had been one as well. She would agree to try again to make the marriage a success if he would agree to stop drinking and seek counseling. Mr. B said to the nurse, "I'll be good and do what she says. You tell her I'll be good."

Selected Nursing Diagnoses:

▼ Ineffective individual coping related to reluctance to be responsible for his behavior, as evidenced by denial of why his wife left

▼ Altered family processes related to alcoholism, as evidenced by cycles of drinking, threats to leave, and promises to change

Mr. B used alcohol to avoid responsibility for his actions and his life. He used his wife in a similar way. When Mrs. B confronted him with her expectations, he responded in a childlike way and tried to place the nurse in the parental role.

Mrs. B appears to be drawn to dependent men. She is probably a very maternal person who likes to take care of others. This increases the possibility that she will assume the role of enabler. The enabler perpetuates the substance abuse problem by not confronting the substance abuser and by helping to cover up the problem. When Mrs. B called Mr.

B's employer to say he was sick, she was being an enabler. When significant others play an enabling role, family counseling or family support groups help the family accept and support the changing behavior of the patient.

GROUP THERAPY. Group psychotherapy is the usual method of treatment in traditional substance abuse treatment programs. Chapter 31 provides detailed information about therapeutic groups.

History sharing and feedback are important elements in traditional program groups. Patients share their substance abuse histories and talk about their daily efforts to stop drinking or taking drugs. The therapist and group members listen closely and give feedback to the patient about his or her recovery efforts. Feedback is the honest reaction of group members to what the speaker says. It is based on the content of what the person says and on previous experiences with the speaker. Although feedback from one person, especially the therapist, may be discounted, it is difficult for the addict to ignore feedback from several group members, especially if they have experienced the same type of behavior at some point. The style of giving feedback varies from person to person. It may be gentle and facilitative or direct and confrontational. The best feedback is that which is focused and shows respect for the person.

In traditional programs, another major group focus is participation in 12-step self-help programs. Patients may be required to attend a certain number of AA or NA meetings each week in order to remain in the group. Patients share their reactions to the meetings they have attended and are encouraged to obtain a sponsor, do service work (such as set up the chairs or make coffee for meetings), and actively work the steps of the program. Successes and difficulties with maintaining abstinence during the past week are shared and discussed. Less traditional groups may encourage trials or active involvement with 12-step programs but not require it. Expectations for work done outside of the group are more individualized. In all groups, homework may be assigned that emphasizes an important recovery topic.

> ❓ *A group member says he has read that studies have found that some alcoholics can learn to drink in a controlled way. How would you respond?*

SELF-HELP GROUPS. The most common type of self-help group for substance abusers is the 12-step group. Alcoholics Anonymous (AA) is the model for 12-step support groups. It is composed entirely of alcoholics who have a desire to stop drinking. They believe that mutual support can give the alcoholic strength to abstain. AA aims for total abstinence. The member must admit to alcoholism openly and publicly by introducing himself at meetings, saying, "My name is John and I am an alcoholic." At speaker meetings,

one or more members share their life histories with the group. This shows that members are more alike than different, removing a common resistance to involvement. AA members also commit themselves to helping each other. Some AA members serve as sponsors, a role that involves availability and accessibility to another member whenever a member feels the need to drink. The sponsor also teaches the person how to work the 12 steps of the program. This reciprocal relationship gives the new member caring support and the sponsor improved self-esteem. AA also involves a strong spiritual orientation that is experienced as supportive by some alcoholics. The 12 steps of AA are listed in Box 24-5. It is easy to see the therapeutic benefit of these steps. For example, admitting the problem, making amends for past behavior, and reaching out to others who need help are sound therapeutic processes.

Some aspects of 12-step programs do not appeal to everyone. One of these is the powerlessness that must be acknowledged. Many people believe that the power to change lies within oneself. Some people are upset by the need to turn over one's will to a higher power. Members are told that this higher power can be the AA group, the sponsor, or

---

Box **24-5** *The 12 Steps of Alcoholics Anonymous*

1. We admitted we were powerless over alcohol—that our lives had become unmanageable.
2. Came to believe that a Power greater than ourselves could restore us to sanity.
3. Made a decision to turn our will and our lives over to the care of God as we understood Him.
4. Made a searching and fearless moral inventory of ourselves.
5. Admitted to God, to ourselves, and to another human being the exact nature of our wrongs.
6. Were entirely ready to have God remove all these defects of character.
7. Humbly asked Him to remove our shortcomings.
8. Made a list of all persons we had harmed and became willing to make amends to them all.
9. Made direct amends to such people whenever possible except when to do so would injure them or others.
10. Continued to take personal inventory and when we were wrong promptly admitted it.
11. Sought through prayer and meditation to improve our conscious contact with God as we understood Him, praying only for knowledge of His will for us and the power to carry that out.
12. Having a spiritual awakening as the result of these steps, we tried to carry this message to alcoholics and to practice these principles in all our affairs.

The Twelve Steps are reprinted with permission of Alcoholics Anonymous World Services, Inc. Permission to reprint this material does not mean that AA has reviewed or approved of the contents of this publication. AA is a program of recovery from alcoholism only; use of the 12 Steps in connection with programs and activities that are patterned after AA, but address other problems, does not imply otherwise.

anything else they want. Although the higher power does not have to be God in the religious sense, the meetings generally have a religious overtone and usually end with the Lord's Prayer. Some members have formed AA groups especially for agnostics.

Other self-help groups have emerged. One of these is Women for Sobriety (WFS).[21] This program shows women how to change their way of life through a change of thinking. The program serves women's needs by teaching them to overcome depression, guilt, and low self-esteem. WFS helps women overcome their drinking problems with the support of other group members who have the same problems and needs. The difference from AA is evident in the first statement of the WFS acceptance program: "I have a drinking problem that once had me." All of the 13 statements of WFS are worded positively.

Another very popular self-help program is the Rational Recovery (RR) movement,[34] which is based on Albert Ellis' Rational Emotive Therapy (see Chapter 3). This program asserts that alcohol dependence is not biologically determined and beyond our control. Rather, it is seen as a way of thinking. Irrational thoughts keep the alcoholic drinking. Rational thoughts can get and keep the alcoholic sober. RR philosophy is one of personal power; there is no reference to a higher power. RR groups have professional advisors who provide occasional rational input and observe members for problems that indicate a need for a higher level of care. Group meetings operate by discussion, also known as cross-talking. This is in contrast to AA, which strongly discourages interrupting or responding to others. Group members read rational literature, learn to think rationally, and become rational counselors to themselves and others.

It should be noted that total abstinence is the goal of each of these programs. Patients who choose to try controlled drinking will get no support for this goal from these programs. Controlled drinking for a person who has experienced the loss of control characteristic of addiction has little support in the research literature.

COMMUNITY TREATMENT PROGRAMS. A variety of community programs are available for drug abusers. Some hospital programs are designed specifically for safe medical detoxification. They have been cut from 1 to 2 weeks in the 1980s to 1 to 2 days currently. Intensive inpatient hospital rehabilitation programs have been drastically cut also. Many have closed, and others have reduced their length of stay from 28 days to 3 to 5 days. Some residential, free-standing rehabilitation programs provide services for 21 to 28 days.

To cut costs, alternatives to expensive hospital and residential programs have developed. Outpatient detoxification programs are becoming more popular. Some offer methadone withdrawal or maintenance for opiate addicts. Methadone programs must have special licensure to operate and follow federal guidelines. Day or evening partial hospitalization programs are also common.[6] The patient spends most of the day in treatment and returns home at night or spends the day at work and several evenings per week in treatment. Regular outpatient programs that are attended once or twice per week are even less intensive. Most programs provide a mix of group, individual, and family therapy, vocational counseling, drug and health education, and involvement with 12-step self-help programs. 12-step programs such as Alcoholics Anonymous may be an adjunct to or substitute for professionally run programs.

EMPLOYEE ASSISTANCE PROGRAMS. Another potential resource for the substance-abusing patient is the employee assistance program that may be part of an employee health service. Many businesses have found that it is profitable for them to help substance-abusing employees. These programs generally offer counseling and health education. Employees with a substance abuse problem are usually required to participate in the program to retain their job. Nurses are often key staff members in employee assistance programs. The health-care system has been rather slow in developing these programs for health-care providers. Because nurses and physicians also have problems with drugs and alcohol, there is a need for programs that can focus on their problems.

A Nursing Treatment Plan Summary for patients who abuse substances is presented on p. 516.

Working with Dually Diagnosed Patients

The dually diagnosed patient needs treatment for both disorders. The problem is that the substance abuse and mental health fields have developed approaches that appear to conflict with each other. For instance, many substance abuse counselors rely on direct confrontation of behavior. Such an approach could be detrimental to a person with severe mental illness. Substance abuse counselors also tend to have a limited understanding of the medications used for psychiatric disorders. In fact, the chronically mentally ill are often excluded from substance abuse programs. Mental health clinicians, on the other hand, often do not understand substance abuse and may overlook symptoms of continued use. They tend to think that the substance abuse will stop when the person's psychiatric illness is under control. Patients can suffer from these differences, either missing out on some important treatments or getting caught in the middle of two different approaches with two different clinicians (called parallel treatment). To avoid this, treatment is sometimes offered in sequence (first psychiatric treatment, then substance abuse treatment or vice versa).

The best possible treatment is an integrated one, with both services offered by program staff qualified in both areas and excellent coordination of other community services. The chronically mentally ill can benefit more from these programs, which generally are less confrontational and more supportive than traditional substance abuse programs. They have professional staff to prescribe and follow medication effectiveness. They often practice assertive case management, in which case workers seek out patients when

Nursing Diagnosis: Ineffective individual coping
Expected Outcome: The patient will abstain from using all mood-altering chemicals.

Short-term Goals	Interventions	Rationale
The patient will substitute healthy coping responses for substance-abusing behavior.	Help the patient to identify the substance-abusing behavior and its consequences. Help the patient to identify the substance abuse problem. Involve the patient in describing situations that lead to substance-abusing behavior. Consistently offer support and the expectation that the patient has the strength to overcome the problem.	Motivation for change is related to recognition of a problem that is upsetting to the patient. Identification of predisposing factors and precipitating stressors must precede planning for more adaptive behavioral responses.
The patient will assume responsibility for behavior.	Encourage the patient to participate in a treatment program. Develop with the patient a written contract for behavioral change that is signed by the patient and nurse. Help the patient to identify and adopt healthier coping responses.	Denial and rationalization are dysfunctional coping mechanisms that can interfere with recovery. Personal commitment will enhance the likelihood of successful abstinence.
The patient will identify and use social support systems.	Identify and assess social support systems that are available to the patient. Provide support to significant others. Educate the patient and significant others about the substance abuse problem and available resources. Refer the patient to appropriate resources and provide support until the patient is involved in the program.	Substance abusers are often dependent and socially isolated people who use drugs to gain confidence in social situations. Substance-abusing behavior alienates significant others, thus increasing the person's isolation. It is difficult to manipulate people who have participated in the same behaviors. Social support systems must be readily available over time and acceptable to the patient.

Nursing Diagnosis: Sensory-perceptual alteration
Expected Outcome: The patient will overcome addiction safely and with a minimum of discomfort.

Short-term Goals	Interventions	Rationale
The patient will withdraw from dependence on the abused substance.	Supportive physical care: vital signs, nutrition, hydration, seizure precautions. Administer medication according to detoxification schedule.	Detoxification of the physically dependent person can be dangerous and is always uncomfortable. The patient's physical safety must receive high priority for nursing intervention.
The patient will be oriented to time, place, person, and situation.	Assess orientation frequently, orient the patient if needed, and place a clock and calendar where they can be seen by the patient.	Cognitive function is usually affected by addiction; disorientation is frightening.
The patient will report symptoms of withdrawal.	Observe carefully for withdrawal symptoms and report suspected withdrawal immediately.	Withdrawal symptoms provide powerful motivation for continued substance abuse; judgment may be impaired by substance use.
The patient will correctly interpret environmental stimuli.	Explain all nursing interventions, assign consistent staff, keep soft light on in room, avoid loud noises, and encourage trusted family and friends to stay with the patient.	Sensory and perceptual alterations related to use of drugs or alcohol are frightening; consistency reduces the need to interpret stimuli.
The patient will recognize and talk about hallucinations or delusions.	Observe for response to internal stimuli, encourage patient to describe hallucinations or delusions, and explain the relationship of these experiences to withdrawal from addictive substances.	Helping the patient to identify delusional or hallucinatory experiences and relate them to withdrawal is reassuring.

they fail to show for treatment and help patients to meet multiple psychosocial needs, including basic living arrangements. Such specialized treatment programs offer special treatment groups for the mentally ill, chemically addicted (MICA) patient (also called mentally ill, substance abusing, or MISA) and refer patients to community self-help groups developed for such people, called double trouble groups. Nurses who understand both conditions are in an ideal position to work with dually diagnosed patients.

Appropriate treatment is linked to correct assessment of coexisting conditions. If the causative disorder can be isolated, it should be the focus of initial treatment unless the secondary disorder has become life-threatening, as when the alcoholic develops a suicidal depression. However, it should not be assumed that resolution of primary psychiatric problems will automatically resolve associated substance abuse problems. If substances are used chronically, substance abuse can develop into a primary disorder, taking on a life of its own. In these cases, the initial emphasis of treatment must be on the most serious problem at the time. Although the relative importance of symptoms may vary with time and influence the focus of treatment, both disorders must be treated.

Comprehensive treatment for co-occurring disorders usually requires a combination of pharmacological treatment, psychosocial treatment, and supportive services. Successful psychosocial programs for patients with psychiatric and substance abuse disorders provide behavioral skill-building interventions as the primary ingredient of active treatment, which has been shown to be more effective than case management or 12-step intervention.[19] In addition, five therapeutic tasks or steps that can serve as guidelines for structuring treatment of dual-diagnosis patients have been identified[7]:

▼ Establish a therapeutic alliance with the patient.

▼ Help the patient evaluate the costs and benefits of continued substance use.

▼ Individualize goals for change with the patient that include harm reduction as an alternative to total abstinence.

▼ Help the patient build an environment and lifestyle supportive of abstinence.

▼ Acknowledge that recovery is a long-term process and help the patient cope with crises by anticipating triggers of relapse and coping with setbacks as they occur.

Because both mental illness and substance abuse are chronic, relapsing conditions, the course of treatment can be expected to take considerable time. Stages of treatment have been identified and are used as the basis for treatment planning in many dual diagnosis treatment programs today. Interventions appropriate to each stage have been identified and are listed along with goals in Table 24-3.[11] Counselors and interdisciplinary teams are also useful, as can be seen in the following clinical example.

TABLE **24-3** *Treatment Stages, Goals, and Interventions for Dually Diagnosed Patients*

Stage of Treatment	Suggested Goals and Interventions
ENGAGEMENT	**Goal:** Development of working relationship between patient and nurse. **Interventions:** Intervene in crises, help with practical living problems, establish rapport with family members, demonstrate caring and support, listen actively.
PERSUASION	**Goal:** Patient acceptance of having a substance abuse problem and the need for active change strategies. **Interventions:** Help to analyze pros and cons of substance use, educate patient and family, arrange peer group discussions, expose patient to double trouble self-help groups, adjust medication, persuade patient to comply with medication regimen (motivational interviewing skills is particularly helpful during this stage).
ACTIVE TREATMENT	**Goal:** Abstinence from substance use and compliance with medication. **Interventions:** Help to change thinking patterns, friends, habits, behaviors, and living situations as necessary to support goals; teach social skills; encourage to develop positive social supports through double trouble self-help groups; enlist family support of changes; monitor urine and breath for substances; offer medication.
RELAPSE PREVENTION	**Goal:** Absence or minimization of return to substance abuse. **Interventions:** Reinforce abstinence, compliance, and behavioral changes; identify risk factors and help to practice preventive strategies; encourage continued involvement in double trouble groups; continue lab monitoring.

Clinical Example Bobby was a 17-year-old who was admitted to the hospital acutely psychotic with a history of recent use of PCP. The emergency room nurse noted scarring of the veins in Bobby's arm and surmised that he also used heroin. Blood and urine testing confirmed this suspicion. Bobby recovered from his psychotic episode in 24 hours but was extremely uncomfortable due to opiate withdrawal. The decision was made to use titrated doses of methadone to help with the withdrawal. Mr. L, a young nurse, established a close relationship with Bobby during this time. Bobby requested the nurse's help in planning for his future, but doubted that he had the strength to stay away from drugs. He was advised to take a day at a time. Mr. L took Bobby on a visit to a drug treatment program, and he agreed to try membership in one of the groups at this center. Bobby did well in the group and was very helpful to new members, describing his experiences and encouraging them to "take 1 day at a time." Bobby expressed an interest in finishing school and said he would like to become a drug counselor. The staff of the drug treatment program agreed that Bobby seemed to have an aptitude for that role and encouraged him to pursue his goal.

Selected Nursing Diagnoses:

▼ Altered thought processes related to PCP use, as evidenced by uncontrolled behavior in the emergency room

▼ Situational low self-esteem related to pessimism about ability to stop using drugs, as evidenced by expressed self-doubt

Mr. L used his relationship with Bobby to communicate his belief that he could successfully give up drugs. This message has a core of positive regard for Bobby's potential strength. The staff of the drug treatment program added to this seed of self-esteem by encouraging Bobby to help others in the program and then to aim higher at becoming a counselor himself. This taught Bobby that there were rewards in life other than those attached to drug use. Gradually, he learned to value the interpersonal rewards more than the drug rewards while making positive use of his past difficulties.

Intervening with Impaired Colleagues

It is usually difficult for nurses to respond to a colleague who is showing signs of a substance abuse problem. This is true of supervisors as well as peers. For the safety of the nurse, as well as the nurse's patients, it is necessary to identify the problem and take action. In addition, many states have laws requiring health-care professionals to report colleagues who show signs of working while impaired. In these states, reporting is both an ethical and a legal obligation.

It is not usually easy to be sure that a nurse's practice is impaired by drug or alcohol use. However, particular patterns of behavior and signs are characteristic of this problem (Box 24-6). The concerned colleague should report incidents of this nature to the supervisor. It is also important that these incidents be documented in writing, with the time, date, place, description of the incident, and the names of others who were present. This documentation will make it easier to intervene.

If the pattern of behavior indicates that impairment exists, an intervention should be planned. An advisor should be selected who has expertise in the area of impaired nursing practice. This advisor could be someone from the state nurse rehabilitation committee, if there is one. A team of people who have meaningful relationships with the nurse should be asked to prepare written statements demonstrating their observations of probable impaired practice. The team should consist of co-workers, the supervisor or other nurse administrator, and perhaps a family member. The team rehearses the statements in a meeting without the nurse present to work out any details and to ensure a non-

moralistic tone. They also anticipate various reactions the nurse may have and decide how to respond to these. Treatment options are discussed and plans made to escort the nurse directly from the meeting to a treatment facility.

After the above preparation, a meeting is called in which the team members read their statements to the nurse, who is informed of the bottom line that the team has decided on. The bottom line is usually that the nurse must enter treatment or resign from nursing and potentially lose the li-

Box **24-6** *Signs of Impaired Nursing Practice*

JOB PERFORMANCE CHANGES
Controlled Drug Handling/Records (potential drug diversion)

Drug counts incorrect
Excessive errors
Excessive wastage, often not countersigned
Medicine signed out to patient who has not been in pain
Two strengths of drug signed out to same patient, same time
Packaging appears to be tampered with
Patient complaints of ineffective pain control
Volunteers to give controlled drugs
Comes in early or stays late
Disappears into the bathroom after handling controlled drugs
Unexplained absences from the unit

General Performance

Medication errors
Poor judgment
Euphoric recall for involvement in unpleasant situations, or confrontations on the job
Illogical or sloppy charting
Absenteeism, especially in conjunction with days off
Requesting leave time just before the assigned shift
Latenesses with elaborate excuses
Job shrinkage (does the minimum work required to get by)
Missed deadlines

BEHAVIOR/PERSONALITY CHANGES

Sudden changes in mood
Periods of irritability
Forgetfulness
Wears long sleeves even in hot weather
Socially isolates from co-workers
Inappropriate behavior
Has chronic pain condition
History of pain treatment with controlled substances

SIGNS OF USE

Alcohol on the breath
Constant use of perfumes, mouthwash, and breath mints
Flushed face, reddened eyes, unsteady gait, slurred speech
Hyperactivity, accelerated speech
Increasing family problems that interfere with work

SIGNS OF WITHDRAWAL

Tremors, restlessness, diaphoresis, pupil changes
Watery eyes, runny nose, stomach aches, joint pains, gooseflesh

cense to practice. The nurse is escorted to either an inpatient treatment program or an outpatient appointment. Because the suicide risk for nurses who have just gone through an intervention is great, the nurse should not be left alone after the intervention.

During treatment the supervisor should maintain contact with the treatment program to see how the nurse is progressing. It is strongly advised that a return-to-work contract be written that clearly describes the nurse's responsibilities upon return. If the state has a nurse rehabilitation or peer assistance program, they can assume some responsibility for monitoring the nurse's progress and developing treatment and return-to-work contracts.[14] This type of intervention makes it possible for the chemically dependent nurse to get the treatment needed, yet remain employed, a situation in which everyone benefits.

> **?** *An enabler is a person who supports someone in maintaining an addiction. Describe behaviors that would enable a colleague to continue drug or alcohol use that impairs performance of nursing roles. What alternative behaviors would be more helpful?*

Preventive Interventions

Primary prevention programs aimed at preventing drug use among children are in place in many elementary schools in this country. School nurses can be involved in education efforts in the schools. Nurses can also support legislation designed to reduce the incidence of use and abuse. Nurses can serve as public speakers in the community on drug abuse issues.

Secondary prevention efforts are aimed at people with mild to moderate drinking problems. For every person with a severe drinking problem, there are several more people with mild to moderate drinking problems. Several brief therapies have evolved to address their special needs. These range from simple advice to stop drinking to more elaborate programs involving early identification, presentation of assessment findings, education (see Patient Education Plan), advice regarding the need to cut down on drinking with an emphasis on personal responsibility, self-help manuals, and periodic follow-up. People with mild to moderate drinking problems are increasingly being referred to treatment programs through the courts following DWI (driving while intoxicated) changes.

Tertiary prevention involves decreasing the complications of addiction. Medical and psychiatric treatment settings still serve a major role here, as do more current case management, community outreach, and dual diagnosis programs.

Evaluation

The evaluation of substance abuse treatment is based on accomplishment of the expected outcomes and short-term goals. The nurse and patient together should evaluate progress toward these goals on a regular basis. If progress is not being made, together they should re-evaluate both the goal and the progress to see where the problem lies and what needs to be done about it.

Relapse does not automatically mean failure. Progress toward a lifelong goal of abstinence from substances of abuse can be measured in many ways. For example, a significant increase in the periods of time that a chronic alcoholic patient stays sober between binges or relapses can be viewed as improvement. A decrease in the amount of time that the alcoholic patient remains in relapse before returning to sobriety can likewise indicate improvement. The patient who returns to treatment after relapse should be commended for

---

📖 **PATIENT EDUCATION PLAN**   **Promoting Adaptive Chemically Mediated Responses**

Content	Instructional Activities	Evaluation
Elicit perceptions of substance use.	Lead group discussion regarding knowledge about chemical use and experience with it; correct misperceptions.	The patient will describe accurate information about substance use.
Demonstrate negative effects of substance abuse.	Show films of physical and psychological effects of substance abuse; provide written materials.	The patient will identify and describe physical and psychological effects of substance abuse.
Interaction with peer who has abused chemicals.	Small group discussion with peer group member who has abused substances and quit because of negative experiences.	The patient will compare advantages and disadvantages of using mind-altering substances.
Obtain agreement to abstain from use of mind-altering substances.	Discuss future plans for refusing abused chemicals if offered.	The patient will verbally agree to abstain from using mind-altering substances.

previous successes and for the decision to keep trying. Then the nurse and patient together can analyze what worked and what did not work in the patient's attempts to maintain sobriety. This information should be used to modify the patient's relapse prevention plan.

It is also recommended that several measures of success toward abstinence goals be used, not just patient self-report. Objective measures such as breath analysis and urinalysis should be used as well as information from collateral sources such as spouses and employers (with a signed release of information). Success toward goals in other areas of living such as obtaining or keeping a job, improvements in health, and improvements in family relationships are interrelated with abstinence goals and important in the total recovery process.

Summary

1. Adaptive chemically mediated responses include "natural highs," which may be related to physical activity or meditation. Maladaptive responses include dependence on tobacco, caffeine, and alcohol and abuse of or dependence on illicit drugs.

2. Although drug use decreased for several years, it has been on the increase since 1992. Deaths and drug-related emergency room visits have increased. Multiple-substance abuse and dual diagnosis continue to be major problems.

3. Patient behaviors related to chemically mediated responses are related to dependence, intoxication, or overdose and vary according to the abused substances. Abused substances may include CNS depressants, alcohol, barbiturates, benzodiazepines, marijuana, stimulants, opiates, hallucinogens, and PCP.

4. Predisposing factors that lead to maladaptive chemically mediated responses are described from the biological, psychological, and sociocultural perspectives. Precipitating stressors include withdrawal from addiction.

5. Coping resources include motivation, social supports, health, social skills, material and economic assets, and intellectual and personality traits. Maladaptive coping mechanisms include denial, rationalization, and minimization.

6. Primary NANDA nursing diagnoses related to maladaptive chemically mediated responses are sensory-perceptual alteration, altered thought processes, ineffective individual coping, and altered family processes related to alcoholism.

7. Primary DSM-IV diagnoses are dependence, abuse, intoxication, or withdrawal related to a particular substance.

8. The expected outcome of nursing care is that the patient will abstain from using all mood-altering chemicals.

9. Planning is based on providing first for safe withdrawal, followed by developing ways to maintain abstinence. Support systems including family, friends, and self-help groups should be involved whenever possible.

10. Interventions include biological, psychological, and social interventions, working with dually diagnosed patients, intervening with impaired colleagues, and preventive interventions.

11. Evaluation criteria for nursing care related to chemically mediated responses include goal achievement, increases in amount of sober time, negative breath and urinalysis tests, and improved psychosocial dimensions.

COMPETENT CARING A Clinical Exemplar of a Psychiatric Nurse

Walter E. Roberson, Jr., RN, MA

One of the most fulfilling experiences I have ever had working with a chemically dependent patient occurred not long ago. This young woman came into the hospital after planning to throw herself into traffic. She had a history of cocaine and alcohol abuse and recently had to give up her son to the Department of Family Services because she had been unable to care for him.

When she first came into the hospital she demonstrated a lot of anger and erratic behavior. I recognized this as part of her withdrawal symptoms and the grief she was experiencing because of the loss of her son. She was unapproachable at first, and much of her conversation was confused and contradictory. Over and over again she refused to talk with me about how she was feeling and what she planned to do in her life. What I finally started to notice was a very subtle change in her affect. It was like very thin layers of an opaque material were being taken away as things inside her began to clear. I was persistent with making myself available for her while giving ongoing support. Finally she reached a point where she said she was ready to talk and she said many things were clear now that she did not understand before. Over the course of the next several days the rest of the treatment team and I began to offer her options. She ended up going into a halfway house for several months, and then she was able to move into an apartment and eventually regain custody of her little boy. She checks back in periodically to say hi and show us how well she is doing.

This has shown me that it is always important to keep trying and that the difference a nurse can make can be very significant in a patient's recovery. Don't ever give up.

your **INTERNET**
connection

Dual Diagnosis Web Site
http://www.erols.com/ksciacca

WEB of Addictions
http://www.well.com/user/woa

Chapter Review Questions

1. **Identify whether the following statements are true (T) or false (F).**

A. ___ Race is an important determinant of substance dependence.

B. ___ Substance abuse invariably leads to substance dependence.

C. ___ Opioids are known to have an acute withdrawal syndrome.

D. ___ Patients with psychiatric disorders have more substance abuse problems than the general population.

E. ___ Mental illness is a primary cause of substance dependence.

F. ___ Most genetic research has been focused on alcoholism.

G. ___ The longer the half-life of the abused drug, the more intense the withdrawal symptoms will be.

H. ___ Newer psychological treatment approaches to substance use disorders emphasize a therapeutic alliance with the patient, avoidance of confrontation, and brevity of treatment.

I. ___ Most patients succeed in abstaining from drugs in their first attempt.

J. ___ Alcoholics Anonymous (AA) uses the 12-step model for recovery from alcoholism.

2. **Fill in the blanks.**

A. The main principle in the treatment of detoxification is _____.

B. Coexistence of psychiatric disorder and substance-related disorder within the same person is called _____.

C. Among adolescents, nicotine, alcohol, and marijuana often act as _____ drugs to substances that are perceived to be more dangerous.

D. The simplest screening tool consisting of only four questions related to alcohol abuse is the _____.

E. The simplest biological measure to obtain a blood alcohol content is by use of a _____.

F. The term _____ was first used to describe people who had become dysfunctional as a result of living in a committed relationship with an alcoholic.

G. The brain's natural opiates are the neurotransmitters called _____.

H. Medically, withdrawal from the _____ drugs is the most dangerous.

I. The process of helping an addict safely through withdrawal is called _____.

J. _____ was the first drug to be approved over 40 years ago for treatment of alcohol dependence and it has been followed by the more recent approval of _____.

3. **Provide short answers for the following questions.**

A. Methadone treatment is available across the country and allows a person to maintain drug abstinence. Why do you think more people do not take advantage of it? Relate your answer to the overall dynamics of addiction and abstinence.

B. Some people believe that treatment programs should only employ as counselors people who have recovered from substance abuse. How would you respond to this?

C. You suspect that one of your friends has a problem with alcohol. How would you go about helping her?

D. Carefully read the 12 steps of Alcoholics Anonymous. Evaluate their content as a treatment approach. How would you respond to a patient who did not believe in a higher power?

E. Design a comprehensive treatment plan for a patient who is dually diagnosed with both bipolar disorder and alcoholism.

REFERENCES

1. American Nurses' Association and National Nurses' Society of Addictions: *Standards of addictions nursing practice with selected diagnoses and criteria,* Kansas City, Mo, 1988, American Nurses' Association.

2. American Psychiatric Association: *Diagnostic and statistical manual of mental disorders,* ed 4, Washington, DC, 1994, The Association.

3. American Psychiatric Association: Practice guideline for the treatment of patients with nicotine dependence, *Am J Psychiatry* 153(suppl):1, 1996.

4. American Psychiatric Association: Practice guideline for the treatment of patients with substance use disorders: alcohol, cocaine, opioids, *Am J Psychiatry* 152:11, 1995.

5. Berg IK, Miller SD: *Working with the problem drinker: a solution-focused approach,* New York, 1992, WW Norton.

6. Block B, Lefkovitz P: Standards and guidelines for partial hospitalization: chemical dependency programs, *Continuum* 3:247, 1996.

7. Carey K: Treatment of co-occurring substance abuse and major mental illness, *New Dir Ment Health Serv* 70:19, 1996.

8. Chandler MC, Mason WH: Solution-focused therapy: an alternative approach to addictions nursing, *Perspect Psychiatr Care* 31(1):8, 1995.

9. Cloninger DR: Neurogenetic adaptive mechanisms in alcoholism, *Science* 236:410, 1987.

10. Doweiko HF: *Concepts of chemical dependency,* ed 2, Pacific Grove, Calif, 1993, Brooks/Cole.

11. Drake RE, Rosenberg SD, Mueser KT: Assessing substance use disorder in persons with severe mental illness, *New Dir Ment Health Serv* 70:3, 1996.

12. Drug Enforcement Administration, Illegal drug price/purity report, United States: January 1992-March 1995, *Drug Intelligence Rep,* October 1995.

13. Dupont R, Gold M: Naltrexone pharmacotherapy for alcohol dependence: an update, *Essential Psychopharmacol* 1:136, 1996.

14. Finke L, Williams J, Stanley R: Nurses referred to a peer assistance program for alcohol and drug problems, *Arch Psychiatr Nurs* 10:319, 1996.

15. Gold MS: Cocaine (and crack): clinical aspects. In Lowinson JH, Ruiz P, Millman RB, editors: *Substance abuse: a comprehensive textbook,* Baltimore, 1992, Williams & Wilkins.

16. Helzer JE, Burnam A, McEvoy LT: Alcohol abuse and dependence. In Robins LN, Regier DA, editors: *Psychiatric disorders in America: the epidemiologic catchment area study,* New York, 1991, Free Press.

17. Henning S et al: Relapse prevention by acamprosate: results from a placebo-controlled study on alcohol dependence, *Arch Gen Psychiatry* 53:673, 1996.

18. Jaffe JH: Opiates: clinical aspects. In Lowinson JH, Ruiz P, Millman RB, editors: *Substance abuse: a comprehensive textbook,* Baltimore, 1992, Williams & Wilkins.

19. Jerrell J: Toward cost-effective care for persons with dual diagnoses, *J Ment Health Admin* 23:329, 1996.

20. King GR, Ellinwood EH: Amphetamines and other stimulants. In Lowinson JH, Ruiz P, Millman RB, editors: *Substance abuse: a comprehensive textbook,* Baltimore, 1992, Williams & Wilkins.

21. Kirkpatrick J: *Turnabout: new help for the woman alcoholic,* ed 3, New York, 1990, Bantam.

22. Marlatt FA, Gordon JR, editors: *Relapse prevention,* New York, 1985, Guilford.

23. Miele G, Trautman K, Hasin D: Assessing comorbid mental and substance-use disorders: a guide for clinical practice, *J Pract Psychiatry Behav Health* 2:272, 1996.

24. Miller NS: Prevalence and treatment models for addiction in psychiatric populations, *Psychiatr Annals* 24:8, 1994.

25. Miller WR, Rollnick S: *Motivational interviewing: preparing people to change addictive behavior,* New York, 1991, Guilford.

26. Mynatt S: A model of contributing risk factors to chemical dependency in nurses, *J Psychosoc Nurs* 34:13, 1996.

27. National Institute on Drug Abuse: *National household survey on drug abuse: main findings 1992,* Rockville, Md, 1995, The Institute.

28. National Institute on Drug Abuse: *Drug use rises again in 1995 among American teens,* Press release, Rockville, Md, December 15, 1995, The Institute.

29. Nobel ET, Parades A: Molecular biology and behavior. In *Recent developments in alcoholism, Volume 11: Ten years of progress,* New York, 1993, Plenum Press.

30. Peachey JE, Lei H: Assessment of opioid dependence with Naloxone, *Br J Addict* 83:193, 1988.

31. Research Developments in Alcoholism: *Alcoholism and women,* New York, 1995, Plenum Press.

32. Sullivan E: *Nursing care of clients with substance abuse,* St Louis, 1995, Mosby.

33. Sullivan JT, Sykora K, Schneiderman J, Naranjo CA, Sellers EM: Assessment of alcohol withdrawal; the revised Clinical Institute Withdrawal Assessment for Alcohol scale (CIWA-AR), *Br J Addict* 84:1353, 1989.

34. Trimpey J: *Rational recovery from alcoholism: the small book,* ed 3, Lotus, Calif, 1989, Lotus Press.

35. Trinkoff AM, Eaton WW, Anthony JC: The prevalence of substance abuse among registered nurses, *Nurs Res* 40:172, 1991.

36. Weddington WW: Methadone maintenance for opioid addiction. In Miller NS, Gold MS, editors: *Pharmacological therapies for drug & alcohol addictions,* New York, 1995, Marcel Dekker.

37. Wesson DR, Smith DE, Seymour RB: Sedative-hypnotics and tricyclics. In Lowinson JH, Ruiz P, Millman RB: *Substance abuse: a comprehensive textbook,* Baltimore, 1992, Williams & Wilkins.

38. Windle M, Searles JS: *Children of alcoholics: critical perspectives,* New York, 1990, Guilford.

ANNOTATED SUGGESTED READINGS

Bachmann K et al: An integrated treatment program for dually diagnosed patients, *Psychiatr Serv* 3:314, 1997.

A Swiss model treatment program is described and the point is made that using conventional approaches in an additive fashion to treat patients with dual diagnoses is inefficient and ineffective.

Humphreys K, Moos R, Cohen C: Social and community resources and long-term recovery from treated and untreated alcoholism, *J Stud Alcohol* 5:231, 1997.

Describes how social and community resources that are readily available for long periods are more likely to have a lasting influence on the course of alcoholism than short-term interventions.

Lowinson J et al: *Substance abuse: a comprehensive textbook,* ed 3, Baltimore, 1997, Williams & Wilkins.

Comprehensive text on substance abuse, including compulsive and addictive behaviors such as gambling, eating, sexual addictions, and sect or cult involvement.

Oumette P, Finney J, Moos R: Twelve-step and cognitive-behavioral treatment for substance abuse: a comparison of treatment effectiveness, *J Consult Clin Psychol* 2:230, 1997.

These two interventions, separately and when combined, showed significant improvements and were equally effective at the 1-year follow-up assessment for patients with substance abuse problems.

Chapter 25

Eating Regulation Responses and Eating Disorders

Carolyn E. Cochrane

© 1998 M.C. Escher/Cordon Art, Baarn, Holland.

Soon her eyes fell upon a little glass box that was lying under the table: she opened it, and found in it a very small cake, on which the words "EAT ME" were beautifully marked in currants. She ate a little bit, and said anxiously to herself, "Which way? Which way?," holding her hand on the top of her head to feel which way it was growing. **Lewis Carroll** ALICE'S ADVENTURES IN WONDERLAND

LEARNING OBJECTIVES

After studying this chapter the student should be able to:

▼ Describe the continuum of adaptive and maladaptive eating regulation responses

▼ Relate the prevalence of anorexia nervosa, bulimia nervosa, and binge eating disorder

▼ Identify behaviors associated with eating regulation responses

▼ Analyze predisposing factors, precipitating stressors, and appraisal of stressors related to eating regulation responses

▼ Describe coping resources and coping mechanisms related to eating regulation responses

▼ Formulate nursing diagnoses for patients related to eating regulation responses

▼ Assess the relationship between nursing diagnoses and medical diagnoses related to eating regulation responses

▼ Identify expected outcomes and short-term nursing goals related to eating regulation responses

▼ Develop a family education plan to promote adaptive eating regulation responses

▼ Analyze nursing interventions related to eating regulation responses

▼ Evaluate nursing care related to eating regulation responses

TOPICAL OUTLINE

Continuum of Eating Regulation Responses
  Prevalence of Eating Disorders
Assessment
  Behaviors
  Predisposing Factors
  Precipitating Stressors
  Appraisal of Stressors
  Coping Resources
  Coping Mechanisms
Nursing Diagnosis
  Related Medical Diagnoses
Outcome Identification
Planning
  Choice of Treatment Setting
  Nurse-patient Contract
Implementation
  Nutritional Stabilization
  Exercise
  Cognitive Behavioral Interventions
  Body Image Interventions
  Family Involvement
  Group Therapies
  Medications
Evaluation

Food is essential to life because it supplies the person with needed nutrients and sources of energy. As such, eating is a crucial self-regulatory activity. However, it can also assume importance and meaning beyond that of nutrition and become associated with biopsychosocial processes that promote or inhibit adaptive functioning.

CONTINUUM OF EATING REGULATION RESPONSES

As a pattern of self-regulation, properly controlled eating contributes to psychological, biological, and sociocultural health and well-being. Adaptive eating responses are characterized by balanced eating patterns, appropriate caloric intake, and body weight that is appropriate for height. Although eating is a common occurrence, society appears to have difficulty understanding the idea of unregulated eating. For example, everyone has at times overeaten, skipped one or more meals, or seen adolescent boys consume large amounts of food at a single meal. Many women have premenstrual cravings for salty, sweet, or other types of foods. These eating behaviors are not viewed as problematic.

However, food can also be used in an attempt to satisfy unmet emotional needs, moderate stress, and provide rewards or punishments. People can also have unrealistic images of their ideal body size and desired body weight. Research has shown that most people think that they should weigh less than they do, and this can result in a range of behaviors from fasting fads to severe dieting. The inability to regulate eating habits and the frequent tendency to overuse or underuse food interferes with biological, psychological, and sociocultural integrity.

Illnesses associated with maladaptive eating regulation responses include anorexia nervosa, bulimia nervosa, and the newly named binge eating disorder (Fig. 25-1). The vast majority of these disorders occur in adolescent and young adult women who are predominantly white and middle to upper class. Although not nearly as widespread, eating disorders are becoming more common among males, minorities, and women of all age groups. These disorders can cause biological changes including altered metabolic rates, profound malnutrition, and possibly death. Obsessions about eating can cause psychological problems including depression, isolation, and emotional lability. Sociocultural ideals concerning body size can cause eating disorders by influencing a person to perceive body size as being larger or smaller than it actually is. This distorted body image may initiate an attempt to attain an unrealistic body size.

Before working with patients with maladaptive eating regulation responses, nurses must closely examine their own feelings and prejudices about weight and body size. Reflecting on the following questions may elicit answers requiring further examination:

▼ What do I believe is the ideal body size and shape?
▼ How do I feel about people who are overweight?
▼ Can a person ever really be too thin?
▼ Do I worry about my weight a lot?
▼ Do I have biases about eating and weight that will interfere with my ability to take care of patients with eating disorders?

If a nurse suspects that she has an eating disorder, she may not be able to provide care for patients who cannot regulate their eating responses. She should seek out professional help for herself before attempting to care for others.

> **?** *Identify three sociocultural factors that influence the type and amount of food you eat and your perception of the ideal body size.*

Prevalence of Eating Disorders

ANOREXIA NERVOSA. Anorexia nervosa occurs in about 1% to 2% of the female population. Its onset is usually between the ages of 13 and 20, but the illness can occur

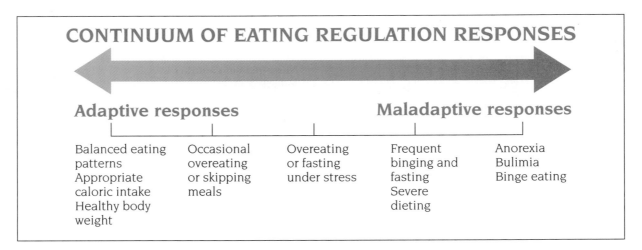

CONTINUUM OF EATING REGULATION RESPONSES

Adaptive responses ←————————————————→ **Maladaptive responses**

Balanced eating patterns	Occasional overeating	Overeating or fasting	Frequent binging and	Anorexia
Appropriate	or skipping	under stress	fasting	Bulimia
caloric intake	meals		Severe	Binge eating
Healthy body weight			dieting	

Fig. 25-1 Continuum of eating regulation responses.

in any age group, including the elderly and prepubertal children. Anorexia nervosa is also seen in males, who are thought to make up only 5% to 10% of the anorectic population. Mortality from anorexia nervosa is estimated to be 5.6% per decade.[27]

BULIMIA NERVOSA. Bulimia nervosa is more common than anorexia, with estimates of 2% to 4% and a prevalence of 4% to 15% in female high school and college students.[27] The age of onset is typically 15 to 18 years of age. It is estimated that men make up 0.4% to 20% of the bulimic population. The gender differences in the prevalence of eating disorders may be attributable to biological, sociocultural, and psychodynamic factors, as well as the fact that men may be more reluctant to seek treatment. Although differences in the prevalence of eating disorders exist between men and women, men are more similar to women than different in characteristics of the illness, rates of comorbid psychiatric disorders, and satisfaction with body image.[18] Interestingly, the incidence for bulimia is lowest in rural areas and highest in large cities; urbanization seems to be a risk factor for bulimia. These differences were not found for anorexia.[11]

Bulimia and anorexia may be present in the same patient. As many as 50% of anorectic patients develop bulimic symptoms, and many people with bulimia can develop anorexia. Bulimia usually occurs in people of normal weight, but it may occur in obese and thin people (Fig. 25-2).

BINGE EATING DISORDER. Binge eating disorder is a new diagnostic category in the fourth edition of the *Diagnostic and Statistical Manual of Mental Disorders,* in which people consume large amounts of calories but do not attempt to prevent weight gain.[2] Previous descriptions of this problem included obese bingers, compulsive overeaters, and pathological overeaters. The differences between people who are obese but do not binge, those who are obese and binge, and nonobese patients with bulimia who both binge and purge are summarized in Table 25-1.

Not all patients with a binge eating disorder are obese. In one national study the incidence of binge eating disorder in females was determined to be 2.3%, with the typical person being of normal weight, any race, and any age.[4] The incidence of binge eating disorder in weight loss programs was found to be 29% to 30%,[22] suggesting that assessing for eating disorders should be an important part of weight management programs.

Assessment

It is essential that patients with maladaptive eating regulation responses receive a comprehensive nursing assessment, including complete biological, psychological, and sociocultural evaluations. A full physical examination should be performed with particular attention given to vital signs, weight for height, skin, the cardiovascular system, and evidence of laxative or diuretic abuse and vomiting. A dental examination may be indicated, and it is useful to assess growth, sexual development, and general physical development indicators. A psychiatric history, substance use history, and family assessment are also needed.

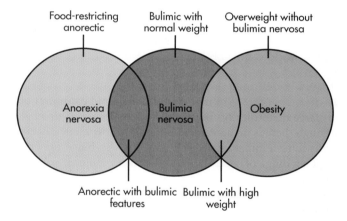

Fig. 25-2 The overlapping relationship between eating disorders and obesity. (Modified from Santmeyer K: Interventions for clients with anorexia nervosa and bulimia nervosa. In Ignatavicius D et al, editors: *Medical-surgical nursing,* ed 2, Philadelphia, 1995, WB Saunders.)

TABLE 25-1 *Differences in Obese Nonbingers, Obese Bingers, and Nonobese Bulimic Patients*

	OBESE NONBINGERS	OBESE BINGERS	NONOBESE BULIMIC PATIENTS
Body image distortion	Low or none	Moderate to low	High level
Amount of binging	Once per month or less	High amount but less than bulimic patients of normal weight	Very high level
Mood disturbance	Same as general population	One third chronic	One third to one half chronic and 75% to 80% lifetime
Purging	Rare	Infrequent (tend to use laxatives)	High level
Degree of control regarding binging	High	Medium to low	Low
Interest in food	Preoccupied at times	Obsessed	Obsessed
Problems with self-esteem	Same as general population	Low self-esteem	Low self-esteem
Substance abuse	Same as general population	Moderate to high	High

Specific attention should focus on the assessment of eating regulation responses. Several questionnaires and rating scales have been developed to screen for the presence of eating disorders. Some of these are listed in Chapter 6. However, a recent study found that asking just two questions may be as effective as more extensive questionnaires in identifying women with eating disorders[10]:

▼ Are you satisfied with your eating patterns?

▼ Do you ever eat in secret?

These questions can be easily incorporated into the nursing assessment of all patients. If a patient is being evaluated for an eating disorder, additional information should be obtained including the following:

▼ Actual and desired weight
▼ Onset and pattern of menstruation
▼ Food restrictions and fasting patterns
▼ Frequency and extent of binging and vomiting
▼ Use of laxatives, diuretics, diet pills, and so on
▼ Body image disturbances
▼ Food preferences and peculiarities
▼ Exercise patterns

It is also helpful to explore the patient's understanding of how the illness developed and its impact on school, work, and social relationships so that a holistic view of the patient's world can be obtained.

Behaviors

BINGE EATING. Binge eating is the rapid consumption of large quantities of food in a discrete period of time, although there is no agreement on exactly how many calories constitutes a binge. Anorectic patients who binge may describe a binge of several hundred calories. Bulimic patients who are not also anorectic may ingest several thousand calories at a sitting. Emphasis on the person's perception of loss of control and perceived excessive caloric intake is more important to the nursing assessment than the total number of calories consumed during a binge. Therefore, it is important that the nurse carefully assess exactly what each patient means by a binge. People usually binge secretively, and there is often considerable shame associated with their binging behavior. The bulimic typically is of average weight or slightly overweight and has a history of unsuccessful dieting. The severity of the binging can vary greatly, ranging from several times a week, to more than 10 times a day, to only occasional binges related to stressful situations.

FASTING OR RESTRICTING. People with anorexia often do not consume more than 500 to 700 calories daily and may ingest as few as 200 calories a day, yet they see their intake as adequate for their energy needs. They may follow an imbalanced vegetarian diet, eliminating all meat, poultry, fish, and dairy products without substituting nonanimal sources of protein and other important nutrients. They may be obsessive-compulsive about their eating habits and choices of foods, such as eating the same foods, or foods in a predetermined order, at the same time every day. They

may have bizarre food preferences, avoid foods considered fattening, and fast for days at a time. Despite these restrictions, many people with anorexia are preoccupied or obsessed with food and may do much of the family cooking or be employed in a food-related occupation. The following clinical example describes the fasting behavior seen in people with anorexia.

Clinical Example Barbara is a 15-year-old white female who has been restricting her food intake for 6 months because she felt too fat. Her weight at the beginning of her food restriction was 128 pounds. This weight was appropriate for her age, her height of 5′5″, and her small body frame. Her current weight is 102 pounds, which is approximately 80% of what she should weigh. The patient denies having any eating problems and feels that her family is overreacting to her weight loss. She is willing to come for treatment only because her family wants her to do so.

Barbara was age 13 at menarche and had regular periods until they stopped 2 months ago. She says that she never tried or planned to lose weight but admits to becoming a vegetarian 6 months ago. Despite her low weight, Barbara thinks that she needs to lose another 10 pounds because she feels her thighs are too large. She is an avid ballet dancer and practices dancing 2 to 3 hours a day. Her family describes her as the perfect daughter.

Selected Nursing Diagnoses:

▼ Altered nutrition related to restricted food intake, as evidenced by weight loss
▼ Body image disturbance related to eating disorder, as evidenced by continued desire to lose weight
▼ Ineffective denial related to eating problems, as evidenced by lack of acceptance of realistic weight parameters

PURGING. A variety of purging behaviors may be used by people with maladaptive eating regulation responses to prevent weight gain. These include excessive exercise, over-the-counter and prescription diuretics, diet pills, laxatives, and steroids. Laxatives are commonly abused by people with eating disorders, yet they are one of the most inefficient ways to lose calories. Laxative abuse often begins gradually, but can increase to 60 a week in some people. Less well-known substances used to counteract weight gain include insulin, cocaine, heroin, thyroid replacements, nicotine, hallucinogens, analgesics, benzodiazepines, antidepressants, ipecac, and sorbitol.[5] Many patients engage in more than one purging behavior.

Exercising for these patients often becomes a grueling, time-consuming affair. Running or participating in high-impact aerobics for 2 to 3 hours each day is typical of the compulsive exerciser. Many patients with an eating disorder exercise so much that they sustain major skeletal injuries, but this still does not deter them from continuing this maladaptive behavior. This is seen in the clinical example that follows.

Clinical Example Bill is a single, 30-year-old man with a 7-year history of anorexia nervosa and bulimia nervosa. Bill exercises compulsively at least 3 hours daily. He was exercising 6 to 7 hours a day from age 23 until age 29. Examples of current and previous exercise rituals include running 25 miles followed by a 2-to 3-mile swim and bicycling 25 miles before allowing himself to eat a meal. His athletic abilities have been rewarded with numerous trophies. He is receiving fewer trophies lately because of damage to his knees from overuse.

In addition to exercising compulsively, Bill also vomits after binging and has periods of fasting lasting 2 to 3 days. When he does eat a regular meal he does so by eating only certain foods and eating these foods in a certain order. Bill also writes obsessively and is methodical about the order of his personal hygiene. He is depressed about the fact that his life revolves around his eating, hygiene, and exercise rituals and is eager to receive treatment.

Selected Nursing Diagnoses:

▼ Altered nutrition related to anxiety about body size, as evidenced by binging and fasting

▼ Body image disturbance related to fears of gaining weight, as evidenced by excessive exercise and food restrictions

▼ Risk for injury related to excessive exercise, as evidenced by knee injuries

> **?** *Binging, fasting, and purging are sometimes described as addictive behaviors. Compare them to smoking, gambling, and substance abuse.*

MEDICAL COMPLICATIONS. Usually every person with maladaptive eating regulation responses has some type of associated physical problem. For example, one study reported that 70% of the bulimic patients admitted for inpatient treatment required medical care, and 90% of the medical complications found on assessment were previously unrecognized.[14] The various complications associated with eating disorders are listed in Box 25-1.

Assessment of the patient's physical status can help reveal the magnitude of the eating problem. Patients 20% below or 40% above their ideal body weight demonstrate more physical abnormalities than those who are closer to their ideal weight. Patients who are 40% below or 100% above their ideal body weight will have clinical and laboratory findings that are often life threatening. People who vomit and use laxatives or diuretics, regardless of their weight, usually have significant and sometimes life-threatening clinical findings and laboratory abnormalities.[14]

In anorexia nervosa, metabolic and endocrine abnormalities result from the body's reaction to malnutrition associated with starvation. All body systems are affected. Most commonly seen are amenorrhea, osteoporosis, and hypometabolic symptoms such as cold intolerance and bradycardia. Starvation may cause hypotension, constipation, and acid-base and fluid-electrolyte disturbances including pedal edema.

In bulimia nervosa, potassium depletion and hypokalemia are often seen as a result of vomiting and laxative or diuretic abuse. Symptoms of potassium depletion include muscle weakness, cardiac arrhythmias, conduction abnormalities, hypotension, and other problems associated with

Box **25-1** *Medical Complications of Eating Disorders*

CENTRAL NERVOUS SYSTEM
Decreased rapid eye movement and shortwave sleep
Cortical atrophy
Thermoregulatory abnormalities

RENAL
Hematuria
Proteinuria

HEMATOLOGIC
Leukopenia
Anemia
Thrombocytopenia

GASTROINTESTINAL
Dental erosion
Parotid swelling
Esophagitis, esophageal tears
Delayed gastric emptying
Gastric dilation
Pancreatitis
Diarrhea (laxative abuse)
Hypercholesterolemia

METABOLIC
Dehydration
Acidosis
Hypokalemia
Hypochloremia
Hypochloremic alkalosis
Hypocalcemia
Hypophosphatemia
Hypomagnesemia
Osteoporosis
Hypercarotenemia

ENDOCRINE
Decreased luteinizing hormone and follicle-stimulating hormone
Decreased triiodothyronine, increased reverse triiodothyronine, rT3, normal thyroxin and thyroid-stimulating hormone
Irregular menses
Amenorrhea

CARDIOVASCULAR
Bradycardia
Postural hypotension
Dysrhythmia, sudden death

electrolyte imbalance. Gastric, esophageal, and bowel abnormalities are common complaints in bulimic patients. Those who vomit are subject to erosion of the dental enamel and parotid enlargement.[12,16]

For those with binge eating disorder and concurrent morbid obesity, serious health problems caused by excess weight or prior health problems exacerbated by increased weight are common. Many have hypertension, cardiac problems, sleep apnea, difficulties in mobility, and diabetes mellitus. Some of the medical consequences of eating disorders are seen in the following clinical example.

Clinical Example Audrey is a 25-year-old black woman with a 4-year history of restrictive intake and a 3-year history of binge eating and laxative abuse. Audrey has been concerned about her weight since high school, when she was a star basketball player, a competitive swimmer, and participant in track, volleyball, and tennis. She bypassed her senior year in high school. She began to diet at age 20, and her severe restriction of food at age 21 led to a 20-pound weight loss and amenorrhea. At age 22 she began to binge eat and use laxatives. Since that time she has binged two to three times a week and used an average of 30 to 60 stimulant-type laxatives each week.

She is constantly preoccupied with food and her weight and has periods of mood lability, sadness, lack of energy, social isolation, anxiety, irritability, and difficulty concentrating. Audrey also reports chronic constipation, bloating, edema of hands, feet, legs, and face, and lightheadedness. She has recently consulted a gastroenterologist for her severe constipation and was advised that her large intestine was grossly oversized. Audrey became very frightened by the report and immediately called a local eating disorder program for help.

Selected Nursing Diagnoses:

▼ Altered nutrition related to fear of gaining weight, as evidenced by binging

▼ Body image disturbance related to anxiety about body size, as evidenced by excessive use of laxatives

▼ Constipation related to maladaptive eating patterns, as evidenced by pain, bloating, and enlarged intestine

PSYCHIATRIC COMPLICATIONS. Many patients seeking treatment for eating disorders have evidence of other psychiatric disorders. Comorbid major depression or dysthymia has been reported in 50% to 75% of people with anorexia and bulimia. Obsessive-compulsive disorder may be found in 10% to 13% of patients with anorexia, with a lifetime prevalence of 25%.[2] Among patients with bulimia, there are increased rates of anxiety disorders, substance abuse, and mood disorders. People with antisocial personality disorders are 6 to 7 times more likely to also have bulimia than the general population.[21] In addition, many bulimic patients have dissociative symptoms, sexual conflicts, and a variety of impulsive behaviors that include overspending, shoplifting, promiscuity, and self-mutilation.[1] Fi-

nally, binge eating disorder has been found to be associated with higher rates of major depression, panic disorder, bulimia nervosa, borderline personality disorder, and avoidant personality disorder.[32]

Predisposing Factors

Biological, psychological, and sociocultural factors have been identified that may predispose a person to the development of an eating disorder. These factors are involved in the regulation and control of food intake. It is generally agreed that the etiological factors are multidetermined and interactive, involving a combination of genetic, neurochemical, developmental, characterological, social, cultural, and familial factors (Fig. 25-3).

BIOLOGICAL. It is generally recognized that eating disorders are familial. There is a higher risk for eating disorders in first-degree female relatives of people with eating disorders than in the general population. Concordance rates for eating disorders in monozygotic twins is 52% and in dizygotic twins it is 11%. There is also a higher risk for other eating disorders and for depression in first-degree relatives of people with eating disorders, suggesting common etiological factors. The development of one or the other in a vulnerable person may be caused by complex relationships among personality traits, environmental and familial factors, and genetic predisposition.[28]

Biological models of the etiology of eating disorders focus on the appetite regulation center in the hypothalamus,

Fig. 25-3 Major peripheral inputs influencing appetite.

which controls specific neurochemical mechanisms for feeding and satiety. In patients with eating disorders it has been hypothesized that the neurotransmitters, neuromodulators, and hormones that control feeding and satiety are dysregulated. Studies in animals and humans indicate that reduced serotonin is associated with reduced satiety and increased food intake and dysphoric mood. For instance, when dietary tryptophan, the amino acid necessary for the brain to manufacture serotonin, was reduced in a recent study of eating disorders, a group of women with bulimia showed a marked increase in eating behavior and mood changes such as irritability, lability, and fatigue not seen in the healthy group of controls, suggesting a disturbance of serotonin activity in this disorder.[3,29] It has also been reported that MHPG, the major metabolite of norepinephrine, is also reduced in eating disorders, suggesting a role for this neurotransmitter as well.

Other hypotheses propose that eating disorders may be variants of mood disorders or may be caused by decreased endogenous opioid activity. This last theory is based on the clinical observations that carbohydrates, particularly sugar, play a role in binge eating and obesity, because many binge eaters preferentially eat sweets during a binge. Beta-endorphin has an appetite-stimulating mechanism, and if sugar stimulates beta-endorphin production, it can eventually lead to increased eating. Positron-emission tomography (PET) scans are also being conducted on anorectic patients, and abnormal findings on computed tomography (CT) scans of the brain have been reported in more than half of patients with anorexia nervosa. All of these models are still in the developmental stage, however, and ongoing research in this area promises to shed more light on the biological factors that may predispose a person to maladaptive eating regulation responses.

> *Analyze the hypothesized role of serotonin in the development of both eating disorders and depressive disorders and the implications this has for the use of selective serotonin reuptake inhibitors as a medication strategy for both disorders.*

PSYCHOLOGICAL. It is well recognized that most patients with eating disorders exhibit clusters of psychological symptoms, such as rigidity, ritualism, and meticulousness. When studied years after treatment, women who had long-term weight recovery continued to show an obsessive need for perfectionism, exactness, and symmetry, and greater risk avoidance, restraint, and impulse control.[23] Early separation and individuation conflicts, a pervasive sense of ineffectiveness and helplessness, difficulty interpreting feelings and tolerating intense emotional states, and fear of biological or psychological maturity may predispose a person to an eating disorder. Additional personality and

psychological characteristics of these patients are identified in Box 25-2.

ENVIRONMENTAL. A variety of environmental factors have been suggested that may predispose a person to develop an eating disorder. Early histories of patients with eating disorders are often complicated by medical and surgical illnesses, separations, and family deaths. Women with bulimia also describe growing up in a conflicted family environment and experiencing more behavioral disturbances such as drug abuse, suicide attempts, truancy, and other emotional problems.[26] Sexual abuse has been reported in 20% to 50% of patients with bulimia, but this rate may be similar to that found in other psychiatric populations.[13,26]

Parents who overemphasize athletics, reward slimness, or express disapproval of overweight people are placing their children at risk for eating disorders. Also, parents who continually skip meals, eat when distressed, and otherwise model poor nutritional habits are not teaching children about the appropriate value of food as nourishment. An important preventive nursing intervention is educating the parents of young children regarding healthy eating behaviors (see the Family Education Plan for preventing childhood eating problems).

SOCIOCULTURAL. In the past 50 years there has been a steady increase in the incidence of diagnosed eating disorders, subclinical eating problems, and body image disturbances. In cultures where plumpness is accepted or valued, eating disorders are thought to be rare. It has also been observed that the sociocultural milieu for adolescent and young women in this country has become progressively unstable, precipitating a range of problems in this age group, including eating disorders.[9,25] Shifting cultural norms for young women have forced them to face multiple, ambiguous, and often contradictory role expectations. Thinness is highly valued, culturally rewarded, and associated with

Box **25-2** *Psychological Characteristics Associated with Eating Disorders*

Anxiety
Compulsivity
Conflict avoidance
Depression
Difficulty expressing feelings, particularly anger
Distorted self-image
Exaggerated sense of guilt
Fear of sexuality and biological maturity
Feelings of alienation
Intolerance for frustration
Low self-esteem
Obsessions
Perfectionism
Poor impulse control
Self-consciousness
Sense of ineffectiveness

FAMILY EDUCATION PLAN Preventing Childhood Eating Problems

Content	Instructional Activities	Evaluation
Describe self-demand feeding and its importance in healthy eating behaviors.	Explore current feeding practices of parents and understanding of healthy eating. Provide information to enhance knowledge of healthy eating behaviors.	Parents will identify healthy eating behaviors and self-demand feeding and begin to explore how their relationship with food influences their children's eating.
Describe physiological and psychological signs of hunger and satiety, as well as the meaning and difference of both types of signs.	Explore parents' own signs of hunger and satiety and have parents describe child's signs.	Parents will keep a hunger diary to record physical and psychological signs of hunger and satiety for themselves and their children.
Describe danger of psychological hunger.	Explain the use of a hunger diary, which is a daily journal regarding signs of hunger.	Parents will be able to distinguish between psychological and physical hunger.
Explore myths about feeding, such as "cleaning the plate" and "eating because other children are starving."	Describe the importance of allowing children to determine their feeding needs and the relationship of healthy eating to the children's ability to differentiate between physical and psychological signs of hunger and satiety. Give homework assignment for each parent to interview three other adults about their current eating practices and memories of eating.	Parents will complete homework assignment, discuss interview experiences, and describe how perpetuating myths about feeding can harm their child.
Implement self-demand feeding at particular developmental stages of children.	Review the eating stages children experience and the potential problems they may have at each stage.	Parents will discuss the developmental stages of their children and plan to implement self-demand feeding.
Discuss parental experiences related to implementing self-demand feeding.	Review parents' expectations and experiences with implementing self-demand feeding.	Parents will relate any problem around self-demand feeding. Nurse will evaluate family for further education and plan for follow-up if necessary.

achievement. The contemporary American ideal woman is lean, strong, graceful, and feminine. One advantage to this profile is its emphasis on fitness and health. A disadvantage is the constant demand this norm places on women to focus on and control their bodies, often as a means for achieving desired goals. The result is intense social pressure on women for self-discipline, rigorous exercise, dieting, and often obsessive concern about weight and body image. The result is that at least 50% of American women are on a diet at any given time, and Americans spend over $5 billion on dieting products alone.

Children, teenagers, and young adults living in communities or going to schools where emphasis is placed on weight and size are often prone to developing eating disorders. Activities or occupations that emphasize beauty or fitness also promote preoccupation with weight and eating behaviors. Ballet dancers, models, actors, athletes, fashion retailers, cooks, and flight attendants all have either tacit or explicit criteria dictated to them concerning body weight and size. These occupations and activities in themselves do not cause eating disorders but they do attract people who may measure their self-esteem, self-worth, and attractiveness by body parameters rather than accomplishments and personal satisfaction.

 Watch television for an evening and count the number of men and women who are overweight. Explain any sociocultural bias you observe.

Precipitating Stressors

Possessing one or more of the predisposing factors previously mentioned puts a person at risk for an eating disorder. People thus predisposed are especially vulnerable to environmental pressures and stress. Lacking an integrated self-concept and realistic body image, they rely on external feedback such as the reactions of others to their appearance and actions. They are unable to perceive or interpret stimuli from within the body, have difficulty describing their feelings and self-concepts, and lack an internal center of initiative and regulation. Thus they must rely on external cues to regulate themselves. Food becomes one of these cues and is used as an external replacement for a deficient internal regulator and inadequate integration of the body and mind.[15]

Appraisal of Stressors

The person is very susceptible to the impact of life stressors, such as the loss of a significant other, interpersonal rejection, and failure. A positive correlation between stress, the severity of binge eating, and one's appraisal of the stressor may also play an important role. Some have suggested that for people predisposed to eating disorders, exercise is not viewed as a way to lose weight but is actually an attempt to experience the reality of their bodies. Controlling their eating or vomiting is another effort at countering the anguish of emptiness, boredom, or tension. Although binge eating may momentarily release this tension, it sets in motion a cycle of binging and purging that, once begun, is very difficult to stop. The importance of a person's appraisal of stressors related to eating disorders is evident in the following clinical example.

Clinical Example Lydia is a 15-year-old female with a 6-year history of binging, a 9-month history of purging, and a 2-year history of restricting her food intake. She is the only child of parents who separated when she was 3 and divorced when she was 6. Her father has a history of frequent mood swings and was later diagnosed and treated for cyclothymic disorder. He had always been overly concerned not only about his bodily appearance but also about the appearance of his family. When Lydia was 9, her father moved to a city 500 miles away, and 2 years later he remarried. Lydia's mother remarried several months after her ex-husband did, but her marriage lasted less than a year. Her husband had concealed an alcohol problem, and Lydia and her mother were verbally abused by this man on many occasions.

After her second divorce, Lydia's mother socialized very little and became overprotective of Lydia. Lydia's mother has often criticized Lydia's father for his extramarital behavior while he was married to her. Lydia's mother had supported the father through college and dental school and was angry about her lowered standard of living since their divorce.

Lydia's parents continue to have a stormy relationship, and she feels caught between them at times. She avoids conflict by siding with her custodial parent, her mother, and avoiding any discussion about her mother with her father. Lydia tries to be the perfect daughter and strives not to displease either parent. She has become very overprotective of her mother and secretly despises her father. She feels that a number of people have hurt her mother and that she and her mother must protect each other. Lydia is afraid to grow up because her mother will be left alone. She states, "I'm the center of my mom's universe. If she's alone, her world will crumble. . . . I'm happiest when I'm worrying about my mom." Lydia does not think she has any eating

problems and is very resistant to treatment. Her parents feel otherwise.
Selected Nursing Diagnoses:
▼ Altered nutrition related to unrealistic self-image, as evidenced by binging, purging, and restricting food
▼ Ineffective denial related to family conflict, as evidenced by overprotection of mother and ambivalence toward father

Coping Resources

One of the most important aspects of the assessment of patients with maladaptive eating regulation responses is their motivation to change behavior. This may be obtained by asking patients to rate their desire for treatment on a scale of 1 to 10, with 10 representing high motivation and 1 low motivation for change. Patients may also be asked to identify the advantages and disadvantages of giving up the behavior, and this information can be used to evaluate a patient's insight, identify coping resources, and stimulate therapeutic issues for future discussion.

The nurse might also inquire into how binging, fasting, and purging serve as a form of coping. Asking patients what precedes these episodes and how they feel afterward are important elements of the nurse's assessment. The patient should also be asked how stress and tension have been handled adaptively in the past and what supports in the environment can be enlisted in the treatment process. These may include family members, friends, work, and leisure activities.

Coping Mechanisms

Anorectic patients are happiest when fasting, losing weight, or achieving their weight goals. Their use of **denial** is severely maladaptive, and they are unlikely to seek help on their own. Concerned family members, primary practitioners, nurses, or school counselors are usually the ones who identify a problem and attempt to obtain help. People with anorexia are usually angry or impatient with the concern shown by others. Interestingly, as the family becomes more distraught about the loss of weight or signs of malnutrition, the anorectic's insistence of normalcy increases. For the patient, the issue is not about weight; it is about control of the anorectic's life and fears. People with anorexia nervosa who fear maturity, independence, failure, sexuality, or parental demands believe they have found a solution to the problem by controlling their food intake and their bodies. With the increasing concerns of the family, the anorectic is now able to control the focus of significant others as well. For the anorectic this seems to be the perfect solution.

The defense mechanisms used by people with bulimia include **avoidance, denial, isolation of affect,** and **intellectualization.** Bulimic patients, regardless of their weight, are usually very upset about their binging and purging behavior. They realize that their behavior is a sign that they are not in control or coping adaptively, but they do not know why. They are more likely to acknowledge that they have a problem than are patients with anorexia nervosa, although they may regard the symptoms as preferable to the prospect of weight gain, and it may be years before the bulimic accepts treatment.

People with binge eating disorder share the bulimic patient's distress about binging, although it is unclear how motivated they are to seek treatment. Obese binge eaters are more likely to seek assistance on their own or be willing to be referred by their primary practitioner.

Nursing Diagnosis

In formulating the nursing diagnosis the nurse should review all aspects of the assessment phase as identified in the Stuart Stress Adaptation Model (Fig. 25-4). Nursing diagnoses related to eating disorders encompass biological, psy-

chological, and sociocultural concerns, and because of the complexity of these disorders, many NANDA nursing diagnoses may be appropriate. Primary NANDA diagnoses for working with patients with maladaptive eating regulation responses include **anxiety, body image disturbance, fluid volume deficit, risk for self-mutilation, altered nutrition, powerlessness,** and **self-esteem disturbance.** The Medical and Nursing Diagnoses box on p. 533 presents nursing diagnoses associated with the range of possible maladaptive eating regulation responses and related medical diagnoses. Primary NANDA nursing diagnoses and examples of complete nursing diagnoses are presented in the Detailed Diagnoses box on p. 534.

Patients with moderate to extreme nutritional deficiencies exhibit symptoms of malnutrition that may be mistakenly related to other causes. Irritability, apathy, depression, obsessiveness, difficulty with concentration, anxiety, de-

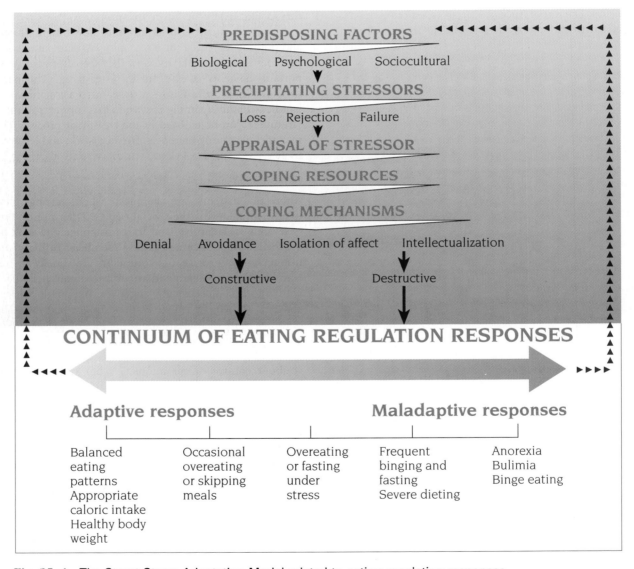

Fig. 25-4 The Stuart Stress Adaptation Model related to eating regulation responses.

creased interest in sex, and negativism are psychological symptoms that usually reverse with adequate nutrition.[14] The nurse may see a very different outward presentation in a patient who is no longer malnourished. Finally, family members may offer important insights into the patient's premorbid functioning and be able to give a clearer picture of the patient's personality before the eating disorder developed.

Related Medical Diagnoses

The medical diagnoses associated with maladaptive eating regulation responses include anorexia nervosa, bulimia nervosa, and binge eating disorder.[2] These medical diagnoses and their essential features are described in the Medical and Nursing Diagnoses box. The key features distinguishing anorexia nervosa from bulimia nervosa are listed in Box 25-3.

Outcome Identification

The expected outcome for the patient with maladaptive eating regulation responses is the following:

The patient will restore healthy eating patterns and normalize physiological parameters related to body weight and nutrition.

For anorectic and bulimic patients, this means that they will be able to eat 100% of all meals, without binging, purging, or engaging in other compensatory behavior. Obese pa-

tients with binge eating disorder should be encouraged to leave something (no more than 5% or less than 2%) on their plate at the end of the meal.

Short-term goals may further specify the steps the patient needs to take to demonstrate adaptive eating regulation responses. These might include the following:

▼ The patient will identify cognitive distortions about food, weight, and body shape.
▼ The patient will develop a week's menu of nutritionally balanced meals.
▼ The patient will accurately describe body dimensions.
▼ The patient will exercise in moderate amounts only when nutritionally and medically stable.
▼ The patient will demonstrate positive family interactions and successful movement toward achievement of separation and individuation issues.

Planning

Choice of Treatment Setting

Nursing care varies to some degree based on the treatment setting of the patient with maladaptive eating regulation responses. A number of factors affect the choice of treatment setting, including the patient's physical and psychological condition, financial resources, availability of treatment specialists, and patient preference. Clinical criteria for inpatient treatment of eating disorders are listed in Box 25-4.

 MEDICAL AND NURSING DIAGNOSES *related to* **Eating Regulation Responses**

Related Medical Diagnoses (DSM-IV)*	Related Nursing Diagnoses (NANDA)†
Anorexia nervosa	**Anxiety**‡
Binge eating disorder	**Body Image Disturbance**‡
Bulimia nervosa	Decisional conflict
	Denial, ineffective
	Family process, altered
	Fatigue
	Fluid Volume Deficit‡
	Growth and development, altered
	Risk for injury
	Risk for Self-mutilation‡
	Hopelessness
	Individual coping, ineffective
	Nutrition, Altered‡
	Personal identity disturbance
	Powerlessness‡
	Role performance, altered
	Self-esteem Disturbance‡
	Sexual dysfunction
	Social interaction, impaired
	Thought process, altered

*From American Psychiatric Association: *Diagnostic and statistical manual of mental disorders,* ed 4, Washington, DC, 1994, The Association.
†From North American Nursing Diagnosis Association: *NANDA nursing diagnoses: definitions and classifications 1997-1998,* Philadelphia, 1997, The Association.
‡Primary nursing diagnosis for eating problems.

DETAILED DIAGNOSES *related to* **Eating Regulation Responses**

NANDA Diagnosis Stem	Examples of Complete Diagnosis
Anxiety	Anxiety related to fear of weight gain, as evidenced by rituals associated with food preparation and eating.
Body image disturbance	Body image disturbance related to fear of weight gain, as evidenced by verbalization of being "fat" while actually being 30% below ideal body weight.
Fluid volume deficit	Fluid volume deficit related to purging activities, as evidenced by weakness, poor skin turgor, hypokalemia, and hypotension.
Risk for self-mutilation	Risk for self-mutilation related to feelings of inadequacy, as evidenced by injuries caused by excessive exercise and self-induced vomiting.
Nutrition, altered	Altered nutrition related to excessive intake of calories, as evidenced by being 40% above ideal body weight, sleep apnea, and difficulty with mobility.
Powerlessness	Powerlessness related to perceived lack of control over eating behaviors, as evidenced by inability to stop binge eating and avoidance of food-related settings.
Self-esteem disturbance	Self-esteem disturbance related to feelings of low self-worth, as evidenced by verbalization of sole standard of success being related to physical attractiveness.
DSM-IV Diagnosis	**Essential Features***
Anorexia nervosa	An intense fear of gaining weight, even when underweight. There is a disturbance in the way the body is experienced and a refusal to maintain body weight above a minimal normal weight for age and height, leading to a body weight 15% below expected. In females there is also the absence of at least three consecutive menstrual cycles.
Bulimia nervosa	Recurrent episodes of binge eating with a feeling of lack of control over the eating behavior and persistent overconcern with body shape and weight. The person also regularly engages in self-induced vomiting, use of laxatives, or rigorous dieting and fasting to counteract the effects of binge eating.
Binge eating disorder	Recurrent episodes of binging that are a cause of distress, with a feeling of lack of control over the eating behavior but without behaviors used to prevent weight gain.

*Modified from the American Psychiatric Association: *Diagnostic and statistical manual of mental disorders,* ed 4, Washington, DC, 1994, The Association.

Box **25-3** *Key Features of Anorexia Nervosa and Bulimia Nervosa*

Anorexia Nervosa	**Bulimia Nervosa**
Rare vomiting or diuretic/laxative abuse	Frequent vomiting or diuretic/laxative abuse
More severe weight loss	Less weight loss
Slightly younger	Slightly older
More introverted	More extroverted
Hunger denied	Hunger experienced
Eating behavior may be considered normal and source of esteem	Eating behavior considered foreign and source of distress
Sexually inactive	More sexually active
Obsessional and perfectionistic features predominate	Avoidant, dependent, or borderline features as well as obsessional features
Death from starvation (or suicide, in chronically ill)	
Amenorrhea	Death from hypokalemia or suicide
More favorable prognosis	Menses irregular or absent
Fewer behavioral abnormalities (these increase with level of severity)	Less favorable prognosis
	Stealing, drug and alcohol abuse, self-mutilation, and other behavioral abnormalities

From Andersen AE: *Practical comprehensive treatment of anorexia nervosa and bulimia,* Baltimore, 1985, Johns Hopkins University Press.

Outpatient treatment may be the best setting because it allows the patient the greatest opportunity for self-control and autonomy. It requires a high level of patient motivation, the active support and involvement of family members, and ongoing physiological monitoring. Contingencies for outpatient treatment should be mutually agreed on expectations of behavioral change, including weight gain and decreased binging or purging, and the acceptance of inpatient or more intense day treatment programs if the patient is not making progress.

Box *25-4* *Clinical Criteria for Hospitalization of Patients with an Eating Disorder*

MEDICAL

Need for extensive diagnostic evaluation
Weight loss greater than 30% of body weight over 3 months
Heart rate less than 40 beats/min
Temperature less than 36° C or 96.8° F
Systolic blood pressure less than 70 mm Hg
Serum potassium less than 2.5 meq/L despite oral potassium replacement
Severe dehydration
Concurrent somatic illnesses (such as infection)

PSYCHIATRIC

Risk of suicide or self-mutilation
Severe depression
Psychosis
Family crisis
Failure to comply with treatment contract
Inadequate response to outpatient treatment

Recently, with the advent of managed care initiatives, outpatient settings, including day treatment or partial hospitalization programs, have become the standard treatment settings. This is because of the unavailability of reimbursement for inpatient programs except under dangerous or severe conditions, such as suicidal intent. Another advantage to inpatient treatment is the availability of 24-hour nursing care to ensure patient safety, support needed behavioral change, and monitor physiological responses. Patients with eating disorders can present a unique challenge to staff, and care requires a high level of interdisciplinary collaboration, coordination, and consistency.

Nurse-patient Contract

Nurse-patient contracts can be formulated for patients with eating disorders who are seen in either inpatient or outpatient settings. The terms of the contract may vary, but the goal is the same: to engage the patient in a therapeutic alliance and obtain commitment to the treatment process.

Before a patient is admitted to an eating disorder treatment program, it is advisable to secure the patient's cooperation in treatment with a nurse-patient contract. By signing such a contract, patients will understand the treatment they will be receiving and be able to make informed decisions about their commitment to the treatment process and their ability to honor the contract.

? *How would you respond to a patient who wants to receive treatment for an eating disorder but does not want to sign the nurse-patient contract because it is "too restrictive"?*

CRITICAL THINKING *about* Contemporary Issues

Should Tube Feeding Be a Component of an Eating Disorders Treatment Program?

The positive and negative consequences of nasogastric tube feeding or even total parenteral nutrition for patients with an eating disorder have been debated among clinicians and researchers. Current guidelines recommend that refeeding interventions should be used only rarely and in life-threatening situations.[1] Specifically, there is recognition of the danger of rapid refeeding, which includes severe fluid retention and cardiac failure, and of forced nasogastric or parenteral feeding. Thus these procedures should not be used routinely. However, some severely malnourished anorectic patients may accept nasogastric feeding more willingly than eating, especially in the early stages of renourishment.

If forced feeding is to be considered, careful thought should be given to the patient's clinical condition, the patient's and family's opinion, and legal and ethical dimensions of the patient's treatment. Each of these areas merits a full discussion by the interdisciplinary health-care team, and treatment decisions should include specific timelines, outcomes, and alternatives.

Implementation

Nutritional Stabilization

Stabilizing the patient's nutritional status is a high priority for nursing intervention. Healthy target weights and expected rates of controlled weight gain or loss should be established. In life-threatening circumstances, patients who are malnourished may need refeeding interventions (see Critical Thinking about Contemporary Issues), but these cases are exceptional. In an inpatient setting, specific nursing interventions to promote weight stabilization and restore healthy eating patterns can be facilitated by program protocols that identify treatment goals, program components, and patient and staff responsibilities.[6] Some of these might include the following:

▼ The time, frequency, and procedure for weighing the patient and whether the patient may see the weight
▼ The time when meals will be served and how many meals are to be eaten each day
▼ How the staff is to interact with the patient during mealtimes to maximize their therapeutic value
▼ The amount of time the patient will be allowed to spend eating each meal, and the consequences if the meal is not completed
▼ Whether diet foods, condiments, or food substitutions are allowed
▼ The amount of water the patient may drink each day
▼ The frequency of obtaining the patient's vital signs, intake and output, and required laboratory work
▼ Times when visitors are allowed on the unit
▼ Conditions regarding bathroom privileges
▼ Indications for close observation by staff

Once inpatients are able to master their meals, they can move toward more independence with eating and food selection. Selecting their own menus with assistance is next. The patient can then progress to selecting food from the hospital cafeteria, followed by shopping for and cooking food with supervision. By discharge the patient should have gained a high level of comfort with food and its preparation.

For anorectic outpatients, stabilizing their nutrition and promoting weight gain usually require a motivated patient and cooperative family. Obtaining the patient's agreement to stop trying to lose weight is the first obstacle the nurse must overcome because patients are often very resistant to such an idea. Getting an anorectic patient to gain weight is an even more difficult task. Nurse-patient contracts can be effective tools with these patients because their need for control of food is so great. For example, the nurse and anorectic patient may set a realistic goal of gaining 1 pound per week. If the patient fails to gain 4 pounds in a month, the contract would stipulate that the patient would agree to enter a hospital, day treatment program, or some other more intensive type of care.

Counseling about healthy eating patterns and behaviors is an essential aspect of nursing care for all patients, regardless of whether they need to gain, lose, or maintain weight. The nurse should also clarify with patients the effect of poor nutrition on the body. Collaboration with a dietitian may be helpful in teaching patients about proper eating habits, as well as in planning menus with patients. Nurses should teach, clarify, and reinforce knowledge about proper nutrition and the importance of planning healthy meals using the recommended servings from each of the five food groups. Patients should be encouraged to make shopping lists, and the nurse may even accompany the patient to the grocery store. Nutritional assessment, education, and ongoing support are essential nursing care activities.

The patient who is struggling with major issues around food will not be ready for intensive psychological interventions. As the patient is feeling less need to be in control of food and eating, issues underlying the eating disorder may start to surface. This can be a difficult time for the patient, who may actually begin to feel worse than when treatment began. If a patient is in the hospital or a partial hospitalization program, there is someone available to talk with, but this is not always true for the outpatient. Thus the outpatient may need more frequent sessions with the nurse or more phone contacts between sessions. However, when sufficient progress has been made toward nutritional rehabilitation, the patient will be better prepared both cognitively and emotionally to begin the next phase of treatment.

Exercise

As the patient's eating increases, the need to increase exercise or engage in a new purging or compensatory behavior also increases. On an inpatient or partial hospitalization unit the patient can be closely monitored to prevent such compensatory activity. However, as the patient stabilizes and responds to treatment it is often appropriate to begin a gradual exercise program. For some patients who exercise compulsively, this can be the most difficult period of treatment. The nurse should initially allow patients limited amounts of exercise, with gradual increases over time. The focus of the exercise program should be on physical fitness rather than working off calories.[33] Consultation with a recreational therapist or exercise physiologist may be helpful to maximize the therapeutic value of the exercise regimen.

Cognitive Behavioral Interventions

Across many studies for a period of 5 years, cognitive-behavioral therapy significantly reduced the binging and purging episodes of patients with eating disorders when compared with other treatment approaches.[17] It is important for the nurse to work with patients around their cognitive distortions and faulty thinking about body shape, weight, and food. Box 25-5 presents a list of cognitive distortions common among patients with eating disorders and an example of each. Cognitive behavioral therapy is discussed in detail in Chapter 30.

Helping the patient to become aware of these thoughts is the first step in changing them. The patient should be asked to monitor and record eating, binging, and purging behav-

---

Box **25-5** *Cognitive Distortions Related to Maladaptive Eating Regulation Responses*

Magnification: Overestimation of the significance of undesirable events. Stimuli are embellished with meaning not supported by objective analysis. "I've gained 2 pounds, so I can't wear shorts any more."

Superstitious thinking: Believing in the cause-effect relationship of noncontingent events. "If I eat a sweet, it will instantly be turned into stomach fat."

Dichotomous or all-or-none thinking: Thinking in extreme or absolute terms such that events can only be black or white, right or wrong, good or bad. "If I gain 1 pound, I'll go on to gain 100 pounds."

Overgeneralization: Extracting a rule on the basis of one event and applying it to other dissimilar situations. "I used to be of normal weight and I wasn't happy. So I know gaining weight isn't going to make me feel better."

Selective abstraction: Basing a conclusion on isolated details while ignoring contradictory and more important evidence. "The only way I can be in control is through eating."

Personalization and self-reference: Egocentric interpretations of impersonal events or overinterpretation of events related to the self. "Two people laughed and whispered something to each other when I walked by. They were probably saying that I looked unattractive. I have gained 3 pounds."

From Garner D, Bemis K: Cognitive therapy for anorexia nervosa. In Garner D, Garfinkle P, editors: *Handbook of psychotherapy for anorexia and bulimia nervosa*, New York, 1985, Guilford.

ior and thoughts and feelings regarding weight, shape, and food.[8] The goal of these exercises is for the patient to better understand the following:

▼ The cues that trigger problematic eating responses
▼ The thoughts, feelings, and assumptions associated with the specific cues
▼ The connection between these thoughts, feelings, assumptions and eating regulation responses
▼ The consequences resulting from the eating responses

CUES. Cues that trigger maladaptive eating behavior can be social, situational, physiological, and psychological. Examples of social cues are loneliness, interpersonal conflict, social awkwardness, and holiday celebrations. Examples of situational cues include observation of diet advertisements and walking by a store that sells a food conducive to binging. Hunger and fatigue are the two most common physiological cues. Memory and mental images are two examples of psychological cues.

Specific cues such as these can trigger cognitive distortions and lead to maladaptive eating regulation responses. For example, when stepping on the scale a patient may see that she has gained a pound. She then may use dichotomous thinking: "Since I've gained 1 pound, I will probably gain 20 pounds in the next week. I better take a package of laxatives so that I can lose the pound by tomorrow."

▼ Stepping on the scale is the cue.
▼ Believing she will gain 20 pounds is the related irrational thought.
▼ Taking the laxatives is the maladaptive eating regulation response connected to the cognitive distortion.
▼ Beginning another purge cycle is the consequence resulting from the maladaptive response.

Cues can be used as a strategy for change. Rearranging cues, avoiding a cue, and changing the response to a cue are ways of altering maladaptive responses. After continued learning about eating, binging, and purging behavior, and thoughts and feelings about food, shape, and weight, it is hoped that the patient will begin to see connections between thoughts and behaviors and recognize the consequences of the harmful activity.

THOUGHTS, FEELINGS, AND ASSUMPTIONS. The nurse helps patients challenge their faulty thoughts, feelings, and assumptions by questioning the evidence supporting or refuting the particular belief. In the previous example, the nurse might ask the patient what specifically happened in the past when she gained a pound. Did she gain 19 more pounds in the same week? If so, how often has it happened in the past? If not, why does the patient believe it will happen this time? It is also important for the nurse to ask the patient about the implications of this type of thinking. Do other people have the same problem if they gain a pound? If so, how do they deal with it? The nurse can help the patient consider alternative explanations for his or her thoughts, and thereby gradually modify the irrational assumptions that underlie these beliefs. This is an example

of the cognitive intervention of decentering.[8] These and other cognitive behavioral techniques may be successfully used in patients with maladaptive eating regulation responses (see A Patient Speaks).

EATING REGULATION RESPONSES. Patients with eating disorders need help in problem solving and making decisions. Rather than resorting to maladaptive responses, the patient must be helped to distinguish between adaptive and maladaptive coping responses and find alternative solutions.

One way of doing this is to encourage the patient to make a list of high-risk situations that cue maladaptive eating and purging behavior. The high-risk situation may be a certain day of the week, time of the day, season of the year, person, group, event, or emotional response, such as anger or frustration. The nurse can then help the patient identify specific alternative ways of handling these high-risk situations that are more adaptive.

Decision-making strategies also may need to be reviewed and modified. Many patients with eating disorders know what they need to do in a given situation but may feel inad-

A **Patient** *Speaks*

Learning to separate my feelings from my eating has been the hardest part but the greatest benefit of treatment for my eating disorder. From early childhood, food had been my main outlet for almost every emotion. When I was sad, I comforted myself by eating. When I was happy, I celebrated by eating. Feelings of loneliness could be diminished by gathering up all my "food friends" and eating. Feeling angry at anyone beside myself was unacceptable, so I would eat and then I had a "good reason" to be angry and focus it all on myself.

Discovering that everything in life is not black or white, good or bad, perfect or imperfect, hungry or full has enabled me to be kinder to myself and more accepting of my imperfections and humanity. I now realize that shades of gray do exist when making a decision, performing a task, feeling an emotion, and even experiencing hunger. Another benefit of this insight is a decrease in my level of anxiety along with feelings of worthlessness.

Each day is no longer a battle to control all aspects of my life, especially my food consumption. The struggle with food and my weight still remains, but now it doesn't completely overshadow everything else that happens in my life. Food is no longer the only friend and enemy life offers. I learned all this from a nurse who took the time to get to know me and in turn helped me to get to know myself. ▼

equate or shy about carrying out a certain plan of action. These people may benefit from assertiveness training and role modeling sessions with the nurse.

Consequences. It is particularly important for the nurse and patient to explore the positive and negative consequences that result from the cognitive distortion and maladaptive response. Consequences can be biological, psychological, and sociocultural, and there are positive and negative consequences resulting from each behavior. Some of these are presented in Table 25-2. A maladaptive behavior such as binging is maintained because positive consequences are more immediate or more valued than the negative consequences.

Strategies for change focusing on consequences involve the use of rewards that increase the likelihood of behavior change. In the example in which the laxatives were taken in response to a 1-pound weight gain, rewards would be given if the person was able to resist taking the laxative. The reward should be received immediately following the desired behavior change. It should be something pleasurable and can be either a material item or a psychological reinforcer, but it should not involve food.

 Should overweight nurses be assigned to care for patients with eating disorders? Why or why not?

Body Image Interventions

Body image distortions are one of the most difficult aspects of the eating disorder to treat. This is partly because researchers disagree on what exactly constitutes a body image distortion. The only agreement is that body image distortion in the eating disorders involves perceptual, attitudinal, and behavioral features[7] (Fig. 25-5). One also needs to distinguish between body image distortion and dissatisfaction.

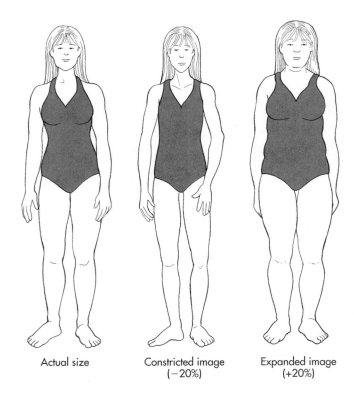

Actual size — Constricted image (−20%) — Expanded image (+20%)

Fig. 25-5 The perception of body shape and size can be evaluated through the use of special computer drawing programs that allow a subject to distort the width of an actual picture of a person's body by as much as 20% larger or smaller. Both anorectic and normal subjects adjusted the figures of other people's bodies to normal dimension. However, anorectic subjects consistently adjusted their own body picture to a size 20% larger than its true form, suggesting that they have a major problem with the perception of self-image. (Modified from Bloom F, Lazerson A: *Brain, mind, and behavior,* New York, 1988, WH Freeman.)

TABLE 25-2 *Consequences of Maladaptive Eating Regulation Responses*

	POSITIVE CONSEQUENCES	NEGATIVE CONSEQUENCES
Biological	Reduced fear of fatness	Weakness, fatigue, dizziness
	Reduced perception of hunger	Poor concentration
	Avoidance of biological maturity	Electrolyte disturbance
		Dental problems
Psychological	Relief from tension, anger, and stress	Depression, guilt, shame
	Relief from boredom	Tendency to overreact emotionally
	Emotional anesthesia	Increase in negative self-reference or guilt-related behavior
	Feelings of nurturance or pleasure	
	Thoughts about avoiding weight gain	
Sociocultural	Avoidance of interpersonal conflict	Social withdrawal
	Social reinforcement for not gaining weight	Lying and lack of trust in relationships
	Distraction from unpleasant tasks	Occupational problems
	Avoidance of responsibility and independence	Financial problems
		Legal problems

Modified from the University of Minnesota's Intensive Group Outpatient Treatment for Bulimia.

Body image distortion is a discrepancy between the patient's actual and perceived body size. Body dissatisfaction is the degree of unhappiness that a person feels in relation to body size.

All people at sometime in their lives may express dissatisfaction with their bodies, but the bulimic or anorectic person's dissatisfaction is constant. People with eating disorders place so much value on their appearance that it begins to exclusively define their self-worth. Behavioral features of body image disturbance are manifested in a lifestyle that revolves around a person's self-concern about the body. Examples of this range from constant weight measurement, wearing baggy clothes, and avoiding social situations in which the person might be scrutinized about appearance. Overestimation of body size or of a body part is a common perceptual distortion in anorexia and bulimia.

A variety of interventions have been suggested for treating body image problems.[7] It is important for the nurse to first determine whether the patient has problems in perception, attitude, or behavior and then devise a treatment program targeting the specific problem area. Cognitive behavioral interventions are effective, as are dance and movement therapies, which create pleasant body experiences and can enhance the integration of mind and body, clarify body boundaries, and modulate negative feelings about the body.[20] Other therapeutic approaches include the use of imagery and relaxation, working with mirrors, and depicting self through art. Researchers agree that body image interventions are crucial to the treatment of eating disorders, and there is much ongoing research in this area.

Family Involvement

Families should be engaged from the beginning of treatment and included in family meetings and treatment planning sessions. The nurse should gather information about the family system and explore how the maladaptive eating response might serve a specific function within the family. Questions the nurse might ask include the following:

▼ What part does the eating disorder serve in stabilizing the family system?
▼ How has the family attempted to deal with the eating disorder?
▼ What is the central theme surrounding the eating behavior?
▼ What would be the consequences of change for each family member?
▼ What is the underlying therapeutic issue from a family perspective?

Many young patients may need intensive family therapy after they have successfully completed the refeeding stage. The initial issue of such therapy is centered on the separation and individuation of the patient within the context of the family. This process requires much openness on the part of the family, and not every family may be able to complete it. However, the nurse should work with family strengths that have been identified and help involved family members work toward change (see A Family Speaks). Family therapy is described in more detail in Chapter 32.

Group Therapies

Many models of group therapy are used for patients with eating disorders, including cognitive behavioral, psychoeducational, psychodynamic, and interpersonal. Reality testing, supporting, and communicating with peers are essential therapeutic factors provided by group intervention. In addition, outpatient support groups may also be helpful if they reinforce social alliances and encourage members to identify and express feelings.[19,24] Therapeutic groups are described in detail in Chapter 31.

Medications

Anorectic patients often resist medication, and no drugs have been found to be completely effective for this disorder. Medications that may be helpful for some patients include antidepressants for patients who are still depressed despite refeeding and antianxiety agents used before meals for anticipatory anxiety concerning eating. An antidepressant

A **Family** *Speaks*

We have a 19-year-old daughter who has had an eating disorder for 8 years. The past 8 years have been most painful for our family as we went from doctor to doctor, counselor to counselor, and therapist to therapist, all with little or no results. What clinicians don't realize is how hard the day-to-day struggle is for families who want so much for their child to be healthy and happy, but who feel so helpless in how to make this happen.

Then we were referred to a nurse who specialized in eating disorders, and slowly our lives began to change. Clearly, this nurse knew about our daughter's illness and together we went about treating it. We went through individual and family therapy, all in an attempt to help our daughter recover. At times it was painful and even frustrating. In the family sessions the nurse helped family members be aware of the part they had to play in our daughter's struggle and helped us realize that it would take a family team effort to help her get well. But the most important part is that all of the hard work of our daughter, each family member, and our nurse has been worth it. Our daughter now knows how to control her eating disorder, she has had very few problems in the last 6 months, and our family has become even closer as we look back on the past with relief and into the future with hope. ▼

NURSING TREATMENT PLAN *Summary* Eating Regulation Responses

Nursing Diagnosis: Altered nutrition
Expected Outcome: The patient will restore healthy patterns and normalize physiological parameters related to body weight and nutrition.

Short-term Goals	Interventions	Rationale
The patient will engage in treatment and acknowledge having an eating disorder.	Help patient identify maladaptive eating responses. Discuss positive and negative consequences of maladaptive eating responses. Contract with patient to engage in treatment.	The first step of treatment is for the patient to acknowledge the illness and see the need for help.
The patient will be able to describe a balanced diet based on the five food groups.	Complete a nutritional assessment including eating-related behaviors and preferences. Teach, clarify, and reinforce knowledge of proper nutrition.	Knowledge of healthy nutrition is essential to establishing and maintaining adaptive eating responses.
The patient's nutritional status will be stabilized by a specified date.	Monitor physiological status for signs of compromised nutrition. Administer medications and somatic treatments for management of symptoms. Monitor and evaluate the patient's response to somatic treatments. Implement nursing activities as specified in the program contract and protocol.	Weight stabilization must be a central and early goal for the nutritionally compromised patient. Medications may assist the appetite regulation center and neurochemical responses to feeding and satiety.
The patient will participate in a balanced exercise program on a daily basis.	Review established exercise routines. Modify exercise patterns, focusing on physical fitness rather than weight reduction. Reinforce new exercise and fitness behaviors.	The focus of a balanced exercise program should be on physical fitness rather than caloric reduction to lose weight.

Nursing Diagnosis: Body image disturbance
Expected Outcome: The patient will express clear and accurate descriptions of body size, body boundaries, and ideal weight.

Short-term Goals	Interventions	Rationale
The patient will correct body image distortions.	Modify body image misperceptions through cognitive and behavioral strategies. Use dance and movement therapies to enhance the integration of mind and body. Use imagery and relaxation interventions to decrease anxiety related to body perceptions.	Body image distortions involve perceptions, attitudes, and behaviors that place so much emphasis on appearance that they define self-worth.
The patient will modify cognitive distortions about body weight, shape, and eating responses.	Help patient identify cues that trigger problematic eating responses and body image concerns; thoughts, feelings, and assumptions associated with each cue; connections between these thoughts, feelings, assumptions and eating regulation responses; and the consequences of the eating responses.	Cognitive distortions result in lowered self-esteem. Behavioral change results from increased awareness of feelings and faulty cognitions.
The patient will identify social support systems that will reinforce accurate body perceptions and adaptive eating responses.	Include family members in the evaluation and treatment planning process. Assess the family as a system and the impact of the eating disorder on family functioning. Initiate group therapy to mobilize social support and reinforce adaptive responses.	Patients with eating disorders benefit from the involvement of family members and supportive group work.

medication may also be helpful with comorbid depression, mood swings or irritability, and obsessions about food and fat.[30] In the treatment of bulimia, studies have shown that antidepressant medications appear to have therapeutic benefit in a majority of patients. Medication-induced benefits include decreases in frequency of binge eating and weight regulatory behaviors such as vomiting. Antidepressants such as TCAs (imipramine, desipramine), SSRIs (fluoxetine), and MAOIs (phenelzine) have been studied and have demonstrated efficacy in the treatment of eating disorders and should be used in conjunction with other therapeutic interventions. Most of the medications that have been used in the treatment of bulimia have also been used in binge eating disorder with some success.[31] More research is needed regarding psychopharmacologic treatments in these patients.

The Nursing Treatment Plan Summary for patients with maladaptive eating regulation responses is presented at left.

Evaluation

Patients with maladaptive eating regulation responses present special challenges to psychiatric nursing care. The evaluation of their care should begin with a focus on the therapeutic nurse-patient relationship. Nurses should determine whether they provided effective role modeling, emotional support, biological monitoring, and reinforcement of the patient's attempts to explore and experiment with new cognitive and behavior patterns. Evaluation activities can then address three specific aspects of care:

▼ Have normal eating patterns been restored?

▼ Have the biological and psychological sequelae of malnutrition been corrected?

▼ Have the associated sociocultural and behavioral problems been resolved so that relapse does not occur?

In answering these questions the nurse should review each aspect of the nursing process and modify care as needed to achieve the identified outcomes.

COMPETENT CARING A Clinical Exemplar of a Psychiatric Nurse

Debra L. Davis, RN

It seemed like a typically busy but uneventful day on our adult inpatient unit. After lunch, patients who had been participating in a group therapy session began returning to the unit. However, one patient was not with the group. Upon inquiring I discovered that Miss G, a 22-year-old patient with an eating disorder, had failed to attend the group session. I told the charge nurse of her absence and, almost simultaneously, the phone rang informing us that someone had been spotted standing on top of our building. I went outside and encountered a security officer, whom I followed to the site of the report. Sure enough, there on top of the three-story building was Miss G, who was saying she intended to jump.

As a staff nurse, I instantly assessed the situation as an emergency and knew that someone had to assume immediate crisis management. I also realized that my considerable tenure as a mental health technician, licensed practical nurse, and now registered nurse, would lend itself to the task. Certainly, I had faced many crises during my years in the mental health field, but none was more perilous than this one, and none had begged for quicker or more decisive action.

In horror, I fixed my gaze on the patient, her toes draped over the edge of the building some 60 feet above the ground. Her precariously positioned frame was teetering, and her state of mind seemed to be of similar disposition. Miss G again

threatened to jump and continued to repeat her desire to "end it all."

I yelled up to her and asked what could I do to reduce her distress. She asked to see Shelley, a staff member who had established a therapeutic relationship with Miss G and was someone she obviously trusted. I successfully bargained with the patient to step back from the edge of the building and sit down while I ran inside to get Shelley. I then directed the security officers to summon the mobile crisis unit to help. In the interim, I knew we had to continue efforts to retrieve the distressed patient. "Someone's got to go in the building and try to reach that roof," I said to Drew, another staff member who was on the scene. He agreed and quickly hurried off to find a way up. Extremely anxious that Miss G would either jump or accidentally fall, Shelley and I, along with some security personnel, dragged mattresses outside and placed them beneath where Miss G was standing.

Shelley began to communicate with the patient via a bullhorn, talking about the progress that Miss G had made and the plans she was looking forward to as they had previously discussed. Suddenly, as we watched, a pair of arms wrapped around Miss G and pulled her back from the edge of the building. Drew had found access to the roof and had snatched the patient back to safety. Applause erupted on the ground, and with the help of the mobile crisis unit and the security officers, Miss G was lowered to the ground and escorted back to the unit.

Those of us involved in the crisis removed ourselves from the scene, and uninvolved staff began postcrisis management interventions on the unit. I breathed deeply and felt the muscles in my neck relax for the first time in hours. So much for a typically busy but eventful day in psychiatric nursing.

Summary

1. Adaptive eating regulation responses include balanced eating patterns, caloric intake, and weight. Maladaptive responses include anorexia nervosa, bulimia nervosa, and binge eating disorder.

2. The majority of the maladaptive eating disorders occur in females and may range from 1% to 4% of adolescent and young adult women.

3. Patient behaviors related to eating regulation responses include binge eating, fasting or restricting, purging, and related medical and psychiatric complications.

4. Predisposing factors for eating regulation responses are described from biological, psychological, and sociocultural perspectives. Precipitating stressors that affect eating responses include peer pressure, interpersonal rejection, and daily solitude.

5. Level of motivation to change behavior is an important coping resource to assess. A variety of maladaptive coping mechanisms may be used including avoidance, intellectualization, isolation of affect, and denial.

6. Primary NANDA nursing diagnoses are anxiety, body image disturbance, fluid volume deficit, risk for self-mutilation, altered nutrition, powerlessness, and self-esteem disturbance.

7. Primary DSM-IV diagnoses are anorexia nervosa, bulimia nervosa, and binge eating disorder.

8. The expected outcome of nursing care is that the patient will restore healthy eating patterns and normalize physiological parameters related to body weight and nutrition.

9. Planning activities involves decisions related to choice of treatment setting and the formulation of a nursing care plan contract.

10. Interventions include nutrition stabilization, exercise, cognitive behavioral interventions, body image interventions, family involvement, group therapies, and medications.

11. The nurse and patient should evaluate whether normal eating patterns have been restored and associated biopsychosocial problems have been resolved.

your **INTERNET**
c o n n e c t i o n

Anorexia Nervosa and Bulimia Association
http://qlink.queensu.ca/~4map/anabhome.htm

The Something Fishy Web Site on Eating Disorders
http://www.something-fishy.com/ed.htm

Chapter
Review
Questions

1. **Match each term in Column A with the correct definition in Column B.**

Column A	Column B
___Maladaptive eating regulation responses	A. Balanced eating patterns, caloric intake, weight
___SSRIs	B. Neurotransmitter implicated in eating disorders
___Adaptive eating regulation responses	C. Anorexia, bulimia, binge eating
___Predisposing factors	D. Treatments for eating disorders
___Serotonin	E. Biological, psychological, environmental, sociocultural

2. **Fill in the blanks.**

A. The majority of eating disorders occur in _____, and they may range from _____% to _____ % of adolescents and young adults.

B. _____ is the rapid consumption of large quantities food in a discrete period of time.

C. Maladaptive coping mechanisms that may affect motivation for change in eating patterns and therefore must be assessed by the nurse include _____, _____, _____, and _____.

D. Several primary NANDA nursing diagnoses for a patient with an eating disorder are _____, _____, and _____.

E. The treatment for eating disorders that targets faulty thinking about food, body shape, weight, and food-related behaviors is _____.

3. **Provide short answers for the following questions.**

A. What are the differences in obese nonbingers, obese bingers, and nonobese bulimic patients regarding amount of binging, purging, and mood disturbance?

B. What is the expected outcome of nursing care for the patient with an eating disorder?

C. Keep a food diary for 1 week and list your thoughts about each meal. Ask a friend/classmate to evaluate it.

D. Design an eating disorder treatment contract that would help to improve your eating patterns and one that you think would be helpful for one of your friends or colleagues. What are the essential differences between the two?

E. How would you explain the differences in cultural support and stigma for the person with obesity and for the person with anorexia nervosa?

REFERENCES

1. American Psychiatric Association: Practice guidelines for eating disorders, *Am J Psychiatry* 150:207, 1993.
2. American Psychiatric Association: *Diagnostic and statistical manual of mental disorders*, ed 4, Washington, DC, 1994, The Association.
3. Brewerton TD: Toward a unified theory of serotonin dysregulation in eating and related disorders, *Psychoneuroendocrinology* 20:6, 1995.
4. Brewerton TD, Dansky BS, O'Neil PM, Kilpatrick DG: *Prevalence of binge eating disorder in U.S. women,* Paper presented at the American Psychiatric Association's Annual Meeting, San Francisco, May 1993.
5. Bulik CM: Abuse of drugs associated with eating disorders, *J Subst Abuse Treat* 4:69, 1992.
6. Cahill C: Implementing an inpatient eating disorders program, *Perspect Psychiatr Care* 30:3, 1994.
7. Cash T, Pruzinsky T: *Body images: development and deviance,* New York, 1990, Guilford.
8. Fairburn C: Eating disorders. In Hawton K et al, editors: *Cognitive behavior therapy for psychiatric problems*, Oxford, 1989, Oxford University Press.
9. Fontaine KL: The conspiracy of culture: women's issues in body size, *Nurs Clin North Am* 26:669, 1991.
10. Freund KM, Graham SM, Lesky LG, Moskowitz MA: Detection of bulimia in a primary care setting, *J Gen Intern Med* 8:236, 1993.
11. Hoek HW, Bartelds IM, et al: Impact of urbanization on detection rates of eating disorders, *Am J Psychiatry* 152:1272, 1995.
12. Hofland SL, Dardis PO: Bulimia nervosa: associated physical problems, *J Psychosoc Nurs Ment Health Serv* 30:23, 1992.
13. Kanter RA, Williams BE, Cummings C: Personal and parental alcohol abuse and victimization in obese bingers and the non-binging obese, *Addict Behav* 17:439, 1992.
14. Kaplin AS, Katz M: Medical illness associated with weight loss. In Kaplin AS, Garfinkle PE, editors: *Medical issues and the eating disorders: the interface*, New York, 1993, Brunner/Mazel.
15. Krueger DW: Eating disorders: a model developmental arrest of body self and psychological self. In *Body self and psychological self: a developmental and clinical integration of the disorders of the self*, New York, 1992, Brunner/Mazel.
16. Laraia MT, Stuart GW: Bulimia: a review of nutritional and health behaviors, *J Child Adolesc Psychiatr Nurs* 3:91, 1990.
17. McGowan A, Whitbread J: Out of control! The most effective way to help the binge-eating patient, *J Psychosoc Nurs* 34:30, 1996.
18. Olivardia R, Pope HG, et al: Eating disorders in college men, *Am J Psychiatry* 152:1279, 1995.
19. Owen SV, Fullerton ML: Would it make a difference? A discussion group in a behaviorally oriented inpatient eating disorder program, *J Psychosoc Nurs* 33:35, 1995.
20. Rice J, Hardenbergh M, Hornyak L: Disturbed body image in anorexia nervosa: dance/movement therapy interventions. In Hornyak L, Baker E, editors: *Experiential therapies for the eating disorders*, New York, 1989, Guilford.
21. Schuckit MA, Tipp JE, Anthenelli RM, et al: Anorexia nervosa and bulimia nervosa in alcohol-dependent men and women and their relatives, *Am J Psychiatry* 153:1, 1996.
22. Spitzer RL et al: Binge eating disorder: a multisite field trial of the diagnostic criteria, *Int J Eating Disord* 11:191, 1991.
23. Srinivasagam NM, Kaye WH, et al: Persistent perfectionism, symmetry, and exactness after long-term recovery from anorexia nervosa, *Am J Psychiatry* 152:1630, 1995.
24. Staples N, Schwartz M: Anorexia nervosa support group: providing transitional support, *J Psychosoc Nurs* 28:6, 1990.
25. Steiner-Adair KS: The body politic: normal female adolescent development and the development of eating disorders. In Gilligan C, Lyons NP, Hammer TJ, editors: *Making connections: the relational worlds of adolescent girls at Emma Willard School*, Cambridge, Mass, 1990, Harvard University Press.
26. Stuart G, Laraia M, Lydiard R, Ballenger J: Early family experiences of women with bulimia and depression, *Arch Psychiatr Nurs* 4:43, 1990.
27. Sullivan PF: Mortality in anorexia nervosa, *Am J Psychiatry* 152:7, 1995.
28. Walters EE, Kendler KS: Anorexia nervosa and anorexic-like syndromes in a population-based female twin sample, *Am J Psychiatry* 152:64, 1995.
29. Weltzin TE, Fernstrom MH, et al: Acute tryptophan depletion and increased food intake and irritability in bulimia nervosa, *Am J Psychiatry* 152:1668, 1995.
30. Wiederman MW, Pryor TL: Overcoming anorexia nervosa, *J Pract Psychiatry Behav Health* 5, 1996.
31. Wolfe BE: Dimensions of response to antidepressant agents in bulimia nervosa: a review, *Arch Psychiatr Nurs* 3:111, 1995.
32. Yanovski S et al: Association of binge eating disorder and psychiatric comorbidity in obese subjects, *Am J Psychiatry* 150:1472, 1993.
33. Yates A: *Compulsive exercise and the eating disorders: toward an integrated theory of activity*, New York, 1991, Brunner/Mazel.

ANNOTATED SUGGESTED READINGS

Garner D, Garfinkel P: *Handbook of treatment for eating disorders*, New York, 1997, Guilford Publications.
  Provides detailed descriptions of all of the major treatments for eating disorders, presented by the leading clinicians and researchers in the field. Highly recommended.

*Stein K: The self-schema model: a theoretical approach to the self-concept in eating disorders, *Arch Psychiatr Nur* 2:96, 1996.
  This article proposes that a limited collection of positive self-schemas available in memory, in combination with an inflexibly accessible body-weight self-schema, lead to the disordered behaviors associated with eating disorders.

Wiederman M, Pryor T: The assessment and treatment of anorexia nervosa, *J Pract Psychiatry Behav Health* 5:162, 1996.
  The authors discuss how anorexia nervosa can be assessed and treated and how to choose the most appropriate setting within the context of a managed care environment.

*Nursing reference.

Sexual Responses and Sexual Disorders

Susan G. Poorman

© 1998 M.C. Escher/Cordon Art, Baarn, Holland.

I locked myself away from you Too long, Tossing aside my feelings For you. Looking for a way out, an excuse Not to touch you; Because I want to, Inciting a riot within me. To reach out for you Is difficult, But less difficult Than turning away. **Leslie Bertel** exuality broadly refers to all aspects of being sexual and is one dimension of the personality. It includes more than the act of intercourse and is an integral part of life. It is evident in the person's appearance and in beliefs, behaviors, and relationships with others. Four components of sexuality have been identified[2]:

▼ **Genetic identity,** which is a person's chromosomal gender

▼ **Gender identity,** which is a person's perception of his or her own maleness or femaleness

▼ **Gender role,** which is the cultural role attributes of one's gender, such as expectations regarding behavior, cognitions, occupations, values, and emotional responses

▼ **Sexual orientation,** which is the gender to which one is romantically attracted

Accepting a broad concept of sexuality allows nurses to explore ways in which people are sexual beings and understand more fully their feelings, beliefs, and actions. Nurses are often called on to intervene in the sexual concerns of patients when providing holistic patient care. Therefore, it is important to develop skills and competence in addressing sexual issues by increasing awareness through education.

As nurses become educated in the basic principles of sexuality, they will better understand sexual needs and problems. If nurses are comfortable with sexual issues, they will convey this to the patient, who will feel more comfortable in discussing such issues. Patients are often experiencing pain and change as a result of threats to health or even as a part of normal growth and development. Thus it is important that the nurse-patient relationship allow for honest discussions about sexuality.

In answering the question, What do nurses need to know about sexuality?, several factors emerge. First, nurses need to know themselves and be aware of their feelings and values regarding sexuality. If nurses are not aware of their feelings, they cannot help patients meet their needs. Second,

nurses need to understand that other people's feelings and values about sexuality are different from their own. Third, all nurses can become educated about sexual health and use sound counseling methods with patients. Specifically, nurses can do the following:

▼ Develop confidence in their ability to discuss sexual issues with patients

▼ Learn interviewing skills for sexual assessment and history taking

▼ Counsel or refer patients for counseling

Education can be gained through nursing courses and continuing education programs. Some nurses pursue additional education and may become sex educators in schools, outpatient clinics, and planned parenthood agencies. Nurses prepared at the graduate level may become sex therapists through postgraduate work in human sexuality and extensive clinical supervision.

CONTINUUM OF SEXUAL RESPONSES

Adaptive and Maladaptive Sexual Responses

Experts in sexuality do not agree on what is normal sexual behavior. For years many people believed that only sexual relations between married heterosexual partners for procreation were normal. Today people view sexual behavior with a wider range of attitudes. Sexuality, on a continuum, ranges from adaptive to maladaptive (Fig. 26-1). The most adaptive responses meet the following criteria: between two consenting adults, mutually satisfying to both, not psychologically or physically harmful to either, lacking in force or coercion, and conducted in private.

Sometimes, however, sexual behavior can meet the criteria for adaptive responses but may be altered by what society deems acceptable and unacceptable. Unfortunately, society often decides this based on fear, prejudice, and lack of information rather than on data and facts (see

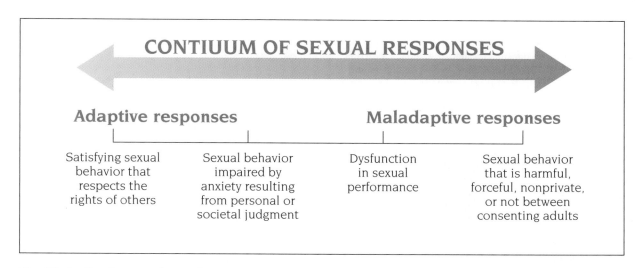

Fig. 26-1 Continuum of sexual responses.

Critical Thinking about Contemporary Issues). For example, the homosexual person may have the potential for healthy responses but be impaired by anxiety about societal disapproval.

Maladaptive sexual responses include behaviors that do not meet one or more of the criteria for adaptive responses.[25] The degree to which these behaviors are maladaptive varies. Some sexual behaviors may not meet any of the criteria mentioned. For example, incest may include force and be psychologically harmful. However, other sexual responses may meet four of the five criteria for adaptive responses but still be maladaptive.

Caution must be used when attempting to label sexual behaviors as adaptive or maladaptive. There will always be disagreements and exceptions to the rule. The continuum shown in Fig. 26-1 is free of moral judgment and was developed to aid the nurse in developing self-awareness and understanding the range of sexual responses.

> **?** *How do you define "normal" sexuality? Compare your views with those of a friend, a family member, and a health care provider.*

Self-awareness of the Nurse

The nurse's level of self-awareness is critical in discussing sexual issues with patients. The first step in developing self-awareness involves clarification of values regarding human sexuality. Foley and Davies[9] identified growth experiences developed around the nursing care of rape victims. Their

---

CRITICAL THINKING *about* **Contemporary Issues**

Does Sex Education in Schools Promote Teenage Promiscuity?

Some people in this country believe that teenagers are sexually active because they are taught sex education in their schools. The issue of sex education for youth in this country has raised a storm of questions and controversy. Unfortunately, much of it is based on values, beliefs, and personal opinion instead of facts. People who oppose sex education fight against comprehensive sex education programs in public schools. In contrast, many parents believe that their children are receiving sex education in school when they often are not.

Research provides some answers to this controversial question. Studies have demonstrated that comprehensive sex education programs can delay the initiation of first intercourse, reduce unprotected intercourse, and decrease unwanted teen pregnancy.[21] Based on these findings, along with the rising incidence of teen pregnancy and sexually transmitted diseases, the more important question this country faces is whether we can afford not to provide comprehensive sex education in our schools.

---

model is also applicable to sexual counseling and consists of four phases of the nurse's growth: cognitive dissonance, anxiety, anger, and action (Fig. 26-2).

COGNITIVE DISSONANCE. The first phase of growth in developing sexual self-awareness is cognitive dissonance, which arises when two opposing beliefs exist at the same time. For example, nurses grow up learning what society, family, and friends believe about sexual issues. If a nurse is raised in an environment that teaches that "it is impolite to talk about sex; it's too personal a subject," the nurse will carry that belief into nursing practice. When a patient wants to discuss a sexual concern, the nurse may feel two opposing reactions simultaneously: "I should not ask questions about such a personal subject as sex" and "As a professional,

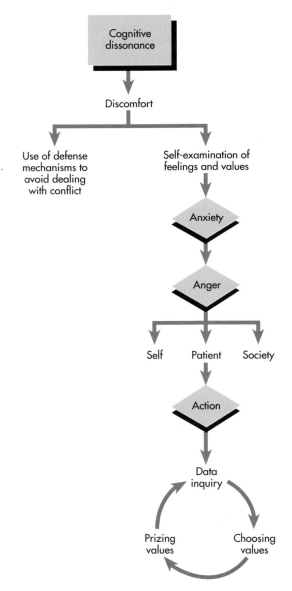

Fig. 26-2 Phases of the nurse's growth in developing awareness of human sexuality.

I should be able to discuss any problem, including sexual problems, with my patient."

These opposing thoughts, based on the different role expectations, make the nurse uncomfortable. However, the discomfort can be positive because it forces the nurse to examine feelings about the issue. The nurse resolves the cognitive dissonance in one of two ways: by continuing to believe that sexual concerns are too personal to discuss with patients or by examining the fact that sexuality is an integral part of being human.

Both of these beliefs have consequences for how the nurse relates to patients who voice sexual concerns. If the nurse continues to believe that sex is too personal to discuss with the patient, the nurse may become uncomfortable and choose not to follow up on sexual issues. This discomfort may be projected onto the patient, with the nurse stating, "The patient seemed too upset to talk about that right now." In this case the nurse should explore personal values and beliefs about sexuality and ask, "Do I believe these ideas about discussing sexual concerns because I have researched the facts and have accurate, current information?" Only when the nurse has examined the available information and made an informed choice on values will clarification of those values occur. If the nurse examines personal and professional values and believes that sexuality is an integral part of being human, a second phase of growth occurs.

ANXIETY. Most people think that anxiety is a negative emotion. However, a mild level of anxiety can be positive because it can promote an awareness of danger, give extra energy, or stimulate professional growth by creating enough discomfort to initiate some type of action. In this second phase the nurse realizes that uncertainty, insecurity, questions, and problems regarding sexuality are normal. The nurse begins to understand that everyone is capable of a variety of sexual feelings and behaviors and that anyone can have a sexual dysfunction or question sexual identity. The nurse experiencing anxiety may exhibit behaviors that hinder discussion of sexual issues such as talking too much (not allowing patients to express their feelings), failing to listen (not picking up on patients' cues and messages), and diagnosing and analyzing (becoming preoccupied with facts rather than feelings). As the anxiety level rises, the nurse becomes more uncomfortable and tries to reduce it. Learning about sexuality and facing conflicting values bring the nurse to the third phase of growth.

ANGER. Anger generally arises after anxiety, fear, and shock subside. It is generally self-directed or directed to the patient or society. The nurse begins to recognize that issues associated with sex or sexuality are emotional and sometimes highly volatile. Rape, abortion, birth control, equal rights, child abuse, pornography, and religious issues all are related to sexuality and give rise to controversy and debate. This realization often breeds anger and contempt in the nurse. For example, the nurse may become angry at a col-

league or a friend who makes judgmental remarks about pro-life or pro-choice activists.

During this phase of anger, the nurse tends to choose words and actions that may be as judgmental as the attitudes the nurse is fighting against. The nurse may lecture other nurses about the need for sex education or critically judge a teenager who does not fear the consequences of having unprotected sex with someone known to be HIV positive. The nurse may also be angry with society for perpetuating ignorance about sexuality. Toward the end of this phase the nurse begins to understand that blaming self or society for lack of proper awareness does not help patients with sexual concerns. This realization helps defuse the anger, and the nurse is ready for the final phase.

ACTION. The final step in the growth experience is the action phase. Several behaviors emerge during this final phase of the growth experience: data inquiry, choosing values, and prizing values. Data inquiry occurs when the nurse seeks out additional information about sexual issues. Once the information is obtained, the nurse may discuss and debate the issues. These are healthy ways of exploring and deciding what to believe, and the nurse will eventually make some choices about a value position.

The final behavior is one of prizing the value position, which consists of an awareness and cherishing of feelings and values and being willing to share them publicly. Although prizing values is considered the final step in a positive growth experience, it does not mean that what is valued will not change. Values are never static; they evolve and shift as a person changes, grows, and acquires new experiences. Thus a person who once opposed abortion may later become understanding and empathetic toward women who have abortions. The following clinical example illustrates the growth health professionals experience while increasing their awareness about sexuality. Chapter 2 has additional content on developing self-awareness and the nurse's therapeutic use of self.

Clinical Example Carol was a new staff nurse at a rehabilitation hospital. At the monthly staff meeting the nursing supervisor asked whether there were any concerns the staff would like to discuss. Carol offered, "I wonder if any of you could help me with a suggestion. Over the past several weeks I've seen a number of patients masturbating. One patient was in the lounge and another was in his room when I came in to give him his meds. I was so embarrassed I didn't know what to do. I just ignored it both times, but part of me wanted to say 'stop that you dirty old man—that's not appropriate for a hospital!' I guess I could use some help with this one." Another staff nurse followed up and said "That's what I feel like saying when I see that kind of behavior." Several other staff in the room began to snicker. The nursing supervisor interrupted and asked, "Can anyone give Carol some suggestions on how to handle this situation therapeutically?" After several moments of silence, other staff members admitted that they too were uncomfortable dealing with patients who were masturbating.

With the help of the supervisor, the staff began to brainstorm about how to handle this situation. Staff agreed that dealing with patients who are masturbating is a difficult issue for many nurses, and that the problem is most often the nurses' rather than the patients' because masturbation is a normal form of sexual expression. They decided that when they observe a patient masturbating in a public area, an appropriate nursing response would be to have the patient return to his or her room for privacy. If a nurse walks in on a patient masturbating in his or her room, the nurse should ensure the patient's privacy by excusing himself or herself and telling the patient he or she will return at a later time.

 In which phase of growth are you in relation to the development of awareness of human sexuality?

Assessment

Any basic health history must include questions about sexual history. A nurse who is comfortable discussing sexuality conveys the message that it is normal to talk about sexual health in a health assessment interview. If nurses are able to eliminate the attitude that sex should not be discussed by being composed and professional, they can ask questions about patients' sexual health naturally. The patient can then discuss sexual matters openly and without embarrassment.

Effective interviewing skills are a necessary part of a sexual assessment. At times, nurses who usually demonstrate effective skills become uncomfortable when addressing sexual issues. However, the principles of effective interviewing are the same for addressing sexual issues. Open-ended questions are one of the most effective ways of promoting a discussion on sexual issues, although some nurses report that direct questions can also be helpful in opening up the subject. Regardless, it is important to remember that questions must be asked at the patient's level of understanding, with sensitivity to the patient's cultural background, because each person is unique. The time and number of questions needed to discuss a problem vary depending on the patient. Often, just a few questions during an interview will obtain the relevant information. Examples of questions nurses may ask related to a patient's sexual health include the following:

▼ Tell me what you understand about (menstruation, sexual changes with aging, menopause).
▼ Since you've been diagnosed, what questions have you had regarding your sexuality?
▼ Are there any changes you've noticed in your sexual patterns since becoming ill?

▼ Have you noticed any differences or problems in your sexual responses since taking this medication?
▼ Often people have questions about (masturbation, sexual frequency, safe sex, alternate positions).
▼ Sometimes it is uncomfortable to talk about sexual issues with your partner. How is this for you and your partner?

Behaviors

There are many modes of sexual expression. Kinsey[20] used a seven-point rating scale to examine sexual preference (Fig. 26-3); 0 represents exclusively heterosexual experiences, 6 represents exclusively homosexual experiences, and 2, 3, and 4 indicate a bisexual orientation. He suggested that most people are not exclusively heterosexual or homosexual. His studies indicated that a substantial percentage of men and women had experienced both heterosexual and homosexual activity.

HETEROSEXUALITY. Heterosexuality can be defined as sexual attraction to members of the opposite sex. It is the predominant sexual orientation among people in American society. The coupling of a man and a woman in a sexual partnership has both legal and religious sanctions. As such, it influences the culture, values, and norms of contemporary American life.

HOMOSEXUALITY. Homosexuality can be defined as sexual attraction to members of the same sex. The term *gay* is used to refer to both male and female homosexuals; however, some use the term to refer only to male homosexuals

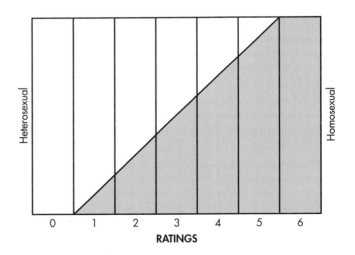

Fig. 26-3 Heterosexual–homosexual rating scale. Definitions of the ratings are as follows: *0,* Entirely heterosexual; *1,* largely heterosexual but with incidental homosexual history; *2,* largely heterosexual but with a distinct homosexual history; *3,* equally heterosexual and homosexual; *4,* largely homosexual but with distinct heterosexual history; *5,* largely homosexual but with incidental heterosexual history; *6,* entirely homosexual. (From Kinsey AC, Pomeroy WB, Martin AC: *Sexual behavior in the human female,* Philadelphia, 1953, WB Saunders.)

and the term *lesbian* to refer to female homosexuals. A person's attraction to people of the same sex, opposite sex, or both sexes is called sexual preference or sexual orientation. Some prefer the term *sexual orientation* over *sexual preference* because *preference* implies that homosexuals choose to be homosexual. Although sexual behaviors do involve choice, sexual orientation includes emotion and erotic attraction and may be genetically determined rather than a matter of free will.[5]

It is difficult to estimate the actual incidence of homosexuality in this country. It is estimated that 3% to 10% of the population are engaged primarily in homosexual activity, which translates to about 7.5 million people. Some studies suggest the smaller numbers of 2.7% of men and 1.3% of women reporting homosexual sex in the past year, and 4.9% of men and 4.1% of women reporting some type of homosexual behavior since age 18.[22] There are three reasons why it is difficult to obtain accurate estimates of the number of people who are homosexual. First, a person's sexual behavior may be transient. For example, a person may have been exclusively homosexual for the past year but have been heterosexual for the previous 20 years. Second, it is hard to distinguish between sexual desire and self-identification. An example of this is the person who may engage in heterosexual sex but have more desire for homosexual sex, even if the desire is not acted upon. Third, there is a tremendous social stigma associated with homosexuality in this country, as evidenced by a 1991 survey in which the majority of Americans reported believing that homosexuality is morally wrong. Thus, many men and women are unwilling to disclose their homosexual identities.[29]

For many years the medical profession, including psychiatry, has searched for causes of homosexuality. Although many psychological and biological theories have been suggested, there is no compelling evidence to support any specific theory.[4] Some experts suggest that there should be less emphasis on determining the cause of homosexuality and more focus placed on learning more about modes of sexual expression. Research findings indicate that gays and lesbians function as well psychologically, emotionally, and sexually as heterosexual people. Heterosexual and homosexual couples have also been found to be similar in that both report a high degree of relationship satisfaction and low amounts of conflict.[28] If current estimates of homosexuality are accurate, nurses come into contact with homosexuals daily but often know little about homosexuality and often assume that all patients are heterosexual.

> ? *How are health care providers' views of homosexuality influenced by social norms and cultural values?*

BISEXUALITY. Bisexuality can be defined as sexual responsiveness to both sexes.[30] A recent study of bisexual men

defined a bisexual as a person who had sex with both a man and a woman in the previous 3 years.[27] Many studies on bisexuality include homosexuals in their research samples and this has made the understanding of bisexuality more difficult. However, the studies that identified bisexuals separately found that data supported basic differences among heterosexuals, homosexuals, and bisexuals. Research in this area showed heterosexuality to be the most common sexual orientation, followed by homosexuality and then bisexuality. Bisexuals reported experiencing stronger orgasms and were more sexually adventurous. They also described higher levels of eroticism and the increased incidence and enjoyment of masturbation.[35]

Although some experts believe that bisexuality is transitional, a recent study of bisexual men found that bisexual activity was stable over time. There has been an increased interest in the behavior and characteristics of bisexual men in light of the AIDS epidemic and the need to design effective preventive interventions for HIV infection. One problem that has been identified with bisexual orientation is that the sexual risk behaviors of bisexual men are quite high. However, their lack of identification with and participation in the homosexual community make them unlikely to be reached by the gay community's safe sex and AIDS prevention programs.[27]

TRANSVESTISM. Transvestism is defined as cross-dressing, or dressing in the clothes of the opposite sex. Most often the transvestite who seeks treatment is a male; very little is known about female transvestism. No reliable statistics concerning the incidence of transvestism are available, but many professionals believe it is more common than generally assumed.

Transvestites tend to be married men who report heterosexual behavior. Although they occasionally or frequently dress in female clothes, they do not want hormonal or surgical sex change. Many transvestites try to find willing partners, and typically their activities of cross-dressing do not prevent sexual relationships with others.

TRANSSEXUALISM. The word *transsexual* simply implies going from one sex to another. More specifically, a transsexual is a person who is anatomically a male or female but who expresses, with strong conviction, that he or she has the mind of the opposite sex, lives as a member of the opposite sex part-time or full-time, and seeks to change his or her sex legally and through hormonal and surgical sex reassignment.[29] Many times the transsexual patient describes himself or herself as "feeling trapped in the wrong body." Transsexuals genuinely believe that they belong to the other sex. Many experience intense emotional turmoil because of stigma from society. There are no accurate estimates of the incidence of transsexualism; however, postoperative transsexuals in the United States now number in the thousands.

Transsexuality is different from homosexuality in that homosexuals are comfortable with their anatomical identity and do not want to change their sex. Many transsexuals are heterosexual and express distaste for homosexual activity. Transsexuals are essentially heterosexual, not homosexual, but are often mistaken by others or themselves as homosexual, as seen in this clinical example.

Clinical Example Mr. L is a 21-year-old biological male who was admitted to the psychiatric unit for evaluation after a serious suicide attempt. Mr. L told his nurse that he tried to kill himself because he has been "sexually mixed up for years" and is tired of feeling like a freak of nature. He said that his friends make fun of him and tell him he is a homosexual. Although he does feel sexually attracted to other men, he does not believe he is a homosexual. "I guess I don't feel like a man, I feel like a woman inside a man's body, and as a woman I am attracted to men."

Selected Nursing Diagnoses:

▼ Altered sexuality patterns related to conflicting sexual feelings, as evidenced by verbalizations of confusion and happiness

▼ Potential for self-directed violence related to sexual identity confusion, as evidenced by suicide attempt

> **?** *Think of a patient you took care of last week. How would your care have been different if you knew this patient was a homosexual, bisexual, transvestite, or transsexual?*

THE SEXUAL RESPONSE CYCLE. In addition to modes of sexual expression or sexual orientation, the physiological and psychological responses to sexual stimulation can also be described. Masters and Johnson[24] were the first to report the physiological changes that occur in men and women during sexual activity. They described the sexual response cycle as consisting of four phases: excitement, plateau, orgasm, and resolution. Kaplan[16] also identified three stages of the sexual response cycle: desire, excitement, and orgasm. Currently, the accepted stages of the sexual response cycle are a combination of those defined by Masters and Johnson and Kaplan and are listed in Box 26-1.

Impairment in sexual response may occur in any one of the phases of the sexual response cycle. For example, when the orgasm stage of the sexual response cycle is disrupted, premature or retarded ejaculation in males or orgasmic inhibition in females may result. If the excitement phase is inhibited, it may produce erectile dysfunction in males and a general sexual dysfunction in females. If the desire phase is absent, it may be evidenced by hypoactive sexual desire disorder or sexual arousal disorders. Although sexual dysfunction can occur when any phase is disrupted, resolution phase inhibition is rarely responsible for specific sexual dysfunctions.

The etiology of sexual dysfunction is varied and complex. Sex therapists agree that many sexual dysfunctions are caused by psychological factors ranging from unresolved

---

Box **26-1** *Stages of the Sexual Response Cycle*

STAGE 1: DESIRE
Sexual fantasies and the desire for sexual activity.

STAGE 2: EXCITEMENT
Subjective sense of sexual pleasure along with physiological changes, including penile erection in the male and vaginal lubrication in the female.

STAGE 3: ORGASM
Peaking of sexual pleasure and the release of sexual tension accompanied by rhythmic contractions of the perineal muscles and pelvic reproductive organs.

STAGE 4: RESOLUTION
Sense of general relaxation, muscular relaxation, and well-being. Females may be able to respond to additional stimulation almost immediately during this stage; however, most males need some time before they can be restimulated to orgasm.

---

childhood conflicts to adult problems such as performance anxiety, lack of knowledge, or failure to communicate with a partner. Sexual dysfunction can also be caused by physiological factors such as vascular and endocrine disorders and medication side effects and is often the result of the interaction of psychological and physiological factors.[34]

Predisposing Factors

No one theory can adequately explain sexual development or predisposing factors of maladaptive sexual responses. Several theories have been proposed, however, and are now briefly described.

BIOLOGICAL. Biological factors are initially responsible for the development of gender, that is, whether a person is genetically male or female. Somatotype includes chromosomes, hormones, internal and external genitalia, and gonads. Sex differentiation is determined by the Y chromosome. Research in humans confirms the general rule that maleness and masculinity depend on fetal and perinatal androgens.

A biological female typically has XX chromosomes, with estrogen as the predominant hormone, appropriate internal and external genitalia, and ovaries. A biological male typically has XY chromosomes, with androgen as the predominant hormone, appropriate internal and external genitalia, and testicles. However, each of these typical configurations may vary. A person may have triple chromosomes, such as XXX, XXY, or XYY, or a single chromosome, XO. There is no YO chromosomal pattern. The triple pattern XXX and the single pattern XO (Turner's syndrome) result in a female body, whereas the triple patterns XXY (Klinefelter's syndrome) and XYY result in male bodies. Assuming no variation occurs, the biological factors result in a single, fully developed gender, either male or female.

Based on family studies and DNA samples of homosexual brothers, it has been suggested that a gene may be related to homosexuality. Early work in the field suggested that homosexuality may be inherited from the maternal side of the family through the X chromosome. Before such research is accepted as definitive, however, it will have to be validated by replication, and similar studies of lesbians have not yet been completed. In addition, such findings cannot account for all cases of homosexuality, but they do support a possible biological basis.

PSYCHOANALYTICAL. Freud saw sexuality as one of the key forces of human life. *In Three Essays of the Theory of Sexuality,*[10] he theorized about the nature of sexuality and sexual development and proposed that sexuality was established before the onset of puberty. He also believed that a person's choice of sexual expression depended on a mix of heredity, biology, and social factors. He wrote extensively about childhood sexuality and believed that sexuality during infancy was central to personality development.

The child, according to Freud, passes through a series of developmental stages in which a different erogenous zone is dominant. The first is the oral stage (birth to 12 or 18 months), in which the infant's chief sense of pleasure is derived from stimulation of the lips and mouth, that is, sucking. In the second, or anal, stage (ages 1 to 3 years), the child's attention is focused on elimination functions and control over body sphincters. The phallic stage follows (ages 3 to 5 years), in which the child's focus is on the genitals. An important occurrence in this stage is the development of the Oedipus complex in boys and the Electra complex in girls.

In the Oedipus/Electra complex the child experiences sexual feelings for the parent of the opposite sex and resents the parent of the same sex. According to Freud, the boy fears retaliation from his father for desiring the mother and fantasizes that the father will cut off his penis (castration anxiety). This fear is the impetus for the young boy's eventually giving up the resentment of the father and identifying with him and the male gender role. The girl, on the other hand, has no penis to fear losing. She believes that at one time she had a penis but it was cut off, and she blames her mother for this.

After the resolution of the Oedipus or Electra complex, the child enters a prolonged stage where sexual impulses are repressed (latency stage). This stage lasts until adolescence, when the child enters the genital stage and sexual urges reawaken. The reemergence of Oedipal/Electra feelings and the need to assert themselves with parents also occur during this phase of development. The adolescent then makes the final transition into mature genital sexuality.

In recent years there has been much criticism of Freud's theory of psychosexual development. Feminists argue that psychoanalytical theory is male centered and views women as anatomically inferior to men (because they have no penis). Lack of scientific evidence is one of the major problems with Freud's theory. Other criticisms include that Freud was a victim of the Victorian era, a time of sexual repression, and that his thoughts and writings were bound by the period in which he lived. Finally, Freud's data were collected from observations of his patients, who were probably not representative of the total population and were to some degree emotionally ill.

 What impact has Freud's theory of psychosexual development had on society's view of women?

BEHAVIORAL. From a behaviorist's perspective, the most legitimate basis for understanding sexual reactions is the observable response to overt, measurable stimuli. Behaviorists are not concerned with the complex intrapsychic process of early childhood and adolescence; rather, they view sexual behavior as a measurable response, with both physiological and psychological components, to a learned stimulus or reinforcement event.

Behaviorists consider the sexual behavior of adults who care for children as important in the children's later sexual development. They are thus interested in sexual difficulties that result from sexual abuse in childhood. Although the research is limited, it appears that adults who were sexually abused as children may have significant adjustment problems. In one study of female survivors of child sexual abuse, 50% or more of the subjects experienced insomnia, sexual dysfunction, overeating, drug abuse, severe headache, and two or more major surgeries. Over 90% of the subjects experienced symptoms such as depression, guilt, low self-esteem, and inability to trust others.[13] Another study found that young adult women who had experienced childhood incest reported less satisfaction with their sexual functioning than did a control group. In this study, 65% of the victims met the DSM-III criteria for one or more of the sexual dysfunctions such as inhibited sexual desire, inhibited orgasm, inhibited sexual excitement, dyspareunia, or vaginismus.[14] Finally, an examination of the aftermath of child sexual abuse in black and white American women found that one of the lasting effects of child sexual abuse was sexual problems for women of both ethnic groups.[37] The care of people who have experienced abuse and violence is described in detail in Chapter 39.

Precipitating Stressors

PHYSICAL ILLNESS AND INJURY. Physical illness may alter sexuality. The patient may find that hospitalization alone changes sexual feelings and behavior. Nurses often care for patients with sexual dysfunctions or altered sexuality patterns; they need to discuss and therapeutically intervene in patients' responses to these changes. A person with rheumatoid arthritis may have body disfiguration and a change in body image caused by swollen areas around joints. The same patient may have decreased sexual interest because of joint pain during intercourse. People who have had a myocardial infarction may have decreased sexual interest because they fear sexual arousal may cause a heart attack.

PSYCHIATRIC ILLNESS. Psychiatric illness affects a person's sexuality as well as the sexual behavior and satisfaction of the person's partner (see A Family Speaks). Depression can be either the result or cause of sexual dysfunction. As many as 70% of depressed patients have decreased sexual desire and decreased frequency of intercourse. Most often, depressed men engage in intercourse less often; depressed women may participate in sex but with less enjoyment. In contrast, hypersexuality may be the first symptom of a manic episode. People with bipolar illness have decreased sexual inhibitions, often impulsively choose sexual partners or begin extramarital affairs, display inappropriate sexual behavior, or act seductively or flirtatiously.

A Family *Speaks*

Our daughter was diagnosed with schizophrenia 5 years ago when she was 17 years of age. Since that time we have received very good care for her. While we understand that she may never be completely well, she has her illness under control and has even started taking some courses at the local community college. She has also met some people her age and seems to enjoy their company.

But ever since she began doing better, we have had the added concern about her sexual needs and activities. As involved parents, we raised this issue with the different health care providers who were managing her care over the years. In each case, almost without exception, we were told "Don't worry about such things; be grateful your daughter is as healthy as she is." While their intentions may have been good, they didn't help resolve our questions or fears. But then our daughter was assigned a nurse who we were told would be her case manager. The first time they met, the nurse took a detailed history and asked our daughter the unthinkable: What sexual feelings did she have and how was she managing her sexual needs? It was as if the floodgate had opened for all of us, and that session marked the beginning of an ongoing discussion we would all have about the very topic we had worried so much about. For the question of that nurse we will always be grateful, and if we could share one thought with future nurses in training, it would be to remember that patients are whole people and that sexuality is as important to those with psychiatric illness as it is to people everywhere. ▼

The sexual expression of patients with psychotic illnesses may be inappropriate and at times intrusive. Delusions and hallucinations may present with sexual content. Mental illness can interfere with one's ability to think coherently and express oneself in a clear and direct manner. Thus a patient's capacity for intimate relationships and sexual expression may be altered. Although having a psychotic illness such as schizophrenia does not imply sexual dysfunction, sexual expression can be affected. The patient may not be able to understand or control sexual thoughts or impulses. For example, a patient may openly masturbate on an inpatient unit or inappropriately touch others. Thinking and judgment may also be impaired, resulting in sexual activity that may be detrimental to the patient's health, such as unsafe sexual practices. This is evident in recent studies that have revealed alarming rates of HIV infection among people with chronic mental illnesses.[18]

The nurse must therefore assess a psychiatric patient's sexual behavior carefully and intervene with inappropriate or dangerous sexual expressions. The nurse can help the patient identify and express needs related to sexuality. This includes helping the patient form healthy relationships with others, learn about safe sex practices, engage in healthy sexual expression, and decrease potentially dangerous sexual encounters.

MEDICATIONS. Some medications contribute to sexual dysfunction and nurses need to be knowledgeable about the medications they administer. The most common side effect of medication is diminished sexual desire, which occurs fairly equally in both sexes. The most common sexual problem is erectile difficulties in men, followed by orgasmic difficulties. The most common sexual problem in women is delayed orgasm.[6] The sexual side effects of psychiatric medications, including antipsychotic and antidepressant drugs, are well documented. Problems with erection, desire, orgasm, and menstruation can occur in 30% to 60% of people taking these drugs.[33] Psychiatric medications and their side effects are described in detail in Chapter 27.

Nurses should be familiar with the sexual side effects of medications, educate their patients about them, and encourage patients to notify a health professional when these effects occur. For example, a patient may not be aware that his medication can cause impotence, yet he may be embarrassed and hesitant to talk with the physician or nurse about the problem. Often the medication itself or the dosage can be changed to correct the problem. Abuse of alcohol or nontherapeutic drugs may also have a debilitating effect on sexuality. Although many people believe alcohol is a sexual stimulant, prolonged use can cause erectile difficulty and other dysfunctions.

HIV/AIDS. Fear of contracting a sexually transmitted disease (STD) may create change in sexual behavior. The most frightening STD is acquired immune deficiency syndrome (AIDS), which is caused by the human immunodeficiency virus (HIV). More than a decade ago the first cases of AIDS were discovered in homosexual men. Since that time, HIV/AIDS has become a leading worldwide health problem despite the attempts by health-care professionals to educate society about safe sex practices. These practices include the following:

▼ Using condoms
▼ Reducing the number of sexual partners
▼ Promoting sexual behaviors that decrease the exchange of body fluids

Although in the United States the majority of those infected with HIV are men, HIV is spreading most rapidly among women. After IV drug use, heterosexual intercourse is the second most common mode of transmission in women.[36] The number of young people in the United States who have AIDS and the number who are infected with HIV also continues to increase.

Today, people in their twenties account for over 20% of all AIDS cases, the majority of whom were probably infected as adolescents, and the number of teenagers who have AIDS has increased more than 70% in the past 2 years.[11] Clearly, this illness has a significant impact on all aspects of society, and it is discussed in more detail in Chapter 40.

? Consider two medications that you commonly administer to patients. Do you know whether they have sexual side effects, and have you talked about this possibility with your patients?

THE AGING PROCESS. In the past, researchers suggested that sexual activity decreased with aging. More recent studies indicate that patterns of sexual activity remain stable over middle and late adulthood years, with only a small decline in later life. In reviewing the studies on sexuality and older adults, Kaplan[17] found that most elders who are in good health remain sexually active until the end of their lives.

There is nothing in the biology of aging that automatically shuts down sexual functioning; however, specific physiological changes do occur. In postmenopausal women there is little to no increase in breast size, and less muscle tension occurs during sexual arousal. Vaginal functioning changes in two ways; there is reduced elasticity in the walls of the vagina and decreased vaginal lubrication. The decrease in vaginal lubrication is the result of decreased blood flow to the vagina, which is caused by low estrogen levels. In men, several physiological changes occur in sexual response. Greater time and more direct stimulation are often needed for the penis to become erect, and erections tend to be less firm. The amount of semen is reduced, ejaculation is less intense, and the physical need to ejaculate is diminished. The refractory period also becomes greater with age.[38]

In Western culture the myth of the older adult as asexual still prevails. Many personality theorists have encouraged the myth of the older adult as an asexual or childlike being, and people have been taught that it is normal for older adults to have little or no interest in sex. Therefore, when health professionals care for older people who express an interest in sex or are sexually active, the professional often judges the older adult to be an exception to the rule. Older adults themselves may accept society's false beliefs about sexuality and aging. Many deny sexual attractions and feelings because they have been socialized to believe that sexual behavior in older people is abnormal or perverted. Older adults are influenced by cultural values of Western society that prize youth and vitality and often disapprove of an elderly person doing anything other than sitting in a rocking chair.

One important variable affecting sexuality in older adults is the lack of knowledge about the normal changes that occur with the aging process. Often nurses and older adults mistake a side effect of a medication or a symptom of a chronic medical illness for an expected part of the aging process. It is important for the nurse to understand the normal changes that occur with aging so that he or she can teach patients about these changes. This allows patients to learn what to expect and how they might compensate for the normal changes related to aging and sexual behavior.

It is equally important for nurses to realize that organic illness can affect sexual functioning. One researcher reports that half of her patients over the age of 50 had some degree of interference with sexual functioning caused by disease states or medication side effects.[17] For example, beta-blockers and diabetes can contribute to impotence in men, and testosterone deficiency can create anorgasmy in women. These can be significant problems and they often can be successfully treated.

Psychological factors, such as self-esteem, can also influence sexual activity in older adults. Older adults may be less inclined to be sexually active if they believe the physical changes that occur with aging make them unattractive. Marital status can also influence sexuality. Because men die at younger ages than women, women are more likely to be widowed and live the last part of their lives alone. Because there are fewer men in the population, it is more difficult for older women to find partners than it is for older men.

Finally, about 5% of people over the age of 65 reside in nursing homes and other long-term care facilities.[7] Many nursing homes restrict physical activity, so residents lack privacy from staff, who tend to care for older adults in a parental way. Physical contact between nursing home residents is often discouraged by nursing home staff, and many residents may feel restricted in their sexual expression. However, nurses are becoming more sensitive about the sexual needs of nursing home residents. By recognizing their sexual needs, nurses can act as advocates and help residents with sexual expression by encouraging discussion of sexual concerns, closing doors to ensure privacy, and allowing socialization with sexual partners.

> **?** *While working in a long-term care facility you walk into a patient's room and see two patients engaged in sexual relations. How would you respond?*

Appraisal of Stressors

Feelings of oneself as a sexual being change throughout the life cycle and they are very much influenced by a person's appraisal of the stressful situation. Sexual identity cannot be separated from self-concept or body image. Therefore, when bodily or emotional changes occur, sexual responses change as well.

Coping Resources

It is important for the nurse to assess the patient's coping resources because these can have a significant impact on sexual health. Resources may include the person's knowledge about sexuality, positive sexual experiences the patient has had in the past, supportive people in the patient's environment, and social or cultural norms that encourage healthy sexual expression. It is also helpful to include the person's sexual partner whenever possible; this allows the nurse to evaluate the quality of this relationship and to frame all nursing interventions within the context of a supportive, loving partnership.

Coping Mechanisms

Coping mechanisms related to sexual response may be adaptive or maladaptive, depending on how and why they are being used. **Fantasy** is a coping mechanism used to enhance sexual experiences. Men and women may escape to erotic fantasies with unknown lovers during sex with their spouse. Although many people fear that fantasies about people other than their sexual partner indicate that they are unsatisfied or unattracted to their partner, this is typically not the case. Fantasies are often a creative way to increase sexual excitement and enjoyment and do not usually indicate dissatisfaction with a current partner. However, excessive fantasy can be maladaptive when used as replacement for actual sexual expression or the development of intimate relationships with others.

Maladaptive coping mechanisms may result from problems with self-concept. Often one member of a sexually dysfunctional couple may use **projection** in blaming his or her partner for the total problem, absolving himself or herself from any responsibility: "I never had a sex problem with any of my previous lovers; I think you are the problem." Projection is also the coping mechanism used when a person's thoughts and feelings are unacceptable and anxiety producing. For example, a wife constantly accuses her husband of wanting to have an affair when actually the wife is contemplating an affair. Because her feelings are unacceptable to her, she projects them onto her husband and accuses him.

Denial and **rationalization** are also common coping mechanisms. Both allow the person to avoid dealing with sexual issues. The following are maladaptive examples:

▼ *Denial:* "I don't have a problem with sex" or "I never feel sexual."
▼ *Rationalization:* "I don't need sex; I'm fine without it. Besides, a good marriage is a lot more than just sex."

To cope with unacceptable feelings about becoming vulnerable and the resulting ambivalent feelings about intimacy, some people withdraw from any form of sexual behavior. Others may engage in increased sexual behavior with multiple partners to protect themselves from one intimate relationship.

Nursing Diagnosis

When developing nursing diagnoses for variations in sexual response, the nurse should consider all the information gathered in the assessment phase and the components of the Stuart Stress Adaptation Model (Fig. 26-4). The identified nursing diagnoses serve as a foundation for future problem solving. There are two primary NANDA nursing diagnoses concerned with sexual response. The first is **altered sexuality patterns,** which include difficulties, limitations, or changes in sexual behaviors or activities. The second is **sexual dysfunction,** which includes lack of sexual satisfaction, alterations in perceived sex role, and conflicts involving values.

Other related nursing diagnoses that address additional behavioral problems may also need to be included. For example, a patient may be sexually functional but sexual identity may be unclear. Nursing diagnoses related to the range of possible maladaptive responses and related medical diagnoses are identified in the Medical and Nursing Diagnoses box on p. 556. The primary NANDA diagnoses and examples of complete nursing diagnoses are presented in the Detailed Diagnoses box on p. 557.

Related Medical Diagnoses

Many people who have transient variations in sexual response do not have a medically diagnosed health problem. Those with more severe or persistent problems are classified into one of three categories of variations in sexual response according to DSM-IV: sexual dysfunctions, paraphilias (sexual perversions or deviations), or gender identity disorders.[1] The medical diagnoses and the essential features of each of these diagnostic classes according to the DSM-IV are described in the Detailed Diagnoses box.

Outcome Identification

Goals must be formulated realistically, remembering the uniqueness of each person. The expected outcome for patients with maladaptive sexual responses is the following:

The patient will obtain the maximum level of adaptive sexual responses to enhance or maintain health.

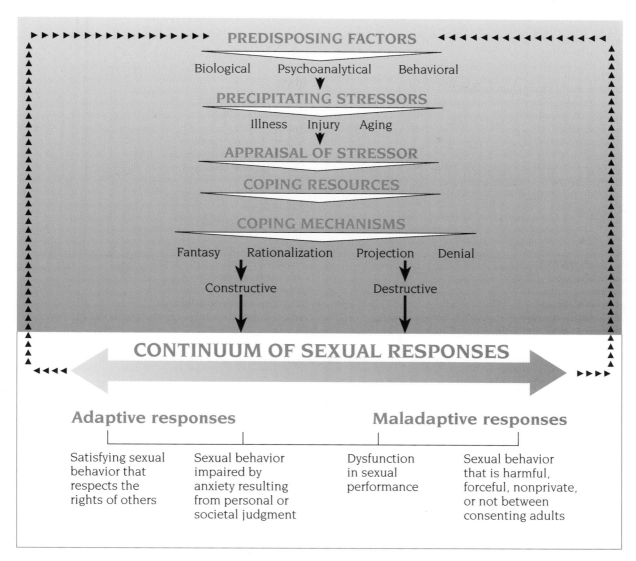

Fig. 26-4   The Stuart Stress Adaptation Model related to sexual responses.

This outcome can be made more specific through the use of short-term goals. These goals must be mutually identified with the patient, priorities must be established, and criteria used to measure progress toward the goals must be defined. Examples of short-term goals include the following:

▼ The patient will describe personal values and beliefs regarding sexuality and sexual expression.
▼ The patient will identify sexual questions and problems.
▼ The patient will relate accurate information about sexual concerns.
▼ The patient will implement one new behavior to enhance sexual functioning.
▼ The patient will report decreased anxiety and greater satisfaction with sexual health.

After identifying goals in partnership with the patient, the nurse begins to implement the appropriate nursing interventions.

Planning

The nurse's level of expertise determines the degree of planning. The planning phase can simply involve reviewing assessment data, exploring options, and making referral sources known and available. This phase can also include sexual instruction for the patient or the patient and partner together. The nurse and patient can discuss a specific sexual issue and approaches that will provide the needed information.

Implementation

Health Education

Primary prevention strives to promote health and prevent problems through specific methods such as teaching and planning, described in Chapter 12. Before engaging in

MEDICAL AND NURSING DIAGNOSES *related to* **Variations in Sexual Response**

Related Medical Diagnoses (DSM-IV)*	Related Nursing Diagnoses (NANDA)†
Hypoactive sexual desire disorder	Anxiety
Sexual aversion disorder	Body image disturbance
Sexual arousal disorder	Decisional conflict
Orgasmic disorder	Fear
Premature ejaculation	Grieving, dysfunctional
Dyspareunia	Health maintenance, altered
Vaginismus	Health-seeking behaviors
Sexual dysfunction due to a general medical condition	Pain
Substance-induced sexual dysfunction	Personal identity disturbance
Exhibitionism	Powerlessness
Fetishism	Role performance, altered
Frotteurism	Self-care deficit
Pedophilia	Self-esteem disturbance
Sexual masochism	Sensory/perceptual alterations
Sexual sadism	**Sexual Dysfunction‡**
Voyeurism	**Sexuality Patterns, Altered‡**
Transvestic fetishism	Social interactions, impaired
Gender identity disorder of childhood, adolescence, or adulthood	Spiritual distress (distress of the human spirit)

*From American Psychiatric Association: *Diagnostic and statistical manual,* ed 4, Washington, DC, 1994, The Association.
†From North American Nursing Diagnosis Association: *Nursing diagnosis: definitions and classifications, 1997-1998,* Philadelphia, 1997, The Association.
‡Primary nursing diagnosis for variations in sexual response.

health education or counseling, however, nurses must examine their values and beliefs about sexual behavior. This can be facilitated by exploring commonly held myths regarding human sexuality. Table 26-1 lists some common sexual myths, the results of believing them, and the facts related to each one.

Education is the most common method of primary prevention of sexual problems. The content and methods of sex education have changed little over the past several decades.[8] Many people receive most of their sex education from friends, who may not provide accurate information. Too few parents discuss sexual issues with their children, and school sex education programs, to avoid discussion of controversial subjects, often focus only on biological factors, which is insufficient for the needs of today's youth.

Recently, because of the epidemic rates of teenage pregnancies and abortion and the spread of AIDS, many experts are suggesting more comprehensive sex education programs, and some are suggesting that these programs begin as early as preschool and kindergarten. Sex education is a lifelong process with the primary goal of promoting sexual health. This includes helping people develop positive views of sexuality, gain information and skills about taking care of their sexual health, and acquire decision-making abilities regarding sexual issues. A comprehensive sex education program has the following four primary goals[31]:

▼ Communicating accurate information about sexuality
▼ Providing an opportunity to develop values, beliefs, and attitudes about sexuality
▼ Helping patients develop relationships and interpersonal skills
▼ Encouraging the exercise of responsibility in sexual relationships

It is also clear that teaching information about sex and sexuality is not enough. For a sex education program to be effective it must promote behavioral change. The most effective sex education programs are comprehensive and skill based. More specifically, it is not enough to teach students to say no to sex, but they must be taught how to say no. This could be done by teaching decision-making and assertiveness skills and by role playing potentially difficult sexual situations.

Sexual Responses within the Nurse-Patient Relationship

SEXUAL RESPONSES OF NURSES TO PATIENTS. A clinical situation in which a nurse feels sexual attraction to a patient is a problem that has received little attention in the nursing literature. One major reason is that nurses often deny sexual feelings for their patients. However, sexual attraction and sexual fantasies are part of the human experience. If these feelings are not examined, they can interfere

DETAILED DIAGNOSES *related to* **Sexual Responses**

NANDA Diagnosis Stem	Examples of Complete Diagnosis
Sexual dysfunction	Sexual dysfunction related to prenatal weight gain, as evidenced by verbal statements of physical discomfort with intercourse
	Sexual dysfunction related to joint pain, as evidenced by decreased sexual desire
Sexuality patterns, altered	Altered sexuality patterns related to financial worries, as evidenced by inability to reach orgasm
	Altered sexuality patterns related to mastectomy, as evidenced by statements such as "My husband won't want to touch me" and "I don't feel like a woman"
	Altered sexuality patterns related to fear of pregnancy, as evidenced by stopping before penetration

DSM-IV Diagnosis	Essential Features*
Hypoactive sexual desire disorder	Persistent or recurrent deficit or absence of sexual fantasies and desire for sexual activity
Sexual aversion disorder	Persistent or recurrent extreme aversion to and avoidance of genital sexual contact with a sexual partner
Sexual arousal disorder	Persistent or recurrent partial or complete failure to attain or maintain the physiological response of sexual activity or persistent or recurrent lack of a subjective sense of sexual excitement and pleasure during sexual activity
Orgasmic disorder	Persistent or recurrent delay in or absence of orgasm following a normal sexual excitement phase during sexual activity that is judged by the clinician to be adequate in focus, intensity, and duration, taking into account the person's age
Premature ejaculation	Persistent or recurrent ejaculation with minimal sexual stimulation before, on, or shortly after penetration, before the person wishes it
Dyspareunia	Recurrent or persistent genital pain before, during, or after sexual intercourse
Vaginismus	Recurrent or persistent involuntary spasm of the musculature of the outer third of the vagina that interferes with coitus
Sexual dysfunction due to a general medical condition	Clinically significant sexual dysfunction etiologically related to a general medical condition
Substance-induced sexual dysfunction	Clinically significant sexual dysfunction that developed during significant substance intoxication or withdrawal
Exhibitionism	A persistent association, lasting at least 6 months, between intense sexual arousal, desire, acts, or fantasies, and exposing one's genitals to an unsuspecting stranger
Fetishism	A persistent association, lasting at least 6 months, between intense sexual arousal, desire, acts, or fantasies, and nonliving objects (such as female undergarments)
Frotteurism	A persistent association, lasting at least 6 months, between intense sexual arousal, desire, acts, or fantasies, and rubbing against a nonconsenting person
Pedophilia	A persistent association, lasting at least 6 months, between intense sexual arousal, desire, acts, or fantasies, and one or more children, aged 13 years or younger
Sexual masochism	A persistent association, lasting for at least 6 months, between intense sexual arousal, desire, acts, or fantasies, and being humiliated, beaten, bound, or otherwise being made to suffer (real or imagined)
Sexual sadism	A persistent association, lasting at least 6 months, between intense sexual arousal, desire, acts, or fantasies, and the affliction of real or simulated psychological or physical suffering (including humiliation)
Voyeurism	A persistent association, lasting at least 6 months, between intense sexual arousal, desire, acts, or fantasies, and observing unsuspecting people who are either naked, in the act of disrobing, or engaging in sexual activity
Transvestic fetishism	A persistent association, lasting at least 6 months, between intense sexual arousal, desire, acts, or fantasies, and cross-dressing
Gender identity disorder of childhood, adolescence, or adulthood	Persistent and intense distress about being a male or a female, with an intense desire to be the opposite sex, a preoccupation with the activities of the opposite sex, and a repudiation of one's own anatomical structures

*Modified from the American Psychiatric Association: *Diagnostic and statistical manual of mental disorders,* ed 4, Washington, DC, 1994, The Association.

TABLE 26-1 *Ten Common Myths and Facts about Human Sexuality*

MYTH	RESULT OF MYTH	FACT
Patients become embarrassed when nurses bring up the subject of sexuality and would prefer that nurses not ask questions about sex.	If nurses believe this, they deny the patient the opportunity to ask questions and clarify concerns related to sexual issues.	Patients prefer that nurses initiate discussions of sexuality with them.
Excessive masturbation is harmful.	People often feel guilty or ashamed about masturbating; some people deny themselves this experience because of uncomfortable feelings perpetuated by society.	There is no evidence that masturbation causes physical problems. If masturbation leads to satisfaction and pleasure, it is unlikely to be a problem.
Sexual fantasies about having sex with a partner other than a lover or spouse indicate relationship difficulties.	People may become uncomfortable about having a fantasy with a different partner. They may feel guilty and view the fantasy as a sign of infidelity.	Imagining sex with a different partner is a common sexual fantasy and does not necessarily indicate a desire to act out the fantasy.
Sex during menstruation is unclean and harmful.	Women often view their bodies as unclean and even unfit or inferior during menstruation. Women use menstruation as an excuse to avoid intercourse rather than simply saying no without a "good reason."	Medically, menstrual flow is in no way harmful or dirty. If women desire, there is no reason to abstain from intercourse during menstrual flow.
Oral and anal intercourse are perverted and dangerous.	Many people refrain from these behaviors or indulge in them only to feel ashamed and guilty afterward.	Oral and anal intercourse are not harmful if certain precautions are taken when performing anal intercourse, such as avoiding contamination of the vaginal tract and wearing a condom to prevent the transmission of disease.
Most homosexuals molest children.	Known homosexuals are often fired from teaching jobs, and many parents do not allow their children to spend any time with anyone who is homosexual.	Research shows that the adult heterosexual male poses a far greater risk to the underage child than does the adult homosexual male.
Homosexuals are sick and cannot control their sexual behavior.	Homosexuals are denied jobs and are sometimes jailed for their homosexuality. Children may be taken away from homosexual parents by courts.	Most homosexuals' social and psychological adjustment is the same as the heterosexual majority, and objectionable sexual advances are far more likely to be made by a heterosexual (usually male to female) than by a homosexual.
Because of sex education programs, most adolescents and young adults are aware of the risks of getting sexually transmitted diseases and practice safe sex.	When health educators believe that young adults have adequate knowledge about sexually transmitted diseases, they may not take the time to assess, add to this knowledge, and correct any misperceptions.	A study of over 500 first-year students at a large university reported that of those who had multiple partners, fewer than 50% used condoms to lower the risk of disease.
Advancing age means the end of sex.	Many older adults become victims of this myth not because their bodies have lost the ability to perform, but because they believe that they have lost the ability to perform.	Sexually, men and women in good health can function effectively throughout their lives.
Alcohol ingestion reduces inhibitions and therefore enhances sexual enjoyment.	Many people use alcohol in the hope that it will increase their sexual pleasure and performance. Alcohol ingestion can also provide an excuse for engaging in sexual behaviors—"I would never have gone to bed with him if I hadn't had all that wine."	Data do not support the belief that alcohol ingestion reduces inhibitions and enhances sexual enjoyment.

with the quality of care by shifting the focus from the patient's needs to those of the nurse.

First, nurses must acknowledge their feelings without judging them. Often nurses try to ignore or deny these feelings because they are uncomfortable and frightening.

They make judgments about themselves, such as, "What's wrong with me? I shouldn't feel this way about my patients. I must be really weird" and "I'm sure I'm the only nurse who ever had these feelings." The nurse who admits these feelings without judging them is able to deal with them. Edelwich and Brodsky[8] offer the following suggestions:

▼ Do not share personal information with patients.
▼ Do not become overly involved in patients' problems.
▼ Do not discuss with the patient feelings of sexual attraction to him or her.
▼ Seek consultation.

Asking for consultation from a more experienced nurse or a supervisor often helps the nurse sort out feelings and, most important, maintain a professional therapeutic relationship with the patient. It is never acceptable for a nurse to engage in sexual behavior of any kind with a patient. Such activity can lead to litigation and loss of the nurse's license to practice.

SEXUAL RESPONSES OF PATIENTS TO NURSES. One of the most common sexual behaviors of hospitalized patients is seductive behavior toward the nurse; this includes making passes and sexual comments, inappropriate touching, asking for their phone numbers, and requesting dates. Nurses are often extremely uncomfortable with such behavior. One recent survey of nursing and occupational therapy students revealed that 40% had been victims of sexual harassment from patients. Of these students, 16% were victims of a forceful physical sexual assault by a patient.[19]

> ❓ *Which sexual myth from Table 26-1 did you believe before reading this chapter? How will knowing the truth affect your nursing practice?*

The first step in intervening is to let the patient know that such behavior is unacceptable. The nurse needs to respond in a firm, matter-of-fact manner that clearly states what limits are being set, such as "Mr. Moore, I am uncomfortable when you suggest that I get into bed with you. Please stop saying that" or "Mr. Dean, take your hand off my breast."

Nurses are sometimes embarrassed or afraid to confront patients and attempt to laugh it off or ignore it with a "boys will be boys" attitude. Patients do not have the right to be verbally offensive or to touch nurses' bodies without permission. Nurses are taught to be accepting of patients' behavior, and this principle is difficult to dispute. However, when the behavior violates nurses' rights, limits must be set.

Nurses have a responsibility as professionals to attempt to understand sexual behaviors and analyze their possible meanings. Patients may show seductive behaviors for various reasons, which may or may not include a serious desire for sex with the nurse. Seductive behavior is often a way of getting the nurse's attention. Hospitalized patients can also feel unattractive or insecure about themselves sexually; thus, seductive behaviors may be a request for reassurance. Sometimes patients confuse their gratitude for and appreciation of the nurse with sexual attraction. These feelings may in turn generate thoughts such as, "Wouldn't my nurse make a wonderful wife. She's so giving and understanding all the time." In this case the patient views professional behavior and concern as self-sacrificing and altruistic.

Finally, patients may have difficulty understanding the difference between a professional and a social relationship. In many ways the nurse-patient relationship is idealized for the patient. The patient receives all the attention and caring and is not expected to give anything in return. It is easy to see how the patient could be confused about his or her relationship with the nurse. The clinical example that follows illustrates this point. Table 26-2 summarizes nursing considerations in sexual responses of patients to nurses.

Clinical Example Mr. P has been hospitalized for an exacerbation of a chronic illness for the past 3 weeks. Ms. S has been his primary nurse during this hospitalization. The following is a conversation between the nurse and patient the day before his discharge.

Mr. P: I wish my wife were more like you, Ms. S.

Ms. S: Mr. P, I'm not sure I understand what you are saying.

Mr. P: Well, it's just that you are always so concerned about me. You always try to make me feel good and want to help me all the time. Sometimes my wife's a grouch; she's so wrapped up in her job and the kids she doesn't always pay as much attention to me as you do.

Ms. S: I'm glad you feel taken care of, but it's impossible to compare my role as your nurse with your wife's role.

Mr. P: I'm not sure I follow you.

Ms. S: They are very different types of relationships. It's nice to have someone take care of us when we can't take care of ourselves, but when we are healthy, we don't need someone to take care of us all the time. Your relationship with your wife is more of a sharing one with mutual benefits. You take care of her needs, and she takes care of your needs in return. If you feel that your relationship with your wife is not a satisfying one, perhaps you need to talk this over with her.

Maladaptive Sexual Responses

ILLNESS. Stress, physical and emotional illness, injury, and aging can lead to changes in sexuality and sexual functioning. These changes and related nursing interventions differ based on whether the illness is acute or chronic. It is important for the nurse to obtain complete information on the nature and course of the illness, the types of medications used in its treatment, the patient's appraisal of the impact of the illness, and any physical limitation imposed by the illness that affects the patient's sexual health.

Several major nursing interventions can then be implemented to facilitate the patient's adaptive sexual responses. The first is for the nurse to act in a supportive way and to help the patient express feelings, fears, and problems. Open communication between the patient and partner should also be encouraged. The nurse can reinforce the positive attributes of the patient, prevent social isolation, mobilize coping resources, and support adaptive coping mechanisms that have helped the patient deal with stressors in the past.

The nurse can also offer anticipatory guidance and give accurate information about the illness or injury, including what the patient may expect from medical or psychiatric treatment and its impact on sexual health (see A Patient Speaks). The nurse can also initiate counseling about sexuality and alternative means of sexual expression. Relaxation techniques, autoerotic activities, and variations in movement and positions may be suggested. The nurse should emphasize that pleasure can be obtained in a variety of ways and stress the importance of a loving relationship. Finally, if the problem is complex and of a long duration, the patient should be referred for psychotherapy or sex therapy from a qualified professional. A Patient Education Plan for patients recovering from an organic illness is presented on p. 562.

> **?** *Should sexual behavior be permitted among patients who are residents of a long-term psychiatric facility? If so, what issues must be addressed by staff? If not, how will the sexual needs of these patients be met?*

SEXUAL ORIENTATION. Most heterosexuals, homosexuals, and bisexuals accept their sexual orientations, although some have difficulty and seek professional help. For example, it is possible that one's sexual behavior may not match one's sexual desire. Someone in a heterosexual relationship may wish to be in a homosexual one, or vice versa, and feel constrained to act because of personal, sociocultural, legal, economic, or religious reasons. This can create internal conflict and distress and the person may seek counseling. The first step in working with a heterosexual, homosexual, or bisexual who views his or her sexual responses as maladaptive is the nurse's acceptance. Most patients are extremely perceptive of their caregiver's values and attitudes toward them. Nurses who believe they are hiding their prejudices are only fooling themselves.

Because nurses have grown up in a homophobic society, it is often difficult to examine the myths and search for facts. Homophobia is a persistent and irrational fear of homosexuals, as well as a negative attitude and hostility toward them. It may also include the person's fear of being homosexual.[26] The homosexual patient has grown up in the same society, where negative attitudes regarding homosexuality still exist, and often experiences the same homophobia as anyone else.

Because of the homosexual element of bisexuality, bisexuals often encounter many of the same difficulties stemming from societal attitudes as homosexuals. Another factor that may present a problem for the bisexual is isolation from a support group. Because bisexuals are often accused

A Patient *Speaks*

It's bad enough to be depressed, but how's a person supposed to feel when the people taking care of them don't give them all the information they need? From what I can see from talking to other patients in my group, my story is not that unusual.

For about 6 months I felt myself slipping deeper and deeper into the black hole of depression. I saw some ads on television and decided that maybe I needed some outside help, since I clearly wasn't getting better by myself. So off I go to a nearby clinic where I see someone who diagnoses me with depression and gives me some pills to take. In the beginning, the drugs made me kind of jittery, but gradually I got over it. In a couple of months I actually almost felt like my old self again—all except for sex, that is. In that one area of my life I simply couldn't experience the satisfaction I used to have and didn't know what was going on. Well, it turns out that the pills I'm on limit my sexual performance, but nobody ever bothered to mention this to me. I guess they thought it wasn't important or something, but they were really wrong.

Now that I understand what's going on I can work around it, since the drugs have helped me in almost every other way. But still, it would have been nice if the people that you turn to for help could give you all the information you need and not just talk about the parts that they think are important or limit themselves to the topics they're comfortable talking about. ▼

of fence-sitting, they can be rejected by heterosexuals and homosexuals. Bisexuals may lack social support; friends and family may pressure them to decide on one sexual orientation (usually heterosexual) so that they will be accepted by society.

An important step in working with homosexual patients is to avoid focusing on the causal factors of homosexuality ("Why did this happen to me?") and to encourage patients to explore their beliefs and values about homosexuality.[32] The patient may have internalized some of society's prejudices, such as "Homosexuality is a sick and abnormal behavior; because I am a homosexual, I am sick and abnormal and should not act on my sexual feelings because they are wrong." Responses can be varied and include denial, confusion, and sexual promiscuity, especially among those trying to prove to themselves that they are not gay. It is helpful to have patients list their beliefs about homosexuality and bisexuality and to discuss each one. However, a review of beliefs about homosexual-

TABLE **26-2** *Summary of Nursing Considerations in Sexual Responses of Patients to Nurses*

GOAL: MAINTAIN A PROFESSIONAL NURSE-PATIENT RELATIONSHIP THAT WILL ENABLE THE NURSE TO PROVIDE THERAPEUTIC NURSING CARE

PRINCIPLE	RATIONALE	NURSING CONSIDERATIONS
Establish a trusting relationship.	An atmosphere of trust allows for open, honest communication between patient and nurse; this enables the nurse to aid the patient in discovering the underlying issues related to sexual feelings and behavior.	Express nonsexual caring and concern for the patient. Be a responsive listener, especially to feelings and needs that the patient may not be able to express directly. Reinforce the purpose of the therapeutic nurse-patient relationship.
Gain awareness of nurse's own feelings and thoughts.	Being aware of his or her feelings and thoughts enables the nurse to understand how they influence his or her behavior; with increased self-awareness the nurse can increase the effectiveness of his or her interactions with patients.	Recognize own feelings and thoughts. Identify any specific patient interaction or behavior that influences the nurse's feelings and thoughts. Identify the influence of the nurse's feelings and thoughts on one's behavior in an attempt to increase the effectiveness of nursing interventions.
Decrease patient's inappropriate expressions of sexual feelings and behavior.	If the nurse is able to help the patient see that his or her sexual interactions and behavior are being expressed to an inappropriate partner (the nurse), the sexual acting out will usually decrease; this allows the nurse to help the patient begin to identify the reasons for his or her behavior.	Set limits on patient's sexual behavior. Use a calm, matter-of-fact approach without implying judgment. Reaffirm nonsexual caring for the patient. Explore the meaning of the patient's feelings and behaviors.
Expand patient's insight into sexual feelings and behavior.	Once the patient begins to identify the reasons for his or her sexual feelings and behaviors, he or she can see that the nurse is not an appropriate outlet for these feelings and behaviors and can move toward a more appropriate and therapeutic relationship.	Clarify misconceptions regarding any feeling patient may have about the nurse as a possible sexual partner. Point out the futile nature of the patient's romantic or sexual interest in the nurse. Redirect patient's energies toward appropriate health-care issues.

ity may not be sufficient. Encouraging the person to read about homosexuality and bisexuality is also helpful. Throughout this process, the patient will be extremely sensitive to the nurse's acceptance or rejection.

Confidentiality is also a central issue. It is helpful for the nurse to demonstrate an appreciation for patients' concerns about unwanted exposure of their homosexuality to family members, friends, or co-workers. The nurse should not encourage or discourage the patient's disclosure of homosexual concerns but rather help the patient to explore and process the choice of disclosure or lack of disclosure with others, as in this clinical example.

Clinical Example Ms. A, a 25-year-old single female, came to the mental health clinic with the complaint of a "sexual problem." Her history revealed that she had been sexually inactive for the past 5 years. At the age of 20, Ms. A had a brief sexual encounter with a man she had been dating for 2 years. She ended the relationship shortly afterward because she had no interest in maintaining a sexual relationship with the man. Recently, she became involved in a relationship with a woman that was very satisfying to her.

She felt she had to end the relationship because she would not tolerate thinking of herself as a homosexual. During one of the initial counseling sessions, Ms. A told the nurse that she must end the relationship before "it" happens again.

Nurse: What are you afraid will happen?

Ms. A: I'm afraid I'll feel attracted to her again.

Nurse: What about that frightens you?

Ms. A: (becoming upset) That will mean I'm homosexual!

Nurse: What does being homosexual mean for you?

Ms. A: It means I'm sick. It's a sin, I couldn't go to church anymore.

Nurse: Are all homosexuals sick?

Ms. A: Yes.

Nurse: How do you know this?

Ms. A: Everybody knows that homosexuality is morally wrong. Homosexuals have a lot of emotional problems.

Nurse: Do you know any homosexual people?

Ms. A: Well, not exactly.

Nurse: What have you read about homosexuality?

Ms. A: Nothing.

PATIENT EDUCATION PLAN **Sexual Response after an Organic Illness**

Content	Instructional Activities	Evaluation
Describe the variety of human sexual response patterns.	Discuss the range of sexual desires, modes of expression, and techniques.	The patient identifies personal sexual orientation and typical level of sexual functioning.
Define the patient's primary organic problem.	Provide accurate information regarding the disruption caused by the organic impairment.	The patient understands the specific organic illness.
Clarify relationship between the organic problem and patient's level of sexual functioning.	Reframe distorted or confused perceptions regarding the impact of the illness on patient's sexual functioning.	The patient accurately describes the impact of the illness on sexual functioning.
Identify ways to enhance patient's sexual functioning and improve interpersonal communication.	Describe additional experiences that would add to the sexual satisfaction and the relationship between the patient and patient's partner.	The patient and partner report reduced anxiety and greater satisfaction with their sexual responses.

Nurse: Then it looks to me like you are basing all of your conclusions on hearsay and not real knowledge. I think that you and I need to explore your beliefs in more detail, then you can do some reading to find out the facts.

Selected Nursing Diagnoses:

▼ Altered sexuality patterns related to questions about sexual preference related to recent interpersonal relationship

▼ Spiritual distress related to conflicting values, as evidenced by questions about religious beliefs

In the preceding clinical example, the nurse and Ms. A developed a plan often used in sexual counseling to explore homosexuality. Some of the interventions included the following:

▼ Ms. A described her beliefs about homosexuality and homosexuals.

▼ The nurse encouraged Ms. A to explore the literature on homosexuality and suggested readings to help dispel the myths.

▼ The nurse then discussed these with Ms. A and suggested that she attend a social gathering for gay people to test out her new knowledge. The nurse suggested the social gathering because many people struggling with a homosexual identity are frightened to test out situations that would dispel the myths.

▼ Finally, the nurse helped Ms. A. explore her responses to these activities and integrate them into a positive view of self.

GENDER IDENTITY. Gender identity is a person's perceptions of his or her maleness or femaleness. Gender identity disorder or gender dysphoria is characterized by a profound discomfort with one's sex and a strong and persistent identification with the opposite gender. It can be experienced along a continuum of responses, with transsexualism being the most severe form of this disorder. Treatment of the transsexual person has been a controversial subject in recent years. In a 5-year follow-up study of people in the process of changing their sex, 70% of the subjects experienced a positive outcome. The authors attribute this to careful selection, close observation over long periods of time, and supportive follow-up treatment. They suggest that sex reassignment surgery is the treatment of choice for true transsexualism.[3]

Most hospitals and clinics that treat transsexuals follow the Harry Benjamin International Gender Dysphoria Association's standards of care.[12] Patients who believe that they are transsexual and request surgical reassignment must meet these standards. They require that two therapists specializing in the treatment of transsexual disorders agree that the reassignment is appropriate. The therapist making the recommendation must have known the patient in a psychotherapeutic relationship for at least 6 months before making the recommendation. The patient must have a 2-year documented history of gender dysphoria and must live in the role of the preferred gender for at least 1 year. The standards also require that certain lab studies be completed and follow-up care provided.

Professionals who care for transsexual patients must be educated in sexuality. The assessment phase of treatment is especially important. The patient and therapist must be certain that implementing the treatment plan is the best approach because the surgery is not reversible.

A Nursing Treatment Plan Summary for maladaptive sexual responses is presented at right.

Dysfunctions of the Sexual Response Cycle

Treating sexual dysfunctions is beyond the scope of the nurse generalist. However, the nurse should be aware of the principles involved and should know creditable sex therapists in the community for referral of patients. Two common models of sex therapy are briefly discussed here:

NURSING TREATMENT PLAN *Summary*   Maladaptive Sexual Responses

Nursing Diagnosis: Altered sexuality patterns
Expected Outcome: The patient will obtain the maximum level of adaptive sexual responses to enhance or maintain health.

Short-term Goals	Interventions	Rationale
The patient will describe values, beliefs, questions, and problems regarding sexuality.	Listen to sexual concerns implied and expressed. Help the patient explore sexual beliefs, values, and questions. Encourage open communication between the patient and partner.	An accepting therapeutic relationship will allow patients to be free to question, grow, and seek help with sexual concerns. Communicate respect, acceptance, and openness to sexual concerns.
The patient will relate accurate information about sexual concerns.	Clarify sexual misinformation. Dispel myths. Provide specific education about sexual health practices, behaviors, and problems. Give professional "permission" to continue sexual behavior that is not physically or emotionally harmful. Reinforce positive attitudes of the patient.	Accurate information is helpful in changing negative thoughts and attitudes about particular aspects of sexuality. It can also prevent or limit dysfunctional behavior. Giving permission allows the person to continue the behavior and alleviate anxiety about normalcy. It allows patients to incorporate sexual behavior in a positive and accepting self-concept.
The patient will implement one new behavior to enhance sexual response.	Set clear goals with the patient. Identify specific behaviors that can be carried out focusing on enhancing self-concept, role functioning, and sexuality. Encourage relaxation techniques, redirection of attention, positional changes, and alternative ways of sexual expression as appropriate. Become familiar with the sex therapy resources available in the community. Refer the patient to a qualified sex therapist as needed.	Giving a patient direct behavioral suggestions can help relieve a sexual problem or difficulty and is a useful intervention when the problem is of recent onset and short duration. While all nurses need to screen for maladaptive sexual responses and provide basic nursing care, complex problems should be referred to qualified sex therapists for further treatment.

the Masters and Johnson and the Helen Singer Kaplan models.

MASTERS AND JOHNSON MODEL. William Masters and Virginia Johnson began pioneering research in sexuality in the 1950s. Their book *Human Sexual Inadequacy*[23] describes their research and counseling methods. Before the work of Masters and Johnson, patients with problems in sexuality were generally referred to a psychiatrist for psychotherapy or psychoanalysis. Health professionals assumed that anyone who had a problem with sexuality was emotionally disturbed. Problems with sexual response are usually not psychiatric problems but are the result of sociocultural deprivation and ignorance of sexual physiology. Masters and Johnson's treatment includes short-term education with step-by-step instructions regarding the physical aspects of sexual activity and supportive psychotherapy. The researchers believe that attitudes and ignorance are responsible for most sexual dysfunctions.

Their approach to patients begins with obtaining a detailed sexual and background history. Then the couple is instructed to carry out a sensate focus exercise in which each partner instructs the other in specific ways of caressing for sensual pleasure without involving the breasts or genitals. The next day the exercise is repeated, including breasts and genital areas, but without coitus. The exercise's purpose is to alleviate performance anxiety and to enhance warm, comfortable feelings between partners. After the sensate focus exercises are completed, the therapy is directed to the sexual dysfunction. The Masters and Johnson model emphasizes education, communication, and cooperation between partners.

HELEN SINGER KAPLAN MODEL. Kaplan's[15] method of treating sexual dysfunctions combines specific tasks with psychodynamic insights, dream interpretations, and gestalt and transactional techniques. Treatment begins with an extensive evaluation, including marital, psychiatric, sexual, medical, and family history from both partners. If serious intrapsychic or interpersonal difficulties are found, the couple may be referred to individual or conjoint therapy and is not accepted for sex therapy at that time.

Like Masters and Johnson, Kaplan uses sensate focus exercises and variations, such as showering together, to begin sex therapy or to further evaluate a client's suitability for sex therapy. Therapy itself consists of erotic tasks performed at home plus weekly or semiweekly meetings with the therapist. Clients and the therapist explore feelings experienced during the erotic exercises. The exercises take into account the motivations and dynamics of the relationship. The role of the therapist includes education, clarification, and support.

Both Kaplan and Masters and Johnson emphasize communication between partners and exploration of the relationship and emotional concerns. The reader is referred to original works of these therapists for more information.[15-17,23,24]

Evaluation

In the evaluation phase the nurse works with the patient to evaluate the effectiveness of the sexual counseling or intervention. Factors to consider include the following:

▼ *Sense of well-being.* How does the person feel about himself or herself? Have these feelings improved during the treatment?

▼ *Functioning ability.* If the person was dysfunctional, is functional ability restored? Somewhat improved? What about the person's ability to function within primary relations at work? With friends?

▼ *Satisfaction with treatment.* Does the patient believe that the treatment was helpful? Were the patient's goals adequately met?

Evaluation of any form of sexual counseling or intervention should be ongoing. The nurse and patient should work together on goals, problems, and alternatives.

Summary

1. Sexuality is defined as a desire for contact, warmth, tenderness, and love. Adaptive sexual behavior is consensual, free of force, performed in private, neither physically nor psychologically harmful, and mutually satisfying.

2. Patient behaviors related to sexual responses include heterosexuality, homosexuality, bisexuality, transvestism, transsexualism, and physiological and psychological responses to sexual stimulation.

3. Predisposing factors for variations in sexual response are described from biological, psychoanalytical, and behavioral perspectives. Precipitating stressors that may change sexuality include physical illness and injury, psychiatric illness, medications, and HIV/AIDS.

4. A variety of coping mechanisms are used with expressions of sexuality: fantasy, projection, denial, and rationalization.

5. Primary NANDA diagnoses are sexual dysfunction and altered sexuality patterns.

6. Primary DSM-IV diagnoses are categorized as sexual dysfunctions, paraphilias, and gender identity disorders.

7. The expected outcome of nursing care is that the patient will obtain the maximum level of adaptive sexual responses to enhance or maintain health.

8. Interventions include sex education and preventive counseling and intervening in sexual feelings and behaviors within the nurse-patient relationship, maladaptive sexual responses, and dysfunctions of the sexual response cycle.

9. The nurse and patient should consider the following factors in evaluating nursing care: the patient's sense of well-being, functioning ability, and satisfaction with treatment.

COMPETENT CARING A Clinical Exemplar of a Psychiatric Nurse

Donald Ribelin, RN, C

Having worked in nursing for over 20 years, I tend to have certain defined responses to almost any given situation. This works well until something comes along that doesn't fit into those preconceived notions of how things should be. I was working as evening charge nurse on an adult acute care psychiatric unit when one of the mental health assistants came to the desk to report that he had seen Mr. B and Mrs. G sneaking into the solarium and that they appeared to be "getting it on." Almost every nurse has had to confront patients, visitors, or both in a sexual situation of one type or another. We'd had our share of such encounters in the past, but the staff reacted very differently this time.

To begin with, Mr. B was a 72-year-old "street" person who had been admitted with a diagnosis of rule-out dementia, and Ms. G was a lovely 70-year-old widow with a diagnosis of situational depression. Mr. B's apparent dementia had proven to be secondary to malnutrition and vitamin B$_{12}$ deficiency. Once he had received treatment for these, we had found him to be a remarkable person whose ready sense of humor lightened many an evening group. Ms. G had been admitted with one of the flattest affects I had ever seen. Her family reported that she had been increasingly depressed since her husband's death 3 years ago. This

COMPETENT CARING A Clinical Exemplar of a Psychiatric Nurse—cont'd

depression increased dramatically around the anniversary of Mr. G's death, which was right around this time of the year.

Over the past week, Ms. G's depression had lifted noticeably. She could be seen talking, laughing, and joking with Mr. B during any free moment. They seemed to always be together, sitting next to each other during groups or meals or walking side by side on outings. We had all commented on how much they had helped each other and what a nice couple they made. Suddenly Mr. B and Ms. G had stopped being a nice "old" couple and had become two psychiatric patients sneaking off to have "sex."

I found myself torn between several reactions to this news. The empathic nurse in me responded, "This is great: Two lonely people in their twilight years of their lives have found love and companionship." The analytical nurse in me wondered whether this relationship would really be therapeutic for Ms. G given Mr. B's background. The cautious nurse in me wondered whether Mr. B could simply be trying to ensure he had somewhere to stay after discharge. But the administrative nurse in me won out, thinking that I don't let other patients behave in this manner, so I have to intercede.

Somewhat loudly I walked down the hall and into the solarium, taking a very long time fumbling for the light switch. The lights revealed Ms. G and Mr. B sitting side by side, holding hands and red faced. Ms. G's blouse was only partially buttoned, and she was obviously upset. I apologized to them, explaining that I had planned to spend my break in the solarium and hadn't meant to startle them. As they quickly stood up and headed toward their rooms, I could see a look of sadness and possibly shame replacing the happy smile that we had been seeing the past few days on Ms. G's face. Mr. B also looked sad, and for a moment I thought I saw the return of the shuffling gait he had at admission. By doing the "right" thing, I now felt like I had done the very worst thing possible.

During my shift report, I gave the incident only brief comment. Talking more about the possible therapeutic benefits of the relationship, I didn't mention the sexual aspects at all. Guilt can be a great censor and rewriter of history, and I was obviously really feeling guilty.

Well, time may heal all wounds, but it only gives rumors time to grow. I was very surprised when, upon returning to work the next evening, my nurse manager asked for the incident report on Mr. B and Ms. G having sex in the solarium. She also wanted to know why I hadn't documented the incident in my nursing notes. By the time I had explained the previous evening's happenings, what had started out as two people wanting to be together had become a major event.

Damage control began with a meeting of all unit staff, where we discussed what had and had not happened. It didn't stop there. A psychiatric unit is often like a small town where there are no secrets. That evening, in group, the patients brought up our hapless couple's "making out." Again I found myself in a position where I felt anything I said could and probably would be wrong. After careful thought I responded by first reminding them that this was a hospital and there were certain rules of conduct that had to be adhered to, even when we might personally disagree with them. Members of the group were asked to share their feelings about these rules and why they were or were not necessary. As the group proceeded, I kept a careful eye on Ms. G and Mr. B. They were sitting about as far from each other as possible and both were very quiet.

As the patients talked, I kept trying to think of something to say or do to alleviate the obvious pain and embarrassment of our elderly, who were now the center of attention. Suddenly Mr. B stood up, smiled at the group, and said, "You know, I've been feeling real bad today. I felt like I had done something wrong and that I was just waiting for my punishment to come." Then he stated, "Yeah! I was feeling real bad until just a moment ago, when I remembered a button I saw once. It said, 'Old people need love too,' and you know that's right because everyone needs to know that someone cares about them, needs them, and loves them. So it really doesn't matter what any of you think because I've found someone to love me and for me to love."

I'll always remember that moment as a time that patients and staff clapped, cried, and laughed together.

your **INTERNET**
connection

Healthy Sexuality
http://www.uiuc.edu/departments/mck...health-info/
sexual/intro/intro.htm

Homosexuality: Common Questions and Statements Addressed
http://www.geocities.com/WestHollywood/1348/

Chapter Review Questions

1. Match each term in Column A with the correct definition in Column B.

Column A

___Bisexuality

___Gender identity

___Gender role

___Genetic identity

___Heterosexuality

___Homophobia

___Homosexuality

___Orgasm

___Sexual orientation

___Transsexualism

___Transvestism

Column B

A. A person's chromosomal gender

B. A person's perception of his or her maleness or femaleness

C. Condition in which there is a profound discomfort with one's own sex and a strong and persistent identification with the opposite gender

D. Condition in which usually a male has a sexual obsession for or addiction to women's clothing

E. Peaking of sexual pleasure and the release of sexual tension accompanied by rhythmic contractions of the perineal muscles and pelvic reproductive organs

F. Persistent and irrational fear of homosexuals along with a negative attitude and hostility toward them

G. Sexual attraction to members of the opposite sex

H. Sexual attraction to members of the same sex

I. Sexual attraction to persons of both sexes

J. The cultural role attributes attributed to one's gender, such as expectations regarding behavior, cognitions, occupations, values, and emotional responses

K. The gender to which one is romantically attracted

2. Fill in the blanks.

A. When a nurse holds two opposing beliefs at the same time it is called _____.

B. A biological female typically has _____ chromosomes, whereas a biological male typically has _____ chromosomes.

C. According to Freud, in the _____ complex the child experiences sexual feelings for the parent of the opposite sex and resents the parent of the same sex.

D. Behaviorists believe that _____ may predispose one to sexual difficulties later in life.

E. _____ is the most common method of primary prevention of sexual problems.

F. The nurse's first step in working with a patient in relation to maladaptive sexual responses is to communicate _____.

3. Provide short responses for the following questions.

A. Identify five criteria for adaptive sexual behavior.

B. Design a sex education program for adolescents that includes a focus on safe sex practices.

C. Critique the assessment form used in your treatment center for its inclusion of information related to a patient's sexual responses.

D. Describe specific ways in which culture defines a society's view of "normal" sexual behavior.

REFERENCES

1. American Psychiatric Association: *Diagnostic and statistical manual of mental disorders,* ed 4, Washington DC, 1994, The Association.
2. Beemer BR: Gender dysphoria update, *J Psychosoc Nurs* 34:13, 1996.
3. Bodlund O, Kullgren G: Transsexualism: general outcomes and prognostic factors: a five-year follow-up study of nineteen transsexuals in the process of changing sex, *Arch Sex Behav* 25:315, 1996.
4. Byne W, Parsons B: Human sexual orientation: the biological theories reappraised, *Arch Gen Psychiatry* 50:228, 1993.
5. Cabas R, Stein T: *Textbook of homosexuality and mental health,* Washington, DC, 1996, American Psychiatric Press.
6. Crenshaw TL, Goldberg JP: *Sexual pharmacology: drugs that affect sexual function,* New York, 1996, WW Norton.
7. Denney NW, Quadango B: *Human sexuality,* ed 2, St Louis, 1992, Mosby.
8. Edelwich J, Brodsky A: *Sexual dilemmas for the helping professional,* New York, 1991, Brunner/Mazel.

9. Foley T, Davies M: *Rape: nursing care of victims,* St Louis, 1983, Mosby.
10. Freud S: *Three essays of the theory of sexuality,* ed 3, London, 1962, Hogarth Press (originally published 1905).
11. Haffner D: Young still at risk, yet barriers to education remain: SIECUS testimony for the National AIDS Commission, *SIECUS Report* 21:10, 1992.
12. Harry Benjamin International Gender Dysphoria Association: Standards of care: the hormonal and surgical reassignment of gender dysphoric persons (revised), Palo Alto, Calif, 1990, The Association.
13. Hulme PA, Grove SK: Symptoms of female survivors of child sexual abuse, *Issues Ment Health Nurs* 15:526-528, 1994.
14. Jackson JL, Calhoun KS, Amick AK, Maddever HM, Habif VL: Young adult women who report childhood intrafamilial sexual abuse: subsequent adjustment, *Arch Sex Behav* 19:211, 1990.
15. Kaplan HS: *The illustrated manual of sex therapy,* New York, 1975, New York Times Book Co.
16. Kaplan HS: *Disorders of sexual desire and other new concepts and techniques in sex therapy,* New York, 1979, Brunner/Mazel.
17. Kaplan HS: Sex, intimacy, and the aging process, *J Am Acad Psychoanal* 18:185,1990.
18. Kelly JA, Murphy DA, Sikkema KJ, Somlai AM, Mulry GW, Fernandez MI, Miller JG, Stevenson LY: Predictors of high and low levels of HIV risk behavior among adults with chronic mental illness, *Psychiatr Serv* 46:813, 1995.
19. Kettl P et al: Sexual harassment of health care students by patients, *J Psychosoc Nurs Ment Health Serv* 31:11, 1993.
20. Kinsey AC, Pomeroy WB, Martin EC: *Sexual behavior in the human female,* Philadelphia, 1953, WB Saunders.
21. Kirby D: Sexuality education: it can reduce unprotected intercourse, *SIECUS Report* 21:19, 1992.
22. Laumann EO, Gagnon JH, Michael RT, Michaels S: *The social organization of sexuality,* Chicago, 1994, University of Chicago Press.
23. Masters WH, Johnson VE: *Human sexual inadequacy,* Boston, 1970, Little, Brown.
24. Masters WH, Johnson VE, Kolodny RC: *Masters and Johnson on sex and human loving,* Boston, 1986, Little, Brown.
25. McConaghy N: *Sexual behavior: problems and management,* New York, 1993, Plenum.
26. McDonald HB, Steinhorn AL: *Homosexuality: a practical guide to counseling lesbians, gay men, and their families,* New York, 1990, Continuum.
27. McKirnan DJ, Stokes JP, Doll L, Burzette RG: Bisexually active men: social characteristics and sexual behavior, *J Sex Res* 32:65, 1995.
28. Metz ME, Rosser BRS, Strapko N: Differences in conflict-resolution styles among heterosexual, gay, and lesbian couples, *J Sex Res* 31:293, 1994.
29. Michael RT, Gagnon JH, Laumann EO, Kolata G: *Sex in America: a definitive survey,* Boston, 1994, Little, Brown.
30. Reinisch JM, Beasley R, Kent D, editors: *The Kinsey Institute new report on sex: what you must know to be sexually literate,* New York, 1990, St Martin's Press.
31. SIECUS fact sheet #3, on comprehensive sexuality education: sexuality education and the schools: issues and answers, *SIECUS Report* 20:13, 1992.
32. Smith GB: Nursing care challenges: homosexual psychiatric patients, *J Psychosoc Nurs Ment Health Serv* 30:16, 1992.
33. Sullivan G, Lukoff D: Sexual side effects of antipsychotic medication: evaluation and interventions, *Hosp Community Psychiatry* 41:1238, 1990.
34. Trudel G, Boulos L, Matte B: Dyadic adjustment in couples with hypoactive sexual desire, *J Sex Educ Ther* 19:31, 1993.
35. VanWyk PH, Geist CS: Biology of bisexuality: critique and observations, *J Homosexuality* 28:369, 1995.
36. Whipple B: Common questions about women and HIV/AIDS, *Am J Nurs* 95:16A, 1995.
37. Wyatt GE: The aftermath of child sexual abuse of African-American and white American women: the victim's experience, *J Fam Violence* 5:61, 1990.
38. Zawid CS: *Sexual health: a nurse's guide,* Albany, NY, 1994, Delmar.

ANNOTATED SUGGESTED READINGS

Augelli A, Patterson C: *Lesbian, gay and bisexual identities over the lifespan,* New York, 1995, Oxford University Press.
  Reviews recent psychological research and theory on lesbian, gay, and bisexual identities, and identifies promising directions for future work.
*Beemer B: Gender dysphoria update, *J Psychosocial Nurs Serv* 31:4, 1996.
  Excellent overview of gender identity disorder, sex reassignment surgery, and the nursing management of gender dysphoric patients.
Butler R, Lewis M: *Love and sex after 60,* New York, 1993, Ballantine.
  This easy-to-read book is excellent as a resource for the older adult. It provides an affirming yet realistic look at the affects of aging on sexuality.
Cabaj R, Stein T: *Textbook of homosexuality and mental health,* Washington, DC, 1996, American Psychiatric Press.
  Comprehensive text that reports on the wide biopsychosocial diversity of sexual variance in men and women. Valuable reference for both expert and lay reader.
Crenshaw T, Goldberg J: *Sexual pharmacology: drugs that affect sexual function,* New York, 1996, WW Norton.
  Comprehensive textbook that examines the sexual side effects of drug classifications such as antihypertensives, psychotropics, and drugs for internal medicine. An excellent resource book for nurses.
*Deevy S: Lesbian self-disclosure, *J Psychosocial Nurs* 31:21, 1993.
  Challenges nurses who are lesbians to share information about lesbian culture with their colleagues and provide healthy role models for their patients and peers.
Hellman R: Issues in the treatment of lesbian women and agy men with chronic mental illness, *Psychiatr Serv* 47:1093, 1996.
  Provides a clinical context for understanding essential issues in the inpatient and outpatient treatment of chronic psychiatric patients who are gay men or lesbian women, a group largely ignored or invisible in the mental health delivery system. Highly recommended.
*Kettl P et al: Sexual harassment of health care students by patients, *J Psychosoc Nurs* 31:11, 1993.
  Reports on a survey of sexual harassment by patients and a training program to deal with this problem.
Miller L, Finnerty M: Sexuality, pregnancy, and childbearing among women with schizophrenia-spectrum disorders, *Psychiatr Serv* 47:502, 1996.
  This study demonstrates that the health care system does not meet the needs of this at-risk group of women, who were found to be less likely to receive screening for pregnancy, HIV, or battering and less likely to be given information about family planning, social skills training, or parenting.
Rowlands P: Schizophrenia and sexuality, *Sex Marital Ther* 10:1, 1995
  Provides a review of sexuality and schizophrenia and discusses the sexual symptoms of schizophrenia and the issues that surface in relationships. For the advanced reader.

*Nursing reference.

Steiner J et al: Psychoeducation about sexual issues in an acute treatment setting, *Hosp Community Psychiatry* 45:4, 1994.
Describes a group educational program for sexual issues in an acute outpatient program for severe psychiatric disorders, including discussion of issues such as sexually transmitted diseases and intimacy in relationships.
*Stewart R: Female circumcision: implications for North American nurses, *J Psychosoc Nurs* 35:35, 1997.

Discusses the history, types, and beliefs surrounding female circumcision with implications for nursing.
*Zawid C: *Sexual health: a nurse's guide,* Albany, New York, 1994, Delmar.
Gives an overview of important sexual issues that aid the nurse in providing quality sexual health care. Sexuality throughout the life cycle and the impact of disease on sexuality are discussed in detail.

*Nursing reference.

Treatment Modalities

4

Maybe there have been times when you've felt that the problems people experience are truly overwhelming and you've wondered how you can ever really help. Sure you're a nurse, but how can one person reduce the world's stress, illness, and social injustice? Although it's true that societal problems are great, it's also true that the contribution of each person is like a ripple in a pool that can eventually turn the tide of life. But to be effective you need to have the right tools for the task, tools that will allow you to help people think about their life situation and change their behavior, tools that will help you work therapeutically with individuals, families, and groups.

In this unit you will be exposed to a wide range of treatment tools, but don't think that these strategies will pertain only to patients with psychiatric illnesses. The fact is that many people take psychotropic medications, and nurses deal with people who struggle with issues of control, aggression, and violence in almost all clinical settings. Also, strategies to change negative thinking patterns and problematic behavior can apply to children and adults throughout their experiences with health and illness. And finally, aren't groups an essential part of every health-care delivery system, and don't all patients have families? As you can see, the skills you will learn in this unit will enhance your nursing practice regardless of setting. So grab your highlighters and get ready to add to your growing repertoire of nursing skills and competencies, because you can and will make a difference.

© 1998 M.C. Escher/Cordon Art, Baarn, Holland.

Chapter 27

Psychopharm-acology

Michele T. Laraia

Medicines are nothing in themselves, if not properly used, but the very hands of the gods, if employed with reason and prudence. **Herophilus**

LEARNING OBJECTIVES

After studying this chapter the student should be able to:

▼ Identify the role of the nurse in psychopharmacological treatments

▼ Describe pharmacokinetics and problems of polypharmacy and drug interactions

▼ Discuss the mechanism of action, clinical use, and adverse reactions related to antianxiety and sedative-hypnotic drugs

▼ Discuss the mechanism of action, clinical use, and adverse reactions related to antidepressant drugs

▼ Discuss the mechanism of action, clinical use, and adverse reactions related to mood-stabilizing drugs

▼ Discuss the mechanism of action, clinical use, and adverse reactions related to antipsychotic drugs

▼ Evaluate the emergence of new psychopharmacological agents

▼ Describe psychiatric nursing practice issues including psychopharmacology guidelines, documentation, patient education, and promoting patient adherence

TOPICAL OUTLINE

Role of the Nurse
  Patient Assessment
  Coordination of Treatment Modalities
  Psychopharmacological Drug Administration
  Monitoring Drug Effects
  Medication Education
  Drug Maintenance Programs
  Clinical Research Drug Trials
  Prescriptive Authority
Pharmacokinetics
  Drug Interactions
  Biological Basis for Psychopharmacology
Antianxiety and Sedative-Hypnotic Drugs
  Benzodiazepines
  Nonbenzodiazepines
Antidepressant Drugs
  Tricyclic Antidepressants
  Selective Serotonin Reuptake Inhibitors
  Monoamine Oxidase Inhibitors
  Other Antidepressant Drugs
Mood-Stabilizing Drugs
  Lithium
  Anticonvulsants
Antipsychotic Drugs
Future Psychopharmacological Agents
Psychiatric Nursing Practice
  Psychopharmacology Guidelines
  Documentation
  Patient Education
  Promoting Patient Adherence

571

The past 50 years have produced a revolution in the treatment of psychiatric disorders and in the theories about the etiologies of these disorders. This revolution was sparked by the introduction of neuropsychopharmacology: drugs that treat the symptoms of mental illness and whose actions in the brain provide models to understand better the mechanisms of mental disorders. This sense of revolution continues as new theories are debated by experts in the neurosciences and as more centers around the world are funded for clinical drug studies.

Amid the growth and controversy, the nurse often is the one professional to integrate these drug treatments with the wide range of nonpharmacological treatments in a manner that is knowledgeable, safe, effective, and acceptable to the patient. Regardless of the nurse's theoretical framework, psychopharmacologic agents are currently among the gold standards of treatment of psychiatric disorders. Nurses should continue to incorporate psychopharmacology into the knowledge base of nursing theory, the arena of nursing research, and the art and science of nursing care. Nurses should also continue to do what nurses do best: lead the patient through the maze of health-care possibilities in a holistic manner, incorporating them into an individualized and effective treatment plan.

This chapter is designed to introduce the nurse to psychopharmacology and describe some of the important principles of drug treatment in psychiatry. The theoretical framework suggested here is one of integration: Drug therapy can complement problem-solving procedures and the wide range of psychodynamic, psychosocial, and interpersonal interventions. Drug therapy should never be viewed as a quick fix or miracle pill. Currently, drug therapy treats symptoms of mental illness with some success, but drugs do not treat the patient's personal, social, or environmental responses to the mental illness. In addition, side ef-

fects and adverse reactions of drug therapy add another level of concern and need for expertise and judgment in nursing care. This is a very exciting time in psychiatric treatment, and nurses are in an excellent position to add new dimensions to their role.

ROLE OF THE NURSE

Psychopharmacological treatment must be integrated with the principles of psychiatric nursing practice presented throughout this text. The psychiatric nurse has a wealth of knowledge and techniques that make nursing unique in the care of people with psychiatric disorders. Following are some examples of the nurse's role in psychopharmacological treatment.

Patient Assessment

Psychoactive drugs treat symptoms of mental disorders. However, not all behaviors are treated by drug therapy, and not every identified personality trait is a symptom of illness targeted for treatment with drugs. It is essential to obtain baseline information about each patient before drug treatment. This information helps distinguish aspects of the patient's psychiatric illness from the patient's personality before the illness. As a result, a list of psychiatric symptoms can be identified as appropriate targets for drug treatment. Residual symptoms of the illness and personality characteristics not related to the illness can be addressed by nonpharmacological treatments. In addition, drug side effects can be identified and appropriately treated as they appear. Symptoms of organ system dysfunction caused by drug treatment can also be identified and treated. Finally, careful assessment of each patient can help identify medical illnesses that are concurrent with psychiatric illness or that possibly cause psychiatric symptoms. Box 27-1 provides a medication assessment tool for the nurse to use in taking a drug history.

Box **27-1** *Medication Assessment Tool*

Obtain the following information from the patient and other sources for each of the following four categories of drugs/substances taken:
1. Prescribed psychiatric medications ever taken
2. Prescribed nonpsychiatric medication taken in the past 6 months or taken for major medical illnesses if more than 6 months ago
3. Over-the-counter medication taken in the past 6 months
4. Alcohol, tobacco, caffeine, and street drugs

1, 2, AND 3

Name of the drug
Reason taken
Dates started and stopped
Highest daily dose
Who prescribed it?
Was it effective?
Side effects or adverse reactions

Was it taken as directed?
If not, how was it taken?
History of drug taken by first-degree relative
Drugs taken prescribed to others

4

Name of substance
Dates and schedule of use
Summarize effects
Adverse reactions/withdrawal symptoms
Attempts to stop/treatments to stop
Assess impact of substance on:
    Quality of life
    Relationships/spouse/children
    Occupation/education
    Health/productivity
    Self-image
    Expense

Coordination of Treatment Modalities

The nurse has an important role in designing a viable treatment program. The most appropriate treatment choices, integrated in a holistic manner and individualized for each patient, should be reflected in the treatment plan. The coordination of treatment modalities is often the primary responsibility of the nurse who works with the patient in an ongoing therapeutic alliance as part of a health-care team.

Psychopharmacological Drug Administration

No one on the health-care team has a greater daily impact on the patient's experience with psychopharmacological agents than the nurse. The nurse administers each medication dose, works out a dosing schedule based on drug requirements and the patient's preferences, and is continually alert for drug effects. This role defines the nurse as a key professional in maximizing therapeutic effects of drug treatment and minimizing side effects in such a way that the patient is a true collaborator in the medication regimen.

Monitoring Drug Effects

The nurse is often the most available professional to the patient and has the important role of consistently monitoring the effects of psychopharmacological drugs, including their effects on target symptoms of illness, side effects, adverse reactions, and the often subtle effects on the patient's self-concept and sense of trust.

Medication Education

The nurse is in a pivotal position to educate the patient and the family about medications. This includes conveying complex information to the patient so that it is understood and accepted.

Drug Maintenance Programs

For some patients the medication maintenance program lasts many years. The nurse can assume the important role of continuing a therapeutic alliance with a patient on drug maintenance in the aftercare setting.

Clinical Research Drug Trials

As a member of the interdisciplinary research team, the nurse can contribute to the body of scientific knowledge, often adding a nursing perspective to team research efforts. The nurse can be included on several levels, from data collector to coinvestigator to principal investigator. The nurse's roles in interdisciplinary clinical research drug trials in the clinical setting are just beginning to be appreciated and defined.

Prescriptive Authority

Within the last 10 years legislation has been passed in most states authorizing advanced practice registered nurses to prescribe medications. Psychiatric nurses who are qualified under their state practice acts are thus able to prescribe

pharmacological agents to treat the symptoms and improve the functional status of patients with psychiatric illness.[3] Specific pharmacological agents can be prescribed by psychiatric advanced practice registered nurses based on clinical indicators of the patient's status, and the role of nurses in psychopharmacological treatments has been expanded once again to increase patient access to high-quality and cost-effective health care.

> **?** *Does your state grant prescriptive authority to psychiatric advanced practice registered nurses? If so, what are the requirements for practice?*

PHARMACOKINETICS

Drugs are chemicals with specific properties that affect treatment. For example, it is important to know a drug's **half-life**. The half-life determines how long it takes to achieve a steady state of concentration. **Steady state** means that the amount of drug excreted equals the amount ingested, and it occurs in approximately four to six half-lives. Until steady state is reached, the drug level continues to build, and it changes after each dosing. This accounts for acute side effects in some patients. It also means that until steady state is reached, the optimum dose for a particular patient cannot be determined, nor is a blood level accurate in determining a proper dose range. It may take longer to reach steady state in the elderly because of slower gastrointestinal activity and liver metabolism.

Another significance of half-life is in the frequency of dosing. Usually a drug with a half-life of 24 hours or more can be administered once a day when steady state is reached; a drug with a shorter half-life should be administered more often to achieve constant clinical effects. Termination of drug treatment is also affected by half-life. In general, the effects of drugs with a long half-life can last a long time (sometimes weeks) after the last dose. Drugs with a short half-life usually must be tapered (discontinued gradually over several days or weeks). In general, most psychoactive drugs should be discontinued by a tapering period.

This chapter focuses on the adult patient under age 55, although children and the elderly are often given psychoactive drugs. Generally, children metabolize drugs more rapidly than adults, although children exhibit a variable response. The elderly and newborns are particularly sensitive to psychotropic drugs. For the elderly, drug distribution, hepatic metabolism, and renal clearance are all affected by age. It is important to start low and go slow (begin with a lower than recommended dose and titrate up slower than the rate recommended for adults under age 55). If a pregnant woman takes psychoactive drugs, the unborn infant may experience drug effects and even withdrawal symptoms at birth unless the baby is detoxified from the drug. The infant whose mother takes psychoactive drugs generally should

Box **27-2** *Guidelines for Polypharmacy*

Identify specific target symptoms for each drug.

If possible, start with one drug and evaluate effectiveness and side effects before adding a second drug.

Be alert for adverse drug interactions.

Consider the effects of a second drug on the absorption and metabolism of the first drug.

Consider the possibility of additive side effects.

Change the dose of only one drug at a time and evaluate results.

Be aware of increased risk of medication errors.

Be aware of increased cost of treatment.

Be aware of decreased patient adherence in the aftercare setting when medication regimen is complex.

In follow-up treatment, eliminate as many drugs as possible and establish the effective dose of the drugs used.

Patient education programs regarding concomitant drug regimens must be particularly clear, organized, and effective.

Patient follow-up contacts should be more frequent.

Box **27-3** *Increased Risk Factors for Development of Drug Interactions*

Polypharmacy
High doses
Geriatric patients
Debilitated/dehydrated patients
Concurrent illness
Compromised organ system function
Inadequate patient education
History of nonadherence
Failure to include patient in treatment planning

not be breastfed.[36] Patients with liver disease are extremely sensitive to most psychoactive drugs, and patients with renal impairment are particularly sensitive to lithium.

Drug Interactions

Drugs can interact with each other on two levels:

▼ **Pharmacokinetic:** One drug interferes with the absorption, metabolism, distribution, and excretion of another drug, thus raising or lowering the levels of the drug in the blood and tissue.

▼ **Pharmacodynamic:** One drug combines with another to increase or decrease the drugs' effects in an organ system.

Concurrent use of drugs, or polypharmacy, can enhance a specific therapeutic action, may be necessary to treat concurrent illnesses, and can counteract unwanted effects of one of the drugs. Unfortunately, a number of problems have been associated with concurrent drug use, including confusion over therapeutic efficacy, side effects, and drug interactions.[4] In general, polypharmacy in psychiatric care should be used only when necessary and with caution. Box 27-2 lists guidelines for polypharmacy, and Box 27-3 alerts the nurse to patients at a higher risk for drug interactions. Table 27-1 is a reference list for the more common drug interactions of psychotropic drugs.

This chapter refers to drugs by their generic names. There is a strong movement in practice to use generic names instead of trade names to be more accurate, to take advantage of price differences, and to prevent confusion when a drug becomes generic (when the patent runs out and the drug can be made by any company, thus reducing cost). Once a drug becomes generic, the patient should be taught to use the same brand of a drug because the bioavailability of psychoactive drugs may vary significantly from one brand to another, thus affecting drug dose and

steady state. The patient can use one pharmacy regularly and can ask the pharmacist to use the same company when filling generic prescriptions of a particular drug.

> **?** *Why do you think patients often fail to report over-the-counter medications when asked about current medications? How can you, as a nurse, be sure to obtain this information?*

Biological Basis for Psychopharmacology

All communication in the brain involves neurons "talking" to each other at synapses. These nerve cells are the basic functional unit of the nervous system, and the study of this communication process forms the basis of much of the neurosciences. The following description presents a very basic frame of reference from which to view the rather overwhelming complexity of neuropharmacological mechanisms.

The synapse is a narrow gap separating two neurons (the presynaptic cell and the postsynaptic cell) at a transmission site (Fig. 27-1). During neurotransmission the chemical neurotransmitter is released from a storage vesicle in the presynaptic cell, crosses the synapse, and is recognized by the receptor on the postsynaptic cell membrane (this recognition is called *binding*). Receptors are the cellular recognition sites for specific molecular structures such as neurotransmitters, hormones, and many drugs. Thus their action is selective for specific chemicals. Neurotransmitters, the chemical messengers that travel from one brain cell to another, are synthesized (manufactured) by enzymes from certain dietary amino acids, or precursors. At the synapse, neurotransmitters act as receptor activators (agonists) or inhibitors (antagonists) and trigger complex biological responses within the cell. The chemical remaining in the synapse is either reabsorbed (through reuptake) and stored by the presynaptic cell or is metabolized (inactivated) by enzymes, one of which is monoamine oxidase.

Many psychiatric disorders are thought to be caused by an overresponse or an underresponse somewhere along the complex process of neurotransmission (called dysregula-

TABLE **27-1** *Interactions of Psychotropic Drugs and Other Substances*

PSYCHOTROPIC CATEGORY	POSSIBLE INTERACTIONS
ANTIANXIETY AGENTS **Benzodiazepines With:**	
CNS depressants (alcohol, barbiturates, antipsychotics, antihistamines, cimetidine)	Potential additive CNS effects, especially sedation and decreased daytime performance.
SSRIs, disulfiram, estrogens	Increased benzodiazepine effects.
Antacids, tobacco	Decreased benzodiazepine effects.
Sedative-Hypnotics With:	
CNS depressants (alcohol, antihistamines, antidepressants, narcotics, antipsychotics)	Enhancement of sedative effects; impairment of mental and physical performance; may result in lethargy, respiratory depression, coma, death.
Anticoagulants (oral)*	Decreased coumarin plasma levels and effect; monitor and adjust dose of coumarin.
ANTIDEPRESSANTS **Tricyclics (TCAs) With:**	
MAOIs*	May cause hypertensive crisis.
Alcohol and other CNS depressants	Additive CNS depression; decreased TCA effect.
Antihypertensives* (quanethidine, methyldopa, clonidine)	Antagonism of antihypertensive effect.
Antipsychotics and anti-Parkinsonians	Increased TCA effect; confusion, delirium, ileus.
Anticholinergics	Additive anticholinergic effects.
Antiarrhythmics (quinidine, procainamide, propranolol)	Additive antiarrhythmic effects; myocardial depression.
SSRIs*	Increased TCA serum level/toxicity through inhibition of cytochrome P-450 system.
Anticonvulsants	Decreased TCA effect; seizures.
Tobacco	Decreased TCA plasma levels.
SSRIs With:	
Clomipramine, maprotiline, bupropion, clozapine	Increased risk of seizures.
MAOIs*	Serotonin syndrome.
Barbiturates, benzodiazepines, narcotics	Increased CNS depression.
Carbamazepine	Neurotoxicity: nausea, vomiting, vertigo, tinnitus, ataxia, lethargy, blurred vision.
MAOIs WITH:	
Many drugs and foods	Hypertensive crisis.
MOOD STABILIZERS **Lithium With:**	
Diuretics,* marijuana	Increased lithium levels/toxicity.
SSRIs	Lithium toxicity; enhanced therapeutic effect.
Nonsteroidal antiinflamatory agents*	Increased lithium blood levels/toxicity.
Antipsychotics	Increased CNS toxicity
Tetracyclines	Lithium intoxication.
Ace inhibitors	Confusion, ataxia, dysarthria, tremor, ECG changes.
Carbamazepine With:	
Lithium	Lithium intoxification; increased effect; inhibits lithium-induced polyuria.
Haloperidol	Decreased effect of either drug.
Calcium channel blockers	Neurotoxicity; dizziness, nausea, diplopia, headache.
Valproate	Decreased valproate serum concentration.
Cimetidine, erythromycin, isoniazid	Somnolence, lethargy, dizziness, blurred vision, ataxia, nausea.
Valproate With:	
SSRIs, erythromycin, cimetidine	Increased valproate serum concentrations.

*Potentially clinically significant.

Continued

TABLE **27-1** *Interactions of Psychotropic Drugs and Other Substances—cont'd*

PSYCHOTROPIC CATEGORY	POSSIBLE INTERACTIONS
ANTIPSYCHOTICS WITH:	
Antacids, tea, coffee, milk, fruit juice	Decreased phenothiazine effect.
CNS depressants (narcotics, antianxiety drugs, alcohol, antihistamines, barbiturates)	Additive CNS depression.
Anticholinergic agents (levodopa)*	Additive atropinelike side effects and increased anti-Parkinson effects.
SSRIs	Increased neuroleptic serum level and extrapyramidal side effects (EPS).
ANTIPSYCHOTICS **Clozapine With:**	
Carbamazepine*	Additive bone marrow suppression.
Benzodiazepines*	Circulatory collapse, respiratory arrest.
SSRIs*	Increased risk of seizures.

tion). For instance, psychosis is thought to involve excessive dopamine neurotransmission. Depression and mania are thought to result from disruption of normal patterns of neurotransmission of norepinephrine, serotonin, and other neurotransmitters. Anxiety is thought to be a dysregulation of gamma-aminobutyric acid (GABA) and other neurotransmitters.

If a particular psychiatric illness is known to result from a dysregulation or imbalance of neurotransmission in a particular neurotransmitter system, and if the mechanism of action of the psychiatric drugs is understood, then some order in the various pharmacological strategies used in psychiatric treatment can be recognized. This process of cell-to-cell communication at the synapse can be affected by drugs in several important ways:

▼ *Release:* More neurotransmitter is released into the synapse from the storage vesicles in the presynaptic cell.

▼ *Blockade:* The neurotransmitter is prevented from binding to the postsynaptic receptor.

▼ *Receptor sensitivity changes:* The receptor becomes more or less responsive to the neurotransmitter.

▼ *Reuptake inhibition:* The presynaptic cell does not reabsorb the neurotransmitter well, leaving more neurotransmitter in the synapse and therefore enhancing or prolonging its action.

▼ *Interference with storage vesicles:* The neurotransmitter is either released again into the synapse (more neurotransmitter) or released to metabolizing enzymes (less neurotransmitter).

▼ *Precursor chain interference:* The process that makes the neurotransmitter is either facilitated (more is synthesized) or disrupted (less is synthesized).

▼ *Synaptic enzyme interference:* Less neurotransmitter is metabolized, so more remains available in the synapse and the presynaptic neuron.

Not all of the above strategies have yielded clinically rel-

evant treatments. Several have, however, and these are emphasized in this chapter (see Fig. 27-1): antipsychotic drugs block dopamine from the receptor site; tricyclic antidepressants (TCAs), selective serotonin reuptake inhibitors (SSRIs), and several other antidepressants block the reuptake of norepinephrine or serotonin and regulate the areas of the brain that manufacture these chemicals; monoamine oxidase inhibitors (MAOIs) prevent enzymatic metabolism of norepinephrine and serotonin; benzodiazepines potentiate (enhance the function of) GABA; and some antidepressants and antipsychotics block specific serotonin receptors.

Understanding this process has led to a variety of treatment approaches in pharmacotherapy that attempt to change one or more of the steps in neurotransmission. It has also led to research efforts to develop drugs with more specificity (drugs that go to areas in the brain specifically targeted for their action, such as the brain regions implicated in mental illness, rather than to nonspecific or untargeted areas, causing drug side effects).

ANTIANXIETY AND SEDATIVE-HYPNOTIC DRUGS

The diagnosis of anxiety is based on the patient's description, the nurse's observation of behaviors, and the elimination of alternative diagnoses. The possibility of a nonpsychiatric cause must also be considered. Hyperthyroidism, hypoglycemia, cardiovascular illness, and severe pulmonary disease are often associated with high levels of anxiety. In addition to a careful physical assessment and a review of laboratory tests, the patient should be asked about use of prescription and over-the-counter drugs, "recreational" substances, alcohol, caffeine, and nicotine. Anxiety also accompanies many psychiatric disorders. In general, the primary disorder should be treated with the appropriate medication. Anxiety may be associated with psychosis or an af-

Neurotransmitters
Dopamine
Norepinephrine
Serotonin
GABA

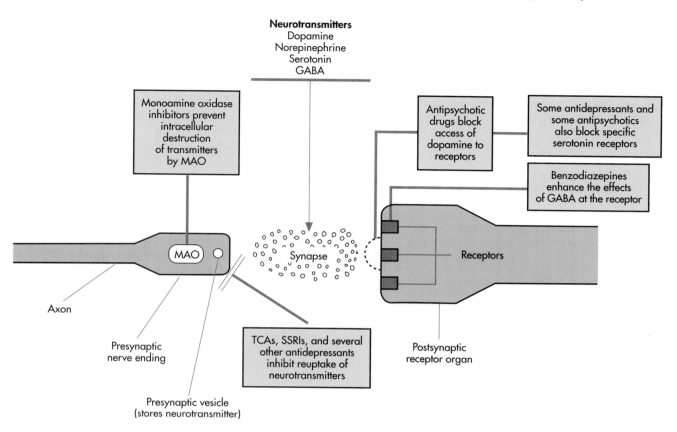

Fig. 27-1 Neurotransmission at the synapse.

fective disorder and often goes away when the target symptoms for the primary disorder subside with appropriate treatment.

This section divides antianxiety and sedative-hypnotic drugs into two categories: the benzodiazepines and nonbenzodiazepines. The latter group includes several classes of drugs. The benzodiazepines are the most widely prescribed drugs in the world, and have almost entirely replaced barbiturates in the treatment of anxiety and sleep disorders. Their popularity is related to their effectiveness and wide margin of safety, and they are the principal drugs used in the treatment of anxiety and insomnia.

Benzodiazepines

MECHANISM OF ACTION. The benzodiazepines are thought to reduce anxiety because they are powerful potentiators of the inhibitory neurotransmitter GABA, although the role of GABA in anxiety is not yet clear. A postsynaptic receptor site specific for the benzodiazepine molecule has been discovered. The benzodiazepine molecule and GABA bind to each other at the GABA receptor site (see Chapter 16). The result is an inhibition of neurotransmission (a decrease in the firing rate of neurons), resulting in a clinical decrease in the person's level of anxiety.

What sociocultural factors may help to explain why benzodiazepines are the most commonly prescribed medications in the United States?

CLINICAL USE. The benzodiazepines are often the drug of choice in the management of anxiety, insomnia, and stress-related conditions. The target symptoms for use of these drugs are listed in Box 27-4. The major indications for their use are generalized anxiety disorder, anxiety associated with other psychiatric diagnoses, sleep disorders, anxiety associated with phobic disorders, posttraumatic stress disorder, alcohol and drug withdrawal, anxiety associated with medical disease, skeletal muscle relaxation, seizure disorders, and the anxiety and apprehension experienced before surgery.[28] High-dose benzodiazepines, particularly alprazolam, appear to have specific antipanic effects in the treatment of panic disorder.

The benzodiazepines have no significant clinical advantages over each other. Differences in half-life (Table 27-2) can be clinically useful. For example, patients with persistent high levels of anxiety should take a drug with a long half-life. Patients with fluctuating anxiety might be better off with short-acting drugs. When used as hypnotics the benzodiazepines should induce sleep rapidly, and their effect should be gone by morning. The rate of absorption of the different benzodiazepines from the gastrointestinal tract varies considerably, thus affecting the rapidity and intensity of onset of their acute effects. Antacids and food in the stomach slow down this process.[28]

Because the benzodiazepines are in the same pharmacological class as alcohol, they can be used to suppress the alcohol withdrawal syndrome. The concomitant use of these two substances can be dangerous because it produces extreme sedation. Any benzodiazepine can be an effective sedative-hypnotic when administered at bedtime.

Although some patients may need to take antianxiety drugs for extended periods, the drugs have their drawbacks and should always be used with nonpharmacological treatments for the patient with chronic anxiety or insomnia. Psychotherapy, behavioral techniques, environmental changes, stress management, and an ongoing therapeutic relationship continue to be important in the treatment of anxiety disorders.

Most experts believe that treatment with benzodiazepines should be brief, used during a time of specific stress. Drugs with a long half-life (longer than 18 to 24 hours) can be given once a day. Drugs with a short half-life (8 to 15 hours) need to be given more often; they can be taken as needed for increased symptoms of anxiety as such symptoms occur. The patient should be observed frequently during the early days of treatment to assess target symptom response and monitor side effects so that the dose can be adjusted. Some patients, such as those with panic disorder, may require long-term antianxiety medication treatment.

Concentrations of benzodiazepines in the blood have not yet been firmly correlated to clinical effects. All benzodiazepines are rapidly absorbed by mouth. The injectable benzodiazepines have been proven reliable when administered in the deltoid muscle and lead to rapid and predictable rises in the blood level when used intravenously. When

---

Box **27-4** *Target Symptoms for Antianxiety and Sedative-Hypnotic Benzodiazepines*

PSYCHOLOGICAL
Vague sense of irritability and uneasiness
Sense of impending doom or panic
Insomnia

PHYSICAL
Flushed skin
Hot or cold flashes
Sweating
Dilated pupils
Dry mouth
Nausea or vomiting
Diarrhea
Tachycardia, palpitations
Dizziness
Shortness of breath
Hyperventilation
Paresthesias
Tremor
Restlessness
Headache
Urinary frequency

TABLE **27-2** *Antianxiety and Sedative-Hypnotic Drugs: Benzodiazepines*

Generic Name (Trade Name)	Active Metabolites	Half-Life (hr)	Days to Steady State	Equivalence (mg)	Usual Adult Dosage Range (mg/day)	Preparations
ANTIANXIETY DRUGS						
Alprazolam (Xanax)	Yes (not significant)	12-20	3	0.5	0.5-4	PO
Chlordiazepoxide (Librium)	Yes	12-100	1-3	10	15-100	PO, IM, IV
Clonazepam (Klonopin)	No	18-50	3-8	—	0.5-10	PO
Clorazepate (Tranxene)	Yes	30-100	5-16	7.5	7.5-60	PO
Diazepam (Valium)	Yes	20-90	4-8	5	2-40	PO, SR, IM, IV
Halazepam (Paxipam)	Yes	20-100	4	20	80-160	PO
Lorazepam (Ativan)	No	10-20	2-3	1	2-4	PO, IM, IV
Oxazepam (Serax)	No	5-15	1-2	15	15-90	PO
Prazepam (Centrax)	Yes	30-200	5-32	10	10-60	PO
SEDATIVE-HYPNOTIC DRUGS						
Estazolam (ProSom)	No	10-24	1-2	1	1-2	PO
Flurazepam (Dalmane)	Yes	30-100	4-8	15	15-60	PO
Temazepam (Restoril)	No	10-20	2-3	15	15-30	PO
Triazolam (Halcion)	No	1.5-4	1	0.25	0.25-0.5	PO

IM, Intramuscular; *IV,* intravenous; *PO,* oral tablet or capsule; *SR,* oral slow-release tablet.

given intravenously, administration should be slow (over 1 minute) and direct, not mixed in an IV infusion, because plastic tubing absorbs the drug and the drug can precipitate when mixed with saline or dextrose.

Another clinical indication for the use of benzodiazepines is as a sedative-hypnotic to improve sleep. Insomnia (poor sleep) includes difficulty falling asleep, difficulty staying asleep, or awakening too early. It is a symptom with many causes and often responds to nonpharmacological strategies such as talking about problems, increased daytime exercise, and physical comfort measures at night. Drugs to induce sleep have their place but are never a substitute for good nursing care.

ADVERSE REACTIONS. Because the benzodiazepines have a very high therapeutic index, overdoses of benzodiazepines alone almost never cause fatalities. Side effects are common, dose related, and almost always harmless. Table 27-3 summarizes these reactions and nursing considerations. The benzodiazepines generally do not live up to their reputation of being strongly addictive if they are discontinued gradually, they have been used for appropriate purposes, and their use has not been complicated by other factors such as chronic use of barbiturates or alcohol.

Tolerance can develop to the sedative effects of benzodiazepines, but it is unclear whether tolerance also develops to induced sleep or antianxiety effects. These drugs should be tapered to minimize withdrawal symptoms (Box 27-5) and rebound symptoms of insomnia or anxiety. If these symptoms occur, the dose must be raised until symptoms are gone and then tapering is resumed at a slower rate.[37]

Elderly patients are more vulnerable to side effects because the aging brain is more sensitive to sedatives. Dosing ranges from one half to one third of the usual daily dose.[35] The benzodiazepines with no active metabolites (see Table 27-2) are less affected by liver disease, the age of the patient,

or drug interactions. Use of benzodiazepines during pregnancy has been associated with infant cleft lip/cleft palate, multiple congenital deformities, and intrauterine growth retardation, especially when used during the first trimester. When used late in pregnancy or during breastfeeding, these drugs have been associated with floppy infant syndrome, neonatal withdrawal symptoms, poor sucking, and hypotonia.

Nonbenzodiazepines

The disadvantages of most older, nonbenzodiazepine antianxiety and sedative-hypnotic agents have led to their greatly decreased use. These drugs, listed in Table 27-4, are often used when alternatives to benzodiazepines are sought or when preferred by clinicians or patients. Some of them, such as the barbiturates, meprobamate, the alcohols, and chloral hydrate have numerous disadvantages: Tolerance develops to their antianxiety effects; they are more addictive;

Box **27-5** *Benzodiazepine Withdrawal Syndrome*

HYPEREXCITABILITY SYMPTOMS
Agitation, anxiety, hyperactivity, insomnia

NEUROPSYCHIATRIC SYMPTOMS
Ataxia, depersonalization, depression, dizziness, headache, hyperventilation, malaise, myalgia, paranoid delusions, paresthesias, pruritis, seizures, tinnitus, tremor, visual hallucinations

GASTROINTESTINAL SYMPTOMS
Abdominal pain, constipation, diarrhea, nausea, vomiting

CARDIOVASCULAR SYMPTOMS
Chest pain, flushing, hypotension, palpitations

GENITOURINARY SYMPTOMS
Incontinence, loss of libido, urinary urgency and frequency

TABLE **27-3** *Benzodiazepine Side Effects and Nursing Considerations*

SIDE EFFECTS	NURSING CONSIDERATIONS
COMMON	
Drowsiness, sedation	Activity helps; use caution when using machinery.
Ataxia, dizziness	Use caution with activity, prevent falls.
Feelings of detachment	Discourage social isolation.
Increased irritability or hostility	Observe, support, be alert for disinhibition.
Anterograde amnesia	Inability to recall events that occur while on drug.
Tolerance, dependency, rebound insomnia/anxiety	Short-term use; discontinue, using a slow taper; contraindicated with drug or alcohol abuse.
RARE	
Nausea	Dose with meals, decrease dose.
Headache	Usually responds to mild analgesic.
Confusion	Decrease dose.
Gross psychomotor impairment	Dose related, decrease dose.
Depression	Decrease dose; antidepressant treatment.
Paradoxical rage reaction	Discontinue drug.

they cause serious, even lethal withdrawal reactions; they are dangerous in overdose and cause central nervous system (CNS) depression; and they can cause a variety of dangerous drug interactions.

Antihistamines, especially hydroxyzine, are usually not as effective as the benzodiazepines; they cause sedation but do not cause physical dependence or abuse. A disadvantage of the antihistamines is that they lower the seizure threshold.

Propranolol blocks beta-noradrenergic receptors centrally and in the peripheral cardiac and pulmonary systems. This drug probably decreases certain physiological symptoms of anxiety, especially tachycardia, rather than centrally acting on anxiety. More research is needed to define a proper role for propranolol in the treatment of anxiety.

Buspirone, a nonbenzodiazepine anxiolytic drug, is a potent antianxiety agent with no addictive potential. Buspirone is effective in the treatment of anxiety and does not exhibit muscle-relaxant or anticonvulsant activity, interaction with CNS depressants, or sedative-hypnotic properties. It is not effective in the management of drug or alcohol abuse or panic disorder. Generally it takes several weeks for its antianxiety effects to become apparent.

Zolpidem is the first of a new class of compounds for short-term treatment of insomnia. Structurally unrelated to benzodiazepines, it binds more selectively to neuronal receptors involved in inducing sleep. It is well tolerated and appears to have little antianxiety, anticonvulsant, or muscle-relaxant properties. Side effects can include daytime drowsiness, dizziness, and diarrhea. Zolpidem is a schedule IV controlled substance.[26]

ANTIDEPRESSANT DRUGS

The 1950s were an important time in the history of psychopharmacology with the discovery of drugs that were effective in treating depression. Early in the 1950s dramatic improvements in mood and well-being were noted in patients with tuberculosis who were being treated with iproniazid before improvement in the tuberculosis lesion was noted. This led to the use of MAOIs as primary drug treatments for depression. At this same time, the first tricyclic antidepressant (TCA), imipramine, was tested for potential antipsychotic activity. It was found to be an ineffective antipsychotic, but depression improved. Imipramine was marketed in 1958 for its significant antidepressant properties.

Research on the biology of depression has led to many new discoveries and even more questions. It has been proposed that serotonin and norepinephrine and perhaps other neurochemicals are dysregulated in depression and mania. The biological understanding of antidepressant drugs supports this theory: MAO inhibitors (MAOIs) inhibit the metabolism of these neurotransmitters, and many antidepressants block their reuptake at the presynaptic neuron. Thus, antidepressant drugs regulate these neurotransmitter systems and their balance with each other.

The primary clinical indication for use of antidepressant drugs is major depressive illness. These drugs are also useful in the treatment of several anxiety disorders and enuresis in children. A variety of preliminary research studies suggest that they are useful in attention deficit disorders, narcolepsy, and bulimia. Table 27-5 lists possible clinical effects of synaptic activity, Table 27-6 presents antidepressant synaptic activity and receptor binding actions, and Table 27-7 presents comparative side effect profiles of antidepressant medicines.

TABLE **27-4** *Antianxiety, Sedative-Hypnotic Drugs: Nonbenzodiazepines*

GENERIC NAME (TRADE NAME)	DOSE (MG)	HALF-LIFE (HR)
BARBITURATES		
Secobarbital (Seconal)	100-200	19-34
Pentobarbital (Nembutal)	100-200	15-48
Amobarbital (Amytal)	100-200	8-42
Butabarbital (Butisol)	100-200	34-42
Phenobarbital	100-200	24-140
PROPANEDIOLS		
Meprobamate (Equanil)	200-800	6-17
ACETYLENIC ALCOHOL		
Ethchlorvynol (Placidyl)	500-1000	10-25
CHLORAL DERIVATIVE		
Chloral hydrate (Noctec)	500-2000	4-10
ANTIHISTAMINES		
Diphenhydramine (Benadryl)	50	unknown
Hydroxyzine (Atarax)	100 tid	unknown
BETA-ADRENERGIC BLOCKER		
Propranolol (Inderal)	10 qid	3
ANXIOLYTIC		
Buspirone (BuSpar)	10-40	2-5
IMIDAZOPYRIDINE		
Zolpidem (Ambien)	10	2.5

> **?** *Your patient who has been taking antidepressant medication for 3 months tells you that he feels better and wants to stop taking it. How would you respond?*

Patients who respond to the initial course of treatment with antidepressants should continue taking the drugs at the same dosage for 9 to 12 months afterward. This is known as continuation treatment. If they are symptom-free during this time, they can then be tapered off the medication. Patients who have relapses after the continuation treatment is ended may require long-term maintenance medication to prevent recurring depression.[12] Patients who have had three or more episodes of major depression have a 90% chance of having another and are therefore potential candidates for long-term maintenance antidepressant medication. The

TABLE 27-5 *Possible Clinical Effects of Synaptic Activity by Psychotropic Drugs*

SYNAPTIC ACTIVITY	POSSIBLE CLINICAL EFFECTS
Serotonin (5HT) reuptake inhibition	Reduced depression, antianxiety effects, GI disturbances, sexual dysfunction
Norepinephrine (NE) reuptake inhibition	Reduced depression, tremors, tachycardia, erectile/ejaculatory dysfunction
Dopamine (DA) reuptake inhibition	Reduced depression, psychomotor activation, anti-Parkinsonian effects
$5HT_2$ receptor blockade	Reduced depression, reduced suicidal behavior, antipsychotic effects, hypotension, ejaculatory dysfunction
Dopamine D_2 receptor blockade	Extrapyramidal movement disorders
Muscarinic/cholinergic (ACh) receptor blockade	Anticholinergic side effects (blurred vision, dry mouth, constipation, sinus tachycardia, urinary retention, cognitive dysfunction)
Histamine (H_1) receptor blockade	Sedation/drowsiness, hypotension, weight gain
$Alpha_1$-adrenergic receptor blockade	Postural hypotension, dizziness, drowsiness, memory dysfunction, reflex tachycardia, potentiation of antihypertensive effect of prazosin and terazosin
$Alpha_2$-adrenergic receptor blockade	Priapism, blockade of the antihypertensive effects of clonidine and α-methyldopa

TABLE 27-6 *Antidepressant Drug Synaptic Activity*

ANTIDEPRESSANT DRUG	PRIMARY SYNAPTIC ACTIVITY
All TCAs	Receptor blockade: H_1, ACh, $Alpha_1$, $5HT_2$
Particularly tertiary amines	Reuptake inhibition: 5HT
Particularly secondary amines	Reuptake inhibition: NE
MAOIs	Receptor blockade: ACh
	Enzymatic inhibition: MAO
SSRIs	Reuptake inhibition: 5HT
Other antidepressants	
Amoxapine	Reuptake inhibition: 5HT and NE
	Receptor blockade: D_2, ACh, H_1
Bupropion	Reuptake inhibition: NE and DA
Maprotiline	Reuptake inhibition: NE
	Receptor blockade: H_1, ACh
Trazodone	Reuptake inhibition: 5HT
	Receptor blockade $5HT_2$, H_1, $Alpha_2$, $Alpha_1$
Venlafaxine	Reuptake inhibition: 5HT, NE, and DA
Nefazedone	Reuptake inhibition: 5HT and NE
	Receptor blockade $5HT_2$, $Alpha_1$
Mirtazapine	Presynaptic autoreceptor inhibition: $Alpha_2$
	Receptor blockade: $5HT_2$ and $5HT_3$

ACh, Acetylcholine; *$Alpha_1$*, and *$Alpha_2$*, norepinephrine receptors; *DA*, dopamine; *H_1*, histamine receptor; *5HT*, serotonin; *$5HT_2$*, serotonin receptor; *NE*, norepinephrine.

TABLE 27-7 *Comparative Side Effect Profiles of Antidepressant Medications*

	CENTRAL NERVOUS SYSTEM			CARDIOVASCULAR			OTHER
	ANTICHOLINERGIC*	DROWSINESS	INSOMNIA/ AGITATION	POSTURAL HYPOTENSION	CARDIAC ARRHYTHMIA	GASTROINTESTINAL DISTRESS	WEIGHT GAIN (OVER 6 KG)
Amitriptyline	4+	4+	0	4+	3+	0	4+
Clomipramine	4+	4+	1+	3+	3+	1+	3+
Desipramine	1+	1+	1+	2+	2+	0	1+
Doxepin	3+	4+	0	2+	2+	0	3+
Imipramine	3+	3+	1+	4+	3+	1+	3+
Nortriptyline	1+	1+	0	2+	2+	0	1+
Protriptyline	2+	1+	1+	2+	2+	0	0
Trimipramine	1+	4+	0	2+	2+	0	3+
Amoxapine	2+	2+	2+	2+	3+	0	1+
Maprotiline	2+	4+	0	0	1+	0	2+
Mirtazapine	1+	4+	1+	2+	0	1+	2+
Nefazodone	1+	3+	1+	2+	0	3+	0
Venlafaxine	1+	1+	3+	0	0	3+	0
Trazodone	0	4+	0	1+	1+	1+	1+
Bupropion	0	0	2+	0	1+	1+	0
Fluoxetine	0	0	2+	0	0	3+	0
Paroxetine	0	0	2+	0	0	3+	0
Sertraline	0	0	2+	0	0	3+	0
Fluvoxamine	0	0	2+	0	0	3+	0
MAOIs	1+	1+	2+	2+	0	1+	2+

Modified from Depression Guideline Panel: *Depression in primary care*, vol 2, *Treatment of major depression. Clinical practice guideline, Number 5* (AHCPR publication no. 93-0551), Rockville, MD, 1993, US Department of Health and Human Services, Public Health Service, Agency for Health Care Policy and Research.

*Dry mouth, blurred vision, urinary hesitancy, constipation.
0, Absent or rare; *1+, 2+,* in between; *3+, 4+,* common.

maintenance medication given is generally the same type and dosage found to be effective in the acute phase of treatment.

Tricyclic Antidepressants

MECHANISM OF ACTION. Although the class of tricyclic antidepressants (TCAs) includes some drugs that are structurally dissimilar, the TCAs are quite similar in their clinical effects and adverse reactions. They are divided into several categories: tertiary tricyclics (or parent drugs), secondary tricyclics (or metabolites), and an "other" cyclic group of drugs dissimilar in many ways.

CLINICAL USE. The antidepressants are listed in Table 27-8. Elderly patients and patients with a concomitant medical illness may require lower doses of these drugs than healthy adults and careful assessments for side effects while they are taking the drugs. An acceptable cardiac history and an ECG within normal limits are particularly important for children and for adults over 40 years of age before initiating tricyclic antidepressants.

Unfortunately, all antidepressants must be taken for 3 to 4 weeks or longer before a therapeutic response is evident. Table 27-9 describes the target symptoms for these drugs in the approximate order of the time it takes for each symptom to begin to improve. When caring for suicidally depressed patients, it is important to remember that they become more motivated and begin to look better long before their subjective depressive feelings and suicidal thoughts are relieved. The nursing care plan must include suicide assessments and suicide precautions for weeks after these patients begin to look less depressed.

Blood plasma levels for most TCAs help keep the dose within the therapeutic range (Table 27-10) and ensure that enough drug is in the patient's system to be effective. Some drugs, particularly nortripyline, have a therapeutic window (the range within which the drug is considered to be therapeutic), and a plasma level below or above the range results in a decrease in antidepressant effectiveness. Blood for a plasma level should be drawn 8 to 12 hours after a single (usually bedtime) dose. Measuring the level soon after drug ingestion results in an artificially high level, representing the

TABLE 27-8 *Antidepressant Drugs*

Generic (trade name)	Usual Adult Dose (mg/day)	Preparations
TRICYCLIC DRUGS		
Tertiary (parent)		
Amitryptiline (Elavil)	50-300	PO, IM
Doxepin (Adapin, Sinequan)	50-300	PO, L
Imipramine (Tofranil)	50-300	PO, IM
Trimipramine (Surmontil)	50-300	PO
Clomipramine (Anafranil)	50-250	PO
Secondary (metabolite)		
Desipramine (Norpramin)	50-300	PO, L
Nortryptiline (Pamelor)	50-100	PO
Protriptyline (Vivactil)	15-60	PO
MONOAMINE OXIDASE INHIBITORS		
Phenelzine (Nardil)	45-90	PO
Tranylcypromine (Parnate)	20-60	PO
SELECTIVE SEROTONIN REUPTAKE INHIBITORS		
Fluoxetine (Prozac)	20-80	PO
Fluvoxamine (Luvox)	50-250	PO
Paroxetine (Paxil)	20-50	PO
Sertraline (Zoloft)	25-200	PO
OTHER ANTIDEPRESSANT DRUGS		
Amoxapine (Ascendin)	50-600	PO
Bupropion (Wellbutrin)	50-600*	PO
Maprotiline (Ludiomil)	50-225*	PO
Mirtazepine (Remeron)	15-45	PO
Nefazedone (Serzone)	200-500	PO
Trazedone (Desyrel)	50-600	PO
Venlafaxine (Effexor)	25-375	PO

*Antidepressants with a ceiling dose due to dose-related seizures.
IM, Intramuscular; *L,* oral liquid; *PO,* oral tablet/capsule.

TABLE 27-9 *Antidepressant Drug Target Symptoms*

Onset of Drug Effect	Symptom
Week 1	Middle and terminal insomnia
	Appetite disturbances
	Anxiety
Week 2	Fatigue
	Poor motivation
	Somatic complaints
	Agitation
	Motor retardation
Week 3 or longer	Dysphoric mood
	Subjective depressive feelings (anhedonia, poor self-esteem, pessimism, hopelessness, self-reproach, guilt, helplessness, sadness)
	Suicidal thoughts

TABLE 27-10 *Therapeutic Plasma Levels for Antidepressant Drugs*

Drug	Therapeutic Range (ng/L)
Imipramine and desipramine	150-250
Desipramine	150-250
Amitriptyline and nortriptyline	100-250
Nortriptyline	50-150
Protriptyline	70-260
Doxepin and desmethyldoxepin	120-250
Maprotiline	150-250
Amoxapine and 8-hydroxyamoxapine	200-600
Trazodone	800-1600

peak of the drug metabolism rather than the steady-state level.

ADVERSE REACTIONS. The nurse should know the common side effects of the antidepressants (Table 27-11) and their nursing treatments (Table 27-12). Most of these side effects cause minor discomfort, but some can produce serious illness. These drugs have no known long-term adverse effects, tolerance to therapeutic effects does not develop, and persistent side effects often can be minimized by a small decrease in dose. Because antidepressants do not cause physical addiction, psychological dependence, or euphoria, they have no abuse potential. Their long half-life (24 hours or longer) allows them to be conveniently adminis-

tered once a day, after steady state is reached, at night for most people. If the bedtime dose interferes with sleeping, the dose should be given in the morning or divided into several doses throughout the day. Patients with bipolar illness may be switched into mania by many of these drugs; they should be watched closely for increased activity, greater difficulty concentrating and eating, and decreased sleeping patterns.

Because the TCAs are highly toxic when taken in excessive amounts, overdoses and suicide attempts using tricyclic antidepressants are extremely serious and require emergency medical attention. Ingestion of 1000 to 3000 mg can be lethal. This may represent barely a 1-week supply of

TABLE 27-11 *Antidepressant Drug Side Effects*

	RECEPTORS/ NEUROTRANSMITTERS	SIDE EFFECTS
ANTIDEPRESSANTS		
TCAs	H_1	Sedation/drowsiness, hypotension, weight gain
	ACh	Anticholinergic side effects: blurred vision, dry mouth, constipation, tachycardia, urinary retention, cognitive dysfunction
	$Alpha_1$	Postural hypotension, dizziness, tachycardia, memory dysfunction
	$5HT_2$	Hypotension, ejaculatory dysfunction
	5HT	GI disturbances (nausea, diarrhea), sexual dysfunction
	NE	Tremors, tachycardia, erectile/ejaculatory dysfunction
MAOIs	ACh	Anticholinergic side effects
SSRIs	5HT	GI disturbances (nausea, diarrhea), sexual dysfunction
OTHER ANTIDEPRESSANTS		
Amoxapine	NE	Tremors, tachycardia, erectile/ejaculatory dysfunction
	5HT	GI disturbance (nausea, diarrhea), sexual dysfunction
	D_2	Extrapyramidal symptoms and tardive dyskinesia (rare)
	ACh	Anticholinergic effects
	H_1	Sedation/drowsiness, hypotension, weight gain
Bupropion	DA	Psychomotor activation
	NE	Tremors, tachycardia, erectile/ejaculatory dysfunction
Maprotiline	NE	Tremors, tachycardia, erectile/ejaculatory dysfunction
	H_1	Sedation, drowsiness, hypotension, weight gain
	ACh	Anticholinergic effects
Trazedone	5HT	GI disturbances (nausea, diarrhea), sexual dysfunction
	$5HT_2$	Hypotension, ejaculatory dysfunction
	H_1	Sedation/drowsiness, hypotension, weight gain
	$Alpha_1$	Postural hypotension, dizziness, tachycardia, memory dysfunction
	$Alpha_2$	Priapism
Nefazedone	5HT	GI disturbances (nausea, diarrhea), sexual dysfunction
	NE	Tremors, tachycardia, erectile/ejaculatory dysfunction
	$5HT_2$	Hypotension, ejaculatory dysfunction
	$Alpha_1$	Postural hypotension; dizziness, tachycardia, memory dysfunction
Mirtazapine	H_1	Sedation, drowsiness, hypotension, weight gain
	ACh	Anticholinergic side effects
Venlafaxine	NE	Tremors, tachycardia, erectile/ejaculatory dysfuntion
	5HT	GI disturbances (nausea, diarrhea), sexual dysfunction
	DA	Psychomotor activation

Additional side effects and adverse reactions of antidepressant drugs less clearly related to receptor effects:

TCAs	ECG changes, dizziness/lightheadedness
	TCA withdrawal syndrome (malaise, muscle aches, chills, nausea, dizziness, coryzia), hallucinations, delusions, activation of schizophrenic or manic psychosis, excessive perspiration
MAOIs	Hypertensive crisis, lightheadedness, drowsiness, insomnia, weight gain, sexual dysfunction
SSRIs	Nervousness, activation, headache, cytochrome P-450 inhibition, serotonin syndrome, insomnia
Venlafaxine	Sweating, nausea, constipation, vomiting, somnolence, dry mouth, dizziness, anxiety, blurred vision, headache, hypertension, insomnia

medication. Accidental overdoses in children whose parents are taking a TCA are common and often lethal. The health teaching and care of these patients should include an assessment of household members, and patients should be cautioned to keep these drugs in the childproof bottles received from the pharmacy, to keep the drugs out of the reach of children, and to discard leftover drugs when pharmacotherapy is completed.

Most patients develop tolerance to side effects, and most side effects are dose related; thus, they can be minimized by increasing the dose gradually when the drug is first prescribed. In the case of severely depressed patients or those who are suicidal, doses are generally increased more rapidly to minimize the time it takes to reach steady state and therapeutic effectiveness.

Antidepressants, like all psychiatric drugs, should be avoided if possible during pregnancy, especially in the first trimester. However, these drugs have been given throughout pregnancy without harmful effects on the fetus and should be considered if a pregnant woman is severely depressed.

TABLE **27-12** *Nursing Considerations for Antidepressant Drug Side Effects*

SIDE EFFECT	NURSING CARE AND TEACHING CONSIDERATIONS
Anticholinergic side effects	
Blurred vision	Temporary; avoid hazardous tasks.
Dry mouth	Encourage fluids, frequent rinses, sugar-free hard candy and gum; check for mouth sores.
Constipation	Increase fluids, dietary fiber and roughage, exercise; monitor bowel habits; use stool softeners and laxatives only if necessary.
Tachycardia	Temporary, usually not significant (except with coronary artery disease), but can be frightening; eliminate caffeine; beta-blockers might help; supportive therapy.
Urinary retention	Encourage fluids and frequent voiding; monitor voiding patterns; bethanecol; catheterize.
Cognitive dysfunction	Temporary; avoid hazardous tasks, adjust lifestyle; supportive therapy.
Cytochrome P-450 inhibition	SSRIs inhibit the liver isoenzyme cytochrome P-450, which is instrumental in the metabolism of a variety of drugs (TCAs, trazedone, barbiturates, most benzodiazepines, carbamazepine, narcotics, neuroleptics, phenytoin, valproate, verapamil). This effect can be potentially life-threatening because it increases serum concentrations as well as therapeutic and toxic effects of these drugs.
Dizziness/lightheadedness	Dangle feet; adequate hydration, elastic stockings; protect from falls.
ECG changes	Careful cardiac history; pretreatment ECG for patients over 40 and children; ST segment depression, T wave flattened or inverted, QRS prolongation; worsening of intraventricular conduction problems; do not use if recent myocardial infarction or bundle-branch block.
Ejaculatory dysfunction	Dose after sexual intercourse, not immediately before.
GI disturbances (nausea, diarrhea)	Take with meals or at HS; adjust diet if indicated.
Hallucinations, delusions, activation of schizophrenic or manic psychosis	Change to another antidepressant class of drug, initiate antipsychotics or mood stabilizers if appropriate.
Hypertensive crisis	See Box 27-7.
Hypotension	Frequent BP; hydrate; elastic stockings; may need to change drug. For postural hypotension: lying and standing BP, gradual change of positions, protect from falls.
Insomnia	Dose as early in the day as possible; sleep hygiene, decrease evening activities; eliminate caffeine; relaxation techniques; sedative-hypnotic therapy.
Memory dysfunction	Temporary; encourage concentration, make lists, provide social support, adjust lifestyle.
Perspiration (excessive)	Frequent change of clothes, cotton/linen clothing, good hygiene; increase fluids.
Priapism	Change dose, change drug.
Psychomotor activation	Take drug in morning rather than HS, adjust lifestyle.
Sedation/drowsiness	Administer drug at HS, avoid hazardous tasks.
Serotonin syndrome (SS)	SS is a life-threatening emergency resulting from excess CNS 5HT caused by combining 5HT-enhancing drugs or administering SSRIs too close to the discontinuation of MAOIs. Symptoms are confusion, disorientation, mania, restlessness/agitation, myoclonus, hyperreflexia, diaphoresis, shivering, tremor, diarrhea, nausea, ataxia, headache. Discontinue all serotonergic drugs immediately; anticonvulsants for seizures; serotonin antagonist drugs may help; clonazepam for myoclonus, lorazepam for restlessness/agitation, other symptomatic care as indicated; do not reintroduce serotonin drugs.
Sexual dysfunction	Dose after sexual intercourse, use lubricant if vaginal dryness is present; bethanecol may help with anorgasmia.
Tachycardia	See anticolinergic side effects.
TCA withdrawal syndrome	Symptoms: malaise, muscle aches, chills, nausea, dizziness, coryzia; when discontinuing drug, taper over several days or weeks.
Tremors	Temporary; adjust lifestyle if indicated.
Weight gain	Increase exercise; reduced calorie diet if indicated; may need to change class of drug.

Note: Always educate the patient, consider decreasing or dividing drug dose, use the techniques in this table, and consider changing the drug only if necessary.

Selective Serotonin Reuptake Inhibitors

The SSRIs inhibit the reuptake of serotonin at the presynaptic membrane. This results in an increase of available serotonin in the synapse, and therefore at the postsynaptic membrane. Thus these drugs promote the neurotransmission of serotonin in the brain. Their selectivity for serotonin means they do not have significant effects at the transmission sites of other neurotransmitters and thus have fewer side effects.[29]

The SSRIs have antidepressant effects comparable to those of the other classes of antidepressant drugs, yet without significant anticholinergic, cardiovascular, and sedative side effects. They usually do not cause weight gain, thus making them more acceptable to patients with bulimia and other patients who are concerned about gaining weight. In addition, they are fairly safe in overdose. These properties have made them very popular in the short period of time they have been available, even though they are more expensive than many of the older tricyclic compounds. Tables 27-11 and 27-12 list the side effects and nursing interventions for the SSRIs and other antidepressant drugs. Particular care must be taken when combining these drugs. Combining serotonergic drugs can cause serotonin syndrome, a life-threatening crisis (see Table 27-12).

Monoamine Oxidase Inhibitors

MAOIs are very effective antidepressant/antipanic drugs. The MAOIs currently used in psychiatry are listed in Table 27-8. Because of the potential for a hypertensive crisis when tyramine-containing foods and certain medicines are taken along with these drugs, careful health teaching of a reliable patient is quite important. The patient must avoid certain foods, drinks, and medicines (Box 27-6), must know the warning signs, symptoms, and treatment of a hypertensive crisis (Box 27-7), and must be taught the more common side effects of MAOIs (see Table 27-11). For various indications these drugs are effective and are safe when used as prescribed. They are nonaddicting, and tolerance does not develop toward therapeutic effects; however, safety in pregnancy has not been established. The patient should be on

Box **27-7** *Signs and Treatment of Hypertensive Crisis on MAOIs*

WARNING SIGNS
Increased blood pressure
Palpitations
Headache

SYMPTOMS OF HYPERTENSIVE CRISIS
Sudden elevation of blood pressure
Explosive occipital headache
Head and face are flushed and feel "full"
Palpitations, chest pain
Sweating, fever, nausea, vomiting
Dilated pupils, photophobia

TREATMENT
Hold MAOI doses
Do not lie down (elevates blood pressure in head)
IM chlorpromazine 100 mg, repeat if necessary (*mechanism of action:* blocks norepinephrine)
IV phentolamine, administered slowly in doses of 5 mg (*mechanism of action:* binds with norepinephrine receptor sites, blocking norepinephrine)
Manage fever by external cooling techniques
Evaluate diet, adherence, and teaching

Box **27-6** *Dietary Restrictions: 1 Day before, during, and 2-6 Weeks after MAOI Therapy*

FOOD AND BEVERAGES TO AVOID
Cheese, especially aged or matured
Fermented or aged protein, meat or fish
Pickled or smoked fish
Chianti and vermouth wines, tap (draft) beer
Yeast or protein extracts
Fava or broad bean pods
Liver, sausages, pepperoni, salami, canned ham
Spoiled or overripe fruit
Banana peel, sauerkraut

FOOD AND BEVERAGES TO BE CONSUMED IN MODERATION
Chocolate
Yogurt, sour cream, cottage and cream cheese
Clear spirits and white wine
Avocado, raspberries
New Zealand spinach
Soy sauce
Aspartame, monosodium glutamate

DRUGS TO AVOID
Most other antidepressant drugs
Nasal and sinus decongestants
Allergy and hay fever remedies
Narcotics, especially meperidine
Asthma remedies
Local anesthetics with epinephrine
Weight-reducing pills, pep pills, stimulants
Other MAOIs
Other medications without first checking with a clinician
Cocaine, amphetamines

MEDICATIONS THAT MAY NEED DOSE DECREASED
Insulin and oral hypoglycemics
Oral anticoagulants
Thiazide diuretics
Anticholinergic agents
Muscle relaxants

Modified from Bernstein JG: *Handbook of drug therapy in psychiatry,* ed 3, St Louis, 1995, Mosby.

the restricted diet several days before beginning the medication, while on the medication, and for 2 weeks after stopping the medication (6 weeks for fluoxetine because of its long half-life). No more than one MAOI should be given at a time. These drugs should not be used along with other antidepressants.

Tyramine is an amino acid released from proteins in food when they undergo hydrolysis by fermenting, aging, pickling, smoking, and spoiling. It is deactivated by monoamine oxidase in the gut wall and liver. When monamine oxidase is inhibited, tyramine may reach adrenergic nerve endings, causing the release of large amounts of norepinephrine and producing a hypertensive reaction. Also, sympathomimetic drugs act on the neurotransmission process by releasing norepinephrine from the storage vesicles in the presynaptic nerve ends. Because monoamine oxidase has been inhibited when MAOIs are used, large amounts of norepinephrine are released and a severe hypertensive reaction can occur. Thorazine, an antipsychotic drug, and the alpha-adrenergic blocking agent phentolamine bind to the norepinephrine receptor sites, preventing norepinephrine stimulation and resolving the hypertensive crisis.

A novel class of MAOIs not yet available in the United States has antidepressant efficacy comparable to that of other antidepressants (moclobamide is available in Canada and Mexico; brofaramine is still in clinical trial testing). These are novel drugs because they are reversible inhibitors of MAO-A (called RIMAs) that have fewer side effects (specifically the absence of severe hypertensive interaction) and do not require the low-tyramine diet that the other MAOIs require. They are short-acting drugs, allowing the recovery of enzyme activity in hours rather than weeks. They may prove to be valuable additions to the list of antidepressant drugs in the future.

Other Antidepressant Drugs

There are a growing number of other antidepressant drugs that differ in their effects at the synapse from each other and from the other categories of antidepressants. They therefore have varying side effect profiles. Efficacy is generally the same, as is the length of time required for efficacy to occur (several weeks at optimal dose). Like SSRIs, they are safer than TCAs and MAOIs in side effects and overdose. Some of these drugs are fairly new, and appear to have more specificity than many of the other antidepressants. Mirtazepine, for example, targets several presynaptic autoreceptors in order to increase levels of norepinephrine as well as serotonin. It also serves as an agonist to the $5HT_1$ postsynaptic receptor, which is thought to be the serotonin receptor implicated in mood disorders. It has fewer receptor actions in other neurotransmitter systems, so it is marketed as having fewer side effects than other antidepressants.[7] The nurse will need to keep abreast of new drugs as they become available and understand their similarities and differences and their appropriateness for each patient.

MOOD-STABILIZING DRUGS

Lithium

Lithium, a naturally occurring salt, was noted to have medicinal properties during the nineteenth century, when it was found to be present in the waters of some European mineral springs. It was described as having antimanic properties in 1949 but was not accepted for use in the United States until 1970 because of reports of its toxic effects. Today it is readily and safely administered under careful clinical guidelines and has an important clinical role as a mood stabilizer in the treatment of cyclical affective disorders.

MECHANISM OF ACTION. The exact mechanism of action of lithium is not fully understood, but many neurotransmitter functions are altered by the drug. It has been suggested that lithium corrects an ion exchange abnormality, alters sodium transport in nerves and muscle cells, normalizes synaptic neurotransmission of norepinephrine, serotonin, and dopamine, increases the reuptake and metabolism of norepinephrine, changes receptor sensitivity for serotonin, and normalizes circadian rhythm dysfunction in bipolar illness.

CLINICAL USE. Acute episodes of mania and hypomania and recurrent bipolar illness are the most common indications for lithium treatment. Other disorders with an affective component, such as recurrent unipolar depressions, schizoaffective disorder, catatonia, and alcoholism, are sometimes effectively treated with lithium, especially when they are periodic or cyclical. In addition, lithium has been reported to be effective in treating nonaffective disorders such as aggressive conduct disorder, borderline personality disorder, and eating disorders. In general, lithium is not as helpful in the initial treatment of an acute depressive episode but can be given with antidepressant drug treatment. Box 27-8 lists the target symptoms of mania and depression for mood-stabilizing drug therapy.

Before treatment with lithium, a complete history and physical examination are required, with special attention to the kidneys (lithium is excreted by the kidneys) and the thyroid. Regular medical checkups are essential while the patient is on maintenance lithium treatment (Box 27-9).

In acute manic episodes lithium is effective in 1 to 2 weeks, but it may take up to 4 weeks or even a few months to treat the symptoms fully. Sometimes additional agents are used as adjuncts in the treatment of acute bipolar episodes because lithium is initially slow acting. In a maintenance regimen lithium decreases the number of affective episodes, their severity, and the frequency of occurrence. However, mild mood swings or the recurrence of affective symptoms are not uncommon while on lithium maintenance. These problems usually respond to a temporary increase in lithium dose or short-term psychotherapeutic support. The maintenance dose for each patient must be individualized and may vary from time to time.

Lithium therapy usually is started with 300 mg tid until steady state is reached, usually in 7 days. Then a blood level

Box 27-8 *Target Symptoms for Mood-Stabilizing Drug Therapy*

MANIA	DEPRESSION
Irritability	Irritability
Expansiveness	Sadness
Euphoria	Pessimism
Manipulativeness	Anhedonia
Lability with depression	Self-reproach
Sleep disturbance (decreased sleep)	Guilt
	Hopelessness
Pressured speech	Somatic complaints
Flight of ideas	Suicidal ideation
Motor hyperactivity	Motor retardation
Assaultiveness/threatening behavior	Slowed thinking
	Poor concentration and memory
Distractibility	
Hypergraphia	Fatigue
Hypersexuality	Constipation
Persecutory and religious delusions	Decreased libido
	Anorexia or increased appetite
Grandiosity	Weight change
Hallucinations	Helplessness
Ideas of reference	Sleep disturbance (insomnia or hypersomnia)
Catatonia	

Box 27-9 *Prelithium Workup*

Renal: urinalysis, blood urea nitrogen (BUN), creatinine, electrolytes, 24-hour creatinine clearance; history of renal disease in self or family; diabetes mellitus, hypertension, diuretic use, analgesic abuse

Thyroid: thyroid-stimulating hormone (TSH), T_4 (thyroxine), T_3 resin uptake, T_4 I (free thyroxine index); history of thyroid disease in self or family

Other: complete physical, history, ECG, fasting blood sugar, complete blood count (CBC)

MAINTENANCE LITHIUM CONSIDERATIONS

Every 3 months: lithium level (for the first 6 months)
Every 6 months: reassess renal status, lithium level, TSH
Every 12 months: reassess thyroid function, ECG
Assess more often if patient is symptomatic

is drawn in the morning, 12 hours after the last dose. Table 27-13 lists the mood-stabilizing drugs. Because of the low therapeutic index of lithium, toxic blood levels can be reached quickly. Also, because lithium is a salt, the sodium and fluid balance of the body affects lithium regulation. It is essential to monitor serum blood levels regularly (every week for the first month, then every 3 to 6 months) to regulate the dose based on these levels and to teach the patient about lithium toxicity symptoms and issues regarding salt and fluid intake.

In general, the serum concentration of lithium should be between 0.6 and 1.4 mEq/L. Treatment at lower or higher serum lithium concentrations is appropriate for some patients who have lithium side effects or fail to achieve ad-

TABLE 27-13 *Mood-Stabilizing Drugs*

GENERIC (TRADE NAME)	USUAL ADULT DOSE (MG/DAY)	PREPARATIONS
Lithium (Eskalith, Lithobid, Lithonate)	900-1800	PO, L, SR
Valproate (Depakene)	10 to 60 mg/kg/day	PO
Divalproex (Depakote)	750 mg/day to 60 mg/kg/day	
Carbamazepine (Tegretol)	200-1600	PO, L, C

C, Chewable tablets; *L*, liquid; *PO*, oral tablet/capsule; *SR*, oral slow-release tablets.

equate mood stabilization. In geriatric patients or those with medical illness, a serum lithium level of 0.6 to 0.8 mEq/L is recommended. Use of lithium in pregnancy is not recommended. Various congenital abnormalities have been reported in babies exposed to lithium in utero, particularly during the first trimester.

> **?** *Your patient's wife calls you and is upset. Her husband says he enjoys his manic highs and does not want to take his medication, which dulls his enjoyment of life. How would you help this family?*

ADVERSE REACTIONS. The use of lithium represents a challenge for nurses and other clinicians. Patients must be taught the difference between side effects and signs of lithium toxicity (Box 27-10). Patients must also be taught the common causes for an increase in the lithium level and ways to stabilize a therapeutic level as described in Box 27-11. Lithium toxicity is an emergency. Management of serious toxic states is outlined in Box 27-12.

Anticonvulsants

Carbamazepine (Tegretol), marketed since the 1960s as an anticonvulsant, was also seen to have mood-stabilizing effects on patients with temporal lobe epilepsy. Carbamazepine is helpful in the treatment of acute mania and in the long-term prevention of manic episodes.[14] Carbamazepine inhibits kindling and enhances the activity of the inhibitory neurotransmitter GABA. Kindling (Chapter 5) is the process by which the brain apparently becomes sensitized by events, such as stressors or injuries, and eventually seems to spontaneously respond in a similar manner without the precipitating events. This is a model used to theorize about cyclical illness such as bipolar illness and intermittent symptoms such as panic attacks or the craving of substance abuse. Carbamazepine has its peak effects within 10 days of administration. Other psychiatric applications of carbamazepine, although still experimental, include the treatment of borderline personality disorder, schizophrenia, and schizoaffective disorder. Side effects include skin rash, sore

Box **27-10** *Lithium Side Effects and Toxicity*

Body image	Weight gain (60% of patients)
Cardiac	ECG changes, usually not clinically significant
CNS	Fine hand tremor (50% of patients), fatigue, headache, mental dullness, lethargy
Dermatological	Acne, pruritic maculopapular rash
Endocrine	Thyroid dysfunction: hypothyroidism (5% of patients); replacement hormone
	Diabetes mellitus: diet or insulin therapy
Gastrointestinal	Gastric irritation, anorexia, abdominal cramps, mild nausea, vomiting, diarrhea (dose with food or milk; further divide dose)
Renal	Polyuria (60% of patients), polydipsia, edema
	Nephrogenic diabetes insipidus: decrease dose; drink plenty of fluids; thiazide diuretics paradoxically reduce polyuria
	Microscopic structural kidney changes (10% to 20% of patients on lithium for 1 year); does not cause clinical morbidity

LITHIUM TOXICITY/USUALLY DOSE RELATED

Prodrome of intoxication (lithium level $\geq$ 2.0 mEq/L): anorexia, nausea, vomiting, diarrhea, coarse hand tremor, twitching, lethargy, dysarthria, hyperactive deep tendon reflexes, ataxia, tinnitus, vertigo, weakness, drowsiness

Lithium intoxication (lithium level $\geq$ 2.5 mEq/L): fever, decreased urine output, decreased blood pressure, irregular pulse, ECG changes, impaired consciousness, seizures, coma, death

Box **27-11** *Stabilizing Lithium Levels*

COMMON CAUSES FOR AN INCREASE IN LITHIUM LEVELS

Decreased sodium intake
Diuretic therapy
Decreased renal functioning
Fluid and electrolyte loss, sweating, diarrhea, dehydration, fever, vomiting
Medical illness
Overdose
Nonsteroidal antiinflammatory drug therapy

WAYS TO MAINTAIN A STABLE LITHIUM LEVEL

Stabilize dosing schedule by dividing doses or use of sustained-release capsules.
Ensure adequate dietary sodium and fluid intake (2 to 3 l/day).
Replace fluid and electrolytes lost during exercise or gastrointestinal illness.
Monitor signs and symptoms of lithium side effects and toxicity.
If patient forgets a dose, a dose may be taken if less than 2 hours have elapsed; if longer than 2 hours, the dose should be skipped and the next dose taken; never double up on doses.

throat, mucosal ulceration, low-grade fever, drowsiness, vertigo, ataxia, diplopia, blurred vision, nausea, vomiting, hepatotoxicity, and a temporary benign 25% decrease in the white blood cell count. A rare but serious problem is carbamazepine-induced agranulocytosis, a significant decrease in the white blood cell count that does not return to normal. Thus blood levels and CBCs are monitored weekly during the first 1 to 2 months of treatment, and at progressively longer intervals throughout the course of treatment.

Another anticonvulsant medicine used in psychiatry is valproate (Depakote). This drug has been shown to be effective in the manic phase of bipolar disorder and schizoaffective disorder, even in patients who did not respond to or were unable to tolerate conventional drug therapy.[6,18] Valproate, like carbamazepine, inhibits kindling and enhances GABA. This drug is well tolerated in general. The most common side effects include gastrointestinal complaints such as anorexia, nausea, vomiting, and diarrhea; neurological symptoms of tremor, sedation, and ataxia; increased appetite; and weight gain. Very rare but serious side effects include pancreatitis and severe hepatic dysfunction. Liver function and hematology levels are

checked monthly during the first 6 months of therapy, and then every 3 to 6 months.

Valproate is usually dosed until a serum level of 50 to 125 µg/l is achieved. Response usually occurs in 1 to 2 weeks. Valproate is not safe for use during pregnancy. It can be used in long-term maintenance alone or with other drugs such as lithium, antipsychotics, or antidepressants. There is no clear evidence of a difference in efficacy between carbamazepine or valproate, so selection is made according to side effect tolerance for individual patients.

Acutely ill patients with bipolar disorder have increased intracellular calcium ion concentration in lymphocytes and platelets, which decreases with resolution of mania. Because lithium reduces platelet calcium ion concentration in manic patients, there is a theoretical basis for considering calcium channel blockers in the treatment of bipolar illness. Calcium channel blockers have been less extensively studied for this indication, and results to date remain mixed.

ANTIPSYCHOTIC DRUGS

The antipsychotic drugs have become a mainstay in the treatment of psychotic disorders and some nonpsychotic conditions. Although they do not offer a cure of psychosis, these drugs are effective in reducing psychotic symptoms. The discovery in 1952 that chlorpromazine produced significant behavioral changes in psychiatric patients revolutionized psychiatric care. Despite the potential for severe side effects, antipsychotic drugs are widely prescribed and offer an alternative for some patients who might otherwise face a lifetime of institutionalization.

Box 27-12 *Management of Serious Lithium Toxicity*

Assess quickly; obtain rapid history of incident, especially dosing; offer support and explanations to patient.

Hold all lithium doses.

Check blood pressure, pulse, rectal temperature, respirations, and level of consciousness. Be prepared to initiate stabilization procedures, protect airway, and provide supplemental oxygen.

Obtain lithium blood level immediately; obtain electrolytes, BUN, creatinine, urinalysis, CBC when possible.

Electrocardiogram; monitor cardiac status.

Limit lithium absorption; if acute overdose, provide an emetic; nasogastric suctioning.

Vigorously hydrate: 5 to 6 l/day; balance electrolytes; IV line; indwelling urinary catheter.

Patient will be bedridden: range of motion, frequent turning, pulmonary toilet.

In moderately severe cases:

Implement osmotic diuresis with urea or mannitol.

Increase lithium clearance with aminophylline and alkalinize the urine with IV sodium lactate.

Ensure adequate intake of sodium chloride to promote excretion of lithium.

Implement peritoneal or hemodialysis in the most severe cases (serum levels between 2.0 and 4.0 mEq/L) with decreasing urinary output and deepening CNS depression.

Ascertain reasons for lithium toxicity, increase health teaching efforts, mobilize postdischarge support system, arrange for more frequent clinical visits and blood levels, assess for depression and suicidal intent.

Box 27-13 *Antipsychotic Drug Target Symptoms*

POSITIVE SYMPTOMS: AN EXCESS OR DISTORTION OF NORMAL FUNCTION*

Psychotic disorders of thinking

Delusions (somatic, grandiose, religious, nihilistic or persecutory themes)

Hallucinations (auditory, visual, tactile, gustatory, olfactory)

Disorganization of speech and behavior

Positive formal thought disorder (incoherence, derailment, illogicality)

Bizarre behavior (catatonic motor behaviors, disorders of movement, deterioration of social behavior)

NEGATIVE SYMPTOMS: A DIMINUTION OR LOSS OF NORMAL FUNCTION†

Affective flattening: limited range and intensity of emotional expression

Alogia: restricted thought and speech

Avolition/apathy: lack of initiation of goal-directed behavior

Anhedonia/asociality: inability to experience pleasure or maintain social contacts

Attentional impairment: inability to mentally focus

*Responsive to traditional and atypical antipsychotics.
†Unresponsive to traditional antipsychotics, responsive to atypical antipsychotics.

Mechanism of Action

Until recently, all the older antipsychotic drugs (now called typical, or conventional, antipsychotics) have been dopamine (DA) antagonists, blocking postsynaptic D_2 receptors in several DA tracts in the brain. This action resulted in their two main effects: a decrease in the positive symptoms of schizophrenia (Box 27-13) and the production of extrapyramidal side effects (EPS; see Table 27-15). Clozapine, the first of the newer antipsychotics (called atypical antipsychotics) exerts both D_2 and $5HT_2$ receptor blocking action. The atypical drugs are DA and 5HT antagonists; they inhibit the reception of these two neurotransmitters, dopamine and serotonin, at specific postsynaptic sites. These new drugs not only improve the positive symptoms of schizophrenia, but also exert therapeutic action in treating the negative symptoms of schizophrenia without significant EPS (one of the major causes of patient nonadherence to the typical antipsychotic drugs).[32]

Clinical Use

The most frequently prescribed antipsychotic drugs are listed in Table 27-14. The typical antipsychotics have been the standard in the field until recently and they are not different from each other in terms of overall clinical response at equivalent doses. Thus, selection from among the typical antipsychotic drugs is determined by the extent, type, and severity of side effects produced, as well as effect of the drug in a first-degree relative. Recent advances in the development of atypical antipsychotic drugs provide new hope for patients with psychosis, particularly those who have not responded well to typical antipsychotics or have suffered dose-limiting side effects from these drugs. They provide better efficacy through the treatment of both the positive and negative symptoms of schizophrenia (see Box 27-13) and they have fewer EPS side effects (Table 27-15).[24]

The major uses for antipsychotic drugs are in the management of schizophrenia, organic brain syndrome with psychosis, and the manic phase of manic-depressive illness. Their occasional use may be indicated in severe depression with psychotic features. Nonpsychiatric uses for antipsychotic drugs include treatment of vomiting, vertigo, and the increased effects of analgesics for pain relief.

The clinical symptoms of psychosis that are considered the major target symptoms for pharmacotherapy with the antipsychotic drugs are listed in Box 27-13. The initial nursing treatment plan should address drug dose, target symptom response, and observed side effects and their treatment, along with patient safety, education, and reassurance. Although the relationship the nurse establishes with the patient who is very psychotic forms the basis for an ongoing therapeutic alliance, active nonpharmacological treatment of the residual symptoms of psychosis is more successful when the patient's behavior, mood, and thought processes begin to show improvement with pharmacotherapy.

Clozapine does not worsen preexisting tardive dyskinesia

TABLE **27-14** *Antipsychotic Drugs*

Generic Name (trade name)	Drug Dosage: Equivalence (mg)	Usual Adult Dosage Range (mg/day)	Preparations
TYPICAL ANTIPSYCHOTICS			
Phenothiazines			
Chlorpromazine (Thorazine)	100	100-2000	PO, IM, L
Thioridazine (Mellaril)	100	100-800*	PO, L
Mesoridazine (Serentil)	50	100-400	PO, IM, L
Perphenazine (Trilafon)	10	8-64	PO, IM, L
Trifluoperazine (Stelazine)	5	5-60	PO, IM, L
Fluphenazine (Prolixin)	4	30	PO, IM, L, L-A (q2-4wk)
Thioxanthene			
Thiothixene (Navene)	5	5-60	PO, IM, L
Butyrophenone			
Haloperidol (Haldol)	4	2-100	PO, IM, L, L-A (q4wk)
Dibenzoxazepine			
Loxapine (Loxitane)	10	30-250	PO, IM, L
Dihydroindolone			
Molindone (Moban)	10	10-225	PO, L
ATYPICAL ANTIPSYCHOTICS			
Clozapine (Clozaril)	50	100-900	PO
Risperidone (Risperdal)	1	1-6	PO
Olanzapine (Zyprexa)	2	10	PO

*Upper limit to avoid retinopathy.
IM, Intramuscular; *L,* oral liquid, concentrate, suspension, or elixir;
L-A, long-acting injectable preparations; *PO,* oral tablet or capsule.

(see Table 27-15), and in some cases symptoms of tardive dyskinesia improved after the standard antipsychotic had been discontinued and clozapine therapy had been initiated.[21] Unfortunately, clozapine may cause orthostatic hypotension, tachycardia, sedation, anticholinergic effects, weight gain, and a paradoxical hypersalivation, especially during sleep. There is a seizure risk that increases with dosage (up to 5% of patients taking 600-900 mg/day) and often a rapid return of psychotic symptoms when the drug is discontinued.

The most serious adverse effect of clozapine is agranulocytosis, which occurs in approximately 1% to 2% of patients (this is 10 to 20 times greater than the risk for standard antipsychotic drugs). This risk continues to increase during the first 6 months of treatment, then declines gradually, but it never entirely disappears. Weekly CBCs to monitor for declines in white cell count and Clozaril prescriptions 1 week at a time are essential to good clinical care.[16] Once a patient has this problem with Clozaril, reinstatement of the drug is contraindicated.[30] Obviously, this adds a significant cost to the treatment of patients taking clozapine. For the schizophrenic patient who needs this drug and can be monitored weekly (the FDA has been petitioned for a less frequent schedule) for agranulocytosis, can afford the additional burden of cost, and does not need concomitant drugs that also lower white blood cell count, such as carbamazepine, Cloz-

aril may make a significant difference in treatment outcome. The other atypical drugs thus far do not have an increased incidence of agranulocytosis thus they do not require frequent lab work. The atypical antipsychotics have potent postsynaptic receptor blocking actions at the dopamine D_2 site. Perhaps the most striking difference of these atypical antipsychotic drugs is their ability to block $5HT_2$ serotonin receptors. These differences in receptor binding by the atypical drugs are thought to account for their lower extrapyramidal side effect profile and greater efficacy in the treatment of the negative symptoms of schizophrenia.

Finally, although the atypical drugs reduce the negative as well as the positive symptoms of schizophrenia, patients taking these medications still need help with other aspects of their psychosocial functioning. Psychoeducation, social skills training, group support, and other rehabilitative interventions are beneficial in improving their overall level of functioning and quality of life.

 How would you help a family evaluate the risk/ benefit ratio for clozapine treatment of their relative?

GENERAL PHARMACOLOGICAL PRINCIPLES. Dosage requirements for individual patients vary considerably

TABLE **27-15** *Nursing Considerations for Antipsychotic Drug Side Effects*

CNS SIDE EFFECTS	NURSING CARE AND TEACHING CONSIDERATIONS
Extrapyramidal symptoms	General treatment principles: Tolerance usually develops by the third month. Decrease dose of drug. Add a drug to treat EPS, then taper after 3 months on the antipsychotic. Use a drug with a lower EPS profile. Patient education and support.
Acute dystonic reactions: oculogyric crisis, torticolis	Spasms of major muscle groups of neck, back, and eyes; occur suddenly; frightening; painful; medicate (Table 27-17), parenteral works faster than po; have respiratory support available; more common in children and young males, and with high potency drugs. Taper dose gradually when discontinuing antipsychotic drugs to avoid withdrawal dyskinesia.
Akathisia	Cannot remain still; pacing, inner restlessness, leg aches are relieved by movement; rule out anxiety or agitation; medicate.
Parkinson's syndrome: akinesia, cogwheel rigidity, fine tremor	More common in males and elderly; tolerance may not develop; medicate with DA agonist amantadine (must have good renal function).
Tardive dyskinesia (TD)	Can occur after use (usually long use) of conventional antipsychotics; stereotyped involuntary movements (tongue protrusion, lip smacking, chewing, blinking, grimacing, choreiform movements of limbs and trunk, foot tapping); if using typical antipsychotics, use preventive measures (see Fig. 27-2) and assess often (AIMS scale; see Box 27-14); consider changing to an atypical antipsychotic drug; there is no treatment at present for TD.
Neuroleptic malignant syndrome (NMS)	Potentially fatal: Fever, tachycardia, sweating, muscle rigidity, tremor, incontinence, stupor, leukocytosis, elevated CPK, renal failure; more common with high-potency drugs and in dehydrated patients; discontinue all drugs; supportive symptomatic care (hydration, renal dialysis, ventilation, and fever reduction as appropriate); can treat with dantroline or bromocriptine; antipsychotic drugs can be cautiously reintroduced eventually.
Seizures	Occur in approximately 1% of people taking these drugs; clozapine has a 5% rate (in patients on 600 to 900 mg/day); may have to discontinue clozapine.

OTHER SIDE EFFECTS OF ANTIPSYCHOTIC DRUGS

Agranulocytosis	This is an emergency; it develops abruptly, with fever, malaise, ulcerative sore throat, leukopenia. High incidence (1% to 2%) is associated with clozapine; must do weekly CBC and prescribe only 1 week of drug at a time; discontinue drug immediately; may need reverse isolation and antibiotics.
Photosensitivity	Use sunscreen and sunglasses; cover body with clothing.
Anticholinergic effects	Symptoms: constipation, dry mouth, blurred vision, orthostatic hypotension, tachycardia, urinary retention, nasal congestion; see Table 27-12 for nursing care.
Sedation, weight gain	See Table 27-12 for nursing care.

and must be adjusted as the target symptom changes and side effects are monitored. Initially the patient is dosed several times a day, and the daily dose can be raised every 1 to 4 days until symptoms improve. Olanzapine is an exception. A starting dose of 10 mg is often needed for the entire course of treatment. Some patients begin to respond in 2 to 3 days, some take as long as 2 weeks. Full benefits from typical drugs may take 4 or more weeks. High parenteral doses can be used initially to control a highly excited or dangerous patient.

When the patient has been stabilized for several weeks, the daily dose can be lowered to the lowest effective dose. The half-life of antipsychotic drugs is greater than 24 hours, so the patient can be dosed once a day after steady state is reached (approximately 4 days). Bedtime dosing allows the patient to sleep through side effects when they are at their peak. After approximately 6 to 12 months of stable maintenance drug therapy, the patient can be slowly tapered from medication to assess the need for continued drug treatment. Some schizophrenic patients require a lifetime of continu-

ous medication management. A patient who is unresponsive to an adequate trial often responds to another chemical class of antipsychotic drug, so a second drug trial usually is given. An adequate trial is 1 month for the typical antipsychotic drugs, and three months (or longer, particularly for clozapine) for the atypical drugs.

Many antipsychotic drugs can be administered by oral and intramuscular routes. Fluphenazine comes in two depot injectable forms that can be given every 7 to 28 days. Haloperidol decanoate is an injectable form of haloperidol that has a 4-week duration of action. It is not appropriate to treat an acute psychotic episode with haloperidol decanoate alone because it takes 3 months to reach steady state drug levels. Thus this drug is more of a long-term maintenance medication.[15] Acute psychotic episodes require a shorter-acting drug. The patient's ability to take these drugs should be tested by first administering the oral form for several days. Long-acting injectables have been important in treating the outpatient who requires supervision of medication

TABLE **27-16** *Acute Side Effect Profile: Antipsychotic Drugs*

DRUGS	SEDATION	EXTRAPYRAMIDAL SYMPTOMS	ANTICHOLINERGIC	POSTURAL HYPOTENSION
LOW POTENCY				
Chlorpromazine	4	2	3	4
Thioridazine	4	1	4	4
Clozapine	4	1	4	3
Olanzapine	2	0	2	2
HIGH POTENCY				
Trifluoperazine	2	3	2	2
Thiothixene	2	3	2	1
Loxapine	2	3	2	2
Molindone	2	3	2	2
Mesoridazine	3	2	3	3
Perphenazine	2	3	2	2
Fluphenazine	1	4	2	1
Haloperidol	1	4	1	1
Risperidone	2	1	1	2

1, Lowest incidence; *4,* highest incidence.

intake because of nonadherence. Most antipsychotic drugs also have antinausea effects.

Contrary to package inserts, there are no ceiling doses for these medicines, with the exception of thioridazine, which can cause pigmentary retinopathy when given in amounts over 800 mg/day. Abruptly stopping antipsychotic drugs can cause dyskinetic reactions and some rebound side effects. The drugs should be tapered slowly over several days to weeks.

Antipsychotic drugs do not cause chemical dependency, nor is there tolerance to their antipsychotic effects over time. Because of their wide therapeutic index, overdoses of these drugs ordinarily do not result in death, so they have a very low suicide potential. Because they do not produce euphoria, they also have a very low abuse potential. Antipsychotic drugs are not respiratory depressants but produce an added depressant effect when combined with drugs that produce respiratory depression. Therefore, patients who also may be taking drugs such as benzodiazepines must be carefully observed. The effects of antipsychotics on the fetus are inconclusive. It is always best to avoid any drug during the first trimester, although what is best for a psychotic pregnant mother must be carefully considered.

Adverse Reactions

The side effects of antipsychotic drugs are varied and require assessment,[33] prevention, and intervention.[34] Table 27-15 is a list of side effects and treatment considerations. Some side effects are merely uncomfortable for the patient, most are easily treated, but some are life threatening. It is important to minimize the patient's fears, increased sense of stigmatization, and possible nonadherence with drug treatment through effective patient education and support.

Most EPS side effects are common with the use of typical antipsychotic drugs (particularly with the high-potency drugs; see Table 27-16), and often painful and disabling.

 TABLE **27-17** *Drugs to Treat Extrapyramidal Side Effects*

GENERIC NAME (TRADE NAME)	ADULT DOSAGE RANGE (MG/DAY)	PREPARATIONS
ANTICHOLINERGICS		
Benztropine (Cogentin)	1-6	PO, IM, IV
Trihexyphenidyl (Artane)	1-10	PO
Biperiden (Akineton)	2-6	PO
Procyclidine (Kemadrin)	6-20	PO
ANTIHISTAMINE		
Diphenhydramine (Benadryl)	25-300	PO, IM, IV
DOPAMINE AGONIST		
Amantadine (Symmetrel)	100-300	PO
BENZODIAZEPINES		
Diazepam (Valium)	2-6	PO, IV
Lorazepam (Ativan)	0.5-2	PO, IM
Clonazepam (Klonopin)	1-4	PO

They are also stigmatizing, can usually be prevented or minimized and effectively treated (tardive dyskinesia is the exception). Because of their efficacy in treating the positive and negative symptoms of schizophrenia and their lower side effect profile, the atypical drugs are coming to be considered the first line of choice in the treatment of psychosis. Drug strategies to treat EPS include lowering the dose of the drug, changing to a drug with a lower incidence of that side effect, or administering one of the drugs in Table 27-17. Because tolerance to most of these side effects usually occurs in the first 3 months, drugs to treat EPS are usually given for up to 3 months and then slowly discontinued. Long-term use is usually not indicated.

Unfortunately, there is no effective treatment for tardive

Box **27-14** *Abnormal Involuntary Movement Scale (AIMS)*

A simple method to determine tardive dyskinesia symptoms. Total score equals the sum of the items.

Patient identification: _____   Date: _____
Rated by: _____   Treatment period: _____

Either before or after completing the examination procedure, observe the patient unobtrusively at rest (for example, in waiting room).

The chair to be used in this examination should be a hard, firm one without arms.

After the patient is observed, he or she may be rated on a scale of 0 (none), 1 (minimal), 2 (mild), 3 (moderate), and 4 (severe) according to the severity of symptoms at time of interview.

Ask the patient whether there is anything in his or her mouth (such as gum or candy) and if there is, ask the patient to remove it.

Ask the patient about the *current* condition of his or her teeth. Ask whether the patient wears dentures. Do the patient's teeth or dentures bother him or her *now*?

Ask the patient whether he or she notices any movement in mouth, face, hands, or feet. If yes, ask the patient to describe such movement and to what extent it *currently* is bothersome or interferes with activities.

0 1 2 3 4   Have the patient sit in a chair with hands on knees, legs slightly apart, and feet flat on floor. (Look at entire body for movements in this position.)

0 1 2 3 4   Ask the patient to sit with hands hanging unsupported. If male, between legs; if female and wearing a dress, hanging over knees. (Observe hands and other body areas.)

0 1 2 3 4   Ask the patient to open mouth. (Observe tongue at rest within mouth.) Have him or her do this twice.

0 1 2 3 4   Ask the patient to protrude tongue. (Observe abnormalities of tongue movement.) Have him or her do this twice.

0 1 2 3 4   Ask the patient to tap thumb with each finger as rapidly as possible for 10 to 15 seconds separately with the right hand then with left hand. (Observe facial and leg movements.)

0 1 2 3 4   Flex and extend patient's left and right arms (one at a time).

0 1 2 3 4   Ask the patient to stand up. (Observe in profile. Observe all body areas again, hips included.)

0 1 2 3 4   Ask the patient to extend both arms outstretched in front with palms down.* (Observe trunk, legs, and mouth.)

0 1 2 3 4   Have the patient walk a few paces, turn, and walk back to chair.* (Observe hands and gait.) Do this twice.

*Activated movements.

---

dyskinesia to date, although it is expected to decrease in incidence with the increased use of the atypical antipsychotic drugs, and clozaril has been reported to minimize it in some patients. Primary preventive measures (Fig. 27-2) should be taken, and the Abnormal Involuntary Movement Scale (AIMS) (Box 27-14) should be administered regularly to patients taking typical antipsychotic drugs.[13]

Another uncommon but potentially fatal (14% to 30% mortality) side effect of antipsychotic drugs is neuroleptic malignant syndrome (NMS; see Table 27-15). It is important for the nurse to assess for NMS and other serious drug side effects. Because many patients are on more than one drug at a time, it can become confusing when symptoms of these side effects are similar. Table 27-18 compares NMS with serotonin syndrome (see Table 27-12).

Because of the importance in managing patients taking psychotropic medications and the problems they cause, medication-induced movement disorders are coded on Axis I of the DSM-IV.[2] Although they are labeled medication-induced, it is often difficult to establish the causal link between medication exposure and the development of the movement disorder because some of these disorders occur in the absence of medication exposure. These disorders are

▼ Neuroleptic-induced Parkinsonism
▼ Neuroleptic malignant syndrome
▼ Neuroleptic-induced acute dystonia
▼ Neuroleptic-induced acute akathisia
▼ Neuroleptic-induced tardive dyskinesia
▼ Medication-induced postural tremor

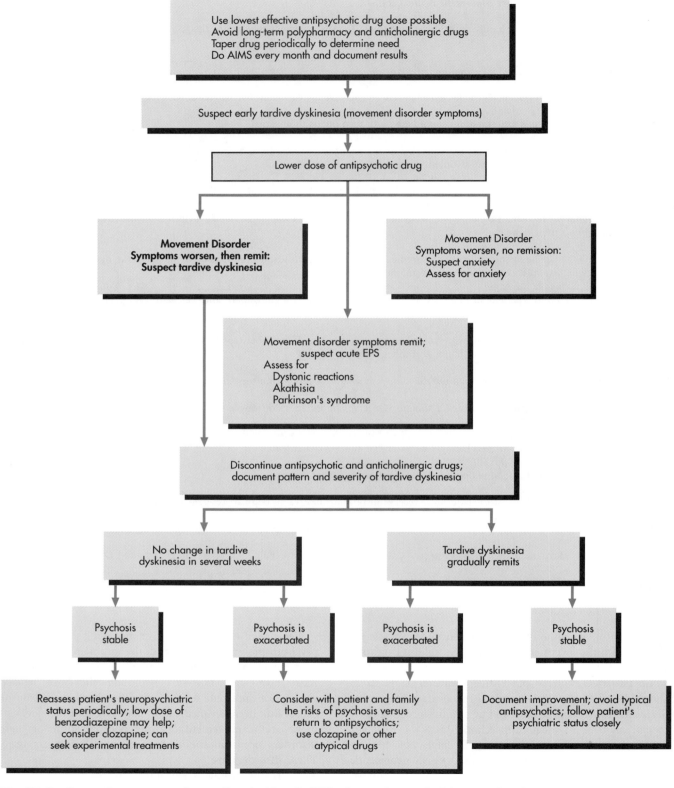

Fig. 27-2 Preventive measure for tardive dyskinesia (TD) when using typical (conventional) antipsychotic drugs.

▼ Medication-induced movement disorder not otherwise specified

▼ Adverse effects of medication not otherwise specified

Currently the correlation between plasma blood levels of antipsychotic drugs or serum dopamine receptor binding and clinical response has yet to be determined, but these tests hold promise for refining drug selection and dosing regimens. Additional classes of antipsychotic drugs that have mechanisms of action highly specific for the target symptoms of psychosis but do not produce a variety of side effects are being tested. Several of these promising new drugs are compared to current antipsychotics in Table 27-19.

FUTURE PSYCHOPHARMACOLOGICAL AGENTS

Based on current trends in psychoactive drug research, the nurse can expect to see new drugs approved for use in mental disorders. Recently, drugs such as tacrine (Cognex) or donepezil (Aricept), both acetylcholinesterase inhibitors, became available. These two drugs enhance the amount of acetylcholine in the brain, which in turn enhances memory and cognition in some people with Alzheimer's disease (Box 27-15). It is important to evaluate new drugs very carefully as they come into clinical use. The nurse should determine the advantages and disadvantages of a new drug as compared to the standard drugs in that class and in relation to the patient's reactions and preferences. The following list is a partial guide to help evaluate new drugs. Ask whether a new drug has

▼ A different mechanism of action more specific to desired biological actions

▼ Quicker onset of action

▼ Fewer drug interactions

TABLE **27-18** *Comparison of Serotonin Syndrome and Neuroleptic Malignant Syndrome*

CLINICAL SYMPTOMS	SEROTONIN SYNDROME	NEUROLEPTIC MALIGNANT SYNDROME
Mental status	Confusion, disorientation, mania	Dazed mutism
Autonomic dysfunction*	50-90%	>90%
Neuromuscular activity		
Muscle rigidity	50%	90%
Hyperreflexia	Common	Rare
Myoclonic jerking	Common	Rare
Ataxia	Common	Rare
Extrapyramidal effects	Rare	Common
Hyperthermia	Mild-marked	Mild-marked
Leukocytosis	Rare	>80%
CPK elevation	Rare	Common
Acute renal failure	Possible	Possible

Modified from Bernstein JG: *Drug handbook in psychiatry*, ed 3, St Louis, 1995, Mosby.
*Tachycardia, labile BP, diaphoresis, tremor, incontinence, dyspnea, shivering, restlessness.

TABLE **27-19** *Comparison of Typical, Atypical, and Newest Antipsychotic Drugs*

	TYPICAL NEUROLEPTIC	CLOZAPINE	RISPERIDONE	OLANZAPINE	QUETIAPINE	SERTINDOLE	ZIPRASIDONE
CLINICAL EFFICACY							
Dosage (mg/day)	Various	300-900	2-10	7.5-20	150-800	4-24	40-160
Acute psychosis overall	+++	+++	+++	+++	+++	+++	+++
Acute positive symptoms	+++	+++	+++	+++	+++	+++	+++
Acute negative symptoms	+	+++	+++	+++	+++	+++	+++
Treatment-refractory psychosis	0	++	?	?	?	?	?
SIDE EFFECT PROFILE							
Agitation	+ to ++	0	+/−	+	+	0	0
Agranulocytosis	Rare	+++	Rare	Rare	Rare	Rare	Rare
Anticholinergic effects	+ to +++	+++	+/−	++	++	0	+
EPS	+ to +++	0	+*	0	0	0	+
Dose-related increase in EPS	Yes	No	Yes	Yes	?	No	?
Nausea/dyspepsia	+	0	+/−	+	0	+	+
Orthostatic hypotension	+ to +++	+++	++	++	+	++	++
Elevation of prolactin levels	+ to ++	0	++	+	0	0	+
Sedation	++ to +++	+++	++	++	++	0	+
Seizures	+	+++ (dose related)	+	+	+	+	+
Tardive dyskinesia	+++	0	?	?	?	?	?

Modified from Jibson MD, Tandon R: A summary of research findings on the new antipsychotic drugs, *Psychiatr Nurs Forum* 2(Summer), 1996.
*Low risk for EPS for risperidone is associated only with low daily doses (< 6 mg).
Efficacy: + = mild, ++ = moderate, +++ = marked, +/− = minimal, ? = uncertain, 0 = none.
Side effects: + = mild, ++ = moderate, +++ = severe, +/− = minimal, ? = uncertain, 0 = none.

B O X **27-15** *Drug Treatment for Alzheimer's Disease*

TACRINE (COGNEX)

Tacrine is the first drug to treat mild to moderate dementia related to Alzheimer's disease.

Tacrine prevents or slows the breakdown of ACh by inhibiting the action of the metabolizing enzyme acetylcholinesterase. An excessive loss of the neurotransmitter ACh is thought to cause the memory problems associated with Alzheimer's disease.

DOSING

10 mg qid po for the first 6 weeks with weekly transaminase levels. Titrate by 10-mg increments to 40 mg qid, at 6-week intervals for each dose, given stable or slightly elevated transaminase levels and patient tolerability. If levels become extreme, stop tacrine until they return to normal and then carefully rechallenge. Measure transaminase levels every 3 months at maintenance doses.

SIDE EFFECTS

Nausea, vomiting, diarrhea, dyspepsia, anorexia, muscle aches, and ataxia. Monitor patients for elevated transaminase levels and abnormal liver function, tacrine-induced bradycardia in patients with sick sinus syndrome, and symptoms of occult or active GI bleeding.

DRUG INTERACTIONS

Can increase theophylline's half-life and plasma concentration. Cimetidine (Tagamet) increases and prolongs blood levels of tacrine. Synergistic effects are expected when given with succinylcholine and other cholinesterase inhibitors or cholinergic agonists.

DRUG LIMITATION

Tacrine's beneficial effects diminish over time as Alzheimer's disease progresses.

DONEPEZIL HYDROCHLORIDE (ARICEPT)

In 1996 the U.S. Food and Drug Administration (FDA) approved donepezil hydrochloride (Aricept) to treat symptoms of Alzheimer's disease. Aricept is only the second approved treatment for Alzheimer's disease.

Like Cognex, Aricept is a palliative that does nothing to slow the progressive neurodegeneration that ultimately leads to dementia and death. By helping the brain retain and use the neurotransmitter acetylcholine, however, both drugs slow the symptomatic progression of the disease, temporarily stabilizing or improving the cognitive state of those taking either drug.

Aricept has a major advantage in its low toxicity compared with Cognex, according to data submitted to the FDA. In addition to lack of liver toxicity, Aricept has a generally more benign side-effect profile than Cognex.

 T A B L E **27-20** *Partial List of New Drugs in Development for Mental Illness*

	INDICATION	MANUFACTURER
ANXIETY DISORDERS		
Flesinoxan	Generalized anxiety disorder	Solvey
Itasertron	Generalized anxiety disorder	Boehringer Ingelheim & Upjohn
Ondansetron	Panic disorder	Glaxo Wellcome
MOOD DISORDERS		
Ipsapirone	Depression	Bayer
Lamotrigine (Lamictal)	Bipolar disorder	Glaxo Wellcome
PSYCHOTIC DISORDERS		
Quetiapine (Seroquel)	Schizophrenia	Zeneca
Iloperidone	Schizophrenia	Hoechst Marion Roussel
Sertindole (Serlect)	Psychosis	Abbott
Ziprasedone	Schizophrenia	Pfizer
DEMENTIAS		
Acetylcarnitine (Alcar)	Alzheimer's disease	Sigma-Tau
Sabeluzole (Reminyl)	Alzheimer's disease	Janssen
Nicergoline (Sermion)	Alzheimer's disease	Pharmacia & Upjohn
SUBSTANCE ABUSE/DEPENDENCE DISORDERS		
Ibogaine (Endabure)	Cocaine dependence	NDA International
Bupropion (Wellbutrin SR)	Smoking cessation	Glaxo Wellcome

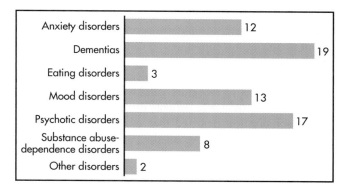

Fig. 27-3 Number of medicines in development for mental illnesses, 1996. (Pharmaceutical Research and Manufacturers of America, Washington, DC, 1996.)

▼ A lower side effect profile
▼ No addictive or abuse potential
▼ No long-term adverse effects
▼ No suicide potential
▼ Permanent or curative effects on neurotransmitter regulation
▼ Several routes of administration, at least by mouth and intramuscularly
▼ A wide therapeutic index
▼ Fewer discontinuation problems
▼ Advantage in cost effectiveness

Table 27-20 lists new drugs currently under review by the FDA or in Phase III (final phase) of clinical testing, soon to be submitted to the FDA for review and approval. There are over 74 psychotropic drugs in clinical trials in the United States (Fig. 27-3). Nurses can expect to see many of these medications approved for use with psychiatric patients in the future.

PSYCHIATRIC NURSING PRACTICE

Psychopharmacology Guidelines

Psychotropic medications are commonly used in the treatment of psychiatric disorders. It is therefore essential for psychiatric nurses to have a complete understanding of psychopharmacology. In response to recent developments in the field, the American Nurses' Association and the National Institute of Mental Health established a task force in 1992 to identify psychopharmacology guidelines for psychiatric–mental health nursing. The result is a document published in 1994 that describes the skills and knowledge psychiatric nurses need to guide them in their work with psychopharmacologic agents.[1] The document identifies specific areas that nurses can review to evaluate their ability to deliver competent nursing care. The complete document on psychopharmacology guidelines can be obtained from the American Nurses' Association; Box 27-16 outlines the major areas.

Box **27-16** *Psychopharmacology Guidelines for Psychiatric–Mental Health Nurses*

NEUROSCIENCES

Commensurate with level of practice, the psychiatric–mental health nurse integrates current knowledge from the neurosciences to understand etiological models, diagnostic issues, and treatment strategies for psychiatric illness.

PSYCHOPHARMACOLOGY

The psychiatric–mental health nurse involved in the care of patients taking psychopharmacological agents demonstrates knowledge of psychopharmacological principles, including pharmacokinetics, pharmacodynamics, drug classification, intended and unintended effects, and related nursing implications.

CLINICAL MANAGEMENT

The psychiatric–mental health nurse applies principles from the neurosciences and psychopharmacology to provide safe and effective management of patients being treated with psychopharmacological agents. Clinical management includes assessment, diagnosis, and treatment considerations.

Assessment

The psychiatric–mental health nurse has the knowledge, skills, and ability to conduct and interpret patient assessments of psychopharmacological agents. Assessments include physical, neuropsychiatric, psychosocial, and psychopharmacological parameters.

Diagnosis

The psychiatric–mental health nurse has the knowledge, skills, and ability to use appropriate nursing, psychiatric, and medical diagnostic classification systems to guide the psychopharmacological treatment of patients with mental illness.

Treatment

The psychiatric–mental health nurse takes an active role in the treatment of patients with mental illness and integrates prescribed psychopharmacological interventions in a cohesive, multidimensional plan of care.

Modified from American Nurses' Association: *Psychiatric mental health nursing psychopharmacology project: ANA task force on psychopharmacology,* Washington, DC, 1994, The Association.

Two other exciting new mechanisms for learning about and keeping up with psychopharmacology are

▼ The Internet, which has hundreds of mental health sites (many of which include psychopharmacology information), journals, research, and user groups. Search on *psychopharmacology* or go to a World Wide Web site that offers links to psychopharmacology pages, such as the home page of The American Psychiatric Nurses Association (http://www.apna.org), click on *Links,* then select a site of your choice.
▼ CD-ROMs such as *Nurses Drug Information: 1996* (by *Facts and Comparisons,* 314-878-2515). This is a fast way to access up-to-date drug information. It covers more than 4500 drugs (not just psychotropics) and includes

over 900 color photographs and 650 audio pronunciations of generic drug names. The many monographs contain pharmacological information, nursing considerations, and patient teaching guidelines.

Documentation

In addition to routine documentation of pharmacological activities, the nurse may have special documentation considerations in the pharmacological treatment of mental illness. The following issues are particularly important to document when working with psychiatric patients:

▼ Drugs administered outside usual recommended levels
▼ Rationale for medication or dose changes
▼ Drugs used for other than the indications approved by the FDA
▼ Continued use of a drug that is causing clinically significant side effects
▼ Polypharmacy rationale
▼ Patient and family knowledge, attitudes, and preferences

Patient Education

Patients taking psychotropic drugs must be knowledgeable about them. Serious consequences can result from what appears to be minor changes in some of the instructions for drug use, such as skipping medication one day, eating cheese, or failing to recognize certain side effects. A recent survey of 253 psychiatric patients discharged from a short-stay hospitalization reported that more than half did not know the name and dosage of the psychiatric medications prescribed for them and why they were taking them, even though they had received both group and individual medication instruction during hospitalization.[8] Results suggest the need for more active forms of medication education, such as supervised self-administration in the final days of hospitalization.[10]

Patients and their families need thorough and ongoing instruction on psychotropic drug treatment. Nursing programs focused on patient education need to address essential elements, such as missed medication doses,[38] focus on

---

Box **27-17** *Teaching Prescribed Medications*

DEFINITION
Preparing a patient to safely take prescribed medications and monitor for their effects.

ACTIVITIES
Instruct the patient to recognize distinctive characteristics of the medications.
Inform the patient of both the generic and brand names of each medication.
Instruct the patient on the purpose and action of each medication.
Instruct the patient on the dosage, route, and duration of each medication.
Instruct the patient on the proper administration of each medication.
Evaluate the patient's ability to self-administer medications.
Instruct the patient to perform needed procedures before taking a medication (for example, check pulse and glucose level).
Inform the patient what to do if a dose of medication is missed.
Instruct the patient on which criteria to use when deciding to alter the medication dosage/schedule.
Inform the patient of consequences of not taking or abruptly discontinuing medications.
Instruct the patient on specific precautions to observe when taking medications (such as no driving or using power tools).
Instruct the patient on possible adverse side effects of each medication.
Instruct the patient on how to relieve or prevent certain side effects.
Instruct the patient on appropriate actions to take if side effects occur.
Instruct the patient on the signs and symptoms of overdosage or underdosage.
Inform the patient of possible drug/food interactions.
Instruct the patient on how to properly store medications.
Instruct the patient on the proper care of devices used for administration.
Instruct patients on proper disposal of needles and syringes at home, as appropriate, and where to dispose of the sharps container.
Provide the patient with written information about the action, purpose, side effects, and so on, of medications.
Help the patient to develop a written medication schedule.
Instruct the patient to carry documentation of prescribed medication regimen.
Instruct the patient on how to fill prescriptions.
Inform the patient of possible changes in appearance or dosage when filling generic medication prescriptions.
Warn the patient of the risks associated with taking expired medication.
Caution the patient against giving prescribed medication to others.
Determine the patient's ability to obtain required medications.
Provide information on medication reimbursement.
Provide information on cost saving programs and organizations to obtain medications and devices.
Provide information on medication alert devices and how to obtain them.
Reinforce information provided by other health-care team members.
Include the family/significant others as appropriate.

From McCloskey J, Bulachek G: *Nursing interventions classification*, ed 2, St Louis, 1996, Mosby.

self-management,[18] and documenting effectiveness. Box 27-17 identifies specific nursing activities from the nursing intervention classification (NIC)[23] related to teaching a patient to take prescribed medications safely.

> **?** *Many chronic mentally ill people have social workers as their case managers. What skills and knowledge would psychiatric nurses bring to this patient population that differ from those of social workers?*

Promoting Patient Adherence

Patients who do not take their medications as prescribed or who do not recognize warning signs of drug problems are at risk for unsuccessful results and adverse reactions. Yet it has been estimated that 30% to 55% of Americans

---

CRITICAL THINKING *about* Contemporary Issues

Is Nonadherence a Patient Problem or a Nursing Problem?

Every nurse and many patients and their families have had the difficult experience of facing relapse in psychopharmacologically treated psychiatric illness. An obvious problem-solving approach includes an assessment of compliance—is the patient taking the drug as prescribed? In the absence of concomitant medical illness, differences in bioavailability among generic brands of a drug, and increases in life stressors, the nurse and family return to the issue of compliance and wonder why the patient deviated from a previously effective drug regimen. Even if patients deny noncompliance, they usually carry the burden of blame for relapse, and their future relationships with mental health care providers may be jeopardized.

The interactions of cultural belief systems and psychotropic drug effects are poorly understood. A relatively unacknowledged but well-documented fact is that the effects of pharmacoactive agents are not solely determined by their pharmacological properties.[20] In the cultural context of care it must be recognized that psychotropic drugs affect diverse populations in diverse ways. Thus cultural differences must be considered in the patient and family medication education plan and in interactions with patients throughout the course of treatment.

The potential incompatibility between lay and professional values and between belief systems and explanatory models of illness often determine patients' satisfaction with treatment, medication compliance, clinical outcome, and most important, self-disclosure in the treatment setting.[19, 31] The understanding, acceptance, and communication necessary to create a culturally competent and effective plan of care for the patient with mental illness rest with the nurse and the mental health team. If treatment planning is individualized and is a mutual and shared responsibility between the nurse and patient, then patient compliance or noncompliance must be viewed as a shared outcome of that responsibility.

---

do not follow their drug regimens properly.[25] The threats to patient adherence are many. Some of them reside primarily with the mental health team, others with the patient, and still others reflect a shared failure of the therapeutic alliance (see Critical Thinking about Contemporary Issues).

The administration of psychotherapeutic drugs places the nurse in a position of control over the patient.[11] The nurse should be aware of this issue and not use the administration of medications to punish or manipulate the patient. The nurse should never withhold a drug that the patient needs and is clinically indicated. It is also the nurse's obligation to be aware of countertransference issues and personal attitudes toward the patient, the prescribing clinician, the patient's diagnosis, and the drug treatment regimen that may negatively affect the patient's care.

Nurses and patients should work together to minimize misunderstandings and unnecessarily complex medication regimens. Too often, however, clinicians blame patients for nonadherence without fully evaluating the treatment plan from the patient's perspective. For example, a consumer of mental health services identified the following common mistakes clinicians make in prescribing medication for psychiatric patients[5]:

▼ Incorrect prescribing as a result of misdiagnosis
▼ Excessive dosages of medications

Box **27-18** *Risk Factors for Patient Medication Nonadherence*

Failure to form a therapeutic alliance with the patient
Devaluation of pharmacotherapy by treatment staff
Inadequate patient and family education regarding treatment
Poorly controlled side effects
Insensitivity to patient beliefs, wishes, complaints, or opposition to the idea of taking medication
Multiple daily dosing schedule
Polypharmacy
History of nonadherence
Social isolation
Expense of drugs
Failure to appreciate patient's role in drug treatment plan
Lack of continuity of care
Increased restrictions on patient's lifestyle
Unsupportive significant others
Remission of target symptoms
Increased suicidal ideation
Increased suspiciousness
Unrealistic expectations of drug effects
Concurrent substance use
Failure to target residual symptoms for nonpharmacological therapies
Relapse or exacerbation of clinical syndrome
Failure to alleviate intrafamilial and environmental stressors that precipitate symptoms
Potential for stigmatization

▼ Too many drugs
▼ Downplaying side effects
▼ Overlooking the consumer's expertise
▼ Discouraging consumer education
▼ Inability of the prescriber to see the consumer from a holistic perspective

In addition, a number of studies have explored reasons given by patients for nonadherence with their medication regimens.[9,17,22,27] Risk factors for potential patient nonadherence are listed in Box 27-18. Understanding this issue from the patient's perspective will allow the nurse to anticipate problems and design nursing interventions that can target areas of potential difficulty.

For example, many patients decrease or completely stop taking their medications as soon as they start feeling better. If they have a bad day, they may take medication again for a day or two. Explaining to these patients how the medication works in the body and the need for therapeutic levels of the medicine in the bloodstream may help patients better understand their illness and adhere to the treatment plan. Still other patients may fear that the medications are addictive, or are embarrassed about the stigma of being on psychiatric medication. Clarifying the use of the medication and the positive impact it can have on all aspects of the patient's life may help to reframe the issue of taking medication in a way that promotes adherence. Most important, patients should be encouraged by the nurse to discuss their questions, fears, problems, and concerns about medication before treatment is altered. Finally, the nurse should realize that the quality of the nurse-patient relationship and the strength of the therapeutic alliance play an extremely important role in whether a patient will adhere to the pharmacological treatment plan and affect the patient's recovery process.

COMPETENT CARING A Clinical Exemplar of a Psychiatric Nurse

Diana Laikam, MS, RN, CS

Even after 25 years in practice as a psychiatric nurse I continue to be surprised at the profound effect nursing interventions can have on patients. I was reminded of that again when I recently conducted a medication education group for psychiatric patients. The group met for six sessions with approximately eight patients in attendance. One older man, Mr. F, paid particularly close attention to the content related to obtaining information about medication, knowing correct self-administration, identifying side effects of medication, and negotiating medication issues with health-care providers. Mr. F did not read very well but followed along as the content of the simple handouts was presented. He was early for each class, asked questions, and did homework with the assistance of the nursing staff.

At the last meeting, the patients were given certificates acknowledging their successful completion of the medication education group. I will always remember that Mr. F had a broad smile on his face as I handed him his certificate and read it to him. Upon leaving the room he turned to me and said with great pride and joy, "I'm going to frame this certificate and hang it over my sofa in the living room."

Before that moment I had really not thought of the emotional impact the medication education group may be having on patients. My goal for the group was that members have increased medication compliance through education. What Mr. F taught me, however, was that completing the class in itself was an accomplishment of which he was extremely proud. Patients such as Mr. F inspire me to put renewed energy into the practice of my profession every day.

Summary

1. Psychopharmacology is the fastest growing treatment in the current practice of psychiatry, and the psychiatric nurse makes a unique contribution to the implementation of this treatment strategy.

2. Various aspects of drug effects include half-life, steady state, polypharmacy, drug interactions, and the role of neurotransmitters in the development of psychiatric disorders.

3. Benzodiazepines, the most widely prescribed class of drugs, have almost completely replaced other classes of antianxiety and sedative-hypnotic agents. They are therapeutic and have a wide margin of safety when taken alone. They can be mildly addictive, especially when taken in high doses over long periods of time or when used with alcohol or barbiturates. Common side effects include drowsiness, dizziness, slurred speech, and blurred vision.

4. Antidepressant drugs are effective, nonaddicting, and some can be lethal in overdose. Tricyclics, selective serotonin reuptake inhibitors, and newer drugs are more commonly used than monamine oxidase inhibitors because they are safer in combination with other substances. Side effects of antidepressants are usually mild.

5. The mood stabilizer lithium is effective in the treatment of bipolar illness in short- and long-term treatment regi-

mens. Lithium is not addictive but can be toxic. The therapeutic dose range is narrow and must be monitored by regularly assessing serum lithium levels. Some anticonvulsants also have mood-stabilizing effects.

6. The various classes of typical antipsychotic drugs have similar therapeutic effects but are dissimilar in side effect profiles. Side effects are varied and can be disabling and life threatening. Clozapine, risperidone, and olanzapine are newer, atypical antipsychotic agents with positive clinical effects and fewer movement disorder side effects. Patients taking clozapine need to be closely monitored for agranulocytosis, which is its most serious side effect.

7. New psychopharmacological agents are being tested in clinical drug trials throughout the United States. Many of them will be beneficial to patients with psychiatric illness.

8. Important issues related to psychopharmacology and psychiatric nursing practice include following ANA psychopharmacology guidelines, documentation, patient education, and promoting patients' adherence to their pharmacological treatment plan.

your **INTERNET**
connection

Psychopharmacology and Drug References on the Mental Health Net
http://www.cmhcsys.com/guide/pro22.htm#A

Psychopharmacology TIPS
http://uhs.bsd.uchicago.edu/-bhsiung/tips/

Chapter Review Questions

1. Match each term in Column A with the correct definition in Column B.

Column A

___Barbiturates

___Selective serotonin uptake inhibitors

___Antianxiety drugs

___Cytochrome P450 inhibition

___Anti-Parkinsonian drugs

___Tricyclics

___Serotonin syndrome

___Sedative-hypnotics

___Atypical antipsychotics

___Hypertensive crisis

___Typical antipsychotics

___Mood stabilizers

Column B

A. SSRIs with MAOIs

B. Clozapine and risperidone

C. MAOIs with decongestants/cold remedies

D. Triazolam (Halcion) and flurazepam (Dalmane)

E. Impramine (Tofranil) and amitryptiline (Elavil)

F. Lithium and depakote

G. Chlorpromazine (Thorazine) and thiothixine (Navane)

H. Fluoxetine (Prozac) and sertraline (Zoloft)

I. Alprazolam (Xanax) and lorazepam (Ativan)

J. Secobarbital (Seconal) and pentobarbital (Nembutal)

K. SSRIs with various other drugs

L. Benztropine (Cogentin) and trihexyphenidyl (Artane)

2. Match each term in Column A with the correct definition in Column B.

Column A

___H_1 receptor blockade

___DA reuptake inhibition

___Alpha$_2$ receptor blockade

___NE reuptake inhibition

___ACh receptor blockade

___5HT reuptake inhibition

___Alpha$_1$ receptor blockade

___5HT$_2$ receptor blockade

Column B

A. Reduced depression, reduced suicidal behavior, antipsychotic effects, hypotension, sexual dysfunction

B. Sedation/drowsiness, hypotension, weight gain effects

C. Reduced depression, antianxiety effects, GI disturbances, sexual dysfunction

D. Postural hypotension, dizziness, tachycardia, memory dysfunction

E. Decreased depression, psychomotor activation, anti-Parkinson effects

F. Priapism

G. Reduced depression, tremors, tachycardia, sexual dysfunction

H. Anticholinergic side effects

3. Fill in the blanks.

A. Patient assessment, coordination of treatment modalities, psychopharmacological drug administration and prescribing, medication education, monitoring and maintenance, and research are all within the _____.

B. Concurrent use of drugs, a sometimes necessary and often

problematic practice in pharmacologic interventions, is called _____.

C. _____is the term used when one drug affects the absorption, metabolism, distribution, and excretion of another drug.

D. Many of the psychiatric disorders are thought to be caused by problems in the regulation of communication in the brain, such as an overresponse or an underresponse somewhere along the complex process of neurotransmission. This hypothesis of mental illness is called the _____.

E. The ANA Psychopharmacology Guidelines for Psychiatric Mental Health Nurses includes three broad categories that are essential content for nurses working with patients on psychotropic drugs. These categories are _____, _____, and _____.

4. Identify whether the following statements are true (T) or false (F).

A. ___ Serotonin syndrome is the enhancement of action of combinations of antidepressant drugs for better efficacy in patients with depression.

B. ___ Neuroleptic malignant syndrome, a common side effect of antipsychotic drugs, responds well to increased doses of any of the psychotropic drugs used to treat mental illness.

C. ___ Hypertensive crisis, a result of MAOIs and tyramine-rich foods, is treated by holding the next dose of drug, elevating the patient's head, and administering a dose of chlorpromazine.

D. ___ Lithium toxicity occurs when blood levels of lithium are raised beyond the therapeutic window by fluid and electrolyte loss, decreased renal functioning, or overdose.

E. ___ Tricyclic antidepressants should be avoided if possible, or prescribed in amounts for 1 week at a time, in patients who are at risk for suicide.

5. Provide short answers for the following questions.

A. List the positive and negative symptoms of schizophrenia, and note which respond better to atypical antipsychotics.

B. Briefly describe the difference between reuptake inhibition and receptor blockade. Identify a psychiatric disorder that might benefit from each of these strategies, and state why it is thought that this is so.

C. Discuss the reasons why suicide assessment should continue for several weeks after the depressed patient appears to be responding to antidepressants.

REFERENCES

1. American Nurses' Association: *Psychiatric mental health nursing psychopharmacology project: ANA task force on psychopharmacology,* Washington, DC, 1994, The Association.
2. American Psychiatric Association: *Diagnostic and statistical manual of mental disorders,* ed 4, Washington, DC, 1994, The Association.
3. Bailey KP: Preparing for prescriptive practice: advanced practice psychiatric nursing and psychopharmacology, *J Psychosoc Nurs* 34(1):16-20, 1996.
4. Bernstein JG: Drug interactions. In Bernstein JG, editor: *Drug therapy in psychiatry,* ed 3, St Louis, 1995, Mosby.
5. Blaska B: The myriad medication mistakes in psychiatry: a consumer's view, *Hosp Community Psychiatry* 41:993, 1990.
6. Bowden CL: The efficacy of divalproex sodium and lithium in the treatment of acute mania, *Psychiatr Nurs Forum* 2(Spring), 1996.
7. Brunello N, Langer SZ, Perez J, Racagni G: Current understanding of the mechanism of action of classic and newer antidepressant drugs, *Depression* 2:119-126, 1995.
8. Clary C, Dever A, Schweizer E: Psychiatric inpatients' knowledge of medication at hospital discharge, *Hosp Community Psychiatry* 43:140, 1992.
9. Conn V, Taylor SG: Medication management by recently hospitalized older adults, *J Community Health Nurs* 9:1, 1992.
10. Coudreaut-Quinn EA, Emmons MA, McMorrow MJ: Self-medication during inpatient psychiatric treatment, *J Psychosoc Nurs Ment Health Serv* 30:32, 1992.
11. Crane K, Kirby B, Kooperman D: Patient compliance for psychotropic medications: a group model for an expanding psychiatric inpatient unit, *J Psychosoc Nurs* 34(1):8-15, 1996.
12. Depression Guideline Panel: *Depression in primary care,* vol 2, *Treatment of major depression. Clinical practice guidelines no. 5* (AHCPR publication no. 93-0551), Rockville, Md, 1993, US Department of Health and Human Services, Public Health Service, Agency for Health Care Policy and Research.
13. Dillon NB: Screening system for tardive dyskinesia: development and implementation, *J Psychosoc Nurs Ment Health Serv* 30:3, 1992.
14. Glod CA, Mathieu J: Expanding uses of anticonvulsants in the treatment of bipolar disorder, *J Psychosoc Nurs Ment Health Serv* 31:37, 1993.
15. Huttunen MO, Tuhkanen H, Haavisto E, Nyholm R, Pitkanen M, Raitasua V, Romanov M: Low- and standard-dose depot haloperidol combined with targeted oral neuroleptics, *Psychiatr Serv* 47(1):83-85, 1996.
16. Jaretz N, Flowers E, Millsap L: Clozapine: nursing care considerations, *Perspect Psychiatr Care* 28:19, 1992.
17. Jibson MD, Tandon R: A summary of research findings on the new antipsychotic drugs: special report, *Psychiatr Nurs Forum* 2(Summer), 1996.
18. Lakshman M, Fernando D, Kazarian SS: Patient education in the drug treatment of psychiatric disorders: effect on compliance and outcome, *CNS Drugs* 3(4):291-303, 1995.
19. Levy RA: Ethnic and racial differences in response to medicines: preserving individualized therapy in managed pharmaceutical programmes, *Pharm Med* 7:139-165, 1993.
20. Lin KM, Poland RE, Nakasaki G: *Psychopharmacology and psychobiology of ethnicity,* Washington, DC, 1993, American Psychiatric Press.
21. Littrell K, Magill AM: The effect of clozapine on preexisting tardive dyskinesia, *J Psychosoc Nurs Ment Health Serv* 31:14, 1993.

22. Lund VE, Frank DI: Helping the medicine go down: nurses' and patients' perceptions about medication compliance, *J Psychosoc Nurs Ment Health Serv* 29:6, 1991.

23. McCloskey J, Bulechek G: *Nursing interventions classification,* ed 2, St Louis, 1996, Mosby.

24. Meltzer HY: New drugs for the treatment of schizophrenia, *Psychiatr Clin North Am* 16:365, 1993.

25. Merkatz R, Couig MP: Helping America take its medicine, *Am J Nurs* 1992:56, 1992.

26. Meyer C: In the realm of the brain, *Am J Nurs* 1993:58, 1993.

27. Mulaik JS: Noncompliance with medication regimens in severely and persistently mentally ill schizophrenic patients, *Issues Ment Health Nurs* 13:219, 1992.

28. Peden JG: Benzodiazepine use at the medicine/psychiatry interface, *Psychiatr Ann* 23:301, 1993.

29. Richelson E: Synaptic effects of antidepressants, *J Clin Psychopharmacol* 16(3), Suppl. 2:1S-18S, 1996.

30. Rifkin A: Pharmacologic strategies in the treatment of schizophrenia, *Psychiatr Clin North Am* 16:351, 1993.

31. Smith M, Lin KM, Mendoza R: Nonbiological issues affecting psychopharmacotherapy: cultural considerations. In Lin KM, Poland RE, Nakasaki G, editors: *Psychopharmacology and psychobiology of ethnicity,* Washington, DC, 1993, American Psychiatric Press.

32. Stern RG, Kahn RS, Davidson M: Predictors of response to neuroleptic treatment in schizophrenia, *Psychiatr Clin North Am* 16:313, 1993.

33. Weiden PJ: How to evaluate for acute medication-induced movement disorders, *J Pract Psychiatry Behav Health* May:176-180, 1996.

34. Weiden PJ: Prevention for acute extrapyramidal side effects, *J Pract Psychiatry Behav Health* July:240-243, 1996.

35. Wengel SP, Burke WJ, Ranno AK, Roccaforte WH: Use of benzodiazepines in the elderly, *Psychiatr Ann* 23:325, 1993.

36. Wisner KL, Perel JM: Psychopharmacological treatment during pregnancy and lactation. In Jensvold MF, Halbreich U, Hamilton JA, editors: *Psychopharmacology and women: sex, gender and hormones,* Washington, DC, 1996, American Psychiatric Press.

37. Woods JH, Winger G: Current benzodiazepine issues, *Psychopharmacology* 118:107-114, 1995.

38. Zind R, Furlong C, Stebbins M: Educating patients about missed medication doses, *J Psychosoc Nurs Ment Health Serv* 30:10, 1992.

Annotated Suggested Readings

Benkert O et al: Public opinion on psychotropic drugs: an analysis of the factors influencing acceptance or rejection, *J Nerv Ment Dis,* 3:151, 1997.

A poll of several thousand people found that psychotropic drugs are less well accepted than cardiac drugs, and negative media reports have a significant negative influence on attitudes.

Carpenter W: The risk of medication-free research, *Schizophr Bull,* 1:11, 1997.

Discussed in detail are issues involved in the need for placebo-controlled drug research and the potential harm this may pose to some patients with progressive psychiatric illness.

*Cornwell C, Chiverton P: The psychiatric advanced practice nurse with prescriptive authority: role development, practice issues, and outcomes measurement, *Arch Psychiatr Nurs,* 2:57, 1997.

Discusses the prescribing role of the advanced practice nurse as a cost effective, high-quality component of comprehensive mental health care delivery.

* Keltner N: Catastrophic consequences secondary to psychotropic drugs, *J Psychosocial Nurs,* Part I and Part II, 35:41, 1997.

Set of articles focuses on a number of the more serious and life-threatening side effects of some psychopharmacological treatments, including agranulocytosis, serotonin syndrome, neuroleptic malignant syndrome, and lithium toxicity.

Lee D et al: Pharmacotherapy of depression in children, *Essential Psychopharmacology* 4:409, 1997.

Comprehensive overview of the drug treatment of depression in this age group, including symptoms, gender, sudden death, research trials, guidelines, and augmentation.

Schnafter L et al: Adolescent psychopharmacology: a brief overview, *Essential Psychopharmacology* 4:435, 1997.

Up-to-date review of specific issues of treatment, current research, rating scales, and general guidelines for drug interventions in this age group.

* Van Dongen CJ: Is the treatment worse than the cure? Attitudes toward medications among persons with severe mental illness, *J Psychosocial Nurs* 35:21, 1997.

Survey of patients taking psychotropic drugs found that patients thought that drugs helped prevent relapse; a positive attitude was important for good compliance.

Weiden P: Psychosocial management of non-compliance, *J Pract Psychiatry Behav Health* 5:169, 1997.

Focus is on interventions that can prevent noncompliance before it happens, including strategies such as psychoeducation, therapeutic alliance, and behavioral interventions.

*Nursing reference.

Somatic Therapies

Gail W. Stuart

© 1998 M.C. Escher/Cordon Art, Baarn, Holland.

Canst thou not minister to a mind diseas'd, Pluck from the memory rooted sorrow,
Raze out the written troubles of the brain, And with some sweet oblivious antidote
Cleanse the stuff'd bosom of the perilous stuff Which weights upon the heart?

William Shakespeare MACBETH, ACT V

LEARNING OBJECTIVES

After studying this chapter the student should be able to:

▼ Describe the use, indications, mechanism of action, and adverse effects of electroconvulsive therapy (ECT) as a treatment strategy for psychiatric illness

▼ Discuss the nursing care needs of the patient receiving ECT

▼ Describe the use, indications, mechanism of action, and adverse effects of phototherapy as a treatment strategy for psychiatric illness

▼ Describe the use, indications, mechanism of action, and adverse effects of sleep deprivation therapy as a treatment strategy for psychiatric illness

TOPICAL OUTLINE

Electroconvulsive Therapy
  Indications
  Mechanism of Action
  Adverse Effects
Nursing Care in Electroconvulsive Therapy
  Education and Emotional Support
  Informed Consent for Electroconvulsive Therapy
  Pretreatment Nursing Care
  Nursing Care during the Procedure
  Posttreatment Nursing Care
  Interdisciplinary Collaboration
  Nursing Staff Education
Phototherapy
  Indications
  Mechanism of Action
  Adverse Effects
Sleep Deprivation Therapy
  Indications
  Mechanism of Action
  Adverse Effects

With the emergence of biological psychiatry and the growing knowledge bases in the neurosciences, interest has increased in somatic therapies for psychiatric illness. The limitations of psychotropic medications, increase in treatment-resistant psychiatric disorders, and refinement in treatment techniques have placed greater emphasis on evaluating the indications for and efficacy of somatic therapeutic interventions.

Psychiatric nurses are usually involved in caring for patients who are receiving somatic therapy. Thus it is essential that all nurses understand how these treatment modalities work and the nursing care that enhances their effectiveness.

This chapter discusses three contemporary somatic therapies: electroconvulsive therapy, phototherapy, and sleep deprivation therapy.

ELECTROCONVULSIVE THERAPY

Electroconvulsive therapy (ECT) was first described by Cerletti and Bini in 1938 as a treatment for schizophrenia. At that time it was believed that epileptics were rarely schizophrenic. It was therefore hypothesized that convulsions would cure schizophrenia. Later research did not support this hypothesis. Further experience with ECT demonstrated that it is much more effective as a treatment for affective disturbances than it is for schizophrenia. It has also been noted that epilepsy and schizophrenia sometimes occur concurrently. ECT is now most often used as a treatment for severe depression.

ECT is a treatment in which a grand mal seizure is artificially induced in an anesthetized patient by passing an electrical current through electrodes applied to the patient's temples. Traditionally the electrodes have been applied bilaterally. More recently, unilateral electrodes have been used. It has been reported that patients have fewer cognitive side effects with unilateral placement, including less disorientation, fewer disturbances of verbal and nonverbal memory, and few pathological electroencephalogram (EEG) changes. However, some data also suggest that unilateral ECT may not always be as effective. Unilateral ECT is most strongly recommended when it is particularly important to minimize cognitive impairment, whereas bilateral ECT should be considered for more severely ill patients.[10]

For the treatment to be effective, a grand mal seizure must occur. The voltage is generally adjusted to the minimum level that will produce the therapeutic effect. The number of treatments in a series varies according to the patient's presenting problem and therapeutic response. For affective disorders, 6 to 12 treatments are normally administered. As many as 30 may be given for schizophrenia. ECT is most commonly given two or three times a week, although it can be given daily.[15]

In some cases, after a successful initial treatment episode, continuation therapy with outpatient ECT may be recommended.[20] The precise timing of continuation ECT varies, but weekly treatments for the first month after remission, followed by a gradual tapering to monthly treatments, appears to be effective.[9] Successful treatment with ECT may also be followed by antidepressant medication to prevent relapse.

> *ECT is sometimes called "shock therapy." Describe how use of this term stigmatizes mental illness and its treatment.*

Indications

The primary indication for ECT is major depression, which probably accounts for about 90% of referrals for ECT in the United States. ECT's response rate of 80% or more is equal to or better than response rates to antidepressant medications. It is particularly useful for people who cannot tolerate or fail to respond to treatment with medication. Box 28-1 lists the primary and secondary criteria for the use of ECT as determined by the American Psychiatric Association (APA) Task Force on Electroconvulsive Therapy.[2]

The primary conditions are ones in which ECT may play a life-saving role, as for the patient who is extremely suicidal or one who is so hyperactive that there is grave danger of self-harm. On occasion, ECT may be used for conditions other than affective disorders. ECT is believed to be quite effective in treating acute mania, and although controversy surrounds its usefulness for treating schizophrenia, some schizophrenic patients with catatonic stupor or catatonic excitement respond well to ECT. Finally, ECT should be considered as an initial intervention when its anticipated side effects are less than those associated with drug therapy, such as with the elderly, for patients with heart block, and during pregnancy. Box 28-2 summarizes behaviors for which ECT is and is not effective.[6]

> *Why would ECT be particularly indicated for depressed patients with heart block?*

Box **28-1** *Criteria for the Use of ECT*

PRIMARY USE

Situations in which ECT may be used before a trial of psychotropic agents include, but are not limited to, the following:
- ▼ When a need for rapid, definitive response exists on either medical or psychiatric grounds
- ▼ When the risks of other treatments outweigh the risk of ECT
- ▼ When a history of poor drug response or good ECT response exists for previous episodes of the illness
- ▼ Patient preference

SECONDARY USE

In other situations, a trial of an alternative therapy should be considered before referral for ECT. Subsequent referral for ECT should be based on at least one of the following:
- ▼ Treatment failure (taking into account issues such as choice of agent, dosage, and duration of trial)
- ▼ Adverse effects that are unavoidable and that are deemed less likely or less severe with ECT
- ▼ Deterioration of the patients' condition to the degree that other treatments have failed

From American Psychiatric Association: *The practice of electroconvulsive therapy: recommendations for treatment, training, and privileging,* Washington, DC, 1990, The Association.

Box **28-2** *Target Behaviors for ECT*

ECT EFFECTIVE	ECT INEFFECTIVE
Hyperemotionality	Severe character pathology
Hypermotility	Substance abuse and dependence
Catatonia	Sexual identification disorders
Severe psychosis with acute onset	Psychoneuroses
Life-threatening psychiatric conditions	Chronic illness without obvious psychopathology
Rigidity of parkinsonism or neuroleptic malignant syndrome	

Mechanism of Action

The specific way in which ECT works has been the subject of extensive research, but the precise mechanism of action is still not known. It is believed that the electric current passing through the brain causes a biochemical response. Most theories about the mode of action of ECT focus on its efficacy with depressed patients. The following theories have been proposed[13]:

▼ *Neurotransmitter theory* suggests that ECT acts like tricyclic antidepressants by enhancing deficient neurotransmission in monoaminergic systems. Specifically, it is thought to improve dopaminergic, serotonergic, and adrenergic neurotransmission.

▼ *Neuroendocrine therapy* suggests that ECT releases hypothalamic or pituitary hormones or both, which results in its antidepressant effects. ECT releases prolactin, thyroid-stimulating hormone, adrenocorticotropic hormone, and endorphins, but the specific hormones responsible for the therapeutic effect are not known.

▼ *Anticonvulsant theory* suggests that ECT treatment exerts a profound anticonvulsant effect on the brain that results in an antidepressant effect. Some support for this theory is based on the fact that a person's seizure threshold rises and the seizure duration decreases over the course of ECT and that some patients with epilepsy have fewer seizures after receiving ECT.

Despite unanswered questions regarding its mechanism of action, ECT is an effective treatment for many psychiatric disorders and is safe when properly administered.

Adverse Effects

The mortality rate associated with ECT is estimated to be the same as that with general anesthesia in minor surgery (approximately 1 death per 10,000 patients). Mortality and morbidity are believed to be lower with ECT than with the administration of antidepressant medications despite the frequent use of ECT in patients with medical complications and in the elderly.[2,10]

Medical adverse effects can to some extent be anticipated and prevented. Patients with preexisting cardiac illness, compromised pulmonary status, a history of central nervous system problems, or medical complications following anesthesia are likely to be at increased risk. Thus a complete medical workup should precede ECT and include a com-

plete blood count, urinalysis, serum chemistry profile, chest and spinal radiographs, electrocardiography, and optional computed tomography scan of the head. Adverse effects can potentially occur in the following categories:

▼ *Cardiovascular effects.* Cardiovascular complications are the major cause of morbidity and mortality associated with ECT, so a cardiovascular evaluation before ECT is essential.

▼ *Systemic effects.* Headaches, nausea, muscle aches and soreness, weakness, drowsiness, anorexia, and amenorrhea occasionally occur after ECT, but they usually respond to supportive management and nursing intervention.

▼ *Cognitive effects.* ECT is associated with a range of cognitive side effects including a period of confusion immediately after the seizure and memory disturbance during the treatment course. These side effects subside after the treatment course, although a few patients report persistent deficits. The onset of cognitive side effects varies considerably among patients. It is believed that patients with preexisting cognitive impairment, neuropathological conditions, and those receiving psychotropic medications during ECT may be at increased risk for more profound side effects.[1] There is no evidence that ECT causes structural brain damage.[4]

NURSING CARE IN ELECTROCONVULSIVE THERAPY*

The effectiveness and limitations of ECT have been the subject of considerable debate within the field of psychiatry (see Critical Thinking about Contemporary Issues). Because it is a somatic therapy for psychiatric illness, nurses have participated in both the debate and the implementation of ECT as a treatment option for their patients. Although sometimes thought to be a seldom-used form of therapy, the increasing number of ECT devices and the volume of recently published articles and books on the subject suggest that ECT usage may be rising.

Although psychiatric nurses have always had a role in helping with the ECT procedure, the nursing functions have historically been limited to supportive and adjunctive care. With the growing sophistication of nursing science and

*Modified from Burns C, Stuart G: Nursing care in electroconvulsive therapy, *Psychiatr Clin North Am* 14:971, 1991.

CRITICAL THINKING *about* Contemporary Issues

Is ECT a Therapeutic Treatment or a Primitive Form of Punishment?

ECT remains a controversial treatment. The controversy is not about its efficacy or safety, because these have been well established in numerous studies. Rather, the controversy is about its presumed effects on the brain, public fears, and health care professionals' lack of education about its beneficial effects. Some people regard ECT as a punishment, believing that it is inhumane. Still others are concerned that permanent brain damage could result.

The opposing view holds that it is more inhumane to allow a person to suffer a severe emotional disorder when ECT provides prompt relief. They believe that the stigmatization related to ECT does considerably more harm than the treatment. Part of the stigma associated with ECT stems from the fact that mental illness is seen as social deviance rather than as a medical disorder. As a result, the treatment of mental illness is seen as a stigmatizing punishment.[7] The second major reason for the stigmatization of ECT is that few people understand the current administration of the procedure. Properly administered, ECT induces far less discomfort and medical complications than most surgical and many psychopharmacological treatments. The third reason rests in the language used to describe the treatment. The fact that it used to be called "shock therapy" conjures up the image of pain that further stigmatizes this treatment option.

It is up to each professional to reach a personal resolution on this issue. This decision should be based on objective data, observation of the treatment, and personal experiences in working with patients who have and have not received ECT.

clinical practice, this role is evolving to include independent and collaborative nursing actions.

Education and Emotional Support

Nursing care begins as soon as the patient and family are presented with ECT as a treatment option. Initially, an important role of the nurse is to allow the patient an opportunity to express feelings, including any myths or fantasies about ECT. Patients may describe fear of pain, dying of electrocution, suffering permanent memory loss, or experiencing impaired intellectual functioning. As the patient reveals these fears and concerns, the nurse can clarify misconceptions and emphasize the therapeutic value of the procedure. Supporting the patient and family in their need to discuss, question, and explore their feelings and concerns about ECT should be an essential component of nursing care before, during, and after the course of treatment.

Once the patient has had an opportunity to express feelings, the nurse can begin ECT teaching, which should take into consideration the patient's anxiety, readiness to learn, and ability to comprehend. Optimally, family teaching should occur at the same time as patient teaching, and the amount of information to be shared should be indi-

vidualized for each patient and family. The nurse should review with the family and patient the information they have received from the physician regarding the procedure and respond to any questions they might have about this information.

During this assessment process, the nurse should also attempt to define specific patient behaviors the family associates with the patient's illness and determine whether the patient or family member has received ECT in the past. Any information about the family's previous experiences with ECT helps the nurse to identify familial beliefs about the patient's illness, the ECT treatment, and the expected prognosis. Both patient and family should also be asked what else they know about ECT, such as through friends who have received it or by reading about it or seeing ECT portrayed in movies. Open-ended questions may give the nurse the opportunity to identify and correct misinformation and address specific concerns the patient or family has about the procedure. These nursing actions may facilitate the family's ability to provide support to the patient during the treatment course and thus further alleviate the patient's anxiety.

Various media may also be used to supplement the teaching of the patient and family about ECT, including written materials and videotape presentations.[5] A tour of the treatment suite itself may help familiarize the patient with the area, procedure, and equipment. Encouraging the patient to talk with another patient who has benefited from ECT may be worthwhile. Finally, the nurse should facilitate flexibility in family arrangements, particularly during the patient's first few treatments, allowing for family presence before and after ECT if the patient and family desire. This serves to allay the family's anxieties and concerns about the treatment while encouraging the family to support the patient.

If the family cannot or does not want to be present, the nurse should contact the family after the treatments to provide information and describe the patient's response. The nurse should also encourage the family throughout the course of treatment to discuss changes they observe or questions that arise. Providing emotional support and responding to the educational needs of both patient and family are essential components of the nursing role.

> *There are many misconceptions regarding ECT. Many of these are perpetuated by movies. Observe ECT in person, then watch the movies* One Flew Over the Cuckoo's Nest, Frances, *and* Ordinary People *and critique the way in which ECT is presented.*

Informed Consent for Electroconvulsive Therapy

Before ECT treatment is begun, the patient should sign an informed consent form (see Chapter 9). If the patient does not have the capacity to consent, it can be signed by a legally designated person. This consent acknowledges the patient's rights to obtain or refuse treatment. Although it is the physician's ultimate responsibility to explain the procedure when obtaining consent, the nurse plays an important part in the consent process.

Informed consent is a dynamic process that is not completed with the signing of a formal document; it is a process that continues throughout the course of treatment. As such, it suggests a number of nursing activities. First, it is helpful if a nurse is present when the information for consent is discussed with the patient. The most appropriate nurse is one who has established a trusting and therapeutic relationship with the patient and who is best able to assess whether the patient comprehends the explanation. The presence of a nurse at this time may enable the patient to feel comfortable asking questions, and the nurse may help to simplify the language if necessary. The nurse can also ensure that the patient has been provided with a full explanation, understands the nature, purpose, and implications of the treatment, including the option to withdraw consent at any time, and has had all questions answered before signing the consent form. After the informed consent is signed, but before the beginning of treatment, the nurse should again thoroughly review this information and discuss the treatment in an open and direct manner, thus communicating that this is an accepted and beneficial form of treatment.

Certain patients pose particular challenges to the nurse in obtaining informed consent. If a patient is unable to make independent judgments and meaningful decisions about care and treatment, the nurse is responsible for acting as a patient advocate. For example, concentration is often impaired in depressed patients, so they are less likely to comprehend and retain new information. For these patients it is essential that the nurse repeat the information at regular intervals because new knowledge is seldom fully absorbed after only one explanation. Then, throughout the patient's treatment course, the nurse should reinforce what the patient already understands, provide reminders of anything that has been forgotten, and be there to answer new questions.

Pretreatment Nursing Care

Providing optimal nursing care for the patient undergoing ECT includes evaluating the pretreatment protocol to ensure that it has been followed according to hospital policy. This involves completing appropriate consultations, noting that any abnormalities in laboratory tests have been addressed, and checking that equipment and supplies are adequate and functional. The treatment nurse is responsible for ensuring that the treatment suite is properly prepared for the ECT procedure. Box 28-3 provides a list of standard equipment needed to provide optimal ECT patient care, as designated by the APA Task Force on ECT. Although not required to be in the treatment room itself,

a crash cart with defibrillator should be readily available for emergency use.

Because ECT is similar to a brief surgical procedure, patient preparation is similar. Because general anesthesia is required, fluids should be withheld from the patient for 6 to 8 hours before treatment to prevent the potential for aspiration. The exception to this NPO status is in the case of patients who routinely receive cardiac medications, antihypertensive agents, or H_2 blockers. These drugs should be administered several hours before treatment with a small sip of water. The patient should be encouraged to wear comfortable clothing, including street clothes, pajamas, or a hospital gown, provided that it can be opened in the front to facilitate the placement of monitoring equipment. The patient should also be reminded to remove prostheses before coming to the treatment area to prevent loss or damage. This includes dentures, glasses, contact lenses, and hearing aids. The patient's hair should be clean and dry for optimal electrode contact. Hairpins, barrettes, hair nets, and other hair ornaments should also be removed for placement of electrodes.

The patient should void immediately before receiving ECT to help prevent incontinence during the procedure and to minimize the potential for bladder distention and damage during treatment. An intramuscular injection of glycopyrrolate (usual dose 0.2 to 0.4 mg) is administered at least 30 minutes before each ECT. Atropine (usual dose 0.3 to 0.6 mg) may be given as an alternative. These medications are administered both to prevent aspiration by decreasing the amount of oral secretions during the treatment and to

Box **28-3** *Equipment for Electroconvulsive Therapy*

Treatment device and supplies, including electrode paste and gel, gauze pads, alcohol preps, saline, EEG electrodes, and chart paper
Monitoring equipment, including ECG and EEG electrodes
Blood pressure cuffs (two), peripheral nerve stimulator, and pulse oximeter
Stethoscope
Reflex hammer
Intravenous and venipuncture supplies
Bite blocks with individual containers
Stretchers with firm mattress and siderails with the capability to elevate the head and feet
Suction device
Ventilation equipment, including tubing, masks, Ambu bags, oral airways, and intubation equipment with an oxygen delivery system capable of providing positive-pressure oxygen
Emergency and other medications as recommended by anesthesia staff
Miscellaneous medications not supplied by the anesthesia staff for medical management during ECT such as labetalol, esmolol, glycopyrrolate, caffeine, curare, midazolam, diazepam, thiopental sodium (Pentothal), methohexital sodium (Brevital), and succinylcholine

minimize cardiac bradyarrhythmias in response to the electrical stimulation.

Nursing Care during the Procedure

The patient should be brought to the treatment suite either ambulatory or by wheelchair, depending on individual need, accompanied by a nurse with whom the patient feels at ease. If possible, the nurse should remain with the patient throughout the treatment to provide support. Because there will be a number of people in the room, including a psychiatrist, the treatment nurse, and the anesthesia staff, the patient should be introduced to each member of the treatment team and given a brief explanation of everyone's role in the ECT procedure.

The patient should then be assisted onto a stretcher and asked to remove shoes and socks. This allows for the placement of a blood pressure cuff on an ankle and clear observation of the patient's extremities during the treatment. Once the patient is positioned comfortably on the stretcher, a member of the anesthesia staff inserts a peripheral intravenous line while the treatment nurse and other members of the treatment team place leads for various monitors. One member of the treatment team should explain the procedure while it is occurring.

EEG monitoring consists of two electrodes, one on the forehead and one on the left mastoid. Two sets of three-lead ECGs, one connected to the ECT machine and the other to the oscilloscope, are placed on the patient's chest (Fig. 28-1). A pulse oximeter is clipped to the patient's finger to monitor oxygen saturation. Blood pressure monitoring throughout the treatment is accomplished by a manual or automatic cuff. A peripheral nerve stimulator, placed on the wrist over the ulnar nerve, serves to determine muscle relaxation.

The treating psychiatrist or nurse cleans areas of the patient's head with alcohol and gel at the sites of electrode contact. The area may be wetted with saline as well. This cleansing process facilitates optimal stimulus electrode contact during treatment, thus eliminating the potential for skin burns and minimizing the amount of electrical stimulus needed for the treatment. The areas being cleaned will be either both temples, if bilateral electrode placement is to be used, or the right temple and top of the head 1 inch to the right of the midline, if unilateral placement is used (Fig. 28-2).

Once the preparation is completed, an anesthetic is administered intravenously at a dosage titrated to the patient's weight, age, and physical status. When the patient is asleep, the blood pressure cuff on the ankle is inflated, allowing it to serve as a tourniquet. A muscle relaxant, succinylcholine (usual dose approximately 0.75 mg/kg), is then administered to minimize the patient's motor response to the ECT treatment. Because the tourniquet is in place on one ankle, the succinylcholine is not effective in that extremity. This is a desired effect because it is used in detecting a motor response to the seizure. Progressive muscle relaxation is monitored by the nerve stimulator, as well as by observing the patient for the cessation of fasciculations. As the muscle relaxant takes effect, the anesthesiologist provides oxygen by mask to the patient through positive-pressure ventilation.

Although most muscles become completely relaxed, the patient's jaw muscles are stimulated directly by the ECT, causing the patient's teeth to clench. This creates the need for a protective device, or bite block, to be inserted in the patient's mouth by the treatment nurse before the electrical stimulus. This disposable or autoclavable device prevents tooth damage and tongue or gum laceration during the stimulus. The bite block should be placed with the thick rubber portion between the upper and lower teeth, with the front rim separating the lips and teeth. The nurse should then support the patient's chin firmly against the bite block during delivery of the brief electrical stimulus. After delivery of the stimulus, the bite block may be removed.

The electrical stimulus causes a brief generalized seizure, the motor manifestations of which can be observed only in the cuffed foot. Characteristic EEG changes may also be observed. One member of the treatment team records the time elapsed during the seizure. A seizure lasting 30 to 60 seconds is generally considered adequate to produce therapeutic effect, and seizures lasting longer than 2 minutes should be terminated using a benzodiazepine, such as diazepam or thiopental sodium (Pentothal), to prevent a prolonged postictal state. Anesthesia staff continuously ventilate the patient with pure oxygen throughout the procedure until the effects of the anesthetic and muscle relaxant subside and the patient is able to breathe spontaneously. Vital signs should

Fig. 28-1   EEG and ECG monitoring during ECT.

Unilateral   Bilateral

Fig. 28-2 Electrode placement in ECT.

be monitored by the nurse both before and after the ECT treatment. Once the patient is stabilized, the anesthesiologist clears the patient for transfer to the recovery area.

Posttreatment Nursing Care

The recovery area should be adjacent to the treatment area to provide accessibility for anesthesia staff in case of an emergency. The area should contain oxygen, suction, pulse oximeter, vital sign monitoring, and emergency equipment. The area should be appropriately staffed and provide a minimal amount of sensory stimulation. Once in the recovery area with pulse oximeter in place, the patient should be unobtrusively observed by a staff member in close proximity until the patient awakens. At this time the staff should be aware of the potential for falls from the stretcher caused by patient restlessness and maintain patient safety.

When the patient awakens, a nurse should discuss the treatment and check vital signs. Most patients do not remember receiving the treatment and may be confused and disoriented, similar to patients recovering from anesthesia. The nurse should provide frequent reassurance and reorientation and repeat this information at regular intervals until the patient retains it. Being postictal, the patient's thinking may also be somewhat concrete. Providing brief, distinct direction is most beneficial.

When the patient is awake and appears ready to return to the hospital room and has maintained a continuous oxygen saturation level of 90% or above, and when vital signs and mental status have returned to an acceptable level, the nurse should help to move the patient from the stretcher to a wheelchair for transport from the recovery area. When a wheelchair is used, the seatbelt should be securely fastened. The patient may be allowed to ambulate if desired.

At this time the ECT treatment nurse should convey as much information as possible about the patient's condition to the unit nursing staff. The most beneficial information includes medications given to the patient that may be evidenced in the patient's behavior or vital signs and any change in the procedure or the patient's response to treatment that may affect the patient's behavior upon return to the unit. Table 28-1 identifies some common problems patients have at this time and related nursing interventions.

The nurse should assess the patient's condition to determine the level of observation required. If desired, the patient may return to bed and sleep, but the nurse should encourage eating breakfast and resuming normal activities as soon as possible. If the patient chooses to return to bed, the siderails should be in an upright position.

The patient should be observed at least once every 15 minutes; if the patient is agitated, confused, or restless, one-to-one observation may be required until the patient's condition has stabilized. Level of orientation should be assessed every 30 minutes if the patient is awake until mental status returns to baseline. If sleeping, the patient should remain undisturbed unless additional nursing intervention is warranted. Sleeping may help the patient return to baseline values more quickly.

The return of the gag reflex should be assessed before administering medication or offering breakfast to the patient. When fully awake, the patient should be observed when getting out of bed for the first time to ensure full muscle functioning after administration of muscle relax-

Table 28-1 *Common Patient Problems and Nursing Interventions Related to ECT*

PATIENT PROBLEM	NURSING INTERVENTIONS
Pretreatment with beta-blockers may cause a decrease in blood pressure, pulse, or both.	Vital signs should be monitored frequently until they return to baseline.
Lengthy seizures (more than 2 minutes) may increase the duration of disorientation or confusion.	Reorientation may need to be repeated for longer periods than usual.
If given a barbiturate or benzodiazepine to terminate the seizure, the patient may be more drowsy than usual.	Patient may need more time to rest after treatment.
Restlessness may increase potential for injury.	Intensity of observation may need to be increased to prevent falls.
Nausea/vomiting creates potential for aspiration.	Increase intensity of observation. Extended stay in the recovery area may be necessary to provide access to suctioning equipment.
Headache creates alteration in comfort.	After assessment for gag reflex return, an analgesic may be administered. If headache is a recurrent problem, a standing order for analgesia to be given as soon as possible after each treatment may be obtained. Change in activity schedule and environment to provide for a darkened room or quiet area may be necessary.

ants. Throughout the posttreatment interval, provision of support and reminders to the patient of having received ECT eliminate patient distress from posttreatment amnesia.

Potential side effects immediately after treatment that may be treated symptomatically include headache, muscle soreness, and nausea. Any confusion or disorientation is likely to be of short duration and may respond well to restricted environmental stimulation and frequent nursing contacts reminding the patient of ECT treatment and providing reorientation. Memory loss affects primarily material that has been recently learned, as well as information acquired during the time of the ECT treatments themselves.

Although memory loss may be distressing for the patient, the nurse should reinforce that such difficulty will pass within several weeks, with a minimal amount lasting up to 6 months. However, some information will not return, including the experience of the treatment itself and events just before the procedure, such as IV placement. In

addition, events during treatment may be unclear. A summary of nursing interventions for patients receiving ECT is presented in Table 28-2.

 What kind of post-ECT environment do you think would be most conducive to the patient's recovery?

Interdisciplinary Collaboration

The nurse is part of an interdisciplinary treatment team that not only administers the treatments but also collaborates to evaluate the effectiveness of ECT and recommend changes in the patient's treatment plan as appropriate. Within the team the nurse identifies patterns of patient behavior and evaluates their implications for treatment. These include behaviors indicative of a positive treatment response, such as improvement in activities of daily living, adaptive changes in social interactions with others, increases in energy, appetite, and weight, or other positive changes in target symptoms. The nurse might also report any adverse behaviors associated with ECT, including prolonged periods of confusion or disorientation, recurrent nausea or headaches, elevation in blood pressure that does not resolve within several hours after treatment, or an increase in the intensity or occurrence of target symptoms. In addition, the nurse's work with the patient's family provides information important for planning treatment.

With these clinical observations and judgments, the nurse becomes an active participant in the decision-making process regarding the patient's illness and proposed plan of care. Together the team evaluates such issues as the length of ECT treatment course, the need for alternative management strategies and adjustments in the frequency of treatments, considerations for maintenance ECT, indications for additional consultations, and other possible modifications in the treatment plan.

Give specific examples of ways in which the psychiatric nurse's role in ECT has evolved from the dependent function of implementing physicians' orders to more independent and interdependent areas of psychiatric nursing practice. How have patients benefited from this change?

Nursing Staff Education

Despite recent increases in the use of ECT and its effectiveness in the treatment of certain psychiatric illnesses, the procedure continues to elicit emotional responses from the public as well as the medical and nursing communities. Some of these responses may be positive. However, many people react negatively to ECT based on outdated ideas and procedures. Also, some patients develop a pathological fear of ECT over the course of treatment.[11] It is critically impor-

TABLE **28-2** *Nursing Interventions for the Patient Receiving ECT*

PRINCIPLE	RATIONALE	NURSING INTERVENTION
Informed participation in the procedure	A patient who understands the treatment plan will be more cooperative and have less stress than one who does not; an informed family is able to provide the patient with emotional support.	Educate regarding ECT, including the procedure and expected effects; teach family about the treatment; encourage expression of feelings by patient and family; reinforce teaching after each treatment.
Biological integrity	General anesthesia and an electrically induced seizure are physiological stressors and require supportive nursing care.	Check emergency equipment before procedure; maintain NPO status several hours before treatment; remove potentially harmful objects, such as jewelry and dentures; check vital signs; maintain patent airway; assist to ambulate; offer analgesia or antiemetic as needed.
Dignity and self-esteem	Patients are usually fearful before ECT treatment; amnesia and confusion may lead to anxiety and distress; patient will need help to function appropriately.	Remain with the patient and offer support before and during treatment; maintain the patient's privacy during and after treatment; reorient the patient; help family members to understand behavior related to amnesia and confusion.

tant that when a patient is referred for ECT, the patient and family be presented with information regarding treatment options in a balanced and unbiased manner. If a nurse has ambivalent or negative feelings about ECT, these feelings will probably be communicated to the patient and render the treatment course less effective. To function as patient advocates nurses need to examine their attitudes and have as much information about the procedure as possible.[8]

Educational efforts should be directed toward nurses who work on units where ECT is implemented as a treatment strategy. Programs should be developed that address both cognitive and attitudinal content because the more knowledge and clinical experience mental health professionals have with ECT, the more positive their attitude will be toward it.

Such programs might be initiated by asking staff to discuss their beliefs and feelings about ECT, including its potential therapeutic value, perceived risks, the nature of the procedure itself, and ethical and legal issues concerning its use. The content can then progress to a discussion of factual material about ECT, including the rationale for the treatment, possible mechanisms of action, its efficacy relative to other treatment options, risks and side effects resulting from ECT, and current research on its indications and benefits. Time should be spent discussing the way in which the procedure has changed over the years, and all nurses should be encouraged to observe the ECT procedure as performed in their institution.

These discussions might be supplemented with written handouts, reference articles, and teaching videotapes about ECT. Finally, this information can be formalized and incorporated into the unit's daily nursing care by the establishment of nursing standards of care for patients receiving

ECT[3] and the development of a standardized nursing care plan that identifies appropriate nursing diagnoses, goals, and interventions.

In addition to informing nurses who care for patients undergoing ECT, there is a need to teach the larger nursing community about ECT. Psychiatric nurses who work with ECT can provide in-services to nurses in other clinical settings, such as geriatrics, neurology, or medicine, to dispel myths, clarify misconceptions, and provide current, accurate information about ECT.

> **?** *What stereotypes did you have about ECT before reading this chapter? How have they changed, and how might this experience help you educate patients and colleagues about this treatment procedure?*

PHOTOTHERAPY

Phototherapy, or light therapy, is a fairly new somatic treatment option. It can be used alone or with medications. It consists of exposing patients to artificial therapeutic lighting about 5 to 20 times brighter than indoor lighting. Patients usually sit, with eyes open, about 3 feet away from and at eye level with a set of broad-spectrum fluorescent bulbs designed to produce the intensity and color composition of outdoor daylight. They then can engage in their usual activities such as reading, writing, or eating (Fig. 28-3). Light boxes currently cost between $350 and $500.

The most recently developed light therapy device is the light visor, a device shaped like a baseball cap and worn on the head, with the light contained in a visor portion suspended above and in front of the eyes. The obvious advantage to such a device is that it allows the person to move

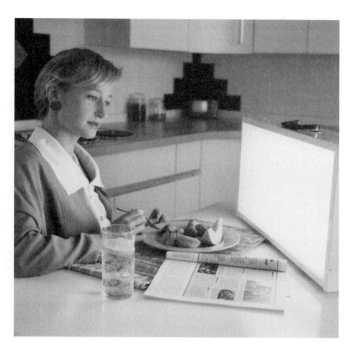

Fig. 28-3   Broad-spectrum fluorescent lamps like this one are used in daily therapy sessions from autumn into spring for people with SAD, who report feeling less depressed within 3 to 7 days. (Courtesy Medlight.)

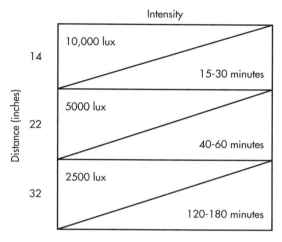

Distance versus intensity versus duration

Fig. 28-4   Timing, dosage, and exposure to light. All times are average durations and may vary with each person. *Lux,* Luminous flux density (unit of illuminance).

about while receiving treatment. However, the results of studies testing the device show great variability in effectiveness and suggest a placebo effect.[21]

The timing and dosage of the light vary from person to person. Some patients respond best to treatment given in the morning, whereas others prefer treatment in the evening. The amount of light to which a person is exposed depends not only on the person but also on the intensity of the light source and the duration of the exposure. The brighter the light, the more effective the treatment per unit of time. For example, 2 hours of treatment with 2500 lux per day appears to have an antidepressant effect equal to that of 30 minutes per day at 10,000 lux (Fig. 28-4).

Light therapy appears to have important positive effects. Treatment is rapid and can be repeated. Most patients feel relief after 3 to 5 days and they relapse equally rapidly after light treatment is stopped. Patients do not appear to develop tolerance to phototherapy, and many have used the treatment for years.[19] Treatment can be received at home, and it need not disrupt daily routine. Light therapy also allows a person to actively participate in the treatment process, which enhances the patient's sense of control in recovering from illness.[12,17] However, the long-term efficacy of light therapy has not been fully evaluated.

Indications

Phototherapy has a 50% to 60% response rate in patients with well-documented, nonpsychotic winter depression or

seasonal affective disorder (SAD). SAD is a cyclical illness characterized by periods of depression that begin in October and subside in April (see Chapter 19). Although people in all latitudes can suffer from SAD, the prevalence of the disorder increases in the northernmost parts of the country. About 6% of the adult population in the United States, or 15 million people, suffer from the symptoms of SAD, which include sadness, irritability, increased appetite, carbohydrate craving, weight gain, hypersomnia, and decreased energy. In addition, 14% of Americans experience a more mild condition called "winter blues."

In a study examining predictors of response to light treatment, responders were characterized by atypical symptoms, especially hypersomnia, afternoon and evening slump, reverse diurnal variation (evenings worse), and carbohydrate craving. In contrast, nonresponders were characterized mainly by melancholic symptoms including retardation, suicidality, depersonalization, typical diurnal variation (mornings worse), anxiety, early and late insomnia, appetite loss, and guilt.[22] Thus light therapy is a safe and satisfactory treatment for many, but may be insufficient for more severely ill patients.[19]

Light therapy should be administered by a professional with experience and training. It is a less conventional treatment that may be of value to patients who do not respond to drug therapy or prefer nonpharmacological treatments, or as an adjunct to drug treatments.

Mechanism of Action

Phototherapy is based on biological rhythms, particularly those related to light and darkness (see Chapter 5).[16] However, scientists are not sure exactly how phototherapy works. The therapeutic effect appears to be mediated primarily by the eyes, not the skin. Ongoing studies of the mechanism of phototherapy are exploring the eye itself, the way in which the eyes send messages to the brain, and the role of brain neurotransmitter systems such as serotonin and dopamine.[18] It also appears that certain people may have a neurochemical vulnerability, possibly inherited, that causes them to develop SAD in the absence of adequate exposure to environmental light.

> ? *Do you think that people who experience common disturbances in body rhythms such as jet lag and shift work can be helped by phototherapy?*

Adverse Effects

Side effects, when they occur, are generally mild. However, light therapy should be carefully monitored. The most common adverse effects of phototherapy are eyestrain, headache, irritability, insomnia, fatigue, nausea, and dryness of the eyes, nasal passages, and sinuses. These can usually be managed by decreasing the duration of therapy or increasing the patient's distance from the light. The long-term effects of phototherapy, if any, are currently unknown. Light therapy should be used with caution with specific ophthalmic conditions.

SLEEP DEPRIVATION THERAPY

It has been reported that as many as 60% of depressed patients improve immediately after one night of total sleep deprivation.[24] Unipolar and bipolar patients appear to do equally well. In addition, partial sleep deprivation that allows for as much as 3 hours of sleep is also effective.[14] Although these findings have been reported in the literature, few randomized controlled clinical studies have been conducted on sleep deprivation. Furthermore, in the existing studies it is difficult to know the effect of the patient's expectations on the treatment outcome. Thus these findings should be considered with caution.

Unfortunately, many patients who respond to this therapy become depressed again when they resume sleeping even as little as 2 hours a night. This disadvantage has tended to discourage the use of sleep deprivation in clinical practice. However, there is some suggestion that improvement can be maintained if the sleep manipulation can be used repeatedly over time, such as by shifting the timing of sleep to earlier in the night. For example, the patient can go to sleep at 5:00 PM and arise at 2:00 AM.

In addition, medications may help prevent relapse after sleep deprivation therapy. It is interesting to note that some antidepressants, especially the monoamine oxidase inhibitors, often interfere with sleep (see Chapter 27). This has led some researchers to wonder whether part of the efficacy of these drugs is a result of their ability to induce partial sleep deprivation.

> ? *How can a patient's expectations of a treatment influence its effectiveness? Can you think of a placebo treatment for sleep deprivation therapy that would control this problem?*

Indications

Evidence suggests that depressed patients with symptoms of marked diurnal variation are most likely to improve after sleep deprivation. Patients who respond favorably to sleep deprivation also appear to have abnormally elevated nighttime body temperatures.

Mechanism of Action

The biological mechanisms of the antidepressant effects of sleep deprivation have not been identified. It has been hypothesized that sleep deprivation works by interrupting REM sleep (see Chapter 5). Another theory proposes that neuroendocrine changes accompanying sleep deprivation account for its antidepressant effects. Yet another hypothesis focuses on the body's thermoregulatory mechanisms and suggests that cold exposure and sleep deprivation may work together to produce antidepressant effects.[23]

Adverse Effects

Unfortunately, sleep deprivation appears to induce mania in some patients with bipolar disorder. Thus, sleep deprivation, like some antidepressant medications, should be used with caution with patients who are susceptible to mania or have a family history of bipolar illness.

On the other hand, the knowledge that sleep deprivation may induce mania can have important preventive applications. For example, people who are biologically vulnerable to bipolar illness might monitor disruptions to their sleep caused by work schedules, travel, drugs, or other life events. Thus for vulnerable people prevention of sleep loss at times of stress might help prevent mania.

Summary

1. Electroconvulsive therapy (ECT) is an effective treatment for major depression with an efficacy rate of 80% or more, which is equal to or better than response rates to antidepressant medications. It is particularly useful for people who cannot tolerate or fail to respond to treatment with medication.

2. Nursing care in ECT involves providing emotional and education support to the patient and family; assessing the pretreatment protocol and the patient's behavior,

memory, and functional ability before ECT; preparing and monitoring the patient during the actual ECT procedure; and observing and interpreting patient responses to ECT with recommendations for changes in the treatment plan as appropriate.

3. Phototherapy, or light therapy, consists of exposing patients to bright, artificial therapeutic lighting for a speci-

fied period of time each day. It is a treatment option for patients with nonpsychotic winter depression or seasonal affective disorder (SAD).

4. Sleep deprivation therapy has been reported to be effective with depressed patients; however, many become depressed again when they resume sleeping even as little as 2 hours a night.

COMPETENT CARING A Clinical Exemplar of a Psychiatric Nurse

Dean Olivet, RN, MS, C

On this particular morning, I arrived at work as usual and performed all the morning rituals that a nurse does before venturing out on the clinical floor. After having several days off, I knew from reports and from listening to my co-workers that the acuity on the unit was high. Not only was the unit psychiatrically tense, but several geriatric patients had been admitted for evaluation and ECT. On a general psychiatric unit, these patients often elicit a variety of feelings from the staff, ranging from mild anxiety to downright fear. Therefore, I opted to take a few of the older, acute patients, including Mr. J, who was 80 years of age. This patient was newly admitted for evaluation of medications and a possible course of ECT. The staff who had contact with him described him as needy, confused, and wanting constant reassurance.

My first contact with Mr. J found him asleep in his bed. He was disheveled, as was his room. I introduced myself to him and found out immediately why he seemed to have caused the staff to be anxious. He grabbed my arm and spoke to me in a high-pitched whine that anyone would want to avoid. My initial reaction was a flight response. To resist this, I began to assess his level of independence, and it became clear in a short period of time that he was unable to make any choices with regard to planning his morning. In organizing my care, the approach I decided on was to outline the morning routine for him in small time increments and assess his ability to make decisions with regard to his basic needs.

We began with his activities of daily living. Mr. J needed help to meet these physiological needs, and his anxiety level made it necessary for me to maximize his safety and security. He told me that his daughter and son had helped him the night before. He assured me that I was too busy and they would help him the next time they visited as well. My nursing pride was somewhat injured, and I was puzzled about the necessity for his family to perform what seemed to be a nursing responsibility. Nonetheless, I carried on with my care and convinced him to bathe while I cleaned up his room and made his bed. Implementing this minor intervention made me feel more comfortable in his room, and he didn't seem quite as overwhelmed.

Since his anxiety was still moderately high, I consulted with the nurse giving his medications and reviewed his chart. Here I learned that this was his second hospitalization, with many years free of symptoms of depression. During his first hospital stay he received a course of ECT that was very successful in helping him get well. I also learned that he was being cared for by his wife and daughter. Their treatment of choice was to medicate him until he slept. Learning this, I sensed the need to evaluate the quality of his experience with his last course of ECT, as well as the need for possible ECT and medication education for the family. These two educational needs became an ongoing process dependent on his and his family's readiness to learn.

My plan of care was quite simple. I would make sure that his activities of daily living were completed each morning, his environment kept orderly, and his introduction to the milieu made in short intervals. This was necessary to keep him safe from patients with less impulse control and avoid overwhelming him or the other patients. The man needed some peer contact as well, and I introduced him to other patients as appropriate.

That afternoon his family came in to visit, and I met with them to assess their need for information and their readiness to learn. I outlined Mr. J's day and apologized for his insistence that they perform his activities of daily living. I thought that perhaps they may be annoyed about this issue and was relieved when they expressed their appreciation for my interest in him. They explained to me that I was the first person they had substantial contact with since he was admitted. In fact, they were quite upset with his condition the night before, and were considering raising the issue to staff. After listening to their concerns, I outlined my plan of care for Mr. J and explained that in my absence the rest of the nursing staff would use the care plan to meet his daily needs. At this point, the family became an ally to the total hospital experience, and I became a resource to the patient and the family. This brought comfort to the family, which in turn allowed Mr. J to meet his basic needs and have the security to meet the challenge of recovering from his illness.

The family members were satisfied with my interventions, and a possible problematic hospital experience was averted. As nurses, we all can relate to experiences when we care for patients only to have family members complain about the care or lack of care their significant other received. We can also describe occasions when it was very rewarding to have a patient respond to our care and to have the family recognize this nursing effort. Given this dichotomy, which do you prefer? The answer really reflects the crux of good psychiatric nursing practice.

your **INTERNET**
connection

Beyond Stigma: ECT and Depression
http://www.frii.com/~hageseth/

Health Care Information Resources:
Alternative Medicine
http://www-hsl.mcmaster.ca/tomflem/altmed.html

Chapter Review Questions

1. **Identify whether the following statements are true (T) or false (F).**

A. ___ For ECT to be effective a grand mal seizure must occur.

B. ___ ECT cannot be followed by antidepressant medications or adverse reactions will occur.

C. ___ There is evidence that ECT causes structural brain damage and permanent memory loss.

D. ___ A seizure lasting 30 to 60 seconds is generally considered adequate to produce a therapeutic effect.

E. ___ The timing and dosage of light therapy vary from person to person.

F. ___ There is substantial research documenting the long-term effectiveness of light therapy.

G. ___ Light therapy is particularly effective as a treatment for more severely ill patients.

H. ___ Partial sleep deprivation is as effective as total sleep deprivation.

2. **Fill in the blanks.**

A. For affective disorders, _____ to _____ ECT treatments are normally administered.

B. For schizophrenia, as many as _____ to _____ ECT treatments many be administered.

C. The primary indication for ECT is _____.

D. ECT's response rate of _____ or more is equal to or better than response rates to antidepressant medications.

E. Preparation for ECT is similar to that implemented for any brief _____ procedure.

F. Potential side effects that may occur immediately after ECT that may be treated symptomatically include _____, _____, and _____.

G. Phototherapy has a _____ to _____ % response rate in patients with winter depression or SAD.

H. Sleep deprivation appears to produce _____ in some patients with bipolar illness.

3. **Provide short answers for the following questions.**

A. You're talking with a nursing colleague and he asks you, "What exactly is ECT?" How would you respond?

B. ECT is often recommended for women with severe depression who are in their first trimester of a pregnancy. Why do you think this is?

C. Obtain the informed consent form used for ECT by your treatment facility. Review it for the elements described in this chapter. Try explaining the procedure to a friend or family member.

REFERENCES

1. Abrams R: *Electroconvulsive therapy,* ed 2, New York, 1992, Oxford University Press.
2. American Psychiatric Association: *The practice of electroconvulsive therapy: recommendations for treatment, training, and privileging,* Washington, DC, 1990, The Association.
3. Burns C, Stuart G: Nursing care in electroconvulsive therapy, *Psychiatr Clin North Am* 14:971, 1991.
4. Devanand D et al: Does ECT alter brain structure? *Am J Psychiatry* 151:957, 1994.
5. *Electroconvulsive therapy: a guide,* Madison, Wisc, 1996, Dean Foundation for Health, Research and Education, Lithium Information Center.
6. Fink M: Who should get ECT? In Coffey C, editor: *The clinical science of electroconvulsive therapy,* Washington, DC, 1993, American Psychiatric Press.
7. Fink P, Tasman A, editors: *Stigma and mental illness,* Washington, DC, 1992, American Psychiatric Press.
8. Fitzsimons L, Mayer R: Soaring beyond the cuckoo's nest: health care reform and ECT, *J Psychosoc Nurs* 33:10, 1995.
9. Fox H: Continuation and maintenance ECT, *J Pract Psychiatry Behav Health* 2:357, 1996.
10. Fox H: Electroconvulsive therapy: an overview, *J Pract Psychiatry Behav Health* 2:223, 1996.
11. Fox H: Patients' fear of and objection to electroconvulsive therapy, *Hosp Community Psychiatry* 44:357, 1993.

12. Hyman J: *The light book,* Los Angeles, 1990, Jeremy P Tarcher.
13. Kellner C, Pritchett J, Coffey C: *Handbook of ECT,* Washington, DC, 1997, American Psychiatric Press.
14. Kuhs H, Tolle R: Sleep deprivation therapy, *Biol Psychiatry* 29:1129, 1991.
15. Lerer B et al: Antidepressant and cognitive effects of twice-versus three-times-weekly ECT, *Am J Psychiatry* 152:564, 1995.
16. McEnany G: Phototherapy & sleep manipulations: an examination of two nondrug biologic interventions for depression, *J Am Psychiatr Nurses Assoc* 2:86, 1996.
17. Rosenthal N: *Winter blues: SAD—what it is and how to overcome it,* New York, 1993, Guilford.
18. Rosenthal N, Wehr T: Towards understanding the mechanism of action of light in seasonal affective disorders, *Pharmacopsychiatry* 25:56, 1992.
19. Schwartz P et al: Winter seasonal affective disorder: a follow-up study of the first 59 patients of the National Institute of Mental Health seasonal studies program, *Am J Psychiatry* 153:1028, 1996.
20. Stiebel V: Maintenance electroconvulsive therapy for chronic mentally ill patients: a case series, *Psychiatr Serv* 46:265, 1995.
21. Teicher M et al: The phototherapy light visor: more to it than meets the eye, *Am J Psychiatry* 152:1197, 1995.
22. Terman M et al: Predictors of response and nonresponse to light treatment for winter depression, *Am J Psychiatry* 153:1423, 1996.
23. Wehr T: Manipulations of sleep and phototherapy: nonpharmacological alternatives in the treatment of depression, *Clin Neuropharmacol* 13(suppl):S54, 1990.
24. Wehr T: Effects of wakefulness and sleep on deprivation and mania. In Montplaisir J, Godbout R, editors: *Sleep and biological rhythms,* New York, 1990, Oxford University Press.

ANNOTATED SUGGESTED READINGS

Electroconvulsive therapy: a guide. Madison, Wisc, 1996, Dean Foundation for Health, Research and Education, Lithium Information Center.
    Excellent booklet on ECT useful for patient and family education.
*Fitzsimons L, Mayer R: Soaring beyond the cuckoo's nest: health care reform and ECT, *J Psychosoc Nurs* 33:10, 1995.
    Update on the usefulness of ECT in the current managed care mental health delivery system.
Fox H: Continuation and maintenance ECT, *J Practical Psychiatry Behav Health* 2:357, 1996.
    Clear, practical article on the latest recommendations regarding continuation and maintenance of ECT.
Fox H: Electroconvulsive therapy: an overview, *J Practical Psychiatry Behav Health* 2:223, 1996.
    Concise and timely update on ECT that is useful for the clinician. Highly recommended.
Hyman J: *The light book,* Los Angeles, 1990, Jeremy P Tarcher.
    Easy-to-read text on how natural and artificial light affect our health, mood, and behavior. Well documented and interesting.
*Kashka M, Keyser P: Ethical issues in informed consent and ECT, *Perspectives in Psych Care* 31:15, 1995.
    The principles of autonomy and beneficence are explored in light of a patient situation. Excellent ethical analysis of a still controversial treatment in psychiatric care.
Kellner C, Pritchett J, Coffee C: *Handbook of ECT,* Washington, DC, 1997, American Psychiatric Press.
    Up-to-date and practical guide to contemporary ECT practice by experts in the field.
Lamburg L: *Bodyrhythms: chronobiology and peak performance,* New York, 1994, William Morrow and Company.
    Comprehensive overview of what is currently known about sleep bodyrhythms. Practical and useful reading for all.
*Loving R, Kripke D: Daily light exposure among psychiatric patients, *J Psychosoc Nurs* 30:15, 1992.
    Describes a study examining the 24-hour light exposure of psychiatric patients and identifies nursing interventions to increase light exposure in therapeutic environments.
*McEnany G: Phototherapy and sleep manipulations: an examination of two nondrug biologic interventions for depression, *J Amer Psych Nurs Assoc* 2:86, 1996.
    Discusses two newer treatments for depression that use biological rhythms as their basis and that result in correction of the rhythm disturbance and the relief of symptoms.
Rey J, Walter G: Half a century of ECT use in young people, *Am J Psychiatry* 154(5):595, 1997.
    Reviews the literature on the efficacy and safety of ECT in young people and examines the evidence for the suggestion that it may be used inappropriately.
Rosethal N: Winter blues: SAD—what it is and how to overcome it, New York, 1993, Guilford Press.
    Best book on the market that describes in layperson terms the illness of SAD and its treatment with phototherapy. Excellent for patient education.

*Nursing reference.

Preventing and Managing Aggressive Behavior

Christine Cahill Hamolia

© 1998 M.C. Escher/Cordon Art, Baarn, Holland.

Healthy children raised in decent conditions among loving people in a gentle and just society where freedom and equality are valued will rarely commit violent acts toward others. **Ramsay Clark** *A Few Modest Proposals to Reduce Individual Violence in America*

LEARNING OBJECTIVES

After studying this chapter the student should be able to:

▼ Discuss the prevalence of aggressive behavior among psychiatric patients and reasons for its increase

▼ Compare passive, assertive, and aggressive behavioral responses

▼ Describe five theories on the development of aggressive behavior

▼ Identify factors useful in predicting aggressive behavior among psychiatric patients

▼ Assess patients for aggressive behavioral responses

▼ Analyze nursing interventions for preventing and managing aggressive behavior

▼ Develop a patient education plan to promote patients' appropriate expression of anger

▼ Describe the implementation of crisis management techniques

▼ Evaluate the need for staff development related to educating staff, working with staff who have been assaulted, and understanding legal implications

TOPICAL OUTLINE

Dimensions of the Problem
Behavioral Responses
  Passive Behavior
  Assertive Behavior
  Aggressive Behavior
Theories on Aggression
  Psychoanalytical
  Psychological
  Behavioral
  Sociocultural
  Biological
Predicting Aggressive Behavior
  Issues of Provocation
Nursing Assessment
Nursing Interventions
  Self-Awareness
  Patient Education

Assertiveness Training
Communication Strategies
Environmental Strategies
Behavioral Strategies
Psychopharmacology
Crisis Management Techniques
  Team Response
  Seclusion
  Restraints
  Terminating the Intervention
Staff Development
  Education
  Staff Assault

Nurses provide care for patients with many types of problems. People who enter the health-care system are often in great distress and may exhibit maladaptive coping responses. Nurses who work in settings such as emergency rooms, critical care areas, and trauma centers often care for people who respond to events with angry and aggressive behavior that can pose a significant risk to themselves, other patients, and health-care providers. Thus preventing and managing aggressive behavior is an important skill for all nurses.

Psychiatric nurses in particular work with patients whose coping mechanisms for dealing with stress have proved to be inadequate. Patients admitted to an inpatient psychiatric unit are usually in crisis, so their coping skills are even less effective. During these times of stress, acts of physical aggression or violence often occur. It is also true that nurses spend more time with patients on an inpatient unit than any other mental health professional. Thus they are more likely to be involved in preventing and managing aggressive behavior and are more at risk for being victims of acts of violence by patients. For these reasons, it is critical that psychiatric nurses be able to assess patients at risk for violence and intervene effectively with patients before, during, and after an aggressive episode.

DIMENSIONS OF THE PROBLEM

High rates of assaultive behavior have been reported in a variety of health-care settings including outpatient clinics, nursing homes, and emergency departments. By far the highest rates of assault occur in psychiatric settings. Injury rates from violence in public sector psychiatric settings are alarmingly high across nursing employment categories, particularly among male technicians, male staff, and on-unit supervisory personnel.[17] In fact, the risk of occupational injury to psychiatric nurses in public sector facilities now exceeds the risk for those working in such high-risk areas as mining, lumber, heavy construction, and manufacturing (Table 29-1).[39]

Much has been written about violence in psychiatric populations in an attempt to describe and predict episodes of violence. Despite the common public misconception,

most mentally ill people do not commit violent acts. In fact, a minority of patients are responsible for a majority of the violent incidents. Differences in research methodology have made it difficult to identify the exact degree of violence in psychiatric facilities. The reported prevalence of both threatened and actual violence on inpatient units ranges from about 6% to 46%, although serious incidents are rare.[6,22] There is also some evidence that the rates of violence may be increasing over time and that rates are higher in the United States than in other countries.[6]

Many reasons help to explain the increasing incidence of violent behavior in psychiatric settings. First, as more emphasis is placed on outpatient and partial hospital treatment programs in the community, an increasing number of patients referred for inpatient care are hospitalized because they display aggressive or dangerous behavior. Before patients can be committed to the hospital, most states require evidence that patients are dangerous to themselves or others (see Chapter 9). This results in a larger proportion of aggressive and violent patients on inpatient units.[37]

Second, the nature of the inpatient milieu has changed because of increasing patient acuity and shortened lengths of stay. In addition, economic constraints have resulted in fewer nurses assigned to inpatient units and limited availability of medical staff to assist in managing patients.

Finally, evolving legal directives and perplexing ethical issues challenge the use of chemical and mechanical restraints and raise questions regarding patients' rights to refuse treatment and the nature of the least restrictive environment. This often results in conflict and confusion for inpatient staff, who try to manage patients effectively at a time of distress and dyscontrol.

> ? *Members of different disciplines sometimes have different views on how to manage aggressive behavior. Talk with nurses and physicians who care for psychiatric patients about their personal experiences and clinical judgments regarding this problem.*

BEHAVIORAL RESPONSES

Within each person lies the capacity for passive, assertive, and aggressive behavior. In a threatening situation the choices are to be passive and fearful and to flee; to be aggressive and angry and to fight; or to be assertive and self-confident and to confront the situation directly. The situation and the characteristics of the people involved determine the appropriate response.

Passive Behavior

Passive people consistently subordinate their own rights to their perception of the rights of others. When passive people become angry, they try to hide it, thereby increasing their own tension. If other people notice the anger by ob-

TABLE **29-1** *Worker Injury Rates from High-Risk Industries*

OCCUPATION	INJURY RATE PER 100 EMPLOYEES
All private sector industries	8.82
Mining	8.3
Manufacturing	13.1
Heavy construction	14.2
Lumber	18.4
Nursing staff (five combined studies)	22.4*

*Injury rates from violence alone. From US Department of Labor, 1991.

serving nonverbal cues, passive people are unable to confront the issue. This can also increase their tension. This pattern of interaction can seriously impair interpersonal growth. The following clinical example illustrates passive behavior.

Clinical Example Ms. J was a staff nurse on a busy surgical unit. She enjoyed her work and liked the patients. She also placed a high value on getting along with her co-workers. Other staff members always spoke positively of her. Ms. C, the head nurse, valued Ms. J as an employee, stating particularly, "She's not like the rest of them. She never complains."

Ms. J made it a practice never to refuse a request made by a patient or another staff member. If a patient who was assigned to another nurse asked her to explain his diet or straighten his bed, she would do so, even if she was then behind in her own work. She never asked for help from others because she felt that her assignment was her responsibility. If a co-worker asked to change days off with her, Ms. J always agreed, even if she had plans, rationalizing that the other person probably had more important plans.

Ms. C began to sense a tenseness when she was around Ms. J. Because she could not think of any problem at work, she assumed that Ms. J must have been having a problem at home. She was concerned and asked Ms. J if she could help. To her amazement, Ms. J recited a long list of angry feelings related to the work situation. Ms. C then felt guilty when she realized that she and the other staff members had been taking advantage of Ms. J.

Although Ms. J had thought that she was acting in a healthy way, she was actually negating her own needs and diminishing her self-respect. Her co-workers, who superficially liked her, in reality felt uncomfortable with her because they were never allowed to reciprocate when she had been helpful. Ms. C's guilty response quickly changed to anger when she realized that she had been a victim of Ms. J's passivity. If Ms. J had informed Ms. C of her feelings, she would have treated her more equitably.

Passivity is also expressed nonverbally. The person may speak softly, often in a childlike manner. There is little eye contact. Body language communicates diffidence and self-denial. The person may be slouched in posture, with arms held close to the body. Fidgeting also communicates passivity. Gestures are seldom used, although the head may be nodded in agreement (even when the person really disagrees).

Sarcasm is another indirect expression of anger. This usually provokes anger in the person who is the target. It is different from assertive behavior because it usually infringes on the rights of the other. A sarcastic remark generally conveys the message "You are not worthy of my respect." Sarcasm may be disguised as humor. Confrontation may then be responded to with a disclaimer such as "Can't you take a joke?" Humor that derogates another person is hostile and

is indulged in for the purpose of self-enhancement. It tends to backfire because the joker is revealed as insecure.

Assertive Behavior

Assertiveness is at the midpoint of a continuum that runs from passive to aggressive behavior. Assertive behavior conveys a sense of self-assurance but also communicates respect for the other person. Assertive people speak clearly and distinctly. They observe the norms of personal space appropriate to the situation. Eye contact is direct but not intrusive. Gestures emphasize speech but are not distracting or threatening. Posture is erect and relaxed. The body language may be symmetrical with that of the other party. The overall impression is that the person is strong, but not threatening.

Assertive people feel free to refuse an unreasonable request. However, they will share their rationale with the other person. They will also base the judgment about the reasonableness of the request on their own priorities. On the other hand, assertive people do not hesitate to make a request of others, assuming that they will inform them if their request is unreasonable. If the other person is unable to refuse, assertive people will not feel guilty about making the request.

Assertiveness also implies communicating feelings directly to others. As a result, anger is not allowed to build up and the expression of feeling is more likely to be in proportion to the situation. If dissatisfaction is verbalized, the reason for the feeling is included. Assertive people also remember to express love to those to whom they are close. Compliments are given when deserved. Assertion also involves acceptance of positive input from others.

Aggressive Behavior

At the opposite end of the continuum from passivity is aggression. Aggressive people ignore the rights of others. They assume that they must fight for their own interests, and they expect the same behavior from others. Life is a battle. An aggressive approach to life may lead to physical or verbal violence. The aggressive behavior often covers a basic lack of self-confidence. Aggressive people enhance their self-esteem by overpowering others and thereby proving their superiority. The next clinical example describes aggressive behavior.

Clinical Example Suzy was a 9-year-old girl brought to the child psychiatric clinic by her mother on referral from the school nurse. She was described as a tomboy who loved active play and hated school. She was the first girl to make the neighborhood Little League baseball team and had proved her right to be there by beating up several male team members. Suzy was sent to the clinic after the teacher caught her forcing younger children to give her their lunch money.

When Suzy came to the clinic, she presented a facade of

toughness. She did not deny her behavior and explained it by saying that the "little kids don't need much to eat anyway. I let them keep some of the money." Suzy was saving money for a new baseball glove. When she was asked about school, she said angrily, "I'm not dumb. I could learn that junk, but who needs it? I just want to play ball."

Psychological testing revealed that Suzy's IQ was slightly below average. She attended school with a group of upper-middle-class college-bound children. Even in fourth grade she was feeling insecure and unable to compete. She masked her insecurity with her bullying behavior, striving for acceptance in sports, where she did have ability. The medical diagnosis was conduct disorder, undersocialized, aggressive. When Suzy's problem was explained to her parents and the school, some of the pressure for academic achievement was alleviated. Her parents spent extra time helping her with her homework. Also, she was given genuine recognition for her athletic ability, demonstrated by the gift of a new baseball glove. Suzy gradually responded to the positive input from others by developing a sense of positive regard for herself. As she did so, she no longer needed to bully other children and began to grow into some real friendships.

Aggressive adults are not unlike Suzy. They try to cover up their insecurities and vulnerabilities by acting aggressive. The behavior is self-defeating because it drives people away, thus reinforcing the low self-esteem and vulnerability to rejection. Aggressive behavior is also communicated nonverbally. Aggressive people may invade personal space. They speak loudly and with great emphasis. They usually maintain eye contact over a prolonged period of time so that the other person experiences it as intrusive. Gestures may be emphatic and often seem threatening (for example, they may shake their fists, stamp their feet, or make slashing motions with their hands). Posture is erect, and often aggressive people lean forward slightly toward the other person. The overall impression is one of power and dominance. Table 29-2 summarizes the major characteristics of passive, assertive, and aggressive behaviors.

> *Do you use passive, assertive, or aggressive behaviors most often in your personal life? How does this compare with your professional life as a nursing student?*

THEORIES ON AGGRESSION

It is useful for nurses to view aggressive and violent behavior along a continuum with verbal aggression at one end and physical violence at the other.[28] Violence is the result of extreme anger (rage) or fear (panic). Specific reasons for aggressive behavior vary from person to person. Nurses need to communicate with patients to understand the events that they perceive as anger-provoking. In general, anger occurs in response to a perceived threat. This may be a threat of physical injury or, more often, a threat to the self-concept. When the self is threatened, people may not be entirely aware of the source of their anger. In this case, the nurse and patient need to work together to identify the nature of the threat.

A threat may be external or internal. Examples of external stressors are physical attack, loss of a significant relationship, and criticism from others. Internal stressors might include a sense of failure at work, perceived loss of love, and fear of physical illness. Anger is only one of the possible emotional responses to these stressors. Some people might respond with depression or withdrawal. However, those reactions are usually accompanied by anger, which may be difficult for the person to express directly. Depression is sometimes viewed as anger directed toward the self, and withdrawal may also be a passive expression of anger.

Anger often seems out of proportion to the event that seemed to cause it. An insignificant stressor may be "the last straw" and result in the release of a flood of feelings that have been stored up over time. Nurses need to be aware of this and not personalize anger expressed by a patient. The nurse may seem to be a safer target than significant others with whom the patient may also be angry.

A number of theories on the development of aggressive behavior have influenced the treatment of violent patients.

TABLE **29-2** *Comparison of Passive, Assertive, and Aggressive Behaviors*

	PASSIVE	ASSERTIVE	AGGRESSIVE
Content of speech	Negative Self-derogatory "Can I?" "Will you?"	Positive Self-enhancing "I can," "I will"	Exaggerated Other-derogatory "You always," "You never"
Tone of voice	Quiet, weak, whining	Modulated	Loud, demanding
Posture	Drooping, bowed head	Erect, relaxed	Tense, leaning forward
Personal space	Allows invasion of space by others	Maintains a comfortable distance; claims right to own space	Invades space of others
Gestures	Minimal, weak gesturing, fidgeting	Demonstrative gestures	Threatening, expansive gestures
Eye contact	Little or none	Intermittent, appropriate to relationship	Constant stare

They can be categorized as psychoanalytical, psychological, behavioral, sociocultural, and biological. Current thinking in the field suggests that aggressive behavior is the result of the interaction of a person's biological, psychological, and sociocultural characteristics and that each of these factors must be considered when determining nursing care.

Psychoanalytical

Psychoanalytical theory suggests that aggressive behavior is the result of instinctual drives. Freud proposed that two primary drives influence human behavior: the life force, expressed through sexuality, and the death force, expressed through aggression. He believed that life was a struggle to maintain a balance between the two drives and that the behavior exhibited by humans was simply the result of the more powerful drive. This theory had a great impact on early thinking in the field. However, little research has supported this theory. It has also been criticized as having limited clinical usefulness because it suggests that humans are innately aggressive and that they do not have a choice in this disposition. Furthermore, it discourages individual responsibility and accountability for behavioral response.

Psychological

According to the frustration-aggression theory, aggression occurs as the result of a buildup of frustration. Frustration results when a person's attempt to achieve a desired goal is blocked. These feelings are then reduced through aggressive behavior. This theory has been criticized for simplifying the complexity of the human spirit and not considering other stressors that might also lead to aggression. In addition, it implies that the absence of aggression is simply caused by the absence of frustration. Thus there is no allowance for alternative ways of handling frustration.

Another psychological view of aggressive behavior suggests the importance of predisposing developmental or life experiences that limit the person's capacity to select nonviolent coping mechanisms. Some of these experiences are listed in Box 29-1. They may limit a person's ability to use

Box **29-1** *Developmental Factors Limiting Use of Nonviolent Coping Techniques*

Organic brain damage, mental retardation, or learning disability, which may impair capacity to deal effectively with frustration
Severe emotional deprivation or overt rejection in childhood, or parental seduction, which may contribute to defects in trust and self-esteem
Exposure to violence in formative years, either as a victim of child abuse or as an observer of family violence, which may instill a pattern of using violence as a way to cope

From Menninger W: Management of the aggressive and dangerous patient, *Bull Menninger Clin* 57:208, 1993.

supportive relationships, leave the person very self-centered, or make the person particularly vulnerable to a sense of injury that can easily be provoked into retaliatory rage. Fig. 29-1 shows how these factors can contribute to an intergenerational transmission of violent behavior. Box 29-2 presents background information about the patient that may also be associated with violence.

Behavioral

Social learning theory proposes that aggressive behavior is learned through the socialization process as a result of

Box **29-2** *Background Information Associated with Violent Behavior*

Childhood cruelty to animals or other children
Fire setting or similar dangerous actions
Recent violent behavior toward self or others
Recent accidents, threats, or poor judgment in potentially dangerous situations
Altered states of consciousness
Escalating irritability, sensitivity, or hostility
Fear of losing control
Efforts to obtain help
Bothering family, neighbors, or police
History of abuse of alcohol or other disinhibiting substances

From Menninger W: Management of the aggressive and dangerous patient, *Bull Menninger Clin* 57:208, 1993.

CRITICAL THINKING *about* **Contemporary Issues**

Does Media Violence Lead to Greater Acts of Aggression in Society?

Some people believe that graphic scenes of violence in television, movies, and video games are directly linked to human aggression. Proponents of this view support measures to decrease media violence and restrict types of programming. Others think that the relationship has not been clearly established. These people believe that violence is more broadly determined by socioeconomic, biological, psychological, cultural, and familial factors.

Research suggests that although many instances of children and adults imitating media violence have been documented, no court has ruled that media violence actually causes harm. However, it has been suggested that although the typical viewer may be mentally resilient and invulnerable to any ill effects, a small group of vulnerable viewers may be more impressionable and therefore more likely to suffer negative effects from violent programming.[15] More research is needed to identify characteristics of such a vulnerable population. It is also important to remember that the public must accept responsibility for the escalation of media violence. If the product were unappealing it would fail. Instead, the entertainment industry appears to exploit a public already fascinated with violence.

internal and external learning. Internal learning occurs through the personal reinforcement received when enacting aggressive behavior. This may be the result of achieving a desired goal or experiencing feelings of importance, power, and control. For example, 4-year-old Johnny wants a cookie just before dinner. When his mother refuses, Johnny has a temper tantrum. If his mother then gives him a cookie, Johnny has learned that an aggressive outburst will be rewarded and he will get what he wants. If similar situations occur, Johnny will continue to use an aggressive approach.

External learning occurs through the observation of role models such as parents, peers, siblings, and sports and entertainment figures. Sociocultural patterns that lead to the imitation of aggressive behavior suggest that violence is an acceptable way of solving problems and achieving social status. According to this view, activities such as violent crime, aggressive sports, and war depicted through the media or witnessed in person reinforce aggressive behavior (see Critical Thinking about Contemporary Issues).

A recent addition to the social learning perspective suggests that violence is a functional behavior that is designed to control others purely for self-gain. There is some evidence that this coercive interactional style may be a strong predictor of violent behavior.[25] It was discovered from direct interviews with patients who when asked "Why are you violent?" responded "Because I'm tired of these people and I want to get them off my back." This theory challenges the notion that violent behavior is most often a symptom of psychiatric illness and that violent patients have a limited ability to control their violent behavior. Rather, it suggests that violence is a method for exerting control over others.[27]

Sociocultural

Social and cultural factors may also influence aggressive behavior. Cultural norms help to define acceptable and unacceptable means of expressing aggressive feelings. Sanctions are applied to violators of the norms through the legal system. By this means, society controls violent behavior and attempts to maintain a safe existence for its members. Unfortunately, this prohibition against violent behavior may also be extended to include any expression of anger. This can inhibit people from the healthy expression of angry feelings and lead to other maladaptive responses. A cultural norm that supports verbally assertive expressions of anger will help people deal with anger in a healthy manner. A norm that reinforces violent behavior will result in physical expression of anger in destructive ways.

Finally, a number of studies have attempted to explore the influences of race, culture, economics, and environmental factors on violent behavior. Physical crowding and heat appear to be related to violent behavior. Other social determinants of violence are linked in a cycle and include[36]:

▼ Poverty and the inability to have basic necessities of life
▼ Disruption of marriages
▼ Production of single-parent families

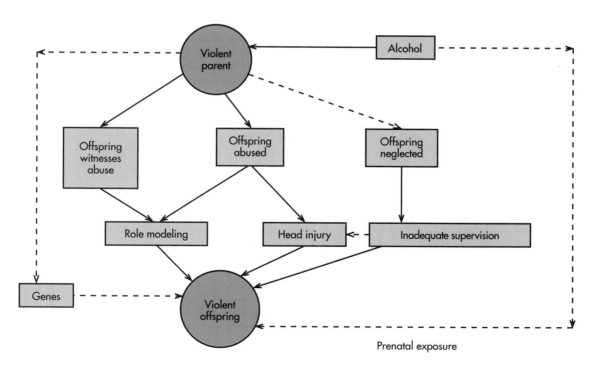

Fig. 29-1   Intergenerational transmission of violence. (From Volavka J: *Neurobiology of violence*, Washington, DC, 1995, American Psychiatric Press.)

▼ Unemployment
▼ Difficulty in maintaining interpersonal ties, family structure, and social control

Biological

Current neurobiological research has focused on three areas of the brain believed to be involved in aggression: the limbic system, the frontal lobes, and the temporal lobe (Fig. 29-2). Neurotransmitters have also been suggested as having a role in the expression or suppression of aggressive behavior.[9,11,40] Each of these areas is described in more detail in Chapter 5.

The limbic system is associated with the mediation of basic drives and the expression of human emotions and behaviors such as eating, aggression, and sexual response. It is also involved in the processing of information and memory. Synthesis of information to and from other areas in the brain influences emotional experience and behavior. Alterations in functioning of the limbic system may result in an increase or decrease in the potential for aggressive behavior.

The frontal lobes play an important role in mediating purposeful behavior and rational thinking. They are the part of the brain where reason and emotion interact. Damage to the frontal lobes can result in impaired judgment, personality changes, problems in decision making, inappropriate conduct, and aggressive outbursts.

The temporal lobes play a role in memory and the interpretation of auditory stimuli. The temporal lobe problem most often linked to aggressive behavior is epilepsy, particularly in people with partial complex seizures. Aggressive behavior may occur during or after seizure activity.

The interaction of the frontal lobes with the limbic system forms an emotional circuit that connects the cognitive processes of the frontal lobes with the emotional processes of the limbic system and with the memory functions of the limbic system and temporal lobes. This emotional circuit determines the meaning given to a particular situation, integrating both current and past experiences with stored memories and beliefs. With aggressive people, meaning given to a particular circumstance may be altered from that person's usual perceptions and memories, or from the norm accepted by the social context. The implication is dysfunction in communication in the areas of the brain responsible for emotional behavior.

Neurotransmitters are brain chemicals that are transmitted to and from neurons through synapses, resulting in communication between brain structures. An increase or decrease in these substances can influence behavior. Changes in the balance of these compounds can aggravate or inhibit aggression. The neurotransmitters most often associated with aggressive behaviors are the four biogenic amines—serotonin, dopamine, norepinephrine, and acetylcholine—and the amino acid GABA (Table 29-3).

PREDICTING AGGRESSIVE BEHAVIOR

Researchers have tried to determine which patients are more likely to become violent. Demographic variables such as age, sex, race, marital status, education, and socioeconomic level have not been useful in predicting violent behavior. In contrast, psychiatric diagnosis has often been correlated with assaultiveness. However, the ability of this variable to predict violence is complicated by the fact that many patients have more than one diagnosis. In addition, patients may have different clinical symptoms depending on the severity and acuity of their illness. Thus a patient's diagnosis is suggestive at best.[21,35] In general, research indicates that two populations of patients are at increased risk of violence[3]:

Fig. 29-2 Structures of the brain implicated in aggression.

▼ Patients with **active psychotic symptoms,** particularly those related to perceived threat or overriding of internal controls, such as delusions of thought control.

▼ Patients with **substance abuse disorders.** The prevalence of violence is 12 times greater for those with alcohol abuse or dependence and 16 times greater for those with other drug dependence compared with those with no psychiatric diagnosis. Comorbid substance abuse has an added effect in increasing the risk of violence for people with major psychiatric disorders.

In recent years research efforts have focused on identifying clinical variables that have been shown to be predictors of violence. The best single predictor of violence appears to be a history of violence.[33] Another significant clinical variable is the length of time spent on an inpatient unit, with more assaultive patients being found to have spent significantly more time than nonassaultive patients on inpatient units since their first admission.[23]

Although knowledge about a patient's history is important in evaluating the risk for violence, it is also important to assess the patient's current clinical condition and situation. High levels of aggression before admission and absence of signs of anxiety at admission are believed to be good predictors of violence. In addition, increased motor activity and indications of poor impulse control or strong aggressive drives in psychological testing may also be sig-

nificant in predicting patient assaultiveness. Other studies report that correlates of violent behavior include a variety of behavioral and cognitive cues such as conceptual disorganization, loud verbalizations, tension, mannerisms and posturing, hostility, suspiciousness, uncooperativeness, hallucinatory behavior, unusual thought content, excitement, and disorientation.[6]

Finally, situational and environmental factors are also believed to play a role in escalating patient behavior from dangerousness to violence. This includes aspects of the physical facilities and the presence of staff and other patients. For example, several studies have found that the number of violent incidents is greater when patients move or gather in groups, are overcrowded, lack privacy, or are inactive. Clinicians may also intentionally or inadvertently precipitate an outbreak of violence because staff attitudes and behavior have a powerful impact on patient behavior. Staff provocation and inexperience, poor milieu management, close physical encounters, inconsistent limit setting, and a norm of violence may all negatively affect the inpatient environment.[2,16]

 What role do you think culture plays in the expression and interpretation of aggressive behavior?

Issues of Provocation

Research suggests that many assaultive patients view their victim as provoking the attack. This is an important issue for nurses to consider. A primary factor of provocation is that of limit setting. Failing to set effective limits may lead to provocation and assault. There is also increased risk of assault when limits are set inconsistently. Taking things away from patients such as food, beverages, or cigarettes also appears to increase the likelihood of an attack.

Staff attitude is another important issue. Aggressive verbal and nonverbal behavior on the part of the staff often escalates the patient's distress and violent behavior. When the nursing staff act in a controlling manner, patients are more likely to use aggression and violence to get control. Staff who are authoritarian, disrespectful, or inflexible in their approach to patients or who have not been trained in crisis management techniques are also more likely to provoke aggressive behavior. Finally, violent behavior may be a way of getting the staff's attention or may lead to a tangible reward.

Finally, locked units, inflexible unit structures, and nontherapeutic milieus can increase the risk for assaultive behavior by suggesting that aggressive behavior is acceptable or even expected. Overly strict unit structure may render staff unable to respond to patients empathically. In turn, patients may perceive the unit as coercive, controlling, and threatening and feel their behavioral options are limited to disruptive, desperate, or violent acts. Such settings often provoke the very behavior they are intended to control.

TABLE **29-3** *Neurotransmitters Implicated in Aggression*

Neurotransmitter	Postulated Relationship with Aggressive Behaviors
Serotonin (5-HT)	Modulates violence, sleep, sensory responses, mood, and performance; case reports of improved behavior in aggressive patients treated with supplemental tryptophan (5-HT precursor); dietary restriction of tryptophan shown to increase aggression.
Dopamine	Increases aggressive behavior and sexual activity, heightens vigilance; elevated levels associated with schizophrenia and organic delusional disorders; L-dopa in treatment of Parkinsonism linked to paranoid psychosis.
Norepinephrine	Increases aggressive behavior, heightens vigilance.
Acetylcholine	Deficiency (as in Alzheimer's disease) may directly increase aggressive tendencies through lowered threshold for confusion and loss of recent memory; aggression, fighting, and killing behaviors in animal studies.
GABA	Inhibits impulsivity and aggression.

Modified from Harper-Jacques S, Reiner M: Aggressive behavior and the brain: a different perspective for the mental health nurse, *Arch Psychiatr Nurs* 6(5):312-320, 1992.

> **?** *Discuss the fine line between talking about ways staff can provoke patients and blaming the staff who are the victims of the aggressive behavior.*

NURSING ASSESSMENT

Although researchers have made progress in determining reliable predictors of violence, a completely accurate prediction of patient violence is not possible.[20] For this reason it is important for psychiatric nurses to be alert for symptoms of increasing agitation that could lead to violent behavior. For example, a correspondence has been shown between nurses' clinical estimates of patients' chances of becoming violent and the number of patients who later displayed some type of aggression.[19]

Some evidence also shows that a hierarchy of aggressive behaviors exists and that lower levels of aggression may lead to more violent behavior (Fig. 29-3).[26] Some of these early behaviors include motor agitation such as pacing, inability to sit still, clenching or pounding fists, and tightening of jaw or facial muscles. There also may be verbal clues such as threats to real or imagined objects or intrusive demands for attention. Speech may be loud and pressured, and posture may become threatening.

Another critical factor in the assessment of a potentially violent patient is the affect associated with escalating behaviors. Anger often is seen in patients who are imminently violent. Inappropriate euphoria, irritability, and lability in affect may indicate that a patient is having difficulty in maintaining control. Changes in level of consciousness may also be an indication of future violent behavior (Box 29-3).

In summary, psychiatric nurses should carefully assess all patients for their potential for violence. A screening or assessment tool such as the one presented in Fig. 29-4 can be useful. Once completed, a violence assessment tool can help the nurse:

▼ Establish a therapeutic alliance with the patient
▼ Assess a patient's potential for violence
▼ Develop a plan of care
▼ Implement the plan of care
▼ Prevent aggression and violence in the milieu

Following the assessment, if the patient is believed to be potentially violent the nurse should:

▼ Implement the appropriate clinical protocol to provide for patient and staff safety
▼ Notify co-workers
▼ Obtain additional security if needed
▼ Assess the environment and make necessary changes
▼ Notify the physician and assess the need for PRN medications

---

Box 29-3 *Behaviors Associated with Aggression*

MOTOR AGITATION
Pacing
Inability to sit still
Clenching or pounding fists
Jaw tightening
Increased respirations
Sudden cessation of motor activity (catatonia)

VERBALIZATIONS
Verbal threats toward real or imagined objects
Intrusive demands for attention
Loud, pressured speech
Evidence of delusional or paranoid thought content

AFFECT
Anger
Hostility
Extreme anxiety
Irritability
Inappropriate or excessive euphoria
Affect lability

LEVEL OF CONSCIOUSNESS
Confusion
Sudden change in mental status
Disorientation
Memory impairment
Inability to be redirected

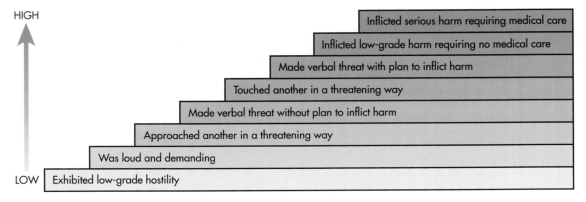

Fig. 29-3 Hierarchy of aggressive and violent patient behaviors.

ASSAULT AND VIOLENCE ASSESSMENT TOOL

Description: This tool is used if a patient
    a. Has a history of violence
    b. Is currently threatening violence
    c. Was threatening violence at the time of the referral.

Directions:
    a. Assess each key factor.
    b. Circle one (of three) descriptor for each factor that best describes the patient.
    c. Add the points for each circled item to obtain the total score.

Key Factors	High Risk	Moderate Risk	No Precautions
History of Violence	Any single episode of violence with injury to others while hospitalized -OR- Multiple assaults with injury while outside hospital **2**	Destruction of property without injury to others while in hospital -OR- A single assault outside the hospital resulting in injury -OR- Multiple assaults outside the hospital not resulting in injury **1**	Violence only when using drugs or alcohol -OR- Destruction of property outside hospital -OR- No history of violence **0**
History of Recent Aggression	Physically threatening at time of referral/admission **2**	Verbally threatening at time of referral/admission **1**	Nonthreatening at time of referral/admission **0**
History of Aggression in Family of Origin	Victim or perpetrator of physical or sexual abuse **2**	Witness of physical or sexual abuse **1**	Witness or victim of verbal aggression -OR- No history of aggression in family **0**
Substance Abuse Status	Recent alcohol/substance abuse actively detoxing -OR- Currently under the influence of alcohol or drugs **2**	Recent substance/alcohol abuse with absence of withdrawal symptoms **1**	Rehabilitated abuser -OR- No history of alcohol/substance abuse -OR- Past history (>3 months ago) alcohol/substance abuse with no rehabilitation **0**
Paranoia/Hostility	Paranoia or hostility generalized to people in the immediate environment **2**	Paranoia or hostility generalized toward inaccessible people **1**	No apparent paranoia No apparent hostility **0**
Impulsivity	Physically impulsive **2**	Verbally impulsive -OR- History of physical impulsivity **1**	No apparent impulsivity **0**
Agitation	Psychomotor agitation with constant pressured physical activity **2**	Psychomotor agitation with intermittent bursts of hyperactivity **1**	No apparent psychomotor agitation **0**
Sensorium	Disoriented with impaired memory **2**	Oriented with impaired memory **1**	Oriented with intact memory **0**

Scoring Key
  9 or more = High-risk precautions
  3-8 = Moderate-risk precautions
  0-2 = No precautions

Total Score: _____
Assessed by (RN): _____
Date: _____
Time: _____

Fig. 29-4 Assault and violence assessment tool. (Courtesy of Psychiatric Nursing, Institute of Psychiatry, Medical University of South Carolina.)

NURSING INTERVENTIONS

The nurse can implement a variety of interventions to prevent and manage aggressive behavior. These interventions can be thought of as existing on a continuum (Fig. 29-5). They range from preventive strategies such as self-awareness, patient education, and assertiveness training to anticipatory strategies such as verbal and nonverbal communication, environmental changes, behavioral interventions, and the use of psychopharmacological agents. If the patient's aggressive behavior escalates despite these actions, the nurse must implement crisis management techniques including seclusion and restraints.

Self-Awareness

The most valuable resource of a nurse is the ability to use the self to help others.[12] To ensure the most effective use of self, it is important to be aware of personal stress that can interfere with one's ability to communicate therapeutically with patients. If the nurse is tired, anxious, angry, or apathetic, it will be difficult to convey an interest in the concerns and fears of the patient. Furthermore, if the nurse is overwhelmed with personal problems, the energy available for patients is greatly diminished.

When dealing with potentially aggressive patients, it is important to be able to assess the situation objectively despite the positive or negative countertransference that might be present. Countertransference is an emotional reaction to some aspect or behavior of the patient (see Chapter 2). Negative countertransference reactions have been found to be a significant factor in the occurrence of violence in hospitals.[6] To prevent this situation the nurse must demonstrate ongoing self-awareness and supervision with the goal of separating personal needs from those of the patient.

Patient Education

Teaching patients about communication and the appropriate way to express anger can be one of the most successful interventions in preventing aggressive behavior (see the Patient Education Plan at bottom right). Many patients have difficulty identifying their feelings, needs, and desires and even more difficulty communicating these to others. Teaching patients that feelings are not right or wrong or good or bad can allow them to explore feelings that may have been bottled up, ignored, or repressed. The nurse can then work with patients on ways to express their feelings and evaluate whether the responses they select are adaptive or maladaptive.[10]

Assertiveness Training

Teaching assertive communication skills is an important nursing intervention (see Chapter 30). Interpersonal frustrations often escalate to aggressive behavior because patients have not mastered the assertive behaviors previously discussed in this chapter. Assertive behavior is a basic interpersonal skill that includes the following:
▼ Communicating directly with another person
▼ Saying no to unreasonable requests
▼ Being able to state complaints
▼ Expressing appreciation as appropriate
For example, the nurse might discuss with the patient how, if the patient talks about angry feelings toward a co-worker with another noninvolved co-worker, it does nothing to solve the problem and may even generate more negative emotions. If the patient pretends to not be angry, the anger is allowed to build up inside. It is likely that the anger will be misdirected at a later time or expressed out of proportion in another unrelated situation.

Patients with few assertive skills can learn them by participating in structured groups and programs. In these settings patients can watch staff demonstrate specific skills and then role play the skills themselves. Staff can provide feedback to patients on the appropriateness and effectiveness of their responses. Homework can also be assigned to patients to help them generalize these skills outside the group milieu. It is expected that aggressive behaviors will diminish as the patient learns new and more effective social skills.

Preventive Strategies   **Anticipatory Strategies**   **Containment Strategies**

Self-awareness
Patient education
Assertiveness training

Communication
Environmental change
Behavioral actions
Psychopharmacology

Crisis management
Seclusion
Restraints

Fig. 29-5   Continuum of nursing interventions in managing aggressive behavior.

How can a nurse who has difficulty being assertive with peers and interdisciplinary colleagues effectively teach assertiveness skills to patients?

Communication Strategies

The psychiatric nurse can often prevent a crisis situation through the use of early verbal and nonverbal intervention. This is sometimes called "talking the patient down." Because it is much less dangerous to prevent a crisis than to respond to one, every effort should be made to carefully monitor patients who are at risk for violent behavior and intervene at the first possible sign of increasing agitation.

Speaking to the patient in a calm, low voice can help to decrease a patient's agitation. Agitated patients often speak loudly and use profanity. It is important that nurses not respond by raising their voice or by using profanity because this will probably be perceived as competition and will only further escalate the volatile situation. The nurse should use short, simple sentences and avoid laughing or smiling inappropriately.

The nurse can also help reduce a rising level of agitation by acknowledging the patient's feelings and reassuring the patient that the staff is there to help. It may be useful to allow the patient to ventilate without interruption. It is important that the nurse communicate expected behavior in a way that encourages the patient to maintain control of any violent impulses. At this early stage, some patients with encouragement may be willing to remove themselves from an overstimulating environment, thus facilitating their self-control.

The specific nonverbal communication used by the nurse can also greatly affect the outcome of the intervention. A calm and relaxed posture that does not tower over the patient is much less intimidating than a posture in which hands are placed on the hips and the nurse looms over the patient. Crossing the arms across the chest is another posture that communicates emotional distance and an unwillingness to help. The nurse's hands should be kept open and out of pockets. Threatening, nervous, and sudden gestures should be avoided. Altering position so that the nurse's eyes are at the same level as those of the patient allows the patient to communicate from an equal rather than inferior position.

The nurse should assume a supportive stance that is at least one leg length or 3 feet from the patient. It is helpful if the nurse remains at an angle to the patient and the pa-

PATIENT EDUCATION PLAN   Appropriate Expression of Anger

Content	Instructional Activities	Evaluation
Help the patient identify anger.	Focus on nonverbal behavior. Role play nonverbal expression of anger. Label the feeling using the patient's preferred words.	Patient demonstrates an angry body posture and facial expression.
Give permission for angry feelings.	Describe situations in which it is normal to feel angry.	Patient describes a situation in which anger would be an appropriate response.
Practice the expression of anger.	Role play fantasized situations in which anger is an appropriate response.	Patient participates in role play and identifies behaviors associated with expression of anger.
Apply the expression of anger to a real situation.	Help identify a real situation that makes the patient angry. Role play a confrontation with the object of the anger. Provide positive feedback for successful expression of anger.	Patient identifies a real situation that results in anger. Patient is able to role play expression of anger.
Identify alternative ways to express anger.	List several ways to express anger, with and without direct confrontation. Role play alternative behaviors. Discuss situations in which alternatives would be appropriate.	Patient participates in identifying alternatives and plans when each might be useful.
Confrontation with a person who is a source of anger.	Provide support during confrontation if needed. Discuss experience after confrontation takes place.	Patient identifies the feeling of anger and appropriately confronts the object of the anger.

tient's need for personal space is respected. It has been noted that violence-prone people need four times more personal space than non–violence-prone people. Intrusion into a patient's personal space can be perceived as a threat and provoke aggression. Finally, when approaching potentially violent patients, nurses should carefully observe their behavior. Clenched fists, tightening of the facial muscles, and movement away from the nurse may suggest that the patient is feeling threatened. The nurse should respond by giving the patient as much distance as possible. These communication strategies are summarized in Box 29-4.

> *Why do you think that standing at an angle to the patient is less threatening than facing the patient full face? Try the two stances with a friend and describe your feelings about each one.*

Environmental Strategies

Violent behavior is more likely to occur in a poorly structured milieu with undefined program rules and a great deal of unscheduled time for patients.[5] Units that are overly stimulating, either visually or aurally, may also increase aggressive behavior. Thus, treatment settings should be structured by unit rules so that levels of sensory stimulation are low to moderate. Televisions, stereos, lighting, temperature, wall colors, and air quality should not be overstimulating.

Inpatient units that provide many productive activities such as reading and group programs reduce the chance of inappropriate patient behavior and increase adaptive social and leisure functioning. Both the unit norms and the rewards associated with such activities may reduce the amount of disorganized patient behavior and the number of aggressive acts. The impact of the environment is seen in the following clinical example.

Clinical Example Mr. T was a 36-year-old man who was admitted for the third time to an acute care unit at a state psychiatric hospital. His medical diagnosis was bipolar disorder, manic. The nursing staff was apprehensive because the patient had a history of assaultive behavior on earlier admissions. At the time of this admission, the unit atmosphere was tense because one of the other patients had made a suicide attempt requiring emergency room treatment.

Mr. I was Mr. T's primary nurse from his previous admission. He was working when the patient arrived on the unit. During the nursing assessment, Mr. I discussed the nursing interventions that had seemed to be helpful in the past. He validated with Mr. T that he was usually able to maintain control of his behavior by participating in a structured physical activity when he was feeling upset. In addition, he recalled that the patient would begin to pace rapidly and sing when he was losing control. Mr. T agreed with these observations.

Mr. T responded very quickly to the tension on the unit. He began to pace up and down the hall and sing in a moderately loud tone of voice. Other patients also began to show signs of increased agitation. The nursing staff held a brief consultation. They decided that the charge nurse would gather the patients for a community meeting to discuss their feelings about the suicide attempt. Meanwhile, Mr. I would take Mr. T to the nearby gym with one of the nurse's aides. They would perform structured calisthenic exercises. The interventions were successful. None of the patients needed to be restrained.

ROOM PROGRAM. In an inpatient setting, the use of a structured room program is another effective tool for the management of agitated patients whose self-control is tenuous and who have not yet decompensated to the point where seclusion or restraints are necessary. A **room program** is the titration of the amount of time patients are allowed in the unit milieu. For example, patients initially may be asked to stay in their rooms for a certain length of time, or conversely be allowed out of their rooms for a specified amount of time every hour. The amount of time in the milieu may then be increased by increments of 15 minutes as patients tolerate the environment. Another way of implementing a room program is to allow patients to come out of their rooms during certain designated hours, such as when the unit is quiet or when other patients are off the unit.

Such a structured program allows patients time away from situations that may increase agitation and provides a way to regulate the amount of stimulation patients receive. Its purpose is the prevention of a crisis that could result in more serious patient complications.

CATHARTIC ACTIVITIES. Many clinicians support the use of cathartic activities as a way of helping patients physically release aggression. These strategies are based on the assumption that some physical activity can be useful in releasing aggression and can prevent more explosive or destructive forms of aggression or violence. However, recent

---

Box **29-4** *Communication Strategies Used in Preventing Aggressive Behavior*

Present a calm appearance.
Speak softly.
Speak in a nonprovocative and nonjudgmental manner.
Speak in a neutral and concrete way.
Put space between yourself and the patient.
Show respect for the patient.
Avoid intense direct eye contact.
Demonstrate control over the situation without assuming an overly authoritarian stance.
Facilitate the patient's talking.
Listen to the patient.
Avoid early interpretations.
Do not make promises you cannot keep.

research suggests that aggressive behavior exists on a continuum and that minor manifestations of aggression can lead to further aggressive behavior.[26] These findings challenge the effectiveness of cathartic activities and call into question some traditional nursing interventions, such as encouraging patients to release tension through the use of punching bags or allowing patients to pace the halls in the expectation that their tension will decrease. Because these strategies are not supported by research and may increase the patient's potential for aggressive behavior, they are not recommended nursing actions. This is also an excellent example of the way in which nursing research can challenge traditional nursing interventions and help psychiatric nurses to base their practice on empirically based data rather than commonly held but untested assumptions.

Behavioral Strategies

Other interventions include applying principles of behavior management with the aggressive patient (see Chapter 30). Effective limit setting is one of the most basic interventions in this area.

LIMIT SETTING. Limit setting is a nonpunitive, nonmanipulative act in which the patient is told what behavior is acceptable, what is not acceptable, and the consequences of behaving unacceptably. Research has shown that it is possible to prevent some of patients' anger by improving nurses' limit-setting styles.[14] The nurse does not assume responsibility for the patient's behavior, adaptive or maladaptive. It is recognized that the patient has the right to choose a behavior and knows the consequences of it. Limits should be clarified before negative consequences are applied.

Once a limit has been identified, the consequences must take place if the behavior occurs. Every staff member must be aware of the plan and carry it out consistently. If staff do not do so, the patient is likely to manipulate staff by acting out and then pointing out areas of inconsistent limit setting. Clear, firm, and nonpunitive enforcement of limits is the goal. It is also important for nurses to understand that when limit setting is implemented, the maladaptive behavior will not immediately decrease. In fact, it may briefly increase. This is consistent with behavioral principles and testing behavior. If staff understand the dynamics of this intervention they will be able to implement this strategy effectively and understand that patient behavior will eventually change.

BEHAVIORAL CONTRACTS. If a patient uses violence to gain control and make personal gains, the nursing care must be planned to eliminate the rewards the patient receives while allowing the patient to assume as much control as possible. Once the rewards are understood, nursing care can be planned that does not reinforce aggressive and violent behavior. Behavioral contracts with the patient can be very helpful in this regard. For example, head-injured patients with low impulse control can be told that staff will take them for a walk if they can refrain from using profanity for 4 hours.

To be effective, contracts require detailed information about the following:

▼ Unacceptable behaviors
▼ Acceptable behaviors
▼ Consequences for breaking the contract
▼ The nurse's contribution to care

Patients should also have input into the development of the contract to increase their sense of self-control. This negotiated process increases the mutuality of the therapeutic alliance and reduces the possibility of aggressive behavior.

TIME-OUTS. Time-out from reinforcement is a behavioral technique in which socially inappropriate behaviors can be decreased by short-term removal of the patient from overstimulating and sometimes reinforcing situations. Time-outs are most effective with patients who feel loss of social contact as a negative consequence. With time-out, patients have more control over the process, and thus this intervention offers an alternative that involves less humiliation and less risk of injury.

With implementation of this intervention, patients who appear to be escalating are prompted to enter time-out, which is usually a quiet, low-traffic area of the unit. They remain there until they have been nonaggressive for a couple of minutes. Patients who do not comply with time-out instructions are told to enter the seclusion room for further protection of themselves and others.

TOKEN ECONOMY. Another effective behavioral strategy is the implementation of a token economy. In this intervention, identified interpersonal skills and self-care behaviors are rewarded with tokens that can be used by the patient to buy items. Behaviors to be targeted are specific to each patient. Guidelines should clearly specify desired behaviors required to receive tokens, the number of tokens to be received for each behavior, and the length of time a desired behavior must be exhibited to receive tokens. Furthermore, in a token economy undesired behaviors can result in the loss of tokens.

Research has shown that inpatient units that have implemented token economies have significantly fewer aggressive episodes than more traditional settings. This strategy for managing aggressive behavior is particularly useful with chronic lower-functioning patient populations. This clinical example describes the use of this intervention.

Clinical Example A regressed patient, Mrs. S, refused to get out of bed in the morning. She would not shower, dress, or wash her clothes. When encouraged to do these things, Mrs. S became agitated, swore, and threatened to hit anyone who tried to help her.

A token store was set up with the number of tokens required to purchase each item. Under her contract, Mrs. S would receive two tokens for each of the following behaviors:

▼ Getting out of bed by 7:30 AM
▼ Showering before 8:00 AM

▼ Dressing before 8:00 AM
▼ Being at breakfast table by 8:15 AM
▼ Eating 100% of breakfast tray by 8:45 AM
▼ Arriving to community meeting by 9:00 AM
Her contract also included the following penalty:
▼ An episode of swearing will result in the loss of 4 tokens.

Psychopharmacology

Pharmacological interventions have proven to be effective in the management of aggressive behavior.[5] They include a variety of therapeutic agents, all of which are discussed in greater detail in Chapter 27.

ANTIANXIETY AND SEDATIVE-HYPNOTICS. These drugs are effective in the management of acute agitation. Benzodiazepines such as lorazepam and clonazepam are often used during psychiatric emergencies to sedate combative patients. They are not recommended for long-term use because they can result in confusion and dependency and may worsen depressive symptoms. Furthermore, some patients have experienced a disinhibiting effect from benzodiazepines that can result in increased aggressive behavior. Buspirone, an antianxiety drug that may be effective in the management of aggressive behavior associated with anxiety and depression, has also been shown to decrease aggression and agitation in patients with head injuries, dementia, and developmental disabilities.

ANTIDEPRESSANTS. Antidepressants have been shown to be effective in controlling impulsive and aggressive behavior associated with mood changes. Amitriptyline and trazodone have been effective in treating aggression associated with head injuries and organic mental disorders.

MOOD STABILIZERS. Studies have shown lithium to be effective in the treatment of aggression resulting from mania. Some evidence also shows that lithium may be useful in decreasing aggression resulting from other disorders such as mental retardation, head injuries, schizophrenia, and personality disorders, and in children with conduct disorder. In patients with temporal lobe epilepsy, lithium may actually increase the frequency of aggressive acts.

Carbamazepine has been shown to be effective in managing aggressive behavior in patients with abnormal electroencephalograms (EEGs). In one study eight patients with schizophrenia with abnormal EEGs demonstrated a decrease in aggressive behavior after being treated with carbamazepine despite a previously negative response to neuroleptics. There is also some evidence that carbamazepine may be effective in managing agitated behavior associated with dementia.

ANTIPSYCHOTICS. These drugs have been commonly used for the treatment of aggression. They cause sedation, and it is this sedation rather than the antipsychotic properties that is often effective for treating acute aggressive behavior. If the agitation is the result of delusions, hallucinations, or other psychotic behavior, the antipsychotic properties may be helpful but may take 1 to 2 weeks before their effects may be evident.

OTHER MEDICATIONS. Several case reports have suggested that naltrexone, an opiate antagonist, may reduce self-injurious behavior. This effect is particularly notable in patients with developmental disabilities.

Beta-blockers such as propranolol have also been shown to decrease aggressive behavior in children, adults, and particularly patients with organic mental disorder. Nurses should be aware of the side effects of beta-blockers including hypotension, bradycardia, and in some cases depression.

> **?** *How do the strategies for managing aggressive behavior relate to the theories of aggression described earlier in this chapter?*

CRISIS MANAGEMENT TECHNIQUES

There are times when attempts at early intervention are unsuccessful and more active intervention is necessary. If the patient is exhibiting behavior that is dangerous either to self or others, it may be unsafe to attempt a verbal intervention. This is evident in the following clinical example.

Clinical Example Mr. B was a 32-year-old man with a medical diagnosis of paranoid personality disorder. He was admitted to the locked ward of a psychiatric hospital because he had been arrested after his neighbors complained that he was letting the air out of their tires. He said that he did this because the neighbors laughed at him and talked about him when he was out walking his dog. He was angry about being arrested and wanted to leave the hospital, but he was held under commitment because he also threatened to burn down the house of the neighbor who had called the police.

Mr. B resisted the admission procedure. He belligerently demanded to be released, threatening to call the governor and "sue everybody in the place." When he was asked to undress for a physical examination, he ran down the hall and barricaded himself in the dining room. As staff forcibly entered the room, he began to lash out. Several staff members removed him to a seclusion room, where he was given intramuscular medication and isolated until he regained control of his behavior. He paced the floor and pounded on the door for 30 minutes before he began to appear calmer.

Several days later, when Mr. B was used to the staff and felt more comfortable in the hospital, he related to a nurse, "I hope I didn't hurt you the other night, but I didn't know what you wanted to do to me. A man has to protect himself, you know."

Experience and wisdom are needed to determine when the time for talking is over and when physical intervention is necessary. Nonviolent physical control and restraint should be used only as a last resort. Like medical emergencies, psychiatric emergencies require immediate action.

Team Response

Effective crisis management must be organized and should be directed by one clearly identified crisis leader (Box 29-5).[4] Because psychiatric nurses are responsible for the management of patient care 24 hours a day, it is most appropriate that the crisis leader be a nurse. The leader may be the charge nurse, the primary nurse, nurse manager, or a staff nurse; however, the person should be decided in advance. Other staff members, including physicians, nurses, and counselors, can be used for support. The crisis leader must decide the intervention necessary to ensure the safety of both patients and staff. This decision can be a difficult one to make, especially when the acuity of the situation does not always allow adequate time to discuss all possible strategies with the entire treatment team.

Once the decision to intervene has been made, the crisis leader must obtain assistance to manage the crisis. All members of the crisis team should be trained in crisis management and have experience working as a cohesive group. The staff should be prepared to intervene under the direction of the crisis leader. In many inpatient facilities, hospital security personnel are also notified when assistance is needed. It is the responsibility of the crisis leader to be acquainted with the security officers, give them a brief description of the situation, describe the intervention, and identify the role of security personnel in managing the crisis. Because security officers are not mental health professionals, their assistance should be used only when the patient cannot be physically managed by the nursing staff. Often, there is little time for planning, and the leader must balance the need to act quickly with the need to be organized so that the safety of the patients and the staff is not jeopardized.

The leader is also responsible for ensuring the safety of the other patients during a crisis. This can be accomplished by assigning a staff member to remove the other patients from the area. Quite often the other patients become more acutely distressed in response to a psychiatric emergency on the unit and require extra nursing attention both during and after the crisis. After the crisis has passed, allowing patients to verbalize their anxiety and concern about the crisis and processing it with them can be helpful. It is not appropriate to encourage this activity during a crisis intervention.

A room without furniture should always be readily available for an emergency. If restraints are necessary, they must be obtained from an easily accessible place. To protect the patient and the staff, the leader must assess the situation quickly and devise a plan. This should include a brief explanation to the staff of the patient's behavior and the intervention necessary. The staff members who will be directly involved in the intervention should each be assigned to secure one of the patient's limbs when directed to do so. The leader must also explain to the team what will be said to the patient and on what signal the staff should secure the patient's limbs. As they approach within 6 to 8 feet from the patient, the leader should express concern for the patient's safety and the behavior demonstrated that has caused such concern. The patient should then be escorted to the appropriate room and informed of the necessary intervention. It should be emphasized that the intervention is not a punishment but is being provided to help ensure the safety of the patient and the rest of the unit.

If restraints are to be used, the patient should be asked to lie on the bed with arms at his or her side. Quite often, the presence of several staff is enough to enlist the patient's cooperation. If the patient is unable to cooperate, the patient should be told that the staff will be assisting. Patients often hesitate at this point in their attempt to remain in control. If patients cannot cooperate within several seconds, they may be unable to cooperate at all, and the leader must then direct the staff to restrain the patient as planned. This can be very frightening for patients and they may need several reminders that they will not be hurt but that the staff will protect them from their impulses.

During this time it is critically important that the leader relate to the patient in a calm, steady voice and manner. Any anxiety or ambivalence will be conveyed to the patient and contribute to a feeling of insecurity. A leader who is anxious will be unable to think clearly about the situation. Many patients are afraid of losing control, and they become assaultive not because they want to frighten people but because they themselves are frightened. If the staff shows control of the situation, the patient's agitation is often defused. When the crisis team is overwhelmed by their own fears of the patient, they cannot be effective in reducing the patient's fear. Consistency is also important so that the patient cannot bargain with or manipulate staff members. If the leader is indecisive, inconsistent, or easily manipulated, the patient

---

Box **29-5** *Procedure for Managing Psychiatric Emergencies*

1. Identify crisis leader.
2. Assemble crisis team.
3. Notify security officers if necessary.
4. Remove all other patients from area.
5. Obtain restraints if appropriate.
6. Devise a plan to manage crisis and inform team.
7. Assign securing of patient limbs to crisis team members.
8. Explain necessity of intervention to patient and attempt to enlist cooperation.
9. Restrain patient when directed by crisis leader.
10. Administer medication if ordered.
11. Maintain calm, consistent approach to patient.
12. Review crisis management interventions with crisis team.
13. Process events with other patients and staff as appropriate.
14. Gradually reintegrate patient into milieu.

will not be assured that the staff can guarantee safety by controlling the situation.

After the crisis is over, the team should discuss any concerns they may have had during the crisis because this type of intervention can be stressful for both staff and patients. The patient's behavior may have evoked feelings of guilt, anger, or aggression in the staff. These issues should be discussed as a team so that care is consistent, interventions are therapeutic, and staff do not become discouraged, negative, or burned out. The final intervention is a reevaluation of the patient's status and the gradual reintegration of the patient into the milieu.

Seclusion

There are times when secluding or separating the patient from others in a safe, contained environment is the most appropriate nursing intervention. It is a useful nursing intervention when the goal is to protect a patient, other patients, and staff from potential harm. As such, seclusion is a therapeutic intervention with specific indications for its implementation and anticipated outcomes.

Often staff members may have negative or conflicting views about using restrictive interventions such as seclusion and restraints. They may believe that they will betray the patient's trust and could jeopardize the relationships between the staff and patient. Some staff may believe that it is unethical or nontherapeutic to restrict a patient's freedom.[34] However, used appropriately, seclusion and restraints are legal, ethical, and therapeutic nursing interventions. Seclusion and restraint have been the subject of much discussion in the field. A review of the literature on these interventions supports the following[7]:

▼ Seclusion and restraint are helpful in preventing injury and reducing agitation.
▼ It is nearly impossible to operate a program for severely symptomatic patients without some form of seclusion or physical or mechanical restraint.
▼ Seclusion and restraint can have negative physical and psychological effects on patients and staff and the psychiatric consumer/survivor movement has emphasized these effects.
▼ Demographic and clinical factors have limited influence on rates of seclusion and restraint.
▼ Nonclinical factors such as cultural biases, staff role perceptions, and the attitude of hospital administration have a greater influence on rates of seclusion and restraint.
▼ Training in violence prediction and prevention, self-defense, and implementation of restraints or seclusion is valuable in reducing rates and untoward effects.
▼ Studies comparing well-defined training programs are potentially useful.

Degrees of seclusion vary. They include confining a patient in a room with a closed but unlocked door or placing a patient in a locked room with a mattress but no linens and with limited opportunity for communication. Patients may be dressed in their clothes or in hospital clothing. A mattress and sheet or blanket are the minimally acceptable conditions for seclusion.

The theoretical and clinical rationale for the use of seclusion is typically based on three therapeutic principles:
▼ Containment
▼ Isolation
▼ Decrease in sensory input

Using the principle of *containment,* patients are restricted to a place where they are safe from harming themselves and other patients. *Isolation* addresses the need for patients to distance themselves from relationships that, because of the illness, are pathologically intense. Some patients, particularly those with paranoia, distort the meaning of the interactions around them. Their distortions create such psychic pain that seclusion may provide some relief and may be the only place they feel safe from their "persecutors." Seclusion also provides a smaller area for these patients to master, allowing for a gradual increase in their interactions with others. The third principle is that seclusion provides a *decrease in sensory input* for patients whose illness results in a heightened sensitivity to external stimulation. The quiet atmosphere and monotony of a seclusion room may provide some relief from the sensory overload. Nursing interventions related to seclusion are presented in Box 29-6.

Legal requirements for the care of the secluded patient vary from state to state. Good nursing care includes optimum fulfillment of basic human needs and concern for personal dignity. The nurse must help the patient to meet biological needs by providing food and fluids, a comfortable environment, and opportunity for use of the bathroom. Frequent observation is essential. The room must be constructed so the patient can be observed without being unnecessarily exposed to those who are not involved in his or her care. Staff should be able to communicate with the patient. Careful records should include all nursing care and observation of the isolated patient. The need for continued isolation should be assessed on a regular basis. It may be necessary for the nurse to initiate this review of the patient's condition with other health team members.

There appears to be a gap between the understanding of staff and patients regarding each other's feelings and intentions related to seclusion.[30,38] Therefore, it is recommended that staff spend more time talking with patients about the issues that led to seclusion and alternative methods of coping that might help the patient avoid seclusion in the future.

The nursing staff should always review the events that led up to the decision to isolate a patient. In particular, staff should be encouraged to give each other feedback about interpersonal relationships involving the secluded patient. Preventive measures that may help the patient to gain control in the future without requiring seclusion should be identified. It is also useful for staff to vent their own feelings following an episode of seclusion. Management of violent behavior is physically and emotionally stressful.

Box 29-6 *Nursing Interventions Related to Seclusion*

DEFINITION

Solitary containment in a fully protective environment with close surveillance by nursing staff for purposes of safety or behavior management.

ACTIVITIES

Obtain a physician's order, if required by institutional policy, to use a physically restrictive intervention.

Designate one nursing staff member to communicate with the patient and direct other staff.

Identify for patient and significant others the behaviors that necessitated the intervention.

Explain procedure, purpose, and time period of the intervention to patient and significant others in understandable and nonpunitive terms.

Explain to patient and significant others the behaviors necessary for termination of the intervention.

Contract with patient (as patient is able) to maintain control of behavior.

Instruct on self-control methods as appropriate.

Assist in dressing in safe clothing and removing jewelry and eyeglasses.

Remove all items from seclusion area that patient might use to harm self or nursing staff.

Assist with needs related to nutrition, elimination, hydration, and personal hygiene.

Provide food and fluids in nonbreakable containers.

Provide appropriate level of supervision/surveillance to monitor patient and allow for therapeutic actions as needed.

Acknowledge your presence to patient periodically.

Administer PRN medications for anxiety or agitation.

Provide for patient's psychological comfort as needed.

Monitor seclusion area for temperature, cleanliness, and safety.

Arrange for routine cleaning of seclusion area.

Evaluate at regular intervals patient's need for continued restrictive intervention.

Involve patient, when appropriate, in making decisions to move to a more or less restrictive form of intervention.

Determine patient's need for continued seclusion.

Document the rationale for use of restrictive intervention, patient's response to the intervention, patient's physical condition and nursing care provided throughout the intervention, and rationale for terminating the intervention.

Upon termination of the restrictive intervention, process with the patient and staff the circumstances that led to the intervention as well as any patient concerns about the intervention itself.

Provide the next appropriate level of restrictive intervention (such as physical restraint or area restriction) as needed.

From McCloskey JC, Bulechek GM: *Nursing interventions classification,* ed 2, St Louis, 1996, Mosby.

One of the best ways to understand the patients' point of view is to "walk in their shoes." Arrange to spend 15 minutes alone in the seclusion room on a psychiatric unit. Dare you try on the restraints? Describe your thoughts and feelings.

Restraints

Restraint involves the use of mechanical or manual devices to limit the physical mobility of the patient. Such an intervention may be indicated to protect the patient or others from injury, particularly if less restrictive interventions, such as environmental change and behavioral strategies, have failed.

The American Psychiatric Association[1] has outlined the following five criteria for the appropriate use of physical intervention, seclusion, and restraint:

▼ To prevent imminent harm to the patient or other persons when other means of control are ineffective or inappropriate

▼ To preclude serious disruption of the treatment program or significant damage to the physical environment

▼ To maintain treatment as part of an ongoing plan of behavioral therapy

▼ To decrease the amount of stimulation a patient receives

▼ To comply with a patient's own request

The primary indication for restraints is the control of violent behavior, either self-directed or directed toward others, that cannot be controlled by medication or psychosocial techniques. Patients who benefit from the use of this technique include those whose physical condition prevents or limits the use of medication. For example, a patient who has developed a toxic reaction to anticholinergic medication may require restraints to control problematic behaviors until the toxicity has resolved. For these patients the use of restraints may be less harmful than additional medications. Other indications for the use of restraints include hyperactivity, insomnia, decreased food and fluid intake, and grossly impaired judgment. Restraints may also be used to reduce disruptive effects of excessive stimulation that have resulted in increased agitation and confusion. Finally, patients sometimes request the use of restraints. Their request for external control should be acknowledged but should be differentiated from attempts to gain excessive attention, ensure dependency gratification, or legitimize regression. Each situation should be assessed carefully for the most appropriate and least restrictive intervention. Nursing interventions related to the use of restraints are presented in Box 29-7.

The patient in mechanical restraint may be confused or delirious and will probably be frightened at the limitation of movement. The nurse should not assume that the patient understands the need for restraint. Support and reassurance are essential. Restraints should be applied efficiently and with care not to injure a combative patient. Adequate personnel must be assembled before the patient is approached. Each staff member should be assigned responsibility for controlling specific body parts. Restraints should be available and in working order. Padding of cuff restraints helps to prevent skin breakdown. For the same reason, the patient should be positioned in anatomical alignment. Privacy is important. If visitors are allowed, the nurse should explain the treatment and the reason for it before they see the patient; this may help them accept the situation. Physical

Box *29-7* *Nursing Interventions Related to Physical Restraint*

DEFINITION

Application and monitoring of mechanical restraining devices or manual restraints to limit physical mobility of patient.

ACTIVITIES

Obtain a physician's order, if required by institutional policy, to use a physically restrictive intervention.

Provide patient with a private yet adequately supervised environment in situations where a patient's sense of dignity may be diminished by the use of physical restraints.

Provide sufficient staff to assist with safe application of physical restraining devices or manual restraints.

Designate one nursing staff member to direct staff and communicate with the patient during the application of physical restraints.

Use appropriate hold when manually restraining patient in emergency situations or during transport.

Identify for patient and significant others the behaviors that necessitated the intervention.

Explain procedure, purpose, and time period of the intervention to patient and significant others in understandable and nonpunitive terms.

Explain to patient and significant others the behaviors necessary for termination of the intervention.

Monitor the patient's response to procedure.

Avoid tying restraints to siderails of bed.

Secure restraints out of patient's reach.

Provide appropriate level of supervision to monitor patient and to allow for therapeutic actions as needed.

Provide for patient's psychological comfort as needed.

Provide diversional activities when appropriate (such as television, reading to patient, visitors, mobiles) to facilitate patient cooperation with the intervention.

Administer PRN medications for anxiety or agitation.

Monitor skin condition of restraint sites.

Monitor color, temperature, and sensation frequently in restrained extremities.

Provide for limited movement according to patient's level of self-control.

Position patient to facilitate comfort and prevent aspiration and skin breakdown.

Provide for movement of extremities in patient with multiple restraints by rotating the removal/reapplication of one restraint at a time (as safety permits).

Assist with periodic changes in body position.

Provide the dependent patient with a means of summoning help (such as a bell or call light) when caregiver is not present.

Assist with needs related to nutrition, elimination, hydration, and personal hygiene.

Evaluate, at regular intervals, patient's need for continued restrictive intervention.

Involve patient, when appropriate, in making decisions to move to a more or less restrictive form of intervention.

Remove restraints gradually (that is, one at a time if in four-point restraints) as self-control increases.

Monitor patient's response to removal of restraints.

Upon termination of the restrictive intervention, process with the patient and staff the circumstances that led to the intervention as well as any patient concerns about the intervention itself.

Provide the next appropriate level of restrictive intervention (such as area restriction or seclusion) as needed.

Document the rationale for use of restrictive intervention, patient's response to the intervention, patient's physical condition and nursing care provided throughout the intervention, and rationale for terminating the intervention.

From McCloskey JC, Bulechek GM: *Nursing interventions classification,* ed 2, St Louis, 1996, Mosby.

needs must be included in the nursing care plan. Vital signs should be checked, and regular observation of circulation in the extremities is necessary. Fluids should be offered regularly and opportunities for elimination provided. Skin care is also essential. Restraints must be released at least every 2 hours to allow exercise of the extremities.

Despite explanations of the therapeutic purpose of the intervention, it is not uncommon for patients to perceive the use of restraints as a punishment. This may result in further discomfort in the staff. Designating an authority figure such as the charge nurse as the crisis leader may help to preserve the therapeutic alliance between the patient and the staff members working more closely with the patient.

Terminating the Intervention

The decision to terminate the use of seclusion or restraints should be well planned. Reviewing the behavior that precipitated the intervention and patient's current capacity to exercise control over his or her behavior are key factors. Patients should be told which behaviors they need to exhibit

and which behaviors or impulses they need to control before the intervention can be discontinued. Communication and careful documentation are critical in making an accurate assessment of a patient's level of control. The difficulty arises when patients appear to be in control for brief periods of time but then quickly decompensate. Their behavior may be subject to diurnal variation and changes in response to different staff members.

Patients should be gradually reintegrated into the milieu. This allows them to test their control without feeling overwhelmed. Patients are initially reintegrated by reducing restraints from four points to three points and then to two points as soon as they begin to regain control. However, a patient should not be left in just a one-point restraint because the risk of injury is high. Once restraints have been discontinued altogether, or once a patient no longer requires locked seclusion, the patient may be given a specified amount of time out of the room. This amount of time will be gradually increased as the patient is able to maintain control in the milieu. The primary nurse, in collaboration with the treatment team, can coordinate this into the inter-disciplinary plan of care.

The success of the patient's reintegration into the milieu depends largely on the consistency of the staff. Some staff members may question the need to follow the time-structured outline if the patient appears to be in control. However, if the staff do not see the importance of the plan, neither will the patient, and cooperation will be more diffi-cult to enlist. Some staff may wish to adhere to a structured room program only if the patient decompensates, but pa-tients who are thrust back into a busy unit can be quickly overwhelmed with the sudden increase in stimulation. Sending them to their room after they have lost control again only reinforces their inability to stay in control and is more likely to be viewed by the patient as punishment. Thus, gradual reintegration into the milieu is more likely to ensure the ability of these patients to maintain control and increase their feelings of achievement.

Finally, debriefing is an important part of terminating the use of seclusion or restraints. Debriefing is a therapeu-tic intervention that includes reviewing the facts related to an event and processing the response to them. It provides staff and patients with an opportunity to clarify the ratio-nale for the seclusion, offer mutual feedback, and promote more adaptive functioning.

Debriefing can be used after any stressful event. De-scribe how talking with your friends after an exam can be seen as a kind of debriefing.

STAFF DEVELOPMENT

Effective management of potentially dangerous patients re-quires highly skilled staff. Nurses, physicians, and other sup-port staff, including security personnel, must be trained in emergency psychiatric care and crisis management tech-niques. The use of least restrictive measures for de-escalating patients' behaviors have been found to be effec-tive in decreasing patient assaults and staff injury and reducing the need for seclusion and restraints when staff re-ceive training in nonviolent self-defense skills, alternative interventions, and crisis management techniques.[18,24,31] Ad-herence to the 1996 Joint Commission on Accreditation of Healthcare Organizations (JCAHO) Standards on Restraint and Seclusion should also be an essential part of a staff edu-cation program.[13] Education should focus on assessment of the patient, particularly mental status, motor behavior, af-fect, and speech. Verbal intervention should be stressed as a way of defusing agitation, and helpful and nonhelpful re-sponses should be reviewed.

Education

All nursing interventions should be grounded in theory and current research, and crisis intervention in psychiatric emergencies is no exception. The theoretical basis and sup-

porting research for various intervention strategies should be discussed as part of the training. Pharmacological inter-ventions should be reviewed with particular attention given to the choice of medication, its purpose, and its potential adverse effects. Ongoing practice sessions in crisis manage-ment should be required of all staff. These sessions should include basic self-protection maneuvers and strategies for restraining assaultive patients. Each member of the staff should be able to function as a leader in the event of a crisis, and the staff as a whole must be able to function smoothly as a cohesive emergency team. The nursing and medical care of these patients should be reviewed as well as the impact of countertransference issues. Finally, it is strongly recom-mended that the current state laws regarding the civil rights of patients be discussed in staff meetings to ensure that care given to patients is proper and respectful of their rights.

Staff Assault

Unfortunately, nurses are sometimes assaulted by patients. It is impossible to predict and prevent all episodes of violent behavior in a psychiatric setting. If a staff member is as-saulted, the support and assistance of colleagues are needed.

Poster and Ryan[32] studied the beliefs and concerns of psychiatric nurses about patient assaults and the safety of the work environment. The majority of those surveyed thought that staff members working with mentally ill pa-tients may be physically assaulted during their careers. In addition, 58% agreed that staff members have a right to take legal action against an assaultive patient. The decision to take legal action appears to be influenced by the degree to which the staff member believes that the patient was re-sponsible for his or her actions and capable of controlling impulses.

Nurses who have been assaulted may experience symp-toms such as anger, anxiety, helplessness, irritability, hyper-alertness, depression, shock, or disbelief that the assault oc-curred. It is not unusual for nurses to blame themselves for the assault or to question their competence in managing potentially violent patients. Nurses can be supported by al-lowing adequate time off from work to address their physi-cal and emotional needs. Discussing the event in a non-blaming manner can also be helpful. Validation from others that assaults occur despite clinical competence and appro-priate interventions can help the assaulted nurse in healing. Acknowledging the nurse's right to take legal action against the patient can also be helpful. In fact, many argue that it is therapeutic to bring criminal charges against assaultive pa-tients. Legal action can help patients take responsibility for their behavior, and perhaps decrease future violent episodes. For the assaulted nurse, taking legal action articulates a po-sition that the personal trauma of being physically assaulted should not be an accepted consequence of caring for others.

Another way of helping nursing staff members who have been assaulted is through a peer support group, which le-gitimizes staff responses and allows for the expression of feelings in a supportive setting. A staff action program can also be developed made up of volunteers who work with staff in critical incident debriefing, run support groups, and offer specialized services such as family and community meetings.[8] A final suggestion is the implementation of a nursing consultation support service that responds to the needs of assault victims and sets the tone for institutional attitudes of nonblaming concern.[29] All of these programs have merit and each organization should select the best way to deal with the problem of staff assault based on the environment, group process, and institutional resources.

Summary

1. High rates of assaultive behavior have been reported in a variety of health-care settings including outpatient clinics, nursing homes, and emergency departments. By far the highest rates of assault occur in psychiatric settings.
2. Within each person lies the capacity for passive, assertive, or aggressive behavior. The situation and the characteristics of the person define the most appropriate response.
3. Theories on the development of aggressive behavior include psychoanalytical, psychological, behavioral, sociocultural, and biological.
4. The best single predictor of violence is a history of violence. It is also important to assess the patient's current clinical condition and situation.
5. Nurses need to assess possible precipitants of violent behavior, issues related to provocation, and biological factors. A screening tool may be useful in this process.
6. Many nursing interventions may be helpful in dealing with aggressive behavior, including self-awareness, patient education, assertiveness training, communication strategies, environmental strategies, behavioral strategies, and psychopharmacology.
7. Effective crisis management must be organized and clearly directed by one team leader. Seclusion and restraint should be used only as a last resort.
8. Staff development issues include educating staff in crisis management techniques, working with staff who have been assaulted, and understanding the implications of possible legal action.

COMPETENT CARING A Clinical Exemplar of a Psychiatric Nurse

Mary Brown, RN

When I think about aggressive behavior, I think back to an incident that could have ended badly, but instead the people involved received the help needed. I was working as a case manager for an agency that provided intensive case management for chronically mentally ill people. The event took place on a weekend. Office hours were 9 AM to 5 PM during the week, and there was someone on call after working hours and on all weekends.

I was on call this particular weekend. One of the agency's patients had been hospitalized and was now ready for discharge. This patient was deaf, and I was to pick him up from the hospital and see that he was settled in his home. After I left the hospital with the patient, my beeper went off and I needed to call the answering service. I was close to the office, so I stopped there to use the phone. The building has two stories, and I had access to only the top floor. I climbed the stairs, the discharged deaf patient behind me, unlocked the door, and turned around to shut the door, but a large hand kept me from doing so.

The owner of this big hand was over 6 feet tall, weighed approximately 250 pounds, and appeared to be psychotic. He forced his way into the building with the patient and me. I was now terrified. He stated, "I came to get my money," in an angry and loud tone of voice.

I then recognized him as a patient I had worked with before and could see the changes in him, which made me feel unsafe to be alone with him. I tried very hard not to let him know how

frightened I was of him. I told him the office was closed and he needed to come back Monday, when the appropriate people could help him. He shouted, "I want my money now!" I became increasingly frightened. There was no panic button to push for help. There were no other staff to distract him to allow me to get my deaf patient and myself to safety. I was the one who needed to protect us.

In a calm tone of voice, I told him I couldn't help him with getting his money. I told him I would need to go to the staff room (he was aware that patients were not allowed in this room) and call someone to help him. He followed me into the room. I firmly told him that he was not allowed to be in the room and to please leave. He sat down anyway. I told him I was only at the office to return an emergency call. I called the service and the doctor who paged me was checking to see whether everything went okay with the discharged patient. I told him about the intrusion from the angry and irrational man who was insisting on not leaving before he got his money. The doctor said he would call the police. While waiting for the police, I kept trying to get the patient to leave the room. He repeatedly refused. He sat at one end of the table and I sat at the other end. The deaf patient was watching our interaction intensely.

The angry patient appeared to be responding to internal stimuli. He was looking at me and began to laugh. He stopped laughing and said, "Why won't you go out with me?" as he proceeded to my end of the table. I told him firmly that this behavior was not appropriate. I reinforced that I was his nurse and again I asked him to leave the room. He stopped, looked at me unexpectedly, and said, "I'll be back on Monday to get my money."

When I heard the door slam, I quickly locked the door. The doctor called back to say that the police were on their way and

COMPETENT CARING A Clinical Exemplar of a Psychiatric Nurse—cont'd

asked whether everything was okay. While shivering, I said yes. The police picked the angry patient up downstairs and found a screwdriver on him. He told them that he was at the office before I arrived and intended to break into the office to take his money. The deaf patient who was watching all this communicated with me by writing on a piece of paper, "Are you all right? I can tell you were afraid of him." I was amazed. Nonverbal communication works both ways.

As a nurse, I am trained to look at what is not being said and make a determination. I realized that the deaf patient also could look at my nonverbal communication and make a determination. I also realized the value of setting firm limits and at all times giving clear, consistent, and nonthreatening messages when managing aggressive behavior.

your **INTERNET**
connection

Anger Management, Trauma, and Dissociation
http://www.kumu.com/~grhoades

Blain Nelson's Abuse Pages
http://www.pacificrim.net/~blainn/abuse/

? *Chapter Review Questions*

1. Identify whether the following statements are true (T) or false (F).

A. ___ Patients who are mildly aggressive should be allowed to pace the halls to decrease tension.

B. ___ Overly crowded and stimulated environments may increase aggressive behavior.

C. ___ The psychoanalytical theory of aggression proposes that it is learned through the socialization process as a result of internal and external learning.

D. ___ A patient's diagnosis is a good predictor of future violent behavior.

E. ___ A minority of psychiatric patients are responsible for a majority of the violent incidents.

F. ___ Failing to set effective limits with patients can lead to provocation and assault.

2. Match each term in Column A with the correct definition in Column B.

Column A

___ Assertive behavior

___ Debriefing

___ Limit-setting

___ Passive behavior

___ Restraint

___ Seclusion

___ Token economy

Column B

A. Acting in a way that conveys a sense of self-assurance but also communicates respect for the other person

B. Nonpunitive, nonmanipulative behavior in which someone is told what is acceptable, what is not acceptable, and the consequences of behaving in an unacceptable way

C. Positive reinforcement in which patients are rewarded for performing desired targeted behaviors

D. Separating a patient from others in a safe, contained environment

E. Subordinating one's own rights to the perception of the rights of others

F. Therapeutic intervention that includes reviewing the facts related to an event and processing the response to them

G. Use of mechanical or manual devices to limit the physical mobility of the patient

3. Provide short answers for the following questions.

A. Identify the three areas of the brain that are believed to be involved in aggression.

B. Identify two preventive strategies, two anticipatory strategies, and two containment strategies for managing aggressive behavior.

C. A patient who appears agitated and potentially threatening approaches you. How should you physically position yourself when interacting with this patient?

D. Do you think that physical restraints are more or less restrictive than the use of chemical restraints (medications) with the aggressive patient? Defend your position.

REFERENCES

1. American Psychiatric Association: *Report of the task force on psychiatric uses of seclusion and restraint*, Washington, DC, 1985, The Association.
2. Bensley L et al: Patient and staff view of factors influencing assaults on psychiatric hospital employees, *Issues Ment Health Nurs* 16:433, 1995.
3. Borum R, Swartz M, Swanson J: Assessing and managing violence risk in clinical practice, *J Pract Psychol Behav Health* 2:205, 1996.
4. Cahill C, Stuart G, Laraia M, Arana G: Inpatient management of violent behavior: nursing prevention and intervention, *Issues Ment Health Nurs* 12:239, 1991.
5. Corrigan P, Yudofsky S, Silver J: Pharmacological and behavioral treatments for aggressive psychiatric inpatients, *Hosp Community Psychiatry* 44:125, 1993.
6. Davis S: Violence by psychiatric inpatients: a review, *Hosp Community Psychiatry* 42:585, 1991.
7. Fisher W: Restraint and seclusion: a review of the literature, *Am J Psychiatry* 151:1584, 1994.
8. Flannery R, Fulton P, Tausch J, DeLoffi A: A program to help staff cope with psychological sequelae of assaults by patients, *Hosp Community Psychiatry* 42:935, 1991.
9. Garza-Trevino E: Neurobiological factors in aggressive behavior, *Hosp Community Psychiatry* 45:690, 1994.
10. Gerlock A: Veterans' responses to anger management intervention, *Issues Ment Health Nurs* 15:393, 1994.
11. Harper-Jacques S, Reimer M: Aggressive behavior and the brain: a different perspective for the mental health nurse, *Arch Psychiatr Nurs* 6:312, 1992.
12. Harris D, Morrison E: Managing violence without coercion, *Arch Psychiatr Nurs* 9:203, 1995.
13. Joint Commission on Accreditation of Healthcare Organizations: *Revised standards and scoring guidelines for restraint and seclusion*, Oakbrook Terrace, Ill, 1996, JCAHO.
14. Lancee W et al: The relationship between nurses' limit-setting styles and anger in psychiatric inpatients, *Psychiatr Serv* 46:609, 1995.
15. Lande R: The video violence debate, *Hosp Community Psychiatry* 44:347, 1993.
16. Lanza M et al: Environmental characteristics related to patient assault, *Issues Ment Health Nurs* 15:319, 1994.
17. Love C, Hunter M: Violence in public sector psychiatric hospitals, *J Psychosoc Nurs* 34:30, 1996.
18. Martin K: Improving staff safety through an aggression management program, *Arch Psychiatr Nurs* 9:211, 1995.
19. McNiel D, Binder R: Clinical assessment of the risk of violence among psychiatric inpatients, *Am J Psychiatry* 148:1317, 1991.
20. McNiel D, Binder R: Correlates of accuracy in the assessment of psychiatric inpatients' risk of violence, *Am J Psychiatry* 152:901, 1995.
21. McNiel D, Binder R: The relationship between acute psychiatric symptoms, diagnosis, and short-term risk of violence, *Hosp Community Psychiatry* 45:133, 1994.
22. Menninger W: Management of the aggressive and dangerous patient, *Bull Menninger Clin* 57:208, 1993.
23. Miller R, Zadolinnyj K, Hafner R, Phil M: Profiles and predictors of assaultiveness for different psychiatric ward populations, *Am J Psychiatry* 150:9, 1993.
24. Morales E, Duphorne P: Least restrictive measures: alternatives to four-point restraints and seclusion, *J Psychosoc Nurs* 33:13, 1995.
25. Morrison E: A coercive interactive style as an antecedent to aggression and violence in psychiatric patients, *Res Nurs Health* 15:421, 1992.
26. Morrison E: A hierarchy of aggressive and violent behaviors among psychiatric inpatients, *Hosp Community Psychiatry* 43:505, 1992.
27. Morrison E: The evolution of concept: aggression and violence in psychiatric settings, *Arch Psychiatr Nurs* 3:245, 1994.
28. Morrison E: Toward a better understanding of violence in psychiatric settings: debunking the myths, *Arch Psychiatr Nurs* 7:328, 1993.
29. Murray M, Snyder J: When staff are assaulted, *J Psychosoc Nurs Ment Health Serv* 29:24, 1991.
30. Norris M, Kennedy C: How patients perceive the seclusion process, *J Psychosoc Nurs Ment Health Serv* 30:7, 1992.
31. Phillips D, Ruderstam K: Effect of nonviolent self-defense training on male psychiatric staff members' aggression and fear, *Psychiatr Serv* 46:164, 1995.
32. Poster E, Ryan J: A multiregional study of nurses and patient assault, *Hosp Community Psychiatry* 45:1104, 1994.
33. Sheridan M, Henrion R, Robinson L, Baxter V: Precipitants of violence in a psychiatric inpatient setting, *Hosp Community Psychiatry* 41:776, 1990.
34. Stilling L: The pros and cons of physical restraints and behavior controls, *J Psychosoc Nurs Ment Health Serv* 30:18, 1992.
35. Tam E, Engelsmann F, Fugere R: Patterns of violent incidents by patients in a general hospital psychiatric facility, *Psychiatr Serv* 47:86, 1996.
36. Tardiff K: *Concise guide to assessment and management of violent patients*, Washington DC, 1996, American Psychiatric Press.
37. Tardiff K et al: Violence by patients admitted to a private psychiatric hospital, *Am J Psychiatry* 154:88, 1997.
38. Tooke S, Brown J: Perceptions of seclusion, *J Psychosoc Nurs* 30:23, 1992.
39. US Department of Labor, Bureau of Labor Statistics: *Occupational injuries and illness in the United States by industry 1989*, Bulletin 2379.
40. Volavka J: *Neurobiology of violence*, Washington, DC, 1995, American Psychiatric Press.

Chapter 30

Cognitive Behavioral Therapy

Gail W. Stuart

© 1998 M.C. Escher/Cordon Art, Baarn, Holland.

But humanism stands for the whole person, the whole individual striving to become as conscious and responsible as possible about everything in the universe. But now you sit there quite calmly and as a humanist you say that due to the complexity of scientific achievement the human being must never expect to be whole, he must always be frightened. **Doris Lessing** THE GOLDEN NOTEBOOK

LEARNING OBJECTIVES

After studying this chapter the student should be able to:

▼ **Define behavior**

▼ **Distinguish between classical and operant conditioning**

▼ **Describe operant conditioning procedures that increase and decrease behavior**

▼ **Relate the role of cognitions in adaptive and maladaptive coping responses**

▼ **Compare cognitive behavioral therapy and the nursing process**

▼ **Identify elements of a cognitive behavioral assessment**

▼ **Apply cognitive behavioral treatment strategies to nursing practice**

▼ **Discuss the role of the nurse in cognitive behavioral therapy**

TOPICAL OUTLINE

Definition of Behavior
Classical Conditioning
Operant Conditioning
  Increasing Behavior
  Decreasing Behavior
Role of Cognition
Cognitive Behavioral Therapy and the Nursing Process
Cognitive Behavioral Assessment
Treatment Strategies
  Anxiety Reduction
  Cognitive Restructuring
  Learning New Behavior
Role of the Nurse

Cognitive behavioral therapy is the application of various learning theories to problems of living. The aim is to help people overcome difficulties in any area of human activity and experience. Often, these problems occur within the context of a medical or psychiatric disorder.[10,13,17] However, the techniques of cognitive

behavioral therapy can be applied to education, the workplace, consumer activities, and sports. In these situations cognitive behavioral therapy can help people achieve personal growth by expanding their coping skills. It can be used by nurses with any background and in any health-care setting to promote healthy coping responses and change maladaptive behavior. Thus, it represents an important area of knowledge for nursing intervention across the health-illness continuum.

Cognitive behavioral therapy is problem focused and goal oriented, and deals with here-and-now issues. It views the individual as the primary decision maker about goals and issues to be dealt with in treatment. This chapter reviews the key concepts of cognitive behavioral therapy, the treatment process, and specific strategies that can be used in nursing practice.

DEFINITION OF BEHAVIOR

Behavior is any observable, recordable, and measurable act, movement, or response. Before a behavior can be measured it must be accurately described, which is done in different ways. For example, the behavior of eating can be broken down into parts such as selecting the food items, preparing the meal, setting the table, eating the meal, and cleaning the dishes when the food is eaten. In contrast, it can be more globally described as eating dinner. This shows that there can be several different and accurate definitions of what appears to be a single, simple behavior. It also points to the need to begin by describing what is seen or heard and then clarifying this information until the participants agree with the description.

A behavior is what is observed, not the conclusion, inferences, or interpretations drawn from observation. For example, hyperactivity is not a behavior; it is a conclusion drawn from a set of behaviors. Hyperactivity cannot be measured. What can be measured is the number of times a child gets out of his or her seat, interrupts a conversation, drops a book, or completes required homework assignments. Thus, treatment for the child should focus not on hyperactivity but on the specific behaviors that interfere with the child's adjustment to school, home, or the community.

Other examples of inferences rather than behaviors are psychiatric diagnoses and the labeling of patients as uncooperative, aggressive, difficult, noncompliant, or hostile. These adjectives globally describe a person but do not reflect the specific behavior that led to such conclusions. Similarly, when formulating a nursing diagnosis it is essential that the nurse identify the specific defining characteristics of the nursing diagnosis that apply to the patient. In this way, treatment can address the patient's specific behaviors and problems at that particular time. In addition, the nurse will have recorded specific behaviors that can be measured over time. These can be used to evaluate the patient's progress toward expected outcomes.

A clear definition of a behavior minimizes subjective interpretations. It is measurable, is not subject to interpretation, and states what the person does.

> **?** *Think about your experiences in psychiatric–mental health nursing. In your view, how much treatment is based on inference rather than behavior? What impact does this have on patient adherence with treatment plans?*

CLASSICAL CONDITIONING

Classical conditioning focuses on the process by which **involuntary behavior** is learned. It is derived from Pavlov's[21] famous work in which he taught dogs to salivate at the sound of a bell by associating the bell with meat presented at the same time. The explanation is that an event occurs when one stimulus, by being paired with another stimulus, comes to produce the same response as the other stimulus. Other examples of classical conditioning include the following:

▼ Blinking in response to directing a puff of air to someone's eye
▼ Salivating at the aroma of cookies baking
▼ Automatically raising the leg when the patellar tendon is struck

A clinical example is when a person becomes conditioned to feel fear in neutral situations that have come to be associated with anxiety, such as heights or traveling in public places. However, inconsistent pairings of the two stimuli lead to less reliable learning, and the response gradually disappears if the pairings are discontinued.

OPERANT CONDITIONING

Operant conditioning has been credited to the work of B.F. Skinner and his co-workers.[23] It is concerned with the relationship between **voluntary behavior** and the environment. Operant behaviors are those that are influenced by the consequences of the action and are regarded as a more complex form of learning. Examples include correcting a spelling mistake when writing a letter or studying class notes before an examination. The basic idea is that behaviors are influenced by their consequences and that operant behaviors are cued by environmental stimuli. Behaviors that have a positive consequence will be stronger and are likely to be repeated. In contrast, behaviors that result in negative consequences will be weakened and are less likely to occur.

For example, if a person tells a joke and everyone who is listening to it laughs heartily, the person will probably repeat that joke in another social setting. However, if the person tells the joke and everyone stares blankly or appears quiet and embarrassed, the person will probably not repeat the joke in the future.

Unlike classical conditioning, operant conditioning is strengthened rather than weakened by inconsistent pairings of the behaviors and consequences. That is, when a certain behavior is followed unpredictably by positive or negative consequences, it is more likely to recur.

Many of the techniques used in operant conditioning fall under the heading of **behavior modification.** They are based on the assumption that high-frequency, preferred activity can be used to reinforce lower-frequency, nonpreferred activity. For example, if a boy enjoys playing with toy racing cars, this high-frequency preferred activity can be used to reinforce the lower-frequency, nonpreferred activity of tidying his room. However, the terms *reinforcement* and *punishment* when used in operant conditioning do not have the same meaning as when used by most laypeople.

> **?** *Give an example of classical and operant conditioning from your work in a psychiatric setting related to either patient or staff behavior.*

Increasing Behavior

Reinforcers are anything that increases the frequency of a behavior. By far the most commonly used form of reinforcement is **positive reinforcement,** or rewarding stimuli—for example, when teachers praise students for remaining in their assigned seats. Because of the praise, the students are likely to remain seated more often. However, what is regarded as a positive reward can be quite subjective, and many times people intending to decrease a behavior actually wind up reinforcing it. For example, when a father yells at his son for fighting with his sibling, the yelling may represent to the son a form of desired parental attention and thus may be interpreted as positive reinforcement. As a consequence, the son is likely to continue fighting with his sibling.

Negative reinforcement also increases the frequency of a behavior by reinforcing the behavior's power to control an aversive, rather than rewarding, stimulus. An example is putting on sunglasses in glaring sunlight. The sunlight is an aversive stimulus; putting on the sunglasses is the behavior; escaping the sun's glare is the negative reinforcer. It is negative because it removes or subtracts something from the environment (sunlight), resulting in an increase in the desired behavior (wearing sunglasses). Other examples of negative reinforcement include the following:

▼ A child who is being scolded by his mother goes up to her and kisses her, and her scolding stops.

▼ An adolescent who is having trouble in school runs away from home, thus avoiding his parents' displeasure.

▼ Drivers maintain the speed limit to avoid receiving a traffic ticket.

Decreasing Behavior

Three techniques are used to reduce the frequency of behavior: punishment, response cost, and extinction. **Punishment** is an aversive stimulus that occurs after the behavior and decreases its future occurrence. An example is a child who has to stay in from recess because of disrupting the class.

Response cost decreases behavior through the experience of a loss or penalty following a behavior. Examples include paying a fine for overdue library books, losing allowance for not keeping a clean room, or not being able to attend the next school dance because of coming home after curfew.

Extinction is the process of eliminating a behavior by ignoring it or not rewarding it. For example, a child who has frequent temper tantrums is sent to summer camp. On the first day at camp, the child has a tantrum because of not being allowed to sleep in a specific bunk. The counselor ignores the child and continues to interact with the other campers. In the next 2 days the child has three more tantrums, and the counselor continues to ignore the outbursts. After the fourth day the child has no more temper tantrums.

The procedures of operant conditioning are summarized in Box 30-1. They are incorporated in many cognitive behavioral treatment strategies, and they can be used by nurses in all areas of practice to help patients overcome a wide range of problems and resume productive lives.

> **?** *Do you think the procedures of operant conditioning can be used by nurses working in medical-surgical settings? Give an example from your experience.*

ROLE OF COGNITION

Cognition is the act or process of knowing. The framework for cognitive therapy proposes that it is not the events themselves but people's expectations and interpretations of events that cause anxiety and maladaptive responses. It suggests that maladaptive behaviors can be altered by dealing directly with a person's thoughts and beliefs.[4,5]

Specifically, cognitive therapists believe that maladaptive responses arise from cognitive distortions. These might include errors of logic, mistakes in reasoning, or individualized views of the world that do not reflect reality. Such distortions may be either positive or negative. For example, someone may consistently view life in an unrealistically positive way and thus take dangerous chances, such as denying health problems and claiming to be "too young and healthy for a heart attack." Cognitive distortions also may be negative, as expressed by a person who interprets all unfortunate life situations as proof of a complete lack of self-worth. Common cognitive distortions are listed in Box 30-2.

The goal of cognitive therapy is to alter irrational beliefs, faulty reasoning, and negative self-statements. Research has shown that cognitive therapy is an effective intervention for a wide range of clinical problems, particularly depression, anxiety, and eating disorders. More recently it has shown to

BOX **30-1** *Operant Conditioning Procedures*

INCREASING BEHAVIOR

Procedure: **Positive reinforcement**
Definition: Adding a rewarding stimulus as a consequence of a behavior, thus increasing the probability that it will occur again
Example: Behavior → Rewarding stimulus → Behavior ↑

Procedure: **Negative reinforcement**
Definition: Removing an aversive stimulus as a consequence of a behavior, thus increasing the probability that it will occur again.
Example: Aversive stimulus → Behavior → Aversive stimulus removed → Behavior ↑

DECREASING BEHAVIOR

Procedure: **Punishment**
Definition: Presentation of an aversive stimulus as a consequence of a behavior, thus decreasing the probability that it will occur again.
Example: Behavior → Aversive stimulus → Behavior ↓

Procedure: **Response cost**
Definition: Loss or withdrawal of a reinforcer as a consequence of a behavior, thus decreasing the probability that it will occur again.
Example: Behavior → Loss of reinforcer → Behavior ↓

Procedure: **Extinction**
Definition: Withholding of a reinforcer as a consequence of a behavior, thus decreasing the probability that it will occur again.
Example: Behavior → Reinforcement → Behavior → No reinforcement → Behavior ↓

BOX **30-2** *Cognitive Distortions*

Distortion: **Overgeneralization**
Definition: Draws conclusions about a wide variety of things on the basis of a single event.
Example: A student who has failed an examination thinks "I'll never pass any of my other exams this term and I'll flunk out of school."

Distortion: **Personalization**
Definition: Relates external events to oneself when it is not justified.
Example: "My boss said our company's productivity was down this year, but I know he was really talking about me."

Distortion: **Dichotomous thinking**
Definition: Thinking in extremes—that things are either always good or all bad.
Example: "If my husband leaves me I might as well be dead."

Distortion: **Catastrophizing**
Definition: Thinking the worst about people and events.
Example: "I better not apply for that promotion at work because I won't get it and I'll feel terrible."

Distortion: **Selective abstraction**
Definition: Focusing on details but not on other relevant information.
Example: A wife believes her husband doesn't love her because he works late, but she ignores his affection, the gifts he brings her, and the special vacation they are planning together.

Distortion: **Arbitrary inference**
Definition: Drawing a negative conclusion without supporting evidence.
Example: A young woman concludes "my friend no longer likes me" because she did not receive a birthday card.

Distortion: **Mind reading**
Definition: Believing that one knows the thoughts of another without validation.
Example: "They probably think I'm fat and lazy."

Distortion: **Magnification/minimization**
Definition: Exaggerating or trivializing the importance of events.
Example: "I've burned the dinner, which goes to show just how incompetent I am."

Distortion: **Perfectionism**
Definition: Needing to do everything perfectly to feel good about oneself.
Example: "I'll be a failure if I don't get an A on all my exams."

Distortion: **Externalization of self-worth**
Definition: Determining one's value based on the approval of others.
Example: "I have to look nice all the time or my friends won't want to have me around."

be of value in working with people who have psychotic disorders.[14] Finally, it can be used in inpatient, outpatient, and psychosocial rehabilitation treatment programs.[27,28] It is also true that psychiatric nurses spend a good deal of time assessing and analyzing patients' cognitions, including how patients view themselves and how they see themselves in relation to their world. Thus, interventions that include principles of cognitive therapy have much to contribute to psychiatric nursing practice.[3,7]

> **?** *Give an example from your personal experiences of each cognitive distortion listed in Box 30-2. What was the consequence of each distortion, if any?*

COGNITIVE BEHAVIORAL THERAPY AND THE NURSING PROCESS

There are many misperceptions about cognitive behavioral therapy. One misperception is that it is controlling of the patient. Another misperception is that relationship factors are neglected in the treatment process. Neither of these perceptions is true.[5] The major characteristics of cognitive behavioral therapy are listed in Box 30-3.

Cognitive behavioral therapy is totally patient centered. It views the person as a unique individual who has a problem of living rather than a psychopathological condition. Cognitive behavioral therapists may seem more accepting of patients because patients' problems are not viewed with suspicion about subconscious motivation or irrational underlying dynamics. Maladaptive behaviors, as well as adaptive coping responses, are believed to be acquired through the process of learning. Thus much emphasis is placed on behavioral monitoring and the completion of homework by the patient. Rather than trying to remove problems by changing subconscious dynamics, the cognitive behavioral therapist works with the patient to plan experiences that encourage the development of new skills.

Another important characteristic is the high degree of mutuality in the treatment process. Cognitive behavioral therapists do not control the patient. Rather, they collaborate with the patient in defining the problem, identifying goals, formulating treatment strategies, and evaluating progress. Because the focus is on the patient's self-control, cognitive behavioral therapy is seen as educational and skill building rather than curative, with the therapist taking a facilitative role. Genuineness, warmth, empathy, and the therapeutic relationship are important, and full recognition is given to their significance in influencing the effectiveness of treatment.

From this overview it is evident that cognitive behavioral therapy has many things in common with the nursing process. The steps of the nursing process closely resemble the steps involved in cognitive behavioral therapy. Similarly, both approaches are patient centered and strongly empha-

---

Box **30-3** *Characteristics of Cognitive Behavioral Therapy*

The patient and therapist focus on defining and solving current problems of living. They discuss the here and now, not the history of the patient.

Dysfunctional behavior is attributed to maladaptive learning. Relearning more adaptive responses is the goal of the treatment.

Collaboration with the patient and active participation by the patient in the treatment process are the norm. Cognitive behavioral therapy helps people to change. The patient does the changing, not the therapist.

The therapeutic process is open and explicit. The patient and the therapist share an understanding of what is going on in treatment.

It is a scientific and patient-centered approach that uses a rigorous assessment process to define the problems and environmental factors that influence the problems.

Explicit treatment goals are identified by the patient and therapist. They are then used to evaluate the patient's progress and treatment outcome.

Treatment strategies are derived from clinical and experimental research. Emphasis is placed on validating the appropriateness of treatment strategies implemented.

The patient is often given homework assignments for data collecting, skill practice, and reinforcement of new responses.

Baseline measurements of the problem behavior are made during the assessment process. These measurements are repeated at regular intervals during and at the completion of treatment. Thus, the treatment process is rigorously monitored.

Change and progress in treatment must be meaningful to the patient and have a positive impact on the quality of the patient's life.

---

size mutuality. Finally, cognitive behavioral therapy places a strong emphasis on an objective assessment process. Specifically, it uses standardized measurement tools, bases treatment strategies on research evidence, and values ongoing evaluation of patient progress.

These characteristics suggest that cognitive behavioral therapy can make a significant contribution to the therapeutic effectiveness of nursing care. Thus, it has relevance for psychiatric nurses practicing in any setting and with any patient population.

COGNITIVE BEHAVIORAL ASSESSMENT

Cognitive behavioral therapy places great importance on assessment.[22,24] In this process there is little interest in personality traits, defensive styles, personality dynamics, or dispositions. Instead, cognitive behavioral therapists assess the patient's actions, thoughts, and feelings in particular situations. Assessment includes collecting information, identifying problems from the data, defining the problem behavior, deciding how to measure the problem behavior, and identifying environmental variables that influence the problem behavior. It also includes a review of the patient's strengths and deficits and minimizes the use of assumptions and unvalidated inferences.

It is noteworthy that nurses most often form conclusions about the physiological problems of patients only after using a variety of tools and tests to collect objective evidence. However, nurses dealing with psychosocial problems often forget to use the scientific approach and base their care on unsubstantiated inferences. The cognitive behavioral assessment, in contrast, is based on validation and supporting evidence through the use of observation, interviewing, and measurement.

It is important that the problem be defined as clearly as possible. Initially the nurse addresses the following questions:
▼ What is the problem?
▼ Where does the problem occur?
▼ When does the problem occur?
▼ Who or what makes the problem occur?
▼ What is the feared consequence related to the problem? The nurse can then assess the problem's frequency, intensity, and duration.

The next step is to find out more about the patient's experience with the problem. This is determined by using a behavioral analysis (Fig. 30-1), which consists of the following three parts (**the ABCs of behavior**):
▼ **Antecedent:** the stimulus or cue that occurs before behavior that leads to its occurrence
▼ **Behavior:** what the person does or does not say or do
▼ **Consequence:** what kind of effect (positive, negative, or neutral) the person thinks the behavior has
Antecedents can include the physical environment, the social environment, or the person's behavior, feelings, or thoughts. Behaviors can also be broken down into discrete actions or series of steps. Finally, consequences can be viewed as powerful rewards or punishments of a person's actions. Thus they are critical elements of the assessment. An example of a behavioral analysis is as follows:
▼ Problem = Anxiety
▼ Feared consequence = Fear of losing control or dying
▼ Antecedent = Leaving the house
▼ Behavior = Avoiding stores, restaurants, and public places
▼ Consequence = Restriction of daily activities
Another way of assessing a person's experiences is to consider the three systems (**the ABCs of treatment**) that are interrelated in this treatment framework:
▼ **Affective:** emotional or feeling responses
▼ **Behavioral:** outward manifestations and actions
▼ **Cognitive:** thoughts about the situation

Fig. 30-2 shows that these three elements are interrelated in explaining human behavior because:
▼ Feelings influence thinking.
▼ Thinking influences actions.
▼ Actions influence feelings.
An assessment of each one of these areas has important implications for understanding the problem and effectively treating it.

Another aspect to be considered in the assessment process is whether the problem is expressed as observable behavior and whether it is current and predictable. Mutually agreed on treatment goals and strategies can then be determined. Finally, throughout the treatment process, cognitive behavioral therapists use various methods to measure problem severity. These may include case-specific measures as well as standardized rating scales. Chapter 6 discusses psychological evaluation and measurement issues in greater detail.

> **?** *Are standardized rating scales used by staff working with patients in your mental health setting? If so, how are they used? If not, how would they influence patient care?*

TREATMENT STRATEGIES

Cognitive behavioral therapy has been shown to be effective for treating a variety of clinical problems across all age groups. These include anxiety, affective, eating, schizophrenic, substance abuse, and personality disorders.[6] It is useful in working with children, adolescents, adults, elderly, and families and may be implemented both individually and in groups. In general, cognitive behavioral treatments include techniques aimed at the following:
▼ Increasing activity
▼ Reducing unwanted behavior

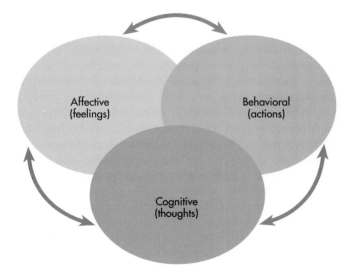

Fig. 30-2 Interacting systems in human behavior.

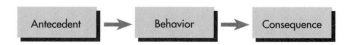

Fig. 30-1 Phases of behavior.

▼ Increasing pleasure
▼ Enhancing social skills

The three groups of cognitive behavioral treatment strategies are listed in Box 30-4. These techniques may be used alone or in combination. They also require practical skills and efforts from both the nurse and patient. This may include activities outside the office setting such as taking a bus ride, riding an elevator, or going to a supermarket.

Anxiety Reduction

RELAXATION TRAINING. As a therapeutic tool, relaxation training effectively decreases tension and anxiety. It can be used alone, in combination with other cognitive behavioral techniques, or in addition to supportive or insight therapy. The basic premise is that muscle tension is related to anxiety. If tense muscles can be made to relax, anxiety will be reduced.

The various relaxation procedures all involve rhythmic breathing, reduced muscle tension, and an altered state of consciousness. Clinical experience suggests that there are individual differences in the experience of relaxation. Not everyone demonstrates all of the characteristics of a relaxed physiological state. The physiological, cognitive, and behavioral manifestations of relaxation are listed in Box 30-5.

Relaxation training involves the tensing and relaxing of voluntary muscles in an orderly sequence until the body, as a whole, is helped. The patient should be seated in a comfortable chair. Soft music or pleasant visual cues may be present. Before beginning the exercises, a brief explanation should be given about how anxiety is related to muscle tension. The relaxation procedure should also be described.

The patient begins by taking a deep breath and exhaling slowly. A sequence of tension-relaxation exercises is then begun. The patient is instructed to tense each muscle group for about 10 seconds while the nurse describes how tense and uncomfortable this body part feels. The nurse then asks the patient to relax this muscle group, as the nurse comments, "Notice how all the hardness and tension is draining from your hands. Now notice how they feel—warm, soft, and calm. Compare this feeling to when they were tense and see how much better they feel now." The patient should be reminded to tense only the muscle group named. The patient then proceeds to the next muscle group in the sequence listed in Box 30-6.

The final exercise asks the patient to become *completely* relaxed, beginning with the toes and moving up through the body to the eyes and forehead. When the patient learns the procedure, exercises can be performed only for the muscles that usually become tense. This is different for each person and may include the shoulders, forehead, back, or neck. Patients may also eliminate the tensing exercises and perform only the relaxation ones.

Systematic relaxation may be followed or replaced by another approach to evoke the relaxation response: *meditation*. The basic components for meditation include the following:
▼ A quiet environment
▼ A passive attitude
▼ A comfortable position
▼ A word or scene to focus on

The first three components are necessary for any relaxation procedure. The fourth component refers to the process in

---

Box **30-4** *Cognitive Behavioral Treatment Strategies*

ANXIETY REDUCTION
Relaxation training
Biofeedback
Systematic desensitization
Interoceptive exposure
Flooding
Vestibular desensitization training
Response prevention
Eye movement desensitization

COGNITIVE RESTRUCTURING
Monitoring thoughts and feelings
Questioning the evidence
Examining alternatives
Decatastrophizing
Reframing
Thought stopping

LEARNING NEW BEHAVIOR
Modeling
Shaping
Token economy
Role playing
Social skills training
Aversive therapy
Contingency contracting

Box **30-5** *Manifestations of Relaxation*

PHYSIOLOGICAL
Decreased pulse
Decreased blood pressure
Decreased respirations
Decreased oxygen consumption
Decreased metabolic rate
Pupil constriction
Peripheral vasodilation
Increased peripheral temperature

COGNITIVE
Altered state of consciousness
Heightened concentration on single mental image
Receptivity to positive suggestion

BEHAVIORAL
Lack of attention to and concern for environmental stimuli
No verbal interaction
No voluntary change of position
Passive movement easy

Box **30-6** *Sequence of Progressive Muscle Relaxation*

1. **Hands.** First the fists are tensed and relaxed, then the fingers are extended and relaxed.
2. **Biceps and triceps.** These are tensed and relaxed.
3. **Shoulders.** They are pulled back and relaxed and then pushed forward and relaxed.
4. **Neck.** The head is turned slowly as far to the right as possible and relaxed, then turned to the left and relaxed. It is then brought forward until the chin touches the chest and relaxed.
5. **Mouth.** The mouth is opened as wide as possible and then relaxed. The lips form a pout and then relax. The tongue is extended out as far as possible and then relaxed, then retracted into the throat and then relaxed. It is pressed hard into the roof of the mouth and relaxed, then pressed hard into the floor of the mouth and relaxed.
6. **Eyes.** They are opened as wide as possible and relaxed, then closed as hard as possible and relaxed.
7. **Breathing.** The patient inhales as deeply as possible and relaxes, then exhales as much as possible and relaxes.
8. **Back.** The trunk of the body is pushed forward so that the entire back is arched, then relaxed.
9. **Midsection.** The buttocks muscles are tensed and then relaxed.
10. **Thighs.** The legs are extended and raised about 6 inches off the floor and then relaxed. The backs of the feet are pressed into the floor and relaxed.
11. **Stomach.** It is pulled in as much as possible and relaxed, then extended and relaxed.
12. **Calves and feet.** With legs supported, the feet are bent with the toes pointing toward the head and then relaxed. Feet are then bent in the opposite direction and relaxed.
13. **Toes.** The toes are pressed into the bottom of the shoes and relaxed. They are then bent to touch the top inside of the shoes and relaxed.

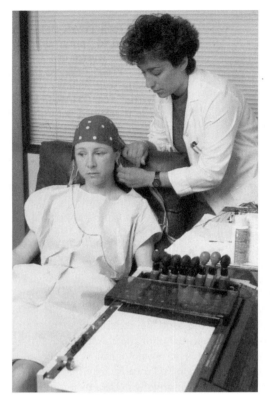

Fig. 30-3 This woman, using biofeedback, can reduce the pain of a migraine headache by learning to lower the temperature of her forehead. (Courtesy Melanie Brown/Photo Edit.)

which the patient selects a cue word or scene with pleasant connotations. The nurse then instructs the patient to close both eyes, relax each of the major muscle groups, and then begin repeating the word silently at each exhalation.

> **?** *Name four clinical settings in which nurses can use relaxation training with patients. Identify whether it would be a primary, secondary, or tertiary prevention activity in each setting.*

BIOFEEDBACK. Biofeedback uses a machine to reduce anxiety and modify behavioral responses. Small electrodes connected to the biofeedback equipment are attached to the patient's forehead (Fig. 30-3). Brain waves, muscle tension, body temperature, heart rate, and blood pressure can then all be monitored for small changes. These changes are communicated to the patient by auditory and visual means. The more relaxed the patient becomes, the more pleasant

sounds or sights are presented. These stop when the patient stops relaxing and resume when the patient reachieves the relaxed state. After developing the ability to relax, the patient is encouraged to apply the technique in stressful situations.

SYSTEMATIC DESENSITIZATION. Systematic desensitization was designed to decrease avoidance behavior linked to a specific stimulus such as heights or airplane travel. The goal of systematic desensitization is to help the patient change the response to a threatening stimulus. It involves combining deep muscle relaxation with imagined scenes of situations that cause anxiety. The assumption is that relaxation is incompatible with anxiety. So if the person is taught to relax while imagining such scenes, the real-life situation that the scene depicted will cause much less anxiety.

With systematic desensitization the patient must first be able to relax the muscles. Additional steps are then taken. Next, a hierarchy of the anxiety-provoking or feared situations is constructed. These are ranked from 1 to 10 in order of difficulty, with 1 evoking little or no anxiety and 10 evoking intense or severe anxiety. Box 30-7 presents a sample hierarchy of a patient with agoraphobia.

With *in vitro*, or imaginal, desensitization, the patient proceeds with the imagined pairing of the hierarchy items

Box **30-7** *Sample Patient Hierarchy for Phobias*

A hierarchy of phobias is a list of your fears and avoidances in order of severity. Your greatest phobia should be at the top of the list and your smallest fear at the bottom. In between, rank your other fears and phobias in order of severity. Try to list 10 but not more than 20 phobias. These activities should be convenient to do, as you will be doing them from several times a day to at least several times per week.

For example, think of yourself standing at the end of a football field marked off in 10 yard lines. Closest to you, at the 0 yard line, is something you are mildly fearful of or avoid doing sometimes but not always; the farthest end of the field is your biggest fear; at the 50 yard line is a medium fear; and on the 10 yard line is a minor fear but one that is stronger than at the 0 yard line.

Remember that everyone's hierarchy will be different. There are no "right" or "wrong" hierarchies. Your hierarchy is a tool to help you approach feared situations in a systematic and controlled way.

SAMPLE HIERARCHY

100	Driving alone across a high bridge in the rain
90	Driving alone on the interstate far from home
80	Driving alone on side streets that are unfamiliar
70	Speaking in front of groups of people
60	Using elevators alone
50	Eating in restaurants alone
40	Going to large public gatherings with safe people
30	Eating with friends or family in familiar restaurants
20	Driving more than several miles from home with a passenger in the car
10	Going shopping with a safe person in big stores and malls
0	Going shopping with a safe person in small stores near home

with the relaxed state, progressing from the least to the most anxiety provoking. *In vivo* desensitization exposes the patient to real rather than imagined life situations. In vivo exposure is widely considered to be the treatment of choice for simple and social phobias, as well as for obsessive-compulsive disorders.

This technique works through a combination of positive reinforcement for confronting anxiety-provoking stimuli and the extinction of maladaptive behavior by realizing that the feared negative consequences never occurred. It is helpful for the nurse to share the following thoughts with the patient during exposure therapy:

▼ Anxiety is unpleasant but is not dangerous; that is, the patient will not die or lose control.

▼ Anxiety does eventually decrease and does not continue indefinitely.

▼ Practice makes perfect, and the more the patient repeats a particular exposure exercise the easier it becomes.

For example, a boy may have a fear of spiders. His daily schedule may then include a series of planned activities involving reading about spiders. He may then begin gradual exposure to pictures and photographs of spiders, followed by looking at real spiders in his yard. Thus the exposure gradually leads to anxiety reduction and more adaptive behaviors.

INTEROCEPTIVE EXPOSURE. This is an exposure technique used to desensitize people to catastrophic interpretations of their internal bodily cues, such as tachycardia, blurred vision, and shortness of breath. A hierarchy is made of the specific symptoms that cause them to have increased anxiety. The patient is then asked to do the things that cause the symptoms in a gradually increasing, repetitive manner in order to desensitize them to these cues. Patients can be asked to jump in place, run up a flight of stairs, or spin in circles. This technique is especially helpful for patients who do not have agoraphobia but have spontaneous, unprovoked panic attacks that cause them increased worry and anxiety.

FLOODING. Flooding is another form of exposure therapy in which the patient is immediately exposed to the most anxiety-provoking stimulus instead of being exposed gradually or systematically to a hierarchy of feared stimuli. If this technique uses an imaginary as opposed to real life event, it is called implosion.

VESTIBULAR DESENSITIZATION TRAINING. This is an exposure therapy for patients whose panic attacks are provoked by environmental cues that cause them to have symptoms of motion sickness such as dizziness, imbalance, vertigo, nausea, tinnitus, blurred vision, or headache. These environmental cues can include a sudden change of position, walking on floors with patterns, walking down a grocery store aisle that is stacked high with products on both sides, or riding in a car on a hilly road. A desensitization hierarchy is created that includes activities that cause these symptoms, such as getting up suddenly from a prone position, sudden head movements, or sudden stop-and-go movements. Patients who get motion sickness when standing in a wide open space with no object to break the horizon are taught to turn in a full circle, keeping their eyes on a selected object for orientation, much like ballet dancers must do when they turn repetitively.

RESPONSE PREVENTION. In response prevention the patient is encouraged to face a particular fear or situation without engaging in the accompanying behavior. It is based on the concept that repeated exposure to the anxiety-producing stimulus without the presence of the anxiety-reducing response will lead to a reduction in the anxiety because the feared consequence does not occur.

For example, a patient may fear using a public restroom and engage in hand washing up to 20 times a day. With response prevention treatment, the patient's daily schedule would include using a public restroom, turning on the water faucets, and washing hands for only 30 seconds. Over time, the maladaptive behaviors would be reduced because the feared consequence of germs and illness did not occur.

EYE MOVEMENT DESENSITIZATION. This therapy is beginning to gain attention, although there are few research reports in the literature to date. The principle behind this treatment is that during early traumatic experiences, the brain lays down biological memory tracks that are provoked later during seemingly unrelated events, causing anxiety and perhaps depression. The patient is asked to think about past traumatic events while the therapist moves his or her hand back and forth in front of the patient's face while the patient's eyes follow. In this way, the neural tracks are hypothesized to become reprogrammed to be less sensitized to anxiety-provoking experiences. Special training is needed before the therapist can use this technique.

> **?** *Do you think a highly anxious nurse can effectively implement anxiety-reduction strategies with patients? Why or why not?*

Cognitive Restructuring

MONITORING THOUGHTS AND FEELINGS. Changing cognitions begins with the identification of what is reinforcing and maintaining the patient's dysfunctional thinking and maladaptive behavior. An important first step is for patients to heighten their self-awareness and monitor their own thinking and feeling. Patients can be helped to do this through the use of the Daily Record of Dysfunctional Thoughts Form. This consists of five columns (Fig. 30-4): the situation, feelings, automatic thoughts in response to the situation, the more rational response, and the outcome or consequence. Through the use of such a form patients are taught to distinguish between thoughts and feelings and to identify adaptive responses to the situation. They also begin to recognize the connection between certain thoughts and maladaptive emotions and behaviors.

QUESTIONING THE EVIDENCE. The next step is for the patient and therapist to examine the evidence that is used to support a certain belief. Questioning the evidence also involves examining the source of the data. Patients with distorted thinking often give equal weight to all sources or ignore all data except those that support their distorted thinking. Having patients question their evidence with staff, family, and other members of their social support network can clarify misinformation and result in more realistic and appropriate interpretations of the evidence.

EXAMINING ALTERNATIVES. Many patients see themselves as having lost all options. This is particularly evident in suicidal patients. Examining alternatives involves working with patients to generate additional options based on patients' strengths and coping resources.

DECATASTROPHIZING. Decatastrophizing is also called the what-if technique. It involves helping patients to evaluate whether they are overestimating the catastrophic nature of a situation. Questions that the nurse can ask include,

Date	Situation Describe: 1. Actual event leading to unpleasant emotion, or 2. Stream of thoughts, daydream, or recollection, leading to unpleasant emotion	Emotion(s) 1. Specify sad, anxious, angry, etc. 2. Rate degree of emotion, 1-100.	Automatic Thought(s) 1. Write automatic thought(s) that preceded emotion(s). 2. Rate belief in automatic thought(s) 0-100%.	Rational Response 1. Write rational response to automatic thought(s). 2. Rate belief in rational response 0-100%.	Outcome 1. Rerate belief in automatic thought(s), 0-100%. 2. Specify and rate subsequent emotions, 0-100.

Explanation: When you experience an unpleasant emotion, note the situation that seemed to stimulate the emotion. (If the emotion occurred while you were thinking, daydreaming, etc., please note this.) Then note the automatic thought associated with the emotion. Record the degree to which you believe this thought: *0%,* not at all; *100%,* completely. In rating degree of emotion: *1,* a trace; *100,* the most intense possible.

Fig. 30-4 Daily Record of Dysfunctional Thoughts. (From Beck A, Rush A, Shaw B, Emery G: *Cognitive therapy of depression,* New York, 1979, Guilford.)

"What is the worst thing that can happen?" "Would it be so terrible if that really took place?" "How would other people cope with such an event?" The goal of this intervention is to help the patient see that the consequences of life's actions are generally not "all or nothing" and thus are less catastrophic.

REFRAMING. Reframing is a strategy that changes a patient's perception of a situation or behavior. It involves focusing on other aspects of the problem or encouraging a patient to see the issue from a different perspective. Patients who dichotomize events may see only one side of a situation. Weighing the advantages and disadvantages of maintaining a particular belief or behavior can help patients gain balance and develop a new perspective. By understanding both the positive and negative consequences of an issue, the patient can attain a broader perspective of it. For example, suggesting that a mother's overinvolvement with her son is actually a sign of her loving concern may help a family see the situation in a new light.

This strategy also creates an opportunity to help challenge the meaning of a problem or behavior because once the meaning of a behavior changes, the person's response will also change.[8] For example, it might involve helping a patient see an adversity as a potentially positive event. The loss of a job may be perceived as a stressor, but it can also be viewed as an opportunity for pursuing a new job or career.

> **?** *Think of a problem you encountered in the past year. How might you have used the technique of cognitive reframing to see the situation in a more positive way?*

THOUGHT STOPPING. Dysfunctional thinking can often have a snowball effect on patients. What begins as a small or insignificant problem can, over time, gather importance and momentum that can be difficult to stop. The technique of thought stopping is best used when the dysfunctional thought first begins. The patient can picture a stop sign, imagine a bell going off, or envision a brick wall to stop the progression of the dysfunctional thought.

To begin, the patient identifies the problematic thought and talks about it as the problem scene is imagined. The nurse interrupts the patient's thoughts by shouting "STOP." Thereafter the patient learns to interrupt thoughts in a similar way. Finally, the patient converts the "stop" into an inaudible phrase or image and thus learns to use the technique quietly in everyday situations.

Learning New Behavior

MODELING. Modeling is a strategy used to form new behavior patterns, increase existing skills, or reduce avoidance behavior. The target behavior is broken down into a series of separate stages that are ranked in order of difficulty or distress, with the first stage being the least anxiety provoking. The patient then observes a person modeling the behavior that the patient finds difficult in a controlled environment. After this, the patient imitates the model's behavior. In participant modeling the model and patient perform the behavior together before the patient does so alone. It is particularly important that the model selected for this treatment be credible to the patient for the treatment to be most effective.

SHAPING. Shaping induces new behaviors by reinforcing behaviors that approximate the desired behavior. Each successive approximation of the behavior is reinforced until the desired behavior is attained. Skillful use of the technique requires that the nurse carefully look, wait, and reinforce. The nurse needs to look for the desired behavior, wait until it occurs, and then reinforce it when it does occur. An example of this strategy is when the nurse notices that an aggressive child is playing cooperatively with a peer and then praises the child for this behavior.

TOKEN ECONOMY. Token economy is a form of positive reinforcement used most often on a group basis with children or psychiatric hospital inpatients.[9,11] It consists of rewarding the patient in various ways, such as with tokens, passes, or points for performing desired target behaviors. Behaviors might include hygienic grooming, attending classes, or verbally expressing frustration rather than striking out at others. Tokens also may be lost for inappropriate behaviors. If tokens or points are used, they may periodically be cashed in for rewards such as free time, off-unit outings, games, or sugarless candy.

ROLE PLAYING. Role playing allows patients to rehearse problematic issues and obtain feedback about their behavior. It can provide practice for decision making and exploring consequences. A related practice is role reversal, in which the patient switches roles with someone else and thus experiences the difficult situation from another point of view.

SOCIAL SKILLS TRAINING. Smooth social functioning is central to most human activity, and social skill problems exist in many psychiatrically ill patients. This technique is based on the belief that skills are learned and therefore can be taught to those who do not have them. The principles of skill acquisition include:

▼ Guidance
▼ Demonstration
▼ Practice
▼ Feedback

These principles must be included in implementing an effective social skills training program, which is often a component of psychiatric rehabilitation programs (see Chapter 14). Guidance and demonstration are usually used early in the treatment, followed by practice and feedback. Treatment typically follows four stages:

1. Description of the new behavior to be learned
2. Learning of new behavior through the use of guidance and demonstration
3. Practice of the new behavior with feedback
4. Transfer of the new behavior to the natural environment

The types of behaviors that are often taught in these programs include asking questions, giving compliments, making positive changes, maintaining eye contact, asking others for specific behavior change, speaking in a clear tone of voice, and avoiding fidgeting and self-criticism. This treatment strategy is most often used with patients who lack social skills, assertiveness (assertiveness training), or impulse control (anger management) and those with antisocial behavior.[1]

AVERSION THERAPY. Aversion therapy helps to reduce unwanted but persistent maladaptive behaviors. Aversive conditioning applies an aversive or noxious stimulus when a maladaptive behavior occurs. An example is for a patient to snap a rubber band on the wrist when being bothered by an intrusive thought. Covert sensitization is an aversive technique in which patients imagine scenes that pair the undesired behavior with an unpleasant consequence. By imagining aversive consequences for a behavior such as overeating, the patient gains control by providing a form of punishment for his or her own behavior.

> **?** *Aversive therapy has sometimes been criticized as unethical and detrimental to patients' well-being. Do you agree? If not, what conditions should be present before implementing aversive therapy with patients?*

CONTINGENCY CONTRACTING. Contingency contracting involves a formal contract between the patient and the therapist, defining what behaviors are to be changed and what consequences follow the performance of these behaviors. Included are positive consequences for desirable behaviors and negative consequences for undesirable behaviors.

ROLE OF THE NURSE

Much of the history of behavioral therapy started in the United States. The first report of nurses functioning as behavioral therapists came in 1959, when Ayllon and Michael[2] taught nurses to use operant skills to modify the behavior of patients in long-term psychiatric institutions. It was believed that nurses were a natural choice because they made up the majority of the staff caring for the patients. Since that time, the practice of behavioral therapy nursing has been more dominant in Britain than in the United States.

In 1975 Isaac Marks, a psychiatrist and researcher in London, established the first program to prepare nurses to be behavioral therapists working with little or no supervision. The clinical outcomes these nurses achieved were at least as good as those obtained by other professionals. Thus it was established that nurses could be prepared to be effective therapists.[19] Marks also calculated the cost-benefit ratio of employing nurses as behavioral therapists. He found that people treated by nurses used fewer health-care resources after treatment than before, resulting in a significant savings of resources.[16] These were impressive findings, and behavioral therapy became an increasingly important component

of the nurse's role in England and Scotland in the years that followed.

In contrast, cognitive behavioral therapy must be more aggressively integrated into the role of the psychiatric nurse in the United States.[25] For example, nurses are the frontline providers of care. They are the group most often called on to carry out selective reinforcement, modeling, extinction, skills training, shaping, and role playing. Because of their direct patient contact, nurses are best able to observe patients, assess problem areas, and recommend targets for cognitive behavioral intervention. However, few nurses are skilled in the principles and techniques of cognitive behavioral therapy.

There are many possible reasons for this (see Critical Thinking about Contemporary Issues). First, nurses may have little formal exposure to cognitive behavioral treatment strategies in the course of their education. Second, nurses have been traditionally reinforced for their unconditional nurturance of patients and their compliance with physicians' orders. In contrast, cognitive behavioral therapy

---

CRITICAL THINKING *about* **Contemporary Issues**

Does Humanistic Nursing Care Promote Maladaptive Patient Behaviors?

Many assume that humanistic nursing care is always therapeutic and health promoting. However, some research that examined the traditional caring orientation of nursing suggests that this notion should be reconsidered. One early study reported that psychiatric patients who demonstrated desirable or nonproblematic behavior were largely ignored by the nursing staff.[15] Conversely, nurses gave a great deal of attention to those who were perceived as sicker or who exhibited disturbed behavior. Another study of the interactional dimensions of the inpatient milieu found that nursing practice in the psychiatric inpatient setting did not regularly promote confirming or open patient-staff interactions.[12] The authors suggest that this interpretation of humanistic care results in the unintentional reinforcement of maladaptive behaviors and the promotion of the sick role.

Two other studies shed further light on this issue. The first examined unit structure on a therapeutic milieu and found that the highest rates of nurse-patient interaction occurred on highly structured units that were based on a behavioral treatment program.[18] The second study compared the effectiveness of the treatment programs of three units: a traditional program, a milieu therapy program, and a social learning program.[20] The social learning program was particularly effective in reducing dangerous and aggressive acts. It also increased the cognitive, social, and instrumental functioning of the patients, prevented rehospitalization in 97% of discharged patients, and was the most cost effective. Although there are few studies in this area, they do suggest the need for psychiatric nurses to reevaluate the basis of their caregiving and treatment activities and to frame their interventions from a more cognitive behavioral and social learning perspective.

requires the use of independent judgment, limit setting, reframing, and selective use of rewards that may not be encouraged for nurses in clinical settings. Third, American nurses have placed great emphasis on the therapeutic use of self, whereas British nurses have assumed a more pragmatic approach to nursing care. The American approach to nursing has sometimes created confusion between the concepts of caring and treatment. It incorrectly suggests that these are different events, with nurses responsible for caring and physicians responsible for treating.

Current changes in the scope and functions of contemporary psychiatric nursing practice underscore the need for all nurses to learn cognitive behavioral therapy skills.[26] Contemporary psychiatric nursing practice includes both caring and treating activities. The reality is that nurses have always been involved with helping patients reduce anxiety, change cognitions, and learn new behaviors. As influential agents of behavioral change, nurses need to be aware of their ability to promote adaptive or maladaptive responses and increase their skills and knowledge in effective treatment strategies.

There are three basic roles for nurses involved in cognitive behavioral therapy. Each of these roles can be performed by all nurses at various levels of expertise, ranging from novice through generalist and specialist. They include

▼ Direct patient care
▼ Planning treatment programs
▼ Teaching others the use of cognitive behavioral techniques

Psychiatric nurses provide direct patient care in both inpatient and community settings, and the value of cognitive behavioral therapy is evident throughout the continuum of care. Most treatments are ideally suited to community settings, and they can include interventions across the continuum of coping responses from promoting health, to intervening in acute illness, to fostering rehabilitation. Nurses also may function as planners and coordinators of complex treatment programs, consultants, and teachers of other nurses, professionals, patients, and their families. It is clear that with the current emphasis on cost-effective treatment and documented outcomes of care, cognitive behavioral therapy will be a growing area of expertise for all psychiatric nurses in the next decade.

Summary

1. Cognitive behavioral therapy is aimed at helping people overcome difficulties in any area of human experience. Behavior is any observable, recordable, and measurable act, movement, or response. It is what is observed, not the conclusions drawn from the observation.

2. Classical conditioning focuses on the processes by which involuntary behavior is learned.

3. Operant conditioning focuses on the processes by which voluntary behavior is learned, including increasing and decreasing behavior.

4. Cognitive therapists believe that maladaptive responses arise from cognitive distortions, and the goal of therapy is to correct faulty thinking that underlies behavioral problems.

5. Cognitive behavioral therapy is similar to the nursing process in that both are patient centered, emphasize mutuality, and place a strong emphasis on measurement of progress and evaluation.

6. Cognitive behavioral assessment includes collecting information, identifying problems, defining the problem, deciding how to measure the problem, and identifying environmental variables that influence the problem behavior.

7. A variety of cognitive behavioral treatment strategies may be used alone or in combination. They focus on anxiety reduction, cognitive restructuring, and learning new behavior.

8. Three basic roles for nurses involved in cognitive behavioral therapy are direct patient care, planning treatment programs, and teaching others the use of behavioral techniques. These roles may be enacted by all nurses in various practice settings.

COMPETENT CARING A Clinical Exemplar of a Psychiatric Nurse

Darcy O'Neill, RN

I first met A, a 13-year-old girl, when she was admitted to our combined child and adolescent psychiatric unit by her mother. Her mother reported that A was becoming increasingly oppositional, refusing to attend school, having sexual relations with multiple partners, running away from home for long periods, and exhibiting destructive outbursts when confronted. A was admitted to our unit following a 3-day runaway. She appeared tired and disheveled, somewhat older than her chronological age, and was extremely angry about hospitalization. However, despite her angry demeanor, it was rapidly apparent that A was a very bright and charming young girl. I was intrigued.

During this hospitalization A continued to have unpredictable violent outbursts. At times the most benign redirection would result in verbal threats, screaming, and cursing, which would often escalate into physical attacks on staff. At other times, a similar or more emphatic directive would be calmly accepted and performed. I was puzzled and rather frustrated by trying to balance

Continued

COMPETENT CARING A Clinical Exemplar of a Psychiatric Nurse—cont'd

this child's need to express some deeply felt anger while maintaining the safety of the milieu.

Our unit uses a token economy as part of a patient's treatment. Patients earn points, or stickers, depending on age and cognitive abilities, for attending activities and participating in treatment. Points are earned as rewards and they may then be exchanged for special privileges. Although we specialize in short-term assessment and evaluation, many children quickly engage in this token economy and are able to address behavioral issues in a direct and timely fashion. Unfortunately, A was not one of these children. Her participation in the point system was as unpredictable and sporadic as her behavior.

The team began to discuss the therapeutic effectiveness of an individually designed behavioral program for A. As a new graduate nurse who knew little about the use of behavioral therapies, I balked. I felt that what A needed was more one-to-one time to process the strong emotions underlying her behavior. A and I were beginning to have regular but brief interactions in which she began to share some of her feelings. I feared that by making a more concrete program, obviously different from the program her peers experienced, we risked alienating a child who already had great difficulties with trust. I also feared that from a position of frustration we were falling into a punitive stance. Unfortunately, A was discharged to an outpatient program before the formulation of a new behavioral program. It seemed that many of my questions concerning the therapeutic value of special behavioral programs would remain unanswered.

After I had been on the unit for 6 months A was readmitted. At this admission her mother reported an increase in the severity and frequency of the behaviors that had precipitated A's first admission. In the time that passed since her first admission, I had had quite a few opportunities to work with individually designed behavioral programs. I had begun to appreciate this therapeutic approach and understand that for many children these programs provided a sense of security and an opportunity to address their problem behaviors more concretely. What I had not understood at the time of A's first admission was that these programs increase the amount of one-to-one while helping children in taking more control of their behavior. I had discovered that behavioral programs provided the framework for increased teaching and learning.

From the outset of her second admission, A was increasingly difficult to reach. She had become more physically and verbally threatening. I continued to try to engage her in the point system, with moderate success.

A was even more unpredictable. At one minute she was willing to discuss her emotions and open to nurturance and support, while at the next she was isolated and violent, with no tolerance of any perceived frustration. I was quickly exasperated. I truly liked this charming, bright young girl who showed me through her behavior that she was in a great deal of pain. Many times after a violent or threatening outburst she would cry inconsolably, curled in the fetal position, appearing much younger than her 13

years. I agonized along with the team members on how to help this child out of a self-destructive downward spiral.

Quickly, the team returned to the discussion of a special behavioral program. Almost as quickly staff became divided on how to best design and implement this program. Individual philosophies, differing levels of appreciation for behavioral therapies, and personal limits and tolerances were shared in numerous discussions. With A's full participation and tenuous acceptance, a preliminary program was designed and implemented. Within 3 days some minor improvements were noted. However, they were buried in continually violent and impulsive behavior. It took a great deal of painstaking discussion for staff to identify the positive behavior changes and suggest appropriate modifications in the behavior plan in an effort to increase these positive behaviors. Unfortunately, this was not effective for A, and within the next few days she needed seclusion to remain safe.

Again, the team reassessed the program and decided to adopt a more concrete contract with A. By either exhibiting new positive behaviors or refraining from old negative behavior, A could earn immediate rewards. The hope was to extinguish the dangerous, self-destructive behaviors while replacing them with new coping strategies. Again, the changes were subtle and erratic, surrounded by what appeared to be setbacks. This program necessitated hypervigilance on the part of staff to be aware of any positive change, no matter how slight.

I recall one time I was attempting to process with A after she was placed in open seclusion after threatening staff. I found myself desperately searching for positive feedback to offer her. All I could immediately identify was total frustration with her behavior and the program, in addition to my own feelings of inadequacy. Yet, as I reviewed her behavioral contract I was able to see a number of significant changes. She had walked to seclusion independently, she needed only one directive to go to the seclusion room, and she was able to sit there without swearing at or threatening me. As soon as I realized all the changes I was witnessing I became elated. Although she was still unable to talk with me, I continued to state how impressed I was by her ability to eliminate these behaviors. I made a point of sharing this information with passing staff, loud enough for A to hear. With time she was able to process what had happened and reintegrate into the milieu.

Through this trying, challenging experience I feel I was able to grow professionally and personally. I learned in a very deep way the therapeutic necessity of a fully functioning interdisciplinary team, and my integral role on that team. But more important, I gained a new respect for behavioral programs and the opportunities they offer not only patients but for nurses. A well-designed behavioral program provides numerous opportunities for teaching, one-to-one relationship building, and a framework for continual assessment, planning, and evaluation. Although the desired outcomes may be slow in coming and the process difficult, I readily look forward to the next opportunity to creatively use my skills in designing and implementing a behavioral treatment program.

your **INTERNET**
c o n n e c t i o n

National Association of Cognitive-Behavioral Therapists (NACBT)
http://www.nacbt.org/

Behavior On Line
http://www.behavior.net

Chapter Review Questions

1. Match each term item in Column A with the correct definition in Column B.

Column A

___ Behavior

___ Biofeedback

___ Contingency contracting

___ Extinction

___ Flooding

___ Punishment

___ Shaping

___ Social skills training

___ Systematic desensitization

___ Reframing

Column B

A. An aversive stimulus that decreases behavior

B. Any observable, recordable, measurable act or response

C. Combines deep muscle relaxation with imagined scenes of situations that cause anxiety

D. Immediate exposure to one's most anxiety-provoking stimulus

E. Induces new behaviors by reinforcing behaviors that approximate the desired behavior

F. Involves a formal contract between the patient and the therapist, defining behaviors to be changed and the consequences

G. Monitors brain waves and body activities, allowing a patient to modify behavioral responses

H. Process of eliminating a behavior by ignoring or not rewarding it

I. Strategy used to modify or change a person's perception of a situation or behavior

J. Technique for learning new behavior that consists of guidance, demonstration, practice, and feedback

2. Fill in the blanks.

A. A person's pupil constricting when exposed to bright sunlight is an example of _____.

B. Putting on sunscreen lotion to avoid a sunburn is an example of _____.

C. The three operant conditioning techniques used to decrease behavior are _____, _____, and _____.

D. Cognitive therapy proposes that it is not the event itself but a person's _____ of the event that causes adaptive or maladaptive responses.

E. A list of a person's fears, avoidances, or maladaptive responses in order of severity is called a _____.

F. The three roles for nurses involving cognitive behavioral therapy are _____, _____, and _____.

3. Provide short answers for the following questions.

A. Analyze the nursing assessment form you use in your clinical work from the perspective of a cognitive behavioral therapist. What changes would you make from this perspective?

B. Describe the ABCs of behavior and the ABCs of cognitive behavioral treatment.

C. For 2 days use the daily record of dysfunctional thoughts and evaluate its value for your work with patients.

D. Try the steps of relaxation training on yourself. Note your thoughts, feelings, and behaviors during the process.

REFERENCES

1. Aschen S: Assertion training therapy in psychiatric milieus, *Arch Psychiatr Nurs* 11:46, 1997.
2. Ayllon T, Michael J: The psychiatric nurse as a behavioral engineer, *J Exp Anal Behav* 2:323, 1959.
3. Barker P: Cognitive therapy model: principles and general application. In Reynolds W, Cormack D, editors: *Psychiatric and mental health nursing,* London, 1990, Chapman & Hall.
4. Beck A: *Cognitive therapy and the emotional disorders,* Philadelphia, 1976, Center for Cognitive Therapy.
5. Beck J: *Cognitive therapy: basics and beyond,* New York, 1995, Guilford.
6. Bellack A, Hersen M: *Handbook of behavior therapy in the psychiatric setting,* New York, 1993, Plenum.
7. Blair DT: Cognitive behavioral therapies within the biological paradigm, *J Psychosoc Nurs* 34:26, 1996.
8. Blise M: Radical positive reframing, *J Psychosoc Nurs* 33:18, 1995.
9. Corrigan P: Use of a token economy with seriously mentally ill patients: criticisms and misperceptions, *Psychiatr Serv* 46:1258, 1995.
10. Deale A et al: Cognitive behavior therapy for chronic fatigue syndrome: a randomized controlled trial, *Am J Psychiatry* 154:408, 1997.
11. Dickerson F et al: Seclusion and restraint, assaultiveness, and patient performance in a token economy, *Hosp Community Psychiatry* 45:168, 1994.
12. Emrich K: Helping or hurting: interacting in the psychiatric nursing milieu, *J Psychosoc Nurs Ment Health Serv* 27:12, 1989.
13. Esterling B: Coping with cancer: psychosocial problems and treatment approaches, *J Pract Psychiatry Behav Health* 2:350, 1996.
14. Fowler D, Garety P, Kuipers E: *Cognitive behavior therapy for psychosis,* New York, 1995, Wiley.
15. Gelfand D, Gelfand S, Dobson W: Unprogrammed reinforcement of patients' behavior in a mental hospital, *Behav Res Ther* 5:201, 1967.
16. Ginsberg G, Marks I: Costs and benefits of behavioral psychotherapy: a pilot study of neurotics treated by nurse therapists, *Psychol Med* 7:685, 1977.
17. Greenberger D, Padesky C: *Mind over mood,* New York, 1995, Guilford.
18. Hodges V, Sandford D, Elzinga R: The role of ward structure on nursing staff behaviors, *Acta Psychiatr Scand* 73:6, 1986.
19. Marks I, Hallam R, Connolly J, Philpott R: *Nursing in behavioral psychotherapy,* London, 1977, Royal College of Nursing.
20. Paul G: Residential treatment programs and aftercare for the chronically institutionalized. In Mirabi M, editor: *The chronically mentally ill: research and services,* New York, 1984, Luce.
21. Pavlov I: *Conditioned reflexes,* London, 1927, Oxford University Press.
22. Richards D, McDonald B: *Behavior psychotherapy: a handbook for nurses,* Oxford, 1990, Heinemann Nursing.
23. Skinner B: *Science and human behavior,* New York, 1953, Free Press.
24. Stern R, Drummond L: *The practice of behavioral and cognitive psychotherapy,* Cambridge, 1991, Cambridge University Press.
25. Stuart G, Laraia M: Panic disorder with agoraphobia. In McBride A, Austin J, editors: *Psychiatric–mental health nursing,* Philadelphia, 1996, WB Saunders.
26. Wakefield M, Pallister R: Cognitive behavioral approaches to panic disorder, *J Psychosoc Nurs* 35:12, 1997.
27. Wright J et al: *Cognitive therapy with inpatients,* New York, 1993, Guilford.
28. Zipple A et al: Cognitive therapy interventions in psychosocial rehabilitation, *Innovations Res* 3:25, 1994.

ANNOTATED SUGGESTED READINGS

Beck J: *Cognitive therapy: basics and beyond,* New York, 1995, The Guilford Press.
    Provides a solid basic foundation for the practice of cognitive therapy. Excellent and highly recommended.
Greenberger D, Padesky C: *Mind over mood,* New York, 1995, The Guilford Press.
    Well-written cognitive therapy treatment manual written especially for patients. Clear and practical.
*Hampton M: Dialectical behavior therapy in the treatment of persons with borderline personality disorder, *Arch Psychiatr Nurs* 11:96, 1997.
    Describes the use of dialectical behavior therapy, which is a form of cognitive-behavioral therapy, and its effectiveness in reducing inpatient hospital days, suicide attempts, and therapy attrition.
*Jensen L, Kane C: Cognitive theory applied to the treatment of delusions of schizophrenia, *Arch Psychiatr Nurs* 6:335, 1996.
    Specific stages and techniques of cognitive therapy in the treatment of schizophrenia are discussed with theoretical underpinnings and suggestions for incorporation in advanced practice psychiatric nursing.
Oumette P, Finney J, Moos R: Twelve-step and cognitive-behavioral treatment for substance abuse: a comparison of treatment effectiveness, *J Consult Clin Psychol* 2:230, 1997.
*Scahill L et al: Inpatient treatment of obsessive-compulsive disorder in childhood: a case study, *J Child Psychiatric Nursing* 6:5, 1993.
    Describes the use of behavioral therapy techniques by nurses working on a child inpatient unit. Clear discussion of theory with a case study.
Wright J et al: *Cognitive therapy with inpatients: developing a cognitive milieu,* New York, 1993, The Guilford Press.
    Explains the use of cognitive therapy with inpatients and their families, adolescents, depressed elderly, alcoholics, and patients with eating disorders. Contains good chapter on the role of psychiatric nurses in implementing a cognitive milieu.
Zipple A et al: Cognitive therapy interventions in psychosocial rehabilitation, *Innovations Res* 3:25, 1994.
    Good description of the application of cognitive therapy interventions in psychosocial rehabilitation programs.

*Nursing reference.

Therapeutic Groups

Paula C. LaSalle and Arthur J. LaSalle

© 1998 M.C. Escher/Cordon Art, Baarn, Holland.

Self and world are correlated, and so are individualization and participation. . . .
Participation means: being a part of something from which one is, at the same time,
separated. **Paul Tillich** *THE COURAGE TO BE*

LEARNING OBJECTIVES	TOPICAL OUTLINE
After studying this chapter the student should be able to:	**Definition**
▼ **Define a group**	**Components of Small Groups**
▼ **Identify and describe the components of a small group**	Group Structure
	Group Size
▼ **Compare the stages of group development**	Length of Sessions
▼ **Describe small group evaluation factors**	Communication
▼ **Discuss the responsibilities and qualities of nurses as group leaders and the types of groups they lead**	Group Roles
	Power
	Norms
	Cohesion
	Group Development
	Pregroup Phase
	Initial Phase
	Working Phase
	Termination Phase
	Evaluation of the Group
	Nurses as Group Leaders
	Groups with Co-Leaders
	Nurse-Led Groups

A group provides nurses with a potentially more therapeutic modality than the two-person nurse-patient encounter. It offers its members a variety of relationships as they interact with each other and with the group leader. Group members come from many backgrounds and must "deal with their likes, dislikes, similarities, dissimilarities, envy, timidity, aggression, fear, attrac-tion, and competitiveness."[21] All of this takes place in the context of the dynamics of the group process in which, with careful leadership, members give and receive feedback about the meaning and effect of their various interactions with each other.

Groups can be conducted in a variety of settings including inpatient units, community and university health centers, schools, churches, and places of employment. Families of people with serious mental illness may join a group for instruction, assistance with coping, mutual support, and crisis intervention. School nurses may lead groups for children who share developmental milestones or life problems, such as parental divorce or death. In each of these situations the format, setting, and goal of the group would vary. Thus group work is an important skill for all nurses to master, regardless of their practice setting or specialty area.

> **?** *Think of some specific patient situations in which a group approach would be more useful than an individual nurse-patient encounter. Discuss the reasons for this. Describe other situations in which a group format would be less helpful.*

DEFINITION

A **group** is a collection of people who have a relationship with one another, are interdependent, and may have common norms. Therapeutic groups have a shared purpose. For example, a group's purpose might be to help members who consistently enter destructive relationships identify and change maladaptive behaviors. Each group has its own structure and identity. The power of the group lies in the contributions of each member and the leader to the shared purpose of the group. These contributions are content and process oriented.

Content functions of the group are met when members share their experiences to help another member. When members share the methods they used to solve a common problem, they are addressing the group's content functions.

Process functions allow the individual to receive feedback from other members and the leader about how the member interacts and is perceived within the group. The group is used as a laboratory or arena to see, experiment, and define relationships and behaviors. For example, a member who complains that his wife is always accusing him of being domineering may receive feedback from the group as to whether others see him acting similarly. Then he has the opportunity to work on changing his behavior in the group before risking the change in the outside world.

The group has primary and secondary tasks. The primary task is necessary for the group's survival or existence; secondary tasks may enhance the group but are not basic to its survival. An example of a primary task for a group of mothers might be to improve mothering skills; a secondary task might be to add to the mothers' social network. Relationships in the group may limit or enhance their willingness to share concerns about mothering.

COMPONENTS OF SMALL GROUPS

To be effective in therapeutic group work, it is necessary to understand the complex processes that occur and be able to

TABLE **31-1** *Components of Small Groups*

COMPONENTS	CHARACTERISTICS
Group structure	The group's underlying order; includes boundaries, communication, and decision-making processes, as well as authority relationships; offers stability and helps regulate behavior and interactional patterns.
Group size	Preferred size is 7 to 10 members.
Length of sessions	Optimum length of a session is 20-40 minutes for lower-functioning groups and 60-120 minutes for higher-functioning groups (divided into time for a brief warm-up, work time, and a brief wrap-up).
Communication	Feedback is used to help members identify group dynamics and communication patterns.
Roles	Determined by behavior and responsibilities assumed by the members of the group.
Power	Ability to influence the group and other members.
Norms	Standards of behavior in the group; influence communication and behavior; communicated overtly or covertly.
Cohesion	The strength of the members' desire to work together toward common goals; related to group's attraction and member satisfaction.

use various approaches to increase the therapeutic potential of the group for its members. The components of small groups are summarized in Table 31-1. This chapter focuses on these processes and approaches only as they relate to small groups. The study of large groups, such as community meetings, is beyond the scope of this chapter.

Group Structure

Group structure is the group's underlying order. It describes the boundaries, communication and decision-making processes, and authority relationships within the group. The structure offers the group stability and helps to regulate behavioral and interactional patterns.

Group Size

The preferred size of an interpersonally oriented group is 7 to 10 members. The group must have enough people to give members the opportunity for consensual validation as well as the expression of different viewpoints. If the group has too many people, not all members will be given enough time to speak and some will feel excluded. There will also be insufficient time to analyze and discuss interactions. If the group has too few members, not enough sharing and interaction may occur.

Length of Sessions

The optimum length of a session is 20 to 40 minutes for lower-functioning groups and 60 to 120 minutes for higher-functioning ones. For the latter groups a few minutes are spent warming to the task of working, then most of the session is spent on group work, and finally the group summarizes and takes care of unfinished business from that session.

Communication

One of the group leader's primary tasks is to observe and analyze the communication patterns within the group. Using feedback, the leader helps members become aware of the group dynamics and communication patterns so that they may realize the significance of these patterns for the group and for themselves. The group or individual members may then experiment and change these patterns if they choose.

Observable verbal and nonverbal elements of the group's communication include:

▼ Individual member communications
▼ Spatial and seating arrangements
▼ Common themes expressed by the group
▼ How often and to whom members communicate
▼ How members are listened to in the group
▼ What problem-solving processes occur in the group

These behaviors help the leader assess resistance within the group, interpersonal conflict, the roles assumed by some of the members, the level of competition, and how well the members understand and are working on the task.

Group Roles

In studying groups it is important to observe the roles that members assume in the group. Each role has certain expected behaviors and responsibilities.

The role a member takes can be determined by observing communication and behavioral patterns. The following factors influence role selection: the member's personality, the interaction in the group, and the member's position in the group. In their classic work Benne and Sheats[2] described three major types of roles people can play in groups:

▼ **Maintenance roles,** which involve group processes and functions
▼ **Task roles,** which deal with completing the group's task
▼ **Individual roles,** which are not related to the group's tasks or maintenance; they may be self-centered and distracting for the group

These roles are summarized in Table 31-2. A person who acts as a harmonizer and peacemaker would be taking a maintenance role. A person in the task role of questioner might clarify and seek new information.

Members may experience a conflict when there is a difference between the role they seek or assume and the role given to them by the group. For example, a member may be expected to be a peacemaker because of having performed that role previously. Now, however, this member may be under additional stress or angry with someone in the group and may choose to start rather than resolve conflict. The group will often be confused and upset by this new role.

TABLE 31-2 *Group Roles and Functions*

Role	Function
MAINTENANCE ROLES	
Encourager	To be a positive influence on the group
Harmonizer	To make/keep peace
Compromiser	To minimize conflict by seeking alternatives
Gatekeeper	To determine level of group acceptance of individual members
Follower	To serve as an interested audience
Rule maker	To set standards for group behaviors (such as time and dress)
Problem solver	To solve problems to allow group to continue its work
TASK ROLES	
Leader	To set direction
Questioner	To clarify issues and information
Facilitator	To keep the group focused
Summarizer	To state current position of the group
Evaluator	To assess performance of the group
Initiator	To begin group discussion
INDIVIDUAL ROLES	
Victim	To deflect responsibility from self
Monopolizer	To actively seek control by incessant talking
Seducer	To maintain distance and gain personal attention
Mute	To seek control passively through silence
Complainer	To discourage positive work and vent anger
Truant/latecomer	To invalidate significance of the group
Moralist	To serve as judge of right and wrong

Modified from Benne KD, Sheats P: *J Soc Issues* 4:41, 1948.

> **?** *Consider the last group of which you were a member. Identify the roles that were taken by each group member. Which helped and which interfered with task accomplishment? Give an example of the behavior that was associated with each role.*

Power

Power is the member's ability to influence the group and its other members. The power structure in the group is usually resolved in its initial stages. To determine the power of various members, it is helpful to assess which members receive the most attention, which are listened to most, and which make decisions for the group.

Resolution of the power struggle does not necessarily mean that everyone will be satisfied with the arrangement. Sometimes a continual struggle for power occurs. This may be functional if the members are trying to gain new leadership that contributes to their therapeutic goals. It can be dysfunctional when it takes the group's energy and attention away from other tasks.

Norms

Norms are standards of behavior. They are expectations of how the group will act in the future based on its past and present experiences. It is important to understand norms because they influence the quality of communication and interaction within the group. The observance of norms results in conforming. The member who does not follow the norms may be considered rebellious or resistant by the other group members. Conforming to group norms is essential to being a fully accepted member. A member who is always late to meetings is not conforming to group norms. The group will decide to what extent it will tolerate this behavior.

Norms are created to:

▼ Facilitate accomplishment of the group's goals or tasks
▼ Control interpersonal conflict
▼ Interpret social reality
▼ Foster group interdependence

Norms may be communicated overtly or covertly. Overt expression of norms may be written or clearly stated. For example, members may tell a new member that smoking is not allowed in the group. Covert expression of norms may be implied through members' behavior. For example, a member who uses foul language may be ignored by the other members. It must be noted that a highly cohesive group may have appropriate or inappropriate norms. For example, a group of patients may unite to help a patient sneak a cigarette when such behavior is contraindicated because of that patient's health problems. The group may also unite to do what it can to prevent that patient from smoking.

One area that is important for a group to address is confidentiality. For a group to be most effective, members will talk about issues that may be painful, embarrassing, or disturbing. The group members need to agree that whatever is discussed in the group belongs to the group. Group content will not be discussed outside of the group unless there is specific discussion and agreement about it. This norm should be communicated overtly and some groups may even want members to sign an agreement of confidentiality.

> **?** *Identify and describe group norms that you have observed in a selected clinical setting and in the classroom. Did anyone deviate from a norm? How did the group respond? How did the leader respond?*

Cohesion

Cohesion is the strength of the members' desire to work together toward common goals. It influences members to remain in the group. It is related to each member's attraction to and satisfaction received from the group. Cohesion is a basic fiber of any group because it affects its life span and success. Many factors contribute to the level of cohesion, including agreement of members on group goals, interpersonal attractiveness between the members, degree to which the group satisfies individual needs, similarities among members, and satisfaction of members with the leadership style. Because cohesion is such an important dimension, some group leader interventions are aimed toward promoting it. These may include encouraging members to talk directly with each other, discussing the group in "we" terms, and encouraging all members to sit within the space reserved for the group. A leader can also promote cohesion by pointing out similarities among group members, helping members listen to each other, and encouraging cooperation among the members.

The group leader continually monitors the level of cohesion in the group. Group leaders might observe how much members express interest in each other and recognize each other for their individuality. Another way to measure cohesion is to find out whether members identify with the group and whether they want to remain in the group.

GROUP DEVELOPMENT

Groups, like individuals, have capacity for growth and development. Likewise, they have the ability to regress and resist working effectively. Stages of development have been described for small groups in several classic works. Bennis and Sheppard[3] theorized that the central concepts of group development are dependency and interdependency.

Schutz[16] stated that every group develops according to a series of three interpersonal stages: inclusion, or being in or out; control, or being top or bottom; and affection, or being near or far. Each stage is characterized by members expressing various aspects of the same interpersonal issue or conflict.

Tuckman[18] believed that any group is concerned with the completion of its task. He referred to the group structure as the interpersonal relationships among the members and task activity as the interactions directly related to the task. Tuckman summarized the various phases of group development as **forming, storming, norming,** and **performing.** Table 31-3 summarizes Tuckman's model.

Group development does not occur in distinct phases. Phases may overlap, and a group may regress to a previous phase. For example, group regression can occur when a new member is added. Phases of group development can be thought of as a path that a group takes to form and accomplish its objectives. The leader's task is to understand and assist the group as it moves along its growth path.

Pregroup Phase

An important factor to consider in starting a group is its goals. The group's purpose will greatly influence many of the leader's behaviors. There may be more than one group

TABLE **31-3** *Developmental Phases in Small Groups*

TUCKMAN PHASE	YALOM PHASE	DEFINITION	TASK ACTIVITY	INTERPERSONAL ACTIVITY
Forming	Initial orientation	Group members concerned with orientation	To identify task and boundaries regarding it	Relationships tested; interpersonal boundaries identified; dependent relationship with leaders, other group members, or preexisting standards established.
Storming	Initial conflict	Group members resistive to task and group influence	To respond emotionally to task	Intragroup conflict.
Norming	Initial cohesion	Resistance to group overcome by members	To express intimate personal opinions about task	New roles adopted; new standards evolved in group feelings; cohesiveness developed.
Performing	Working	Creative problem solving done; solutions emerge	To direct group energy toward completion of task	Interpersonal structure of group becomes a tool to achieve its task; roles become flexible and functional.

Modified from Tuckman B: *Psychol Bull* 63:384, 1965.

goal; if so, the primary goal should be clear. To guarantee success, the group's goals must be understood by all people involved, including the members and sponsoring agencies. It is the leader's role to clarify the task and help the group achieve it. An example of a group goal for survivors of spouse abuse would be to provide support for each member.

Once the purpose is established, the leader must be sure that the group has administrative permission. A written group proposal is one effective way to request this. Box 31-1 lists information to include in a group proposal. To avoid possible problems, the leader should explore any administrative limitations. For example, an agency may not permit a group to meet beyond its physical facilities or may prefer that the leader not use certain techniques in the group. Also, any potential cost to the agency should be clearly identified.

The leader is also responsible for finding physical space for the group. The leader identifies the room requirements of the group. For example, in a patient education group resources such as a blackboard or movie projector may be needed. A psychotherapy group may need space for comfortable chairs to be placed in a circle without a table. In a group that plans to use human relations exercises, a more spacious room will probably be needed. In all cases the group room should be comfortable, private, and quiet. The same room should be used for each meeting. Leaders often have to adapt inadequate space to fit the needs of the group. The session itself is more important than where it is conducted.

The next responsibility of the group leader is to select members. The selection is based on the purposes of the group, referrals to the group, and interviews with potential members. The leader or the agencies must provide information about the group to potential sources of referrals. All information should clearly identify the group's purpose and

Box **31-1** *Group Proposal Guideline*

List the group goals, primary and secondary.
List group leaders and their related expertise.
List theoretical frameworks used by the leaders to meet the group goals.
List criteria for membership.
Describe the referral and screening process.
Describe the structure of the group.
   Meeting place _____
   Meeting time _____
   Length of each meeting _____
   Number of members _____
   Length of group _____
   Expected member behaviors _____
   Expected leader behaviors _____
Describe the evaluation process for members and the group.
Describe resources needed for the group, such as coffee, a movie projector, or audiovisual equipment.
If pertinent, describe the expected cost and financial benefits incurred by the group.

state the criteria for membership eligibility and the time, place, and duration. The leaders' names and professional credentials should be provided.

Membership will greatly influence the group's outcome. In selecting members, the leader should consider group cohesion and therapeutic problem solving. Selection criteria include problem areas, motivation, age, sex, cultural factors, educational level, socioeconomic level, ability to communicate, intelligence, and coping and defensive styles. Homogeneous groups will share preselected criteria (for example, all members will be women who suffered incest as children). Heterogeneous groups will include a mixture of people, such as a group for men and women who want to build their self-esteem.

If possible, the leader should decide whether the membership of the group will be closed or open before screening members. A group is closed if no new members are added once the group is started. In an open group, members leave and new members are added throughout the duration of the group. Open groups may maintain the same purpose, with both members and leaders changing. They usually continue indefinitely with no termination date. The closed group offers the advantage of consistency of leadership, norms, and expectations. The open group, on the other hand, continually brings fresh ideas and opportunities for learning to its members.

The screening interview's primary purpose is to determine the appropriateness of the potential member to the group. Secondary purposes accomplished during the screening interview include:
▼ Beginning to develop a relationship between the leader and the member
▼ Determining the motivation of the possible member
▼ Determining whether the candidate's goals are in agreement with the group goals
▼ Educating the candidate about the nature of the group
▼ Determining the type of group experience the person has had
▼ If appropriate, beginning to review the group contract

In addition to or instead of the screening interview, some clinicians use group intake meetings. Several new members meet in a group for one to three sessions to learn about the group process and identify some possible treatment goals. This approach is less costly and has the same objectives as the screening interview.

As soon as possible a decision should be made about group membership. Candidates not selected should be referred to other treatment options. The reasons for not being selected should be explained to the candidate and, if appropriate, to the person who made the referral.

> **?** *You are asked to develop a group treatment program for victims of discrimination. What membership characteristics will you list as necessary for inclusion in the group? What will you say to the patients who are not selected for inclusion in your group?*

Initial Phase

The initial phase includes meetings in which the group's members begin to settle down to work. This phase is characterized by anxiety about being accepted by the group, the setting of norms, and the casting of various roles. Curative factors such as catharsis and universality begin to operate. This phase has been subdivided into three stages by Yalom[21]:

the orientation, conflict, and cohesive stages. The stages correspond to Tuckman's[18] first three stages of group development (see Table 31-3).

ORIENTATION STAGE. This stage corresponds to Tuckman's **forming** stage. The leader is more directive and active than in other stages. The leader orients the group to its primary task and helps the group arrive at a group contract. Some common factors that may be included in the group contract are goals, confidentiality, meeting times, honesty, structure, and communication rules (for example, only one person may talk at a time). Because an important part of this phase is norm setting, the leader should ensure that the norms will help the group achieve its goals. Another task of the leader in this stage is to foster a sense of belonging or cohesion among the members. To accomplish this, the leader encourages interaction among members and maintains the group at a working level of anxiety. For example, the leader could refer to the group as "our" group and suggest how members can help each other. Members could be encouraged to state what they hope to learn from the group. The leader would then reinforce realistic expectations and give examples of how the group might meet them.

During the first stage the members are evaluating each other, the group, and the leader. They are deciding whether they are going to be a part of the group and how much they will participate. Some common conscious or unconscious concerns of members during this stage are fear of being rejected, fear of self-disclosure, and fear of not being seen as an individual. Social behaviors are important, and the members are attempting to develop their social roles. The roles members assume during this stage are often renegotiated during other stages. The group is dependent, and members will often test out their dependency needs and wishes on the leader. They look to the leader for structure, approval, and acceptance, and may try to please the leader with reward-seeking behaviors. The leader must not meet all the dependency wishes of the members but must encourage them to interact more with one another. This supports members in becoming more interdependent and less dependent on the leader. The dependency issue between the leader and the members may lead the group into conflict and thus into the second stage.

CONFLICT STAGE. This stage of the group corresponds to Tuckman's[18] **storming** stage of group development. Issues related to control, power, and authority become primary. Members are concerned about the pecking order or deciding who is top or bottom in control and decision making. The dependency conflict may be openly or covertly expressed, with members polarized between independent and dependent issues. Bennis and Sheppard[3] describe this stage as a struggle between the counterdependent and dependent members, with the counterdependent members wanting to assume the leader's role. For example, a group may be divided over the issue of whether members can telephone each other. Some members may want the leader to decide, whereas others may think that the leader's statements are irrelevant. During this phase the counterdependent members might sit in the leader's chair and let the leader know that the directions have been unsuccessful or unheard. The dependent members might ask the leader for more directions. Other members who are neutral (neither dependent nor counterdependent) eventually may help the group resolve this conflict.

Subgroups usually form within the group, and hostility may be expressed. Often the hostility is directed toward the leader, but it may also be expressed toward other members. The leader's tasks are to allow expression of both negative and positive feelings, help the group understand the underlying conflict, and prevent or examine nonproductive behaviors such as scapegoating. This phase is usually the most difficult for the new leader because some members may lead the leader to believe that he or she has failed the group by not living up to its unrealistic expectations.

The leader must be careful not to avoid or suppress the group members' anxiety and, at times, should encourage the expression of hostility. If hostility toward the leader is expressed indirectly, such as anger toward other authority figures (such as staff members, teachers, or parents), the leader should help the group express its anger more directly. A useful technique is for the leader to give the group permission to discuss its anger by acknowledging that the group may be disappointed or angry at the leader.

By the end of the conflict stage the leader may be dethroned, and his or her omnipotent role, with its "magical" solutions, may be discarded. Slowly the leader becomes humanized. Members learn that responsibilities for the group are shared. Members may also learn that expressions of anger and disappointment do not destroy the leader and may help the group assess its resources and limitations more accurately. The group's resources can then be used to achieve its tasks. Members may realize that conflicts need not be avoided; instead, through discussion, conflicts may increase the group's maturity and usefulness.

COHESIVE STAGE. Tuckman's **norming** phase[18] is closely related to the cohesive stage. Group members, after resolving the second stage, feel a strong attraction toward one another and a strong attachment to the group. Positive feelings toward one another and the group are often expressed, and negative feelings are usually not shared.

At this stage, members feel free to give self-disclosing information and share more intimate concerns. However, the group's problem-solving ability is restricted because negative communication is usually avoided in order to maintain the high group morale. The leader's task is to make a connection between the members' disclosures and the group's primary task. The leader should not interfere with the group's basic cohesion but should encourage the group to use its problem-solving ability. The leader shows how a group member can have individual concerns and values and still be productive within the group. In other words, the leader demonstrates that differing and opposite opinions may not destroy the group identity.

At the resolution of this stage, members may learn that self-discoveries and differences should not be feared. They also learn that similarities and differences between the members may help the group achieve its tasks. At the end of the cohesive stage the group begins to see task achievement as a reality. The members gain a more realistic and honest view of their ability to work together and accomplish their primary and secondary tasks.

> **?** *Compare behaviors that would indicate that a group is in the orientation stage, the conflict stage, and the cohesive stage. Give specific examples. What leader interventions would be appropriate at each stage?*

Working Phase

The working phase of a group can be compared with Tuckman's **performing** stage of group development. During this stage the group becomes a team. It directs its energy mainly toward completing its tasks. Although they are hard at work, this phase is enjoyable for both the leader and the members. Responsibility for the group is more equally shared, anxiety is usually decreased and tolerated better, and the group is more stable and realistic.

Yalom and Vinogradov[20] have described some of the positive forces that occur in group therapy. They listed 11 curative factors that may occur (Table 31-4). Although these factors were identified in relationship to therapy groups, they are relevant to experiences in all types of groups. In addition, seven therapeutic factors that are important in promoting positive change in short-term groups have been identified[7]: self-responsibility, self-understanding, instillation of hope, group cohesiveness, catharsis, altruism, and universality. The last five are also included in Yalom's factors.

The leader's major role is to help the group complete its tasks by maximizing effective use of its curative properties. Because the members are fully participating in the group's work, the leader's activity level decreases. The leader now acts more as a consultant to the group. The leader helps to keep the group goal-directed and tries to decrease the impact of anything that may regress or retard the group.

Because this phase is the group's creative problem-solving and resolution phase, there are few, if any, specific guidelines for the leader. The leader's interventions are based primarily on theoretical frameworks, experiences, personality, and intuition, as well as the needs of the group and its members. In addition to fostering group cohesion, maintaining its boundaries, and encouraging the group to work on its tasks, the leader may help the group solve spe-

TABLE **31-4** *Yalom's Curative Factors*

FACTOR	DEFINITION
Imparting information	Receiving didactic information and advice
Instillation of hope	Increasing hopefulness of group members
Universality	Realization that others experience similar thoughts, feelings, and problems
Altruism	Experience of sharing part of oneself to help another
Corrective reenactment of primary family group	Ability of members to alter learning experience previously obtained in their families
Development of social interaction techniques	Opportunity to increase awareness of social interactions and develop social skills
Imitative behaviors	Opportunities to increase skills by imitating behaviors of others in group
Interpersonal learning	Ability to engage in wider range of interpersonal exchanges, thereby increasing each member's understanding of responsibility and complexity of interpersonal relationships and decreasing members' interpersonal distortions
Existential factors	Ability of group to help members deal with meaning of their own existence
Catharsis	Opportunity to express feelings previously unexpressed
Group cohesion	Attraction of member for group and other members

Modified from Yalom ID, Vinogradov S: *Group psychotherapy,* Washington, DC, 1989, American Psychiatric Press.

cific problems. Because these problems are unique to the group, many are not predictable. Some of the more common problems are the formation of subgroups, the management of conflict, and determining the optimum level of self-disclosure.[20]

Subgroups that conflict with the group's goals and are not acknowledged by the group can restrict its work. Other members may feel excluded, and loyalties will be divided between the subgroup and the whole group. For example, in a women's group, two of the members may become close friends, keeping secrets from the group and engaging in private conversations during the session. Other members may feel excluded from this pair and be ineffective in working with them. To decrease the negative impact of a subgroup, its consequences and the group's reactions should be openly discussed.

Conflict is unavoidable and can be used to foster growth. However, expression of conflict may need to be controlled so that the intensity does not exceed the group's tolerance. Examples of conflict are competition among members for the leader's attention and a disagreement between two members. A leader may manage conflicts by identifying the conflict, explaining that conflicts are natural and can lead to growth, and encouraging members to discuss the reasons for the conflict. Successful conflict resolution is related to the amount of group cohesion, trust, and acceptance among the members.

The amount of *self-disclosure* is usually related to the amount of acceptance and trust the member feels. Self-disclosure is always risky. If people give private information too quickly, they will feel vulnerable. On the other hand, if people disclose too little during the working phase they may not be able to form supportive interpersonal relationships. Their growth potential in the group may be decreased.

Resistance, or holding back the therapeutic process, can be expected in therapy groups. Resistance to working on the therapeutic goal can occur at both an individual and a group level. It is one matter to agree on goals and another to work on obtaining the actual therapeutic outcomes. Resistance by individual members may take many forms, such as avoiding discussion of a conflict, frequent or prolonged silences, attempting to become an assistant leader, absence from the group, pairing between two members, and prolonged or unusually intense expression of hostility. Resistance by the group or a majority of its members may be expressed in ways similar to those used by individuals. Other examples of group resistance include shared silence among the members, unusual amounts of dependency on the leader, scapegoating, subgroup formations, and the wish for magical solutions to resolve group conflict.

Resistance to group psychotherapeutic efforts can have a demoralizing effect on the therapist. With experience in handling resistance, it will become less threatening. The nurse will realize that resistance is a signal that treatment is progressing—that the therapist and the group members are getting close to crucial issues.[9] Resistance may occur because of increased anxiety related to conflict or change. The management of resistance depends on the type of group, the group contract, and the therapist's theoretical framework. Some methods of decreasing resistance are to establish trust, make observations regarding the group process or individual behaviors, offer interpretations, counteract the resistant behavior, and demonstrate more adaptive behavioral patterns.

By the end of the second phase, members have made significant progress toward goal achievement. They have a sense of their own productivity and accomplishments. The need for the group or their involvement in the group is less apparent. The group must begin to deal more actively with its final task: separation.

Termination Phase

The work of termination begins during the first phase of the group. However, as the group or individual members approach termination, certain processes are more likely to occur. The termination phase is not always discussed as a definite phase in the literature. It is discussed as a separate phase here because of the significance it may have for the members.

There are two types of termination: termination of the group as a whole and termination of individual members. A closed group usually terminates as an entire group; in an open group, members (and perhaps the leader) terminate separately. Members and groups may terminate prematurely, unsuccessfully, or successfully.

Termination is a highly individual process. Members and groups will terminate in unique ways. If the group has been successful, termination may be painful and involve grieving or a sense of loss. It may cause the group to experience increased anxiety, regression, and a feeling of accomplishment. Permitting members to avoid discussing termination would deprive them of a possible growth experience. Leadership behaviors include encouraging an evaluation of the group or its terminating members, reminiscing about important events that occurred in the group, and encouraging members to give each other feedback. Evaluation usually focuses on the amount of achievement of the group's or individual's goals. Leaders must be careful not to collude with members in denying termination; rather, they should encourage full discussion. Termination should be talked about several sessions before the final session to allow members time to work through issues that surface. Termination may lead to discussion of many related topics, such as other separations, death, aging, and the use and passage of time. If terminated successfully, members may feel a sense of resolution about the group experience and use these experiences in many other life situations.

Premature termination means that the group ends before its tasks are completed or a member leaves the group before his or her work is finished. Premature termination may occur for appropriate and inappropriate reasons. Appropriate reasons include moving to another city before the group is terminated. Inappropriate reasons might include a member's unwillingness to discuss an issue central to the group but painful to that person.

> **?** *As a staff nurse you are given the responsibility for developing a transition group for patients who are to be discharged from a day treatment program. Outline the points you will need to consider and the steps you would take to establish the group.*

Box **31-2** *Group Session Note Outline*

Date _____ Group Meeting No. _____
Membership:
    List members attending (state whether new member).
    List members who were late.
    List absent members.
List individual members' pertinent issues or behaviors discussed in the group.
List group themes.
Identify important group process issues (such as developmental stage, roles, and norms).
Identify any critical leadership strategy used.
List proposed future leadership strategies.
Predict member and group responses for the next session.

EVALUATION OF THE GROUP

Evaluation of the group and the group members' progress is an ongoing process that begins in the selection interview. Notes describing group sessions should be descriptive to help identify goal achievement. To make record keeping easy, it is usually helpful to have a group notebook. In this notebook leaders can write pertinent data on individual members such as their goals, their telephone numbers, their addresses, the screening note, any individual comments, and a termination summary note. In another section of the group notebook the leaders can describe each group meeting. One format for quickly recording each group meeting is provided in Box 31-2. In most agencies summary notes are also included in individual members' clinical records.

In addition, it is helpful to determine each member's goal attainment periodically during the course of the group. This can be done using subjective ratings by the group leaders and by obtaining individual members' perceptions on how they are meeting their goals. For a slightly more objective evaluation, members are asked to rate their goal achievement on a Likert scale (one that allows members to rate their response along a continuum, with 1 being low, 5 being high, for example). Members' goal achievement should always be evaluated at termination.

Along with the descriptive evaluation the clinician may decide to administer before- and after-group written tests. The tests selected should be related to the expected changes in the group. For example, an anxiety scale could be administered to members attending a group whose major goal is to reduce anxiety. If this type of evaluation is used, it is critical that the clinician use the most appropriate standardized scale available and that the agency's and the members' permissions are obtained. Commonly used rating scales are described in Chapter 6. It is very important that all parties involved know the intent of such tests and the disposition of test results.

It is also essential to identify outcomes so that the impact and validity of nursing group interventions can be communicated to consumers and health-care organizations. For example, vanServellen et al.[19] identified possible short-term outcome measures for nurse-led groups including increased knowledge of coping skills and increased insight into the members' own effective and ineffective coping behaviors. These were measured by a pregroup and postgroup coping test. Longer-term outcomes included a decrease in hopelessness measured by the Beck Hopelessness Scale, decreased depression measured by the Beck Depression Scale, and decreased manic behavior measured by the Young Manic Scale. In contrast, a nursing staff support group model identified the following measurable outcomes[6]:

▼ Use of a problem-solving approach
▼ Development of a communication tool
▼ Assertive handling of conflict
▼ Seeking assistance from each other when stressed
▼ Decreased patient complaints
▼ Decreased staff turnover

NURSES AS GROUP LEADERS

Nurses who are group leaders must be concerned about the many previously discussed factors regarding the group. The group leader must be able to study the group and participate in it at the same time. The leader must constantly monitor the group and, whenever necessary, help the group achieve its goals.

The qualities of an effective nurse leader are the same qualities that are important in the therapeutic relationship (see Chapter 2). In particular, these include the responsive and active dimensions of empathy, genuineness, and confrontation. In addition, creativity and opportunism are helpful qualities for leaders to possess. While they are listening to members' words, leaders also need to be aware of the group process. They must be alert to opportunities for the group to use themes and behaviors and see how these are related to individual issues. Leaders may be likened to an orchestra conductor who seeks to focus on the sound of a particular instrument for the appreciation and reaction of the total orchestra. The leader may encourage examination of the music from different perspectives and look for possible variations that would create a new piece of music. Opportunities for creativity may also lead to the development of innovative group techniques (see Critical Thinking about Contemporary Issues).

Group leaders must make it safe for members to challenge their authority. In examining the interplay between the leader and the members, there are opportunities to practice conflict management, confrontation, and assertive communication. The leader needs to accept confrontation without taking it personally.

Leaders also need to have assertive communication skills so that they can foster independence in the group but also help the group focus to reach its goals. Achieving this balance requires a blend of skills and judgment that

CRITICAL THINKING *about* Contemporary Issues

Do Computer Networks Provide a New Way for Nurses to Interact with Groups of Patients?

Interaction through computer networks is growing in popularity. Nurses have begun to identify opportunities to establish patient groups using this technology. Nurses have reported on the effectiveness of facilitating computer network groups for people with AIDS and for caregivers of people with Alzheimer's disease.[15] They found that all of Yalom's curative factors could be identified during the course of these groups. Advantages to the members included convenience, ability to relate to a variety of people in similar situations, and ready access to peer support. This approach also offers the option of anonymity to group members.

Psychiatric nurses need to consider the implications of this new way of conducting groups. The inability to perceive nonverbal communication removes an important dimension from the communication process. Because interaction among members is not simultaneous, time gaps occur between interventions and the responses of various members. Spontaneity may also be lost. The development of trust among group members could proceed differently than in traditional groups. Confidentiality may be even more of a concern to members than it is in face-to-face groups.

Identifying and exploring the dimensions of computer network groups offer a challenge to psychiatric nurses. Nurses who lead groups need to adapt their skills to enhance the advantages of the technology and minimize the disadvantages. As more people become computer-literate and accustomed to online relationships, the potential for this new form of group support will evolve.

can be gained with practice in group leadership, supervision by an experienced group facilitator, and study of group process.

It is also critical for leaders to be able to organize a great deal of information and to identify themes for the session. Novice leaders usually need to review the group experience with a supervisor after the session so that they can identify and analyze the important events.

Finally, a nurse leader also needs a sense of humor. Laughter helps reveal truth and enables participants to share and empathize about serious matters without the high levels of tension that often accompany such discussions. For example, in a women's codependent group, humor and laughter were regularly used. The group adopted this technique to talk about their "rescuing" and controlling behaviors. This group was composed of fragile women who grew up in abusive families. They worked hard at seeing, understanding, and changing their contribution to the destructive relationships they developed. The members brought examples of their "setting themselves up" to the group weekly and laughed as they were able to find humor in recognizing behavior that was similar to their own. The humor also allowed the members to give feedback in a less confrontive manner.

Groups with Co-Leaders

For a group, the presence of co-leaders may have advantages and disadvantages. When two clinicians share the leadership, the breadth of observation and the choice of interventions are greater than with one. For example, a male and female team may represent the family and offer the group members an opportunity to deal with issues related to parents or other significant male and female figures.

A male-female team also offers group members opportunities to observe a man and a woman working together with mutual respect and without exploitation, sexualizing, or putting each other down. A variety of transference reactions are available with experienced co-leaders to assist in learning and the resolution of problems. Exploration of the members' fantasies regarding the relationship between the leaders can give them a chance to see conflict and resolution. This can contribute significantly to the group's openness and power.

Disadvantages of the leadership team are often related to difficulties between the leaders. When there is competition, a major philosophical difference, or great variance in strategy or style, the group will not work effectively. Differences in levels of experience are handled if both are comfortable with their roles of apprentice and senior leader. Conflict between co-leaders could lead to the splitting of the group or the group developing an alliance with one of the leaders, which could be very damaging. Splitting must be openly interpreted in the group and dealt with by the group members and leaders.

Nurse-Led Groups

Nurses lead groups in a variety of health-care settings. Some types of groups that may be led by nurses are task groups, self-help groups, teaching groups, supportive/therapy groups, psychotherapy groups, and peer support groups. The type of group intervention provided by an individual nurse is determined by the needs and goals of the patients and by the education and experience of the nurse.

TASK GROUPS. Task groups are designed to accomplish a particular task. Nursing care planning meetings and committees are examples of task groups. The emphasis of these groups is on decision making and problem solving. They often have specific goals to accomplish and a deadline for completion of the work.

SELF-HELP GROUPS. Groups organized around a common experience are labeled self-help groups. Some examples include smoking cessation groups, Overeaters Anonymous, Alcoholics Anonymous, Parents and Friends of Lesbians and Gays, Parents Without Partners, and numerous groups related to specific health problems. They may or may not receive consultation from a health-care provider, such as a professional nurse. Although some are established and organized by professionals, they are run by the members and often do not have a designated leader. Leadership evolves within the group depending on the need that arises. Nurses can support self-help groups by referring members and by offering advice and assistance if it is requested. They can also promote links between the self-help group and the health-care system.

TEACHING GROUPS. The goal of teaching groups is to provide information. Examples are childbirth preparation and parent education groups. In-service education groups for staff are also included in this category. The nurse leader is able to educate more people more efficiently using a group format. The members themselves often become co-teachers as they share their information and experiences. Humphrey,[8] a school nurse, organized an Asthma Club to address the problems of asthmatic students who were doing poorly academically and felt stigmatized by their condition. Children discussed the disease and treatment. Positive outcomes included decreased absenteeism among the group members, use of inhalers in the classroom without embarrassment, and positive parent feedback. The group helped break the chain of illness, isolation, and self-perceived failure.

Psychoeducation groups are designed for 20 or more people who complete a series of structured educational sessions. These sessions are designed to teach symptom identification, symptom management, and recovery planning skills. Mohr[12] developed a curriculum for a psychoeducation program for a heterogeneous group of inpatients. The only patients excluded from the group were those who were so narcissistic or psychotic that they would inhibit the work of the other group members. The groups were taught in six subject areas:

▼ Stress management
▼ Medication management
▼ Life enrichment
▼ Social skills development
▼ Assertiveness skills
▼ Identification of feelings and coping skills

Nurse leaders took the roles of teacher and facilitator. They thought the groups added concreteness and substance to the treatment program.

SUPPORTIVE THERAPY GROUPS. The primary goal of supportive therapy groups is to help the members cope with life stress. The focus is on dysfunctional thoughts, feelings, and behaviors. Nehls[13] identified successful interventions used with a group of community mental health center patients who had a psychiatric diagnosis of borderline personality disorder. Giving and receiving information was used to provide structure for the group. This enabled these patients, who had problems with appropriate limit-setting, to practice effective problem-solving techniques.

Koontz, Cox, and Hastings[10] implemented a short-term support group to work with families of patients briefly hospitalized for evaluation and treatment on a general hospital psychiatric unit. During 10 months, over 120 people attended these sessions an average of three times. The leaders discovered major gaps in information about illness and treatment. There was also a great need for family support. The short-term group provided emotional support and critical information to increase members' coping and problem-solving abilities, thereby strengthening patients' support systems.

PSYCHOTHERAPY GROUPS. The goal of a psychotherapy group is the treatment of emotional, cognitive, or behavioral dysfunction. Group techniques and processes are used to help members learn about their behavior with other people and how it relates to core personality traits. The intent is for the members to change their behavior, not just understand or seek support for it. Members also learn that they have responsibilities to others and can help other members achieve their goals.

An example of a nurse-led psychotherapy group is a reality-based, ego-supportive therapy group for mothers of incest victims.[4] The nurses identified four strategies that they used to develop and maintain the group: noncritical acceptance and listening, appropriate nurturance and modeling of behaviors, restatement or reframing of paradoxical statements, and clarification. The effectiveness of the interventions was demonstrated by changes in the women's perceptions and behaviors. Another example is a group for women who were survivors of incest.[11] Through the group these women were able to learn and experience positive self-esteem, give up the victim role, and feel empowered. In a similar fashion, nurse-led outpatient therapy groups have been shown to be effective treatment modalities for women survivors of trauma with varying presentations of dissociative symptoms.[1]

BRIEF THERAPY GROUPS. Many managed care organizations are placing a new emphasis on group therapy as a cost-effective alternative to individual therapy. Most recently, the focus on cost containment and outcome evaluation in the treatment of health-related problems has been a major influence on the increasing importance of time-limited or brief therapy groups that are linked to individual treatment plans. The purpose of brief therapy groups is to focus on the actions participants can take to improve their current situation. Far less importance is given to the causes of the patient's problems or the accompanying emotional reactions. These groups target what can be done now to change a patient's problem-solving approach and help the patient implement more adaptive coping skills. The establishment of a recognized and self-sustaining group program is greatly facilitated by advanced planning, well thought-out structure, and clearly stated goals. A planning checklist for establishing time-limited psychotherapy groups is included in Box 31-3.

INTENSIVE PROBLEM-SOLVING GROUPS. Intensive problem-solving groups are designed for 6 to 10 patients, each working on the identification and resolution of spe-

---

Box **31-3** *Planning Checklist for Time-Limited Psychotherapy Groups*

Check for the following planning factors:

___*Clear administrative mandate:* Establish achievable annual goals for the number of therapy groups and the number of patients seen in these groups in a particular setting.

___*Clinical group coordinator:* Determine need for groups and guidelines for referrals, identify group therapists, conduct staff training, market the group, and establish pregroup and postgroup tests and outcome evaluations.

___*Population-based approach:* Identify the main diagnostic categories to be included and the needs of the target population that could be met by group therapy.

___*Group screening:* Pregroup orientation and screening ensures that patients understand how the group will operate and that the patient's needs will be addressed.

___*Clear referral criteria:* Clearly written referral guidelines help reduce clinician resistance to making referrals, promote effective use of the group, and increase patients' acceptance of the referral.

___*Regular status reports:* A weekly status report reminds referrers of the availability of groups. It should include the dates and times when groups meet, the types of groups, openings in groups, and the contact person.

___*Testing and evaluation:* Pretesting and posttesting help clarify the patient's response to treatment and allow for assessment of the effectiveness of the group.

___*Treatment models:* Use of a variety of group models (psychoeducational, social skills, relapse prevention, crisis intervention, cognitive-behavioral, and so on) matches patients with their presenting problems and increases patient receptivity.

___*Training:* A group therapy apprenticeship (clinicians observe and assist the group and are observed by experienced therapists) increases clinician effectiveness, acceptance of group modality, and appropriateness of referrals.

___*Adequate resources:* A reasonable fee schedule, adequate clinician time to develop and conduct groups, and appropriate physical space are essential for the group's success.

Modified from Crosby G, Sabin JE: A planning checklist for establishing time-limited psychotherapy groups, *Psychiatr Serv* 47:25, 1996.

cific target problems, goals, and problem-solving strategies related to an individual treatment plan. They are based on cognitive, behavioral, and affective therapy models implemented in a structured problem-solving format. The goal is to identify and clarify the problem, explore alternative solutions, and get action-oriented commitments for change. The therapist acts as a leader, teacher, and coach, whose purpose is to teach group members the interpersonal skills needed to solve the problems identified in their treatment plans. There are several keys to developing effective problem-solving groups[5]:

▼ Screen and match patients for entry into groups. Research shows that group members do best when they can easily relate to other members.

▼ Open each session with group members systematically reporting their reactions to the last session and their progress and problems in completing assignments.

▼ Use a standard group process. An example is one in which one patient presents a problem and the other members ask clarifying questions and give feedback.

▼ Use a standard closure procedure that identifies what members learned during the session, how this will help them solve their target problems, and the assignments they have given themselves to work on for the next session. This allows the therapist to identify progress made by members who did not directly work on their own issues, but developed insight into their own target problems by becoming involved in the problem-solving processes of other members.

MEDICATION GROUPS. Clinical studies show that the combination of psychotherapy and psychopharmacology can produce better results in groups of patients than the use of either treatment alone. Thus, it has become standard practice in mental health treatment settings to view psychotropic medication as an integral part of psychotherapeutic treatment rather than something to be tried only when psychotherapy is failing. A time-limited therapy group can be an important modality for the combination of these therapies. Allowing patients to deal with their feelings regarding the taking of medication in a group setting not only facilitates compliance but also allows important psychodynamic issues to emerge, such as acting out, dependence, and authority conflicts, encouraging the resolution of these issues for all the patients in the group. The prescription of medications can take place outside of the group setting for each patient or within the group itself. Having both a prescriber and a group leader in the group helps keep their roles from becoming blunted and confusing. The medication prescriber often fills an authoritarian or directive role, in contrast to the role of the group leader, which is more facilitative.[14]

ACTIVITY GROUPS. Activity group therapy is designed to enhance the psychological and emotional well-being of long-term psychiatric patients. These patients of-ten exhibit cognitive dysfunction, complacency, negativism, anxiety, disinterest, low self-esteem, poor interpersonal relationships, and isolation. Activity group therapy is a combination of group psychotherapy and remotivation therapy that stimulates interaction among members by focusing on simple tasks that encourage members to focus on group goals rather than their individual issues.[17] Tasks can include drawing, exercising to music, baking, community trips, arts and crafts, and reviewing current events. As health care moves away from the more costly inpatient setting toward community-based programs for the serious and persistently mentally ill, nurses are in a good position to serve these patients with creative and effective interventions.

PEER SUPPORT GROUPS. Finally, peer support groups are an effective way for professionals to share the stresses and problems related to their work. An example of a peer support group is a group of advanced practice psychiatric nurses who meet monthly. Group purposes may include case consultation, sharing information about educational opportunities, providing information about management skills, and decreasing professional isolation. Another example is a group of nurses who work with people with HIV/AIDS. They meet regularly for nursing consultation and support in coping with the continual loss associated with this disease.

> **?** *As a head nurse, you decide to form a staff support group. How would this differ from a therapeutic group? Discuss in terms of the roles of the leader and the members. Would there be any similarities?*

Summary

1. A group is a collection of people who are interrelated and interdependent and may share common purposes and norms.

2. Components of a small group including structure, size, length of sessions, communication, roles of members, norms, and cohesion were identified and described.

3. The phases of group development (pregroup, initial phase with orientation, conflict and cohesion stages, working phase, and termination) were presented.

4. Small group evaluation is based on accomplishment of individual goals and expected group outcomes. Careful documentation of each group session is required.

5. The responsibilities and qualities of nurse group leaders include empathy, nurturance, genuineness, creativity, acceptance of confrontation, assertive communication skills, organization, and a sense of humor. Types of nurse-led groups including task, self-help, teaching, supportive therapy, psychotherapy, brief therapy, intensive problem solving, medication, activity, and peer support groups were described.

COMPETENT CARING A Clinical Exemplar of a Psychiatric Nurse

Lynn Klair, MS, RN

While I was working as a clinical nurse specialist in an inpatient psychiatric setting, I co-led a predischarge group. Five of the group members went to the same domiciliary care home. I was concerned about their adjustment to a community setting, so I arranged to continue providing group therapy in the community setting.

The group consisted of three women and two men. We met early in the morning, in part so I could stop on my way to work and in part so we could meet before the members became involved in their daily activities. All of the members attended the group on a fairly regular basis; two of them are particularly memorable to me because of the progress they made.

P was a former nurse who had depression and anorexia nervosa. One of her goals was to get some new clothes, but her finances were very limited. I obtained some used clothing that I brought to her to replace her old clothes, which were several sizes too large for her. It took her a long time to try the new clothes because she believed that they were too tight on her. This was evidence of her distorted body image. P's greatest accomplishment was to reestablish contact with her family, who lived in another state. The group provided support to her as she struggled with the decision to write to them. They all felt a sense of accomplishment when she wrote and then later talked to family members on the telephone. By the time the group terminated, P was beginning to gain confidence and had stayed out of the hospital longer than she had after any previous hospital discharge.

R was a middle-aged man who had been hospitalized for 15 years following an arrest for a serious assault. He was college educated and had been employed in the past. He was a very large man, and I thought of him as a "gentle giant." He was very kind to the other group members and was liked by all of them, even the most paranoid member. R needed to learn to manage money; he carried his money in his sock. He also needed new clothing, but resisted the group's encouragement to go shopping. When I brought some catalogs to the group, I discovered that R had great difficulty making choices. He finally decided that he would give me money to use to buy clothing for him. Although I felt somewhat uncomfortable with this, I agreed because I knew that it was difficult for him to develop this much trust in another person. When he wore his new clothing to the group, the other members complimented him and I could see his self-esteem improving. R eventually moved into a smaller group home. The group mourned his loss, but felt good about their role in helping him progress.

After several months of meeting at the house, we decided to have some of our meetings at a nearby fast-food restaurant. This was done to help members to feel more comfortable out in the community, as well as to address their wish to have refreshments during the meetings. This change worked out well because we could work on socialization and community survival skills.

My experience leading this group was rewarding and resulted in professional growth for me. I gained a new understanding of what was required for patients to live successfully in the community and also developed an appreciation for the difficulties they face in doing this. I never stopped being impressed by their strength and courage as they met the challenges presented to them.

your **INTERNET**
connection

Group Psychotherapy Home Page
http://freud.tau.ac.il/~haimw/group2.html

The International Association of Group Psychotherapy
http://www.psych.mcgill.ca/labs/iagp/IAGP.html

Chapter Review Questions

1. Match each term in Column A with the correct definition in Column B.

Column A	Column B
E. Follower	A. Determines level of group acceptance of individual members
C. Moralist	B. Keeps the group focused
H. Truant	C. Serves as judge of right and wrong
A. Gatekeeper	D. States current position of the group
J. Encourager	E. Serves as an interested audience
G. Questioner	F. Discourages positive work and vents anger
B. Facilitator	G. Clarifies issues and information
I. Leader	H. Invalidates significance of the group
F. Complainer	I. Sets direction
D. Summarizer	J. Acts as a positive influence on the group

2. Fill in the blanks.

A. ___Power___ is the member's ability to influence the group and its other members.

B. The stage of group development in which the leader is more directive and active than in other stages is the ___orientation___ stage.

C. The optimum length of a session is ___60–120 min.___ for higher-functioning groups and ___20–40 min___ for lower-functioning groups.

D. The four phases of a group's development identified by Tuckman are ___forming___, ___storming___, ___norming___, and ___performing___.

E. According to Yalom, the realization that others experience the same thoughts, feelings, and problems is called ___universality___ and the experience of sharing part of oneself to help another is called ___altruism___.

3. Provide short answers for the following questions.

A. Define a group and list eight components of small groups as described in this chapter.

B. Compare psychoeducational, intensive problem-solving, and activity groups.

C. Describe four functions that group norms serve.

D. Assess your own level of comfort working in groups. What roles do you usually assume? What additional skills would you need to be an effective group leader?

REFERENCES

1. Applegate M: Outpatient group therapy for dissociative trauma survivors, *J Am Psychiatr Nurses Assoc* 2:37, 1996.
2. Benne KD, Sheats P: Functional roles and group members, *J Soc Issues* 4:41, 1948.
3. Bennis W, Sheppard H: A theory of group development, *Hum Relations* 9:415, 1956.
4. DelPo KG, Koontz MA: Group therapy with mothers of incest victims: II. Therapeutic strategies, recurrent themes, interventions, and outcomes, *Arch Psychiatr Nurs* 5:70, 1991.
5. Gorski TT: Making group therapy work in the age of cost containment, *Treatment Today* Spring:16, 1996.
6. Guillory BA, Riggin OZ: Developing a nursing staff support group model, *Clin Nurse Spec* 5:170, 1991.
7. Hoge MA, McLoughlin KA: Group psychotherapy in acute treatment settings: theory and technique, *Hosp Community Psychiatry* 42: 153, 1991.
8. Humphrey E: The politics of asthma: a lesson in confidence, *Nurs Times* 88:31, 1992.
9. Kemper BJ: Dealing with resistance in group therapy, *Perspect Psychiatr Care* 30:31, 1994.
10. Koontz E, Cox D, Hastings S: Implementing a short-term family support group, *J Psychosoc Nurs Ment Health Serv* 29:5, 1991.
11. Kreidler MC, Carlson RE: Breaking the incest cycle: the group as a surrogate family, *J Psychosoc Nurs Ment Health Serv* 29:28, 1991.
12. Mohr WK: A nurse-led educational program in psychiatric settings: developing a curriculum, *J Psychosoc Nurs Ment Health Serv* 31:34, 1993.
13. Nehls N: Group therapy for people with borderline personality disorder: interventions associated with positive outcomes, *Issues Ment Health Nurs* 13:255, 1992.
14. O'Kelly JG, Piper WE: Group dynamics and medication in evening treatment, *Continuum* 3:85, 1996.
15. Ripich S, Moore SM, Brennan PF: A new nursing medium: computer networks for group intervention, *J Psychosoc Nurs Ment Health Serv* 30:15, 1992.
16. Schutz W: Interpersonal underworld, *Harvard Bus Rev* 36:123, 1958.
17. Smith MK, Harty KM, Riggin OZ: Working with the patient with a chronic mental impairment: an activity group approach, *J Psychosoc Nurs* 34:28, 1996.
18. Tuckman B: Developmental sequence in small groups, *Psychol Bull* 63:384, 1965.
19. vanServellen G et al: Methodological concerns in evaluating psychiatric nursing care modalities and a proposed standard group protocol format for nurse-led groups, *Arch Psychiatr Nurs* 4:117, 1992.
20. Yalom ID, Vinogradov S: *Group psychotherapy*, Washington, DC, 1989, American Psychiatric Press.
21. Yalom ID: *The theory and practice of group psychotherapy*, ed 4, New York, 1995, Basic Books.

ANNOTATED SUGGESTED READINGS

Crosby G, Sabin JE: A planning checklist for establishing time-limited psychotherapy groups, *Psychiatr Serv* 47:25, 1996.
Presents a useful explanation of 10 essential factors for setting up brief therapy group programs in both clinic practices and managed care settings.

*Dallam S, Manderino M: Peer group supports patients with MPD/DD, *J Psychosocial Nurs* 35:22, 1997.
Describes the value of group therapy for relatively stable patients with MPD/DD that focuses on the here-and-now and is supportive and psychoeducational in nature.

Hamilton I et al: Quality assessment and improvement in group psychotherapy, *Am J Psychiatr* 150:316, 1993.
These authors developed a monitoring and evaluation program for the group therapies used in a large general hospital psychiatric unit.

*Hastings-Vertino K, Getty C, Wooldridge P: Development of a tool to measure therapeutic factors in group process, *Arch Psychiatr Nurs* 10:221, 1996.
Describes a tool developed by nurses to measure Yalom's therapeutic factors that will allow therapists to study these factors objectively rather than subjectively.

*Nursing reference.

*Lanza M, Satz H, Stone J, Kayne H: Developing psychodynamic group treatment methods for aggressive male inpatients, *Issues Ment Health Nurs* 17:409, 1996.
Explores relevant literature and clinical applications for conducting a psychodynamic psychotherapy group for aggressive patients.

Scheidlinger S: An overview of nine decades of group psychotherapy, *Hosp Community Psychiatry* 45:217, 1994.
Provides a thorough history and literature review of group therapy since its inception, with a look to the role this modality is likely to play in the future of a changing health care environment.

Shields J, Lanza M: The parallel process of resistance by clients and therapists to starting groups: a guide for nurses, *Arch Psychiatr Nurs* 7:300, 1993.
Delineates several ways in which group therapy trainees and patients who have been referred to groups resist initial group involvement.

Yalom ID: *The theory and practice of group psychotherapy*, ed 4, New York, 1995, Basic Books.
An informative and easy-to-read book that includes not only the basic principles of therapy and group work and the various roles of the therapist but also a full review of the scientific literature on clinical effectiveness.

Family
Interventions

Patricia E. Helm

© 1998 M.C. Escher/Cordon Art, Baarn, Holland.

We are truly heirs of all the ages; but as honest men it behooves us to learn the extent of our inheritance. **John Tyndall** "MATTER AND FORCE," IN VOL. 2, *PRAYER AS A FORM OF PHYSICAL ENERGY*

LEARNING OBJECTIVES

After studying this chapter the student should be able to:

▼ Describe the characteristics of adaptive and maladaptive family functioning

▼ Discuss nonclinical interventions useful in working with families of the mentally ill, including psychoeducation

▼ Relate indications for the use of clinical interventions with families

▼ Analyze the theoretical basis, components, and interventions associated with family systems therapy

▼ Analyze the theoretical basis, components, and interventions associated with structural family therapy

▼ Analyze the theoretical basis, components, and interventions associated with strategic family therapy

TOPICAL OUTLINE

Psychiatric nurse generalists, without master's degrees, are exposed to families at all levels of functioning. Understanding principles of family intervention can allow nurses to make more acute observations, thus enhancing their assessment of families' needs and resources. It can also suggest new ways in which to promote adaptive family functioning and enhance a family's use of positive coping skills. It can help nurses more readily identify problems within family systems and may help the nurse generalist in initiating appropriate referrals.

Clinical training programs in family therapy are open to psychiatric nurses across the United States. They vary in duration, theoretical framework used, and the level of knowledge required. Usually they are limited to clinicians with graduate degrees in mental health. The psychiatric nurse doing family therapy should have a master's degree with didactic content and clinical seminars focused on family work. The nurse also needs to obtain individual or group supervision to refine clinical skills and deepen theoretical understanding of family systems and interventions.

FAMILY FUNCTIONING

Nurses encounter all different types of families in their clinical work. Fig. 32-1 presents an overview of four dimensions that can be used to describe families in contemporary society: biological tie, marital status, sexual orientation, and gender roles or employment status. There are other ways in which families differ as well. Many families face special challenges because a member has experienced something out of the ordinary. Some of these families include families with a mentally ill member, families who have a member with AIDS, or families affected by violence within the household.

Contact with patients' families is a natural part of nursing care. For many years nurses have been making intuitive observations about functional and dysfunctional families. They have been intervening with families without formal training in family therapy. A well-functioning family can shift roles, levels of responsibility, and patterns of interaction as it experiences stressful life changes. A well-functioning family may, under acute or prolonged stress, produce a symptomatic member. This family rebalances in such a way that function of all members is restored and symptoms fade. A functional family has the following characteristics[28]:

▼ It completes important life cycle tasks.
▼ It has the capacity to tolerate conflict and to adapt to adverse circumstances without long-term dysfunction or disintegration of family cohesion.
▼ Emotional contact is maintained across generations and between family members without blurring necessary levels of authority.
▼ Overcloseness or fusion is avoided, and distance is not used to solve problems.
▼ Each twosome is expected to resolve the problems between them. Bringing a third person in to settle disputes or to take sides is discouraged.
▼ Differences between family members are encouraged to promote personal growth and creativity.
▼ Children are expected to assume age-appropriate responsibility and to enjoy age-appropriate privileges negotiated with their parents.
▼ The preservation of a positive emotional climate is more highly valued than doing what "should" be done or what is "right."
▼ Within each spouse there is a balance of affective expression, careful rational thought, relationship focus, and care taking; each spouse can selectively function in the respective modes.
▼ There is open communication and interactions among family members.

The above characteristics represent an ideal family that may be more fictional than real. Most families have some but not all of these elements and still operate with integrity and respect. It is also important to remember that culture affects families in a number of ways. Specifically, culture determines:
▼ The definition of family
▼ The conflict and tensions present in a family and the adaptive or maladaptive responses to them
▼ The norms of a family
▼ How outside events are perceived and interpreted
▼ When, how, and what type of family interventions are most effective

At the opposite end of the continuum are dysfunctional

Biological Tie

• Biologically both parents related

• One parent biologically related (artificial insemination, surrogate parenting, lesbian families, blended families)

• Neither parent biologically related (adoption)

Marital Status

• Single parent (by choice, heterosexual or insemination, or due to divorce)

• Married parents (parents married to each other, or stepfamily)

• Cohabiting parents (heterosexual or gay or lesbian)

Sexual Orientation

• Heterosexual

• Gay or lesbian

Gender Roles/ Employment Status

• Traditional

• Nontraditional

Fig. 32-1 Dimensions of the contemporary family.
(From Harway M, Wexler K: Setting the stage for understanding and treating the changing family. In Harway M, editor: *Treating the changing family,* New York, 1996, Wiley.)

families. Some of the more common dysfunctional family patterns include the following:

▼ The overprotective mother and distant father (distant through work, alcohol, or physical absence)
▼ The overfunctioning "superwife" or "superhusband" and the underfunctioning passive, dependent, and compliant spouse
▼ The spouse who maintains peace at any price and denies difficulties in the marriage but suddenly feels wronged and self-righteous when the mate is discovered to be in legal trouble or having an affair
▼ The child who evidences poor peer relationships at school while attempting to parent younger siblings to compensate for ineffective or emotionally overwhelmed parents
▼ The overclose three generations of grandparent, parent, and grandchild in which lines of authority and generational identity are poorly defined and the child acts out because of a lack of effective limit setting by an agreed-upon parental figure
▼ The family with a substance-abusing member
▼ The family subjected to physical, emotional, or sexual abuse by one of its members

> ? *Watch a popular television show that depicts a family situation and evaluate the family's level of functioning.*

Competence Paradigm

The concepts of family functioning just discussed have most recently given way to a competence paradigm for professional practice.[17,18] This new approach was derived from the fact that older conceptual models tended to focus on pathologic states and dysfunction as opposed to family strengths, resources, and competencies. The competency paradigm values empowerment instead of a helper-helpee ideology and stresses the importance of treating people as collaborators who are the masters of their own fate (Table 32-1).

An empowerment model has been used increasingly as a framework for professional practice with families who are coping with a member who is mentally ill or mentally retarded. Its use is likely to increase the understanding of familial attributes that are relevant to coping with mental illness, facilitate the assessment of positive attributes among family members, offer a blueprint for designing effective interventions for families, and advance efforts to evaluate the outcome of family-oriented services. In addition, unlike pathology models that may stigmatize and alienate families, a competence paradigm attempts to foster positive alliances between families and health-care providers and enhance the delivery of services.

The competence paradigm emphasizes the following[7]:

▼ Focus on growth-producing behaviors rather than on treatment of problems or prevention of negative outcomes
▼ Promotion and strengthening of individual and family functioning by fostering the acquisition of prosocial, self-sustaining, self-efficacious, and other adaptive behaviors
▼ Definition of the relationship between the help seeker and help giver as a cooperative partnership that assumes joint responsibility
▼ Encouragement of assistance that is in line with the family's culture and congruent with the family's appraisal of problems and needs
▼ Promotion of the family's use of natural support networks

In this framework it is expected that families will play a major role in deciding what is important to them, what options they will choose to achieve their goals, and whether they will accept help that is offered to them.[24,25]

NONCLINICAL INTERVENTIONS

Critically important to psychiatric nurses is the development of nonclinical family interventions that are designed primar-

Table **32-1** *Paradigms in Working with Families*

	PATHOLOGY PARADIGM	COMPETENCE PARADIGM
Nature of paradigm	Disease-based medical model	Health-based developmental model
View of families	Pathological, pathogenic, or dysfunctional	Basically or potentially competent
Emphasis	Weaknesses, liabilities, and illness	Strengths, resources, and wellness
Role of professionals	Practitioners who provide psychotherapy	Enabling agents who help families achieve their goals
Role of families	Clients or patients	Collaborators
Basis of assessment	Clinical typologies	Competencies and competence deficits
Goal of intervention	Treatment of family pathology or dysfunction	Empowerment of families in achieving mastery and control over their lives
Modus operandi	Provision of psychotherapy	Strengthening of the relevant competencies
Systemic perspective	Family systems framework	Ecological systems framework

From Marsh D: Working with families of people with serious mental illness. In VandeCreek L, Knapp S, Jackson T, editors: *Innovations in clinical practice: a source book,* vol 2, Sarasota, Fla, 1992, Professional Resource Exchange.

ily to educate and support.[17] They are the result of the emergence of the family self-help movement in psychiatry.

In the 1970s some families began forming local self-help and consumer advocacy groups for families of the mentally ill. In 1979 about 100 such groups together formed the National Alliance for the Mentally Ill (NAMI). This strong and politically active group is organized with the following goals[14]:

▼ Educating and informing families of services and treatment available

▼ Supporting families and friends of those with severe and disabling mental illness

▼ Advocating improved treatment and services for the chronically mentally ill

▼ Promoting support for research into the neurophysiological, neurochemical, and genetic factors important in prolonged mental illness

▼ Improving training for mental health professionals to foster a more enlightened understanding of the nature of prolonged mental illness

▼ Working with the media to share accurate information and challenge stereotypes to overcome stigma about the mentally ill and their families

As enlightened consumers, NAMI members advocate for information about services needed for their ill family members and themselves. For participating families, local self-help and support groups offer mutual aid, intimacy with others, and involvement beyond the immediate family.[6,23]

> **?** *Families of the mentally ill believe some family therapy theories stigmatize and blame families for their relatives' illness. Evaluate family systems, structural, and strategic therapies as presented in this chapter based on this criticism.*

Psychoeducational Programs for Families

Due mainly to the efforts of NAMI and other family groups, a variety of psychoeducational programs have been developed for families of the mentally ill.[19] Although these programs vary, they share certain features. The program approach is mainly educational and pragmatic, and its aim is to improve the course of the family member's illness, reduce relapse rates, and improve the patient's and family's functioning. These goals are achieved through educating the family about the illness, teaching families techniques to cope with symptomatic behavior, and reinforcing family strengths. Not all programs include the ill family member, but they do promote regular contact of the family with other affected families.

In general, a comprehensive program of nonclinical family intervention should include the following components[17]:

▼ A didactic component that provides information about mental illness and the mental health system

▼ A skill component that offers training in communication, conflict resolution, problem solving, assertiveness, behavioral management, and stress management

▼ An emotional component that provides opportunities for ventilation and sharing and mobilizing resources

▼ A family process component that focuses on coping with mental illness and its sequelae for the family

▼ A social component that increases use of informal and formal support networks

Although no single program works equally well in all situations, it is possible to describe a general structure that can be modified to meet individual needs. The educational program outlined in Box 32-1 is time limited and didactic and is designed to primarily meet the cognitive and behavioral needs of families.[17] It is important that psychoeducational programs for families meet a range of needs and that there be an opportunity for families to ask questions, express feelings, and socialize with each other and mental health professionals.

CLINICAL INTERVENTIONS

Deciding when family therapy is appropriate, or indicated over individual or group therapy, is not always easy. Resource availability is a factor; many settings do not have anyone trained in family therapy. When the resources are available, the therapist's bias may have an influence. Some family therapists conceptualize all emotional problems within the family framework. Others recommend certain guidelines in determining which problems should be treated in family therapy. They suggest that family therapy is indicated in the following situations:

▼ The presenting problem appears in system terms, such as marital conflicts, severe sibling conflicts, or cross-generational conflicts (parents versus offspring, parents versus grandparents).

▼ Various types of difficulty and conflict arise between the identified patient and other family members.

▼ The family is experiencing a transitional stage of the family life cycle, such as beginning a family, marriage, birth of the first child, entrance of children into adolescence, the first child leaving home, retirement, or the death of a spouse.

▼ Individual therapy with one family member results in symptoms developing in another family member.

▼ No improvement occurs with adequate individual therapy. Enlarging the conceptual field to include the family in therapy may produce therapeutic movement.

▼ The person in treatment seems unable to use an intrapsychic or interpretive mode of individual therapy but uses therapy sessions primarily to talk about or complain about another member.

This chapter provides an overview of three theoretical approaches to clinical interventions with families: family systems therapy, structural therapy, and strategic therapy. It describes some of the major techniques that are derived

Box 32-1 *10-Week Educational Program for Families of the Mentally Ill*

NATURE AND PURPOSE OF PROGRAM
Introductions of family members and staff
Purpose and scope of program
Description of treatment program, policies, and procedures
Brief, written survey of specific family needs and requests

THE FAMILY EXPERIENCE
Family burden and needs
The family system
Family subsystems
Life-span perspectives

MENTAL ILLNESS I
Diagnosis
Etiology
Prognosis
Treatment

MENTAL ILLNESS II
Symptoms
Medication
Diathesis-stress model
Recent research

MANAGING SYMPTOMS AND PROBLEMS
Bizarre behavior
Destructive and self-destructive behavior
Hygiene and appearance
Negative symptoms

STRESS, COPING, AND ADAPTATION
The general model
The stressor of mental illness
The process of family adaptation
Increasing coping effectiveness

ENHANCING PERSONAL AND FAMILY EFFECTIVENESS I
Behavior management
Conflict resolution
Communication skills
Problem solving

ENHANCING PERSONAL AND FAMILY EFFECTIVENESS II
Stress management
Assertiveness training
Achieving a family balance
Meeting personal needs

RELATIONSHIPS BETWEEN FAMILIES AND PROFESSIONALS
Historical context
New modes of family-professional relationships
Barriers to collaboration
Breaking down barriers

COMMUNITY RESOURCES
The consumer-advocacy movement
Accessing the system
Legal issues
Appropriate referrals

from each of these theories. The principles and strategies proposed by these theories are distinct and sometimes conflicting, yet each defines a theoretical framework developed from clinical research with families, and each has some utility in clinical practice.

FAMILY SYSTEMS THERAPY

Family systems therapy was developed by Bowen[3] in the 1950s and continues to evolve.[30] A premise of this therapy is that a family is a homeostatic system. A change in functioning of one family member results in a change in the functioning of other family members. It resembles a centerless web in which, when one strand moves, the tensions in the entire web readjust.

Systems therapy explains emotional dysfunction in human relationships, specifically in the family system. Symptoms in any member of the family, whether social (such as child abuse or delinquency), physical (such as drug abuse, alcoholism, or chronic illness), emotional (such as depression or schizophrenia), or conflictual (such as marital conflict), are viewed as evidence of dysfunction in the family relationship process. Although the family is only one emotional system in which a person is involved, it is probably the most intense and influential one. Extrafamilial relationships rarely have the intensity of the family emotional system. The family system fosters or inhibits function but it

does not totally determine behavior. Individuals are responsible for their own actions within the family system.

The purpose of any theory is to understand, predict, and gain some control of the phenomena being studied. Understanding, as applied to family systems therapy, does not entail uncovering intrapsychic motivations. It identifies the functional facts of a relationship: what happened, when, where, how, and who was involved. These observable facts are more important than the reasons why the problematic behavior occurred. A systems therapist gathers from family members descriptions of behavior rather than feeling states. Conventional psychodynamic jargon is not present in family systems writing. Systems therapy uses simple, descriptive words.

Bowen[3,12] has described in detail the team research he conducted in the early 1950s on schizophrenic families in a live-in hospital setting. A new theory of family psychotherapy evolved from this live-in research. This theory, based on clinical observations of the research families' behavior, also applies to relationship patterns in more functional family systems. Bowen believed that "patterns originally thought to be typical of schizophrenia are present in all families some of the time and in some families most of the time."[3]

A cornerstone of systems therapy developed from a central pattern observed in research families. Some families failed to distinguish between the intellectual process of thinking and the more subjective process of feeling. It was as if the thinking processes were so flooded with feeling that members were unable to separate intellectual belief from subjective feelings. Routinely a person would say, "I feel that . . ." when "I think that . . ." would have been more accurate. The families focused on feelings in an attempt to foster togetherness and agreement. They avoided statements of

TABLE **32-2** *Central Concepts of Family Systems Therapy*

CONCEPT	DEFINITION
Differentiation	Sufficient separation between intellect and emotions so that one is not dominated by the reactive anxiety of the family's emotional system.
Triangle	A predictable emotional process that takes place when difficulty exists in a significant relationship.
Nuclear family emotional system	Patterns of interaction between family members and the degree to which these patterns promote emotional fusion.
Multigenerational transmission process	The assumption that relationship patterns and symptoms in a family have their origin several generations earlier; a four- or five-generation genogram reveals such patterns.
Family projection process	The projection of spouses' problems onto one or more children to avoid intense emotional fusion between the spouses.
Sibling position	Birth order and sex are seen as determining factors in a person's personality profile.
Emotional cutoff	A dysfunctional way in which some family members deal with intense family conflict by using either emotional isolation or geographical distance.

opinion or belief that would make one member different or separate from the family "party line."

A key goal of systems therapy is to clarify and distinguish thinking and feeling in family members. The observation of this fusion between thinking and feeling led to the concept of the undifferentiated family ego mass. People with the greatest fusion between feeling and thinking function poorly. They inherit a high percentage of life's social, psychiatric, and medical problems.

Family systems theory consists of seven interlocking concepts. Three concepts apply to overall characteristics of family systems: differentiation of self, triangles, and the nuclear family emotional system. The remaining four concepts are related to the central family characteristics: the multigenerational transmission process, the family projection process, sibling position, and the emotional cutoff (Table 32-2).

All these concepts refer to family processes that inhibit or promote individual family members' rising out of the emotional "we-ness," or fusion. Bowen believes that a member's movement toward increased emotional closeness or distance is reflexive and predictable. The higher the level of differentiation in a person, the higher the level of functioning. Differentiating the self from the "we-ness" is the ultimate goal of treatment.

Differentiation of Self

The concept of differentiation of self is Bowen's attempt to measure all human functioning on a continuum. The continuum proceeds from the greatest emotional fusion of self boundaries to the highest degree of differentiation or autonomy (Fig. 32-2). A concise description of the differentiated person is one who is less anxious than the family system. This person is able to bring up emotion-laden issues in a nonassaulting way without anxiety. In his earlier work, Bowen refers to the undifferentiated family ego mass that exists in varying degrees of intensity in families. The intensity of emotional closeness in a family may allow members to know each other's thoughts, feelings, and fantasies.

There is a cyclical quality to this closeness. As the emo-

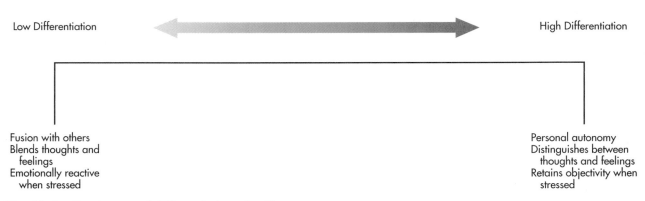

Low Differentiation → High Differentiation

Fusion with others
Blends thoughts and
 feelings
Emotionally reactive
 when stressed

Personal autonomy
Distinguishes between
 thoughts and feelings
Retains objectivity when
 stressed

Fig. 32-2 Continuum of differentiation of self.

tional intensity or fusion between two people increases and the self of one is incorporated into the other self, becoming enmeshed, the relationship is perceived to be uncomfortably close. This is usually followed by distance-creating behavior characterized by hostile rejection of the overcloseness. The two people actively repel each other. Relationships can cycle through these phases because anxiety in the relationship ebbs and flows. Relationships can also become fixed at an angry, repelling standoff. People who operate at the lower reactive end of the continuum are so fused that they are dominated by the automatic emotional system. These people are less adaptable, less flexible, and more emotionally dependent on those around them. They are easily stressed into dysfunction. People at the higher end of the continuum maintain a degree of separation between thought and emotion. In periods of stress they can retain intellectual functioning. They are more flexible, adaptable, and more independent of the reactive emotionality around them.

The concept of differentiation eliminates the notion of normalcy. It has no direct connection to presence or absence of symptoms, although Bowen believes people at the lower end of the scale tend to inherit more of life's problems. People at the higher end of the continuum recoup rapidly if they are stressed into dysfunction.[2,3]

> **?** *How might a parent's level of self-differentiation affect their child's growth and development from infancy through adolescence?*

Triangles

The concept of triangles is the key to understanding the systems approach to emotional function. Many techniques evolve from this concept. The idea of triangles is not new. Freud's theory of the Oedipal complex describes a sexual triangle. Bowen has called the triangle the basic building block of an emotional system. A triangle is a predictable emotional process that takes place in any significant relationship experiencing difficulty. The three corners of the triangle can be composed of three people; two people and a group, such as a religious affiliation or Al-Anon; two people and an issue, such as drinking or success; or two people and an object, such as a house or drugs. The possible list of groups, issues, or objects is endless; it must have an emotional significance equal to that of a person.

All people seek closeness in emotional systems. Emotional closeness but separateness is difficult for two people to maintain; the tendency is to fuse, to lose self, or parts of self, in the other. A natural urge exists to seek completeness of self by accumulating parts of the other. The old adage "opposites attract" reflects this assumption. It is difficult for two people to maintain sufficient emotional closeness without fusion. The inevitable result is emotional distancing.

The system is then ripe for the formation of a triangle. For example, the husband wants more expression of affection from an emotionally constricted wife. The more he pursues her, the more she withdraws, most often into preoccupation with her child. The husband starts working longer hours. Husband and wife then start arguing circularly: "You care more about making a new account than you do about your wife and children!" "You expect to have nice things and then blame me for working extra hours!" Triangles stabilize by maintaining the status quo while avoiding tension, conflict, or talking about sensitive emotional areas. The two people can then focus on the new issue (or person or object) and avoid discussing the painful issues between them. Feelings are thus drained off, and the focus is removed from the self and one's own part in the problem. Change in self is avoided.

The reciprocal function of a triangle and the idea of equal responsibility can be difficult to convey to a couple. This is especially true when the distancing mechanism used by one spouse is as emotionally charged as an extramarital affair. Suppose the wife distances from the painful issues in the relationship. By "triangling" his wife's affair, the husband makes it difficult to relinquish his self-righteous position of the "wronged husband." He does not see his behavior of working 14 to 16 hours a day as serving the same distancing function in the relationship. The nature of the distancing mechanism has meaningful content, whether it is overwork, extramarital affairs, homosexuality, psychotic symptoms, religious preoccupation, suicidal gestures, depression, or psychoanalysis. All serve the same function in a triangular relationship.

The concept of a family scapegoat originally broadened the individual pathological view to include the part the family played in the symptomatic behavior. However, the tendency was to view the scapegoat as the helpless victim of a persecuting family. For example, a husband and wife who are unable to settle their differences and wish to avoid their marital discord may focus on the "victim child." This leads to blaming the parents. In contrast, the concept of triangles from the systems view holds each person in the triangle responsible, as evident in Fig. 32-3. Father and mother avoid conflict by focusing on the son. Mother and son avoid dealing with their overcloseness by having a common enemy in

Fig. 32-3   Example of a family triangle.

the father. Father and son avoid awareness of their emotional distance by relating through the mother as go-betweens. Thus, the "victim" is eliminated. All members of a triangle participate equally in maintaining the triangle, and no triangle can persist without the active cooperation of all its members.

It is not a problem to be in a triangle; in fact, it is impossible to stay out of all triangles. Triangles form and reform rapidly and are the daily way most people handle conflict or tension. Problems arise if a triangle becomes fixed and involves significant relationships of deep friendship, blood ties, or marriage. Triangles are not static but form and reform around emotion-laden issues such as money, sex, child rearing, religion, alcohol, and education. A person's position in a triangle alters depending on the issue. A mother and father may be distant on the highly charged issue of how to spend their money. They may be close and in accord about their adolescent daughter's sexual activity. However, judgments about these issues are often based on emotion rather than careful thought.

> *?* *Many people marry thinking that they can change the parts of their spouse that they don't like after the honeymoon. What would a family systems therapist say about this?*

OPERATING PRINCIPLES. A person's operating principles are the laws that govern personal conduct. They must be inferred from what the person does in regard to an emotion-laden issue rather than what the person says. Operating principles vary from valuable ones based on conscious conviction to more immature, reactive, impulsive principles. Immature principles are other-focused rather than self-focused; they lead to a loss of freedom or self-determination. Any behavior that is predictable, such as behavior operated by a triangle, is not free. The loss of freedom impairs self-functioning, perpetuates problems, causes a deterioration in family functioning, and promotes symptom development.[15]

Other-focused, triangle-promoting operating principles are reflected in various ways. These include declaring feelings "right" or "wrong"; using plural pronouns *we* or *us* rather than *I;* accusing the other person, as in "You made me do it"; stepping in to settle, side taking, or blaming in two other people's conflict; telling or holding secrets; telling the other person what to do; and assuming responsibility for the other person's feelings, for example, "I want to make her happy" or "I couldn't tell him because it would hurt him." These statements are typically interpreted as thoughtful or responsible. In fact, avoiding one's own feelings by focusing on the other person is irresponsible. Everyone falls into this pattern, especially in a marriage or parent-child relationship. When a person becomes anxious, it is more comfortable to project the problem onto the other person and then work to change the other. The implicit assumption here is, "I can't help my behavior, but he is behaving that way deliberately."[15]

In more dysfunctional, closed family systems, interaction between family members is determined by fixed interactional patterns. These fixed triangles are an effort to maintain a homeostatic balance and avoid stress. When an additional stress occurs outside or within the family, such as a job change or the birth of a child, symptoms may arise in a dysfunctional attempt to reduce stress and restore balance. This is evident in the following clinical example.

Clinical Example Mr. and Mrs. D, who already had six children, had a seventh unplanned child. The family was financially strained, and Mr. and Mrs. D had a conflictual and distant relationship. When the last child was born, a middle sibling, 13-year-old Andy, developed symptoms and became school phobic. The school insisted that the child receive treatment. Late in the treatment the mother finally revealed that one of the reasons for the family's financial strain was the husband's work phobia and occasional gambling sprees. The wife had covered for him for years, calling his boss to make excuses and taking part-time work herself. Until the birth of the last child, the family was able to maintain a precarious, minimally functional balance. However, the additional stress produced symptoms that caused an outside agency, the school, to become involved.

INTERVENTIONS. Treatment encourages key figures in key triangles to identify their emotional triggers. The person identifies the verbal or behavioral cues of the other person, to which he reacts with a predictable behavior. When the person pinpoints these cues, he can take control of his part in the process. Once one person takes control and changes his part in a triangle, the whole system changes.

An example of this was a mother who was overclose to her 16-year-old daughter. The daughter had become school phobic and stayed home from school for a year before the family sought treatment. The father would come home from work, see that the daughter had missed school another day, and angrily attack her with "shape-up speeches." The mother bitterly complained about the daughter being home all day doing nothing. However, when the father began his verbal attacks, she became protective of the daughter and launched an attack on the father: "How can you say those things to her; you know how upset she gets." When the mother was able to identify her emotional trigger (she had always been terrified of her "drill sergeant" father), she was able to step back and permit the father to become more effective with his daughter.

Nurses must identify key triangles in a family and operating principles of its members. They must understand what sets off their emotional triggers and assume that the family will attempt to triangle them into its own emotional system to reestablish equilibrium. The nurse's job is to maintain sufficient emotional distance to watch the process unfolding between family members while maintaining emotional contact with each family member.

Therapist reactions that indicate that the therapist is part of a triangle include feeling sorry for or pitying the other, feeling angry at the system or member, being overly positive about the system, wanting to correct behavior, and finding oneself without questions or responses in the session. The nurse must limit the action to the two family members and avoid becoming involved. Once the therapist steps in to take sides, progress stops and status quo is reestablished. Side taking should be a planned strategy in which the nurse maintains the freedom to realign with specific family members.[13]

Systems therapists do not believe they can change family members; change is possible only when it is generated within the self. Family members are encouraged to take responsibility for the self and not try to change the other. The therapist must avoid becoming part of a triangle in the system. To get out of an emotional process in the session, the nurse may elicit the members' responses. For example, if the nurse becomes irritated at a critical, intrusive husband, the nurse can ask the wife, "What happens to your insides when your husband interrupts with criticism?" This feeds the process back into the system, keeping it between the spouses.

One area of controversy is the importance of the family therapist's working on his or her own family of origin. Systems therapists believe that it is a major aspect of training. "Working on" means that the nurse differentiates herself in her own family of origin. She identifies the issues in her family that she is reactive to and with whom she is part of a triangle around these issues. She then works to get out of the triangle by gaining control of her reflexive distancing and fusing. This way she has the freedom of emotional closeness and of some emotional distance with each family member (without using geographical distance to create emotional space). Unless a therapist is conscious of the triangles she is a part of in her own family, she will be vulnerable to the same roles and behaviors in the families she is treating.

Nuclear Family Emotional System

The nuclear family emotional system refers to patterns of interaction between family members and the degree to which these patterns promote emotional fusion (see Critical Thinking about Contemporary Issues). These patterns of interaction are the ways the person behaves in most significant relationships. All marriage relationships reflect a balance, or complementarity, of operating principles and reciprocal function.[3] For example, the reasonable, object-oriented, and emotionally distant spouse is married to the affectively expressive, relationship-oriented, emotional pursuer. These differences provide the attraction and the balancing stability to the marriage relationship. One spouse is the object-oriented overfunctioner, the other the emotion-oriented overfunctioner. Difficulty arises when dependence on attributes of the spouse reduces acquiring those at-

---

CRITICAL THINKING *about* **Contemporary Issues**

Does a Strong Mother-Daughter Attachment Imply Low Self-Differentiation?

Much attention has been given to the impact of the mother-daughter relationship on the development of women, particularly focusing on issues related to mental health and self-efficacy. Some theorists emphasize self-differentiation and devalue interpersonal attachment as a feminine behavior. Others analyze the concepts of caring, intimacy, closeness, and emotional reciprocity only when their absence is evident in intergenerational conflict, delinquency, broken homes, or family violence.

However, recent research suggests that a daughter's attachment to mother and her level of self-differentiation are not causally related, and that the concepts of self-differentiation and attachment appear to be separate variables in personality development.[5] Specifically, these researchers found that daughters' levels of self-differentiation were positively related to positive energy, and women who were mentally healthy and functioning effectively also showed high levels of attachment. The findings from this research affirm the value of attachment behaviors and self-differentiation in adulthood, challenge the traditional bias against attachment behaviors of women, and provide psychiatric nurses with a focus for mental health promotion when working with women.

---

tributes in the self. The self borrows on the functioning of the spouse, and self-boundaries are blurred. This is called ego fusion. When there are fixed positions of overfunction-underfunction, symptoms can occur, such as chronic depression or physical illness. In such a relationship, to view one spouse as strong and independent and the other as weak and dependent fails to recognize the overfunctioner's dependence on the underfunctioning of the other spouse. The underfunctioner must be one-down for the other to appear one-up.

Emotional fusion operates in all marriages. When the relationship is unstressed, the reciprocal function works smoothly; however, when stress occurs, each spouse becomes more as one self. The distancer seeks space and objects (work, hobbies, alcohol); the pursuer seeks togetherness and expression of personal feelings. Both are efforts to avoid personal anxiety. The pursuer takes the distancer's withdrawal as personal rejection and reactively withdraws. No longer feeling crowded, the distancer then moves in emotionally, only to be met with, "Where were you when I needed you? Get lost." The distancer then pulls back, baffled and angry at the rejection. A fixed emotional distance sets in.[13] These are the relationships often seen just before a couple decides on a divorce. These relationships are ripe for triangulation with an affair or with an unsuspecting therapist.

People tend to pick spouses who have similar levels of differentiation of self.[3] The greater the undifferentiation, the greater is the tendency toward fusion and potential problems. If there is a high degree of ego fusion and intensity in the nuclear family, this intensity can be diffused and reduced through active contact with the family of origin. In periods of stress, contact with the extended family or family of origin can stabilize the nuclear family. Promoting such contact can be an effective therapeutic strategy.

Kerr and Bowen[15] have identified two patterns in the nuclear family emotional system, labeled the explosive family and the cohesive family. Family units of a cohesive family are geographically close, in frequent contact and communication. The person who geographically separates from his family of origin because of the fusion or intensity of attachment may marry a spouse from a cohesive family. The person's unresolved attachments to his own family of origin lie dormant until ritualized contact (at a wedding or funeral) stirs them up. In a nuclear family in which both spouses are detached from their families of origin, the spouses tend to be more dependent on each other. The process between them is more intense and these can be explosive families.

Bowen[3] proposes three mechanisms by which spouses maintain sufficient emotional distance from each other to handle the anxiety associated with fusion. All three mechanisms may be used by the couple, or tension may be focused in one area. If tension is great enough, it will spill over into other social systems, such as mental health centers or school counselors. The three mechanisms used are marital conflict, dysfunction in one spouse, and projection of the problem onto one or more children.

> ? *How might the concept of emotional fusion explain why some people stay married to spouses who are physically or sexually abusive?*

MARITAL CONFLICT. Conflictual marriages are built on a constant struggle between spouses. They want "their fair share" of needs met, freedom, love, attention, or control. Neither spouse is willing to compromise. A high percentage of the self is wrapped up in the "happiness" of the other. Functioning of the self is enmeshed in the function of the other. These relationships tend to be stable, whether positive ("Anything to make her happy") or negative ("I sacrificed the best years of my life helping him be a success; I'll never let him go now"). They endure predictable cycles of intense closeness, distance-creating conflict, making up, then renewed closeness. It is commonly believed that this amount of conflict would harm the children of such marriages. However, Bowen believes that the children are protected because tension is focused between parents.

Intervention in conflictual marriages usually involves working with the most motivated spouse first. If both spouses are seen together, often the uproar between them is too great to tolerate. They are very reactive to each other. Limit setting, such as prohibiting interruptions, and strategies such as using a "listening chair" or turning one spouse's chair to the wall to listen are ineffective. In such situations spouses must be seen separately initially. The approach is to get the focus on the self and decrease efforts to change the other. The nurse focuses on what part the spouse plays in the situation. This spouse gains some self-control over reactive triggers. Once blaming is reduced, the spouse reevaluates beliefs and values without the need to attack the other. Such reevaluation entails contacting the family of origin by phone, letters, or planned visits. The goal is to understand better the source of the nuclear family conflict and to work to establish more personal relationships with the family of origin. Bowen calls this process "coaching." Usually, before this point is reached in the treatment, the absent, less motivated spouse seeks to join the sessions because of the changes that have occurred in the other spouse.

Significant changes in the marriage system occur when one spouse reduces overinvestment in the other and focuses on self. The spouse making changes must be warned of predictable efforts by the other to reestablish status quo. These efforts may include an escalation of anger-provoking behavior, threats to leave, and so on. If the spouse making changes can maintain a self-focused position through the resistance, both partners may become active in the treatment. While temporarily working with one spouse, nurses must guard against becoming part of a triangle. They may emotionally side with the spouse initially in treatment or become the spouse's only support. This can be especially difficult for nurses when the unexpressed plan of the unmotivated spouse is to deposit the husband or wife in treatment and obtain a divorce. Nurses may then be expected to "take care of" the spouse.

SPOUSE DYSFUNCTION. The second mechanism used by spouses to maintain emotional distance is the dysfunction of one spouse. As mentioned earlier, one spouse may be emotionally, socially, or physically disabled to varying degrees. The degree to which the one underfunctions is the degree to which the other overfunctions. This ensures that emotional equilibrium is maintained because both partners are locked into a mutually dependent relationship. Interventions with such a relationship are similar to those used with the conflictual marriage. Herz Brown[13] suggests working with the overfunctioning spouse by first helping him or her to pull back. The underfunctioning spouse then moves in to take up the slack, as evidenced in this clinical example.

Clinical Example Mr. and Mrs. S sought treatment because the husband was missing many days at work. The couple had extensive arguments about Mr. S not wanting to work and Mrs. S feeling outraged at the financial stress he was creating. It became apparent that Mrs. S treated Mr. S as one of their adolescent boys. She overfunctioned to the point of cleaning up after her husband's destructive temper tantrums. Over time, with considerable coaching, she was able to pull back in several areas, refusing to wake her husband or clean up after him, leaving it up to him to pay the bills, and generally holding back her critical nagging. The first sign of progress was at Mr. S's next temper tantrum (he did delicate electrical work and had a low frustration tolerance). He carefully selected which objects he would throw or smash in his workroom, for example, not throwing a box of small nuts and bolts. He cleaned up his own workroom and began going to work regularly. As Mr. S's functioning improved, Mrs. S became depressed and began addressing unresolved issues in her family of origin. This couple demonstrated the reciprocity in the mechanism of underfunctioning and overfunctioning in a marriage.

PROJECTION ON CHILD.   The third distancing mechanism used by spouses to control the intensity of fusion between them is the projection of the problem to one or more of the children. Before the development of a family pathology theory, the parents of a symptomatic child were excluded from therapy. This further reinforced the dysfunction in the family by focusing on the child as the problem. Child-focused families either view the problem as exclusive to the symptomatic child or deny the existence of a problem entirely. When the school or probation officer recommends treatment, they passively comply but participate reluctantly. When a couple centers on their children, it is easier to avoid marital confrontations because there is always something to worry, criticize, or complain about with the children. These families strongly depend on the children's symptoms and resist exploring broader issues in therapy.

How one child becomes a parental concern is a complex process. It may have its roots in several previous generations. Key triangles tend to repeat themselves over generations; thus the parent's natural tendency is to put one child in the parent's past position in the triangle. Nodal events are the normative events that occur in every family life but generate anxiety because change ensues. These include such events as birth, death, sickness, marriage, job changes, school changes, divorce, and family relocation. The amount of stress generated around a nodal event depends on the amount of resultant change. If a significant developmental stage of the child (for example, in utero, birth, entering school for the first time, or adolescence) coincides with the occurrence of a nodal event, this child may be vulnerable to the focus of family stress and to impairment. The first-born and last-born children are also particularly vulnerable to family focus.

The primary goal of treatment is to remove the focus from the child and place the conflict between the parents where it belongs. The child's dysfunctions must be placed within the context of the family system by taking a family history and drawing a family genogram. A three-generation **family genogram** is a structured method of gathering information and graphically symbolizing a lot of the factual and emotional relationship data in the initial interview.[20] A sample genogram is presented in Fig. 32-4. Drawing a family genogram in full view of the family on large easel paper or a blackboard broadens the family's focus. The therapist's questions and comments are geared toward change of self rather than changing the child.

The therapist may identify problematic behavior in other family members to remove blame from the child. Another therapeutic strategy is to discuss how grandparents might handle the problem. With some families the nurse can coach the overinvolved parent, such as the mother, to pull back from the focused child and send a note to her own mother telling her one thing about herself that she had not wanted her to know. This reveals the three-generational aspect of the presenting problem. It may also be helpful to work with the siblings at times, separately from the parents. This promotes a more positive support system among the siblings. Siblings often mimic their parents' negative behavior toward the focused child. They may also resent the excessive attention he receives from parents and act aggressively toward him.

Families with an acting-out child and two parents in the ineffective helpless position (or one parent set up as the "heavy" and the other as "the nice one") need a direct approach initially. The parents may have given up their authority to the child. This may be determined by asking them the following extreme questions: "If your child had third-degree burns, could you get her to take the horribly painful treatments?" or "If your child had heart disease, could you limit her activities?" Following are five guidelines for parents locked in a triangle with the acting-out child:

▼ The person who sets the rule must be present to enforce it.

▼ With two parents in the home, divide the areas of responsibility (such as allowance, bedtime, and nights out) so that when a dispute comes up, it is clear with whom the child must negotiate.

▼ Yelling is ineffective and inhibits thinking. Parents need to control their reactions and act as adults.

▼ Decide the logical consequences of repeated disobedient behavior and inform the child of them in advance. When the behavior occurs, without yelling, carry out the consequence even if the parents' personal plans must be changed to do so.

▼ Always give reassurance that the child is loved unconditionally.

As soon as the child focus is sufficiently reduced, the child is removed from the sessions. The therapist then becomes the third corner of the triangle, actively relating to both spouses without taking sides and thereby keeping conflict between the spouses.

Multigenerational Transmission Process

The roots of the family emotional system extend back through generations. When emotional dysfunction occurs, it can be scattered throughout the family tree. Drawing a three-generation family genogram often reveals certain relationship patterns otherwise believed to be peculiar to one

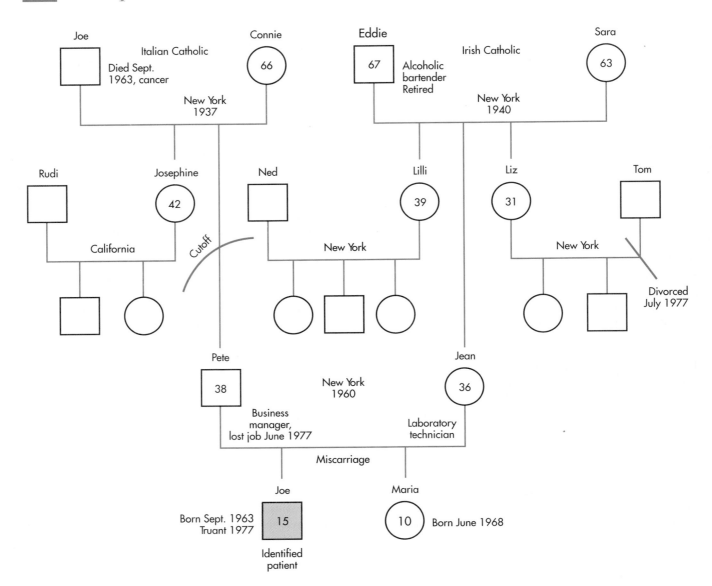

Fig. 32-4 Example of a family genogram.

nuclear family. Coloring in these problems on the genogram can help track them across generations. For example, suicide of younger brothers, divorce among female siblings, or alcoholism might be a pattern across a family system when four or five generations are mapped out on a genogram. In family therapy, a symptom in one family member in one generation has its origin several generations before.[3,12] This differentiates it from other forms of family therapy. However, families seeking treatment usually present symptoms as a nuclear family problem.

Family Projection Process

The family projection process is the way in which anxiety about specific issues is transmitted through the generations. These are emotionally powerful issues, such as money, sex,

child rearing, religion, work or school achievement, alcohol, politics, illness, and death, around which a rigid "party line" develops. Family members polarize around these issues, taking the family position or the direct opposite. Neither position allows freedom or flexibility of thought. Positions are reactive and fixed. Studying the family of origin helps identify a person's predictable position in family triangles involving specific issues. If individuals think about the issues they normally react to emotionally, they can plan strategies that will free them from triangled positions.

The family projection process also refers to the process that labels and assigns characteristics to certain family members. These labels may be overpositive ("Mary Sunshine," "The Genius") or overnegative ("The Crazy One," "Dummy"). They are equally unrealistic and confining. After years of family labeling, the labeled person will come to volunteer for the label and earn it.

> ? *Identify two emotionally powerful issues in your family of origin and think about your position related to them. Describe family labels you also heard while growing up.*

Sibling Position

The concept of personality profiles based on sibling position is borrowed from Toman,[27] who believes that important personality characteristics are determined by the sex of one's siblings and one's birth order. For example, the younger brother of two older sisters is quite different from the older brother of a brother. The personality profiles Toman developed can suggest marital discord or harmony on issues of rank or sex. For example, a younger brother of brothers may have more difficulty relating to his spouse than a younger brother of sisters. If this younger brother of brothers married a younger sister of sisters, they may both have discomfort with the opposite sex. In addition, they might struggle for juniority rights (who's going to take care of whom). The couple who recognizes sibling rank and each sibling's sex as a possible source of their conflicts can help each other to cope with their differences.

Emotional Cutoff

The emotional cutoff is a way to deal with intense unresolved attachment between children and parents. The cutoff is emotional isolation, although members may still live geographically close. It also may be physical distance from the family of origin. The cutoff creates the illusion of separation from parents. The more intense the emotional cutoff, the more likely this problem will be reestablished in the next generation. Reconnecting emotionally with the cutoff family may prevent the same process from occurring with the parents and children of the next generation because such patterns tend to be repeated.

Modes of Therapy

Several modes of therapy have been mentioned thus far, including therapy with both spouses. Another mode of family therapy involves only one family member. This is most often used with the young adult who is single and self-supporting. This method includes learning about the functioning of family systems and triangles. It also involves keeping an active emotional relationship with important family members by planned phone calls, letters, and visits. This therapy requires developing an ability to control emotional reactiveness to avoid becoming part of an emotional triangle during visits with the family.[26] The goal is to achieve more self-differentiation from the family of origin.

The person must also develop a person-to-person relationship with important family members. This therapy is called coaching. Once the person is knowledgeable about triangles and methods of detriangling within the family, coaching sessions can be held as needed to supervise ongoing self-differentiation efforts.

The last mode of therapy is multiple family therapy (MFT), developed in the late 1960s. MFT is different from multiple family group therapy. The latter uses role playing and psychodrama and promotes interfamily group processes to change family interaction and increase its sensitivity to the family environment.[1] MFT, from a family systems framework, is different. Sessions are structured to ensure against emotional exchange between families. Bowen believes that this emotional exchange encourages a fusion of other families into a large, undifferentiated ego mass. The idea behind MFT is:

▼ To conserve teaching time of families
▼ To provide contact with a greater volume of families
▼ To allow the opportunity for families to learn from the efforts and experiences of other families

While other families observe, the nurse therapist works with each family as if only one family were receiving therapy. While the family answers detailed questions about its problem, the nurse defocuses feelings and addresses one spouse while the other spouse listens. Then the silent spouse is asked to share thoughts or reactions to what the other spouse has said. The family members observing can talk to the therapist about another family but cannot directly talk to the other family.

STRUCTURAL FAMILY THERAPY

Structural family therapy is theory and techniques based on the individual within a social context that is clearly described by Minuchin.[21,22] The assumption is that behavior is a consequence of the family's organization and the interactional patterns between members. Changing the family organization and the feedback processes between members changes the context in which a person functions. Thus the person's inner processes and behavior change.

The basic question of a structural family therapist is, "In what way is this family structure maintaining this maladaptive symptom?" Family structure is the invisible set of demands that determine the way in which family members interact. A family is a system that operates through transactional patterns. Repeated transactions establish patterns of how, when, and to whom to relate, and these patterns determine whether the system is functional or dysfunctional.

> ? *What impact would sociocultural factors have on the effectiveness of a structural therapist's interventions with a family?*

Components

FAMILY IN TRANSITION. In this model the family is a social system in transformation. The family system must maintain its continuity so that family members can grow. At the same time it must adapt to internal and external stresses to the system. Normal anxiety occurs during transitional stages. Traditional therapists call this anxiety pathological. This is described in the following clinical example by Minuchin.[21]

Clinical Example An elderly widow decided to move from her apartment where she had lived for 25 years because she came home one day and found it had been robbed. Soon after moving, she sought treatment from a psychiatrist. She complained that the people who moved her were trying to control her and had purposely lost precious possessions. They left sinister messages for each other on her furniture, and when she went outside, people followed her and signaled to each other. The psychiatrist diagnosed her as psychotic with paranoid delusions and prescribed tranquilizers. When this did not help, she sought a second psychiatrist, who recommended hospitalization. The third therapist she saw was a context-related therapist. He understood her symptoms as an ecological crisis. It was precipitated by feeling forced to move into an unfamiliar environment. He explained to her that she had lost her shell: the familiarity of objects in her apartment, the neighborhood, the neighbors. Like any crustacean that has lost its shell, she felt vulnerable and was experiencing reality differently than before. He instructed her to go home, unpack, and place her familiar objects, books, and pictures in the new apartment. He told her to do her daily chores routinely, go to the same shops and checkout counters, and for 2 weeks make no effort to meet neighbors. She was to visit old friends and family but not discuss her recent experiences. If anyone asked, she was to explain that those had just been the problems of an illogical, fearful old woman.

Structural family therapists change the relationship between a person and the familiar context in which the person functions. This changes the subjective experience and enables more functional behavior to emerge. In the preceding clinical example, the therapist's interventions protected the woman from the unfamiliar and frightening environment until she could "grow a new shell." He blocked the environmental feedback that confirmed her paranoid fears as friends and family secretly discussed her frightening behavior. As her experience of her environment changed, her symptoms disappeared.

STAGES OF FAMILY DEVELOPMENT. Every family undergoes predictable stages of development over time. These stages require adaptive restructuring. Each stage involves a process of transition and requires changes in family functioning for adaptive growth and development. The stages of the family life cycle are presented in Table 32-3.[4]

FAMILY STRUCTURE. A third component of Minuchin's model of a functioning family relates to the family structure. The major elements of structure are:
▼ Power and influence within the family
▼ Sets and family relationships, including subsystems
▼ Family boundaries that may be individual, sexual, or generational

Structure can become dysfunctional in any or all of these areas.[8]

First, as in any organization, the family system must have a power hierarchy with different levels of authority to function efficiently. Functions must be complementary because the family needs to work together as a team. Over the years, mutual expectations of particular family members evolve. These expectations may be openly negotiated but are often implicit, with patterns of behavior developing around minor daily events. Critics of this aspect of structural therapy point out that too often, restoring the parent-child hierarchy means restoring a traditional male authority structure, which supports damaging gender inequalities existing in the family and society.[9] The nurse who focuses only on generational (parent-child) differences may ignore differences in power, resources, and needs among all family members. Thus the nurse could inadvertently promote gender-based power inequities that can result in destructive behavior. This dilemma highlights the need for family therapists to be particularly careful not to bring personal and sociocultural bias into their work with families.

> **?** *Describe how wife abuse and childhood incest can arise from a family structure that is based on male power and authority and female dependence and submission.*

Second, the family system differentiates and functions through sets of relationships or subsystems. Subsystems can be made up of individuals or dyads. They are formed by generation, sex, interest, or function. Each person belongs to many subsystems. Each subsystem has different levels of power in which differentiated skills are learned.

Third, boundaries of a subsystem are the rules defining who participates in subsystem functions and how. Boundaries must be free of intrusion. Each subsystem has specific functions and interpersonal developmental tasks to be accomplished. Patterns of mutual accommodation and healthy competition cannot develop among siblings if parents or grandparents constantly interfere. Subsystem boundaries must be clear for proper family functioning but must also permit emotional contact among members.

Minuchin[21,22] describes families with extreme boundary problems as either enmeshed or disengaged. Enmeshed boundaries are weak and fluid; personal space and subsystem boundaries rapidly change and affect all subsystems.

TABLE **32-3** *The Stages of the Family Life Cycle*

STAGE	EMOTIONAL PROCESS OF TRANSITION: KEY PRINCIPLES	SECOND-ORDER CHANGES IN FAMILY STATUS REQUIRED TO PROCEED DEVELOPMENTALLY
Leaving home: single young adults	Accepting emotional and financial responsibility for self	Differentiation of self in relation to family of origin Development of intimate peer relationships Establishment of self regarding work and financial independence
The joining of families through marriage: the new couple	Commitment to new system	Formation of marital system Realignment of relationships with extended families and friends to include spouse
Families with young children	Accepting new members into the system	Adjusting marital system to make space for children Joining in child rearing, financial, and household tasks Realignment of relationships with extended family to include parenting and grandparenting roles
Families with adolescents	Increasing flexibility of family boundaries to include children's independence and grandparents' frailties	Shifting of parent-child relationships to permit adolescent to move in and out of system Refocus on midlife marital and career issues Beginning shift toward joint caring for older generation
Launching children and moving on	Accepting a multitude of exits from and entries into the family system	Renegotiation of marital system as a dyad Development of adult-to-adult relationships between grown children and their parents Realignment of relationships to include in-laws and grandchildren Dealing with disabilities and death of parents (grandparents)
Families in later life	Accepting the shifting of generational roles	Maintaining own or couple functioning and interests in face of physiological decline; exploration of new familial and social role options Support for a more central role of middle generation Making room in the system for the wisdom and experience of the elderly, supporting the older generation without overfunctioning for them Dealing with loss of spouse, siblings, and other peers and preparation for own death; life review and integration

From Carter E, McGoldrick M: *The changing family life cycle: a framework for family therapy,* ed 2, Boston, 1989, Allyn & Bacon.

This diffuseness of boundaries prevents the development of autonomy and competence. Perceptions of self and others are poorly differentiated. A child in such a family might be so sensitized to conflict between parents that school performance may decline. The parents in such a family can become upset because the child refuses to eat vegetables at dinner. Such families flood with anxiety at times of stress and adapt poorly to change.

Disengaged families have rigid boundaries. Communication between subsystems is poor; supportive or protective contact is minimal. Members of such systems may function autonomously but have a skewed sense of independence. They lack feelings of loyalty and belonging and the capacity for interdependence. Some suggest that the product of a disengaged family is the sociopath. Because of the rigidity of subsystem boundaries, members may fail to respond adequately when one member is stressed. In such a family, a child's reading disorder might go unnoticed or a husband's suicidal behavior may be disregarded.

In this model of family therapy the nurse often functions as a boundary maker and may clarify diffuse boundaries by discouraging interruptions and encouraging shutting bedroom doors. The nurse may also open overly rigid boundaries by recommending that a distant parent and child spend time together or by calling attention to a member's feeling that would otherwise go unnoticed by other members. The nurse's assessment of family subsystems and boundary functioning provides a rapid diagnosis of the family. It indicates the direction and goals of therapeutic interventions.

As mentioned earlier, each subsystem has specific functions and interpersonal developmental tasks to be accomplished. The spouse subsystem must develop patterns of mutual support. Couples must make decisions and settle arguments without domination or relinquishing of self by either spouse. Ideally, they will bring out the best in each other, with each promoting personal growth and creativity in his or her spouse.

Spouses typically engage in an "other-improvement program." They bring into the marriage certain expectations of their spouse and work hard to have the spouse meet them. Interpretations in this area should be directed to both spouses. The part each plays in the destructive process should be pointed out. A mutual interpretation would be to say to the wife, "In your efforts to make contact with your husband, you are driving him away," and to the husband, "Your strong, silent style is alluring but elicits nagging." Balanced interpretations emphasize the complementarity of the system. Both positive and negative qualities are recognized in each spouse.

The parental subsystem socializes the children without sacrificing mutual support and accommodation between the spouses. Children must have access to each parent but be excluded from spouse functions. Minuchin advocates parental authority in an era that promotes "pure democracy" between parents and children. He recognizes the difficulty of parenting. Many parents are not satisfied with their own functioning. Parenting processes are different depending on the child's age. Part of promoting differentiation in the family is making the differentiation in ages clear. Adolescents have responsibilities and privileges that 12-year-old siblings do not. Children must learn to negotiate with their parents to live in a world of unequal power relationships.

Children first learn about peer relationships in the sibling subsystem. They learn to make friends, compete, negotiate, cooperate, and gain recognition of their skills. Knowledge of growth and development of children is valuable for the nurse, who at times must translate age-appropriate skills, needs, and values to parents. The nurse should support the child's right to growing autonomy and the parents' responsible authority at the same time.

Interventions

A vital component to structural family therapy is the process of joining the family.[21,22] Nurse therapists temporarily become part of the family system. They adapt their behavior to the particular family's rules and manner. The aim is to accommodate to the family to gain experiential entrance into the family system. Unless this is accomplished at the outset, restructuring and change are impossible. Methods of joining the family are described in Table 32-4.

Another initial task of nurse therapists is to assume leadership in the session. They must join the family while still retaining the freedom to confront and challenge by presenting themselves as experts, gaining the family's confidence, and instilling hope. The nurse establishes the rules of the system by determining who attends the session, allowing no one to talk for another, and prohibiting interruptions. The nurse controls the flow and direction of communication.

At the beginning of the session, the nurse contacts each member. More than 15 to 20 minutes must not be spent with an individual or the nurse will become part of the system. Very soon the nurse asks two people to interact directly to enact a problem they have been describing. The nurse can now directly observe dysfunctional interactions. Rather than going from content issue to content issue, the nurse therapist can introduce the conflict inherent in small events and make conflictual events from nonevents.

Minuchin is a master of intensifying minute, simple nonevents for therapeutic intervention. For example, in a demonstration videotape, a father is "helping" the identified patient, the adolescent son, adjust his microphone wire. Minuchin turns this into a therapeutic intervention focusing on the family's infantilization of the son. This occurs in the first 5 minutes of the tape. The amount of knowledge needed about the family to diagnose and begin restructuring dysfunctional interactions is available quickly. Structural family therapy does not explore or interpret the past; it is active and immediate.

Diagnosis in family therapy depends on the observation of how the family affects the nurse's behavior. It is also based on the nurse's impact on the family. The interactional diagnosis changes according to the family's acceptance or resistance of the therapist's restructuring interventions. It also varies depending on which family subsystem is active

TABLE **32-4** *Methods of Joining the Family*

METHOD	DESCRIPTION
Mirroring or mimicking	Matching the family's mood, pace, or communication patterns, such as becoming jovial, somber, fidgety, or terse in conversing with them
Respecting family values	Supporting family hierarchies, such as by addressing all communication through the spouse that appears to be the "central switchboard"
Finding common elements	Keying in culturally or establishing areas of kinship, such as by offering "I have an adolescent boy, too"
Searching for strength	Observing for the smallest positive aspect of each family member that the nurse can use to confirm that person's sense of self, such as by appreciating a clever phrase or a sense of humor
Supporting family subsystems	Confirming important family subsets, such as by giving small children toys to play with while talking with older ones, or by having parents sit together as they discuss their difficulty with the children
Tracking	Asking for elaboration with concrete details and examples of specific content in the family's discussion; this confirms people who are speaking and explores family structure, such as in tracking a mother's mentioning that she and her son are close by asking what time of the day and in which part of the house they are closest, thus learning that the mother and son sleep together while father sleeps in another room

in the therapeutic situation at any one time. In this way, diagnosis and therapy are inseparable.

Intervention strategies transform the dysfunctional transactional patterns that maintain symptomatic behavior. The nurse is concerned about symptom removal and changes the family's organization to ensure that the symptom is not passed on. However, if an area of organization such as the parents' relationship does not contribute to the symptom, the therapist does not enter there. Therapy should be limited to the family's presenting symptom.

Minuchin identifies seven categories of restructuring operations: enacting family transactional patterns, marking boundaries, escalating stress, assigning tasks, using symptoms, manipulating mood, and supporting, educating, or guiding.[21]

ENACTING TRANSACTIONAL PATTERNS. Enacting transactional patterns involves family members actively discussing an event that they might otherwise be describing to the nurse. Instead, the nurse instructs specific members to discuss the matter between themselves. The nurse disengages from the interaction to observe nonverbal confirmation or contradiction of the content, patterned sequences, interruptions, distractions, alliances, and coalitions.

It may be difficult to stay outside these transactions, and the family may drag the nurse back into direct discussion. Going behind a one-way mirror after giving the family directions is a way to avoid this temptation. Manipulating space by rearranging seating or position can be an effective way of encouraging or intensifying dialogue. The seating pattern a family assumes when it first walks into a session provides clues to alliances, coalitions, centrality, and isolation. The nurse's manipulation of seating and space can be a diagnostic probe to see how flexible the family is to such change. It is also a graphic indication to the family of a therapeutic goal. For instance, the nurse may seat the spatially isolated father next to his son, where the mother was seated. The wife is placed next to the nurse. This encourages more direct involvement between father and son, with the mother outside that relationship.

MARKING BOUNDARIES. Boundaries must be marked in both individuals and subsystems. This promotes clarity in enmeshed families and reduces rigidity in disengaged families. Rules promote individual autonomy and include insisting that family members speak to each other and not about each other. No one speaks for another, no one may interrupt, and no one acts as another's memory bank. The nurse encourages subsystem boundaries by including or excluding various subsystems attending a session. She would ask children to leave or not attend a session about spouses' sex life. The nurse may assign tasks to promote subsystem boundaries. She might instruct the father and daughter to go out for a pizza once a week without the mother or younger siblings. Having the sibling subsystem interact in a session, with the mother behind a one-way mirror, helps the children find alternative ways to resolve conflicts normally interrupted by mother's interventions. At the same time, this lets mother identify more positive interaction among the children. Previously, she could only reflexively react to their anger, rebelliousness, and selfishness by intruding on their boundaries. Rigid triads involving cross-generational interactions can be especially resistant to boundary marking.

ESCALATING STRESS. Increasing stress in a family forces members to develop more functional ways of resolving stress. In families seeking treatment, dysfunctional patterns have developed around the symptomatic member. To escalate stress, the nurse may block usual transactional patterns and emphasize differences the family ignores. Asking for the silent spouse's opinion following the dominant spouse's statements highlights unspoken family disagreements. Developing implicit conflict involves making covert conflict overt.

Families develop methods for diffusing conflict rapidly. For example, siblings may tease and shove each other noisily just before their parents argue. This prevents the parents' conflict from surfacing. Blocking the sibling conflict forces the parents to contact directly. The nurse can polarize conflict to increase stress. If the mother and father appear equally concerned about their son's delinquent activities, the nurse may ask the husband if he had ever tried telling his wife she was "messing up" with the son. The positions of the overprotective mother and the "reasonable" distant father develop.

The nurse can also produce stress by temporarily joining one member or subsystem. This operation must be carefully planned and requires the nurse's ability to disengage, which can be done serially to help members take differentiated positions. Also, a coalition can be formed, usually with a spouse, when the system rigidly resists open conflict. Joining a husband's attack on the wife makes the conflict too intense for the wife to diffuse stress onto the son; she is forced to address the conflict between herself and the husband.

ASSIGNING TASKS. Task assignment structures the setting for alternative interactions and behavior. In designing tasks, the nurse must have a clear idea of the family's structure and dysfunctional patterns. Specific interactional goals to accomplish through the task must be outlined. Tasks can be simple. The nurse may ask a husband and wife to sit next to each other as they discuss an issue. In a family in which the wife disciplines the children, the father is assigned the job. The mother handles only emergencies; otherwise, the father learns of infractions he does not directly observe. The wife may not interfere with her husband's disciplinary tactics. She takes notes. Both parents become active and effective.

In assigning tasks the nurse should give all critically involved members a portion of the task to complete. This reduces the likelihood of one member sabotaging another's new behavior if each member must remain self-focused. This also makes it easier to relinquish a fixed behavior if another behavior is assigned to replace it. Whether the task is completed or not, the family and nurse have new information about family patterns and progress.

USING SYMPTOMS. Symptoms can be used in restructuring operations in various ways. Symptoms may be focused on, as in a family Minuchin describes in which the daughter was a fire setter. The focus remained on the daughter, but the mother was instructed to spend time daily teaching the daughter how to light matches safely. This promoted a closer mother-daughter relationship, which was previously obstructed. A helpful focus remained on the symptom. Symptoms can be exaggerated to increase their intensity and mobilize family resources. A symptom can be relabeled, as in the case of a mother who continually nagged the son. Redefining her nagging as concern encouraged caring interactions. A new symptom shifts the family's focus onto another family member temporarily. For example, the husband fails to go to work and the wife alternately protects and threatens to leave him. Identifying her behavior as seriously depressed reduces her intense focus on the husband. A symptom's affect can also be changed, thereby altering interactions around it. For example, the mother who interacts positively with her fire-setting daughter evokes a new affect with the symptom.

MANIPULATING MOOD. Manipulating the family's mood is another restructuring operation. For example, by exaggerating the common family mood, the family reacts by showing a wide range of expressions. The nurse can also model a more appropriate affect for the family, for example, by reacting with strong indignation to a young boy's criticism of his mother. This promotes respect and clarifies the boundaries of a passive, enmeshed parental subsystem.

SUPPORTING, EDUCATING, GUIDING. Support, education, and guidance can be a restructuring operation. They can take the form of modeling, assigning tasks, or sharing concrete information. Minuchin shows families how they program each other in the circular process of a family system.

The goal of structural family therapy is not a change in behavior but a change in the whole family's organization. This allows individual members a new experience in the family. Using a model of an effectively functioning family, the therapist joins the family in a therapeutic system, hoping to restructure the family. The restructuring helps to maintain functional subsystems or form new subsystems that will promote healing and growth.

STRATEGIC FAMILY THERAPY

Strategic family therapy developed out of communication theory.[29] Communication theorists, such as Haley, contend that all behavior, not only verbal acts, is communication. They recognize that most communication consists of many levels between sender and receiver, and that the significance of any message depends on how it is reinforced, contradicted, or framed by other messages. These, along with the setting and the relationship between sender and receiver, constitute the context that must be considered in interpreting any message (see Chapter 2).

Another basic tenet of communication theory is that communication is an ongoing process. There is no beginning point or end point in the stimulus-response-reinforcement pattern of human interaction. In most relationships the behavior of each participant depends on the other's behavior. In families, complex, highly patterned, repetitive interactions become established. When a two-person (or more) system is dysfunctional in its communication, potential exists for problems. Three types of common communication problems are disqualification, disconfirmation, and incongruent communication.[29]

Disqualification includes self-contradictions, inconsistencies, subject switches, incomplete sentences, misunderstandings, obscure mannerisms of speech, and literal interpretation of metaphor. An example of disqualification is a question an older brother used to baffle his younger sister: "Do you walk to school or carry your lunch?"

Disconfirmation involves ignoring or invalidating essential elements of a significant other's self-image. It involves saying that you do not feel the way you feel, need what you need, or experience what you experience. An example is when a spouse says, "I know you don't mean that. You're just upset and getting angry doesn't suit you."

Incongruent communication is delivering two conflicting messages at the same time. In responding to either message, the receiver will be charged with "badness or madness." This is the basis of the double bind. An example is the command "Be spontaneous!" or the direction to "Be assertive, and don't make waves."

Components

Strategic therapists make a distinction between difficulties and problems. Difficulties are either undesirable states of affairs that can be removed by a logical solution or undesirable, common life problems that must be lived with. Problems arise from small difficulties that escalate. They are maintained by mishandling attempts to solve them. Mishandling often occurs around adaptation to ordinary life events and ranges from ignoring or denying difficulties that require action, to attempting to resolve an ordinary life difficulty that is unnecessary (such as a husband who would not talk to his wife before breakfast) or impossible to resolve (such as the generation gap), to difficulties where action is needed but the wrong kind is taken.[11,16]

Strategic family therapists are not concerned with the history of the problem or the motivation behind it. They are not interested in characteristics of people, and they place no importance on insight. Little distinction is made between acute and chronic problems. Chronic problems are ones that have been mishandled longer. The presenting problem behavior and the problem-maintaining behavior are the primary focus of treatment.

Communication theorists have identified a positive feedback loop in human interaction. This is the vicious cycle that develops from efforts by family members, or the identified patient, to stop or "help" undesirable behavior. For example, the rebellious teenager, when faced with parental discipline, becomes increasingly rebellious. As discipline becomes harsher, the boy's behavior escalates further. Thus the action that is meant to alleviate the behavior of the other party aggravates it. From this view, the cause and the nature of a problem are essentially the same process. People try to change behavior in the most logical way possible. Common sense suggests prevention or avoidance of undesirable behavior by means of opposite behavior. If this does not work, they try harder with the same behavior. The resolution of problems therefore requires changing the problem-maintaining behaviors. This interrupts the vicious positive feedback cycles.[16]

Interventions

Intervention occurs with the identified patient, another family member, or both, depending on who is most concerned with the problem. This is the person most willing to change. Effective intervention can be made through any member of the system to break the positive feedback loop. This is illustrated in the following two clinical examples.

Clinical Example A colonel was being militarily strict with his son, and the boy was becoming increasingly defiant. The therapist told the father that his son was "going to the dogs." The therapist suggested that the father hold back on his discipline to get a baseline measurement of how bad the boy's behavior would become. As pressure on the boy was reduced, his behavior improved.

Clinical Example A woman had problems with urinary frequency. She was isolated at home, feeling unable to leave the house to socialize. She was also isolated at work because she had her desk by the bathroom door where there were no co-workers. She worked from 12 to 8 PM. The therapist instructed her to urinate as many times as she felt she had to each morning before going to work but to use the toilet only three times; after that she was to urinate sitting in the tub. She was to make no effort to change her pattern at work. The next week the woman reported she had been in agony the first morning but was unable to urinate sitting in the tub. She then figured that if she could limit herself at home, she could do so at work, and had no further problems with urinary frequency.

These examples demonstrate the use of reversal or symptom prescription. They stop the family or patient from trying to change. Persuading people to change behavior that they believe is correct often requires treatment strategies that appear weird, illogical, or paradoxical.

The nurse's first task is to obtain a statement from the patient of the presenting complaint in specific, concrete terms. After obtaining this statement, the nurse determines what about the behavior makes it a problem. The nurse asks what solutions the family has tried. This identifies which remedies to avoid and indicates the problem-maintaining behavior.

Next, the nurse asks what the family's or patient's minimum goal of treatment would be—what smallest identifi-

able change would signify progress or some success. General goals such as "improved communication" are not acceptable. Changes such as "feeling happier" or negative goals such as "stopping certain behavior" are equally unacceptable. Rather, the nurse seeks positive, specific behavioral goals that reflect an attitude or feeling change, such as "the father will engage in one positive activity with his son each week." If a small but significant change can be made in what appeared to be a hopeless situation, a ripple effect may occur. That is, once a patient is mobilized and regains confidence in the ability to solve a small problem, sometimes other difficulties can be surmounted.[16]

As soon as possible, the therapist attempts to grasp the patient's language and main ideas and values. Tuning in to the family's view and then extending that view is a critical step known as **reframing**. It precedes the therapist's strategic intervention. To reframe means to change the conceptual or emotional setting or viewpoint in which a situation is experienced. Using language common to the family's world view, the therapist places the experience in another frame that fits the "facts" of the same concrete situation equally well. The situation's entire meaning changes.[10,11]

An example of reframing includes using hostility when it is present in a woman's frigidity. The therapist may reframe the problem as one produced by her overprotecting the male. Assuming that there is hostility and protecting the husband is the last thing the woman would want to do, the new frame to the problem uses hostility as an incentive to release her inhibited sexual feelings. Tom Sawyer reframed whitewashing the picket fence as an artistic, entertaining enterprise rather than a dreary chore. He used his friends' competitiveness to vie for the opportunity to whitewash. Reframing causes an attitudinal change and a change in emphasis of a situation's facts. This changes the situation's meaning to permit new behavior. The concrete facts remain unchanged.

Strategic therapists place no importance on the therapist undergoing therapy, as family system therapists do. Nurses can be trained in this theoretical framework without understanding their involvement with their families. Structural therapists share this view.

Strategic therapists are sometimes attacked as having a manipulative, insincere approach. They acknowledge that this is the case. Communication research stresses that it is impossible not to communicate. Likewise, it is impossible not to influence. A nondirective, dynamically oriented therapist influences the patient's communication in hundreds of subtle ways. These ways include body movement, intonation, and leading responses. The insight school and the nondirective school of therapy influence patients outside the patient's awareness. Strategic therapists do so openly. The patient's awareness of the manipulation itself is irrelevant as long as the strategy is given and followed. The difference between the insight school and the strategic school of psychotherapy is conceptual rather than ethical. The insight school believes that change in people occurs

TABLE 32-5 *Models of Family Therapy*

	FAMILY SYSTEM (BOWEN)	STRUCTURAL (MINUCHIN)	STRATEGIC (HALEY)
View of normal family function	Differentiation of self in relation to others Balance between thinking and feeling	Generational hierarchy with strong parental authority Clear boundaries Flexibility of system for autonomy, interdependence, and adaptive change	Flexibility Large behavioral repertoire for problem solving and life cycle passage
View of symptoms/ dysfunction	Functioning is impaired by relationship with family of origin Poor differentiation Emotional reactivity Triangulation Emotional cutoff	Symptoms result from current structural imbalance and malfunctioning generational hierarchy or boundaries Enmeshed or disengaged style Maladaptive reaction to internal or external demands	Symptom is embedded in interaction pattern Origin of problem not significant Symptoms are maintained by unsuccessful problem solving Impasse at life cycle transition
Goals of therapy	Greater self-differentiation Increased thinking Decreased emotional reactivity Detriangulate self	Reorganize family structure to achieve strengthened parental hierarchy, clear, flexible boundaries, and more adaptive patterns	Interrupt rigid feedback cycle Change symptom-maintaining sequence to attain new outcome
Role of the nurse in change	Stays detriangulated Change can occur only within the self Change in one member can bring about systemic change	Joining the family is prerequisite for restructuring Nurse is responsible for change while crediting the family for beneficial changes	If treatment fails, the fault lies with the nurse Success is credited to the family, thus enhancing its confidence in future problem-solving skills
Interventions	Teach how family systems work Coach individual to establish person-to-person relationship with key members of family of origin Use genogram to track triangles, myths, and themes across the generations Ask factual who, what, when, where, and how questions to promote thinking and reduce emotionally reactive behavior	Joining Enacting Marking boundaries Escalating stress Assigning tasks Using symptom Manipulating mood Supporting Educating Advocacy	Detailed questions to track behaviors surrounding the problem Symptom prescription Reframing Strategies designed to interrupt self-reinforcing behavioral sequence maintaining the symptom

through a change in their understanding of themselves. The strategic school persuades a person to change "spontaneously." It arranges a situation so that the person initiates the change in behavior.

The strategic therapist is an active and deliberate change agent. The therapist creates a strategy to bring about the change the patient wants to achieve. The responsibility for success or failure therefore rests on the nurse. The nurse never takes the credit for change in the patient's eyes. In this therapy, the point at which termination takes place is clear. It occurs when the patient is satisfied with the improvement that has been made.

The theoretical views of family therapy presented in this chapter are summarized in Table 32-5. These models reflect current thinking in family therapy.

 Compare strategic family therapy with cognitive behavioral therapy, as described in Chapter 30.

Summary

1. Characteristics of the functional and dysfunctional family were described. The competence paradigm was also introduced, with its emphasis on family strengths, resources, and competencies.
2. Nonclinical family interventions are designed primarily to educate and support. They are the result of the family self-help movement in psychiatry. Components of a comprehensive psychoeducational program were described.
3. Family systems theory conceptualizes all family systems on a continuum ranging from total dysfunction to high levels of functioning. Separating the thinking and feeling processes of family members is foundational to this therapy. The goal of systems therapy is for individual members to differentiate themselves from the family emotional "we-ness" system.
4. Structural family therapy assumes that behavior and the family's level of function are consequences of the family's organization and the interactional patterns between

members. The major elements of a family structure that enable viable family functioning are a power hierarchy with different levels of authority, differentiated sub-systems with different functions and levels of power, and subsystem boundaries sufficiently well defined to prevent intrusion but also able to allow emotional contact between members.

5. Strategic therapists are concerned with the removal of problematic behavioral patterns or symptoms. The goals of strategic therapy include obtaining a clear statement from the family of the presenting complaint in specific, concrete terms. The therapist reframes the problem, thereby changing the situation's meaning, permitting new behavior to occur.

COMPETENT CARING A Clinical Exemplar of a Psychiatric Nurse

Carole Bennett, MN, RN, CS

As a psychiatric nurse, I have always found it difficult to describe the rewards I experienced for the years of hard work I have dedicated to my profession. Sometimes, the rewards elude even me. Then, quite unexpectedly, I have the opportunity to really help someone and I remember why I have been a psychiatric nurse for such a long time.

Recently, a nurse working on our youth unit was having difficulty with teaching parenting skills to a mother. It seemed that no matter how many times she demonstrated limit setting and reinforcement, this mother seemed unable to use these skills. The nurse asked me to see the mother and intervene using the family genogram and I agreed. The next day the family anxiously appeared: the mother, the father, and an aunt who flew down from New York. When I heard that the father's older sister from New York was waiting to be in family therapy, I thought that this would be a rough one. So I drew a deep breath, offered coffee all around, poured myself a big cup, and began the meeting. Yes, they all knew why they were there. Yes, they all knew it might get uncomfortable. Yes, they all wanted to stay.

The father and his sister began with their family. They grew up in the projects, had different fathers, described years of struggle, related how the older sister was sent to New York to live with her natural father, and how their mother managed all the while to raise them from a wheelchair. But she had done it; she had shown them how to do it, too.

Then the mother began. She too was raised in the projects, but by her grandparents. Her mother never really visited often, and

her grandmother was an alcoholic. Yes, she had a grandfather, but he was an alcoholic, too. She also lived with other family members at various times, but they were all heavy drinkers. In fact, every adult in her childhood was an alcoholic. But it was hard for her to recall facts. Had she been sexually abused? Well, she remembers being told something about that but she couldn't remember any details. She does remember being beaten regularly by various people, but that didn't seem unusual to her.

Everyone was quiet. It was hard for me to know quite what to say. By this time the husband was patting his wife lovingly. He had known only parts of the painful story he just heard his wife describe. And his sister from New York moved closer to her sister-in-law on the couch. They were very supportive while I suggested that perhaps no one had ever shown the wife how to be a mother. No one had ever shown her what to do, and so she really didn't know how to take care of the seven boys she was now raising.

As a group, we continued to talk until we came up with a plan. The sister was leaving for home soon, but there would be two other sisters who could help. The father said he could shorten his work day, and perhaps the mother could look for a job, which was something she wanted to do. The unit nurse said she could arrange for the mother to spend entire days on the unit so that she could begin to learn how to do this thing called "child rearing." And finally, we discussed the issue of therapy. Well, no thank you. The mother didn't think she was ready to talk to someone about what had happened to her so long ago, but maybe she would be sometime in the future.

We all stood up and shook hands, smiling and sensing the partnership among us. The sister from New York gave my hand an especially firm squeeze and looked me right in the eye. I think she was saying she was glad I was there, and I was sending the same message back to her. At that moment I knew exactly why I have been a psychiatric nurse for such a long time.

your **INTERNET**
c o n n e c t i o n

The WholeFamily Center
http://www.wholefamily.com/

Magic Stream
http://fly.hiwaay.net/~garcon/

Chapter Review Questions

1. Identify whether the following statements are true (T) or false (f).

A. ___ Triangles should be avoided at all costs.

B. ___ Triangles distance a person from a painful issue and allow one to avoid change.

C. ___ There is always a third person in a triangle willing to deflect emotional intensity.

D. ___ Therapists can be most effective by becoming part of the triangle and thereby effecting change.

E. ___ Participants of a triangle shift in a family depending on the emotional issue at stake.

2. Fill in the blanks.

A. Using the competency paradigm, a family's _____ are emphasized in therapy, as compared with older conceptual models, which emphasize a family's _____.

B. Nonclinical interventions with families are designed primarily to _____ and _____.

C. The largest self-help and consumer advocacy group in the United States is _____.

D. Family systems therapy was developed by _____.

E. A basic premise of family systems therapy is that families fail to distinguish between _____ and _____.

F. When self-boundaries are blurred it is called _____.

G. Structural family therapy seeks to interrupt the sequence of _____.

H. To _____ means to change the conceptual or emotional setting or viewpoint in which a situation is experienced.

I. The first task of the strategic family therapist is to _____.

3. Provide short answers for the following questions.

A. Discuss how a person with high differentiation of self differs from someone with low self-differentiation.

B. Define a genogram and sketch one for your own family.

C. Critique the adaptive and maladaptive family functioning portrayed in a novel by Pat Conroy (*Prince of Tides, Lords of Discipline*), Ann Tyler (*Accidental Tourist, Dinner at the Homesick Restaurant*), or another author of your choice.

REFERENCES

1. Bender PJ: Multiple family therapy for adolescents: a case illustration, *J Child Adolesc Psychiatr Nurs* 5:27, 1992.
2. Bohlander J: Differentiation of self: an examination of the concept, *Issues Ment Health Nurs* 16:165, 1995.
3. Bowen M: *Family therapy in clinical practice*, ed 2, Northvale, NJ, 1988, Jason Aronson.
4. Carter E, McGoldrick M: *The changing family life cycle, a framework for family therapy*, ed 2, Boston, 1988, Allyn & Bacon.
5. Davis B, Jones L: Differentiation of self and attachment among adult daughters, *Issues Ment Health Nurs* 13:321, 1992.
6. Doornbos M: The strengths of families coping with serious mental illness, *Arch Psychiatr Nurs* 10:214, 1996.
7. Dunst C, Trivette C: *Enabling and empowering families: principles and guidelines for practice*, Cambridge, Mass, 1988, Brookline.
8. Fishman HC: *Intensive structural therapy: treating families in their social context*, New York, 1993, Basic Books.
9. Goodrich TJ, editor: *Women and power: perspectives for family therapy*, New York, 1991, WW Norton.
10. Haley J: *Problem solving therapy*, San Francisco, 1987, Jossey-Bass.
11. Haley J: *Learning and teaching therapy*, New York, 1996, Guilford Press.
12. Herz Brown F: The multigenerational model. In Herz Brown F, editor: *Reweaving the family tapestry*, New York, 1991, WW Norton.
13. Herz Brown F: The therapeutic relationship. In Herz Brown F, editor: *Reweaving the family tapestry*, New York, 1991, WW Norton.
14. Howe C, Howe J: *The national alliance for the mentally ill: history and ideology, New directions for the mental health services*, no. 34, San Francisco, 1987, Jossey-Bass.
15. Kerr M, Bowen M: *Family evaluation: an approach based on Bowen theory*, New York, 1988, WW Norton.
16. Madanes C: Strategic family therapy. In Gurman A, Kniskern D, editors: *Handbook of family therapy*, vol. 2, New York, 1991, Brunner/Mazel.
17. Marsh D: *Families and mental illness: new directions in professional practice*, New York, 1992, Praeger.
18. Marsh D: Working with families of people with serious mental illness. In VandeCreek L, Knapp S, Jackson T, editors: *Innovations in clinical practice: a source book*, vol. 11, Sarasota, Fla, 1992, Professional Resource Exchange.
19. McFarlane W: Multiple family groups and psychoeducation in the treatment of schizophrenia, *Arch Gen Psychiatr* 52:679, 1995.
20. McGoldrick M, Gerson R: *Genograms and family assessment*, New York, 1986, WW Norton.
21. Minuchin S: *Families and family therapy*, Cambridge, Mass, 1974, Harvard University Press.
22. Minuchin S, Fishman H: *Family therapy techniques*, Cambridge, Mass, 1981, Harvard University Press.
23. Mueser KT, Gingerich S: *Coping with schizophrenia: a guide for families*, Oakland, 1994, New Harbiner.

24. Parker B: Living with mental illness: the family as caregiver, *J Psychosoc Nurs Ment Health Serv* 31:19, 1993.
25. Peternelj-Taylor C, Hartley V: Living with mental illness: professional/family collaboration, *J Psychosoc Nurs* 31:23, 1993.
26. Schwartzberg N: Single young adults. In Herz Brown F, editor: *Reweaving the family tapestry,* New York, 1991, WW Norton.
27. Toman W: *Family constellation,* ed 4, New York, 1993, Springer.
28. Walsh F: Conceptualizations of normal family processes. In Walsh F, editor: *Normal family processes,* ed 2, New York, 1993, Guilford.
29. Watzlawick P, Beaven J, Jackson D: *Pragmatics of human communication,* New York, 1967, WW Norton.
30. Wylie MS: Family therapy's neglected prophet: Bowen's legacy, *Fam Ther Networker* Mar/Apr:25, 1991.

Annotated Suggested Readings

Annunziata J, Jacobson-Kram P: *Solving your problems together,* Washington, DC, 1994, American Psychological Association.
   A "family-friendly" text, designed to answer common questions about family therapy, that can be used by child and adult family members to help evaluate whether family therapy is right for them.

Ascher-Svanum et al: Education need of families of mentally ill adults, *Psychiatric Serv* 48:1072, 1997.
   Describes the response by family members to a survey about preferences for family psychoeducation programs, including type of information, format, presenter, frequency, and length of educational programs, setting, and cost.

*Bohlander J: Differentiation of self: an examination of the concept, *Issues Men Health Nurs,* 16:165, 1995.
   Excellent discussion of the concept of differentiation of self, including theoretical background, concept uses, defining attributes, antecedents, consequences, measurement, empirical referents, and implications for clinical practice.

*Nursing reference.

*Cox R: Systemic circularity: working with individuals, *J Psychosoc Nurs,* 32:33, 1994.
   Describes the concept of circularity in empowering individual patients to make their own family system interventions and improve family functioning.

*Doornbos M: The strengths of families coping with serious mental illness, *Arch Psychiatric Nurs,* 10:214, 1996.
   Outlines a descriptive study that documents the strengths of families with members suffering from mental illness. These included family coping, adaptability, and conflict management.

Harway M: *Treating the changing family,* New York, 1996, John Wiley & Sons.
   A "must read" text for nurses who work with families. Separate chapters review challenges to traditional and nontraditional families and the role of the clinician.

Marsh D, Dickens R: *Troubled journey: coming to terms with the mental illness of a sibling or parent,* New York, Tarcher/Putnam, 1997.
   Draws on the voices of siblings and adult children to tell of the pain brought by mental illness to all members of the family. Helpful in structuring a sibling support group.

Mikesell R, Lusterman D, McDaniel S: *Integrating family therapy,* Washington, DC, 1995, American Psychological Association.
   Unique in its review of broad classes of core family therapy interventions and their application to clinical cases. Practitioners will find this text most useful.

Nichols W: *Treating people in families,* New York, 1996, Guilford Press.
   Written for the student and practitioner of family therapy, this is a practical synthesis of what works in the field. Accessible, logical, and very helpful.

Wasow M: *The skipping stone: ripple effects of mental illness on the family,* Palo Alto, Calif, Science and Behavior Books, 1995.
   Content of this text is based on findings from interviewing family members of people with severe mental illness about the effects of the illness on members of the immediate and extended family. Meaningful drawings reflect the mood of each chapter.

UNIT 5

Treatment Settings

You may think that most people with emotional and psychiatric problems spend many days of their lives in an acute or long-term psychiatric hospital being cared for by specially trained staff. Years ago you would have been correct, but today, most people with such problems live in the community and receive their mental health care in outpatient settings. These are the people you pass on the street, see at the mall, and laugh with at the movies. Today, we no longer try to separate and isolate the mentally ill in large, impersonal institutions. Rather, we ask our caregivers to reach out to these people and their families in the neighborhoods in which they live, love, and learn.

In this unit you will discover how contemporary psychiatric hospitals take care of patients. You will read how inpatient psychiatric nurses protect and stabilize people in crisis and then turn their care over to a variety of community-based mental health care providers. As psychiatric treatment grows in the community, new and expanded roles are opening up for psychiatric nurses. These tap into nurses' spirit of innovation, creativity, and resourcefulness. Finally, you'll learn about home care and the way in which psychiatric nurses are returning to their roots in public health and crossing the hearths and homes of the patients they treat. So step up, step out, and step into the current practice settings of psychiatric care.

Hospital-Based Psychiatric Nursing Care

Joan M. Herbert and Victoria A. Queen

© 1998 M.C. Escher/Cordon Art, Baarn, Holland.

"We're all mad here. I'm mad. You're mad." "How do you know I'm mad?," said Alice. "You must be," said the Cat, "or you wouldn't have come here." Alice didn't think that proved it at all. **Lewis Carroll** *Alice's Adventures in Wonderland*

LEARNING OBJECTIVES

After studying this chapter the student should be able to:

▼ Describe recent changes in hospital-based psychiatric care

▼ Identify the components of the therapeutic milieu and their implications for hospital-based psychiatric nursing practice

▼ Discuss the caregiving activities of the psychiatric nurse in structured treatment settings

▼ Analyze the psychiatric nurse's role in integrating and coordinating hospital-based patient care

▼ Evaluate outcomes related to hospital-based psychiatric nursing practice

TOPICAL OUTLINE

The Psychiatric Hospital in Transition
  Inpatient Programs
  Partial Hospital Programs
Managing the Therapeutic Milieu
  The Therapeutic Community
  The Therapeutic Milieu
  Nursing Implications
Implementing Caregiving Activities
  Assessing and Intervening in Potential Risks
  Patient and Family Education
  Activities, Groups, and Programs
  Meeting Physical Needs
  Discharge Planning
Integrating Care Delivery
  Teamwork and Coordinated Care
  Resource Allocation
  Nursing Care Delivery Modalities
  Professional, Regulatory, and Accreditation Standards
Evaluating Outcomes
  Quality Improvement Programs
  Risk Management
  Utilization Review

The treatment of the mentally ill has always reflected social values and public policy. Before World War II, effective medications were largely unavailable, and the mentally ill were separated from the community and housed in institutions for the protection of patients as well as society. Nursing care for these patients was primarily custodial. With changing social perspectives and the move toward more humane treatment, the psychiatric hospital came to be seen as a possibly powerful force that could influence patient behavior and help people recover from mental illness. More recently, scientific advances in biomedical practice have led to the use of effective medications and somatic therapies to treat symptoms of psychiatric illness. These, used in conjunction with therapeutic principles and management strategies of the treatment milieu, offer hospital-based psychiatric nurses valuable tools for the comprehensive care of the mentally ill.

THE PSYCHIATRIC HOSPITAL IN TRANSITION

Health-care costs, changing reimbursement trends, and problems with accessibility of care among vast numbers of citizens have prompted major changes in how health care is delivered in the United States.[31] As efforts to reduce the growth of health-care expenditures have shortened inpatient lengths of stay, less expensive treatment alternatives have become increasingly important. Today, considerably more treatment options are being offered. Many hospital facilities have become integrated clinical systems and provide a full range of services, including partial hospitalization, ambulatory, and even home care programs.

Inpatient Programs

In recent years the focus of psychiatric care has moved away from extended care in predominantly inpatient settings toward shorter lengths of inpatient stays and a wider choice among continuum of care options.[19,30] For example, in 1988 the average length of stay for acute psychiatric inpatient treatment was about 25 days, as compared with 15 days in 1994 (Fig. 33-1). More recently, many inpatient psychiatric settings have an average length of stay of 5 to 10 days, and crisis stabilization inpatient programs may involve only a 2- or 3-day length of stay.

The major psychiatric diagnoses of patients admitted to inpatient and partial hospital programs are listed in Table 33-1.[5] In previous years, most patients with maladaptive coping responses entered the psychiatric hospital in the **acute** treatment stage and were able to stay in the hospital until the goal of symptom **remission** was attained (Fig. 33-2). Today, however, the majority of patients are admitted to hospitals in the **crisis** stage, with the treatment goal of **stabilization** rather than symptom remission.[17,22] The indications for inpatient hospital use have become more focused in recent years and include:

▼ Prevention of harm to self or others

Fig. 33-1 Hospital stays for psychiatric patients.

Note: All figures for treatment in an acute care psychiatric hospital

TABLE **33-1** *Major Diagnoses of Patients Admitted to Inpatient Programs and Partial Hospital Programs*

DIAGNOSIS	PERCENTAGE
INPATIENT PROGRAMS	
Affective disorders	32
Schizophrenia	23
Substance use disorders	21
Adjustment disorders	7
Organic mental disorders	3
Personality disorders	2
PARTIAL HOSPITAL PROGRAMS	
Schizophrenia/affective	61
Personality	17
Disruptive behavior	4
Substance abuse	4
Developmental disability	1
Other	13

▼ Stabilization to allow treatment at a less restrictive level of care

▼ Initiation of a treatment process with safety risks that must be monitored by specially trained personnel

▼ Management of severe symptoms resulting in significant confusion, disorganization, and inability to care for self

▼ Need for a rapid, multidisciplinary diagnostic evaluation that requires frequent observation by specially trained personnel

As the goals of hospitalization have shifted, treatment objectives have also become more focused and include:

▼ Rapid evaluation and diagnosis

▼ Decreasing behavior that is dangerous to self or others

▼ Preparing the patient and significant caregivers to manage the patient's care in a less restrictive setting

▼ Arranging for effective aftercare to facilitate continued improvement in the patient's condition and functional level

CONTINUUM OF COPING RESPONSES

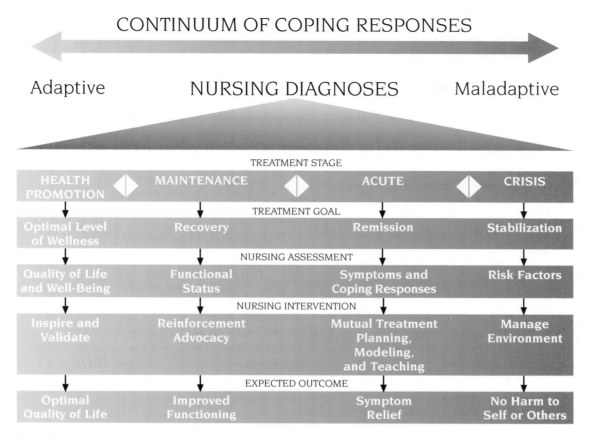

Adaptive   NURSING DIAGNOSES   Maladaptive

TREATMENT STAGE

| HEALTH PROMOTION | MAINTENANCE | ACUTE | CRISIS |

TREATMENT GOAL

| Optimal Level of Wellness | Recovery | Remission | Stabilization |

NURSING ASSESSMENT

| Quality of Life and Well-Being | Functional Status | Symptoms and Coping Responses | Risk Factors |

NURSING INTERVENTION

| Inspire and Validate | Reinforcement Advocacy | Mutual Treatment Planning, Modeling, and Teaching | Manage Environment |

EXPECTED OUTCOME

| Optimal Quality of Life | Improved Functioning | Symptom Relief | No Harm to Self or Others |

Fig. 33-2 Continuum of coping responses and treatment stages from the Stuart Stress Adaptation Model.

In some locations brief admissions have been scheduled for patients with severe, persistent illness in order to prevent decompensation and maintain optimal functioning.[25]

Partial Hospital Programs

Partial hospital or day treatment programs have become an important part of the continuum of care for mental health and chemical dependency treatment. Partial hospital programs are medically oriented, with a focus on providing specific treatments such as medication and individual, group, and family therapy in a highly organized, structured program. These programs are similar to inpatient programs without the room and board provided by hospitals. The services provided by partial hospital programs are listed in Table 33-2.[6]

Partial hospital programs are designed to perform two major functions: crisis stabilization and intermediate-term treatment.[4]

▼ Crisis stabilization is used to avert psychiatric hospitalization or to offer transitional treatment back to the community in order to shorten an episode of acute inpatient care.

▼ Intermediate-term treatment provides more extended, daily, goal-directed service for patients at high risk for hospitalization or readmission because of the serious and persistent nature of their disorder.

Indications for use of partial hospitalization are very similar to those for inpatient admission; the primary differences are related to the stability and supportiveness of the patient's living environment that are necessary to maintain safety during treatment. Length of stay is determined by the treatment team, with input from the patient. Typically, the patient is in treatment all day, every day for the first week or two. As the crisis stabilizes and the level of functioning improves, there is a reduction in the number of days the patient attends. This allows the patient to gradually make the transition back to work, home, or school.

The partial hospital psychiatric team is multidisciplinary and generally includes a psychiatrist, psychiatric nurse, social worker, activity therapist, and vocational counselor. Each member of the team has discipline-specific functions as well as some overlapping ones. For example, group therapy is an important component of most partial hospital programs and psychiatric nurses, social workers, and activity therapists may all function as group psychotherapists or lead activity groups. Unlike inpatient settings where the psychiatrist is expected to see patients daily, in most partial hospital programs the patient is usually seen weekly. The psychiatric nurse in most partial hospital programs assumes primary responsibility for assessing and identifying medical issues that may be contributing to the patient's psychiatric condition.

TABLE **33-2** *National Profile of Partial Hospitalization Programs*

SERVICE	% PROGRAMS PROVIDING
MENTAL HEALTH TREATMENT	
Group psychotherapy	85.5
Adjunctive therapy	82.1
Specialty group therapy	80.7
Life skills training	70.7
Individual psychotherapy	61.9
Family therapy	44.8
Psychological assessment	24.1
Speech and language	8.4
MEDICAL SERVICES	
Nutrition	57.6
History and physical	56.9
Psychiatric assessment	88.2
24-hour emergency services	60.8
Medication management	82.7
SERVICES TO FAMILIES	
Individual psychotherapy	40.3
Marital therapy	42.4
Multifamily group	33.3
Parent self-help or support	39.4
Parent and family education	70.1
EDUCATION SERVICES	
Assessment	44.7
Schooling	28.7
Prevocational	40.5
Vocational	21.2
Adult education	16.6
Transportation	50.1

n = 580.

From Culhane D, Hadley T, Kiser L: A national profile of partial hospitalization programs, *Continuum* 1:81, 1994.

Partial hospital programs have been demonstrated to be an effective treatment modality for a variety of patient diagnoses and more cost-effective than inpatient care.[16,32] Studies have also shown that combining inpatient care with an active, treatment-intensive partial hospital program can reduce symptoms and improve social functioning.[15]

> **?** *How do you think the changes in inpatient psychiatric care affect the families and support systems of the mentally ill? How can nurses help them with the problems they now face?*

Today the majority of psychiatric nurses work in inpatient and partial hospital psychiatric settings. Hospital-based psychiatric nursing practice is rich in history and tradition. Psychiatric nurses are the only group of mental health professionals who are responsible for meeting the needs of inpatients 24 hours a day, 365 days a year. In partial hospital programs, it is not uncommon for psychiatric nurses to be in contact with patients throughout the full day of treatment as other disciplines move in and out of the program to provide specific treatments.

To deliver cost-effective, high-quality inpatient or partial hospital care, psychiatric nurses must manage the one-to-one nurse-patient relationship within a complex social and organizational environment. The scope of contemporary psychiatric nursing practice requires knowledge and expertise in four broad areas:
▼ Managing the therapeutic milieu
▼ Implementing caregiving activities
▼ Integrating and coordinating care delivery
▼ Evaluating outcomes

Through the integration of these four components, psychiatric nurses can improve a patient's overall treatment outcome.

All psychiatric nurses, regardless of education or experience, engage in these activities every day. To do so requires that the nurse be aware of and value the full range of psychiatric nursing activities (see Chapter 1) and know about the changing mental health care delivery system (see Chapter 9). This chapter is organized around these four areas of functioning because they represent both the structure and the process of hospital-based psychiatric nursing care.

MANAGING THE THERAPEUTIC MILIEU

The basic difference between inpatient, partial hospital, and outpatient psychiatric care is the controlled environment, or milieu, in which it occurs. Hospital-based treatment facilities generally provide a milieu that physically shelters patients from what they perceive to be painful and frightening stressors. This respite, although brief, provides patients with an opportunity to begin to stabilize while being protected from factors that would interfere with their treatment progress. Similarly, partial hospital treatment provides structure and respite for part of the day and intensive support and intervention to promote a home environment that supports positive therapeutic outcomes.

Understanding the concepts of the therapeutic milieu is an essential part of effective psychiatric nursing care. The aim of the therapeutic milieu is to provide patients with a stable and coherent social environment that facilitates the development and implementation of an individualized treatment plan. Many people have studied different aspects of the inpatient psychiatric environment and identified structures and principles that make it helpful in treating the mentally ill.

The Therapeutic Community

In 1953 Maxwell Jones[18] first described the inpatient environment as a **therapeutic community** with cultural norms for behaviors, values, and activity. He saw patients' social interactions with peers and health-care workers as treatment opportunities. For example, he believed that interpersonal

TABLE **33-3** *Managing Disturbing Behaviors in the Milieu*

DISTURBING BEHAVIOR	INTERVENTION
Destructiveness: Physically destructive behavior. It is a response to a variety of feelings, such as fear or anger.	In working with destructive behavior, the goal is to control or set limits on the maladaptive response but support the feeling underlying the behavior. Validation is essential to help the patient recognize the feeling and ultimately regain control of maladaptive behavior.
Disorganization: Distorted or unusual behavior a psychotic patient may exhibit as symptomatic of the illness. It may be triggered by elevated anxiety, profound depression, or organic dysfunctions.	Reassure and help the patient while reducing the degree to which these behaviors inhibit therapeutic processes.
Deviancy: Behaviors often described as acting out. They are the result of the patient expressing conflicts overtly in the environment. It is often difficult to determine precisely what acting out behavior is, as well as what is justifiable or even tolerable, because much of it may be influenced by sociocultural factors.	The therapeutic goal in working with deviancy is to analyze how the behavior affects the milieu and how it inhibits the patient's progress. Examining the behavior with the patient and identifying consequences and alternatives are useful approaches.
Dysphoria: Patients with mood alterations may be dysphoric, which is evident in maladaptive responses such as withdrawal from the environment, obsessional behaviors, intrusiveness, or hyperreligiosity.	Establishing a therapeutic alliance is the first task. From there, the nurse and patient can explore feelings and dysfunctional thoughts and begin to modify behavioral responses.
Dependence: Evidenced by patients who do not identify and meet their own needs despite being able to do so. The avoidant nature of dependency interferes with therapeutic progress.	The initial therapeutic goal is to work with the patient to draw on any remaining areas of independence and strength. Then, situations can be identified in which the patient can apply these independent behaviors successfully.

difficulties between patients provided fertile material for psychodynamic intervention. He also believed that the clinical staff should share community governance with the patient group on an equal basis. He further emphasized the benefit of mutual participation of patients in each others' treatment, predominantly through sharing of intimate information and feedback in group settings such as the community meeting.

Since its introduction, the concept of the therapeutic community seems to have lost some of its credibility and popularity. One reason for this is that its philosophy of democracy and egalitarianism among patients and clinical staff is not compatible with the medical model. Others point out that the concept of the therapeutic community was developed when patients spent months and even years in the hospital. This is in sharp contrast to the short-term nature of most current inpatient psychiatric hospitalizations.

> **?** *The therapeutic community is an example of the social model of psychiatric care described in Chapter 3. Discuss how it differs from the medical model in the roles of patient and therapist and the therapeutic process.*

The Therapeutic Milieu

More than a decade later, Abroms[1] introduced the idea of the **therapeutic milieu.** He said that it serves two main purposes:

▼ It sets limits on disturbing and maladaptive behavior
▼ It teaches psychosocial skills

He described five categories of disturbing behaviors and related interventions that would help patients keep maladaptive behaviors under control and thus allow treatment to progress. These are listed in Table 33-3.

Once maladaptive behaviors were limited, Abroms stressed the use of the therapeutic milieu to foster the development of four important psychosocial skills in mentally ill patients.

▼ **Orientation:** All patients could achieve a greater level of orientation and reality awareness. Orientation is the patient's knowledge and understanding of time, place, person, and purpose. Awareness of these elements can be reinforced through all patient interactions and activities. For example, introducing oneself, one's role, and the rationale for an interaction helps disoriented patients attend to their surroundings. Another intervention would be a "current events" group conducted with patients.

▼ **Assertion:** The ability to express oneself appropriately can be modeled and exercised in a variety of ways in the treatment setting. Supporting patients in expressing themselves effectively and in a socially acceptable manner on a specific topic or issue is the overall goal. Some example interventions include assertiveness training groups, focus groups for lower-functioning patients, or any facilitated, interactive patient group.

▼ **Occupation:** Patients can feel a sense of confidence and accomplishment through industrious activity. Many therapeutic opportunities are provided through completion of individual or group hands-on activities. Spending time working with patients on something as simple as a jigsaw puzzle can provide purposeful activity, physical skill development, and the added benefit of practiced social interaction.

▼ **Recreation:** The ability to engage in and enjoy constructive leisure activity is a beneficial outlet for pleasure and relaxation. Providing a variety of recreational opportunities helps patients apply many of the skills they have learned, including orientation, assertion, social interaction, and physical dexterity. Some examples include informal games such as cards, charades, bingo, or brief walks outdoors.

These are useful and practical ideas related to the therapeutic environment that continue to have value in both inpatient and partial hospital settings today. They support the use of some of the different therapies patients receive in structured settings, such as recreation therapy, occupational therapy, and art therapy. However, their appropriateness in short-term inpatient settings is being reevaluated given the acute nature of contemporary inpatient psychiatric care in many settings.[29]

Perhaps the most important contribution to the concept of the therapeutic milieu came in 1978 when Gunderson[12] described five functional components of a therapeutic milieu: containment, support, structure, involvement, and validation. These components are commonly used to evaluate the therapeutic value of the treatment setting.

> **?** *How would you respond to a patient's wife who asks you why her husband is spending time in a fitness program and making crafts when he has only 5 days of insurance to pay for his hospitalization for severe depression?*

CONTAINMENT. The function of containment is to sustain the physical well-being of patients and to remove the patient's feelings of omnipotence. It includes the provision of food, shelter, and medical attention, as well as the steps necessary to prevent the patient from harming self or others. Thus it includes a continuum of interventions, with the use of seclusion and restraints being the most extreme. It is intended to reinforce temporarily the internal controls of patients, allowing them to reality test their omnipotent beliefs.

Containment is necessary to provide safety and foster trust. Therapeutic use of containment communicates to patients that the nurse will impose external controls as necessary to keep them and the environment safe. Appropriate and consistent limit setting is essential to meeting this goal. Nursing examples of therapeutic containment include the use of time-outs, room programs, specified observation periods, and seclusion (see Chapter 29).

Planning for containment in partial hospital settings poses additional challenges. The nurse must not only attend to the structured therapeutic milieu of the treatment pro-

gram but also plan how containment can be enacted in the patient's living environment outside program hours. The nurse must assess the patient's home environment, both physical and interpersonal, to identify supports and potential problems. This assessment may be based on data collected from interviews with the patient and family members or living companions or may be based on data collected by direct observation during a home visit. The knowledge from the home assessment can then be analyzed in conjunction with knowledge about the patient's triggers for disturbing behaviors and productive coping mechanisms that work best for the patient. In collaboration with the patient and others from the home environment, the nurse can develop an effective plan for reducing the triggers as much as possible and defining coping mechanisms for use in avoiding or managing disturbing behaviors.

SUPPORT. Support includes the staff's conscious efforts to help patients feel better and enhance their self-esteem. It is the unconditional acceptance of the patient, whatever his or her circumstances. The function of support is to help patients feel comfortable and secure and reduce their anxiety. It may take many forms, but it falls under the general heading of paying attention to the patient.

Support can be communicated through empathy, being available, appropriately offering encouragement and reassurance, giving helpful direction, offering food or beverages, and engaging patients in activities that they are reluctant to do. Other nursing examples include giving direction, suggestions, and education; promoting reality testing; and modeling healthy relationships and interactions. To best accomplish this task, nursing staff activity must be coordinated, cohesive, and consistent with the patient's treatment goals. Supportive nurturance enhances self-esteem. Milieus that offer support also provide nurturance and encourage patients to become engaged in other therapeutic efforts.

In both inpatient and partial hospital programs it is essential to coordinate support with others in the home so that they understand the behavioral changes the patient is attempting, how difficult it is to make such changes, the improbability of complete success in initial attempts, and the importance of recognition and support for all attempts.

STRUCTURE. Structure refers to all aspects of a milieu that provide a predictable organization of time, place, and person. This dependability in activity, staff, and environment helps the patient feel safe. Having a predictable timetable of meetings, group sessions, and other activities is one feature of structure. Other nursing examples include the setting of limits and the use of contracts, token economies, and required meetings. The more these uses of structure are planned with the patient according to shared ideas of what is adaptive and maladaptive, the more the structure becomes therapeutic in itself. For partial hospital programs this also involves planning with the patient how he or she will structure his or her activities while outside the hospital.

The patient can then begin to accept responsibility for behavior and its consequences. Providing structure helps the patient control maladaptive behaviors. The nurse uses appropriate consequences if the patient is unable, for whatever reason, to impose or honor effective limits. As natural consequences are consistently applied, the patient learns to delay impulsive and inappropriate responses through consistent expectations and behavioral responses.

INVOLVEMENT. Involvement is a part of the structure that goes beyond compliance with rules and activities. It refers to processes that help patients to actively attend to their social environment and interact with it. The purpose is to strengthen a patient's ego and modify maladaptive interpersonal patterns. Interpersonal communication and shared activity provide patients with opportunities to interact with others in their community.

Nursing examples of involvement include the use of open doors and open rounds and facilitating patient-led groups, activities, and self-assertive experiences. Programs that emphasize involvement encourage the use of cooperation, compromise, and confrontation. In addition, patients' patterns of involvement and interaction in their social environment can be identified. Progressively demanding opportunities for practicing these skills can then be planned and the results evaluated to help the patient to build the skills necessary to develop the level of social involvement needed to support continued therapeutic progress.

Through this involvement, patients learn appropriate interaction patterns and experience the consequences of unacceptable behaviors. For example, a patient who displays anger or offensive behavior that distances others can participate in activities that will help in verbalizing feelings, working out differences, and receiving feedback. This supportive experience strengthens the patient's sense of self, behavioral control, and social interactive skills. Thus encouraging involvement provides corrective experiences for the patient.

VALIDATION. Validation means that the individuality of each patient is recognized. It is the act of affirming a person's unique world view. Validation can help patients develop a greater capacity for closeness and a more consolidated identity. The psychiatric nurse communicates this through individual attention, empathy, and nonjudgmental acceptance of the patient's thoughts, feelings, and perspective. Other nursing examples of validation include individualized treatment planning, showing respect for a patient's rights, and providing opportunities for the patient to fail as well as succeed. Therapeutic listening and acknowledging the feelings underlying the patient's personal experience reinforce individuality. Clarification of these feelings helps the patient to understand and accept his or her own unique experience. This strengthens the patient's sense of individuality and encourages the integration of pleasant and unpleasant aspects of personal experience.

? *Visit an inpatient psychiatric unit. Which of the five components of a therapeutic milieu did you observe? Which ones were missing? What barriers prevented the unit from fully implementing this concept?*

Nursing Implications

One of the earliest advocates of the importance of the environment for nursing care was Florence Nightingale. She believed that the essential responsibilities of nursing included the provision of pure air and water, efficient drainage, cleanliness, and light. In addition, the "prudent" nurse prevented unnecessary noise and attended to the aesthetics and nutritional value of food and the comfort of bedding.[27] Since Nightingale's time, the inpatient environment and the therapeutic management of the milieu have continued to be important aspects of the role of all nurses and this has now been expanded to provide direction for nurses working in partial hospital settings.

Managing the therapeutic milieu remains the domain of the psychiatric nurse. It is essential that psychiatric nurses working in structured settings realize the potential impact that the environment can have on the patient and consciously use it for the patient's benefit.[24] The challenge is for psychiatric nurses to adapt to changes in the patient population and the mental health delivery system by evolving new approaches to managing the milieu as needed.[20,33,34]

Milieu management is a deliberate decision-making process. The psychiatric nurse should first identify what each patient needs from the therapeutic milieu, taking into consideration the needs of the larger patient group. Weighing individual needs against group needs can be difficult, but it is essential for the successful implementation of a therapeutic milieu. The nurse can then engage aspects of the therapeutic milieu to meet the patient's needs by providing:

▼ Limits and controls (containment)
▼ Education about the patient's illness and treatment plan (support)
▼ Therapeutic and predictable activity schedules (structure)
▼ Opportunities for social interaction (involvement)
▼ Acknowledgment of the patient's feelings (validation)

Activities related to each component of the therapeutic milieu can be incorporated in the nursing plan of care, thus maximizing the therapeutic effect of the environment.

The nature of psychiatry and the focus of treatment will continue to change with the influence of health-care reform and advances in the nursing and biomedical sciences. The principles of patient participation in decision making and the belief that the environment can be a treatment agent continue to be a part of most hospital-based settings. To be successful, however, the culture of the setting must have a value system that is congruent with the therapeutic milieu concept. The management team and interdisciplinary staff must have common goals, respect each other's contributions, and communicate openly to truly enact the components of the therapeutic community.

> **?** *Compare the components of the therapeutic milieu with the responsive and action dimensions of the therapeutic nurse-patient relationship described in Chapter 2.*

IMPLEMENTING CAREGIVING ACTIVITIES

Hospital-based psychiatric nurses must have clinical knowledge and skills and apply them for the benefit of patients and their families. The atmosphere created by the psychiatric nurse strives to provide patients with activities and interactions carefully designed to meet their needs. This includes both direct and indirect psychiatric nursing care functions as well as dependent, independent, and interdependent aspects of psychiatric nursing practice. A few of these caregiving activities in the hospital-based setting merit special discussion.

Assessing and Intervening in Potential Risks

One of the most important aspects of psychiatric nursing practice is physical safety for the patient and others. This process begins with a thorough assessment of risks at the time of admission and throughout the course of treatment. Common areas of risk for psychiatric patients include potential for aggression or violence, suicide attempts, elopement, seizures, falls, allergic reactions, and communicable diseases. Based on assessment findings, the nurse is responsible for selecting and implementing the appropriate safety precautions or treatment protocols. Implementation includes not only enacting the prescribed nursing care but also explaining the assessed risk and nursing care plan to the patient, as well as notifying other members of the nursing staff and treatment team of the identified risk.

Patient and Family Education

Education of patients and significant others consumes a considerable portion of a psychiatric nurse's time and is essential for sustained therapeutic progress. The process of education must begin with an assessment of the patient's barriers to learning. Such barriers may include lack of insight or denial related to the illness, illiteracy, sensory deficits such as visual or hearing impairments, limited concentration and attention span, or impaired memory. Once barriers have been identified, particular strategies can be incorporated in the teaching plan to facilitate the patient's retention and use of the information. As with any learner, repetition of information, providing information through multiple sensory avenues, and opportunities for practice and feedback promote learning for psychiatric patients. Common topics for education include symptom recognition and management, desired effects and potential side effects of medication, relapse prevention, and importance of and plans for aftercare.

Almost every interaction provides an opportunity for informal education. For example, meal selection provides an opportunity to learn about nutrition as well as to practice decision making and communication skills. Conflicts between patients provide opportunities to learn about and practice problem solving, anger management, negotiation, cooperation, and assertive communication. In addition to these impromptu opportunities for learning, more formal educational activities may be structured into patient care.

Activities, Groups, and Programs

Therapeutic nursing activities, groups, and programs provide a wide variety of opportunities for the nurse to influence the patient's progress toward treatment goals. In providing these corrective experiences, the psychiatric nurse must be clear on the purpose of these activities. They should be designed to accomplish specific nursing and patient goals in a constructive, efficient, and supportive way. The nurse's challenge is to plan these events to integrate the desired patient outcomes, the interests of the patients, and the ability of the patients to participate with feelings of pleasure and accomplishment.

Structured activities can accomplish several goals of the nursing process at the same time. For example, encouraging a cognitively impaired patient to play a common table game, such as cards, allows the nurse to assess the patient's concentration, orientation, memory, and abstract thinking. Based on these observations, the nurse can better understand the patient's learning needs and incorporate them in the plan of care. This same activity can help the socially withdrawn patient try out newly learned interactive skills, experience the role modeling of the nurse, and receive supportive feedback. In addition, the nurse can use these activities to evaluate the effect of nursing, somatic, and psychopharmacologic treatments. Thus, planned nursing activities offer endless possibilities as supportive and corrective experiences for the psychiatric patient.

Therapeutic nursing groups and programs provide a cost-effective way to implement psychiatric nursing care. Nursing interventions applied in a group allow one or two nurses to work with many patients at the same time. Such interventions are productive not only in hospital-based settings but across the continuum of care. For example, day treatment patients may join inpatients in the same groups or programs. This heterogeneity adds breadth of experience and perspective to the group. Each patient may accomplish a different goal within the same group or program, and such offerings can provide valuable structure to the therapeutic milieu. Some examples of psychiatric nursing groups are described in Box 33-1.

With the focus of psychiatric care shifting away from extended inpatient stays, opportunities for activity, group, and program development by psychiatric nurses are great. Nursing programs in social skills development, assertiveness, community-based support, crisis intervention, family preservation, and general health teaching are growing areas of psychiatric nursing responsibility.

> **?** *Ask an inpatient psychiatric nurse whether you can "shadow" him or her for a day. Group the nursing functions you see performed as direct or indirect and as dependent, independent, or interdependent. Did this experience change your perception of the inpatient psychiatric nursing role?*

Meeting Physical Needs

Studies have documented the prevalence of physical illness among psychiatric patients in both inpatient and outpatient treatment settings.[10] Yet too often, physical illness is undetected in this patient population. Physical illness may:

▼ Be the causative factor in a patient's presumed psychiatric illness

▼ Exacerbate a psychiatric illness

▼ Have no direct relationship to the psychiatric illness but still require medical and nursing intervention for the patient's well-being

The increase in medical and psychiatric comorbidity among psychiatric patients emphasizes the need for psychiatric nurses to stay current with their physical assessment and medical-surgical nursing skills. It is not uncommon for patients in psychiatric programs to need dialysis, hyperalimentation, intravenous therapy, or dressing changes. Thus completing a physical assessment on admission and monitoring the patient's physical and psychological status throughout the hospitalization are essential functions of the psychiatric nurse.

Discharge Planning

The most obvious goal for inpatient or partial hospital care is to discharge the patient to outpatient status. Thus discharge planning must begin on admission and be a focused nursing activity throughout the patient's stay. The nurse must be knowledgeable about the patient's environment. Potential needs and resources should be identified on admission. Once the nurse has decided what knowledge, skills, and behaviors will help the patient adapt to the discharge environment, creative and purposeful activities can be planned to provide the needed resources.

Throughout this process, the nurse should include family members, friends, significant others, and any other support system of the patient. Information regarding supportive resources and medications should be provided to

---

Box **33-1** *Examples of Psychiatric Nursing Groups or Programs*

MEDICATION EDUCATION GROUP

In this group basic concepts related to medication can be discussed. Providing general information about taking medications, such as the influence of slight dosage or schedule changes, serum levels, the therapeutic window, or how some medication potentiates the effect of other medications, can help the patient and family understand the specifics of the prescribed regimen. Common problems encountered by patients taking psychotropic medication can be discussed, and strategies for dealing with these potential barriers can be shared.

COMMUNITY RESOURCE GROUPS

These can be ongoing groups with rotating topics. Topics should be selected based on the learning needs of the group members and their ability to share knowledge about and experiences with varied community resources. For example, a pertinent topic might be the public transportation system of the city. Using maps and information from the local transit authority, exercises can be constructed where patients go from destination to destination practicing getting around the area independently. Another topic may be how to use the newspaper, library, or telephone book to learn about and contact nonprofit, social service, health-care, philanthropic, or other agencies, thus teaching the patient how to mobilize resources after discharge.

NUTRITION GROUPS

Nutrition groups can be helpful in teaching patients the importance of balanced diets and how to recognize and prepare healthful and appetizing meals for themselves. Food ingredients also provide excellent topics for discussion with psychiatric patients. For example, caffeine can be discussed, pointing out its subtle but pervasive effects on the body and its ability to interfere with the effectiveness of some medication. Other topics can include the basic food groups, shopping strategies, and the role of exercise in promoting health and balanced body weight.

SLEEP IMPROVEMENT PROGRAMS

Sleep improvement programs are often needed by psychiatric patients. Relaxation techniques such as simple yoga positioning, progressive muscle relaxation, and deep breathing may be helpful for some patients. The importance of a healthy sleep-wake cycle can be discussed. Group members can be encouraged to share their sleep-inducing secrets. Commonly used ideas for encouraging sleep can be shared with the group, such as spending time in a soothing bath, sipping warm milk, or reading with a soft light. Behaviors and influences that inhibit sleep may be discussed as well. Group members can be encouraged to try out the ideas and report back to the group on their effectiveness.

patients and their families to encourage functional independence and decrease the chances of relapse once discharged. This can significantly influence patients' abilities to maintain adaptive coping responses.

Psychiatric discharge planning can be considered part of the psychiatric rehabilitation model that addresses biopsychosocial needs in a manner similar to the physical rehabilitation process. A discharge checklist can be used as an interdisciplinary tool to review the patient's discharge needs and include the patient in the planning process.[14] Areas pertinent to discharge planning that should be included are medications, activities of daily living, mental health aftercare, residence, and physical health care. Special education and the need for financial assistance should also be reviewed with the patient and family.

Finally, research studies have found that transitional care services for mentally ill patients leaving the hospital are often inadequate.[9] Strong communication linkages between hospital-based and community-based providers are essential in order to ensure continuity of care, maximize the value of hospital-based services, and minimize future admissions.[3,17] Some of the caregiving activities of hospital-based nursing practice can be seen in the following clinical example.

Clinical Example Ms. R was a 17-year-old, single high school student who was admitted to an inpatient psychiatric unit with the diagnosis of bipolar disorder. She was admitted for uncontrollable behavior (sexual promiscuity, running away from home, hyperverbalization, and extreme irritability).

The initial nursing assessment provided a data base that revealed a chaotic family system with a long history of mental illness on both sides of the family, a social and cultural environment in which drug and alcohol abuse were prevalent, and a community that, because of its low socioeconomic status, had limited mental health resources. However, the patient was very bright, cooperative, and motivated to benefit from her hospitalization.

The initial nursing actions were to administer the prescribed medications, including lithium carbonate, and check blood levels three times a week until a therapeutic level was reached. The nurse assessed that there was an immediate need to protect the patient from her impulsive, uncontrollable behavior. The patient was placed under close nursing observation at all times until she was able to control her own behavior.

Once the patient's mood had stabilized, she was presented in nursing rounds. During this time the patient was able to identify a great need for the nurse to teach her and her family about bipolar disorder and the importance of continued lithium treatment. The patient and staff agreed that a home visit would explore the pressures that the family placed on the patient to function as a surrogate mother to her eight siblings. The patient also believed that it was important that her illness not be viewed in exactly the same manner as that of her sister, who was diagnosed as schizophrenic. The patient viewed her intellectual ability and the love that existed in her family system as her best resources. She thought that, with the help of the nursing staff, she and her family could develop more understanding of her illness and decrease the chaos within the family. After discharge the patient was followed up in outpatient therapy by her primary nurse.

INTEGRATING CARE DELIVERY

The integrative function of the hospital-based psychiatric nurse is very important, although it is often overlooked or taken for granted. It includes all activities involved in the coordination of patient care such as managing nursing resources, balancing costs and outcomes in decision making, evaluating nursing care delivery modalities, ensuring compliance with professional and regulatory standards, and encouraging communication, participative problem solving, and conflict resolution among mental health team members. In addition, the clinical practice of the nurse involves ongoing implementation of new ideas and approaches for improving quality and decreasing costs.

Teamwork and Coordinated Care

Almost all programs use a multidisciplinary team to deliver treatment. To integrate and coordinate patient care the psychiatric nurse must collaborate with professionals from other disciplines and manage a group of nursing care providers. If therapeutic outcomes are to be optimized, team members must work together to address targeted behaviors and treatment goals. In order to achieve this level of coordination, team communication must be open and active. Psychiatric nurses can facilitate this process by organizing their observations and interactional data into useful assessment findings that reflect such things as the patient's responses to medications and other interventions, patterns of behavior indicating escalation, interventions that are found to be effective, and the patient's beliefs about what will help him or her progress toward treatment goals.[7]

The degree of cooperation and cohesion among disciplines may vary widely. Interdisciplinary problems have been identified that could interfere with the quality of psychiatric care (see Critical Thinking about Contemporary Issues). Problems between providers may involve poor communication, professional self-doubt, role confusion, and conflict, all of which may be increased by work-related stress.

Whenever multiple people, each with a unique perspective, are working together there is the potential for conflict. Handling conflict productively is an ongoing challenge for the psychiatric nurse. When poorly handled or avoided, conflict can interfere with the continuity of patient care and

CRITICAL THINKING *about* Contemporary Issues

Do Nurses and Psychiatrists View Patients in the Same Way?

It has been suggested that different members of the mental health care team perceive patients differently, and that this can create problems in developing cohesive treatment plans and maintaining a therapeutic milieu. One recent study compared characteristics attributed by nurses and residents to difficult-to-treat patients in a short-stay setting.[11] The researchers found that both groups identified self-harm behaviors, violence toward others, and treatment sabotage as characteristics of difficult patients, although these behaviors posed more problems for the nurses. Lack of response to medication and patient manipulation were the most important problems identified by the residents. Nurses found difficulty with patients who were unable to form therapeutic alliances.

The researchers suggest that this may be because psychiatric nurses have seen their role as shaping the therapeutic milieu. Thus their interventions center on providing opportunities within the unit for improving interpersonal and coping skills and maximizing healthy aspects of the patient's ego functions. If the patient fails to engage or withdraws, these treatment goals are thwarted and the nurse's role as a therapeutic agent is blocked. Such findings suggest that differing perceptions of difficult patients may create communication problems for the treatment team. If the different disciplines do not share common concerns, they may not recognize the significance of their observations and not respond to them.

the management of a therapeutic milieu. However, effective management of conflict can facilitate stronger professional working relationships, model positive communication skills for patients, and contribute to the nurse's professional development.

> *Observe a multidisciplinary treatment team in the inpatient psychiatric setting. Did you see any areas of team conflict, role blurring, or turf struggles? If so, how did the team handle these issues?*

Resource Allocation

Psychiatric nurses must be able to justify the type and level of personnel needed to provide high-quality nursing care. Allocation of numbers and types of personnel based on patient care needs is an essential consideration for achieving positive outcomes.[13] Thus attention to the most appropriate and efficient use of personnel and other resources is an important part of the psychiatric nurse's role. The assignment of nursing resources must be based on identified patient care needs, clinical competencies, and available resources. This requires that all nurses become actively involved in ex-

amining patient needs, identifying realistic outcomes of care, and assessing the strengths and weaknesses of available nursing personnel.

> *You report to work one evening and discover that you and one other staff member have been assigned to cover the 20-bed psychiatric unit. You realize that the hospital has been reducing costs, but you believe that this is unsafe staffing. How would you present your case for more staff to nursing and hospital administration?*

Nursing Care Delivery Modalities

The nursing care delivery modality reflects the professional values of the organization. It also influences the cost and quality of the nursing care provided and the outcomes achieved. Nurses prefer autonomous practice environments in which participation is elicited, professional competency is formally recognized, and administration is decentralized.[23,26] A professional practice environment encourages professional accountability and involves those who deliver the care in the decision making process regarding care delivery.

Many nursing care delivery modalities have been described in the literature. Examples include primary nursing, team nursing, modular nursing, functional nursing, and case management.[28] Each has distinct advantages and disadvantages, affects personnel costs differently, and varies in its application to the hospital-based setting (Table 33-4). Other factors to be considered are: the needs of the patient population served by the facility, goals and objectives of the nursing department, level of the nurses' education and experience, the organization's structure and governance, amount of staff turnover, nursing and nonnursing care priorities, professional expectations, and the presence or absence of union activity.[2] Finally, selection of a delivery model is also influenced by the type of treatments and services given to patients and the number of activities provided in the particular setting.

> *What nursing care delivery modality is used in your hospital-based psychiatric facility? Do you think another modality would be better? Defend your position based on a cost-benefit approach.*

Professional, Regulatory, and Accreditation Standards

Professional standards of the American Nurses' Association (ANA) for psychiatric–mental health clinical practice provide a basis for evaluating nursing care. In addition to the standards of care (see Chapter 10) and professional perfor-

TABLE **33-4** *Comparison of Nursing Delivery Modalities*

DELIVERY MODALITY	DESCRIPTION	ADVANTAGES	DISADVANTAGES
Primary nursing	The nurse assumes 24-hour accountability for an identified number of patients. The primary nurse is responsible for determining and evaluating all aspects of care for those primary patients. The nurse assumes accountability for the care of these same primary patients if later readmitted. The nurse helps to implement the prescribed care for other nurses' primary patients. Other nurses and adjunct staff help to implement the primary nurse's care plan. These providers are accountable for this care to the patient's primary nurse.	Opportunity for continuous care is greater. Patients and their primary nurse are able to establish a more profound nurse-patient relationship. Lines of accountability for clinical outcomes are clearer.	Motivation for assumption of this level of accountability varies among nurses. Higher personnel costs often result.
Team nursing	A group of nursing personnel, called a team, works together to deliver comprehensive care to a larger number of patients. The team is led by a registered nurse who may supervise other nurses and adjunct staff. The whole team, and ultimately the registered nurse leading the team, is accountable for the care delivered to the patients for that shift.	Enables group cohesiveness to develop. Enables different types and skill levels of providers to share knowledge and expertise. Develops leadership abilities.	May fragment care delivery by dividing holistic care into tasks delegated to a number of providers.
Modular nursing	Similar to team nursing in that a group of patients receives care from a mixed group of providers. The patient group is designated by close geographic proximity, as on one hallway. Modules are often organized with access to all materials and documents needed for that team to care for those patients in that geographically distinct module.	Concentrates activity in a smaller area. Allows quicker, easier access to materials. Helpful with patients staying in their hospital rooms.	Not helpful in psychiatric settings where physical mobility and group activity are encouraged and access to materials is not a major concern.
Functional nursing	Functional nursing relegates nursing activity by task; one nurse may distribute medications, another may take vital signs and participate in somatic treatments.	Enables tasks to be done quickly and simultaneously.	Difficult to determine lines of accountability. Patient care is fragmented.
Case management	As in primary nursing, the case manager assumes responsibility for all aspects of care for a group, or caseload, of patients. With this modality, the care accountability extends before and beyond the inpatient phases of treatment. Coordination of the patient's providers, medications, treatments, and resources is organized, evaluated, and often determined by the case manager. All decisions are made with knowledge of all aspects of the patient's clinical and personal situation.	Greater opportunity for continuity of care. Accountability is clear. Greater emphasis on patient participation. Active, ongoing negotiation with the patient and significant others is integral to this modality.	Areas and agencies vary widely in application of this modality. Success of this method is closely linked with the amount of authority and autonomy associated with this role.

mance (see Chapter 11), other ANA standards are available to guide nursing activities in administrative and educational areas.

Regulatory and accreditation standards must also be considered by the hospital-based psychiatric nurse. These include the state laws and regulations governing nursing practice and facility licensure, the laws and regulations determining the payment of federal and state insurance funds (Medicaid and Medicare), and standards set forth by accrediting bodies. A health-care facility may be required to show how any of these standards are met, including those pertaining to the condition of the physical facility, credentialing of employees, or the documentation of patient care. Requirements vary depending on the type of facility, state regulations, and types of services offered.

The Joint Commission on Accreditation of Healthcare Organizations (JCAHO) has become a leading accrediting agency for many different types of health-care facilities. Their standards have served as a benchmark for many other regulatory agencies. JCAHO standards are a helpful and comprehensive guide for all aspects of health-care delivery in this country.

The Health Care Financing Administration (HCFA) is the federal agency that oversees the spending of Medicare and Medicaid funds. Each state has an identified agency that implements HCFA policies locally. Often, for the care and treatment delivered by health-care agencies to be reimbursed by Medicare or Medicaid, HCFA consultants or representatives of the state agency conduct surveys of the facility. They may review patient records, inspect the physical plant, interview staff, and evaluate programs to ensure that their specific regulations are met. Once the facility has shown that all required standards are met, it is eligible to receive payment for treating patients insured by Medicaid and Medicare. These standards are often similar to those of other regulatory and credentialing bodies and focus mainly on the sanitation and safety of the facility, competency of the personnel, and the adequacy and pertinence of the care delivered and documented.

EVALUATING OUTCOMES

A crucial aspect of psychiatric nursing practice involves the evaluation of the care provided. Continuous evaluation is mandatory for professional nursing practice (see Chapters 10 and 11). Evaluation is an ongoing activity that ranges from simply raising questions to engaging in formal clinical research. At a minimum, it involves evaluating the effectiveness of care provided based on the patient's response to particular interventions and the level of achievement of treatment goals. All aspects of inpatient nursing care involve evaluation, from the staff assigned to work with a certain group of patients, to the value of a particular nursing group activity, to the piloting of a new nursing care delivery modality. From this perspective, evaluation is the validating activity of the psychiatric nurse's practice.

More facilities are implementing formal outcome measurement systems so that objective data are available for assessing and reporting the organization's ability to achieve desired therapeutic outcomes. Common areas of measurement for such systems include symptom reduction, improvements in the patient's quality of life, and levels of satisfaction with the services received. Nurses often are responsible for components of the evaluation process.

The psychiatric nurse is ultimately accountable for the outcomes of the nursing care provided. It is the responsibility of the nurse to analyze pertinent data and negotiate with the patient and other health-care providers to identify outcomes and a means of achieving them. Other staff work with the psychiatric nurse to accomplish this task. Given the varied education, skills, experience, and priorities of the other providers, success in achieving and evaluating patient care outcomes can often be difficult.

> **?** *Determine the bed charge for 1 day of care in your psychiatric inpatient unit. How does that compare with the bed charge in a medical-surgical unit? How much of that charge do you think is related to nursing services?*

Quality Improvement Programs

Evaluating outcomes and key processes is an essential element in improving organizational performance in both inpatient and partial hospital programs.[21] An emphasis on continuous performance improvement is reflected in the standards of JCAHO. These standards require that health-care agencies select and monitor key indicators of performance. Continuous monitoring of these performance indicators and feedback from patients and staff allow the organization to identify opportunities for improvement. Because of the complexity of patient care and work processes, an interdisciplinary team is formed to collect information and analyze the systems and processes that influence the outcomes achieved, incorporating the unique perspectives of the various team members. The team then designs and implements new processes and collects data to evaluate the effectiveness of the new activities. Psychiatric nurses place essential roles in identifying opportunities for improvement, collecting data for analysis of the current process, evaluating the effectiveness of new processes, and representing nursing's perspective in the improvement team's deliberations.

Risk Management

Evaluation also involves the assessment of **risk management** activities. These usually relate to situations that could result in legal action involving patients, families, the hospital, or the health-care provider. Issues related to involuntary admission, refusal of treatment, informed consent, confidentiality, duty to warn, least restrictive environment, and seclusion and restraint are confronted daily by the psychiatric nurse (see Chapter 9). All nurses should become aware of the statutes governing the care of the mentally ill in their state and ensure that systems are established to recognize, intervene in, and report any actual or potential breaches of the legal standard.

Utilization Review

Utilization review is a final but important aspect of evaluating outcomes in inpatient and outpatient psychiatric settings.[8] It is carried out by most hospitals and many health-care agencies, government-sponsored local agencies, third-party payers, managed care companies, and private insurers. The utilization review process is intended to ensure that health-care resources are used appropriately. However, many believe that it primarily involves saving money. If this is true, it is unfortunate because utilization review has the potential to improve the quality and efficiency of health care.

Utilization review typically occurs in three stages. Before admission, the patient or clinician requests approval to hospitalize the patient. This is called *preauthorization*. This approval is usually good for a certain number of days. It is not done with court-ordered admissions. Next, *concurrent review* takes place after admission but before discharge. The reviewer looks at cases in which the patient has been hospitalized the approved number of days and may need authorization for additional days. The reviewer may also look at cases that exceed some statistical norm, such as the average length of stay for that diagnosis in that hospital. The treatment team must justify the need for continued stay or any deviations from the norm. Finally, *retrospective review* occurs after discharge, when the entire chart can be reviewed.

Psychiatric nurses need to be aware of this process because they must document patient symptoms and responses to interventions that justify continued treatment or support discharge. In addition, nurses should continually evaluate all patients' needs for care and the most appropriate use of limited mental health care resources to meet those needs.

Summary

1. The treatment goals, processes, expected outcomes, and length of stay related to hospital-based psychiatric care are changing. The majority of psychiatric nurses currently work in inpatient or partial hospital settings, but they must be ready and able to provide their services throughout the continuum of care.
2. The aim of the therapeutic milieu is to provide patients with a stable and coherent social environment that facilitates the development and implementation of an individualized treatment plan. Components of the therapeutic milieu include containment, support, structure, involvement, and validation.
3. Hospital-based psychiatric nursing includes both direct and indirect nursing functions as well as dependent, independent, and interdependent aspects of practice. Assessing and intervening in potential risks, providing patient and family education, implementing activities, groups, and programs, meeting patients' physical needs, and planning discharge are important caregiving activities.
4. The integrative function of the hospital-based psychiatric nurse includes all activities involved in the coordination of patient care such as those related to managing nursing resources, evaluating nursing care delivery modalities, ensuring compliance with professional and regulatory standards, and facilitating teamwork and coordinated care.
5. Continuous evaluation of outcomes is essential to psychiatric nursing practice. Relevant activities include quality improvement programs, risk management, and utilization review.

COMPETENT CARING A Clinical Exemplar of a Psychiatric Nurse

Simmy Palecko, RN

One of the true rewards of psychiatric nursing is that many patients get better and return to functional lives in which they can again experience pleasure and increased self-esteem. It is unbelievably fulfilling to see patients regain a sense of independence and renewed control over their own destinies.

Ms. M was an example of how an intensive short-term psychiatric hospitalization can remarkably improve the quality of a patient's life. She was a 72-year-old woman who was admitted to our adult unit with electrolyte imbalance. She was psychotic and delusional, refusing to eat or drink, not sleeping, highly anxious, and refusing to perform her activities of daily living (ADLs). She believed that her body was rotting away. She was also extremely paranoid, insisting that the clients in the boarding home where she lived were plotting to kill her and that the staff were laughing and talking about her outside her door during the night. She complained of auditory hallucinations and how she felt tortured. Ms. M was extremely irritable and argumentative, and physically and verbally threatening. She refused to get out of bed and even ambulate. She insisted that we leave her alone so that she could die.

COMPETENT CARING A Clinical Exemplar of a Psychiatric Nurse—cont'd

Ms. M was a recurrent patient on our unit. Her diagnoses were Axis I, bipolar affective disorder; Axis III, colon cancer status postresection, hypertension, degenerative joint disease, peptic ulcer disease, neurogenic bladder, and recurrent urinary tract infections. She was a particular challenge to the nursing staff that we were more than willing to undertake. We were able to use our medical-surgical skills with repeat blood draws, IVs, ECGs, urinary catheterizations for residuals, accurate intake and output calculations, and range-of-motion activities. Safety and emotional support were also a major focus of our patient care. Ms. M was placed on fall precautions with continued teaching and reinforcement, even though she was minimally receptive.

Within a few days of admission, her physical condition stabi-

lized and she was scheduled for electroconvulsive therapy (ECT), which had been successful for her in the past. The staff impatiently waited for Ms. M's mood to improve, her appetite to increase, her nighttime sleeping to improve, her interest in her ADLs to increase, and her auditory hallucinations, negativism, and anxiety to decrease. After the fourth ECT treatment, the staff began to see Ms. M's return to her baseline. She was smiling more and her humor was returning. She no longer stated that her body was rotting. She even began to joke with the nursing staff.

Ms. M was discharged to the boarding home approximately 10 days after her admission. The change in the patient's mental and physical condition was remarkable and I was again reminded of the intrinsic rewards of psychiatric nursing.

your **INTERNET connection**

Planning and Designing Today's Mental Health Institution
http://www.tiac.net/users/hfp/mhealth/site.htm

Joint Commission on Accreditation of Healthcare Organizations
http://www.jcaho.org/

? Chapter Review Questions

1. Match each example in Column A with the correct component of the therapeutic milieu in Column B.

Column A

___Allows for predictable organization of time, place, and person

___Affirming the patient's world view

___Offering education and encouragement

___Promoting the patient's attention and interaction with the social environment

___Provision of food, shelter, medical care, and safety from harm

___Unconditional acceptance, nurturance, and promotion of self-esteem

___Use of contracts, token economies, and required meetings

___Use of individualized treatment plans and showing respect for patients' rights

___Use of open doors, open rounds, and patient-led groups

___Use of time-outs and room programs

Column B

A. Containment
B. Involvement
C. Structure
D. Support
E. Validation

2. Fill in the blanks.

A. Today the majority of patients admitted to psychiatric hospitals are in the _____ stage, with the treatment goal of _____.

B. The partial hospital psychiatric team is _____ in nature.

C. Maxwell Jones first described the inpatient environment as a _____ with cultural norms for behaviors, values, and activity.

D. One of the earliest advocates of the importance of the environment for nursing care was _____.

E. _____ is the leading accreditation agency for hospital-based facilities.

F. Situations that can result in legal action involving patients, families, the hospital, or the provider are the focus of _____ activities.

G. The _____ process is intended to ensure that health-care resources are appropriately used.

3. Provide short answers for the following questions.

A. What are the two major functions of partial hospitalization programs?

B. Describe the three stages of the utilization review process.

C. Describe how patient teaching would need to be modified in an inpatient setting where patients are in the most acute stages of their illnesses.

D. In many hospital-based facilities, psychiatric nurses rotate between inpatient and partial hospital programs. Discuss how this can benefit both patients and the nursing staff.

REFERENCES

1. Abroms G: Defining milieu therapy, *Arch Gen Psychiatry* 21:553, 1969.
2. Armstrong D, Stetler C: Strategic considerations in developing a delivery model, *Nurs Econ* 9:112, 1991.
3. Behner N: Establishing linkages in a changing mental health practice environment, *Issues Ment Health Nurs* 17:51, 1996.
4. Block B, Lefkovitz P: *Standards and guidelines for partial hospitalization adult programs*, ed 2, Alexandria, Va, 1994, AABH Publications.
5. Center for Mental Health Services and National Institute of Mental Health: *Mental health, United States, 1992*, Washington, DC, 1992, US Government Printing Office.
6. Culhane D, Hadley T, Kiser L: A national profile of partial hospitalization programs, *Continuum* 1:81, 1994.
7. Delaney K, Ulsafer-Van Lanen J, Pitula C, Johnson M: Seven days and counting: how inpatient nurses might adjust their practice to brief hospitalization, *J Psychosoc Nurs* 33:36, 1995.
8. Dolwart R, Epstein S: Issues in psychiatric hospital care, *Curr Opin Psychiatry* 4:789, 1991.
9. Dorwart R, Hoover C: A national study of transitional hospital services in mental health, *Am J Public Health* 84:1229, 1994.
10. Felker B, Yazel J, Short D: Mortality and medical comorbidity among psychiatric patients: a review, *Psychiatr Serv* 47:1356, 1996.
11. Gallop R, Lancee W, Shugar G: Residents' and nurses' perceptions of difficult-to-treat short-stay patients, *Hosp Community Psychiatry* 44:352, 1993.
12. Gunderson I: Defining the therapeutic process in therapeutic milieus, *Psychiatry* 41:327, 1978.
13. Harkness G, Miller J, Hill N: Differentiated practice: a three-dimensional model, *Nurs Management* 23:26, 1992.
14. Hochberger J: A discharge check list for psychiatric patients, *J Psychosoc Nurs* 33:35, 1995.
15. Hoffman F, Mastrianni X: Partial hospitalization following inpatient treatment: patient characteristics and treatment outcome, *Continuum* 2:247, 1995.
16. Hueller J: Partial hospitalization: a study of outcomes and efficiency, *Continuum* 3:59, 1996.
17. Hughes K, Ashby C: Essential components of the short-term psychiatric unit, *Perspect Psychiatr Care* 32:20, 1996.
18. Jones M: *The therapeutic community*, New York, 1953, Basic Books.

19. Kizer L, Lefkovitz P, Kennedy L, Knight M: The continuum of ambulatory mental health services, *Continuum* 1:7, 1994.
20. LeCuyer E: Milieu therapy for short-stay units: a transformed practice theory, *Arch Psychiatr Nurs* 6:108, 1992.
21. Mahler C, Mahler R: Quality improvement in the field: what are partial hospitalization programs actually doing? *Continuum* 3:23, 1996.
22. McGihon N: Health care reform: clinical implications for inpatient psychiatric nursing, *J Psychosoc Nurs* 32:31, 1994.
23. McGinn N: Restructuring patient care delivery systems through empowerment, *J Nurs Admin* 22:21 1992.
24. Melle I et al: The importance of ward atmosphere in inpatient treatment of schizophrenia on short-term units, *Psychiatr Serv* 47:721, 1996.
25. Merchant D, Henfling P: Scheduled brief admissions: patient "tuneups," *J Psychosoc Nurs* 32:7, 1994.
26. Moritz P: Innovative nursing practice models and patient outcomes, *Nurs Outlook* 39:111, 1991.
27. Nightingale F: *Notes on nursing: what it is and what it is not,* New York, 1960, Dover.
28. Ryan J et al: A comparative study of primary and team nursing models in the psychiatric care setting, *Arch Psychiatr Nurs* 2:3, 1988.
29. Santos A, McLeod-Bryant S: Strategies for operational efficiency in a general hospital inpatient unit, *Hosp Community Psychiatry* 42:66, 1991.
30. Schreter R: Ten trends in managed care and their impact on the biopsychosocial model, *Hosp Community Psychiatry* 44:325, 1993.
31. Sharfstein S, Stoline A, Goldman H: Psychiatric care and health insurance reform, *Am J Psychiatry* 150:7, 1993.
32. Sledge W et al: Day hospital/crisis respite care versus inpatient care, part II: service utilization and costs, *Am J Psychiatry* 153:1074, 1996.
33. Tuck I, Keels M: Milieu therapy: a review of development of this concept and its implications for psychiatric nursing, *Issues Ment Health Nurs* 13:51, 1992.
34. Watson J: Maintenance of therapeutic community principles in an age of biopharmacology and economic restraints, *Arch Psychiatr Nurs* 6:183, 1992.

ANNOTATED SUGGESTED READINGS

*Behner N: Establishing linkages in a changing mental health practice environment, *Issues Ment Health Nurs* 17:51, 1996.
    Relates the role of the inpatient program in the establishment of communication linkages with community providers and regional care delivery systems to ensure continuity of patient care.
Berger L, Vuckovic A: *Under observation: life inside a psychiatric hospital,* New York, 1994, Ticknor & Fields.
    A collaboration between a family member and a neuroscientist produced this book to educate the general public about a state-of-the-art inpatient unit and how the staff combats mental illness.
*Bultema J, Getzfrid M, Slade M: Defining professional practice: the evolution of the RAMA model, *J Am Psychiatric Nurses Assoc* 2:117, 1996.
    Describes the development and implementation of a patient-centered care model in a psychiatric hospital that involved unit-based leadership with 24-hour accountability, responsibility, and authority. Good example of inpatient reengineering and restructuring done by nurses.

*Nursing reference.

Cohen N, Gantt A, Sainz A: Influences on fit between psychiatric patient's psychosocial needs and their hospital discharge plan, *Psychiatr Serv* 48:518, 1997.
    Reports on a method to systematically evaluate discharge planning by tracking progress toward securing relevant posthospital care and support.
*Delaney K: Milieu therapy: a therapeutic loophole, *Perspect Psychiatric Care* 33:19, 1997.
    Chronicles the decline of milieu therapy and concludes that nurses should focus on clarifying how specific nursing interventions are operationalized and tied to patient outcomes.
*Delaney K et al: Seven days and counting: how inpatient nurses might adjust their practice to brief hospitalization, *J Psychosocial Nursing* 33:36, 1995.
    Strategies to provide patient care with less time and resources include the precise articulation of nursing functions, data systems that integrate services, and preservation of a unit's "culture of caring."
*Goren S: Pursuit of the ordinary: short-term inpatient treatment, *Arch Psychiatr Nurs* 11:82, 1997.
    Offers a set of norms and expectations appropriate for the pursuit of effective treatment within the mandate of short-term inpatient care.
*Hughes K, Ashby C: Essential components of the short-term psychiatric unit, *Perspect Psychiatric Care* 32:20, 1996.
    Suggests that nurses reorganize their caregiving to stabilize patients in crisis and form linkages with aftercare services to maximize therapeutic gains of clients in a minimum period of time.
Kiser L et al: The continuum of ambulatory mental health services, *Continuum* 1:7, 1994.
    Describes a continuum of care model for ambulatory mental health services with three levels of structure and intensity designed to encompass both patient needs and cost-containment approaches.
Laskey C, Johnson J: Inpatient case management within the treatment team, *J Pract Psychiatry Behav Health* 5:184, 1997.
    Relates a system that takes into account managed care reimbursement parameters and individual patient treatment needs to decrease the number of denied hospital days. Timely reading.
*McGihon N: Health care reform: clinical implications for inpatient psychiatric nursing, *J Psychosocial Nurs* 32:31, 1994.
    Explores the need for the rapid incorporation of new modalities to remain competitive and give quality care while attempting to meet the changing needs of today's health care environment.
Polcin D, Guterman T: Working with deinstitutionalized patients in milieu treatment: issues for novice therapists, *Continuum* 3:111, 1996.
    Good discussion of the ways in which novice therapists must adapt to the demands of the "new" milieu in community settings for the treatment of patients with serious mental disorders.
*Vaugh K et al: Brief inpatient psychiatric treatment: finding solutions, *Issues Ment Health Nurs* 16:519, 1995.
    Describes how solution-focused therapeutic modalities are used in the continuum of care to meet the needs of patients within the managed care-shortened hospital length of stay.
*Webster D et al: Modeling the client's world through brief solution-focused therapy, *Issues Ment Health Nurs* 16:505, 1995.
    Identifies the shift in philosophical assumptions that must underlie hospital programs to meet the managed care dictate for brief lengths of stay with focused goals and measurable outcomes.

Community Psychiatric Nursing Care

Nancy K. Worley

© 1998 M.C. Escher/Cordon Art, Baarn, Holland.

What life have you if you have not life together? There is no life that is not in community. **T. S. Eliot** CHORUSES FROM "THE ROCK"

GOALS OF COMMUNITY MENTAL HEALTH

The Community Mental Health Centers Act of 1963 marked the beginning of a major federal effort to provide comprehensive community-based mental health services to all people in need regardless of income. Each community mental health center was mandated by law to provide five essential mental health services. Four of these services—inpatient, emergency, partial hospitalization, and outpatient—were to provide psychiatric care in the community to reduce the number of admissions to state hospitals. The goal of the fifth essential service, consultation and education, was to provide information about mental health principles to other community agencies, reduce the number of people at risk for mental illness, and increase community awareness of mental health practices through education. The dual nature of this mission, care of those with diagnosed mental illness and prevention of mental illness, has led to controversy in defining the purpose of community mental health.

Four models have dominated the community mental health movement since 1963. Each one has been influenced by the political, social, and economic climate of the time. They have contributed much to the field, and the best parts of each model continue to be used today. They are summarized in Table 34-1.

PUBLIC HEALTH MODEL

Mental health professionals who believed in primary prevention through social change dominated the community mental health movement in its early years, using the public health model of service delivery. In this model the "patient" is the community rather than the individual, and the focus is on the amount of mental health or illness in the community as a whole, including factors that promote or inhibit mental health. The emphasis in this model is on reducing the risk of mental illness for an entire population by providing services to high-risk groups. Use of the public health model required that mental health professionals be familiar with a range of skills that were not a traditional part of their training. These included community needs assessment, identifying and prioritizing target or high-risk groups, and intervening with new treatment modalities such as consultation, education, and crisis intervention.

 Do you believe it is possible to prevent mental illness in an individual or a community?

Community Needs Assessment

In the public health model services are developed and delivered based on a culturally sensitive assessment of community needs. Because it is not possible to interview each person in the community to determine mental health needs, four techniques are used to estimate service needs.

SOCIAL INDICATORS. Social indicators infer need for service from descriptive statistics found in public records and reports, especially statistics that are highly correlated with poor mental health outcomes. Examples of statistics most commonly used are income, race, marital status, population density, crime, and substance abuse.

KEY INFORMANT SURVEYS. Key informants are people knowledgeable about the community's needs. Typical key informants are public officials, clergy, social service personnel, nurses, and primary care physicians.

COMMUNITY FORUMS. In a community forum, members of the community are invited to a series of public meetings where they can express their ideas and beliefs about mental health needs in their community.

EPIDEMIOLOGICAL STUDIES. Epidemiological studies examine the incidence and prevalence of mental disorders in a defined population. Because they are expensive to carry out, most community needs assessments use results from previously published studies and apply these findings to their situation. For example, several large epidemiological

TABLE 34-1 *Models of Community Mental Health Services*

MODEL	CONCEPTUAL FRAMEWORK	INTERVENTION STRATEGIES	NURSING ROLE
Public health (1960-1970)	Focuses on prevention Community as patient Services target high-risk groups	Community needs assessment Identifies high-risk groups Consultation Education Crisis intervention	Some group and family involvement Caring for people with chronic mental illness Limited preventive work
Biological-medical (1970-1980)	Focuses on those with diagnosed mental illness Stimulated by deinstitutionalization Views mental illness as brain disease	Medical management Psychotherapy Aftercare programs	Medication administration and monitoring Coordination of aftercare programs Psychotherapy
System (1980-1990)	Focuses on the role of the biological, psychological, and environmental in rehabilitation Developed comprehensive systems of care	Community support systems Service coordination Case management	Coordination of community services Case management activities
Patient centered (1990-present)	Focus on patients who overlap service systems Culturally relevant services Consumer participation	Assertive community treatment	Medication management New initiatives such as home health, outreach, collaborative practice, prevention, and family preservation

studies have estimated that the impairment rate (the number of people with some form of emotional disorder) in the United States ranges between 15% and 30%.[32] These studies have shown that high impairment rates in a population are correlated with certain demographic and socioeconomic characteristics such as poverty, low educational status, and a high number of people who are divorced, separated, or widowed. Applying this information to a particular community allows for an estimation of the impairment rate. It has been common to assign an impairment rate of 15% to a population that includes few high-risk people, 22.5% to populations with moderate risk factors, and 30% to populations with many high-risk people.

Identifying and Prioritizing High-Risk Groups

When the data from the various community needs assessments are analyzed, specific high-risk groups begin to emerge. For example, socioeconomic data might show that a large number of elderly widows live in the community. Community forums and surveys of key informants may find that there are few services and programs for the elderly, and epidemiological studies might suggest that elderly widows living alone are at high risk for depression. Therefore, elderly widows might become a target group for program development and intervention.

Demographic data might also show that a community has many preadolescent females, and socioeconomic indicators may suggest that many of these young women live in single-parent households and in poverty. Community forums and surveys of key informants may reveal few recreational and social services for children and adolescents. Finally, epidemiological studies may report high correlations among poverty, single-parent households, and adolescent pregnancy. Therefore, community mental health administrators might consider adolescents in this community to be at risk for mental health problems and target them for intervention.

> **?** *Describe the characteristics of a group that was at high risk for developing mental illness in the community in which you grew up.*

Intervention Strategies

Intervening with high-risk groups in the community can include primary, secondary, or tertiary prevention activities.

▼ **Primary prevention:** Targets people at risk for developing psychiatric illness and promotes their adaptive coping mechanisms

▼ **Secondary prevention:** Targets people who show early symptoms of an emotional disorder but regain pretreatment level of functioning through aggressive treatment

▼ **Tertiary prevention:** Targets those with mental illness and helps to reduce the severity, discomfort, and disability associated with their illness

The public health model of community mental health required the development of new interventions. Before the community mental health movement of the 1960s, most mental health outpatient services consisted of expensive, office-based, individual psychotherapy sessions. Although this may have been a good secondary prevention strategy, it did not promote mental health or prevent emotional problems on a communitywide basis. New treatment strategies that were developed to fulfill the goals of community mental health included mental health promotion (Chapter 12) and crisis intervention (Chapter 13).

Role of Nurses

The public health model had major consequences for the role of psychiatric nurses in community mental health. Social workers and psychologists who had years of experience in the public sector dominated administrative and management positions in this model. Theoretically, nursing should have been readily accepted as one of the mental health disciplines because of public health nurses' long-standing presence in community care; however, public health nurses were seen as closely allied with secondary and tertiary prevention activities, the medical model, and care of the sick. Therefore, although patients with chronic mental illness were referred to public health nurses, few nurses were invited to join psychiatry, psychology, and social work as professional staff in most community mental health centers.[9] A 1962 national survey of nurses' roles in outpatient psychiatric clinics found that fewer than 10% of these facilities included a nurse on the professional team.[15] The passage of the Community Mental Health Centers Act in 1963 did little to change that pattern. Specifically, the number of psychologists and social workers in community mental health centers increased between 1970 and 1980, whereas the number of psychiatrists and nurses declined.

In addition, nursing education was slow to revise curricula and change clinical practice to reflect this shift in care from the hospital to the community. As a result, nurses felt unprepared to function in the community and were unable to create a role for themselves. With few exceptions, the nurse's role in community mental health centers was limited to traditional nursing tasks such as medication monitoring and caring for patients with chronic mental illness.

BIOLOGICAL-MEDICAL MODEL

In the mid-1970s several events turned public attention to the second mission of the community mental health movement: the care of those with diagnosed mental illness. A new political administration, the waging of an expensive war in Vietnam, and a general economic downturn stimulated a national discussion regarding the best use of scarce health-care resources. At the same time, public disillusionment with the deinstitutionalization of people with chronic mental illness led to questions about the cost effectiveness of community mental health centers, with their focus on prevention rather than care of those who were already ill.

Families of people with mental illness had also become a political force in the late 1970s. Their agenda was to force as many resources as possible toward the care of those with severe and persistent mental illness and to direct federal research dollars toward finding a biological basis for the major mental illnesses. Psychiatrists, with their new focus on the biological model of psychiatry, and family groups thus became allies and formed a coalition that put biological psychiatry in a strong leadership position in the mental health field.

Financial pressures also brought about a change in the focus of mental health centers. At the beginning of the community mental health movement the federal government had promised to pay 75% of the cost of each center. Regulations stated that federal support would decrease by 15% each year; by the eighth year of their existence the centers were expected to be self-supporting through a combination of state funds and third-party reimbursement. By the early 1970s many centers faced the end of federal funding and state governments were unable or unwilling to take on the burden of funding them. The centers then had to rely heavily on third-party reimbursement through fee-for-service mechanisms, which were typically physician directed and illness oriented. Centers thus began to focus on the diagnosis and treatment of the deinstitutionalized people with severe and persistent mental illness, primarily through the reimbursable services of medication management and psychotherapy.

These factors led to major amendments of the Community Mental Health Centers Act in 1975, requiring centers to offer services for people with serious mental illness who had been discharged from the state hospitals. These services included screening admissions to inpatient services, aftercare services, and transitional housing. Because centers were not allowed to reduce the five original essential services and were not given sufficient funds to add these new services, decisions about priorities had to be made. Because of political and social pressure to care for those who were being discharged into the community in large numbers, the community mental health centers reluctantly decreased their preventive efforts and moved toward the increased use of the medical model and the care of people with diagnosed mental illness.

Deinstitutionalization

Between 1965 and 1975 nearly 500,000 patients were either discharged or diverted from state hospitals to care in the community. It was hoped that psychiatric treatment in community centers, combined with living arrangements provided by family or board and care homes, would allow these people to live more humane lives in their own communities. However, it rapidly became clear that policymakers had seriously miscalculated both the service needs of this population and the ability of communities to accommodate the large numbers of people with mental illness who had been discharged from the state hospitals. Often,

these former patients had to be readmitted to state hospitals. In the early days of deinstitutionalization, as many as 70% of the patients discharged from state hospitals had to be readmitted within 1 year. Others who could not meet the increasingly strict admission criteria of state hospitals drifted into the criminal justice system or into homelessness. Many who were elderly were admitted to nursing homes.

In reviewing the failures of this early attempt to move patients into community care, mental health experts agree that the following problems contributed to the lack of success:

▼ Poor coordination between state hospitals and community mental health centers
▼ Underestimation of the support systems needed to enable people with mental illness to live in the community
▼ Lack of knowledge about psychiatric rehabilitation
▼ Underestimation of community resistance to deinstitutionalization
▼ Shortage of professionals trained to work with this population in the community
▼ Reimbursement systems that rewarded hospitalization

It was apparent by the 1980s that the biological-medical model of community mental health might not be able to provide the psychological and social supports that were needed to allow people with severe and persistent mental illness to live successfully in the community. Professionals began to search for a more comprehensive model of care that would take into account all aspects of a person's life.

> **?** *Do you think that all psychiatric patients are better off living in the community rather than in public or private hospitals?*

Role of Nurses

Nurses began to play a more important role in community mental health care during the 1970s and 1980s. This was partly because traditional nursing roles in the medical model were well known and readily accepted by physician team leaders and administrators of community mental health centers; also, the number of deinstitutionalized patients was growing. Initially, nurses worked in aftercare programs providing support, coordination of care, and health teaching. Gradually, those responsibilities grew to those of nurse therapists in individual, group, and family therapies with a variety of patients, not just those with chronic mental illness. Many psychiatric nurses with master's degrees opened private practices and initiated creative and innovative mental health services.

Nursing's expansion into less traditional roles in community mental health can be attributed to the influence of the National Institute of Mental Health (NIMH). In 1975 a NIMH task force examined the staffing needs in mental health and existing training programs. The result was a new NIMH policy mandating that to be eligible for NIMH training grants, educational programs had to address the needs of unserved and underserved populations including children, people with chronic mental illness, minorities, and women. By the fall of 1979 training grants were awarded only to educational programs that focused on one or more of these priorities, particularly those that focused on providing clinical training in community mental health centers.[7]

The outcome of this mandate was that nursing school faculty began to reach out to community mental health centers to develop clinical placements for nursing students. In this process, faculty were able to educate center administrators about the scope of nursing practice and the variety of skills, in addition to medication administration and monitoring, that nurses could bring to the community setting. At the same time, curricula in nursing schools were revised to reflect this new practice setting. Crisis intervention, brief therapy, counseling, assessment, and diagnosis were emphasized as nurses began to take their place as members of the interdisciplinary teams in community mental health centers while striving to keep their unique identity.[29]

> **?** *Why is the role of the psychiatric nurse on an interdisciplinary mental health care team more difficult to define in community settings?*

SYSTEMS MODEL

The systems model of community mental health emerged in the 1980s and operated on the philosophy that all aspects of a person's life needed to be cared for—basic human needs, as well as needs for psychiatric treatment and rehabilitation. The focus of this model was on developing a comprehensive system of care and coordinating needed services into an integrated package. This model of community mental health emerged as it became apparent that mental health treatment alone would not enable people with severe and disabling mental illnesses to live successfully in the community. A special federal initiative was launched in 1977 to help states and communities to develop comprehensive services for this population. This initiative was led by NIMH, which began to fund demonstration programs for community support systems in all states.

Community Support Systems

Community mental health centers were given primary responsibility for the development and implementation of community support systems for people in their service areas. These systems were to be guided by the principles listed in Box 34-1.[39] In implementing these systems, case management became the primary means for ensuring that the components of the service system were available to every person with a chronic mental illness who needed them (Fig. 34-1). These components included client identification and outreach, mental health treatment, crisis response services,

Box 34-1 *Principles of Community Support Systems*

People with long-term mental illness should have access to specialized mental health services and the supports needed by all people.

The community is the best place to provide long-term care. Inpatient care is part of the needed community-based services and should be used for short-term evaluation, stabilization, and occasional long-term hospitalization.

Services should be consumer centered and based on the needs of the consumer rather than those of the system or provider.

Services should empower people. Services should include consumer self-help approaches and allow people to retain the greatest possible control over their lives.

Services should be racially and culturally appropriate.

Services should be flexible. Services should be available whenever they are needed and for as long as they are needed.

Services should focus on strengths.

Services should be offered in the least restrictive and most natural settings possible.

Services should meet special needs, including those of people with severe mental illness, the homeless, the elderly, people with substance abuse problems, and people with mental illness who have been inappropriately placed in the criminal justice system.

Service systems should be accountable. Services should be monitored by the state to ensure quality of care and continued relevance. Consumers and families should be involved in planning, implementing, monitoring, and evaluating services.

Services should be coordinated. Written agreements and linkages between participating agencies and various levels of government should be developed. Mechanisms should be in place to ensure continuity of care and coordination between hospitals and other community services.

health and dental care, housing, income support and entitlement, peer support, family and community support, rehabilitation services, and protection and advocacy.[2] These services are discussed in Chapter 14.

Case Management

Case management services are aimed at linking the service system to the consumer and coordinating the service components so that he or she can achieve successful community living. It includes problem solving to provide continuity of services and overcome problems of rigid systems, fragmented services, poor use of resources, and problems of inaccessibility. The six activities that form the core of case management are:

▼ Identification and outreach
▼ Assessment
▼ Service planning
▼ Linkage with needed services
▼ Monitoring service delivery
▼ Advocacy

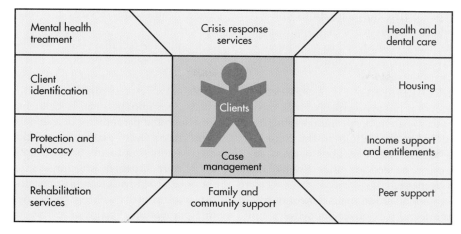

Fig. 34-1   Components of a community support system. (Department of Health and Human Services: *Toward a model plan for a comprehensive community-based mental health system,* October 1987.)

In addition, four components and thirteen interventions related to clinical case management have been identified.[21] These are listed in Table 34-2.

> **?** *Which interventions of clinical case management listed in Table 34-2 should be provided by a mental health professional and which ones, if any, can be carried out by a lay person?*

IDENTIFICATION AND OUTREACH. To encourage states to provide case management services, the federal government passed the State Comprehensive Mental Health Services Plan, which required that case management services be provided to every person with mental illness in a state that receives a significant amount of public funds or services. A comprehensive mental health service plan must have strategies to locate potential clients, inform them of available services, and ensure their access to these services. Establishing and maintaining close working relationships with potential referral sources such as public and community hospitals, community mental health centers, and social service agencies were essential to meeting this goal. Some case management agencies specialize in working with a particular target population, such as the homeless or those with a dual diagnosis of mental illness and substance abuse. These case managers establish contacts with potential clients in homeless shelters, soup kitchens, drug treatment centers, and emergency facilities.

ASSESSMENT. A thorough assessment of a person's strengths and deficits is required for an effective service plan. Assessments address all aspects of a person's life, including psychological, emotional, financial, medical, educational, vocational, social, and housing needs. Particular emphasis is placed on identifying patient strengths that can be

TABLE 34-2 *Components and Interventions of Clinical Case Management*

COMPONENT	INTERVENTION
Initial phase	Engagement
	Assessment
	Planning
Environmental interventions	Linkages with community resources
	Consultation with families and caregivers
	Maintenance and expansion of social networks
	Collaboration with physicians and hospitals
	Advocacy
Patient interventions	Individual psychotherapy
	Training in independent living skills
	Psychoeducation
Patient-environment interventions	Crisis intervention
	Monitoring

used to compensate for weaknesses and understanding patients' cultural and health-related values and beliefs. The knowledge and skills needed for a comprehensive assessment are generally beyond the ability of one case manager and often require a multidisciplinary approach. The expected outcome of the assessment is a detailed outline of the person's present functioning, highest level of functioning, and needed services.

SERVICE PLANNING. A comprehensive service plan guides all case management activities and must be carefully formulated with individual and family involvement. The goal of the service plan is to help the person to live in the community successfully. Because many of these people have histories of numerous psychiatric hospitalizations, the service plan should include new approaches that might interrupt the chain of events that previously led to rehospitalization. Treatment objectives and specific actions that will be taken should also be clearly stated.

LINKAGE WITH NEEDED SERVICES. A major component of case management is linking the people with mental illness with the various social, medical, and rehabilitative services that they need to live successfully in the community. Once again, this activity often requires a team approach because the services needed are often diverse and span a broad range of agencies.

Mental Health Treatment. Clinical management of psychiatric disorders is an integral part of service delivery and may be provided on a long-term basis if needed. Clinical care should be directed at helping the patient manage symptoms, understand medications, recognize signs of relapse, and cope with daily living. Clinical care should also include diagnostic evaluation and ongoing monitoring of the patient's psychiatric condition. Supportive counseling and individual, family, or group intervention should be offered as appropriate.

An essential component of clinical management is medication management. Medication management services include prescribing medications, ensuring that needed medications are available, carefully monitoring medications to ensure maximal benefits and minimal side effects, and educating the patient and family about the medications.

Crisis Response Services. Despite the provision of ongoing clinical care, people with serious and long-term mental illness tend to have crises. The primary goal of crisis services is to help those in psychiatric crisis to maintain or quickly resume functioning within the community. Emergency services offered 24 hours a day must be provided by community mental health centers, and this can be accomplished in a variety of ways. It is common in large urban areas for this service to be provided by the emergency room of a local hospital. Other community mental health centers provide this service on site. In rural areas, where travel time and distance make a central crisis location unfeasible, mobile crisis outreach services visit the patient in the setting in which the crisis is occurring. Some community agencies provide 24-hour hotlines staffed by professionals or volunteers who offer crisis counseling or referral services over the telephone. However, when these services do not resolve the crisis, crisis residential services should be available in a residential nonhospital setting on a short-term basis.

Health and Dental Care. Psychiatric patients have been found to have higher mortality rates from both natural and unnatural causes than the general population.[13] Numerous studies have also shown that psychiatric patients have higher rates of comorbid medical illnesses, which are largely undiagnosed and untreated. These medical illnesses may cause or exacerbate psychiatric symptoms. Thus adequate health care services for this population are very important.

Despite the fact that people with psychiatric illnesses also have serious medical problems, their use of general health-care services is often limited because of barriers to access and availability.[45] Access problems often result from active psychiatric symptoms, such as hallucinations regarding body functions and paranoid or delusional thinking. These symptoms may prevent people from seeking appropriate health care or adhering to treatment. Another factor is that psychiatrically ill people who do seek medical care are sometimes regarded with fear, hostility, and suspicion by healthcare professionals who are inexperienced in working with this population. Finally, access and availability of general health care are also affected by the current health-care delivery environment, which is oriented toward specialization and episodic treatment of acute conditions (see Chapter 9).

Housing. An important goal of the community support system is to locate, secure, and maintain affordable housing for people with long-term mental illness. Group homes where three to six people with mental disabilities live together with minimal supervision are becoming available, as well as apartment complexes that have several units rented to people with mental illness scattered throughout the complex.[6] Training, supports, and services are provided to allow people with mental illness to live as independently as possible. Commonly offered services include social and recreational activities, on-site crisis intervention, and client advocacy. A variety of more structured residential settings are being used for more disabled people. Finally, foster care homes that provide accepting, normalized settings for people with severe mental disabilities are also becoming more common.

Although great strides are being made to provide adequate and appropriate housing for people with severe mental illness, the greatest barrier continues to be community resistance to the placement of such people in residential settings. In many places the outcome of this resistance has been psychiatric ghettos in which large numbers of people with psychiatric impairment live in poorly supervised board and care homes in low-income areas or on the streets.

> **?** *How would you and your family feel about a group home for people with mental illness being built in your neighborhood?*

MONITORING SERVICE DELIVERY. Monitoring is an important part of case management and is often difficult to implement. The monitoring function of case management serves two basic purposes: It ensures that the objectives of the service plan are being met and it provides the information necessary for an ongoing reevaluation of the plan. The case manager helps the patient obtain the services identified in the service plan. Because the needs of people with mental illness are usually complex and require the services of multiple agencies, the case manager must develop coordinating and facilitating skills. Periodic review of the person's progress with each of these service providers is part of the case manager's duties. Information gained from these contacts should also be documented in regular reviews of the overall service plan.

ADVOCACY. Helping people to receive the available services and influencing providers to improve existing services and develop new ones are important roles of the case manager. Psychiatric patients and their families struggle with issues of discrimination, stigma, compromised rights, and inadequate resources on a daily basis. Advocacy activities address these injustices proactively. They include political negotiation as well as consumer and professional collaboration. Finally, it is essential for advocacy efforts to be sensitive to the cultural background of the consumer and the norms and values of the community.

MANAGED CARE AND CASE MANAGEMENT. At present, case management is an ambiguous concept without a clear base in any one professional discipline. Early definitions stressed the linking, brokering, and advocacy functions of the role. These roles evolved into a more clinically oriented definition. Furthermore, there are various models or types of case management, including service broker, clinical, intensive, collaborative, aggressive, and problem-focused. The work of the case manager is very complex, covering a broad array of activities. Recently, with the advent of managed care, case management has come to reflect two basic but apparently contradictory underlying goals: increasing access to services and limiting costs. In the public sector, case management is intended to increase access to care and make more services available to those eligible and underserved. In the private sector, case management has become synonymous with utilization review, where the emphasis is placed on cost control and limitation of resource use.

Clearly, functions resembling case management will be an increasingly prominent part of mental health care in the future as attempts are made to balance cost, access, and effectiveness (see Chapter 9). Resources of patients, families, providers, and society must be managed in order to carry out these complex goals. However, important questions remain, including what the tasks of case managers are, who should be doing case management (what personal qualities and training are needed), to whom the case manager is accountable, and how the work of case management should be organized.[36]

Role of Nurses

The systems model of community mental health was based on a holistic approach that focused on the caring and the curative aspects of service delivery. Nurses, with a similar focus, thus had an opportunity to perform a variety of roles in this model. Case management, in particular, allowed nurses to assume direct care, supervisory, and consulting roles while working with patients and families by:

▼ Serving as their gatekeepers and facilitators in accessing the health-care system
▼ Helping them make informed decisions about their health-care needs
▼ Monitoring their health and human service plan of care
▼ Educating them to enhance their self-care ability

The American Nurses' Association states that[1]:

> Psychiatric and mental health nurses are highly qualified to function as both case managers and providers within managed care systems. Psychiatric and mental health nurses are positioned to have a maximum impact on the managed care of psychiatric clients because:
>   They are committed to improving access, quality, and cost containment.
>   They understand prevention and wellness and know how to educate patients to improve health.
>   They know how to triage and assess the needs of patients.
>   They know how to accurately evaluate the necessity for inpatient admissions and continued hospital stays.

There is great opportunity for nurses to expand their roles and develop new career directions by functioning as case managers who can address the physical and psychiatric needs of patients.[26,37] This can include people with chronic mental illness as well as general psychiatric patients in outpatient settings.[19] The following clinical example illustrates the contributions a psychiatric nurse can make in providing case management services.

Clinical Example Jane M is single, 33 years old, and has a history of multiple psychiatric admissions. She was referred to the community mental health center case management unit upon discharge from a 6-month stay at the state hospital. She had a diagnosis of undifferentiated schizophrenia in remission and was discharged to the care of her family on thioridazine 400 mg daily. Jane has occasional auditory hallucinations, is somewhat suspicious, and has a long history of disruptive family relationships and noncompliance with medications.

The psychiatric nurse case manager volunteered to take the case and made an appointment with the family for a home visit. When she arrived, the family was visibly upset and related that in the week since Jane had been home, she slept much of the day and roamed around the house during the night, taking long showers, slamming kitchen cabinet doors, and playing loud rock music. When she was awake during the day, she would disappear for hours at a time, causing great anxiety for the family. The mother was tearful and wringing her hands in an agitated manner while the father sat on the sofa with his head bowed. Jane sprawled in a chair and intermittently swore at her mother as the mother described these events.

The nurse recognized that Jane's illness dominated the household, essentially putting her in control of the rest of the family. The nurse worked intensely with this family to restore generational boundaries by supporting the parents in making mutually agreed upon rules about behavior that would be tolerated in their household. She helped the family identify ways to support Jane while setting limits that would promote adaptive family functioning. The family found this exchange to be very helpful and they called on the nurse to validate their ideas and provide them with ongoing information on Jane's illness. The nurse also evaluated the impact of the medication on Jane's behavior. She arranged to have the time of Jane's medication changed so that she received a dose at bedtime.

Over the next few weeks, Jane began to sleep at night. With continued support from the nurse, the parents became skilled and comfortable at presenting a united front. Although Jane initially resisted, she adapted rather quickly to the new norms in the house, and a family crisis that might have resulted in Jane's readmission to the hospital was averted.

Despite these expanding clinical services, the trend among psychiatric nurses with advanced training and education in the 1980s was to remain in inpatient settings rather than to work with people with serious mental illness in the community. Thus many challenges remained for nursing as the community mental health movement moved to the next model of care.

> **?** *What factors influence whether psychiatric nurses work in inpatient settings or community-based psychiatric programs?*

PATIENT-CENTERED MODEL

Although the systems model of community mental health contributed to an improved and more coherent service delivery system, new problems and populations began to emerge (see Critical Thinking about Contemporary Issues). Many patients' problems did not fit well in any service system, but instead required intervention by more than one of these systems simultaneously. Examples of such groups include people with HIV/AIDS (discussed in Chapter 40) and patients who are dually diagnosed with both substance and psychiatric disorders (discussed in Chapter 24). Complex problems also emerged in two other groups: homeless people with mental illness and mentally ill people in jail.

Homeless People with Mental Illness

Homeless people are an inescapable presence in American society, where they live in subway tunnels and on steam grates and die in cardboard boxes on windswept corners in communities throughout the country. To most Americans, homelessness seems neither invisible nor insurmountable (Box 34-2). People who are mentally ill and homeless reflect the tension between a mental health system that views housing as a social welfare problem and public housing

CRITICAL THINKING *about* Contemporary Issues

How Many State Hospital Beds Are Needed in This Country?

Controversy surrounds the impact of deinstitutionalization on the quality of life of people in need of psychiatric care. In 1955 there were 559,000 state hospital beds for a population of 165 million. Today there are 103,000 state hospital beds for a population of more than 248 million. Thus state hospital beds per 100,000 population have dropped from 339 to 41. In some states the statistics are even more drastic. For example, California has 14 state hospital beds, including forensic beds, per 100,000 population and only 8.3 nonforensic beds per 100,000.

The question that has been raised is how many state hospital beds are really needed. Specifically, what will happen to people with chronic and severe mental illness who experience such problems as assaultive behavior, overt major psychopathology, lack of internal controls, resistance to medication, inability to adjust to open settings, serious problems with drugs and alcohol, and self-destructive behavior? Many of them are lost to the mental health system and wind up in jail or on the streets. Perhaps even more important, what moral obligation does society have to assess quality of life issues when formulating health-care policy?

Although state mental hospitals have been replaced by community-based service structures in some parts of the United States, they continue in general to occupy a critical place in systems of care.[3] It has been argued that long-term care is an important part of a mental health system, specifically for people with severe mental illness. The state mental hospital can provide that care and be made to function more efficiently.[4] However, renewed efforts to integrate them as full partners within those systems must be undertaken.

agencies that believe that this population needs specialized residential programs provided by mental health agencies. Thus the needs of this population are underserved as services are fragmented and inaccessible. However, a number of studies have shown that when homeless people with mental illness are given the opportunity to participate in treatment programs that address their needs for services in areas such as housing, health care, substance abuse, and income support, many can be helped to find homes and achieve substantial improvements in their lives. Thus mental health professionals have begun to explore the use of new approaches to providing treatment, rehabilitation services, and housing to homeless people with mental illness, who often avoid contact with traditional mental health programs because of past difficulty in gaining access to care, demands from clinicians for treatment compliance, or past involuntary hospitalization.[27,44] Key components of this new treatment approach have been identified as[33]

▼ Frequent and consistent staff contact through assertive outreach

▼ Meeting the client where he or she is, both geographically and interpersonally

Box 34-2 *What Americans Say about the Homeless*

A national survey conducted for *Parade* magazine in 1994 found the following:

70% saw homeless people in their own communities.

76% said something should be done to reduce homelessness in America.

36% can imagine a situation in which they might become homeless.

84% thought that at least half of the homeless could be helped enough to reenter society.

82% said the homeless should not be prohibited from public places.

77% thought homeless people are not adequately helped by the government.

69% did not want a legal procedure that would forcibly remove homeless people from the street.

7% thought homeless people were violent but 60% said the homeless contribute to the rising crime rate.

56% thought homeless people were not responsible for the situation they were in.

30% said a homeless person who is nonviolent but with a diagnosed mental illness should be institutionalized against his or her will.

16% said they would go out of their way to avoid homeless people.

▼ Help with immediate survival needs such as food, emergency shelter, and clothing

▼ Gradual treatment through the development of trust

▼ An emphasis on client strengths

▼ Client choice of services and the right to refuse treatment

▼ The delivery of comprehensive services including mental health and substance abuse treatment, medical care, housing, social and vocational services, and help in obtaining entitlements

One particularly innovative program is the Access to Community Care and Effective Services and Supports (ACCESS) demonstration program. It was initiated in 1993 by the US Department of Health and Human Services as part of a national agenda to end homelessness among people with serious mental illness. Demonstration projects are ongoing in nine states, which are developing integrated systems of care for this population. The purpose of the ACCESS program is to determine whether integration initiatives implemented at the program, policy, and organizational levels will improve outcomes for the homeless people with mental illness beyond those obtained by integration at the direct service delivery level—that is, by case management.[31] Demonstration programs such as these hold hope for better care for this vulnerable population.

  Should people be allowed to choose to be homeless if they are not dangerous to themselves or others?

Mentally Ill People in Jail

A nationwide survey reported that 1 of every 14 jail inmates in this country has a mental illness. This does not include inmates with mental illness in state or federal prisons. Twenty-nine percent of jails surveyed house people with serious mental illness who have not committed crimes. These people are often jailed because no other facilities are available to respond to their psychiatric emergencies.[40]

However, there are model programs to deal with this problem in various parts of the United States, including counties in Ohio, Virginia, Washington, and New York. A community model for services (Fig. 34-2) has been proposed by Laben and Blum that includes methods for preventing incarceration of people with mental illness and intervening effectively when such a person is jailed.[22] This model is based on the formation of a community board and includes both preventive and postrelease interventions.

Have jails become today's substitute for yesterday's state hospitals for people with mental illness? If so, which alternative is better?

As the needs of these groups illustrate, it is clear that if contemporary American society is to deal effectively, compassionately, and humanely with people with psychiatric illness, several factors must be taken into account.[16] First, those with mental illness include people with very different disorders, prognoses, and needs. Second, outcomes for these patients vary over time, as some people recover fully whereas others remain disabled for the rest of their lives. Third, serious mental disorders are often exacerbated by poverty, racism, and substance abuse. Finally, although psychiatric treatment can alleviate symptoms and permit patients to live in the community, there is no magic bullet that will cure all cases of serious mental illness. Rather, these illnesses require both therapy and management.

These system problems were frustrating to health-care providers, consumers, families, and the public, and consumers of mental health services and their families became increasingly vocal about their lack of participation in the planning of mental health services. Thus in the 1990s a patient-centered model of community mental health emerged, focusing on outreach clinical services. In this model, consumer participation in planning culturally relevant services is a guiding principle of service delivery.

Outreach Clinical Services

Outreach implies that mental health workers reach out to patients wherever they are in the community, including family homes, board and care homes, group homes, fast-food restaurants, homeless shelters, street corners, or prisons. This kind of assertive treatment is usually reserved for people with one of the following characteristics:

▼ *Unwillingness to seek out services.* Some patients are un-

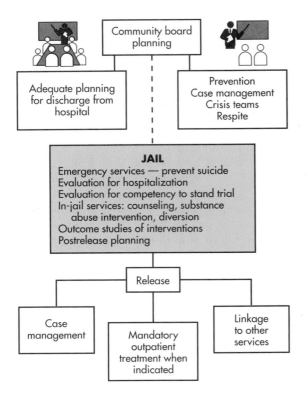

Fig. 34-2 **Community model for services.** (From Laben J, Blum J: Persons with mental illness in jail. In Worley N, editor: *Mental health nursing in the community,* St Louis, 1997, Mosby.)

willing to go to community mental health centers for treatment. Others often miss appointments. This behavior is seen as part of the illness and requires more intensive outreach by the provider.

▼ *Medication nonadherence.* Patients who are not willing, lack the money, or are too disorganized to take their medications require a treatment approach that can determine the problem, monitor the patient, and implement strategies to ensure that needed medication is taken. Sometimes this can be accomplished by education, encouragement, titrating dosages, or switching medications. Depot injections of long-acting psychotropic medication may also be useful. Packaging medications in daily doses with the date and time to take each pill can be an effective compliance tool. Sometimes legal procedures may be implemented by the treatment team because many states have outpatient commitment laws in which patients are legally required to comply with outpatient treatment.

▼ *Inability to self-monitor symptoms.* Patients sometimes respond to hallucinations and delusions by discontinuing their usual social and treatment contacts. They become isolated and withdrawn and must be visited frequently and encouraged to resume regular activities.

▼ *Inability to structure daily activities.* Some patients have a social network and the ability to structure their daily ac-

tivities, but others have difficulty and need to be provided with structured daily activities by a professional team. Many are strongly encouraged to participate in day treatment programs or other community activities.

▼ *Frequency of crises.* Patients who have frequent or severe crises need treatment from a program that provides intensive crisis intervention.

ASSERTIVE COMMUNITY TREATMENT. Assertive Community Treatment (ACT) was developed in Wisconsin in the early 1970s as a program originally called Training in Community Living (TCL). It was created as a way of organizing outpatient mental health services for patients who were leaving large state mental hospitals and were at risk for rehospitalization. This model program provides a full range of medical, psychosocial, and rehabilitative services by a community-based team that operates 24 hours a day, 7 days a week. Treatment takes place in natural settings: patients' homes, neighborhoods, and places of work. Staff members teach and help patients in daily living activities such as laundry, shopping, cooking, grooming, budgeting, and use of public transportation. In addition, patients are given intensive assistance in finding jobs or sheltered workshop placements. Staff have daily contact with patients and patient supervisors or employers to help resolve on-the-job problems. Staff also guide the patients in constructive use of leisure time and the development of social skills.[38]

The original TCL model has been replicated in thousands of communities under names such as Continuous Treatment Teams (CTTs), Programs for Assertive Community Treatment (PACT), and Intensive Case Management (ICM). The overall goals of treatment and desired outcomes for patients in these programs include:

▼ Reduced symptoms and relapse

▼ Increased community tenure

▼ Enhanced satisfaction with life

▼ Reduced subjective distress

▼ Improved functioning at work, at home, and in social settings

ACT uses an interdisciplinary team-oriented approach that typically includes up to 10 staff members (nurses, psychiatrists, social workers, activity therapists) who meet regularly to plan individualized care for a shared caseload of about 120 patients. More than 75% of staff time is spent in the field providing direct treatment and rehabilitation. In a recent national survey of assertive outreach programs, it was found that 88% had a psychiatric nurse as an integral member of the treatment team.[10] ACT teams function as continuous care teams who work with patients with serious mental illness and their families over time to improve their quality of life. In effect, these programs function as a community-based "hospital without walls," providing a high-intensity program of clinical support and treatment.

Controlled clinical trials have been conducted with a wide range of people with severe mental illness, including patients with schizophrenia, veterans, dually diagnosed patients, and homeless people. These studies report that patients spent less time in hospitals and more in independent community housing. Their symptoms were reduced and their satisfaction with treatment increased.[5,25] The ACT model has been disseminated unevenly in various settings across 33 states, with the highest concentration of programs in midwestern and eastern states.[10] Implementation has been slowed by the self-interest of established community mental health systems, the resistance of clinicians to change traditional hierarchical role relationships, and the substantial cost per patient of the program. However, the potential for ACT to reduce problems related to homelessness and rehospitalization is a compelling reason for states to continue adopting this approach.

MULTISYSTEM THERAPY. Multisystemic therapy (MST) is a highly flexible treatment approach that addresses the multiple, interrelated needs of youths with serious behavioral and emotional problems and their families.[17] It is usually delivered through the family preservation model of service delivery to provide interventions in home, school, and neighborhood settings. The primary goal of family preservation has been to prevent out-of-home placement by providing home-based, intensive, and time-limited services to families whose children are at immediate risk of such placement. The goal of MST is to develop parent skills and resources needed to address the difficulties of raising teenagers and to teach youths to cope with family, peer, school, and neighborhood problems. At the peer or school level, a goal of treatment is to decrease the youth's involvement with deviant peers and to increase involvement with prosocial peers.

MST uses existing pragmatic and goal-oriented treatment strategies, and interventions are guided by nine principles that reflect the nature of MST (Box 34-3). MST is usually delivered by master's-level clinicians with caseload ratios of one staff to four to six families. Service duration usually ranges from 3 to 5 months, with an average of 40 to 60 hours of direct clinical contact over the course of treatment. Staff are available 24 hours a day, 7 days a week during the active treatment phase. Studies provide strong support for MST as a viable approach to adolescents and their families who have traditionally been regarded as unresponsive to treatment. It has also been shown to improve communication in families of juvenile offenders and parent-child interaction in abusive or neglecting families. Other reported outcomes include improved family relations and peer relations and the prevention of expensive out-of-home placements.[18]

> **?** *ACT and MST programs are new models of psychiatric care. Determine whether they are being used in your community and the impact they may be having on vulnerable populations where you live.*

Box 34-3 *Nine Basic Principles of Multisystem Therapy*

The primary purpose of assessment is to understand the fit between the identified problems and their systemic context.

Therapeutic contact should emphasize the positive and interventions should use systemic strengths as levers for change.

Interventions should promote responsible behavior and decrease irresponsible behavior.

Interventions should be present focused and action oriented, targeting specific and well-defined problems.

Interventions should target sequences of behavior within and among systems.

Interventions should be developmentally appropriate and fit the developmental needs of the young person.

Interventions should be designed to require daily or weekly effort by family members.

Intervention efficacy should be continuously evaluated from different perspectives.

Interventions should promote treatment generalization and long-term maintenance of therapeutic change.

Modified from Henggeler SW, Schoenwald SK, Pickrel SG, Brondino MJ, Borduin CM, Hall JA: *Treatment manual for family preservation using multisystemic therapy,* Charleston, 1994, South Carolina Health and Human Services Finance Commission.

Assertive community treatment, used for adults with severe mental illness, and multisystem therapy, used for adolescents with serious emotional disorders, share common elements that differ from traditional systems and that have important implications for mental health policy (Table 34-3).[34] They both use a social-ecological model of behavior applied to mental health patients. In addition, therapeutic principles emphasizing pragmatic (outcome-oriented) treatment approaches, home-based interventions, and individualized treatment goals are key elements of their success. Most importantly, both systems embody a therapeutic philosophy demanding therapist accountability, in which staff are rewarded for clinical outcomes and therapeutic innovation rather than for following a prescribed plan. As empirically tested approaches they provide a scientific foundation for continued mental health care reform and illustrate the critical elements needed in designing new community treatment initiatives for behavioral as well as medical conditions.

Role of Nurses

Current trends of shortened stays in psychiatric hospitals, use of alternatives for hospitalization whenever possible, increased focus on patients with complex treatment problems, and the growth of consumer and family movements have had major impacts on the ways in which mental health care is delivered in the United States. A number of new approaches are being implemented to overcome the clinical and system problems that have interfered with providing patient-centered care. These represent unique opportunities and challenges for nursing and the literature reflects the in-

TABLE **34-3** *Differences between Traditional Mental Health Care Systems, Assertive Community Treatment, and Multisystem Therapy*

SERVICE ELEMENT	TRADITIONAL SYSTEM	ASSERTIVE COMMUNITY TREATMENT	MULTISYSTEM THERAPY
Primary locus of care	Hospital, residential programs, day programs, offices	In the field (community, home, neighborhood, workplace)	In the field (community, home, neighborhood, school)
Provider of care	Individual clinician for individual outpatients, multidisciplinary teams for inpatients; treatment time highly variable; outpatient caseloads high, inpatient caseloads low; fragmented continuity of care across loci of care	Generalist teams share fixed case load; ratio of staff to patients = 1:10-15; treatment time unlimited; direct services continuously available	Generalist teams share temporary caseload; treatment time averages 4 months; ratio of staff to patients = 1:6; continuous services and emergency response available around the clock for treatment period
Treatment approach	Specific individual or group psychosocial therapies and biological treatments provided mostly in a health-care facility; providers not held directly accountable for outcomes	Medication monitoring and social support (help with housing, health, basic needs) in natural community environment; providers held accountable for outcomes	Pragmatic approach addresses problems identified in the child, family, peer, school, and neighborhood; family taught to sustain benefits, providers held directly accountable for outcomes

From Santos A et al: Research on field-based services: models for reform in the delivery of mental health care to populations with complex clinical problems, *Am J Psychiatry* 152:1111, 1995.

creasing participation of psychiatric nurses in assertive community treatment teams.[8,24,30,46]

On the other hand, psychiatric nurses continue to struggle with their involvement in community psychiatric care. Many community mental health centers are reluctant to hire psychiatric nurses because they are "too expensive" compared with other mental health care workers. Psychiatric nurses have also been slow to articulate the range and quality of services they can provide in community settings, thus demonstrating their cost effectiveness as health-care providers. In addition, community settings have difficulty differentiating among nurses based on education and experience, and they often underuse psychiatric nurses by confining their activities to medication administration. Finally, psychiatric nurses have not been active enough in designing, organizing, and administrating mental health delivery systems, so they are often viewed as implementers rather than decision makers.

NEW PSYCHIATRIC NURSING ROLES

Despite these problems, psychiatric nurses are beginning to play pivotal roles in emerging treatment modalities. They are fulfilling vital functions in day treatment facilities, psychotherapy clinics, vocational and rehabilitation centers, psychopharmacology clinics, psychiatric emergency rooms, and other community settings that provide care for people with mental illness. Other areas of role development are described here.

Primary Mental Health Care

Many people are not receiving the mental health care they need. Some are undiagnosed in general medical settings.

Others are correctly diagnosed but lack a consistent care provider. Still others have problems with their prescribed treatments and have relapses that could have been prevented.

Psychiatric nurses are moving into the domain of primary care and working with other nurses and physicians to diagnose and treat psychiatric illness in patients with somatic complaints. Cardiovascular, gynecological, respiratory, gastrointestinal, and family practice settings are appropriate for assessing patients for anxiety, depression, and substance abuse disorders. As health-care initiatives continue to move into schools and other community settings, psychiatric nurses can assume a leadership role in providing expertise through consultation and evaluation.

Psychiatric nurses are very well suited to provide comprehensive health care to patients in both psychiatric settings and primary care environments.[11] In particular, advanced practice psychiatric nurses acting as consultants to nonpsychiatric providers in hospital-based or outpatient clinics are in a unique position to assess and triage these patients on the basis of the immediacy of their needs. Early assessment and triage can minimize the length of time between psychiatric referral and intervention. By identifying patients in crisis and intervening in a timely fashion, they may reduce failed appointments and enhance the efficacy of treatment.[42]

Collaborative Practice Models

Psychiatric nurses are providing medical and medication management for selected groups of patients in collaborative practices. For example, patients who are having difficulty being stabilized on their medications or who have comorbid medical illnesses are seen in a psychiatric nursing clinic in which nurses and physicians collaborate

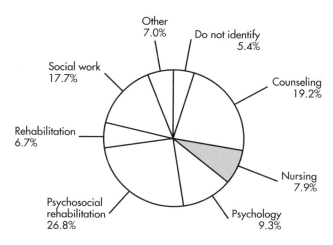

Fig. 34-3 The national survey of PSR workers, 1993.
(Modified from Blankertz LE, Robinson S: Who is the PSR worker? Psychosoc Rehab J, 1995.)

to provide high-quality patient care.[28,35,41] Psychiatric nurses who obtain prescriptive authority can further expand the services they provide and deliver cost-effective psychiatric care to communities that do not have access to a psychiatrist.

Psychosocial Rehabilitation Programs

Psychosocial rehabilitation encompasses the principles, practices, and programs that help people with severe mental illness lead more independent and satisfying lives in the community (see Chapter 14). Psychosocial rehabilitation is a young field that is expanding rapidly. There are many opportunities for nurses to use their clinical skills in a creative way and to practice autonomously in these programs.[12] Fig. 34-3 shows the percentage of psychosocial rehabilitation workers from each of the mental health disciplines. Only 7.9% of workers in this field are nurses. Nonetheless, with the advent of managed care, a large percentage of nurses are shifting from traditional inpatient care to work with consumers and their families in rehabilitation-oriented, community-based settings.[14] A recent study conducted in England suggested that community psychiatric nurses in the United Kingdom can provide the backbone for a system of mental health care that is continuous, community based, and rehabilitation oriented.[23] Psychiatric nurses have much to learn from and offer to the field of psychosocial rehabilitation and it promises to be a rich area of future psychiatric nursing practice.

> ? *Describe an innovative psychiatric nursing service that you could provide to people with mental illness in your community.*

Prevention and Wellness Programs

Prevention and wellness programs are increasing as society moves away from a focus on illness to a focus on the maintenance of health and quality of life. Many serious, expensive, and chronic illnesses are lifestyle disorders, including obesity, smoking, lack of exercise, unhealthy diets, drug use, and unsafe sexual practices. Preventive programs that promote healthier lifestyles have been found to be effective, and many corporations provide their employees with fitness and weight management centers and smoking cessation and stress management classes. These efforts have proved to be cost effective in the prevention of lost work days and expensive outpatient treatment and hospitalizations. Because they are partly educational and partly motivational, they are well within the expertise of psychiatric nurses.

In addition, certain groups who are at high risk and have been underserved in the past will receive more attention, and psychiatric nurses will be asked to expand the services they provide to these targeted populations. Psychiatric nurses are currently involved in a number of innovative community-based preventive initiatives. Examples include nurses who support high-risk adolescent mothers during the early postpartum period[43] and those who conduct community-based psychoeducational groups to promote and enhance effective coping in children who live in communities with chronic violence.[20] Mental health prevention is only now receiving the attention is has long deserved, and it holds exciting opportunities for psychiatric nurses.

Summary

1. The goals of community mental health are to care for those with diagnosed mental illness and prevent mental illness. There have been four models of community mental health.
2. The public health model (1960-1970) focused on the community and emphasized reducing the risk of mental illness for a population by providing services to high-risk groups. Intervention strategies included community needs assessment, identification of high-risk groups, consultation, education, and crisis intervention. The role of the nurse was minimal and often limited to caring for patients with chronic mental illness.
3. The biological-medical model (1970-1980) focused on people with diagnosed mental illness and viewed mental illness as brain disease. Interventions included medication management and psychotherapy. Nurses became more involved in community roles ranging from medication administration to coordinating aftercare programs and functioning as therapists for individuals, families, and groups.
4. The system model (1980-1990) focused on developing a comprehensive system of care and coordinated services. Interventions included community support systems, service coordination, and case management. Nurses began

to assume roles as coordinators of community services and case managers.

5. The patient-centered model (1990-present) focuses on patients who overlap service systems and emphasizes consumer participation and culturally relevant services. Interventions include outreach clinical services, assertive community treatment, and multisystem therapy. Nurses are demonstrating the range and quality of their services in this system of care.

6. New psychiatric nursing roles include initiatives in primary mental health care, collaborative practice models, psychosocial rehabilitation and prevention, and wellness programs.

your **INTERNET**
connection

Community Mental Health Management Information Systems Resource Center
http://www.chmis.org

National Mental Health Association
http://www.nmha.org/

COMPETENT CARING A Clinical Exemplar of a Psychiatric Nurse

Suzanne Smith, MSN, RN

An experience I'll always remember involved a patient who was being discharged from the state psychiatric hospital and whom I interviewed for admission into an intensive case management program. R had been in and out of the state hospital for 3 years with the diagnosis of chronic schizophrenia. His frequent readmissions were related to the system's inability to place him in the community, which was due in part to his history of setting fires. Before this admission, he had burned down his residence during a psychotic episode. However, his psychosis had resolved quickly after he was admitted to the hospital and started on a regimen of neuroleptics.

R was admitted into the intensive case management program, and his first 6 months had been very busy. He had been placed in an apartment with a roommate and became responsible for managing the apartment, cooking his own food, balancing his checkbook, and paying his bills. His adjustment to life in the community was progressing well. I was able to work with R on almost a daily basis, and all was going well.

On this specific day, I had called R to let him know that I would be coming to take him to the bank. We discussed in detail his checking account balance and financial obligations for that month. When I arrived at his home, R's roommate informed me that R had gone to the store to get a cup of coffee. While waiting, I walked into the hallway to check on a problem thermostat. As I glanced into R's room, I noticed that something was amiss. There were several cigarette burns in the carpet. On the bed there were a number of cigarette lighters. Propped on the pillows were cover photos from several women's magazines. The mouths on the models had been enlarged and a cigarette had been placed through the hole. In the bedside table I found several more ciga-

rette lighters. I noted all of these things, as well as the fact that R did not smoke.

On his return, we discussed some problems R was having with his roommate and banking affairs. His conversation was calm and rational. I then talked with him about what I had seen in his bedroom. Initially he was silent and refused to discuss the matter. I realized that one of his greatest fears was returning to the state hospital to live for the remainder of his life, so I assured him that if something was wrong and he needed to go back to the hospital, it would be for a short-term hospitalization. At that point he began to explain that he had not taken his medication in a week and that recently he drank a six-pack of beer with several other patients in the program. Since then, he had been hearing messages from God in which she told him to smoke cigarettes because carbon monoxide was needed to clear all the pollution on the earth.

After a consultation phone call, I told R that I thought he was ill again and needed some time in the hospital. He agreed and we left in my car for an admission assessment at a local hospital. On the way, we stopped at the bank and R completed his banking business. When we arrived, several of my peers were astonished that I had let R ride in my car and go to the bank when he was obviously psychotic. They exclaimed that they would have certainly called for backup from the office or the mobile crisis unit. I explained to them that I had assessed R and felt that this decision would not endanger him or me. My decision was based on my skills as a psychiatric nurse, my experience in working with psychotic patients for a number of years, and my evaluation of R, with whom I had worked closely for 6 months.

When I think back to this experience, I realize that it captured some of the critical essence of psychiatric nursing decision making. I believe that it is calculated thinking woven into a fabric of clinical experience that guides psychiatric nursing practice. For R it was also a nursing act that expressed both caring for and caring about. After 10 days in the hospital, R was stabilized once more and returned to the life he so wanted to live.

Chapter Review Questions

1. Match each descriptor in Column A with the mental health model in Column B.

Column A

___Aimed at linking and coordinating needed services.

___Consumer participation and culturally relevant care were guiding principles.

___Defined the patient as the community.

___Developed and implemented community support systems.

___Emphasized preventive services to high-risk groups.

___Focused on outreach clinical services.

___Nurses played more active role in meeting the needs of underserved populations.

___Shifted clinical priorities to treatment as a result of deinstitutionalization.

Column B

A. Public health model

B. Biological-medical model

C. System model

D. Patient-centered model

2. Fill in the blanks.

A. _____ studies examine the incidence and prevalence of mental disorders in a defined population.

B. Interventions that target those who have mental illness and help to reduce the disability associated with the illness are called _____ prevention.

C. _____ is a system in which services are aimed at linking the resources and coordinating care to achieve successful community living.

D. Interventions that target those at risk for illness and promote their adaptive coping are called _____ prevention.

E. _____ is a type of program that functions as a community-based hospital without walls to provide intensive clinical support and treatment.

F. Interventions that target people who show early signs of an illness and help them receive prompt treatment are called _____ prevention.

G. A treatment approach that addresses the needs of youth with behavioral and emotional problems and their families is called _____.

3. Provide short answers for the following questions.

A. Describe common elements of ACT and MST programs.

B. What groups are at high risk for developing mental illness in your community? How many resources are devoted to prevention activities with these groups? How can you help to better match community needs with community resources?

C. Most case managers in this country are social workers. Describe how you as a nurse and a social worker might differ in implementing the case manager role.

D. What new roles that you read about in this chapter appeal to you as a potential career option?

REFERENCES

1. American Nurses' Association: *Position statement on psychiatric mental health nursing and managed care,* Washington, DC, 1993, The Association.
2. Anthony W, Blanch A: Research on community support services: what we have learned, *Psychosoc Rehab J* 12:55, 1989.
3. Bachrach L: The state of the state mental hospital in 1996, *Psychiatr Serv* 47:1071, 1996.
4. Belcher J, DeForge B: The appropriate role for the state hospital, *J Ment Health Admin* 24:64, 1997.
5. Burns B, Santos A: Assertive community treatment: an update of randomized trials, *Psychiatr Serv* 46:669, 1995.
6. Carling P: Housing and supports for persons with mental illness: emerging approaches to research and practice, *Hosp Community Psychiatry* 44:439, 1993.
7. Chamberlin J: The role of the government in development of psychiatric nursing, *J Psychosoc Nurs Ment Health Serv* 21:11, 1983.
8. De Cangas J: A comprehensive evaluation of the effectiveness and outcomes of hospital based treatment versus a nurse directed assertive case management program, *Int J Psychiatr Nurs Res* 1:72, 1995.
9. De Young C, Tower M: *The nurse's role in community mental health centers: out of uniform and into trouble,* St Louis, 1971, Mosby.
10. Deci P et al: Dissemination of assertive community treatment programs, *Psychiatr Serv* 46:676, 1995.
11. Dyer J et al: The psychiatric–primary care nurse practitioner: a futuristic model for advanced practice psychiatric–mental health nursing, *Arch Psychiatr Nurs* 11:2, 1997.
12. Farrell S, Deeds E: The Clubhouse model as exemplar, *J Psychosoc Nurs* 35:27, 1997.
13. Felker B, Yazel J, Short D: Mortality and medical comorbidity among psychiatric patients: a review, *Psychiatr Serv* 47:1356, 1996.

14. Furlong-Norman, Palmer-Erbs V, Jonikas J: Strengthening psychiatric rehabilitation nursing practice with new information and ideas, *J Psychosoc Nurs* 35:35, 1997.

15. Glittenberg J: The role of the nurse in outpatient psychiatric clinics, *Am J Orthopsychiatry* 39:713, 1963.

16. Grob G: Mad, homeless and unwanted: a history of the care of the chronic mentally ill in America, *Psychiatr Clin North Am* 17:541, 1994.

17. Henggeler S, Borduin C: *Family therapy and beyond: a multisystemic approach to treating the behavioral problems of children and adolescents,* Pacific Grove, Calif, 1990, Brooks/Cole.

18. Henggeler S, Melton G, Smith L: Family preservation using multisystemic therapy: an effective alternative to incarcerating serious juvenile offenders, *J Consult Clin Psychol* 60:953, 1992.

19. Jambunathan J, Van Dongen C: Use of RN case management and costs and utilization of outpatient mental health services: a pilot study, *Issues Ment Health Nurs* 16:407, 1995.

20. Jones F, Selder F: Psychoeducational groups to promote effective coping in school-age children living in violent communities, *Issues Ment Health Nurs* 17:559, 1996.

21. Kanter J: Clinical case management: definition, principles, components, *Hosp Community Psychiatry* 40:361, 1989.

22. Laben J, Blum J: Persons with mental illness in jail. In Worley N, editor: *Mental health nursing in the community,* St Louis, 1997, Mosby.

23. Lancashire S et al: Effects of training in psychosocial interventions for community psychiatric nurses in England, *Psychiatr Serv* 48:39, 1997.

24. Liefland L et al: A crisis intervention program, *J Psychosoc Nurs* 35:32, 1997.

25. McGurrin M, Worley N: Evaluation of intensive case management for seriously and persistently mentally ill persons, *J Case Manage* 2:59, 1993.

26. Mound B et al: The expanded role of nurse case managers, *J Psychosoc Nurs* 29:21, 1991.

27. Murray R et al: Components of an effective transitional residential program for homeless mentally ill clients, *Arch Psychiatr Nurs* 9:152, 1995.

28. Nehls N et al: A collaborative nurse-physician practice model for helping persons with serious mental illness, *Hosp Community Psychiatry* 43:842, 1992.

29. Osborne O et al: The rise of public sector psychosocial nursing, *Arch Psychiatr Care* 7:133, 1993.

30. Primm A, Houck J: COSTAR: flexibility in urban community mental health. In Cohen N, editor: *Psychiatry takes to the streets,* New York, 1990, Guilford.

31. Randolph F et al: Creating integrated service systems for homeless persons with mental illness: the ACCESS program, *Psychiatr Serv* 48:369, 1997.

32. Regier D, Kaelber C: The Epidemiologic Catchment Area (ECA) program: studying the prevalence and incidence of psychopathology. In Tsuang M, Tohen M, Zahner G, editors: *Textbook in psychiatric epidemiology,* New York, 1995, Wiley-Liss.

33. Rowe M, Hoge M, Fisk D: Critical issues in serving people who are homeless and mentally ill, *Admin Policy Ment Health* 23:555, 1996.

34. Santos A et al: Research on field-based services: models for reform in the delivery of mental health care to populations with complex clinical problems, *Am J Psychiatry* 152:1111, 1995.

35. Saur C, Ford S: Quality, cost-effective psychiatric treatment: a CNS-MD collaborative practice model, *Arch Psychiatr Nurs* 9:332, 1995.

36. Sledge W et al: Case management in psychiatry: an analysis of tasks, *Am J Psychiatry* 152:1259, 1995.

37. Smith G: Hospital case management for psychiatric diagnoses: focusing on quality and cost outcomes, *J Psychosoc Nurs* 32:3, 1994.

38. Stein L, Test M: The training in community living model: a decade of experience, *New Dir Ment Health Serv* 26:7, 1985.

39. Stroul B: *Community support systems for persons with long-term mental illness: questions and answers,* Rockville, Md, 1988, National Institute of Mental Health.

40. Torrey E, Wolfe S, Flynn L: *Criminalizing the seriously mentally ill: the abuse of jails as hospitals,* Arlington, Va, 1992, NAMI.

41. Wilkinson L: A collaborative model: ambulatory pharmacotherapy for chronic psychiatric patients, *J Psychosoc Nurs Ment Health Serv* 29:26, 1991.

42. Wilkinson L et al: Mental health problems in hospital-based clinics: patient profile and referral patterns, *J Am Psychiatr Nurses Assoc* 1:140, 1995.

43. Williams-Burgess C, Vines S, Ditulio M: The parent-baby venture program: prevention of child abuse, *J Child Adolesc Psychiatr Nurs* 8:15, 1995.

44. Wolff N et al: Cost-effectiveness evaluation of three approaches to case management for homeless mentally ill clients, *Am J Psychiatry* 154:341, 1997.

45. Worley N, Drago L, Hadley T: Improving the physical health-mental health interface for the chronically mentally ill: could nurse case managers make a difference? *Arch Psychiatr Nurs* 4:108, 1990.

46. Worley N, Sloop T: Psychiatric nursing in a rural outreach program, *Perspect Psychiatr Care* 32:10, 1996.

ANNOTATED SUGGESTED READINGS

Bachrach L: The state of the state mental hospital in 1996, *Psychiatr Serv* 47:1071, 1996.
Identifies the critical place state hospitals currently still have in mental health systems of care and advocates for better integration of them with community-based services.

D'Ercole A et al: Effects of diagnosis, demographic characteristics and case management on rehospitalization, *Psychiatr Serv* 48:682, 1997.
Reports on a randomized controlled clinical trial to assess the effects of case management and patient characteristics on the use of inpatient services, with findings supporting the need for appropriate and effective outpatient services to truly reduce rehospitalization.

Dickerson F: Assessing clinical outcomes: the community functioning of persons with serious mental illness, *Psychiatr Serv* 48:897, 1997.
Describes the challenges to measuring the community functioning of persons with serious mental illness including the many domains that must be measured, the conflicting interests of the various stakeholders, the limitations of self-report data and other methodological problems. Excellent discussion of this timely topic.

Hopper K et al: Homelessness, severe mental illness and the institutional circuit, *Psychiatr Serv* 48:659, 1997.
Research study that describes four distinctive ways that shelters effectively substituted for more stable and appropriate housing for those who are mentally ill.

*Jambunathan J, Van Dongen C: Use of RN case management and costs and utilization of outpatient mental health services: a pilot study, *Issues Ment Health Nurs* 16:407, 1995.
Good example of nursing research on outcomes associated with nursing case management of patients in an outpatient psychiatric setting. More research like this is needed in the field.

*Nursing reference.

Morse G et al: An experimental comparison of three types of case management for homeless mentally ill persons, *Psychiatr Serv* 48:497, 1997.

Reports on research that found that assertive community treatment is superior to broker case management in assisting those who are mentally ill and at risk for homelessness.

*Murray R: Stressors and coping strategies of homeless men, *J Psychosocial Nurs* 34:16, 1996.

Interesting nursing study on the major stressors commonly experienced by homeless men and the strategies they use to cope.

Rowe M, Hoge M, Fisk D: Critical issues in serving people who are homeless and mentally ill, *Administration and Policy in Mental Health* 23:555, 1996.

Highly recommended discussion of issues related to serving the homeless mentally ill with good ideas on strategies and practical nontraditional approaches to care.

*Nursing reference.

*Saur C, Ford S: Quality, cost-effective psychiatric treatment: a CNS-MD collaborative practice model, *Arch Psychiatr Nurs* 9:332, 1995.

Case study showing decreased costs and enhanced quality of life for a patient whose psychotherapy was provided by a CNS. Such outcomes must be studied in larger, randomized, controlled clinical trials.

Wolff G, Pathare S, Leff J: Who's in the lion's den? *Psychiatr Bull* 20:68, 1996.

A report worth reading about a survey of the perceptions and attitudes of a community regarding community care for the mentally ill.

*Worley N: *Mental health nursing in the community,* St Louis, 1997, Mosby.

The only psychiatric nursing text that exclusively focuses on the community.

Home Psychiatric Nursing Care

Beth Gage Greco and
Joan Kenerson King

© 1998 M.C. Escher/Cordon Art, Baarn, Holland.

We shall not cease from exploration And the end of all our exploring Will be to arrive
where we started And to know the place for the first time. **T. S. Eliot** *Four Quartets*

The first home care agencies were established in the United States in the 1800s by nurses who provided care to people in their community. Since then, home care has undergone many changes. Rapid growth occurred in home care after initial Medicare legislation passed in 1965 allowed reimbursement for home care services to the elderly. The number of home care agencies has increased dramatically, from 1100 in 1963 to greater than 17,500 in June 1995.[1] However, psychiatric home care had a slower start. Before 1987 there were few psychiatric home care programs in the United States. In 1987 a class action lawsuit against the Health Care Financing Administration (HCFA) resulted in the revision of the Medicare home care payment laws. This revision added to the growth of home care and led to further expansion of psychiatric home care programs.

GROWTH OF PSYCHIATRIC HOME CARE

National Association of Home Care statistics for 1993 show that 3.4% of all patients receiving home care services had a primary psychiatric diagnosis.[1] Psychiatric home care is now available to a broad segment of the population.[6] In addition to regulatory changes, other factors have contributed to the development of this treatment setting:

▼ Continued trend toward deinstitutionalization
▼ Availability of Medicare reimbursement for home care
▼ Growth of managed care, which focuses on cost, outcomes, and earlier hospital discharges
▼ Advocacy by consumer groups to find less restrictive and more humane ways of delivering care to people with mental illness

Psychiatric home care programs are changing rapidly in response to the increased numbers of acute psychiatric patients in the community and the newly created competitive health-care market. Thus the psychiatric home care industry has seen tremendous growth within the last few years. Some of this growth is a result of the proven efficacy of psychiatric home care programs in meeting the needs of the psychiatric patient in a cost-effective manner. For example, a program in Connecticut reduced hospital admissions, shortened hospital stays, and reduced hospital readmissions. This study of 600 patients over a 2-year period found that 81% of patients who were referred for hospitalization could be successfully treated at home. Hospital stay, when indicated, was reduced from approximately 12 days to 7 days with the addition of home care to the treatment plan, and only 12% of home care patients required readmission. Of the patients without psychiatric home care services, 46% required readmission to the hospital.[19] Another study of psychiatric home care conducted in 1991 by the Visiting Nurse Association in Kentucky showed 72% patient compliance with outpatient follow-up care, 68% compliance with medications, and an average reduction in the annual hospitalization rate after home care of 76%.[23] Clearly, these are impressive outcomes and they speak strongly to the benefits of this emerging treatment setting.

However, it should be noted that cost effectiveness is not the only rationale for home care. In fact, the best argument for psychiatric home care is that it is a humane and compassionate way to deliver health care and supportive services. Home care reinforces and supplements the care provided by family members and friends and maintains the recipient's dignity and independence—qualities that are all too often lost in even the best institutions.

Psychiatric home care ranges from serving as an alternative to hospitalization to functioning as a single home visit for the purposes of evaluating a specific issue. Psychiatric home care programs receive and refer patients from the entire community's general medical and mental health care services. The advantages of home care in relation to inpatient treatment involve its ability to serve as[21]:

▼ An alternative to hospitalization by maintaining a patient in the community
▼ A facilitator of an impending hospital admission through preadmission assessment
▼ An enhancement of inpatient treatment through integration of home issues in the inpatient treatment plan
▼ A way to shorten inpatient stays while keeping the patient engaged in active treatment
▼ A part of the discharge planning process by assessing potential problems and issues

Examples of other gains obtained by psychiatric home care include its outreach capacity and emphasis on patient participation, responsibility, autonomy, and satisfaction.

 What specific kind of patients do you think would benefit most from psychiatric home care?

Reimbursement Issues

Reimbursement for psychiatric home care is largely provided by Medicare, Medicaid, managed care companies, and private insurance. Each payer has requirements for services covered and some require advance authorization for psychiatric nursing services in the home. The majority of home care is paid for by Medicare (Table 35-1). The Medicare population with mental illnesses falls into two broad categories. One group is patients over 65 who may have a history of mental illness or a newly diagnosed mental illness, usually depression. The second group is composed of people under 65 who qualify for Medicare because of their disability. The most common diagnosis in this group is schizophrenia.

Medicare guidelines (HCFA Pub. 11, 1996) do not provide very specific information on psychiatric nursing services that are covered on home visits (Box 35-1). They do require that the patient:

▼ Be homebound
▼ Have a diagnosed psychiatric disorder
▼ Require the skills of a psychiatric nurse

TABLE **35-1** *Sources of Payment for Home Care, 1992, National Home and Hospice Care Survey*

Source of Payment	% Home Health Care
Medicare	59
Medicaid	16.8
Private insurance	8.1
Out-of-pocket	2.7
Other	13.3

Box **35-1** *Medicare Guidelines for Psychiatric Home Care Nursing*

PSYCHIATRIC EVALUATION, THERAPY, AND TEACHING

The evaluation, psychotherapy, and teaching activities needed by a patient suffering from a diagnosed psychiatric disorder that requires active treatment by a psychiatrically trained nurse and the costs of the psychiatric nurse's services may be covered as a skilled nursing service. Psychiatrically trained nurses are nurses who have special training and/or experience beyond the standard curriculum required for a registered nurse. The services of the psychiatric nurse are to be provided under a plan of care established and reviewed by a physician.

HCFA Publication 11, 1996.

It is largely left up to the home care agencies to interpret the Medicare guidelines and apply them to psychiatric home care. This has created many problems in the field and psychiatric home care programs continue to struggle with this reimbursement issue.

Psychiatric **homebound status** is qualitatively different from medical homebound status. In determining psychiatric homebound status, a useful definition is a patient who is unable to independently and consistently access psychiatric follow-up. This definition is broad enough to encompass a person who is physically healthy and mobile, but too depressed to get out of bed. It also allows inclusion for agoraphobic patients as well as patients with psychotic thinking processes who are vulnerable in the community. Medicare considers a person to be homebound if:

▼ The condition restricts his or her ability to leave home without an assistive device or another person.

▼ The effort required to leave the home is considerable and taxing.

▼ It is medically contraindicated to leave the home.

▼ If the patient does leave home, absences are infrequent, of short duration, or attributable to the need to receive treatment.

Each patient is individually evaluated with regard to homebound status. Box 35-2 lists some conditions that might make a patient psychiatrically homebound.

Medicare is a retrospective payer and records are reviewed by fiscal intermediaries to determine the necessity and appropriateness of psychiatric nursing care. It is important for the psychiatric home care nurse to concentrate on Medicare-recognized reimbursable skilled nursing services such as teaching, assessment, skilled management of the care plan, and direct care activities when planning and delivering service. As managed care companies control an increasing share of the market, psychiatric home care programs are beginning to develop specific programs for these companies.[11,13] Some examples are in-home substance abuse programs, crisis intervention programs, and hospitalization prevention programs. Managed care companies' requirements for psychiatric home care services vary and preauthorization for services is the norm.

Box **35-2** *Conditions That Might Make a Patient Psychiatrically Homebound*

Confusion, disorientation, poor judgment
Immobilizing depression
Severe anxiety that interferes with independence
Agoraphobia with or without panic attacks
Vulnerability in the community
Psychosis or paranoid delusions that interfere with safety
Need for 24-hour supervision

PSYCHIATRIC HOME HEALTH NURSING

Role Definition

More psychiatric nurses are choosing psychiatric home care as their practice setting and conferences on psychiatric home care are held nationwide. In order to work in home care the nurse must have a clear sense of one's role in the patient's life and be able to articulate what help can be offered and what cannot. The psychiatric home care nurse will be confronted with extremely complicated social and economic situations in addition to the complexity present in the psychiatric and medical evaluation. The nurse must be able to identify what the priorities are for care, what change can be brought about, and what situations, no matter how unpleasant or uncomfortable they may be for the nurse, are outside of the nurse's power or the patient's desire to change.

One particularly effective role for the psychiatric home care nurse is case management (see Chapter 34).[4,7,20] Case management promotes self-care and encourages cost-effective use of resources (Fig. 35-1). Other roles for the psychiatric home care nurse include teacher, counselor, therapist, resource coordinator, consultant, staff educator, supervisor, researcher, direct caregiver, and discharge planner.[2,9,15] Participation in some role aspects requires advanced practice preparation. Other role aspects, such as assessment, direct care, patient-family education, supervision of home health aides, counseling, coordination of services, collaboration with multidisciplinary team members, and management of the care plan are a part of every psychiatric home care nurse's role. Finally, psychiatric home care nurses function as members of an interdisciplinary treatment team and must have a clear understanding of the contributions each person can make to the comprehensive treatment plan of a patient (see Critical Thinking about Contemporary Issues).

Qualifications of the Psychiatric Home Care Nurse

Psychiatric home care is a subspecialty that calls for a nurse with certain kinds of skills, education, and experience. On any given day the nurse will be confronted with the extremes of the human condition and with multiple problems that have no obvious solution. In the face of these realities,

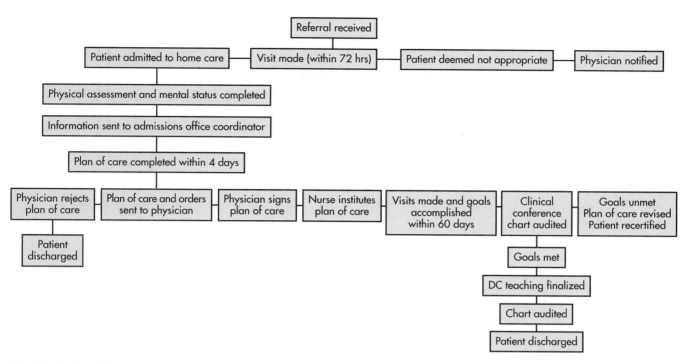

Fig. 35-1   Psychiatric nursing case management. (© North Mississippi Medical Center Home Health Agency.)

Is There Conflict between Social Workers and Psychiatric Nurses in the Field of Psychiatric Home Care?

Clinical territory can be a potential area of conflict among health care providers. Medical social work, although somewhat focused on brief counseling, is primarily responsible for referral to community resources, financial assistance, and transportation. In contrast, psychiatric nursing is focused on biopsychosocial interventions that include specific cognitive and behavioral strategies. In a well-functioning home health agency the introduction of psychiatric nurses may actually result in increased rather than decreased social work referrals because psychiatric nurses can identify people needing the services of the medical social worker.[16]

The goal in home health is to provide care in a cooperative manner and to use the strengths of the various disciplines with minimal overlap. Overall, this collaborative approach can strengthen the home health agency and provide needed services to the most challenging psychiatric patients.

Box **35-3** *Medicare Requirements for Psychiatric Nurses in Home Care*

A registered nurse with a master's degree in psychiatric or community mental health nursing

A registered nurse with a BSN degree and 1 year of related work experience in an active treatment program for adult or geriatric patients in a psychiatric health-care setting

A registered nurse with a diploma or AD degree and 2 years of related work experience in an active treatment program for adult or geriatric patients in a psychiatric health-care setting

ANA certification in psychiatric or community health nursing

Other qualifications may be considered on an individual basis

Any nurse can be hired to work in an inpatient psychiatric unit, but Medicare has specific requirements for a psychiatric home care nurse. Discuss the implications of this from the point of view of the patient, the nurse, and the employing health care organization.

the ability to laugh and find humor is critical to maintaining perspective. Assertiveness, flexibility, respect for the patient's right to choose, curiosity, and an awareness of one's own humanity are other important personal qualities needed by the psychiatric home care nurse. Medicare outlines additional specific requirements for the psychiatric nurse practicing in the home care setting (Box 35-3).

CONTEXT OF PSYCHIATRIC HOME CARE

Psychiatric home care nursing provides unique challenges and opportunities to the nurse. In an inpatient clinic or office setting the provider has the control and power that come with ownership. The patient is a guest and the nurse is the host. In the home setting the nurse is the guest and the patient sets the rules. This raises four key issues for the nurse: cultural sensitivity, flexibility in boundary setting, trust, and safety.

Cultural Sensitivity

Awareness of the patient's ethnic and cultural background is critical to effective care in all settings but nowhere is it more obvious to the attentive eye and more critical to treatment outcome than in the home care setting. The nurse is exposed to the patient's culture and the patient will observe the nurse's reaction. Ways of addressing members of the family, views of health and mental illness, the role of the nurse and health care providers in general, and the importance of alternative therapies are just a few of the issues that vary across cultures. All of these differences must be considered by the nurse planning care with the patient in the home. Recognition and use of the patient's cultural beliefs in delivery of nursing care can positively influence the patient's participation in recovery.[22]

It is important that the nurse also have an understanding of one's own cultural background and the prejudices related to socioeconomic status, gender, family structure, and ways of dealing with emotion rising out of that background. Self-awareness gives the nurse the ability to step back from a judgmental stance and ask whether a certain behavior, opinion, or way of coping stands in the way of the patient's ultimate health.

> **?** *How should a nurse address alternative therapies, acupuncture, vitamin therapy, or folk remedies in home care?*

Boundary Issues

Closely related to cultural issues are the differences in boundary issues. In the home setting it may be appropriate for the nurse to sit and share a cup of tea with the patient or eat a piece of cake. If the patient's culture is one that sees hospitality as connected closely to the sharing of food and refusal of food as an affront, then being willing to share in this ritual can build trust in the relationship between the nurse and patient. Differing opinions exist regarding boundary issues in psychiatric home care,[6,8,18] but the experienced psychiatric home care nurse knows that nursing care must be adapted to each patient's needs and environment. This area requires further nursing research and clinical review.

Trust

The psychiatric home care nurse must consider many different factors when planning and implementing nursing care. Unlike nursing practice in the hospital or outpatient mental health center, psychiatric home care nurses have little control over their patients' environments. It is therefore essential to establish trust in the initial evaluation home visit. Trust then becomes a vital part of the nurse-patient relationship as the patient and nurse work together to solve problems and achieve goals. The nurse trusts the patient to be home at scheduled visits, take medications, and participate fully in all aspects of the plan of care. The patient trusts the nurse to be reliable, clinically knowledgeable, competent, and caring. Methods to establish and build trust in home care patients include[24]:

▼ Cultivate the patient's trust with the first contact
▼ Establish credibility with the patient
▼ Use an empathic, nonjudgmental approach
▼ Guard the patient's privacy
▼ Expect testing behavior from patients
▼ Learn to trust the patient
▼ Persevere with the nurse-patient relationship, demonstrating commitment to the patient despite any noncompliance or resistance

Safety

In general, psychiatric home care patients are not at greater risk for violence than the general home care patient population. However, the assessment of the environment should include issues of safety for the patient and the nurse. Strategies must be identified for dealing with suicidal or aggressive behavior. In this way, home health nursing does have its limitations. The nurse and patient must work together to achieve an acceptable plan, given the reality of having intermittent visits. If the situation becomes unsafe, the nurse must leave the home. Patients' families, caregivers, and other community resources should be urged to notify the police or take the patient to the hospital for an evaluation if the patient becomes dangerous.

NURSING PROCESS IN THE HOME SETTING

The nursing assessment of the home care patient is a comprehensive look at the many facets of a person's life. Areas of assessment include physical, emotional, spiritual, environmental, economic, and cultural factors. All of these factors can affect a person's health and well-being. The psychiatric home health nurse must be adept at interviewing the patient, family, and, if indicated, friends, neighbors, and members of the patient's social support system to gain a thorough understanding of the patient's problems, possible solutions, and available resources.

Although home care agency policies differ, the initial assessment can include standardized rating scales and tools to target and quantify symptoms and to allow easier identification of progress toward goals once nursing care has begun.[7] Bay Area Health Care, a Medicare-certified home health care agency in Baltimore, Maryland, identifies 19 assessment tools that psychiatric nurses can use in the formulation of the care plan.[3] Other data gathered during the assessment visit include a health history, a full set of vital signs, history of present illness, current medication regimen, all concurrent medical diagnoses, patient/family's understanding of psychiatric home care, home and patient safety issues, patient's functional status, social, spiritual, and financial needs, and patient's and caregivers' knowledge and skill level.

Careful attention is needed to identify patients with chaotic family or social situations or multiple medical diagnoses so early interventions by other disciplines are planned at the start of care. As patient problems and needs are identified, the psychiatric home health nurse formulates nursing diagnoses, collaborates with the patient's physician, and establishes an individualized plan of care. Home visit patterns are determined by the patient's needs and financial resources, with more frequent visits scheduled until the patient's condition stabilizes. Preauthorization for psychiatric home care may be required by some health insurance plans and services could be limited to a few visits. In these cases it is critical that the nurse set priorities and plan obtainable goals.

The plan of care in psychiatric home care must identify measurable and attainable outcomes. This is vital to attaining patient goals in a timely manner. One way to ensure this is to use clinical pathways in planning patient care in the home setting. There are a few clinical pathways that are specific to psychiatric home health care.[14] Chapter 19 presents a clinical pathway for depression used by one home health agency.[7] In a cost-conscious health-care industry, proven cost-effective strategies make psychiatric home health nursing a viable mental health treatment option. The use of clinical pathways in planning psychiatric home care can improve accountability, predict outcomes, and reduce costs.[5] Because clinical pathways in psychiatric home care are in the developmental stage, most psychiatric home health nurses develop more traditional care plans for their patients. Nursing interventions most appropriate and adaptable to the psychiatric home care setting are then selected.

Nursing interventions in the home include assessment, teaching, medication management, administration of parenteral injections, venipuncture for laboratory analysis, and skilled management of the care plan. All of these interventions are recognized as reimbursable skilled nursing services by Medicare. In actuality, psychiatric home care nurses provide numerous additional skilled nursing services (Box 35-4). They act as case managers, coordinating an array of services including physical therapy, occupational therapy, social work, and community services such as home-delivered meals, home visitors, and home health aides. They collaborate with all of the patient's health-care providers and often facilitate communication among the psychiatrist, therapist, physician, and others in the multidisciplinary team. Psychiatric home care nurses make appropriate referrals to community agencies and help their patients to access community resources independently. They educate families and patients, provide supportive counseling and brief psy-

---

Box 35-4 *In-Home Behavioral Health Services*

In-home behavioral health services include but are not limited to:
   Direct patient care
   Development and implementation of specific mental health assessment tools
   Coordination of care or visits by other disciplines
   Joint visits with the primary nurses
   Consultation with the home care staff related to the psychosocial needs of patients
Services specifically include the following:
   Assessment of mental health status and evaluation of the patient's response to illness and treatment
   Assessment of the home environment
   Development and implementation of an individualized treatment/care plan through consultation with the primary psychiatrist or physician in regard to:
   Therapeutic interventions
   Safety issues
   Medication compliance
   Physical exercises
   Education and support of the patient's caregivers
   Medication instruction, monitoring, and administration
   Provision of supportive psychotherapy
   Development of individualized education plans regarding all aspects of the illnesses and how to develop coping skills
   Collection of lab specimens and monitoring of results (lithium, Tegretol, antidepressants)
   Referrals to and follow-up with community resources
   Support for patients with absent or inadequate family and community support to help prevent recidivism
   Provision of 24-hour on-call service for crisis intervention and referrals

Courtesy National Association for Home Care. From *Caring*, 14(7), November 1995.

---

chotherapy, promote health and prevent illness, and, above all, document everything in precise detail so that their agency is reimbursed for the services they provide.

Documentation is the nemesis of the home care industry. If the nurse's documentation does not reflect the skilled service given, the payment for that service can be denied by Medicare or other payers. Few guidelines are available for documentation of psychiatric home care and agencies have developed elaborate and often complex documentation systems.[3,4] The psychiatric home care nurse must be very organized and detail oriented to successfully manage the seemingly endless paperwork.

Finally, the psychiatric home care nurse continuously reviews the patient's progress toward goals and revises the care plan. The evaluation process is an ongoing collaborative task between the patient and the nurse. The patient's family and support system play a vital role in recovery. As goals are met or outcomes achieved, the patient moves increasingly closer toward his or her highest level of functioning. When the patient reaches maximum potential, discharge from psychiatric home care is indicated. A patient may be discharged to the care of the family, a day or partial hospital program, a skilled nursing facility, a personal care facility, or self-care. The psychiatric home care nurse terminates one's relationship with the patient and caregivers and provides specific written instructions for follow-up care.

> ? *How might the use of a laptop computer facilitate more concise and timely documentation in the home health setting?*

SPECIAL POPULATIONS

Many types of patients can benefit greatly from psychiatric home health care (Box 35-5). Chapters 36-40 address nursing interventions related to some of these special groups in more detail.

Children and Adolescents

Psychiatric home care is often successful for children and adolescents in the home.[12,15,21] Children and adolescents have a unique set of needs that can be addressed by the psychiatric home care nurse. Providing care in the home gives the nurse immediate access to the family, the home environment, and the community surrounding the child or adolescent. This contextual understanding opens up new possibilities for intervention and new understandings of the complexity of the problem the youth and family may be experiencing. Multisystem therapy, as described in Chapter 34, is one type of home-based intervention that is effective with youth.

Box **35-5** *Who Can Benefit from In-home Psychiatric Nursing Services?*

Patients with repeated inpatient or crisis unit admissions
Patients with a history of medication or treatment plan noncompliance or lack of follow-through with aftercare plans
Patients with combined diagnoses of a medical and psychiatric nature (such as elderly or HIV-positive patients)
Patients with combined substance abuse and psychiatric diagnoses
Patients receiving injectable medications who are homebound or do not follow through with scheduled outpatient appointments
Patients in need of laboratory monitoring who are homebound or do not follow through with outpatient laboratory appointments
Patients who are depressed and who neglect self-care
Patients who suffer from anxiety or panic and have difficulty leaving the home

Courtesy National Association for Home Care. From *Caring* 14(7), November 1995.

Older Adults

Older adults make up the majority of the home care caseload and present many challenges to the psychiatric home care nurse.[10] There is a high incidence of comorbidity in this group and the nurse often must address both psychiatric and medical diagnoses in these patients. Care must be taken not to overlook the impact of the body on the mind and of the mind on the body. Older adults often do not use available mental health services.[25] They may be unable to access these services or may consider them embarrassing. However, psychiatric home care overcomes these obstacles and can bring a much-needed service to the older adult. For the older adult living in an unsafe inner-city neighborhood, a visit from a psychiatric nurse can help bring order to chaos. For the older adult living in an isolated rural environment, a psychiatric home care nurse can provide support and education and decrease the impact of social isolation.

Clinical Example Ms. P, a 78-year-old woman, was referred to psychiatric home care by a local hospital discharge planner. She had been hospitalized for an acute MI and during her hospital stay had developed depressive symptoms with severe anxiety that necessitated a transfer to the hospital's inpatient psychiatric unit. After 5 days on the inpatient psychiatric unit, Ms. P was discharged to her home.

Ms. P lived alone in a second-floor apartment and had functioned independently before her MI. Her functional status on discharge from the hospital was much diminished. She could no longer climb a flight of stairs and became easily fatigued during ADLs. She was on several medications to improve her cardiac status and she was also on medication for her depression and anxiety. She had five children who were supportive from a distance. She was also very determined to maintain her independent status and wanted very much to regain her previous lifestyle.

The psychiatric home care nurse completed an assessment and initiated a care plan with the patient and the physician. The patient's family was included in the planning process because it was necessary that they take an active role in their mother's care. Initial goals were established, with functional independence identified as the outcome of care. A physical therapist and a home health aide were essential to the patient's recovery and were provided by the home care agency.

Unfortunately, the patient fell during her second week of home care services. The focus of care changed as it became increasingly obvious that the patient would not regain independent function. The psychiatric nurse and the physician made a referral to the agency's social worker and the process of locating appropriate placement for the patient began. The family was very supportive and helpful with the placement process. However, Ms. P was not.

The nurse recognized that placement in a nursing home was an assault to this patient's self-esteem. She also knew that Ms. P was no longer safe alone in her own apartment.

She encouraged Ms. P to discuss her concerns, identify her fears, and participate in the placement process. Gradually, through tears and smiles, Ms. P grieved the loss of her health, her independence, and her home. The nurse discharged Ms. P to a local nursing home a few blocks from her home. Ms. P said, "At least I'll be in the same neighborhood," as she accepted her circumstances on that final visit.

Patients with Serious and Persistent Mental Illness

Patients with serious and persistent mental illness are particularly suited to home care interventions.[15] This population often does not follow through with medications and scheduled outpatient appointments. Repeated hospitalizations are often needed to restart medications and stabilize symptoms. Noncompliance is a complicated issue but it can be more readily addressed in the home setting. The nurse can create an alliance with the patient and family in the nonthreatening environment of the home. Assertive community treatment, described in Chapter 34, is one type of home-based intervention documented to be effective with patients with serious and persistent mental illness.

The psychiatric home care nurse can identify obstacles to patient compliance such as financial issues, transportation problems, and inadequate knowledge. The nurse can work with the patient to find solutions to these and other problems and help prevent relapse. The psychiatric home care nurse can also administer long-acting neuroleptic injections when the patient is unable to follow a medication administration schedule. Many of the complications of living with a chronic mental illness can be alleviated through proper medication, patient-family education, and continued supportive therapy by a caring mental health professional. The psychiatric home care nurse can provide these services in the patient's home on a time-limited basis. The nurse can also act as the vital link between hospital and community services for patients with serious and persistent mental illness, whose needs have been underserved since deinstitutionalization began in the 1960s.[17]

Clinical Example Sonia, a 49-year-old woman, was referred by a managed care company to psychiatric home care after a 2-week inpatient stay at a local psychiatric hospital. She had a long history of psychiatric admissions for stabilization of her schizophrenia. Most hospitalizations were preceded by the patient's noncompliance with her medications and follow-up care at the mental health center.

Sonia lived with her sister and elderly mother in a small row house in the Hispanic section of a large city. The family's native language was Spanish. They spoke English as a second language and understood some written English. Sonia's sister was the family's caregiver. She cared for their bedridden mother and helped with Sonia's care. Sonia's sister could not understand why Sonia was all right for long periods and then would become "crazy" and not listen. So-

nia agreed to psychiatric nursing visits but initially would not agree to treatment at the mental health center. Paranoia was a major component of her illness. Other barriers were financial concerns, lack of knowledge about her illness, and cultural and language issues.

The psychiatric nurse's plan of care included administration of Haldol decanoate every 3 weeks, education of the patient and her sister on the disease process, signs and symptoms of relapse, the importance of continued medical care, medication actions and side effects, and the correct administration of the prescribed medication, Cogentin. As care progressed and Sonia became stable, the nurse helped the patient and her sister to make and attend a follow-up appointment at the mental health center. Sonia was discharged from home care and agreed to go to the mental health clinic for her Haldol decanoate injections and follow-up medical care.

Patients with HIV/AIDS

Psychiatric disorders associated with HIV/AIDS include adjustment disorder, anxiety disorder, depression, and central nervous system dysfunction. Central nervous system dysfunction can include delirium symptoms, dementia, agitation, or confusion. Patients with HIV/AIDS have many mental health needs (see Chapter 40). They sometimes have chronic mental illnesses. They struggle with the stigma of AIDS and try to cope with the tremendous losses and grief. Psychiatric home care nurses can make a significant contribution by helping these patients with their many physical and emotional needs.

Clinical Example Mr. J was referred by an outpatient medical clinic nurse to the psychiatric home care program of the local Visiting Nurse Association. He had missed several of his scheduled appointments and was displaying increased anxiety about his health and future. He had been HIV positive for several years and was beginning to show symptoms of AIDS.

The psychiatric home care nurse arrived at the patient's home for the evaluation visit and was greeted by the patient, his brother, and his sister-in-law. Mr. J had just told his family of his AIDS diagnosis and was hoping the nurse could act as an intermediary for the family. Mr. J had not told the nurse of his intentions for her first visit. The nurse quickly sized up the family situation, intervened, and provided essential education about HIV/AIDS for the family.

Later home visits focused on teaching the patient about assertive communication, coping skills, and relaxation exercises to decrease his anxiety. Brief cognitive psychotherapy was used to help Mr. J to identify his thoughts and feelings. Grief counseling was initiated and the patient was encouraged to find a long-term therapist in his community who was sensitive to his needs. Mr. J made an appointment with a psychologist and attended his first session, but he canceled his final visit with the psychiatric home care nurse. The nurse was left to wonder about Mr. J's first visit with the psychologist. Did he have a surprise for that mental health provider too?

Summary

1. Psychiatric home care programs are being developed in response to the changing health-care industry. Measures are being introduced to identify patient outcomes and control the use of resources. Reimbursement for services is dependent on meeting medical necessity and appropriateness guidelines and the demonstrated effectiveness of nursing services.

2. The home care setting offers autonomy and flexibility in nursing practice. Nursing roles in psychiatric home care are in part determined by the education, experience, and abilities of the nurse. Psychiatric nurses practice in the home care setting at basic and advanced levels. All psychiatric home care nurses are required to have experience with psychiatric patients.

3. Issues of importance to psychiatric home care nurses include cultural sensitivity, flexibility in boundary setting, trust, and safety.

4. Psychiatric home care patients may have comorbid illnesses, few support systems, inadequate housing and finances, and variable levels of motivation for change. Comprehensive assessment, outcomes identification, use of clinical paths, and case management techniques are important aspects of the nursing process in home settings.

5. Special populations that can benefit from psychiatric home care include children and adolescents, older adults, patients with serious and persistent mental illness, and patients with HIV/AIDS.

your **INTERNET**
connection

Home Care Nurse Page
http://junior.apk.net/˜nurse/

Middle Tennessee Home Health Care
http://www.medi.com/homecare/

COMPETENT CARING A Clinical Exemplar of a Psychiatric Nurse

Royce Sampson, MSN, RN, CS

When I first saw this patient in his home, he was withdrawn and rarely spoke. He remained in his room all the time because he required total care and was incontinent of bowel and bladder. The medical history indicated that the patient had suffered a severe closed head injury several years before, he was aphasic, and he had a neurogenic bladder and bowel. His rehabilitation potential appeared poor. Through my multidimensional assessment of him and conversations with his family and home health aide, I identified multiple needs and strengths. By establishing a rapport with him and gaining his trust, I was able to identify what he thought he needed to feel better. He wanted adequate food, care, security, and safety. He wanted nursing home placement. I knew through my experience that many months would pass before nursing home placement could be obtained, if at all. After discussing all the alternatives with the patient and his family, we agreed on a few additional goals and selected a possible nursing home. I would help the family through the nursing home placement process, and in the meantime would coordinate additional services to meet his needs and maximize his ability to care for himself.

Through the assessment process, I identified that this patient was alert and oriented. He could communicate adequately and had through necessity (although unsafely) learned to transfer himself to his wheelchair. The home health aide also identified that the patient was capable of remaining continent if reminded. I talked to the patient about rehabilitation services in response to his remarks about his desire for increased independent mobility and function. He agreed that he would like to try these services. We decided that adult day-care services would be the best option to meet many of his needs with the limited community resources available.

Through negotiations with his physician and the other health-care providers, I arranged for the home health aide to get him ready for adult day care and for the bus to pick him up and take him to the center, where he would receive hot meals, group socialization, physical therapy, occupational therapy, and speech therapy. I also counseled his family about how they could better meet his needs at home. The patient had very limited social supports and financial resources and lived in a rural area, which complicated and sometimes thwarted the process of meeting his needs. Home-delivered meals were unavailable, and the adult day-care bus did not usually travel to the patient's home.

Over the next few months the patient made tremendous progress. At day care, he met friends his own age from the boarding home that was attached to the center. These friends provided him with much-needed socialization. An added advantage was the motivation for self-care and independence that the peer group evoked in the patient. When he was with his peer group, he wheeled his wheelchair independently and toileted himself. Periodically, he stopped going to the day-care center, and the staff called me to intervene. The expense of going to the patient's home when he refused to go to the center after the bus arrived at

COMPETENT CARING A Clinical Exemplar of a Psychiatric Nurse—cont'd

his home, combined with his loss in function when therapy was missed, might have led to termination of all services. Sometimes recoordination of services was needed, but many times it was psychological support and counseling that were indicated.

Therapy was painful, frustrating, and difficult for the patient. At times he was afraid of what his increasing independence would mean for him. If he became too independent, he would not be eligible for nursing home placement, and he did not want to remain in his home environment. We discussed the possibility of placement in a less restrictive environment, such as the boarding home where the day-care center and his friends were located, but the patient was afraid that he would not be able to maintain the level of independence the facility required. By spending much time counseling and helping him identify his abilities and the progress he had made, and negotiating with the boarding home for a trial placement, I was able to help him gain enough self-confidence to try the boarding home placement. I maintained contact with the patient and the facility for the next month to ensure that he was appropriately placed and happy. The placement was a huge success.

Although I have always advocated maintaining a patient in his or her own home if possible, in this instance the patient's safety and security needs could not be adequately satisfied at home. Boarding home placement not only met those needs, but also helped him to meet higher needs of socialization through his peer group, increased self-esteem through the confidence he gained by being able to function in a less restricted environment, and self-actualization through reaching for his maximum potential.

I learned a great deal from my involvement with this patient as I constantly reevaluated my own values and goals for him. I wanted the patient to reach his maximum potential, and I had faith in his ability, but, as he taught me time and time again, it was his goals on which I had to focus, and his belief in himself that I had to foster. My skills in collaboration, advocacy, coordination of services, counseling, and clinical nursing enabled me to attain a successful and satisfying outcome for my patient and a rewarding experience for me.

Chapter Review Questions

1. Identify whether the following statements are true (T) or false (F).

A. ___ The growth of managed care has contributed to the development of psychiatric home care programs.

B. ___ As long as a patient is able to leave the house regardless of circumstances, he or she is ineligible for homebound status under Medicare guidelines.

C. ___ Most managed care companies require preauthorization for psychiatric home care.

D. ___ Medicare is a prospective payer.

E. ___ If a home situation is identified as unsafe for the nurse, he or she must leave the home.

F. ___ The use of clinical pathways in psychiatric home care is well established and used extensively throughout the field.

2. Fill in the blanks.

A. For Medicare to approve psychiatric home care, it is required that the patient _____, _____, and _____.

B. A patient who cannot independently and consistently access psychiatric follow-up can be described as _____.

C. One particularly effective role for the psychiatric home care nurse is that of _____.

D. The majority of home care is paid for by _____.

E. The two categories of the Medicare population with mental illness are _____ and _____.

F. The initial home health care assessment should include the use of _____ to target and quantify symptoms and allow easier identification of progress toward goals.

G. The use of _____ can be one way to ensure the successful attainment of patient goals in a timely manner.

H. _____ is the nemesis of the home care industry.

3. Provide short answers for the following questions.

A. Describe the advantages of home care in relation to inpatient psychiatric treatment.

B. Some people say that with home care, psychiatric nurses are "going back to their roots." Explain what is meant by this.

C. Many nurses believe that there are few career options in psychiatry. Challenge this notion based on the expanding growth of psychiatric home and community care.

REFERENCES

1. *Basic statistics about home care,* Washington, DC, 1996, National Association for Home Care.
2. Blazek L: Development of a psychiatric home care program and the role of the CNS in the delivery of care, *Clin Nurse Specialist* 7:164, 1993.
3. Carson V: Doing psych but talking med-surg language, *Caring* 4:32, 1994.
4. Carson V: Bay area health care psychiatric home care model, *Home Healthcare Nurse* 13:26, 1995.
5. Corbett C, Androwich I: Critical paths: implications for improving practice, *Home Healthcare Nurse* 12:27, 1994.
6. Daudell-Strejc D, Murphy C: Emerging clinical issues in home health psychiatric nursing, *Home Healthcare Nurse* 13:17, 1995.
7. Duckworth C, Kitchens B: *An overview of psychiatric home health,* Tupelo, Mississippi, 1996, North Mississippi Medical Center Home Health Agency.
8. Duffy J, Miller M: Toward resolving the issue: in-home psychiatric nursing, *J Am Psychiatr Nurses Assoc* 2:104, 1996.
9. Duffy J, Miller M, Parlocha P: Psychiatric home care. A framework for assessment and intervention. *Home Healthcare Nurse* 11:22, 1993.
10. Kozlak J, Thobaben M: Psychiatric home health nursing of the aged: a selected literature review, *Geriatr Nurs* 15:148, 1994.
11. Lapierre E, Soileau J: In-home behavioral health services establishing a program, *Caring* 5:7, 1995.
12. Lima B: In-home psychiatric nursing, *Caring* 5:14, 1995.
13. Lockhart C et al: The paradigm shift: behavioral home care, *Caring* 4:10, 1994.
14. Marrelli T, Hilliard L, editors: *Home care and clinical paths: effective care planning across the continuum,* St Louis, 1996, Mosby.
15. Mellon S: Mental health clinical nurse specialist in home care for the '90s, *Issues Ment Health Nurs* 15:229, 1994.
16. Miller M, Duffy J: Planning and program development for psychiatric home care, *JONA* 23:35, 1993.
17. Morris M: Patients' perceptions of psychiatric home care, *Arch Psychiatr Nurs* 10:176, 1996.
18. Peplau H: Some unresolved issues in the era of biopsychosocial nursing, *J Am Psychiatr Nurses Assoc* 1:92, 1995.
19. Pigot H, Trott L: Translating research into practice: the implementation of an in-home crisis intervention triage and treatment service in the private sector, *Am J Med Quality* 8:138, 1993.
20. Quinlan J, Ohlund G: Psychiatric home care, *Home Healthcare Nurse* 13:20, 1995.
21. Soreff S: Psychiatric home care revisited: its scope and advantages, *Continuum* 1:71, 1994.
22. Spruhan J: Beyond traditional nursing care: cultural awareness and successful home healthcare nursing, *Home Healthcare Nurse* 14:445, 1996.
23. Visiting Nurse Association: *Study shows in-home mental health nursing reduces hospitalizations of the mentally ill,* Louisville, Ky, 1994, news release.
24. Wendt D: Building trust during the initial home visit, *Home Healthcare Nurse* 14:93, 1996.
25. Wykle M:. Geriatric mental health interventions in the home, *J Psychosoc Nurs* 33:50, 1995.

ANNOTATED SUGGESTED READINGS

*Boland D, Sims S: Family care giving at home as a solitary journey, *Image J Nurs Sch* 28:55, 1995.
    Burden, responsibility, isolation, and commitment shaped the context of nonpsychiatric caregiving from the perspective of 17 families in a metropolitan area.

Brown L: Legal and ethical issues in psychiatric home care, *Continuum* 3:187, 1996.
    A law review of the full continuum of health care services with a specific focus on the minimal information regarding lawsuits in the new field of psychiatric home care.

*Carson V: Doing psych but talking med-surg language, *Caring* 6:32, 1994.
    Describes a "denial-proof" documentation system for behavioral home care services in response to the need to document services in acceptable medical language.

*Daudell-Strejc D, Murphy C: Emerging clinical issues in home health psychiatric nursing, *Home Healthc Nurse* 13:17, 1995.
    Explores the unique clinical concerns of the home health psychiatric nurse, clinical issues specific to home health psychiatric care programs, and offers a theory-based model for practice.

*Duffy J: Beyond how to: theory-based management practice considerations for psychiatric home care, *Continuum* 3:163, 1996.
    Lack of policies, procedures, and resources affecting psychiatric home health care are solved using principles of total quality management and Covey's seven principles of highly successful people.

*Duffy J et al: Psychiatric home care: a framework for assessment and intervention, *Home Healthc Nurse* 11:22, 1993.
    Discusses the theories of crisis intervention, self-care, and behavior, and uses case examples to illustrate their application to a psychiatric home care situation.

Klebanoff N: Mental health home care services: A review of current clinical issues, *Continuum* 3:147, 1996.
    While mental health home care services offer a full range of care options, specific clinical concerns include program development, in-home assessment and high-risk intervention, and reimbursement.

*Lapierre E, Soileau J: In-home behavioral health services: establishing a program, *Caring* 7:7, 1995.
    Discusses strategies for developing an in-home behavioral health care service, and evaluates the success of the first year of such a service.

*Lima B: In-home psychiatric nursing: the at-home mental health program, *Caring* 7:14, 1995.
    Outlines a home care program that bridges the gap between traditional models of inpatient and outpatient treatment of mental illness, providing a more comfortable, less costly alternative.

*Mellon S: Mental health clinical nurse specialist in home care for the 90s, *Issues Men Health Nurs* 15:229, 1994.
    Explores the role of the CNS in psychiatric home care as a key point of entry and intervention in the mental health delivery system with a focus on prevention and wellness care.

Soreff S: Psychiatric home care revisited: its scope and advantages, *Continuum* 1:71, 1994.
    Evaluates psychiatric home care: its cost-effectiveness, outreach capability, and emphasis on patient participation, and its ability to enhance, shorten, facilitate, and even replace hospitalization.

*Nursing reference.

UNIT 6

Special Populations in Psychiatry

Life is unfair. It is unfair that many people who are very young or very old may have to suffer in ways they are not even responsible for. But that is a reality of life that nurses, more than many others, need to understand and incorporate in their practice. It has been said that a society can be judged by how it treats its most vulnerable populations. Given that criterion, how would you rank American society? What level of compassion, protection, and caring is needed to make a society humane? What resources are given to health-care providers to educate, empower, and help heal these vulnerable groups? These are questions you may wrestle with the rest of your professional life.

In this unit you will enter the world of children, adolescents, and adults who are vulnerable to developing or being disabled by psychiatric illness. You will learn about their special needs and begin to search your heart and mind for ways to reach out and help them. In that sense, you have come to the end of your journey in this textbook. Your next passage as a professional nurse will be in other pages of your life. Good luck and godspeed.

Child Psychiatric Nursing

Carole F. Bennett

© 1998 M.C. Escher/Cordon Art, Baarn, Holland.

Youth's love Embracingly integrates Successfully frustrates And holds together, Often unwittingly, All that hate, fear, and selfishness Attempt to disintegrate.

R. Buckminster Fuller *And It Came to Pass—Not to Stay*

LEARNING OBJECTIVES

After studying this chapter the student should be able to:

▼ Discuss issues related to the care of children with psychiatric illnesses, including a framework for child psychiatric nursing practice

▼ Assess nine ego skills and adaptive responses necessary for children to become competent adults

▼ Identify nursing diagnoses and interventions related to ego competency skill deficits

▼ Implement therapeutic treatment modalities with children

TOPICAL OUTLINE

Recent epidemiological estimates suggest that approximately 14% to 20% of all children from birth to 18 years of age have some type of psychiatric disorder, and about 3% to 5% of this group have a serious disorder.[5,9] These children have significant difficulty coping with the demands of family, school, and community life. However, less than one fifth of the children who need treatment receive it.[29] As a reflection of recent changes in health care, some states now offer psychiatric services to children in a wide variety of settings that together make up systems of care.

These systems of care can improve access to service for children and their families and provide high-quality, appropriate, and cost-effective care.[35] Such systems are organized to be child centered and family focused, with the needs of the family dictating the types of services that are offered to each child. Systems of care for children are comprehensive and community based, offering a broad array of services, including some combination of those listed in Box 36-1. They are sometimes called wrap-around services because they are meant to encompass all aspects of a child's life. The major goals of these treatment systems are to:

▼ Develop and provide a full array of community-based services for children with psychiatric illnesses and their families
▼ Reduce reliance on restrictive treatment environments and out-of-home placements
▼ Facilitate interagency coordination and collaboration in planning, developing, and delivering services
▼ Increase education to families and promote appropriate parenting skills
▼ Provide flexible, individualized services tailored to the unique needs of each child and family
▼ Contain costs and demonstrate the cost-effectiveness of systems of care for children

In each of these settings, whether they are hospital based or community based, nurses are crucial members of the treatment team. Nurses function as team members, team leaders, milieu managers, case managers, therapists, prescribers, and program directors. They participate in assessment, treatment planning, and implementation of care in children's mental health services in all settings.

PSYCHIATRIC ILLNESS IN CHILDREN

Historically, the debate over the etiology of mental disorder has dominated the field, and discovering the cause of a mental illness in large part determined the approach to treatment. Etiological theories have proposed both genetic factors (nature) and childhood experiences (nurture) as predisposing and precipitating causes for the development of a psychiatric illness. It is now recognized that both nature and nurture play a role in the development of health and illness. With the current understanding of the roles of neurotransmitters and brain development, the effect of experience combined with genetic predisposition begins to explain the complexity of the development of psychiatric illnesses.[22]

Traumatic events, for example, have been recognized to have a profound impact on children. The symptoms that are characteristic of posttraumatic stress disorder (PTSD) in children are those of increased arousal, including hypervigilance, irritability, anxiety, physiological hyperactivity, impulsivity, and sleep difficulty. These symptoms are often also diagnosed as attention-deficit hyperactivity disorder, conduct disorder, anxiety disorder, and mood disorder.[30] It is also now recognized that the particular constellation of symptoms a child experiences are often related to the family history. Specifically, if a family member has a history of anxiety disorder, the child may experience symptoms that are more anxious in appearance. However, if family members have a strong history of alcoholism and sociopathy, symptoms may pertain more to conduct disorder. Thus, it is now believed that there is a genetic predisposition to certain symptoms and that these symptoms can be stimulated as a response to an event in the environment.

Following traumatic events, many factors are important in the development of the intensity of symptoms, including the nature of the trauma, the degree to which body integrity is threatened, the threat posed by the event to the child's self-system and security, and the nature of the family support system. The neurophysiology that is activated during acute stress is usually rapid and reversible. The brain has mechanisms that down-regulate the stress reaction after the threat has passed, returning the brain to its prior level of functioning. However, if the stress is prolonged, severe, or repetitive, the resulting increases in neurotransmitter activity are often not reversible. This process has a significant impact on the development of the child's brain. A trauma-induced brain response would probably result in abnormal patterns, time, and intensity of catecholamine activity in the developing brain. Young children who are exposed to a high rate of stress-induced trauma are at risk for developing permanent changes in neuronal organization, making it more difficult for them to learn and to control their behavior.

Box **36-1** *Services Offered to Children in Systems of Care*

RESIDENTIAL SERVICES
Therapeutic foster care
Therapeutic group care
Crisis residential services
Residential treatment services
Inpatient hospital services

NONRESIDENTIAL SERVICES
Assessment
Psychological testing
Outpatient therapy (individual, family, group)
Home-based services
Day treatment
Crisis services
After-school and evening programs
Therapeutic respite services
Behavioral aide services

Other psychiatric illnesses, such as attention-deficit hyperactivity disorder (ADHD), also illustrate the interplay of genetics and environment.[32] Children with ADHD are usually characterized as having excessive activity and difficulty paying attention. These behaviors are often tolerated by a family. However, when these children begin school, they are identified as problematic as these behaviors interfere with the child's academic performance and peer relationships. As in PTSD, children with ADHD often have differing constellations of symptoms, including symptoms that overlap with anxiety disorders, oppositional defiant disorder, and conduct disorder. Although the precise etiology of ADHD remains unclear, it is believed that environmental factors such as lead ingestion, prenatal and perinatal complications, socioeconomic factors, genetic factors, and brain dysfunction resulting from brain damage may contribute to the development of the illness. No one finding has adequately explained this complex disorder, but there is agreement that it has a neurobiological basis. However, by the time a child and family seek treatment, the child may have developed secondary mental health problems such as low self-esteem and poor socialization. Thus, the effect of this illness on the child is significantly mediated by its severity, the ability of the family to cope with the illness, and the secondary symptoms that result.

As these two examples illustrate, psychiatric illness in children is complex and can be debilitating for both the child and the family. Treatment involves the combination of several modalities, including medication to improve brain function, milieu therapy to improve socialization, behavior management to learn impulse control, cognitive therapy to practice problem solving and communication, and parent education to integrate the new behaviors and skills into the child's home life.

In order to help organize this complex approach and individualize care to each child's needs, a skill development framework is presented in this chapter. This approach can be used in both hospital and community treatment settings, is applicable to any psychiatric diagnosis that a child may have, and can be individualized to meet each child's needs. It also includes the parents as essential to the treatment plan as they work with the child to incorporate these learning skills into family interactions.

> **?** *Do you think that the incidence of child abuse is increasing in this country or that it is the same as in years before, and is simply being discussed more openly?*

A Framework for Nursing Practice

Child psychiatric nurses must have an organizing framework to conceptualize, implement, and research effective care of children with psychiatric illnesses. Nurses are challenged to derive realistic, well-defined goals, respond to the complex social needs of the child, understand and advocate for the child, and develop a comprehensive treatment plan that identifies and integrates the child's needs and resources. All of this must be done with the realization that the behavior of children is largely culturally based and must be viewed from a sociocultural perspective.[18,25]

Children with psychiatric illness experience disabling symptoms that are responses to biological alterations, traumatizing situations, and maladaptive learning. The DSM-IV classifies disorders usually first evident in infancy, childhood, or adolescence by separating them into 10 major groups.[2] These diagnostic categories and their essential features are listed in Table 36-1. Children can also experience the broad range of psychiatric illness listed in Appendix A (DSM-IV).

In addition to being knowledgeable about psychiatric diagnoses, child psychiatric nurses must also be able to implement nursing care that has as its goal modifying a child's coping responses and strengthening a child's competency skills. Nursing care requires a comprehensive nursing assessment and the identification of treatment outcomes measured by a child's ability to adapt and function in life. Child psychiatric nurses should refer to the ANA *Standards of Child and Adolescent Psychiatric and Mental Health Nursing Practice* when implementing care.[1]

Regardless of the child's psychiatric diagnosis, nursing care must be focused on the child's response to illness and the nursing interventions designed to teach and model to the child and family more adaptive coping responses and improved methods of functioning. Thus nursing diagnosis and intervention proceed independently of and concurrently with psychiatric diagnosis and treatment. Although nursing and medicine have collaborative roles, nursing has a critical and distinct contribution to make in the care of the child with psychiatric illness.

Organizing child psychiatric nursing care around ego competency skills is an effective and culturally sensitive way of planning and implementing nursing interventions for children regardless of psychiatric diagnosis or setting. Strayhorn[34] has identified the following nine skills that all children need to become competent adults:

▼ Establishing closeness and trusting relationships
▼ Handling separation and independent decision making
▼ Negotiating joint decisions and interpersonal conflict
▼ Dealing with frustration and unfavorable events
▼ Celebrating good feelings and experiencing pleasure
▼ Working for delayed gratification
▼ Relaxing and playing
▼ Cognitive processing through words, symbols, and images
▼ Establishing an adaptive sense of direction and purpose
These skills give the psychiatric nurse a framework with which to evaluate and intervene with children with emotional illnesses.[14]

Often a child's maladaptive responses are expressed

differently from those of an adult. To develop the nursing plan, the nurse must learn to recognize and describe symptomatic behavior in children. It is helpful to use a specific assessment form, such as the one presented in Fig. 36-1, that identifies both competency skills and nursing diagnoses related to particular skill deficits to more fully describe the child's response or experience. Such a form would be used in addition to a standard nursing assessment tool completed by the nurse for each child (see Chapter 6).

The nurse should talk with the child about the child's strengths and then discuss the skills that need further development. Strategies used to teach these skills can be explained to the child and the parents, which allows them to become active participants in the planning of nursing care. Children will be more motivated to cooperate if they are encouraged to sign a copy of their care plan after it has been explained to them. Even if they cannot write, a mark that represents their name is sufficient to signify their participation in the process. Nursing interventions can then be designed to improve the maladaptive responses and teach the accompanying skill.

ASSESSING EGO COMPETENCY SKILLS

The nursing assessment focuses on the specific skills that all children need to become competent adults. Regardless of psychiatric diagnosis, a child should be assessed for mastery of each of the following skill areas (see Fig. 36-1).

Skill 1: Establishing Closeness and Trusting Relationships

A basic skill for positive growth and development is the child's ability to establish close and trusting relationships with others. The following questions are used to evaluate this skill:

▼ Does the child enjoy making friends?
▼ Does the child often feel picked on by other people?
▼ Does the child not know what to say when getting to know someone?

To reinforce this skill, nursing staff should encourage interaction and be attentive to the child without being intrusive. Talking with the child in a face-to-face position and offering nurturance are beginning nursing actions. Trust can then be demonstrated by the staff in their interactions with the child. If a child violates a trust, a discussion of the issue should take place, allowing trust to be reestablished. In this way, children learn about acknowledging mistakes and the importance of forgiveness in developing trusting relationships.

Skill 2: Handling Separation and Independent Decision Making

Individuation is an important mental health process. Being able to identify and express feelings and make independent decisions is critical to becoming a competent individual. The following questions are used to evaluate this skill:

▼ Does the child get upset or worry when away from his or her mother?

TABLE **36-1** *DSM-IV Disorders of Infancy, Childhood, and Adolescence*

DISORDER	ESSENTIAL FEATURES
Mental retardation	Significantly subaverage intellectual functioning with an IQ of approximately 70 or below. Mild retardation = 55-70 Moderate retardation = 40-55 Severe retardation = 25-40 Profound retardation = below 25
Learning disorders	Functioning that is below that expected given the person's chronological age, measured intelligence, and age-appropriate education. May be evident in the areas of reading, mathematics, or written expression.
Motor skills disorder	Motor coordination is substantially below that expected given the person's chronological age and measured intelligence.
Pervasive developmental disorders	Impairment in a variety of indicators related to normal growth and developmental milestones, including social interaction, communication, and the display of restricted, repetitive, and stereotyped patterns of behavior, interest, and activities (autistic disorder).
Disruptive behavior and attention-deficit disorders	Behaviors related to inattention that are maladaptive and inconsistent with the child's developmental level (attention deficit or hyperactivity disorder); violation of the basic rights of others (conduct disorder); or negativism, hostility, and defiance (oppositional defiant disorder).
Feeding and eating disorders of infancy and early childhood	Behaviors related to eating of nonnutritive substances (pica), regurgitation and rechewing of food (rumination disorder), and failure to eat adequately (feeding disorder).
Tic disorders	An involuntary, sudden, rapid, recurrent, nonrhythmic, stereotyped movement or vocalization (Tourette's disorder).
Communication disorders	Difficulty with receptive or expressive language or the articulation of speech.
Elimination disorders	Repeated passage of feces in inappropriate places after 4 years of age (encopresis) or voiding of urine into bed or clothes after 5 years of age (enuresis).
Separation anxiety disorder	Inappropriate and excessive anxiety concerning separation from home or from those to whom the child is attached.

▼ Does the child get upset or worry if he or she thinks someone does not like him or her?

▼ When upset, is there something the child can do to feel better?

Nursing interventions that focus on helping the child identify and clarify aspects of the self are critical exercises for promoting individuation. This may be done in many ways, such as by encouraging children to draw self-portraits, interview staff members regarding their opinions on an issue, or identify personality differences between themselves and others. Any experience that clarifies differences between individuals helps the child to identify himself or herself as a unique individual in a social context. In the therapeutic milieu, opportunities also can be provided for the child to make choices and decisions, further supporting the child's growing sense of individuality and ego competency.

Skill 3: Handling Joint Decision Making and Interpersonal Conflict

Children who have not been allowed to participate in joint decision making or who have not been rewarded for cooperating may be deficient in this skill. However, this skill is critical for success in interpersonal relationships. The following questions are used to evaluate this skill:

▼ When the child has a problem, can he or she usually think of several solutions?

▼ Does the child get angry if he or she does not get his or her way?

▼ Do other people make the child agitated or easily upset?

The therapeutic milieu can provide an opportunity for the child to learn and practice these skills. For example, the nurse can set up opportunities for problem solving. Exercises may be developed for making group decisions in which cooperation and collaboration are rewarded. The child should be helped to identify fears related to cooperating with others, and assertiveness can be modeled and taught. It is important that the nurse not resolve conflicts for the child. Rather, these situations should be used to teach negotiating skills and shape appropriate socialization through the use of reinforcement.

> **?** *Games can be useful in teaching cooperation and compromise to children. What games can you identify that would be particularly helpful in teaching children this important skill?*

Skill 4: Dealing with Frustration and Unfavorable Events

Tolerating frustration, although difficult, is critical to becoming a competent adult. The following questions are used to evaluate this skill:

▼ Does the child feel bad if he or she has hurt someone's feelings?

▼ If someone disagrees with the child, does it make him or her angry?

▼ Does the child not like playing a game if he or she loses? Children who have little frustration tolerance become angry easily and are often unable to complete tasks. Children typically learn this skill through cooperation and competition in playing childhood games. However, if a child has not had the opportunity to play games in this way and if tolerance has not been modeled for the child, he or she probably has not developed this skill. The child will experience numerous frustrations during the course of treatment. The nurse should use these opportunities to think through the process with the child and help increase the child's frustration tolerance and anger control.

> **?** *Do you think that a child's ability to handle frustration and stressful events is influenced by biological makeup? If so, does biology excuse people from being responsible for their actions?*

Skill 5: Celebrating Good Feelings and Feeling Pleasure

Children who are raised in a healthy environment naturally experience good feelings and pleasure. However, in a maladaptive environment shame is often used to control children's behavior, with the result that they feel guilty for having angry or unacceptable thoughts. Consequently, they may lose the ability to celebrate life and feel pleasure. The following questions are used to evaluate this skill:

▼ Does the child worry about the future a lot?

▼ Does the child not like it when people say good things about him or her?

▼ Does the child feel good about the things he or she does well?

A healthy environment is one in which celebrating good feelings and feeling pleasure are natural, spontaneous occurrences. Celebrating and having fun are important nursing interventions. These activities should not be confined to holidays but should be part of the child's weekly activities. Children's families can be invited to participate in these celebrations, where nursing staff model having fun with the children. In this way, children and their families learn the skill of celebrating good feelings and feeling pleasure.

> **?** *How often and in what ways did your family celebrate good feelings and experience pleasure when you were growing up? How do you incorporate this in your life today?*

Skill 6: Working for Delayed Gratification

As children grow they are expected to delay needed gratification by following rules and waiting their turn. This skill is

Questions used to evaluate competency skills are presented on the left. Nursing diagnoses related to these skills appear at the right. The screened response (N = 0 or Y = 1) represents the appropriate competency skill. A patient score of 2 or 3 indicates a skill deficit, and the nurse should then select an appropriate nursing diagnosis based on the child's history and presenting problem.

		Establishing Closeness and Trusting Relationships	
SCORE 1._____			
N Y		1. I like making friends.	Fear
N Y		2. People pick on me a lot.	Anxiety
N Y		3. I don't know what to say when I am getting to know someone.	Posttrauma Response
			Family Processes Altered
			Growth and Development Altered

		Handling Separation and Independent Decision Making	
SCORE 2._____			
N Y		1. I'm upset when I am away from my mom and worry about her.	Self-Esteem, Chronic Low
N Y		2. If I think someone does not like me, I worry and get upset.	Anxiety
N Y		3. When I am upset, there is something I can do to feel better.	Thought Processes Altered
			Coping, Ineffective Individual

		Handling Joint Decisions and Interpersonal Conflict	
SCORE 3._____			
N Y		1. When I have a problem, I can usually think of several solutions.	Social Interaction Impaired
N Y		2. If I do not get my way, it makes me mad.	Communication Impaired, Verbal
N Y		3. Other people get on my nerves a lot.	Violence, Potential for
			Decisional Conflict

		Dealing with Frustration and Unfavorable Events	
SCORE 4._____			
N Y		1. If I have hurt someone's feelings, I think about it and feel bad.	Social Interaction Impaired
N Y		2. If someone disagrees with me, it makes me mad.	
N Y		3. I do not like playing a game if I lose.	

		Celebrating Good Feelings, Feeling Pleasure	
SCORE 5._____			
N Y		1. I worry about the future a lot.	Hopelessness
N Y		2. When people say good things to me, I don't like it for some reason.	Body Image Disturbance
N Y		3. There are things I do well, and it makes me feel good.	

		Working for Delayed Gratification	
SCORE 6._____			
N Y		1. Most rules are reasonable and I don't mind following them.	Growth and Development Altered
N Y		2. I find it hard to be honest; sometimes, lying is the only thing I do.	Sexuality Patterns Altered
N Y		3. I get mad if my mother dosen't get me what I want.	

Fig. 36-1 Competency skills assessment form.

Continued

SCORE 7. _____		**Relaxing and Playing**	
N	Y	1. There are some things I really enjoy doing.	Social Isolation Grieving-Anticipatory Sleep Pattern Disturbance
N	Y	2. I have lots of fun.	
N	Y	3. I enjoy sitting around and thinking about things.	

SCORE 8. _____		**Cognitive Processing through Words, Symbols, and Images**	
N	Y	1. It is hard for me to describe how I feel to someone.	Growth and Development Altered Social Interaction Impaired Thought Process Altered Anxiety
N	Y	2. I never know how something is going to turn out for me.	
N	Y	3. I know what my strengths are.	

SCORE 9. _____		**An Adaptive Sense of Direction and Purpose**	
N	Y	1. I feel my life is going to get better.	Personal Identity Disturbance Family Coping, Potential for Growth Hopelessness
N	Y	2. I am confused about growing up and don't know what to do about it.	
N	Y	3. I know school is important and going is my job in life right now.	

Fig. 36-1, cont'd   Competency skills assessment form.

often difficult for anxious children to achieve. The following questions are used to evaluate this skill:
▼ Does the child believe that most rules are reasonable and does he or she not mind following them?
▼ Does the child find it difficult to be honest and think that lying is the only thing to do?
▼ Does the child get angry if his or her mother doesn't give what he or she wants?

Delayed gratification can be taught by the nurse through the earning of points for daily expectations, such as tidying one's room or completing homework assignments. Children's games, such as Red Light, in which they respond to "stop" and "wait" commands, are also useful in teaching this skill to younger children. As a child's behavior improves, the reward for the points earned can require the accumulation of many points or tokens. Thus the child is given the opportunity to delay the reinforcer for a reward of higher value to be received at a later time. As the child learns greater self-control, he or she will be better able to delay gratification for longer periods of time.

Skill 7: Relaxing and Playing

Given the stressful environment of current family life, many children may have little opportunity to learn the skill of relaxing and playing. For children and adults, learning to re-

lax and play is an important skill. The following questions are used to evaluate this skill:
▼ Are there some things the child really enjoys doing?
▼ Can the child have lots of fun?
▼ Does the child enjoy sitting around and thinking about things?

Time should be devoted to learning this skill. Children should be given unstructured play time in which the staff participate with them in playing games. Having spontaneous talent shows or other forms of fun can contribute to a child's well-being. In this way, relaxing and playing become part of the therapeutic experience and children learn to value and master this skill.

Skill 8: Cognitive Processing through Words, Symbols, and Images

Children with psychiatric illnesses may not have developed the important skill of cognitive processing. The following questions are used to evaluate this skill:
▼ Is it difficult for the child to describe how he or she feels?
▼ Does the child feel as if he or she never knows how something is going to turn out?
▼ Can the child identify his or her strengths?

A responsive environment should be created to stimulate children's cognitive development. Furnishings and toys, communications and interactions, and group experiences should all be designed to support the child's cognitive processing. The nurse can help the child learn this skill by encouraging abstract thinking whenever possible, such as by asking "What is the moral of the story?" or "What point do you think the movie was trying to communicate?" Children who are encouraged to express themselves in a responsive environment will gain greater competency in this important area of development.

Skill 9: Adaptive Sense of Direction and Purpose

Children, even as preschoolers, begin to think about their adult life. As they view adult life from watching those around them, they begin to draw conclusions about themselves in the world. The following questions are used to evaluate this skill:

▼ Does the child feel that his or her life is going to get better?

▼ Is the child confused about growing up and doesn't know what to do about it?

▼ Does the child believe that school is important and see it as his or her job in life at present?

Having role models for healthy, meaningful adult experiences is essential to healthy growth and development. Feeling valued as an individual provides the child with an opportunity to learn to value others. Nurses should actively listen to children in their interactions, and even young children should be encouraged to express their needs and feelings. The child's importance as a person can be shown through the approach the nurse uses in providing basic care. Older children can benefit from more in-depth discussions and the use of journals to gain perspective on the direction of their lives. Above all, the nurse should actively help all children to realistically assess their abilities and potential to contribute to a better world.

> ? *Many people believe that youth in contemporary society lack a sense of hope, direction, and purpose in life. Do you agree with this, and if so, what sociocultural factors might influence the learning of this skill?*

NURSING DIAGNOSES AND RELATED INTERVENTIONS

Once the nurse has completed the ego competency skill assessment, the appropriate nursing diagnosis should be formulated. Nursing interventions can then be identified for each skill deficit, developmental stage, and related nursing diagnoses as summarized in Table 36-2.

Altered Family Processes

The family should be included in the child's treatment process as soon as possible. Psychiatric illness in any one family member affects all other family members. In addition, the most common problem that precipitates hospitalization in children is the inability of the family to control the child at home.[16] When the need for hospitalization is identified, the parents have usually exhausted all immediately available resources. A combination of reflective thinking with the parents about their child, clarifying problems, and behavioral parent training provides the best results in reducing family stress.[36]

The nurse should focus on the needs of each family and either promote family competence through education and support or engage the family in specific clinical interventions, such as family therapy (see Chapter 32). In addition, some children with psychiatric problems may not have had consistent nurturing or may come from families that display maladaptive responses. Therefore, activities that are less threatening should be used initially to teach the child about family relationships. Pictures of families cut out from magazines can provide opportunities for a child to interpret emotional content in the picture and describe what he or she thinks is happening in the picture. The nurse can then describe a healthy family scenario for the child to learn about adaptive family functioning.

> ? *Many people believe that families are in crisis in this country. Describe the evidence for this conclusion and give specific ways to address each problem identified.*

Altered Growth and Development

Normal growth and development in childhood require a supportive, nurturing environment. A child with a psychiatric illness often has delayed physical and emotional development (see Table 36-2). However, through carefully planned nursing interventions, a child can be taught the skills that have not yet been developed. For example, for the child to achieve independence in dressing, grooming, and room cleaning, a checklist can be made using pictures instead of words. Points can then be given for each accomplished task. Using similar behavioral interventions (see Chapter 30), the nurse can help the child to make significant gains in the area of growth and development.

When considering altered growth and development, delays are often the presenting problem. However, many children who are unprotected by their parents and have early exposure to abuse or violence can develop a pseudomaturity. At times, they may have experienced a role reversal with their parents; the child may have become the more responsible person while the parent assumed the dependent role. These children appear to be overcompliant with adults. Although this behavior may seem well adapted, it is inappropriate developmentally and should not be reinforced. Rather, the child should be encouraged to choose developmentally appropriate play activities, and the parent encouraged to resume appropriate adult role responsibilities.

TABLE **36-2** *Ego Competency Skills Summary*

COMPETENCY SKILL	DEVELOPMENTAL STAGE AND TASKS	RELATED NURSING DIAGNOSIS	NURSING CARE FOR SKILL DEFICIT
Trusting, closeness, relationship building	**Infancy** Trust Attachment Learning to walk, talk, and feed self	Fear Anxiety Posttrauma response Altered family processes Altered growth and development	Encourage interaction. Use face-to-face positioning. Use touch (when appropriate) and nurturance. Offer food and transitional objects. Be attentive without being unnecessarily intrusive. Offer nurturance to the child's mother. Make attempts to connect family to child. Take time to develop relationship through play.
Handling separation and independence	**Toddlers** Autonomy Separation Toilet training Learning right from wrong	Chronic low self-esteem Anxiety Altered thought processes Coping, ineffective individual	Offer frequent exercise and motor activities. Allow child opportunities to make choices. Offer transitional object. Take control if child is out of control; otherwise let child have some control. Set limits and boundaries to help the child feel secure.
Handling joint decisions and interpersonal conflicts	**Preschoolers** Initiative Tolerance of others Sexual identity Socialization Developing a conscience	Social interaction, impaired Impaired verbal communication Violence, potential for Decisional conflict	Set up opportunities for problem solving and cooperative thinking. Help child to identify fears through books, art, play. Shape appropriate socialization using reinforcement. Become model for conflict resolution.
Dealing with frustration and unfavorable events	**Middle childhood** Industry Physical skill development	Social interaction impaired Hopelessness	Help the child to cope with frustration using stories and plays. Model cooperation and reinforce cooperative behavior.
Celebrating good things, feeling pleasure	Peer relationships Learning to read, write, and calculate Development of morality and values	Body image disturbance	Do not use shame or humiliation to gain control. Have fun with the child. Use community meetings for peer support and modeling. Use positive reinforcement for child's strengths and abilities.
Working for delayed gratification	**Early adolescence** Identity Role acceptance	Altered growth and development Altered sexuality patterns	Use daily expectations and games to teach delayed gratification. Encourage self-reinforcement.
Relaxing and playing	New relations with peers of both sexes	Social isolation Anticipatory grieving Sleep pattern disturbance	Encourage playfulness at appropriate times.
Cognitive processing	**Later adolescence** Emotional and economic independence from parents	Altered growth and development Social interaction, impaired Altered thought process Anxiety	Offer games that use cognitive processing. Discuss abstractions such as the moral of stories or movies. Actively listen to and encourage the expression of needs and goals.
Adaptive sense of direction and purpose	Preparation for occupation Civic responsibility	Personal identity disturbance Family coping, potential for growth Hopelessness	In community meetings discuss relevant issues and life events. Help the child to realistically assess his or her ability and potential.

Altered Sexuality Patterns

Children who are exposed to sexual behavior prematurely may exhibit precocious sexuality. Research has shown that overt sexual behavior that is inappropriate for the child's age is an indication of sexual abuse.[33] Appearing seductive, they then may become vulnerable to additional abuse. Children who have been sexually abused may reenact the abuse experience by sexually acting out with other children. If the other child involved is considerably younger or coercion is used, this behavior is abusive and the other child then becomes the victim. These issues must be discussed openly with a supportive nurse. The nurse can provide the child with needed insight about his or her behavior, information about prevention, and protection from future abuse[4,6] (see Chapter 39).

Reporting of sexual abuse is a legal and ethical issue for nurses.[26] Although they are required by law to report suspected abuse, nurses are not required to prove that the abuse actually occurred. Nurses are permitted to enter evidence and testify on behalf of the victim, especially if the abuse is harmful or traumatic to the child. However, frequent interviewing can retraumatize a child and distort the child's perception of what occurred and must be carefully considered.[27] Because it is unclear during this process whether a child will be returned to a parent's custody, the nurse needs to be able to maintain a relationship with both the child and the parent. This process may be difficult for a nurse, who may experience a kind of vicarious trauma.[10] Therefore, when working with sexually abused children it is critically important for the treatment staff to meet regularly to express their feelings and support each other in this difficult work.

Altered Thought Processes

Under stress, children often have difficulty thinking, identifying options, and making decisions. They become easily frustrated and may respond to their frustration with aggressive behavior. The most effective intervention for the school-aged child with this problem is to help the child think through options in a nonthreatening way. This thinking process can be practiced throughout the day by inventing a hypothetical situation that is potentially threatening and helping the child think through possible options. The created situations can gradually become more and more similar to the child's current life situation, and actual problems on the unit can be processed in a similar way. Through practicing identifying options and making decisions in nonstressful situations, the child can learn to respond more adaptively to stressful situations.

Although rare, children may have psychotic episodes. It is important that the psychiatric nurse be able to discriminate between normal and abnormal thought processes in children. Healthy preschool and school-aged children typically have vivid imaginations, and their normal fears can become quite intense; however, these responses should not be confused with psychotic delusions or hallucinations. Children who are psychotic rarely discuss these experiences. Their symptoms are distinguished by their level of intensity, distress, and duration. For example, a child may hallucinate seeing the devil or animals. These psychotic episodes are terrifying and should be treated as psychiatric emergencies. Antipsychotic medications are usually indicated to control these episodes.

Anticipatory Grieving

Children in chaotic families often experience many losses. With the chronic nature of life stressors, these children may experience the loss of stability, loss of security, and in many ways the loss of childhood. Children who have experienced repetitive losses begin to anticipate the future with grief. They may lose interest in playing and become withdrawn. Children who are withdrawn generally do not cause any disturbance in the milieu, so their needs can easily be overlooked. However, they need to be encouraged to actively express their grief by drawing or participating in play therapy, and then to join the other children in unstructured play. Rumination is discouraged, and participation is encouraged. Most importantly, the significance of their grief should not be minimized.

Anxiety

Children who are anxious may become very active and appear to be uncooperative. Gentle touch and redirection is often effective in restoring a child's self-control. If this is insufficient, a child may need to be moved to a less stimulating environment, such as a small empty room, to reduce anxiety and regain self-control. This must not be done in a punitive manner, but presented in a way to help the child. Also, children may have separation anxiety related to particular people, often their parents.[11] The child may have difficulty separating from a parent, and the parent may similarly be ambivalent about leaving the child. Each may require a great deal of reassurance to tolerate separation when hospitalization is needed. The nurse can help the child reduce anxiety by providing some attachment object, such as a small cuddly toy or other object the parent brings from home. Often, drawing pictures of home, a family gathering, or the family's reaction to the hospitalization can be reassuring to a young child (Fig. 36-2). The nurse can also help the parent by having frequent telephone contact to report the child's progress. Nursing interventions are then planned to help the child and parent anticipate the future, reduce anxiety related to each other, and focus on further development of the child's sense of self.

Body Image Disturbance

Some children with emotional illness may have distorted ideas about their body and experience gender identity confusion. This is usually identified in drawings in which a child consistently deletes important body parts or covers

Fig. 36-2   **A,** Child's drawing of himself at home before entering the hospital: "I'm sad about the things I do and how people feel about me." **B,** Same child's drawing of himself entering the hospital.

them up by marking through them with dark colors. They may also draw gender-specific details that are incorrect, such as breasts on a boy or male genitalia on a girl. An effective nursing intervention is to have a child recline on a large piece of paper and draw a body outline. The child then draws in features, clothes, and other accessories. The child can separate himself or herself from the drawing and be more explicit about details than when asked to verbalize about the problem. The children as a group may then have

discussions about differences between boys and girls. At this time, open discussion can clarify any distortions or misperceptions. Also, children who have been sexually abused are often confused about body invasion for themselves and others. These children are often intrusive and need to be taught about appropriate and inappropriate touching and respect for body boundaries. Nurses, male and female, can improve a child's body image disturbance through thoughtful, supportive care.

Chronic Low Self-Esteem

Children with psychiatric illness often have low self-esteem. It may be expressed by infrequent eye contact, lack of motivation, withdrawal, or the use of negative behavior to seek attention. Specific therapeutic activities can be planned to improve a child's self-esteem. Accomplishment of a goal, no matter how small, is very rewarding, and incremental goal setting can be an effective way to provide opportunities for success. For example, a child who is a chronic complainer could be rewarded for refraining from complaining for 15 minutes. The time can then be gradually increased. At the same time, new methods of communication, such as initiating a conversation, can be taught and rewarded. A bedtime review of accomplishments of the day in which the child lists personal strengths can also be positively reinforcing. Finally, the nurse can provide information and guidance to parents to help them enhance their child's self-esteem (Table 36-3).

Decisional Conflict

Children who have been abused or otherwise traumatized often respond to their experience by appearing defiant and oppositional. In evaluating a child's ability to handle interpersonal conflict, the child's developmental level should be considered. There are many tasks that are difficult for children to complete, particularly if they are developmentally delayed or anxious. Therefore, expectations must be carefully evaluated to determine whether they exceed a child's capability. After a careful nursing assessment, an intervention should be planned to reward or positively reinforce a child's appropriate decision-making ability. For example, a point system in which a child earns points and then exchanges them for privileges may be very helpful.

Family Coping: Potential for Growth

Each family has an extensive history that has shaped the development of each family member. This collective family history and its adaptability for change have a powerful influence on a child's prognosis for learning, practicing, and applying new skills. Therefore, the family's willingness to participate in the therapeutic process and interest in making change should guide the nursing intervention for the child. For example, if the child is returning home after discharge, the parents should be asked to participate in a parent education program early in the hospitalization process.[36] During the parent education, a nurse models the effective use of reinforcement, communication, and behavior management techniques identified in Box 36-2, while another nurse watches the modeling of these skills with the parents and provides instruction about them (Fig. 36-3). The parents are then expected to practice these techniques with their child

TABLE **36-3** *Enhancing a Child's Self-Esteem*

Targeted Area	Strategy
Caregiver expectations	Describe expectations for the child.
	Assess anticipated developmental milestones.
	Review family patterns and influences.
Personal value	Communicate confidence in the child.
	Structure situations to promote success of the child.
	Implement effective ways of praising the child.
	Role model self-value.
Communication	Listen attentively.
	Encourage openness to feelings.
	Avoid using judgmental statements.
	Elicit different points of view.
Discipline	Use effective methods of limit setting.
	Discuss and implement appropriate consequences.
	Review problem-solving techniques.
	Teach that physical punishment should not be used.
Guidance	Encourage open exchanges with the child.
	Know the child's activities away from home.
	Plan family time and activities together.
	Express interest in school events.
	Become familiar with the child's friends.
Autonomy	Demonstrate respect for the child.
	Promote the child's responsible decision making.
	Expect reciprocal respect.

Box **36-2** *Strategies for Behavior Management of Children*

Respond warmly to a child's positive behaviors.
Communicate approval by facial expression, tone of voice, and touch.
Express excitement around a child's accomplishments.
Ignore negative behavior whenever appropriate.
Refrain from giving unnecessary commands.
Respond calmly but effectively to negative behaviors. (Example: "No yelling," stated in a calm tone of voice.)
Use time-outs when necessary and appropriate. (30 to 60 seconds per year of a child's age.) This should be done in a nonpunitive manner and presented as a way to help the child gain control or use problem-solving techniques.
Avoid making unrealistic demands of a child.
Avoid negative remarks about the child.
Communicate often, using the following techniques:
  The parent or staff member telling about personal experiences.
  The parent or staff member listening, paraphrasing, and asking follow-up questions.
  Nightly review of positive behaviors noted during the day that the parent wants to be repeated. (Negative behaviors should not be mentioned at this time.)

Modified from Strayhorn J, Weidman C: *J Am Acad Child Adolesc Psychiatry* 28:888, 1989.

during the course of treatment. Throughout this time the parents are encouraged to function more and more independently in managing their child's behavior while being supported by the nursing staff. Before the child is discharged, specific plans are made for adapting these skills in the home.

> **?** *Do you think the strategies for behavior management of children described in Box 36-2 are culture bound or culture free? Defend your position.*

Fear

Excessive or maladaptive fear in children may be displayed by aggressive or oppositional behavior. If children have been abused by someone they trusted, they will have fear associated with establishing close, trusting relationships. To minimize fears during hospitalization, consistent schedules should be maintained and children should be prepared for changes in activities. For example, sometimes during shift changes for the nurses children can suddenly become agitated as the oncoming staff is beginning to organize activities. The change of personnel is often difficult for young children to understand and tolerate. Therefore, staggered scheduling and discussion about the changing of personnel may be helpful in reducing children's fears. If unexpected symptoms of fear or agitation appear, an assessment should be made to determine whether this behavior is related to a change that has taken place in the nursing milieu.

Hopelessness

Many children live in chaotic and dangerous environments. Communities are often unsafe, and schools may be plagued with violence. Children in these situations may feel very

Fig. 36-3 A parent training program. The nurse with the child is modeling behavior management techniques, while a second nurse is providing instruction to the parent about them.

hopeless. Play therapy and bibliotherapy are effective in helping a child cope with these experiences. Setting small goals that a child can accomplish may help to reduce feelings of hopelessness. Nurses also have an opportunity to teach these children and families about community helping agencies, to find advocates for the child, and to teach the child about self-protection. Trips to the police station, fire station, or community centers may help reduce the child's sense of hopelessness. Often a relative, teacher, guidance counselor, or church member can provide the child with a concerned adult in the community. Contact with some individual or agency that can provide safety for the child is an essential nursing intervention.

Children who are frequently hospitalized or who live in foster care or residential facilities often experience hopelessness. It can be helpful to make a scrapbook about the child's life. It should begin with the child's birth and biological family. By drawing pictures or using pictures from magazines, the child can create a book. The current hospitalization should be included with a picture of the nursing staff. Accomplishments from the treatment program are featured as important life events. Autographs and words of encouragement may be written by staff members to the child. The child can then take this record to the next treatment facility or foster home. In this way the child begins to record life events so that hope for the future can be created.

> **?** *Imagine you are taking one of your school-age patients on a trip to the community. What helping agency would you visit, and what would you like the child to learn from the experience?*

Impaired Social Interaction

Children with emotional problems often have not learned basic social skills that help them relate to others. The therapeutic nurse-patient relationship can be used to learn these skills. Group therapy (see Chapter 31) and behavioral therapy strategies (see Chapter 30) such as social skills training and modeling socially appropriate responses that demonstrate respect for other people are also effective nursing interventions. Children can practice these skills by enacting plays or creating stories that demonstrate socially appropriate solutions to normal childhood dilemmas. Through guidance, demonstration, practice, and feedback, social interaction can be improved.

Some children may not be able to control their behavior in a group setting. A child with this level of impairment requires intensive social training by a nurse with whom a positive relationship exists. This nurse models socially appropriate behavior and then asks the child to repeat the behavior. This game is played, gradually incorporating other staff members into it. Slowly, the child is incorporated into the milieu and becomes attached to other role models.

Eventually the child begins to internalize these socialization behaviors and is able to become part of the group.

For children with cognitive impairment, early social skills training is essential. These children are often small in stature. Consequently, they are often infantilized by their parents and the nursing staff. However, a cognitively impaired child needs to be encouraged to function as independently as possible. Therefore, a plan of care should be developed and adhered to precisely. Because of the child's limited cognitive ability, exact repetition by all members of the nursing staff to the child's behavior is crucial. With repetition of responses from others, the cognitively impaired child who is poorly socialized will learn appropriate age-related behavior.

Impaired Verbal Communication

Being able to describe personal experience and express feelings is important to a child's mental health. The nurse can model clear communication by initiating a conversation with a child about a recent life experience, such as something that happened on the way to work. The nurse can then prompt the child to tell about some personal life experience. As the child begins, the nurse reinforces communication with a smile, nod, and touch.

After the child has mastered the skill of talking about external experiences, the nurse can change the intervention to talking about an internal experience or feeling. Once again, the nurse may begin by describing a feeling that has become

associated with an event, and then prompt the child, wait, and reinforce. A child who has never been encouraged to talk about feelings may require the use of therapeutic play involving dolls to express feelings or may be better able to talk about feelings by drawing. This is evident in the artwork shown in Fig. 36-4, in which a 6-year-old boy was able to draw his different feelings.

> **?** *Have you ever tried to talk with a shy or unresponsive child? What techniques did you find to be effective in drawing the child out, and could these strategies be applied to a child in a psychiatric setting?*

Ineffective Individual Coping

Children with psychiatric illness often have chronic overwhelming family stress with inadequate coping resources and support. The resulting dysfunctional behavior is often observed in a structured situation, such as school, where compliance is required. These children need to learn more effective methods of coping. School-age children may use a variety of coping strategies. Boys often report engaging in physical activities, such as riding bicycles, to cope with stress, whereas girls often find talking to friends to be helpful. Once a child learns to use more adaptive skills, the focus should shift to integrating them into the daily routines of home or school.

Fig. 36-4 Drawing by a hospitalized 6-year-old boy of his different feelings.

Personal Identity Disturbance

As children approach adolescence they begin to struggle with an individual identity. Without role models for finding meaning in life, a child's personal identity formation becomes a crisis. If a child does not have successful adult models in life, fictional models can be used to help children imagine success in their own life. For example, nursing staff may select a movie, such as one of those listed in Box 36-3, that provides positive role models. After the group views the movie, the nurse can lead a discussion about the hero's or heroine's life, talking about the obstacles the person had to confront and overcome. It is useful to discuss the skills the characters applied in their efforts to overcome problems. The discussion will naturally flow into finding direction and purpose in life. Within the context of important discussions such as this, a child with personal identity disturbance can develop a competent identity of self and meet the challenges of the adult world.

Posttrauma Response

Children who have been traumatized may have sudden and dramatic mood changes. Often, some unexpected event reminds them of a previous abuse episode, and they experience the anxiety associated with the earlier abuse. At that time their behavior may change without any identifiable cause. Nursing interventions such as art therapy and play therapy can be very useful in helping a child to cope with a previous abuse incident and reduce a posttrauma response.[21,28] Through a guided process using play or drawings, a child may be able to identify the things that are associated with the trauma, such as certain types of weather, body features such as mustaches, or experiences such as hearing loud voices. With this awareness, a child can learn to anticipate responses and may be able to gain some control over them.

Potential for Violence

Being able to handle conflict without becoming aggressive toward oneself or others is very important for children to learn. In contemporary American culture, violence is widespread, and children may perceive it to be an acceptable way of dealing with conflict. Also, with widespread media and television coverage of violent events, children may become numb to feelings related to violence. Therefore, alternatives must be taught so that a child will have a repertoire of solutions to use in conflict situations (see Chapter 29).

For a younger child, a brief time-out may be effective in interrupting behavior that is escalating or becoming out of control. Older school-age children may benefit from an intermittent room program in learning self-control. During these periods alone it may be helpful for a child to read a story about a similar conflict or for an older child to write thoughts and feelings in a journal.

Another useful strategy is to establish a contract with a child who is capable of understanding, writing, and adhering to it.[19] Such a contract would specify the level of precautions and restrictions that the child would face, based on the specific behavior. Contracts allow the child to play an active role in the treatment process and provide immediate and constructive feedback about the child's actions.

As a last resort, seclusion may be needed. Seclusion should never be used as punishment, for the convenience of staff, or as a substitute for individualized treatment (see Critical Thinking about Contemporary Issues). During seclusion the child should be encouraged to express feelings so that the nurse can help the child gain insight into the interconnectedness of emotions, actions, relationships, and alternatives to aggressive behavior.

Sleep Pattern Disturbance

Children who are experiencing anxiety may have sleep disturbances and nightmares. If a child is receiving psychostimulants, such as methylphenidate (Ritalin), and has disturbed sleep, the dosage or time of administration may need to be changed. Sleep disturbances can also be treated with various nursing interventions. Warm milk helps to induce sleep in some children. Back massage can also be helpful in encouraging relaxation. Many children's stories that deal with nightmares and fears related to bedtime can be read and discussed. In general, however, the most effective way to make a successful transition to bedtime and subsequently to sleep is to develop a consistent, predictable bedtime ritual, such as taking a bath followed by quiet time and a bedtime story. The consistent application of these activities usually reduces this maladaptive response in children.

Social Isolation

Dysfunctional families often isolate themselves from others. Young children may not have had normal socialization experiences with other children or adults. Therefore, the opportunity for teaching positive social skills during hospitalization is critical. The simplest activity, such as looking out a window with a child, can become an opportunity for learning. Cars and people provide an endless array of

Box **36-3** *Movies with Positive Role Models*

Black Beauty	*Man without a Face*
The Black Stallion	*Milo & Otis*
Charlotte's Web	*My Girl*
The Cure	*The Neverending Story*
D.A.R.Y.L.	*Old Yeller*
Fern Gully	*Radio Flyer*
Free Willy	*School Ties*
Home Alone	*The Secret Garden*
Huckleberry Finn	*Star Wars*
Indian in the Cupboard	*Three Wishes*
Jumanji	*Where the Red Fern Grows*
The Karate Kid	*White Fang*
The Last Starfighter	*White Wolves*
The Lion King	*The Wizard of Oz*

CRITICAL THINKING *about* Contemporary Issues

Is the Use of Seclusion and Restraints with Children Therapeutic?

The use of seclusion and restraints in the care and treatment of children with psychiatric problems has been the subject of considerable debate.[15] Advocates of these techniques cite the widespread problem of violent behavior among psychiatric patients, including children, and describe the clinical efficacy of these interventions.[3] In fact, seclusion and restraint appear to be widely used in inpatient settings by nurses who are the front-line professionals responsible for initiating emergency procedures and supervising the actions taken to prevent violent outbursts. On the other hand, these interventions have also been associated with punishment, custodial care, and institutional abuse and neglect. Some even view seclusion as a violation of a patient's civil liberties.

In examining the issue, Wong and colleagues[37] recommend a three-pronged approach to the reduction of dangerous, inappropriate behavior by children, including aggressive, destructive, and highly disruptive behavior. First, they recommend teaching and reinforcing acceptable ways for children to express themselves and satisfy their needs. Second, the authors advocate the use of procedures such as time-outs, room programs, or open-door seclusion to reduce inappropriate behavior. Third, they stress the need to evaluate the effect of these interventions on the child and to continuously monitor the efficacy of these interventions in research studies using objective measures and experimental controls. As with all other nursing interventions, the therapeutic value of seclusion and restraints for children is determined by the treatment goals, context of care, and respect shown by the nurse for the needs of the child and family.

TABLE 36-4 *Therapeutic Aspects of Play*

THERAPEUTIC FACTOR	BENEFICIAL OUTCOME
Overcoming resistance	Working alliance
Communication	Understanding
Competence	Self-esteem
Creative thinking	Problem solving
Catharsis	Emotional release
Abreaction	Perspective on traumatic event
Role playing	Learning new behaviors
Fantasy	Compensation and sublimation
Teaching through metaphors	Insight
Relationship enhancement	Trust in others
Mastering developmental fears	Growth and development
Game play	Socialization

Modified from Schaefer C: *The therapeutic powers of play*, Northvale, NJ, 1993, Jason Aronson.

speculation and imagined scenarios about life. A trip for a diagnostic test can also be an adventure for a child. A sensitive nurse capitalizes on the opportunity to interest the child in people and the surroundings at all times. These experiences turn ordinary events into occasions for learning, relaxing, and playing.

THERAPEUTIC TREATMENT MODALITIES

Once a thorough assessment has been completed and nursing diagnoses have been formulated, the nurse can implement a variety of individualized interventions that are effective in treating maladaptive responses in children.[7]

Therapeutic Play

Because play is normal and fun for children, it is a very effective tool for nurses to use in individual interventions. Interventions that are enjoyable, arouse curiosity, and stimulate the imagination will capture the child's attention and interest. Many children with psychiatric problems may have lost interest in play or may have never experienced the joy

of spontaneous play. Learning to play is critical not only to a child's development but also to mental health. Therapeutic aspects of play and their beneficial outcomes are listed in Table 36-4. The nurse should keep these elements in mind when incorporating play therapy into the plan of care.

The first step is for the nurse to develop a therapeutic alliance and trust with the child so that life can be perceived from the child's perspective and the child's concerns can be anticipated. When a child feels understood and safe, participation in therapeutic play with the nurse is common. If the child is anxious, his or her developmental level may fluctuate rapidly, and this should be continuously assessed by the nurse. However, care must be taken to ensure that the child does not fail at the activity, either because the developmental level is too advanced or because of the severity of the child's symptoms. Children will become easily frustrated with play that is too difficult and thus feel a sense of failure at a time when their self-esteem is already compromised. Nursing interventions therefore must be adapted to the child's presenting developmental level and gradually change as the child's anxiety is reduced.

Toys that are age appropriate and imaginative should be offered to a child. These may include blocks, a play house, family characters, soldiers, trucks, and rescue vehicles. The child is then encouraged to begin play without specific direction from the nurse. The nurse may ask the following clarifying questions:
▼ What is this person doing?
▼ How does this little boy feel?
▼ What is happening now?

The nurse can then follow up with some clarifying and validating statements such as, "This little girl looks afraid." The nurse refrains from guiding the play, making unnecessary remarks, or making interpretations that may link the play to the child's life experience. The play should continue

Fig. 36-5 Self-image drawings by two boys. **A,** Drawing by a 7-year-old boy. **B,** Drawing by a 13-year-old boy. Differences related to age, body perceptions, and interests are evident.

until the child is no longer engaged. The nurse can then evaluate the play intervention by considering the following questions:

▼ What did the play activity communicate about the child's development level?

▼ What emotions and behavioral responses were evidenced by the child while at play?

▼ What information can be added to the child's assessment or treatment plan based on observations during play therapy?

Art Therapy

Drawing is a valuable tool for children to use in describing an event or expressing a feeling. Children often do not have the vocabulary to express themselves, and they feel pressured to answer questions they do not understand. Drawings provide the nurse with the child's perspective of an experience. Through drawings, a child can provide information about behavior and developmental maturity that the nurse can then use to help the child in preparing for future change (Fig. 36-5).

Art is particularly useful in assessing a child's therapeutic

needs. The nurse may begin by asking the child to draw a picture of something that happened before he or she was admitted to the hospital. Children also can be asked to draw a picture of their family, a person or object that they are afraid of, or where they are going after they leave the hospital. Children may find drawing stressful if they have been criticized about it in the past. However, with some encouragement they will usually produce an interesting and often revealing picture. The nurse might ask the child what is happening in the picture or to name the people. The nurse should make notes about whatever the child reports the people are saying or thinking. This process can be continued until the child becomes disinterested in the activity or the child's anxiety level becomes too great. In evaluating the effectiveness of this intervention, the nurse should consider the following:

▼ What was learned about the child's experience and perceptions from this intervention?

▼ What do the pictures reveal about the child's view of the world?

▼ Is there any gender confusion evident?

▼ Is there any distortion between the child's perception of personal experience and that which was reported?

Children's Games

Children with behavioral or emotional problems often have difficulty with motor control. These symptoms may be developmental or may be caused by anxiety. In either case, games that teach motor control can help the child. These games include Simon Says, Red Light, Musical Chairs, and many others. Games can also be used to increase a child's concentration and frustration tolerance. Games such as Candy Land, Hide and Seek, and Find the Button can be played with gradually increasing difficulty to teach these skills.

When initiating these activities the nurse should consider the child's motor development and level of anxiety and choose among games that engage large or small muscle groups. Thought should also be given to the child's tolerance for frustration and competition. Games may then be modified to meet the specific therapeutic needs of the child. Games can also be played with increasing demands placed on concentration and cognitive processing; however, it is important to stop playing a game that is too difficult or stressful for a child.

During the game it is important to keep in mind the therapeutic goal and for the nurse to be flexible about the rules. Although the goal is to challenge the child, it is also important to have fun and to use the game to shape and reinforce new adaptive behaviors for the child. The nurse should consider the following questions at the completion of the game:

▼ Was the game developmentally appropriate for the child?

▼ Was playing the game a pleasurable experience?

▼ If not, why not?

▼ Was the nurse's therapeutic goal met?

▼ How should the game be modified in the future to further the child's skill development and adaptive coping responses?

Bibliotherapy

Bibliotherapy is the use of literature to help children identify and express feelings within the structure and safety of the nurse-patient relationship[8] (Box 36-4). Because children actively engage in imaginary thinking, they can easily identify with the fictional characters in a story and gain insight into their own lives.

In implementing this activity, the nurse should carefully consider the child's age and attention span. To be effective, the story should have illustrations that capture the child's interest. The nurse should also think about the child's situation and try to select a book that describes a situation or issue relevant to the child's life situation. For example, hospitalized children who are separated from their families may be comforted by a story about a kitten who gets lost. It is often helpful to offer a choice of two books to the child. One book could be directly related to the child's experience and the other one less directly related, because the child may not be ready to confront life situations directly. This also gives the child the opportunity to make choices and be included in decision making.

While reading the story the nurse should be sensitive to the child's response. If the text is wordy, the child may become bored or distracted. If this occurs, paraphrasing the story or asking what the child thinks is happening to the characters may be helpful. In this way the child's imagination becomes engaged and the experience will have value. It is also important to give the child an opportunity to reflect on the story and discuss any thoughts or feelings about the characters because it is often easier to talk about the feelings of the characters than one's own.

After reading the story, the nurse should evaluate the usefulness of the intervention and assess the following:

▼ Was the story appropriate to the child's developmental age?

▼ Was the child engaged with the story?

▼ Did the child enjoy the experience?

▼ What was learned by the child and about the child as a result of this intervention?

? *Traditional fairy tales are based on and convey many gender stereotypes. Do you think this is a problem, and how might you go about dealing with this issue in working with children?*

Box **36-4** *Suggested Books for Bibliotherapy*

ABUSE
Stanek M: *Don't Hurt Me, Mama,* Niles, Ill, 1983, Albert Whitman.

ANGER
Hapgood M: *Martha's Mad Day,* New York, 1977, Crown.
Sendak M: *Where the Wild Things Are,* New York, 1963, Harper & Row.
Sharmat M: *Attilla the Angry,* New York, 1985, Holiday House.
Viorst J: *Alexander and the No Good Horrible Terrible Very Bad Day,* New York, 1972, Atheneum.

DIVORCE AND STEP-PARENTS
Brown L and M: *Dinosaurs Divorce,* Boston, 1986, Little, Brown.
Schuchman J: *Two Places to Sleep,* Minneapolis, 1977, Carolrhoda.
Vigna J: *She's Not My Real Mom,* Niles, Ill, 1980, Albert Whitman.

FEARS
Mayer M: *There's A Nightmare in My Closet,* New York, 1968, Dial.
Viorst J: *My Mother Says There Aren't Any Zombies, Ghosts, Vampires, Creatures, Demons, Fiends, Goblins, or Things,* New York, 1974, Atheneum.

GRIEF
Bryan M, Ingpen R: *Lifetimes,* New York:, 1983, Bantam.
Gaffney P: *The Seasons of Grief: Helping Children Grow through Loss,* New York, 1988, Penguin.

IDENTITY
Mayer M: *A Silly Story,* Italy, 1972, Publishers Group West.

SEPARATION
Brown M: *The Runaway Bunny,* New York, 1942, Harper & Row.

SIBLING RIVALRY
Alexander M: *Nobody Asked Me if I Wanted a New Baby Sister,* New York, 1971, Dial.
Keats E: *Peter's Chair,* New York, 1967, Harper & Row.
Sendak M: *Outside Over There,* New York, 1981, Penguin.
Viorst J: *I'll Fix Anthony,* New York, 1969, Harper & Row.

SLEEP AND BEDTIME
Brown M: *Goodnight, Moon,* New York, 1942, Harper & Row.
Holabird K: *Alexander & the Dragon,* New York, 1972, Clarkson N. Potter.
Sendak M: *The Night Kitchen,* New York, 1970, Harper & Row.

SOCIALIZATION
Lobel A: *Frog and Toad,* New York, 1970, Harper & Row.
Marshall J: *George and Martha: Back in Town; George and Martha: Tons of Fun; George and Martha: Round and Round,* Boston, 1972, Houghton Mifflin.

TRUST
Berry J: *Let's Talk about Breaking Promises,* Newark, NJ, 1982, Peter Pan.

Storytelling

The therapeutic use of storytelling for relieving distress and teaching new coping skills is a valuable intervention. Because children do not separate imaginary experiences from real experiences, stories that teach appropriate problem-solving skills can serve as models for real situations.

Initially the nurse must identify a social skill that the child needs to learn, such as assertiveness. The nurse may make up a story about a character who needs that particular skill, giving the hero or heroine similar characteristics to the child. It is important to select an ending to the story that will guide the child in learning the skill. Next, the nurse should plan a time and place for storytelling that is free from distractions and interruptions. Bedtime is often a natural time for individual storytelling. The story should be told using animated facial expressions and expressive voice inflections, and the child should be actively involved in the story as much as possible. At the end of the story the nurse should ask the child about the story and how it made the child feel. This may then lead to a broader discussion of other aspects of the child's life. In evaluating the outcome of the intervention, the nurse should consider the following questions:

▼ Could this character be used to teach this child other skills through other stories?

▼ Could the child add to the story or make up one of his or her own?

▼ What was the moral of the story, and how did it apply to the child?

▼ Could the story be used in other creative ways, such as by having the child enact the story or by including others?

Autogenic Storytelling

A similar version of storytelling is **autogenic storytelling**, a therapeutic activity in which the child participates in creating the story. Nurses may find this activity particularly valuable in helping children explore fears related to traumatic events. This intervention is particularly useful for a school-age child who has been traumatized or is having nightmares. A child will often reenact anxiety-related experiences in a story portrayed by animals or other fictional characters. Unlike real life, the child can have control over the experience if it is relived in play or storytelling.

Children often like audiotaping the story and then listening to their voice telling the story. The nurse should discuss the general structure of the story with the child, and together they can decide on the main characters and the beginning plot. The nurse should begin the story with the introduction and then stop, allowing the child to add the next event. The nurse picks up the storytelling when the child runs out of material or becomes anxious or overstimulated. At the end of the story, if the child has chosen an unhealthy ending, the nurse begins the storytelling intervention again. In the retelling, however, the nurse takes on a more active role and adds adaptive responses at important moments in the story. This allows the child to explore a traumatic event while learning healthy coping responses.

This intervention can be very useful for children who have had traumatic and abusive experiences. However, it is critical that the nurse implementing this intervention be attentive to clues from the child indicating increased anxiety. The nurse should also avoid interpreting the story to the child, and this intervention should not be used to coerce the child to reveal information about an experience of abuse. Instead, the child should be allowed to explore the experience through storytelling with as much freedom as possible. At the conclusion the nurse should evaluate the following:

▼ What emotions and behaviors did the child portray in the story?

▼ What were the predominant themes?

▼ How did the child resolve the story, and what does it suggest about the child's ability to solve problems and resolve conflicts?

Enacting Plays

Enacting plays gives children the opportunity to practice new behaviors with peers in a structured activity. Using a story with a simple and familiar plot, the nurse can choose a play for social skill development. It can be performed by groups of children or by one child using a set of toy characters.

In designing this activity, the nurse should consider a recurring social problem in the group or a symptom that has caused or is causing a child difficulty. The nurse can then find a book or write a story that depicts the problem and teaches an appropriate and adaptive response. The children should be allowed to select the characters, and dress-up props are particularly helpful to engage the children's imagination. The play may then be performed with the nurse prompting the children with the lines. Often, children will ask to repeat the performance and change characters. Each child must be given the opportunity to play each part so that all of the character options the story offers can be enacted. If a video camera is available, it can be therapeutic to videotape the performance and replay it for the children. At the conclusion the nurse should review the intervention considering how it affected each child:

▼ Was enacting the play fun for the children?

▼ Are there other social skills that the children need to practice in this format in the future?

Medication Management

Many children with a psychiatric illness receive psychotropic medication as part of their treatment.[20,24,31] Tables 36-5 and 36-6 list some of the drugs commonly used with children and adolescents, along with their indications and dosages. See Chapter 27 for a more extensive discussion of these drugs. Psychiatric nurses must be knowledgeable about these medications and develop interventions to monitor, educate, and evaluate medication effects with children and their families. Nurses should also be aware that

TABLE **36-5** *Child and Adolescent Psychiatric Disorders and Drug Treatments*

DISORDER	DRUG CLASS	COMMENTS/NURSING CONSIDERATIONS
Affective disorders: depression, bipolar disorder	Antidepressants Mood stabilizers	Careful diagnosis is necessary to differentiate depression from normal feeling states.
Anxiety, transient insomnia, acute extrapyramidal symptoms (EPS)	Antihistamines (Benadryl) Benzodiazepines	Tolerance to sedative effects may develop.
Attention deficit–hyperactivity disorder (ADHD)	Stimulants	Used when primary symptoms are manifest in school. Less reliable in preschoolers and adolescents.
	Antidepressants	Once-a-day dose and improved monitoring of compliance and toxicity using plasma levels. Monitor cardiac status and signs of overdose.
	Antipsychotics	Sometimes used in combination with stimulants for symptomatic relief.
Conduct disorders (aggressive and nonaggressive)	Antipsychotics, stimulants, antidepressants, mood stabilizers	May improve a child's capacity to benefit from social and educational interventions.
Eating disorders	Antihistamines (cyproheptadine), antipsychotics, TCAs	Anorexia nervosa.
	Antidepressants (imipramine), SSRIs	Bulimia.
Functional enuresis	Antidepressants (imipramine)	Used when an immediate therapeutic effect is necessary because of severe emotional distress.
Impulsivity	Antipsychotics, mood stabilizers	Help to increase behavioral control
Mental retardation with psychiatric symptoms and behavioral problems	Antipsychotics	Used to control behavioral and psychiatric complications.
	Antidepressants	Treat affective symptoms.
	Stimulants	Treat ADHD.
	Lithium	Helps control aggression.
	Carbamazepine	Anticonvulsant that can help control aggression.
Obsessive-compulsive disorder (OCD)	Antidepressants (clomipramine, SSRIs)	Reduce OCD symptoms.
Panic and school phobia	TCA, MAOI, SSRI	Concurrent behavioral interventions recommended.
Pervasive developmental disorders	Antipsychotics	Used to treat agitation, stereotypic movements, destructive behaviors.
	SSRIs	Stereotypic movements and OCD-like symptoms.
Psychosis	Antipsychotics	Assess for EPS and tardive dyskinesia.
Rage	Haloperidol, mood stabilizers	Require careful education and laboratory monitoring.
Schizophrenia	Antipsychotics	As with adults, choice of drug depends on prior efficacy and the spectrum of pharmacological properties.
Separation anxiety disorder	Antidepressants (imipramine, SSRIs)	Effective at high doses. Speculative: panic disorder symptoms.
Tic disorders: Tourette's disorder	Antipsychotics (haloperidol), SSRI	Stimulants are avoided because they worsen symptoms.
	Alpha-adrenergic agonist (clonidine)	Hypotension, dizziness, dry mouth, drowsiness.

promoting a child's knowledge of medications can have a positive effect on self-esteem and feelings of control and self-worth. Thus numerous therapeutic outcomes can be achieved by effective medication teaching.

This area allows for many creative nursing interventions.[23] A variety of puppet play, art, graphics, and audiovisual materials can be used to successfully teach and prepare children for managing their medications and their illness. Posters created by nurses to teach children about medications are presented in Fig. 36-6. Peer group participation is

particularly effective in helping children describe common experiences, decrease their sense of isolation, and enhance their responses to the teaching materials. Through imaginative but goal-directed nursing interventions, children can learn important information and experience greater control over the treatment of their illness and their future mental health.

Finally, it is important for nurses to realize that children metabolize and eliminate medications more rapidly than adults. Although initial doses should be low, doses may ul-

TABLE 36-6 *Drugs Commonly Used in Children and Adolescents with Psychiatric Disorders*

Drug	Description	Daily Dose (mg/kg of body weight)	Side Effects
STIMULANTS: GENERIC (TRADE)			
Dextroamphetamine (Dexedrine)	Short-acting (2-4 hr)	0.3-1.5,* 1-3 doses daily	*Short term:* Decreased appetite, sleep disturbances
Methylphenidate (Ritalin)	Short-acting (2-4 hr)	0.3-1.5,* 1-3 doses daily	*Long term:* Possible minor effects on growth; associated with onset of Tourette's syndrome in children with family history of tics
Pemoline (Cylert)	Long-acting (2-4 wk delay in therapeutic effect)	0.5-3.0,* 1 daily dose	*Abrupt discontinuation:* Behavioral deterioration
ANTIDEPRESSANTS			
Clomipramine (Anafranil)	20-40 hr half-life		TCA: metabolized more rapidly in children, necessitating higher doses
Imipramine (Tofranil)	10-17 hr half-life; immediate response with enuresis or ADHD; 2-4 week delay in response with depression	Usual daily dose should not exceed 5 mg/kg/day	*Short term:* Dry mouth, blurred vision, constipation, electrocardiogram changes, insomnia *Abrupt discontinuation:* Gastrointestinal (GI) symptoms, drowsiness, headaches
Fluoxetine (Prozac)	6-week half-life	5-20 mg/day	*Short term:* Insomnia, GI symptoms, agitation
MOOD STABILIZERS			
Carbamazepine (Tegretol)	Peak effect in 7-10 days	10-30; maintain plasma level at 4-12 mm/L	*Short term:* GI symptoms, polyuria, polydipsia, tremors, sleepiness, impaired memory
Lithium	12-hr half-life	Maintain plasma level at 0.6-1.2 mm/L	*Long term:* Decreased calcium metabolism and thyroid function; possible kidney changes, blood dyscrasias, and hepatotoxicity
ANTIPSYCHOTICS			
Chlorpromazine (Thorazine)	Low potency	8-6	*Short term:* Drowsiness, weight gain, dry mouth, blurred vision, nasal congestion, acute dystonia, parkinsonism, postural hypotension, hyperpyrexia
Haloperidol (Haldol)	High potency	0.05-0.15	
Thioridazine (Mellaril)	Low potency	0.5-3.0	
Trifluoperazine (Stelazine)	High potency	0.1-0.5	*Abrupt discontinuation:* Withdrawal dyskinesias
Atypical drugs			Use in children is anecdotal
ANTIANXIETY AGENTS			
Diphenhydramine (Benadryl)		37.5-50 mg/day, children ≤20 lb 37.5-100 mg/day, children >20 lb	*Short term:* Drowsiness; may cause excitation in young children *Contraindications:* Bronchial asthma, narrow-angle glaucoma, pyloroduodenal and bladder neck obstruction

*Doses are lower for younger children.

timately be as high as adults, requiring frequent clinical and laboratory follow-up. Although psychopharmacological treatment is increasingly used in children, with some reports of significant benefit, it should be remembered that there are very few studies of these drugs in children and limited indications for their use with children approved by the Food and Drug Administration (FDA).

Milieu Management

A final important role of the child psychiatric nurse is the organization, management, and integration of multi-ple treatment interventions with the child throughout the continuum of care, such as in the inpatient setting, day treatment program, or intensive in-home intervention. With escalating aggression among children, the management of a therapeutic milieu in any of these settings is very challenging.[12,13,16] The child's day must be organized into manageable time units that are age appropriate, with specific but varied activities assigned to each time unit. For example, younger children's development requires that they be assigned shorter time units and large motor activities should be scheduled to follow

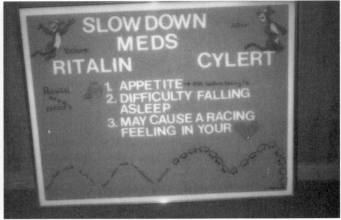

Fig. 36-6 Posters created by nurses to teach children about medications.

periods of sitting or after therapy sessions, which might produce anxiety.

Whenever possible, children should be assigned to a small group with specific staff members. A schedule should be set up in advance that is predictable from one day to the next. Consistency and predictability are very important in the treatment of children with psychiatric illness. Transitioning from one activity to the next is often difficult for children; therefore, a transitional object such as a reward sheet of stickers that is carried from one activity to the next can be helpful. Before leaving one activity, the child should be prepared for the next activity. Helping children to anticipate what is expected of them in the next time period will help them better manage their anxiety.

Anxiety and aggression in any setting can be contagious and they can escalate abruptly. Nurses should be prepared to act quickly and decisively if a child becomes aggressive. If this occurs, the child who is aggressive or anxious must be separated from children who are in control of their behavior. When the child is isolated, the aggressive behavior will begin to de-escalate, the child can be brought under control, and the process of learning about why this occurred can begin.

These problems can be minimized by having a well-planned schedule and implementing it consistently. Whenever tension in the milieu begins to rise, the staff must be very visible and engage the children in activities while being vigilant for potential problems. A carefully planned milieu schedule anticipates problems, creates solutions, and capitalizes on the strengths and energy of the children. Keeping the milieu safe and therapeutic is a high priority for child psychiatric nursing intervention. Ongoing clinical supervision and peer review improve communication and collaboration among staff members.[17] These activities allow staff to evaluate and refine their therapeutic skills and facilitate goal-directed interactions with children.

Summary

1. Today, 14% to 20% of all children from birth to age 18 have some type of mental disorder, of which 3% to 5% are serious psychiatric disorders. Psychiatric services are now being offered to children in a wide variety of settings that together make up systems of care. Nurses function in these settings by assessing a child's competency skills and providing interventions to teach the skills that are deficient.

2. Strayhorn identified nine skills that all children need to become competent adults. All of these skills and ways to assess a child's mastery of them were described.

3. Nursing diagnoses used by child psychiatric nurses were discussed and related nursing interventions were presented.

4. Psychiatric nurses can also implement a variety of therapeutic treatment modalities when caring for children, including therapeutic play, art therapy, games, bibliotherapy, storytelling, autogenic storytelling, enacting plays, medication management, and milieu management.

COMPETENT CARING A Clinical Exemplar of a Psychiatric Nurse

Evelyn Middleton, BSN, RN, C and LeeAnn Welsh, RN

L, a 9-year-old black girl, was admitted to our 25-bed combined child and adolescent psychiatric unit because of recent suicidal attempts and homicidal ideation. L was extremely depressed and had a difficult time talking about the situations that brought her to the hospital. Her family was dysfunctional. Her father was physically and sexually abusive to both her and her mother.

Early in her hospitalization, L didn't trust anyone. She had suffered numerous traumatic events. She would lie in a fetal position, suck her thumb, and periodically talk about wanting to jump off a large bridge in the downtown section of our city. Working as a team on evening shift, we (with other members of the nursing staff) were able to assess the chronically low self-esteem and sadness this child was feeling. With a lot of one-to-one attention and the therapeutic use of touch, we developed a bond with this child, who viewed us as caregivers, and we were able to establish a trusting relationship with her. She asked questions about our childhood and how we were brought up by our parents. She also asked about how we treated our children. From this conversation, she understood she was not to blame for the beatings and the sexual abuse she endured. L continued talking to us with tears in her eyes and her hands clenched while hitting her pillow in an effort to control her anger. She would talk about a dream she often had, and we encouraged her to vent her feelings about this dream. The more this child spoke, the clearer it became to us that it was not only her father who repeatedly violated her, but also her grandfather. She constantly referred to these memories as dreams because she did not want to believe a grandfather could do this to his own flesh and blood. We continued to sit with L at night, consoling and reassuring her that she was not to blame and how great it was that she was finally able to release these ghosts.

During these conversations L had decided that she no longer wanted to be home with her father because she felt the beatings would continue. We prepared her for discharge by discussing different options for placement, her responsibility to keep herself safe, and other ways besides suicide to express her anger. At one point, the Department of Social Services failed to substantiate any sexual misconduct on the father's part toward L. It was their recommendation that she be returned to her father. This disappointment encouraged L to feel betrayed by the adults she had begun to trust. She cried, exclaiming that she told us everything and we had let her down. She stated she would kill her father if she went home. We again reassured her that we would help see that she not be returned home.

Because of the time factor and lack of support from the Department of Social Services, L had to be prepared to go to the state hospital. With a team effort, we were honest and positive about this placement at the state hospital. L was informed as to how she would be transported. We then called the state hospital and gathered some general information to share with her about the facility and different activities that went on there. On the day of discharge, L wanted to meet our children. LeeAnn brought her little boy in to have lunch with L. While interacting with us, L was able to see a healthy parent-child relationship. Once she was settled at the state hospital, she called the unit, requesting to speak to Evelyn and LeeAnn. We encouraged her to trust the staff there and mentioned that she was welcome to call us anytime to let us know how she was doing.

Working as a team, we shared the hurt and love this child was feeling. As two experienced psychiatric nurses, we were able to assess, implement, and plan care for this suicidal patient. Together we established a trusting relationship and created a safe environment for her. Our expertise allowed this child to grow, develop self-esteem, and reclaim the will to live. For us, it truly reflected the essence of child psychiatric nursing practice.

your **INTERNET**
connection

The Child Advocate
http://itsa.ucsf.edu/~mww/

ParentNews: A Unique Opportunity
for Parent Information
http://parent.net/

Chapter Review Questions

1. Indicate whether the following statements are true (T) or false (F).

A. ___ Mental disorders are rare in children (less than 1% of the population).

B. ___ Nursing care of children with psychiatric disorders is focused on skill development regardless of psychiatric diagnosis.

C. ___ Nurses who take care of children who have been abused can be traumatized vicariously.

D. ___ Young children who exhibit overt sexual behavior should be ignored in order not to reinforce the behavior.

E. ___ In order to avoid aggression in the milieu, the nurse should make strict rules and follow them without exception.

2. Fill in the blanks.

A. Less than _____ of the children who need psychiatric treatment in the United States currently receive it.

B. If a child becomes upset when away from his or her mother, it may indicate problems mastering the competency skill of _____.

C. If a child gets mad when he or she doesn't gets his or her way, it may indicate problems mastering the competency skill of _____.

D. _____ is the use of literature to help children identify and express feelings.

E. A therapeutic activity in which the child participates in creating the story is called _____.

F. The most common problem that precipitates hospitalization in children is the _____.

G. Reporting child abuse is a _____ and _____ issue for nurses.

3. Provide short answers for the following questions.

A. What competency skills are associated with middle childhood?

B. Identify areas that parents can target to enhance a child's self-esteem.

C. Television networks are now rating television programs for violence and nudity, and new technologies are allowing parents to block the viewing of certain programs. Do you think this will have a significant impact on the upbringing of children? Why or why not?

D. It has been said that children have a low priority in contemporary American society. Learn about how two other countries provide for the health, education, and welfare of their children and compare them to the United States.

REFERENCES

1. American Nurses' Association: *Standards of child and adolescent psychiatric and mental health nursing practice,* Kansas City, Mo, 1985, The Association.
2. American Psychiatric Association: *Diagnostic and statistical manual,* ed 4, Washington, DC, 1994, The Association.
3. Barlow D: Therapeutic holding: effective intervention with the aggressive child, *J Psychosoc Nurs Ment Health Serv* 27:10, 1990.
4. Bennett C: Sexually abused boys: awareness, assessment, and intervention, *J Child Adolesc Psychiatr Nurs* 6:29, 1993.
5. Brandenberg N, Friedman R, Silver S: The epidemiology of childhood psychiatric disorders: prevalence findings from recent studies, *J Am Acad Child Adolesc Psychiatry* 29:76, 1990.
6. Carrey N, Adams N: How to deal with sexual acting-out on the child psychiatric inpatient unit, *J Psychosoc Nurs Ment Health Serv* 30:19, 1992.
7. Clunn P: *Child psychiatric nursing,* St Louis, 1991, Mosby.
8. Cohen L: Bibilotherapy: using literature to help children deal with difficult problems, *J Psychosoc Nurs Ment Health Serv* 25:20, 1987.
9. Costello E et al: How can epidemiology improve mental health services for children? *J Am Acad Child Adolesc Psychiatry* 32:1106, 1993.
10. Crothers D: Vicarious traumatization in the work with survivors of childhood trauma, *J Psychosoc Nurs* 33:9, 1995.
11. Dashiff C: Understanding separation anxiety disorder, *J Child Adolescent Psychiatr Nurs* 8:27, 1995.
12. Delaney K: Calming an escalated milieu, *J Child Adolesc Psychiatr Nurs* 7:5, 1994.
13. Delaney K: Nursing in child milieus, Part I: what nurses do. Part 2: mapping conceptual footholds, *J Child Adolesc Psychiatr Nurs* 5:10, 1992.
14. Division of Psychiatric Nursing: *Competency in childhood: healthy development,* Charleston, SC, 1993, Medical University of South Carolina (videotape).
15. Fassler D, Cotton N: A national survey on the use of seclusion in the psychiatric treatment of children, *Hosp Community Psychiatry* 43:370, 1992.
16. Goren S, Abraham I, Doyle N: Reducing violence in a child psychiatric hospital through planned organizational change, *J Child Adolesc Psychiatr Nurs* 9:27, 1996.
17. Hallberg I: Systematic clinical supervision in a child psychiatric ward: satisfaction with nursing care, tedium, burnout and the nurses' own report on the effects of it, *Arch Psychiatr Nurs* 8:44, 1994.
18. Hendren R, Berlin I: *Psychiatric inpatient care of children and adolescents: a multicultural approach,* New York, 1991, Wiley.
19. Jones R, O'Brien P, McMahon W: Contracting to lower precaution status for child psychiatric patients, *J Psychosoc Nurs Ment Health Serv* 31:6, 1993.

20. Joshi P, Coyle J, Walkup J: Pharmacotherapy in children and adolescents. In Ghuman H, Sarles R, editors: *Handbook of adolescent inpatient psychiatric treatment,* New York, 1994, Brunner/Mazel.

21. Kaufman B, Wohl A: *Casualties of childhood: a developmental perspective on sexual abuse using projective drawings,* New York, 1992, Brunner/Mazel.

22. Keltner N: Neuroanatomy and physiology in modern child psychiatric nursing, *J Child Adolesc Psychiatr Nurs* 9:5, 1996.

23. Knight M et al: Medication education for children, *J Child Adolesc Psychiatr Nurs* 3:25, 1990.

24. Laraia M: Current approaches to the psychopharmacologic treatment of depression in children and adolescents, *J Child Adolesc Psychiatr Nurs* 9:15, 1996.

25. Leininger M: Transcultural mental health nursing assessment of children and adolescents. In West P, Evans C, editors: *Psychiatric and mental health nursing with children and adolescents,* Gaithersburg, Md, 1992, Aspen.

26. Lewin L: Child abuse: ethical and legal concerns, *J Psychosoc Nurs* 32:15, 1994.

27. Lewin L: Interviewing the young child sexual abuse victim, *J Psychosoc Nurs* 33:5, 1995.

28. Malchiodi C: *Breaking the silence: art therapy with children from violent homes,* New York, 1990, Brunner/Mazel.

29. National Advisory Mental Health Council: *National plan for research on child and adolescent mental disorders,* Rockville, Md, 1990, US Department of Health and Human Services.

30. Perry B: Neurobiological sequelae of childhood trauma: PTSD in children. In Murberg M, editor: *Catecholamines in post-traumatic stress disorder: emerging concepts,* Washington, DC, 1994, American Psychiatric Press.

31. Scahill L, French P: Nonstimulant medications in the treatment of attention deficit hyperactivity disorder, *J Child Adolesc Psychiatr Nurs* 9:39, 1996.

32. Shealy A: Attention-deficit hyperactivity disorder: etiology, diagnosis, and management, *J Child Adolesc Psychiatr Nurs* 7:24, 1994.

33. Slusser M: Manifestations of sexual abuse in preschool-aged children, *Issues Ment Health Nurs* 16:481, 1995.

34. Strayhorn J: *The competent child: an approach to psychotherapy and preventive mental health,* New York, 1989, Guilford.

35. Stroul, B: Systems of care for children and adolescents with emotional disorders: what are the results? *Continuum* 1:29, 1994.

36. Violand M, Williams J: Clinical forum: parent teaching in inpatient child psychiatry, *J Child Adolesc Psychiatr Nurs* 7:41, 1994.

37. Wong S, Martinez-Diaz J, Thorne-Henderson M: How therapeutic is therapeutic holding? *J Psychosoc Nurs Ment Health Serv* 28:24, 1990.

ANNOTATED SUGGESTED READINGS

*Bennett L: Projectile methods in caring for sexually abused young people, *J Psychosocial Nurs* 35:18, 1997.
Emphasizes the value of projectile methods, particularly the use of poetry and pictures, as clinical tools for assessment and treatment of verbally unresponsive children.

*Nursing reference.

Burns B: What drives outcomes for emotional and behavioral disorders in children and adolescents? *New Dir Ment Health Serv* 71:89, 1996.
An overview of factors that may influence treatment outcomes for children with behavioral problems, with an examination of the potential of research technology to document these outcomes.

*Canuso R: Rethinking behavior disorders: whose attention has a deficit? *J Psychosocial Nurs* 35:24, 1997.
Using nursing theory as a framework to assess children's behavior issues, describing the key role nurses can play in designing and implementing interventions that promote a healthy child and family.

*Carpenter M et al: Indicators of abuse or neglect in preschool children's drawings, *J Psychosocial Nurs* 35:10, 1997.
Family drawings by preschool children can be indicative of abuse or neglect. This emphasizes the particularly advantageous use of art with children too young to communicate their feelings clearly.

*Delaney K: Parents' perceptions of their child's emotional illness and psychiatric treatment needs, *J Child Adolesc Psychiatr Nurs* 9:15, 1996.
Describes parents' efforts to control the crisis caused by illness, acceptability of treatment, needs, and future concerns for the child, as well as implications for facilitating communication.

Dubuque N, Dubuque S: *Kid power tactics for dealing with depression,* King of Prussia, Penn, 1996, The Center for Applied Psychology.
A unique workbook for children written by a mother and son who have first-hand experience in coping with depression.

*Goren S, Curtis W: Staff members' beliefs about seclusion and restraint in child psychiatric hospitals, *J Child Adolesc Psychiatr Nurs* 9:7, 1996.
Findings indicate a low to moderate level of confidence regarding the efficacy, and the use of seclusion and restraint, suggesting the need for an accepted standard for this intervention.

*Richardson L et al: Identification and treatment of children's mental health problems by primary care providers: a critical review of research, *Arch Psychiatr Nurs* 10:293, 1996.
Impressive review of research showing that primary care providers underidentify mental health problems in children and adolescents and that those identified did not receive needed treatment.

Schaefer C, Cangelosi D: *Play therapy techniques,* Northvale, New Jersey, 1993, Jason Arenson.
Serves as a resource book for commonly used play therapy techniques, including which modalities are most effective and practical, how-to advice for using them.

Adolescent Psychiatric Nursing

Audrey Redston-Iselin

© 1998 M.C. Escher/Cordon Art, Baarn, Holland.

I'm so mixed up and lonely Can't even make friends with my brain.
I'm too young to be where I'm going But I'm too old to go back again.

John Prine "Rocky Mountain Time"

LEARNING OBJECTIVES

After studying this chapter the student should be able to:

▼ List the developmental tasks of adolescence
▼ Compare the various theoretical views of adolescence
▼ Identify the major areas that should be included when assessing adolescents
▼ Describe maladaptive responses evident in adolescence
▼ Analyze nursing interventions useful in working with adolescents
▼ Evaluate nursing care provided for adolescents

TOPICAL OUTLINE

Developmental Stage
Theoretical Views of
  Adolescence
  Biological Theory
  Psychoanalytical Theory
  Psychosocial Theory
  Attachment Theory
  Cognitive Theory
  Cultural Theory
  Multidimensional
    Theory
Assessing the Adolescent
  Body Image
  Identity
  Independence
  Social Role
  Sexual Behavior
Maladaptive Responses
  Inappropriate Sexual
    Activity

Unwed Motherhood
Suicide
Runaways
Conduct Disorders
Violence
Drug Use
Hypochondriasis
Weight Problems
Occult Involvement
Parental Divorce
Working with Adolescents
  Health Education
  Family Therapy
  Group Therapy
  Individual Therapy
  Medication Management
  Talking with Adolescents
  Parents of the Adolescent
Evaluating Nursing Care

Adolescence is a time of transition—an age when the person is not yet an adult but is no longer a child. The intense feelings experienced at this time are meaningful and the issues raised during adolescence are central to personal development. Psychiatric nurses treating adolescents focus on their movement toward adulthood, considering social, emotional, and physical aspects of their adjustment in their family, school, and peer groups. These nurses concentrate on helping adolescents move successfully toward adulthood, and they have special expertise in identifying problems in the developmental process and working with support systems to enhance growth.

DEVELOPMENTAL STAGE

Adolescence is a unique stage of development that occurs between the ages of 11 and 20, when a shift in growth and learning occurs. The developmental tasks that emerge during adolescence threaten the person's defenses. They can either stimulate new adaptive ways of coping or lead to regression and maladaptive coping responses. Old problems may interfere with the adolescent's coping abilities, and environmental factors may help or hinder the adolescent's attempts to deal with these issues. Previous coping skills, if used successfully, can promote healthy adaptation and integrated adult functioning.

An earlier, but still popular view of adolescence described it as a time of conflict and upheaval that was necessary for later personality integration. More recent research suggests that this is not true; the complex changes in biological, social, and emotional development do not necessarily lead to psychological conflicts.

During adolescence major events occur, and attempts are made to deal with them. This results in behavior uniquely "adolescent." Havighurst[10] identified the following tasks that should be accomplished during adolescence:

▼ Achieving new and more mature relations with age mates of both sexes

▼ Achieving masculine or feminine social roles
▼ Accepting physical build and using the body effectively
▼ Achieving emotional independence from parents and other adults
▼ Preparing for marriage and family life
▼ Preparing for a career
▼ Acquiring a set of values and an ethical system as a guide to behavior and developing an ideology

Different theories describe these developmental tasks and how their positive resolution moves the adolescent toward adulthood. They will be briefly reviewed and are summarized in Table 37-1.

THEORETICAL VIEWS OF ADOLESCENCE

Biological Theory

One of the most fundamental features of the adolescent period is the series of biological changes known as puberty. These changes transform the young person physically from a child into a reproductively mature adult. This process is a universal feature of human life and is so basic to adolescent development that many people identify puberty as the beginning of adolescence. Puberty involves a set of biological events that produce change throughout the body. The changes fall into two categories: hormonal and somatic. In both sexes, increases in hormone production lead to the development of reproductive capability and a mature physical appearance. Physical changes include pubic hair growth, breast development, and menarche in girls, and genital development, pubic hair growth, voice change, and the emergence of facial hair in boys. A spurt in height and weight occurs in both sexes. Although all adolescents experience the changes of puberty, there are large individual differences in the timing of these changes, as well as the pace at which they take place.

There is substantial evidence that brain growth contin-

TABLE **37-1** *Summary of Theoretical Views of Adolescence*

THEORY	DESCRIPTION
Biological	Emphasis is on physical growth, behavior, and the environment, which influence feelings, thoughts, and actions.
Psychoanalytical	Puberty is called the genital stage, in which sexual interest is awakened. Biological changes upset the balance between the ego and id, and new solutions must be negotiated.
Psychosocial	Adolescents attempt to establish an identity within the social environment. They seek to coordinate self-security, intimacy, and sexual satisfaction in their relationships.
Attachment	Focuses on the quality of attachments as defining one's vulnerability to developmental changes and sees insecure attachments as a risk factor that can result in maladaptive responses to loss or trauma.
Cognitive	Adolescence is an advanced stage of cognition in which the ability to reason goes beyond the concrete to more abstract thinking, described as formal thought.
Cultural	Views adolescence as a time when a person believes that adult privileges are deserved but are withheld. This stage ends when society gives full power and status of an adult.
Multidimensional	Adolescence is seen as adaptation on a continuum of development. There is less emphasis on age and more on the developmental level and timing of biological, psychological, and environmental influences.

ues into adolescence as well. Although the number of neurons does not increase, there is a proliferation of the support cells that brace and nourish the neurons. In addition, growth of the myelin sheath around nerve cell axons continues at least until puberty, enabling faster neural processing. Simultaneously, the number of interconnections between adjacent neurons decreases, probably reflecting the disappearance of redundant or inappropriate neural connections. This fine tuning of the neural system coincides with the development of formal operational thought.

Psychoanalytical Theory

Freud believed that human development was biological and was marked by stages. During puberty (ages 13 to 18), Freud's genital stage, a reawakening of sexual interest occurs. The adolescent with new sexual urges looks for gratification outside the home. This renewal comes from physiological maturing. The genitalia mature, and the release of sex hormones increases. Sexual exploration and maturation often occur. Freud stressed that the first years of life were important in establishing traits that become permanent in adolescence.

More modern psychoanalytical theories define adolescence as the stage between childhood and adulthood correlated with the biological changes of puberty. Increased drives or impulses due to hormones cause a personality reorganization in adolescents as they attempt to adjust to their new physical status. These increased impulses confront a weak ego. Adolescents therefore return to earlier coping skills in an effort to reestablish mastery over the environment.[1]

Psychosocial Theory

The classic psychoanalytical description of adolescence has been modified by Erikson, Sullivan, and others, who emphasize the effect of social factors on these developmental processes. Erikson[7] describes ego identity, or the relationship between a person's self-perception and how a person appears to others. To Erikson, adolescence represents an attempt to establish an identity within the social environment. This search is described as normal adolescent identity crisis. He calls the stage of adolescence identity versus identity diffusion, which is followed in young adulthood by the stage of intimacy versus isolation. He stresses that identity must be established before intimacy can occur.

In Sullivan's[32] developmental model, psychological growth is driven by an integrating tendency that compels people to seek increasingly intimate personal relationships. Sullivan suggests that adolescents strive to coordinate needs of self-security and self-esteem, closeness and intimacy, and general activity and satisfaction of sexual strivings. If these needs become conflicting rather than integrated, emotional problems may result.

Attachment Theory

This theory proposes that attachment is the prominent developmental issue in adolescence.[27] It views development as a process of reorganizing previous personality patterns and structures, and holds that the adolescent's attachments with others play a major role in defining one's vulnerability to developmental changes. In this theory, insecure attachment is a risk factor in the development of adolescents. Autonomous adolescents value attachment relationships and regard experiences with attachment as important. Adolescents who have difficulty with attachments may have experienced rejection in the past or may not have had caretakers who were physically and emotionally available to them. The result is that they may have maladaptive responses to loss or trauma and be insecure in their relationships with others.

> **?** *What problems might adolescents face if they decide to get married as teenagers, and what resources may be helpful to them?*

Cognitive Theory

Cognitive theory views adolescence as an advanced stage of cognitive functioning in which the ability to reason goes beyond concrete objects to symbols or abstractions, or what Piaget called formal thought.[23] Piaget believed that the adolescent has the ability to deal with logic, metaphors, and rational thought. This develops continuously from the concrete thinking of childhood to about age 12, when the concern with realities, tangible objects, and action is transferred to an ideational plane. This allows for conclusions to be made and for reflection to take place without the reality or object being present. Piaget called this ability the logic of operations.

Cultural Theory

Anthropologists who have studied adolescents in different cultures report that primitive cultures have less stressful periods than those experienced by American teenagers and conclude that adolescent rebellion is culturally determined and not biologically based. They view adolescence as a period when the person believes that adult privileges are deserved but are being withheld. It ends when society gives the person the social status of an adult. Anthropologists see growth as a continuous process and a cultural phenomenon, with people reacting to social expectations. The more clearly defined these expectations, the less stressful and ambiguous the adolescent period. The more culture changes, the greater the generation gap becomes.

Several issues in contemporary American society directly influence the support an adolescent can obtain from the environment. Blurring sexual roles is one such issue. Women have less traditional attitudes, expectations, and behaviors. Men have become more involved in functions that were previously believed to be women's, and vice versa. Another social issue is the current concern about the economy. There are fewer jobs, particularly for adolescents. The cost of higher education has increased dramatically, which has resulted in prolonged economic dependency. These changes increase the complexity of society and add new pressures to adolescents, who are becoming adults and attempting to define their role in today's cultural milieu.

Multidimensional Theory

Multidimensional theory proposes that no singular view of adolescent development and mental health exists. Rather, these issues are related to the wide variation in adolescents' social relationships, behaviors, and attitudes and revolve around three main themes[20]:

▼ Profiles of ego and moral development are used to characterize adolescents for rates of progression, regression, and stability in age-related development.

▼ Attention is given to biological, sociological, psychological, and cultural integration. These variables change rapidly during adolescence and affect the adolescent's behavior and view of self.

▼ The developmental issues of both psychological and biological maturation are viewed as affecting the adolescent's adaptation and functioning. For example, the timing of the adolescent's physical development in relation to a peer group has a direct influence on the teenager's self-esteem.

These issues may vary widely, not only individually but also by culture and society.

The multidimensional view of adolescence sees adaptation on a continuum of development. Less emphasis is placed on specific age and more is put on developmental level and the timing of various biological, psychological, and environmental influences. This theory also proposes that severe family conflict need not necessarily occur. Rather, the degree and nature of conflicts change from childhood through adolescence and reflect both the diversity and the functional and dysfunctional aspects of family life.

ASSESSING THE ADOLESCENT

Nursing care of adolescents begins with a thorough assessment of their health status. Data collection by the nurse is based on current and previous functioning in all aspects of an adolescent's life. A variety of approaches and tools may be used,[33] but data collection should include the following information:

▼ Appearance

▼ Growth and development (including developmental milestones)

▼ Biophysical status (illnesses, accidents, disabilities)

▼ Emotional status (relatedness, affect, and mental status, including mood and evidence of thought disorder and suicidal or homicidal ideation)

▼ Cultural, religious, and socioeconomic background

▼ Performance of activities of daily living (home, school, work)

▼ Patterns of coping (ego defenses such as denial, acting out, withdrawal)

▼ Interaction patterns (family, peers, society)

▼ Sexual behaviors (nature, frequency, preference, sexually transmitted diseases)

▼ Use of drugs, alcohol, and other addictive substances (tobacco, caffeine)

▼ Adolescent's perception and satisfaction with health (functional problems or complaints)

▼ Adolescent's health goals (short- and long-term)

▼ Environment (physical, emotional, ecological)

▼ Available human and material resources (friends and school and community involvement)

These data are collected from adolescents and significant others through interviews, examinations, observations, and reports. In addition, the nurse may ask the following questions of the adolescent's family:

▼ What concerns you about your adolescent?

▼ When did these problems start?

▼ What changes have you noticed?

▼ Have the problems been noticed in school as well as home?

▼ What makes the behavior better or worse?

▼ How have these problems affected your adolescent's relationship with you, siblings, peers, and teachers?

▼ Has your adolescent's school performance changed?

One outcome of the nursing assessment should be the identification of teenagers at high risk for problems.[6] Nurses need to understand the difference between constructive and age-appropriate exploration and engagement in activities that are potentially dangerous and threaten the adolescent's physical and emotional well-being. A profile of the high-risk adolescent is presented in Fig. 37-1. A number of factors combine to affect the potential for adolescent risk-taking behavior, including age, socioeconomic status, education, race, gender, self-esteem, autonomy, social adaptation, vulnerability, impulsivity, and thrill-seeking activity.[4] Nurses who work in schools and community settings can engage in screening and early nursing intervention with high-risk teenagers to promote adaptive responses and prevent the development of future problems.

In summary, an examination of typical adolescent behaviors reveals that adolescence is a time of change. The issues of body image, identity, independence, social role, and sexual behavior can produce adaptive or maladaptive responses as the adolescent attempts to cope with the developmental tasks at hand.

? *Many nursing students are adolescents themselves. How might this positively and negatively affect their work with adolescent patients?*

Body Image

Chronological age is not a true guide for physical maturation because growth often occurs in spurts and individual differences exist. Because school classes and extracurricular

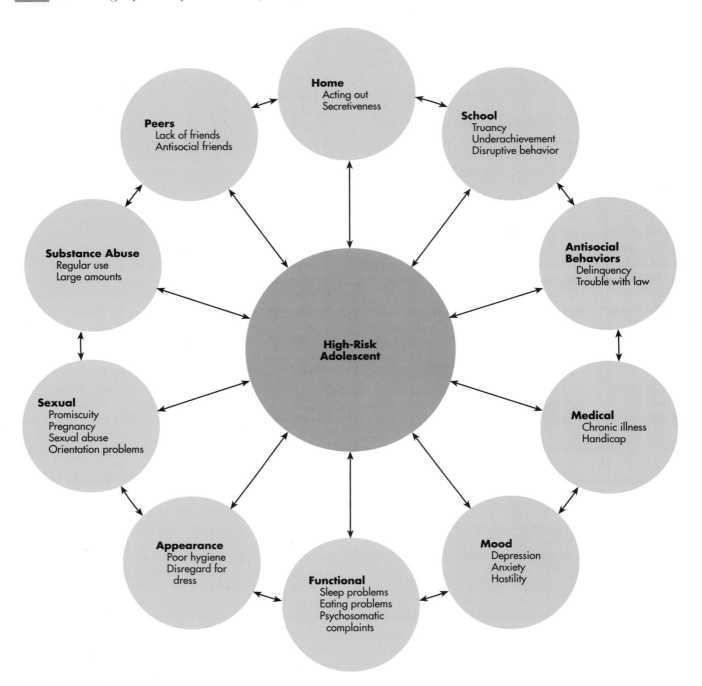

Fig. 37-1 Profile of the high-risk adolescent.

activities are usually grouped by age, the adolescent must face being with others who vary greatly in physical development and interests. This explains why adolescents often imitate behavior as an effort to keep within the expected range of conduct and be compatible with peers. The greater the divergence from the rest of the group, the greater the adolescent's anxiety. The lack of uniformity of growth often puts great demands on physical and mental adaptability. Growth is uneven and sudden, rather than smooth and gradual, and causes a change in body image.

Adolescents reevaluate themselves in light of these physical changes, particularly the onset of primary and secondary sex characteristics, which are so pronounced. They tend to compare themselves and their physical development to that of their peers. They are very concerned about the normality of their physical status. The physical changes of puberty cause adolescents to be self-conscious about their changing bodies. Often they are reluctant to have medical examinations because they fear abnormalities will be found. Examinations may intensify masturbatory conflicts, sexual fantasies, and guilt feelings. The early and middle phases of puberty may also give rise to increased conflict, distance, and dissatisfaction in parental relationships.

Identity

In response to the physical changes of puberty, adolescents experience heightened periods of excitement and tension. They use defenses against these feelings that were helpful in childhood and experiment with new, more adultlike attempts at mastery. Thus in their attempt to cope, adolescents sometimes act like adults and at other times behave like children. For example, adolescents show behavior marked with experimentation and test the self by going to extremes. This can be useful in establishing self-identity. The rebelliousness or negativism of the adolescent shows a movement toward individuation and autonomy that is more complex than but also similar to the 2-year-old's "no." Adolescents may also assert themselves by acting in a negative or contrary manner when relating to parents and other authority figures who they believe are not allowing them to be separate and unique. This is seen in the following clinical example.

Clinical Example Scottie, an avid football fan for several years, suddenly switched his interest to basketball. He quit his local football team despite his father's urgings to continue. His father, also a football fan, could not understand Scottie's sudden negative attitude toward football and newly found interest in basketball.

The individuation process of adolescence is accompanied by feelings of isolation, loneliness, and confusion because it brings childhood dreams to an end and attributes them to fantasy. This realization of childhood's end can create intense fears or panic. Many adolescents attempt to remain in this transitional stage. The awakening of emotional ties with the family also occurs in the establishment of new, more interdependent relationships. This fearful yet exciting entrance into adulthood is a profound experience that is not resolved in adolescence but is confronted throughout life. Adolescents mourn the loss of childhood, and the feelings of loneliness and isolation that accompany this loss create an intense need for closeness, love, and understanding. If they are unable to obtain support during this struggle, depression may result.

Exploratory behavior allows the adolescent to try on new roles and find what fits as identity is formed. Adolescents with poor identity formation are vulnerable for engaging in high-risk behaviors because there is a link between an adolescent's self-concept and the use of adaptive coping responses.[19] Parenting styles that encourage individuality and relatedness to families are associated with support of adolescent identity exploration. Adolescents expressing high levels of identity exploration have parents who express mutuality and separateness, encourage member differences, and are aware of clear boundaries between themselves and their teenagers. These adolescents are also more likely to have competent approaches to peer and social relationships and more developed skills in initiating, diversifying, sustaining, and deepening peer friendships.

Independence

Adolescents have an unconscious longing to give in to their dependency needs. Adolescence is also a time of movement toward independence. Adolescents show this ambivalence by responding to petty annoyances and irritations with intense outbursts. They see the process of gaining independence as being free of parental control. They do not see gaining independence as a gradual learning process but as an emancipation accomplished by acting "differently." If one acts adult, then one is adult. Therefore, they expose themselves to situations beyond their capabilities and then become overwhelmed and frightened. They seek reassurance in an attempt to reduce their anxiety by returning to childlike ways and being dependent on those with whom they feel most secure, usually their parents. This accounts for the inconsistency of adolescent behavior.

Well-adjusted adults usually use a problem-solving approach and do not feel as threatened when inexperience requires dependency on others. However, adolescents who are already tempted to give in to dependency needs feel as if they are regressing to childhood, which deflates their self-esteem. They must deny their need for their parents. Sometimes they criticize their parents for treating them as a child and then remark that their parents are not helpful enough. When adolescents seem to be rebelling against their parents, they may be rebelling against their own childhood conscience or superego. They project their ambivalence onto their parents because they were the original source of restrictions. This projection actually reveals a movement toward a more mature standard and also indicates their insecurity about giving up childhood standards. By blaming their parents for their childish actions, they can avoid blows to their fragile self-esteem and protest that their actions result from parental demands, not their own.

The interaction between adolescent changes in autonomy and family relationships is an important consideration. Three parenting styles have been described in relation to whether they help or hinder independent functioning in adolescence.[24]

▼ Traditional parents tend to value a sense of continuity and order. They accept the patterns of understanding and value judgments that come from previous generations. Adolescents from these families tend to be more attached to their parents, conforming, and achievement oriented. Often they avoid major conflicts in their teenage years.

▼ Authoritarian parents are oriented toward shaping, controlling, and restricting the adolescent to fixed standards. Obedience is seen as a virtue. Power and responsibility are not shared with the adolescent. Harsh discipline is used to curb autonomous strivings that are viewed as willfulness. The approach here is often punitive and it can result in problems with the adolescent's development of autonomy.

▼ Democratic parents do not believe that their standards are always right. They tend to be supportive and respond to the specific situation with solutions that promote the adolescent's autonomy. The environment fostered is one of stimulation and challenge. This parenting style combines limit setting with negotiation, thus encouraging the teenager's participation in the disciplinary process. It is shown to predict greater independent functioning in adolescents.

> ? *Did your parents have a traditional, authoritarian, or democratic parenting style, and what would you do differently in raising children of your own?*

Social Role

Adolescents respond intensely to people and events. They may be totally invested in one interest and then suddenly change to something different. These intense and unstable feelings can account for their extreme sensitivity to the response of others. They are easily hurt, disappointed, and fearful of others. There is a tendency toward hero worship and crushes, but with little evaluation of the people to whom these feelings are directed.

Adolescent relationships serve many functions. Often adolescents relate to a friend as if neither person were a separate individual. They often mimic each other's dress, speech, language, and thoughts. These relationships help in the development of self-identity and establishment of a social role. The peer group is also very important because within the security of the peer group, adolescents can attempt to resolve conflicts. With peers they can test out their thoughts and ideas. Their thoughts may differ, but through mutual sharing, they can try to find an answer. The peer group can also explore other ways of dealing with problems and offer its members companionship, protection, and security. In the peer group, adolescents can accept dependency, not as a child but as one of the gang, testing out ideas and trying new values. Within the safety of the peer group, they can observe, comment on, and evaluate the activities of others. Adolescents usually are very loyal to their group of friends. Sometimes group security is so important that it is pursued at all costs, even if it involves destructive behavior.

Adolescents react to many stimuli and drain off the tension created by new drives and impulses by investment in many interests. They do this with great intensity, which is why adolescents are susceptible to fads. This is often seen in their dress, music, or hobbies. Close relationships with the opposite sex provide adolescents with security (often by "going steady") and a person with whom to discuss problems and evaluate solutions. Often the partner may take on similar characteristics. This reciprocal relationship enhances self-esteem by demonstrating sexual attractiveness to the self and to the world, and it indicates that one is lovable. It also allows for bisexual expression because the girl expresses her partner's feminine parts and her boyfriend represents her masculine parts.

> ? *Think about a current television program that is a favorite among adolescents and describe why it is popular, based on adolescent norms and developmental tasks.*

Sexual Behavior

Adolescents use fantasy to discharge sexual tension. However, they may feel guilt and shame about sexual feelings or fantasies. Fantasies usually are an attempt to find solutions and evaluate consequences. They may indicate a disturbance if they continually occupy the adolescent's thoughts, are not converted into constructive actions, or are not modified by reality. Then they may disrupt other activities important to adolescent functioning and indicate a withdrawal from reality.

Masturbation is another way in which adolescents discharge sexual tension. The value of masturbation may be lessened if shame and guilt accompany it. Male adolescents often fear discovery of evidence of ejaculation, and females often fear changes in their genitalia as a result of masturbation. Fears are not limited to discovery by others. They may also result from the loss of ego boundaries experienced during orgasm. Mutual masturbation can serve the purposes of tension release and fusing of identity. It can help to dispel anxieties about sexuality by assuring adolescents that they are sexually adequate.

Although 5% to 10% of American youth acknowledge homosexual experiences and 5% feel that they could be gay, homosexual experimentation is common during late childhood and early adolescence.[28,31] Experimentation may include mutual masturbation and fondling of the genitals and does not by itself cause or lead to adult homosexuality. Theories about the cause of homosexuality include genetic, hormonal, environmental, and psychological models; however, there is no definitive explanation for causality (see Chapter 26). Thus nurses need to be aware of the following:

▼ Not all homosexual adolescents are sexually active.
▼ Many homosexual adolescents are heterosexually active.
▼ Many heterosexual adolescents are homosexually active.
▼ The relationship between sexual identity and sexual behavior is variable during adolescence.
▼ Sexual issues produce stress and anxiety for adolescents of all sexual orientations.

MALADAPTIVE RESPONSES

Behaviors that impede growth and development may require nursing intervention. The nurse should consider the nature of the adolescent's maladaptive responses and the harm resulting from them.[13] If the difficulty is significant and ongoing, intervention may be needed. Adolescents may also be diagnosed with the various DSM-IV psychiatric illnesses described in Chapters 16 through 26 of this text.[22] The nursing interventions described in these chapters can be implemented with adolescents, as well as the various treatment modalities described in Chapters 27 through 32. Empirically based treatment strategies for adolescents have been identified for clinical practice that take into consideration their particular developmental issues and the unique challenges of establishing a therapeutic alliance with an adolescent.[11,15]

Inappropriate Sexual Activity

Sexual behaviors are the cause of many teenage problems, as evidenced by the facts presented in Table 37-2. Sexual activity is often not as much an outlet for sexual passion as an attempt to achieve closeness with another person. Adolescents tend to use their sexuality to sublimate other needs, such as those of love and security, and personal anxiety about sexual adequacy and peer group pressure may lead the adolescent to have inappropriate sexual relations. For example, some adolescents engage in sexual relations as a means of punishing themselves. Their promiscuity elicits external control and criticism from others. This is especially true when there is an exhibitionistic quality and subtle efforts to "get caught" are seen. This is evident in the following clinical example.

Clinical Example Isabel, a 14-year-old girl, had been sexually active since age 12. She was brought to the clinic by her parents when a neighbor told them Isabel had bragged of her sexual ventures. Two years before referral, her parents had placed her in a more controlled parochial school because they were concerned she was "acting wild." It became apparent that Isabel wanted her parents to know about and put limits on her behavior. She admitted to not enjoying sexual

intercourse very much. She seemed to be trying desperately to get approval from her distant mother. She described her father, who was a policeman, as "a hopeless case," secretly wishing that he would be a better policeman for her.

However, it is important to differentiate between inappropriate behavior and defects in socialization that may result from the absence of an adequate parental role model, physical disabilities, sexual abuse, and personality temperament.

The additional risk of sexually transmitted diseases, including HIV, makes sexual experimentation more problematic because of its potential short-term and long-term effects. Adolescent needs for exploration and sexual gratification, as well as their feelings of invincibility, put them at great risk for HIV infection and other sexually transmitted diseases. Despite educational efforts, many adolescents are misinformed about the transmission of these illnesses and effective preventive strategies. Some believe "it can't happen to me" or think that having only one partner ensures their safety. Unprotected sex is the area of highest risk. Oral, anal, and vaginal contacts all pose a risk because they involve the transfer of body fluids that can contain viruses. Alcohol and drug use increases the risk potential of adolescents because they are more likely to have unplanned sex and not use a condom, and in the case of drug use, there is the additional risk from contaminated needles.

The nurse must explore the meaning of the adolescent's sexual behavior by asking the following questions:

▼ Does the adolescent desire sexual gratification or punishment?
▼ Do the adolescent's goals match the situation, or is self-deception present?
▼ Is the adolescent demanding adult privileges while acting irresponsible and dependent?
▼ To what extent is the sexual behavior experimentation, a defense against depression, or a way of expressing anger toward others?
▼ Is the sexual behavior a way to avoid anxiety-producing fantasies?
▼ How close is the relationship to a mature one?

Interventions related to sexual responses are discussed in Chapter 26 and care of the patient with HIV/AIDS is discussed in Chapter 40.

Unwed Motherhood

Pregnancy in adolescence is a complicated issue. Some adolescent girls have low self-esteem and fears of inadequacy. To ease these fears, they may become pregnant. Sometimes pregnancy is an effort to escape a difficult family situation or to force the parents to agree to a marriage that may be inappropriate, as shown in the following clinical example.

Clinical Example Susie, a 15-year-old girl, had run away for the second time, only to return home to the same chaos. She had tried to run away with her boyfriend. Her alcoholic mother and angry 19-year-old brother were making life un-

---

TABLE **37-2** *Adolescent Reproductive Health Issues*

▼ Once every 10 seconds, a teenager has sexual intercourse for the first time.
▼ One third of all males and one fourth of all females have had sexual intercourse by age 15.
▼ Once every 104 seconds, a teenager becomes pregnant.
▼ Almost 60% of those who become teenage mothers are living in poverty when they deliver.
▼ Over $120 billion of public money was associated with teenage pregnancy between 1985 and 1990.
▼ It is estimated that consistent and appropriate condom use among teenagers is as low as 10% to 20%.
▼ Adolescents have the highest rates of human papilloma virus, chlamydial cervicitis, other sexually transmitted diseases and hospitalization for pelvic inflammatory diseases.
▼ AIDS is the leading killer of adults aged 24 to 45, many of whom became infected with HIV as adolescents.
▼ Once every 9 hours a person under the age of 24 dies of AIDS.

bearable. Her mother was surprised to learn about 3 months after her return that Susie was pregnant. Susie was delighted because she had hopes that she could get out of the house, knowing her mother would now approve of her marriage to her boyfriend.

Occasionally, emotionally deprived adolescents hope to give their child what they believe they have never received (or, perhaps more accurately, receive from the child what they have not received). Sometimes pregnancy appears to be a way to allow parents to give up parental responsibility for the adolescent. In other cases the adolescent has lived out a scapegoat role as the bad one in the family, thereby justifying parental neglect and hostility. The pregnancy can then improve family relationships because, with the adulthood the pregnancy implies, parents may be freed of guilt and may not need to encourage the adolescent to act in ways that make her unlovable.

Pregnancy in adolescence may have other origins. It can occur accidentally after sexual exploration. The adolescent may be unaware of contraceptive methods or may have delayed obtaining contraceptives. Research suggests that most teenage girls delay seeking contraceptives and become pregnant either because they are unwilling or unable to make conscious decisions about their sexual and contraceptive behavior or because they do not mind becoming pregnant.[6] Thus regular contraceptive use among sexually active adolescents requires that they believe that they can become pregnant and that using contraceptives is safe and the only way to prevent pregnancy. They must also have access to reliable, affordable contraceptives and must have a positive self-concept that allows them to make conscious decisions about their sexual and contraceptive behavior. Finally, they must want to postpone childbearing.

Pregnancy for unmarried adolescents may also be associated with sexual promiscuity. If it is, the girl may be ostracized. Sometimes pregnancy occurs within a close, caring relationship. Peer groups can be supportive to a girl who becomes pregnant as a result of a meaningful relationship but intolerant of one whose pregnancy is the result of promiscuity. Both the circumstances and the adolescent's level of maturity need to be assessed. In some cultures, out-of-wedlock pregnancies are an accepted part of adolescence.

Decisions involving abortion, placement of the baby, and marriage are difficult. Attitudes and laws influencing these decisions are diverse. Many believe that to force the adolescent to have the baby and then give the infant up is more traumatic for her than abortion. Others believe that abortion can be more disturbing. Marriage is another alternative. Forcing a marriage to avoid societal stigma usually adds to the adolescent's problems, but a mature couple might do well in marriage. All the alternatives should be presented to the adolescent, with the consequences clearly stated. The adolescent should make her decision with the aid and support of her partner, her family, the nurse, and other involved health-care professionals.

> ? *Pregnancy among adolescents is increasing in the United States. Why is this, and what, if anything, should be done about it?*

Suicide

Suicide is the second leading cause of death among adolescents and the suicide rate for people 15 to 24 years of age has more than tripled in the past 30 years. Adolescent suicide completers use firearms, hanging, jumping, carbon monoxide, and drug overdose. Males 15 to 19 years of age are nearly five times more likely to kill themselves than females in the same age group, although female adolescents attempt suicide two to three times more often than their male counterparts. Although adolescent suicide victims are more likely to be white than black, the rate for black and other minority males has increased markedly since 1986.[30] Depression has been shown to be significantly related to suicidal behavior, as have diagnoses of conduct disorder and bipolar disorder. Finally, findings from research studies indicate that only 25 to 33% of adolescent suicide completers have ever received mental health treatment.[14]

One of the most common factors in adolescent suicide is lack or loss of a meaningful relationship. Many researchers think suicide is an attempt for attention and does not necessarily represent a true desire to die. Regardless, it is a bid for help that must be recognized. Subtle references, as well as attempts, should always be taken seriously and explored. Suicidal gestures are more often seen in girls, with boys expressing their depression by bravado that results in accidents, as in the following clinical example. It is often difficult to distinguish between risk-taking behavior, accidents, and suicidal gestures, thus requiring a careful nursing assessment.

Clinical Example John, a 12-year-old depressed adolescent, had just gotten a dirt bike. Six months earlier John's grandfather, his only friend, had died. John's father had died when he was 2 years old, and he had lived with his mother and grandparents ever since. John, feeling hopeless, had ridden his bike into a car. After medical treatment for his broken arm and rib and multiple bruises, John began to receive therapy. He described feeling helpless and lonely, especially without his grandfather.

Parent-adolescent relationships can influence suicidal behavior.[3] For example, the adolescent may be prevented from acting on suicidal feelings by parental concern and the establishment of new relationships. In contrast, feelings of helplessness and worthlessness can be caused by threatened abandonment, being asked to take the adult role, and lack of opportunities to be dependent. Sometimes these adolescents perceive themselves to be expendable because they believe that the family unconsciously wishes them dead.

The nurse must make it clear to the adolescent that suicidal behavior is not confidential and that parents must be told. Family involvement is essential to avoid angry, hostile, and hopeless feelings of abandonment and to create support and caring.

In working with suicidal adolescents, the nurse should explore the following areas:

▼ The seriousness of the attempt
▼ The mental status of the adolescent
▼ The extent of environmental stress, especially family problems
▼ The adolescent's wider social environment and the strength of support systems (social isolation, school performance, parental loss, disruption of friendship or romantic alliance)
▼ The likelihood of repeated suicidal attempts, especially if conditions remain the same

Nursing interventions related to suicide are described in detail in Chapter 20. The next two clinical examples illustrate suicide attempts by adolescents.

Clinical Example   Maria, a 15-year-old girl, was referred to her local community mental health center from the neighborhood emergency room after ingesting pills. Maria had taken five of her mother's "arthritis pills" after an argument with her father about her 17-year-old boyfriend, José. Her father, who came home only on weekends, told her to stay away from him. After he left, the other family members noticed that Maria became sleepy while playing cards in the living room. Maria admitted to taking the pills and was rushed by her mother to the emergency room.

She had performed poorly in school in the year since her father had left the family. Maria had always been her father's favorite. When she reached puberty at age 13, that relationship changed. Maria's position as her father's favorite was delegated to a younger female sibling, causing Maria to feel angry and rejected. Her father left the family a year later and returned for weekend visits, during which he mainly disciplined the children. Maria's attempt to get close to José as a replacement for her father was sabotaged by her father as well. She thought her only recourse was to elicit her father's caring and concern through a suicide attempt.

Clinical Example   Donald, age 13, was brought to the emergency room after cutting his wrists one evening when he thought his family was asleep. His mother had awakened and found him bleeding. She rushed him to the local emergency room, where he received medical treatment. It was then revealed that this was Donald's second suicide attempt. The first attempt occurred a year ago, when he ingested pills. Donald had received therapy for about a month. It was then discontinued because the family moved to a new location, despite recommendations to continue with a new therapist. Donald was always an isolated child. He was never very close with anyone but had two friends. Since the move he had become more withdrawn. He had done well in school in the past but now had given up and was failing almost every subject. The youngest of nine children, Donald had little contact with his siblings, who were all older than he and not at home much. Donald's parents, both ap-

proaching old age, seemed not to notice that he had become increasingly upset. Donald was hospitalized because the risk of his attempting suicide again was high.

Runaways

The number of adolescents who run away or are forced from their homes and become homeless is growing. Many of these young people have left or been forced from dysfunctional or abusive families only to face a life on the streets that can bring more problems such as poverty, substance abuse, physical and sexual assault, pregnancy, injury or illness, HIV infection, psychological and emotional problems, trouble with the law, and suicide. In addition, their prospects for a healthy and productive adulthood are reduced by the health risks they face and the lack of educational and employment opportunities for homeless youth.

Running away might be a cry for help or an attempt to escape from an unbearable living situation, including child abuse and family violence.[16] It is sometimes a solution for an unmotivated youth who has little self-direction, drive, or ambition, and conduct disorder and severe aggression are common among runaway and homeless youth.[2] Finally, it is common in inner cities, where an unknown number of older children and adolescents move among the homes of friends or relatives, the streets, and abandoned buildings. Usually victims of poverty and overburdened single-parent homes, these teenagers may have had little opportunity to gain any sense of security or loving discipline or to have a vision of a hopeful future.

Adolescent runaways often have been rejected by their parents since birth, and the parent may alternate between extreme punitive measures and a laissez-faire attitude toward the adolescent. Adolescent runaways are often conflicted, especially regarding dependence and independence, and feel embarrassed, helpless, and defeated by their dependency wishes. This can result in a panic that motivates running away to prove autonomy and escape painful circumstances. They usually run away from disappointment toward something viewed as favorable and supportive. Parents often feel guilty and ashamed and have difficulty acting on practical issues, although some, relieved of their responsibility, are secretly pleased. Often the adolescent becomes involved in dangerous activities after running away. Most runaway adolescents want to return home if they believe their parents really want them. The following clinical example illustrates home conditions that may lead to an adolescent's running away.

Clinical Example   Karen, age 14, ran away from home to a friend's house. Her mother had often expressed a desire to leave; in fact, she had once left the family to the charge of Karen's father when Karen was 9 years old. Karen's mother had suddenly told her she could not see her boyfriend for a month because she had come in late the night before. This caused a tremendous scene because Karen had been out late every night the week before without her mother even noticing. Karen's friend's mother was different. She spent a lot of money on her children, talked to them, and never limited their activity; thus, the friend's home appeared attractive to Karen.

> ❓ *How would you design a community-based program to prevent adolescents from running away from home?*

Conduct Disorders

Adolescents with conduct disorders display behavior that violates the basic rights of others or societal norms and rules. Examples include fighting, cruelty, lying, truancy, and destroying property. Conduct-disordered adolescents often have poor relationships with their parents. Antisocial acts allow the adolescent to express anger toward parents, who are often punished for the adolescent's acts. Children are socialized mainly by their parents and, it is hoped, learn from their parents' acceptable behaviors that become part of the internalized self or conscience. A good relationship between parent and child facilitates this process.

However, adolescents learn not only from their parents but also from others. The school and peer groups are influencing factors, as are the social, economic, and cultural environments. The self-destructive behaviors seen in conduct-disordered adolescents may indicate the need for punishment, anger at the family, peer group pressure, depression, feelings of self-defeat, a search for opportunities to take what they feel emotionally deprived of, and testing omnipotence through exciting experiences. Alignment with delinquents gives a defeated adolescent a feeling of self-respect and companionship through a sense of belonging to a subculture.

Clinical Example Levar, 13 years of age, was referred by the juvenile court for therapy because he had been picked up for the second time after breaking into a store with another boy. Levar's parents were separated for the past 2 years, after his father served a sentence in jail for possession of drugs. Levar was extremely upset when his parents separated and rarely saw his father. His antisocial acts caused his father to become more involved with him because his father claimed he did not want his son to go through what he had experienced in prison. Levar gained his father's attention during these times, even though his father was angry. His delinquent actions enabled Levar to express his anger at his father's leaving, as well as to fantasize about having his father return.

This clinical example illustrates the many factors that may lead to adolescent delinquency. Adolescents may not differentiate between their stealing and their parent's business dealings. Stealing may also be an effective way to rebel against parents. Adolescents may perpetuate childhood by indulging in immediate gratification through stealing rather than working for things. Sometimes adolescents steal in hopes of getting caught and obtaining help. Parents may consciously or unconsciously condone stealing. Adolescents may also act out their anger with the justification that they deserve the stolen items.

Finally, the conflict of dependence and independence can be expressed in poor school adjustment. Some adolescents view teachers as parental surrogates who do not help or who merely apply rules of attendance and homework. Dependent feelings are sometimes elicited by these rules, and adolescents, in proving their independence, may become negative about learning. They may think that schoolwork is secondary to more important activities they are attempting to master. Daydreaming may interfere with schoolwork as adolescents concentrate on and fantasize about achieving independence.

Adolescents may drop out of school for financial reasons, or they may be rebelling against education laws. The adolescent may be part of a peer group that denounces school attendance and involvement. Parents may overtly or covertly discourage education. This is conveyed through lack of support and approval for education or by their making it difficult for the adolescent to follow through with school expectations, as illustrated by the following clinical example.

Clinical Example Debbie, a 15-year-old girl, dropped out of school after several years of poor school performance and truancy. She occasionally went shopping with her mother on a school day. Her mother never knew the names of her teachers or guidance counselor, and did not provide her with a place or time to study.

Violence

Most adolescents displaying aggression have experienced frustration and have had violent role models during their childhood. Aggression is a human impulse that must be channeled constructively by a learned process that occurs within a supportive, loving relationship. Under favorable conditions, a child learns the healthy expression of aggression by involvement in activities that result in pleasure and active problem-solving attempts. Under less favorable conditions, aggression can result in destructive activities that are harmful to self and others. Violence can also be a maladaptive way of coping with adolescent anxiety and frustration, as evident in a "rage response."

However, not all violence in adolescence comes from violent impulses. Many teenagers are violent because of periods of overstimulation or strong desires for emotional contact. Empathic responses are most helpful with these teenagers. Some adolescents express hostility and violence to others who fail to live up to their idealized expectations. They try to rebuild a disintegrating self by turning the violent attack into a psychic victory.[17]

Much anxiety of adolescents is related to the fear that they may be unable to control their destructive aggression.

Adolescents often have violent dreams and fantasies that they express in threats, even though in some the potential for violence is minimal. Pointing out the harmlessness of these thoughts is helpful to adolescents because it shows them that these thoughts are not as powerful as they fear. However, some adolescents are genuinely fearful that they will be unable to stop their thoughts from becoming actions. They require the recognition of their fear and the reassurance of external limits. Pointing out to the adolescent the necessity of self-responsibility and control is very important. Their defenses against aggressive outbursts should be reinforced and supported. Focus should be on the behavior and feared loss of control, not on the roots of the anger. The following clinical example illustrates the management of a violent adolescent.

Clinical Example Ricky was a 14-year-old boy referred for treatment for violent outbursts at home. When frustrated, he would break and destroy objects in his path. Ricky was an only child, adopted shortly after birth by a couple in their forties who were unable to have children. Now Ricky's parents, who were about 55 years of age, were increasingly frightened by his aggressive outbursts. They had also felt powerless with his childhood temper tantrums and had consistently responded to outbursts by attempting to limit frustrating situations. They felt guilty and inadequate about his being an adopted child and continually made attempts to reassure Ricky of their love for him. They consequently reinforced his lack of control by assuming that these outbursts were results of his fear of being unloved and would offer gifts and rewards to make peace. Ricky assumed he was omnipotent, successfully controlling his parents, but was afraid that he could not control his anger. Acknowledging Ricky's fear of loss of control, applying external controls, and pointing out areas of Ricky's ability for responsibility and control resulted in a gradual decrease in outbursts.

Adolescents who have committed extreme acts of violence or homicide are often from families in which violence is the norm. These adolescents may have experienced physical or sexual abuse, as described in Chapter 39, or they may have witnessed violence between their parents. Behavior toward them has often alternated between seductiveness and physical brutality, adding to the adolescent's confusion and arousing intense frustration. Often these adolescents are encouraged to be violent. Sometimes parents can predict the adolescent's ability to injure or kill. Often there is a history of dangerous assaults on family members and pets. In severely violent adolescents, violent acts can be followed by a calmness and lack of sorrow or guilt, or they may claim that outside forces provoked them. Many homicidal adolescents freely discuss their violent plans or fears. These should be explored and homicidal intent evaluated. Does the adolescent have a victim, weapons, or a plan? This information,

along with the history, shows the level of success or failure in controlling feelings and delaying gratification.

 What do you think society can do to decrease gang violence among adolescents in this country?

Drug Use

Nationwide, drug use and abuse is a significant problem for adolescents (Fig. 37-2). The 1993 survey of US high school students reported a sharp rise in marijuana use in eighth-, tenth-, and twelfth-grade students. In addition, there were significant increases in stimulant, LSD, and inhalant use at all three grade levels.[12] Of greatest concern was that the survey noted decreased perceived dangers and decreased disapproval of people using illicit substances.

Alcohol is the most commonly used and abused substance by youth. Nearly all high school seniors report some experience with alcohol. Although not all youth who drink have a drinking problem, nearly one third of seniors report being intoxicated in the past 30 days. Higher levels of adolescent alcohol use are associated with the three most frequent forms of mortality among adolescents: accidental deaths, homicides, and suicides. Nearly 9 out of 10 teenage automobile accidents involve the use of alcohol. Risk factors for adolescent alcohol use are presented in Table 37-3.[6] Alcohol use has also been characterized as a gateway substance, preceding the use of marijuana and then other illegal substances such as cocaine and heroin.

The onset of drug use before age 20 predicts more sustained use over time. From 70 to 90% of males and 50 to 60% of females who abused drugs in adolescence continue to do so in adult life. Chemical dependency is the result of a gradual process. Table 37-4 presents the stages of adolescent substance abuse. It is important for the nurse to remember that not all adolescents progress through these stages, but the younger the user, the greater the risk for chemical dependency. Substance abuse is discussed in detail in Chapter 24.

The meaning of drug use in adolescence is a complex question. The adolescent's motivation must be explored. The nurse must keep in mind that it may be an expression of rebelliousness with support of a peer group, as well as a way of obtaining gratification. It may also indicate an effort to come to grips with feelings of vulnerability and emptiness.

Adolescents often report a wish for closeness that is satisfied by sharing a drug experience with friends. Drug users can experience an illusion of closeness because drugs decrease anxiety and users can share anticipation of drug use. Some adolescents fill the void of isolated loneliness with drugs and would otherwise feel suicidally depressed. Drugs can be crippling and delay healthy maturity by promoting the avoidance of developing an adult identity in a real world, as illustrated in the following clinical example.

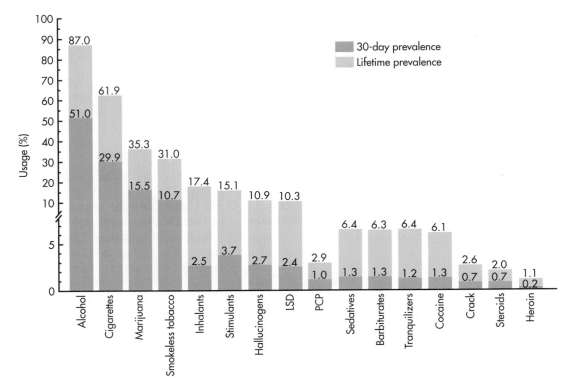

Fig. 37-2 Percentage of high school seniors reporting substance use. (Data obtained from Johnston LD, O'Malley PM, Bachman JG: *National survey results on drug use from the Monitoring the Future study, 1975-1993*, vol 1, Rockville, Md, 1994, National Institute on Drug Abuse.)

TABLE **37-3** *Risk Factors for Adolescent Alcohol Use*

RISK FACTOR	EXAMPLE
SOCIETAL-COMMUNITY	
Laws and normative behavior	Encouragement of youthful drinking in the media, absence of legal enforcement of underage drinking.
Availability	Easy access via the home or adults (such as siblings) purchasing liquor for minors.
Extreme economic deprivation	Escapist drinking to cope with harsh realities of everyday life.
Neighborhood disorganization	Undermine sense of security and purpose in life.
SCHOOL	
Low commitment to school	School expectations and career expectations very low.
Academic failure	Poor attendance, poor grades, underachievement.
Early persistent behavior problems	High aggression, attentional problems.
FAMILY	
Family members alcohol users (abusers)	Role modeling influences.
Family management practices	Failure to monitor children; inconsistent parenting practices or harsh discipline.
Family conflict	Marital dysfunction or partner violence.
Low bonding to family	Lack of reciprocal nurturing and open communication.
PEERS	
Peer rejection in elementary grades	Rejection or neglect by peers undermines positive self-concept.
Associating with alcohol-using peers	Peer selection fosters cycles of negative behaviors.
Friends with attitudes favorable to alcohol use	Peer selection fosters cycles of negative attitudes and beliefs.
INDIVIDUAL	
Physiological	Genetic susceptibility to alcohol via enhanced tension reduction or misjudgment about level of intoxication.
Alienation and rebelliousness	Removed from normative attitudes and values of society and commitments toward societal goals.
Early-onset deviant behavior	Early-onset deviant behaviors consolidate and perpetuate negative spiraling cycles.
Problem-solving coping skills	Absence of strong problem-solving skills may contribute to adaptation of less desirable negotiating strategies (such as an aggressive coercive interpersonal style).

TABLE **37-4** *The Five Stages of Substance Abuse in Youth*

STAGE	DRUGS	SOURCES	FREQUENCY	FEELINGS	BEHAVIOR	TREATMENT
1. Curiosity	None	Available but not used	—	Curiosity	Risk taking, desire for acceptance	Optimal time, anticipatory guidance to develop good coping skills and strong self-esteem, clear family guidelines on drug and alcohol use, drug education
2. Experimentation	Tobacco, alcohol, marijuana	House supply, friends, siblings	Weekend use for recreational purposes	Excitement, pleasure, few consequences; learning how easy it is to feel good	Lying, little change	Drug education; attention to societal messages; reduction of supply; strict, loving rules at home; establishment of drug-free alternative activities
3. Regular use	As above, plus hashish or hash oil, tranquilizers, sedatives, amphetamines	Buying	Progresses to midweek use; purpose is to get high	Excitement followed by guilt	Mood swings, faltering school performance, truancy, changing peer groups, changing style of dress	Drug-free self-help groups (Alcoholics or Narcotics Anonymous), family involvement, psychiatric counseling unhelpful unless family therapy and aftercare provided
4. Psychological or physical dependency	As above, plus stimulants, hallucinogens	Selling to support the habit, possibly stealing or prostitution in exchange for drugs	Daily	Euphoric highs followed by depression, shame, guilt and perhaps suicidal thoughts	Pathologic lying; school failure; family fights; involvement with the law over curfew, truancy, vandalism, shoplifting, driving under the influence, breaking and entering, violence	Inpatient or foster care programs that require family involvement and provide aftercare
5. Using drugs to feel "normal"	As above; any available drug, including opiates	Any way possible	All day	Euphoria rare and harder to achieve; chronic depression	Drifting, with repeated failures and psychological symptoms of paranoia and aggression; frequent overdosing, blackouts, amnesia; chronic cough, fatigue, malnutrition	Inpatient or foster care programs that require family involvement and provide aftercare

Modified from MacDonald D: *Pediatr Rev* 10:89, 1988.

Clinical Example Carlos was a 16-year-old boy who had been school phobic since age 10. He had been receiving home instruction since that age and was referred for a yearly assessment to obtain approval for a continuation of home instruction services. Carlos proudly spoke of his drug episodes. He and his small group of friends were close and had many exciting experiences induced by various hallucinogens and amphetamines. Carlos had little support in the real world because he had been isolated at home and developed interpersonal relationships primarily by obtaining drugs and experiencing their effects.

> **?** *You're concerned about your best friend's increasing use of drugs, but she denies that it is a problem. How can you best help her?*

Hypochondriasis

Adolescents are preoccupied with their bodies and body sensations. They are uncomfortable with their bodies because of the rapid changes in size, shape, and functioning. To establish their identity, adolescents try to become familiar with their changing bodies. They respond to sensations with increased intensity. When an adolescent appears overly concerned, it may indicate underlying difficulties in formation of self-image.

Hypochondriasis occurs when the adolescent has intense anxiety about personal health. This anxiety may be diffuse or directed toward one specific area. Adolescents' concern that their bodies are inadequate, that they will be rejected by others, or that they are unable to reach adulthood may predominate. Hypochondriasis may be a way of avoiding activities that expose these and other stressful fears. Fears such as inadequacy at school, either socially or in schoolwork, may be a projection of general fears of inadequacy. Lack of knowledge of normal body changes may be a simple precipitating factor. This can be tackled by reassurance that these changes are normal. If reassurance does not alleviate anxiety, more intense fears may be involved.

It is important to communicate to adolescents that people are aware something is wrong and that their concerns will be taken seriously until the core problem is alleviated. Intense body concern is a signal that something is wrong and help is needed. Physical status must be assessed first before a psychological basis for concern is assumed. Sometimes body preoccupation is an effort to recreate childhood dependency by eliciting caregiving. This is particularly seen in adolescents who experienced early emotional deprivation, as shown in the following clinical example.

Clinical Example John, age 12, was referred for treatment from the local hospital after having been seen for chest pains. The physician found no medical problems. John was embarrassed and angry about the episode, insisting that the physician was wrong. The chest pains had disappeared, but he now had injured his arm. He also was often plagued by attacks of tonsillitis and middle ear infections. John had experienced early emotional deprivation because he was often moved around in his living arrangements. He was born out of wedlock and lived occasionally with his mother, often with his maternal grandmother, and infrequently with his father. He generally had the feeling that no one really cared for him. Further exploration revealed that John's body concerns were vocalized to initiate caregiving by those around him, who, he feared, really were not there for him. He performed well in school and had friends, but none of these compensated for his feelings of inadequacy.

Weight Problems

Eating disorders are another group of problems often seen in adolescence. They include anorexia nervosa, bulimia nervosa, and obesity. The sociocultural milieu for female adolescents in the United States has precipitated identity and body image confusion and anxiety in this age group. The emphasis on thinness, athletics, and physical attractiveness suggests that these are highly valued achievements for young women. These traits demonstrate self-control and social success and are culturally rewarded. The result is that fear of fat, restrained eating, binge eating, and body image distortion are common problems among teenage girls.

Recent understandings suggest that eating disorders represent a complex of issues related to many possible causes. Psychodynamics, family characteristics, physiology, and biochemical interactions all play a part in the development and treatment of these disorders. They are discussed in detail in Chapter 25. The following clinical example illustrates the development of anorexia nervosa in a young girl.

Clinical Example Janet, age 15, was admitted to the hospital because it was feared that her extreme weight loss was endangering her life. Exploration revealed that Janet was afraid of her sexual feelings and the response of others to her budding sexuality. Her father, provocative and teasing toward Janet, was continually kidding her about her oncoming sexual attractiveness and implied that he really preferred her to her mother. This created panic, and Janet refused to eat. She liked her thinness, which was a protection from sexual desires. In the hospital, the area of concentration was not the behavior of not eating, but rather the underlying feelings about her sexuality and her relationship with her father. This provided freedom for normal sexual growth and development.

Occult Involvement

Adolescent risk-taking behavior is also evident in the involvement of teenagers in the occult.[8] People particularly prone to this involvement tend to be alienated from their family, be socially isolated, and have poor skills for interacting with others. They are cognitively curious and seek attention; they have their own belief system and are attracted to the bizarre. They are often negative, fatalistic, sensation seeking, and poor judges of danger, and have low self-esteem. They rely on superstition to deal with their feelings of powerlessness and their fear of making decisions. In this way, their belief system establishes a sense of control for them. These adolescents depend on external rewards to make them feel good, and they conjure up spells to help them make decisions.

Satanism, the worship of Satan, is the dark side of the occult. Satanists do not necessarily believe in a personal devil, but rather that Satan symbolizes evil. Witchcraft includes a variety of magic, with the goal of manipulating the spirits to do the will of humans. Astrology uses the earth-centered view of the solar system to interpret the influence of the heavenly bodies on human affairs. Witchcraft and astrology can be used for good or evil purposes.

Adolescent behaviors that are often associated with involvement in the occult include the following:

▼ Sleep disturbances, including insomnia and nightmares
▼ Suicidal ideation with overwhelming feelings of guilt
▼ Chemical dependency and drug use
▼ Voyeurism, nudity, and sexual activity that includes thrill seeking
▼ Feelings of learned helplessness
▼ Excessive fantasy role play, including Dungeons and Dragons and various computer games
▼ Ritualistic use of objects such as knives and black clothing
▼ Strong preference for heavy metal music with hidden messages that ridicule society

Family systems that predispose adolescents to participate in occult practices may have unresolved conflicts and may use distancing to solve problems. A tolerance for deviance and a disengaged family structure may be present. Often the family structure has recently changed because of death or crisis. The adolescent's peer relations are often characterized by isolation and peer group rejection. Involvement in the occult therefore provides the teenager with an opportunity for acceptance. Environmental factors may include frequent exposure to the supernatural in movies, books, and games. These suggest magical solutions to life's problems. Finally, the adolescent may experience a disenchantment with formal religion and contempt for social norms and values.

Parental Divorce

Nearly one fourth of all children and adolescents in the United States live in single-parent homes. Nearly half of all youngsters born in the past decade will experience a parental divorce. The effect of divorce on children varies with the child's age and developmental level. Adolescents are particularly vulnerable, and their initial reactions include depression, anger, and identification of one parent as the victim and rejection of the other. Over time, adolescents may become anxious or pessimistic about their own future in-

volvement in intimate relationships. However, some adolescents become more mature and independent in perceiving that they have helped their parents in this time of crisis.

The most favorable outcome of divorce is seen when the divorced parents are able to put aside old conflicts and anger and return to meaningful caretaking relationships with their children. The adolescent's adaptation is also influenced by the amount of relief the divorce provides from predivorce marital strife and the young person's own emotional strengths, vulnerabilities, coping resources, and support systems. Major goals in the treatment of adolescents of divorced parents include helping the adolescent[29]:

▼ Grieve the loss of the family unit
▼ Maintain distance from parental conflicts
▼ Express age-appropriate involvement in developmental tasks
▼ Decrease anger, anxiety, depression, and acting out
▼ Assess both parents realistically
▼ Improve communication with both parents
▼ Continue the separation-individuation process
▼ Control overly aggressive and sexual drives

 How might growing up in a single-parent household positively and negatively affect an adolescent?

WORKING WITH ADOLESCENTS

Knowledge of normal adolescent development is necessary to differentiate between age-expected behavior and maladaptive responses. Although there is some controversy over whether adolescent turmoil is normal (see Critical Thinking about Contemporary Issues), studies suggest that professionals view normal adolescents as being more disturbed than they really are.

When dealing with an adolescent, it is advisable for the nurse to have an initial contact directly with the adolescent. Many adolescents are concerned that the nurse is aligned with the parents. Other adolescents take a passive role, letting the adults straighten things out for them. By initiating contact with the adolescent, the nurse aligns with the patient's independent, mature aspects. Parents asking for advice on how to approach the adolescent about seeking treatment should be advised to be honest, stating the true nature of the visit and their reasons for requesting it. Many agencies and institutions use a child guidance approach, seeing the parents first to obtain a full developmental history. Family sessions have also been used in diagnostic evaluation, helping to reveal family interaction and later being helpful in establishing family support.

Health Education

The psychiatric nurse is in an excellent position to educate the adolescent, the parents, and the community. Basic health information can be given in such areas as drugs, sex

CRITICAL THINKING *about* Contemporary Issues

Is Adolescent Turmoil Normal?

Although it is a commonly held belief that adolescence is a time of conflict and turmoil, research disputes the notion that teenagers must experience a difficult adolescence.[24] Nonetheless, nurses should not underestimate the severity of adolescent problems. The National Adolescent Student Health Survey of more than 11,000 eighth and tenth graders in 20 states revealed many threats to the health and well-being of teenagers[5]:

- 56% of students did not wear a seat belt the last time they rode in a car and 44% rode with a driver who had used alcohol or drugs before driving.
- 50% of the boys and 25% of the girls had been involved in at least one physical fight in the past year.
- 25% of the girls reported that someone had tried to force them to have sex in the past year.
- 23% of the boys carried a knife at least once in the past year and 7% carried one daily.
- 42% of the girls and 23% of the boys reported having seriously considered suicide at some time during their lives.
- 60% of the girls had dieted during the past year, 16% had used diet pills, 12% had induced vomiting, and 8% had used laxatives.

and contraception, suicide prevention, and crime prevention. A recent nursing research study found that adolescents wanted information about what activities were healthy and unhealthy, including facts about exercise, nutrition, and expressing feelings. The barriers they perceived to receiving health-care services included not enough money, inconvenient schedules, not wanting parents to know about it, lack of transportation, and not being aware of available resources.[25] The nurse can also provide information on healthy emotional functioning. Defining adolescent mental health is a difficult task, but two dimensions of positive mental health have been identified for adolescents[21]: coping with stress and anxiety and pursuing personally meaningful activities. Coping with stress includes:

- Skills and motivation to manage acute, major life stressors and recurring daily stressors
- Skills to solve problems (problem-focused coping) and skills for emotion management (emotion-focused coping)
- Personal flexibility and the ability to meet the demands of varying types of stress

Involvement in personally meaningful activities includes:

- Skills and motivation to engage in instrumental and expressive activities that are personally meaningful
- Behaviors and activities that are experienced as autonomous and self-determined

By educating them on normal adolescent behavior and by interpreting the underlying conflicts, the nurse prepares parents, teachers, and other community members to support

adolescents and encourage healthy independent functioning. Often parents and other adults become frustrated, angry, and confused by the independent strivings of adolescents. Encouraging independence and lessening power struggles can produce a positive change in adolescents' relationships with adults and in their feelings about themselves.[26] However, adults should still set limits. Setting limits and providing structure can be done in a way that encourages the adolescent's independent functioning. Many parents are conflicted about their children becoming adults. This, together with the adolescent's own ambivalence and fears about independence, can create havoc.

One of the best ways to educate parents on adolescent development is through a parents' group. The nurse can inform parents on normal adolescent functioning and provide them with much needed support from other parents in the same situation. Sharing mutual experiences and searching for solutions in a supportive environment can be extremely helpful to parents. It is important to remember that parents have nurtured children to reach this juncture of adolescence, moving toward adulthood. Many believe that "showing them how" is their primary parental responsibility. It is a difficult change for them to suddenly switch from the "how to" of the child to the "try to" of the budding adult. Parents can learn the process of providing increased responsibilities based on a gradual progression of independent functioning. Despite their fears of their teenagers getting into trouble, they can be educated to promote self-reliance. The next two clinical examples show the need to educate parents and community members.

Clinical Example Mr. and Mrs. B came to the attention of the psychiatric nurse by their distressed calls to the community mental health center. Mrs. B tearfully explained that they had lost all control of their 14-year-old daughter. She had become arrogant and hostile, locking herself in her bedroom after an argument they had about her going to the movies with a 14-year-old boy she had met at school. Further exploration revealed that Emily was an honor student at school, maintaining a solid A average. She had many friends at school, was on the volleyball team, and babysat regularly on weekends for the neighbors' two children. She had always been pleasant, happy, and friendly. Suddenly this boy that the parents did not know called her at home. After many phone conversations he asked Emily to join him on a weekend evening at the movies. Mr. and Mrs. B felt that Emily was much too young to date, that she could get involved with drugs, sexual promiscuity, and so on. They were sad and worried that they had lost their little girl who always did what she was told. Emily was hurt and furious. She thought her parents were being totally unreasonable and that they did not trust her. Further exploration revealed that Mrs. B had gotten into trouble sexually as a young girl. She did not want Emily to make the same mistake. Mrs. B's parents had been very lenient, and she blamed their lack of guidelines for her error. Mrs. B became aware of her overreaction.

After discussion with a psychiatric nurse, she was able to understand that dating was a normal part of adolescent development. A compromise was arranged when she recognized Emily's competent and responsible functioning. After Mr. and Mrs. B met the boy, Emily was able to go to the movies with him and two other friends on a Saturday afternoon.

Clinical Example Lui Lee, an adolescent girl starting high school, had always functioned well. Beginning high school was a totally different experience. She became overwhelmed by the large building, increased academic responsibilities, and complex peer relationships. She began school in September with much anxiety. By October she began having numerous illnesses that prevented her from attending school. This came to the attention of the school guidance counselor, who noticed her increased absences. The guidance counselor saw her and, after no medical problems were found, invited Lui Lee to come to her office whenever she felt sick at school. When this did not help, she suggested that Lui Lee receive some home instruction until she felt less anxious. This suggestion validated Lui Lee's fears that she could not handle high school and its increased pressures. Her solution of retreat was supported. Fortunately, her parents sought the help of a psychiatric nurse, who encouraged immediate return to school with entry into a peer support group, with individual sessions initially as needed. This enabled her to talk out her fears and receive support from her peers. This also strengthened her confidence and fostered healthy functioning. She found she could handle high school after all. The nurse educated the guidance counselor on ways to be supportive while encouraging independent functioning.

> ❓ *What teaching methods or aids would be particularly effective when implementing a health education program with adolescents?*

Family Therapy

The nurse needs to assess the level of family functioning and determine how to best interact with and help the family of the adolescent. Family therapy is particularly useful when disturbed family interaction is interfering with the adolescent's development.[18] Sometimes a series of family sessions may be enough, and the adolescent may benefit from either individual or group approaches to support the effort to separate emotionally from the family. Occasionally, after a few family sessions, it may become clear that the adolescent may not need the intervention directly. Engaging the parents may free the adolescent to progress on the developmental continuum.

The techniques used in family therapy are reviewed in detail in Chapter 32. Whatever modality is selected in working with the adolescent, a family orientation and the adolescent's attempt to separate from the family and become an independent adult should be considered.

Group Therapy

Group therapy addresses adolescents' need for peer support. The conflict between dependence and independence with adults becomes somewhat diluted by the presence of other adolescents. Conflicts, especially about authority, can be detected by peers rather than adults, making group therapy particularly helpful for adolescents. It is valuable in teaching skills in relating and dealing with others. Group therapy also helps fulfill the adolescent's need for a positive, meaningful peer group for ego identity formation.

Adolescent groups, in contrast to other groups, are difficult to manage because many adolescents react to peers defensively. Sibling rivalry often disrupts group cohesion. Many groups suffer from poor attendance, a high dropout rate, antisocial behavior, and a lack of group cohesion. However, group therapy with adolescents has proved to be successful in many community mental health centers, outpatient clinics, and hospital settings.

Often, beginning group sessions with some activity provides a stabilizing factor for young adolescents. The number of members to include in the group depends on the type. For example, it may not be feasible to limit an outpatient walk-in group. Because of the age spread among adolescents, it is usually preferable to form at least two groups. A possibility is an early adolescence group consisting of 13- to 15-year-olds who have conflicts of separation from parents. An older adolescent group, ages 15 to 17, would probably consider issues such as the further establishment of identity, the beginning of dating, sex, experimentation with drugs, handling money, responsibilities of driving, and vocational plans.

Conflict between therapists, if there is an open and honest discussion, can provide a corrective experience because adolescents can see adults disagree without devastating consequences. If therapists are of the opposite sex, a parental similarity is often apparent; members often play on the therapist's feelings and try out tactics as they would with their own parents. Even if both therapists are of the same sex, one is usually more active, and a member may project a good or bad image onto each therapist that corresponds with how the parents are viewed. Group process with adolescents is often similar to that with adults, and specific aspects of working with groups are reviewed in Chapter 31.

> ❓ *When might a same-sex adolescent therapy group be most helpful? Compare this to the value of a mixed male and female group.*

Individual Therapy

Individual therapy done by the psychiatric clinical nurse specialist can consist of brief goal-directed therapy, behavioral therapy, or insight therapy. A description of insight therapy is presented here because the principles are helpful in other types of individual therapy. Once the decision to engage in individual therapy is made, a pact or contract between the nurse and adolescent is established.

THERAPEUTIC ALLIANCE. This contract is described by Meeks[20] as a therapeutic alliance in which nurses align themselves with the healthy, reality-oriented aspect of the adolescent's ego and move toward an honest and critical understanding of the adolescent's inner experience. This alliance is created through the interpretation of the adolescent's feeling states and defensive behavior, especially toward the nurse.

Adolescents' alliances are focused on links between their feelings and behavior in the present. The alliance is a central aspect of individual therapy. Once it is established, a feeling of working together is apparent. Meeks[20] gives specific hints to establish and maintain this alliance:

▼ Point out that behavior is motivated by feelings. Often, early in treatment, adolescents express feelings of impatience, helplessness, and failure at having to seek treatment. Defenses are often seen in rebelliousness, passivity, shyness, negativism, and intellectualization. Adolescents generally have a tendency to act out and avoid examining their feelings.

▼ Limit acting out by pointing out how it interferes with the therapeutic process and that it must be controlled to proceed. Maintain a neutral but interested attitude toward all behavior.

▼ Point out the adolescent's tendencies to be judgmental and self-critical. This is supportive and helps to encourage the adolescent to look for sources of behaviors, attitudes, and feelings.

▼ Establish that the adolescent's behavior is the result of many inner feelings. Some of these unknown feelings are interfering with the adolescent's happiness. This knowledge strengthens motivation for therapy and maintains an alignment with the adolescent's wishes for autonomy.

▼ Point out the adolescent's tendency to see things in extremes; the desire to be complete master opposes the feelings of total helplessness. Reveal areas of strength and competence that are often unrecognized. Avoiding exclusive focus on problems and weaknesses shows neutrality and is supportive. Giving the adolescent as much information as possible, to be prepared to make decisions, helps the adolescent work toward self-direction.

▼ Distinguish between thought and action, discouraging impulsiveness. Encourage open expression of strong feeling but not strong action. For example, anger does not mean killing; sexual feeling does not mean intercourse. Adolescents sometimes confuse discussion with permission to experiment with action, especially with sexual issues.

▼ Encourage emotional catharsis in sessions by expressing interest in and acceptance of feelings involving the nurse and events outside the session. Point out the importance of feelings.

▼ Be alert to the defenses of denial and reaction formation.

▼ Maintain neutrality and encourage objectivity without directly attacking needed defenses.

▼ Adolescents often act provocatively to force punishment by adults. This puts the nurse in alignment with the self-hatred aspect of the adolescent's conscience and should be avoided. The nurse provides support by continuing therapy even during these difficult periods.

The work of the nurse is to recognize the adolescent's anxiety and help assist in finding ways to deal with emerging impulses. Accepting any healthy and adaptive responses of the adolescent strengthens the sense of ego mastery. Adolescents often have wishes that they regard as crazy and frightening. Open discussion of fears helps adolescents realize that these feelings are uncomfortable but harmless thoughts.

TRANSFERENCE. Transference often occurs in adolescent treatment. The nurse must point out that these projections originate in the adolescent's mind and not in reality and that they usually represent a meaningful person such as a parent. It often helps to mention this is a common response. Several common transference patterns have been identified[20]:

▼ Erotic-sexual, especially if the nurse is young and of the opposite sex. This transference typically is shown by awkward blushing and agitated confusion by the adolescent. It is usually best to emphasize the mutual work of emotional growth while tactfully establishing the nurse's unavailability as a sexual object. Focusing on origins or encouraging elaboration of these feelings is not helpful and provokes anxiety.

▼ Omnipotent, expecting that the nurse will have answers to all questions. It is easy for the nurse to drift into this pattern because often the adolescent appears to be helpless. The adolescent's secret desire for personal omnipotence is somewhat fulfilled by granting it to the nurse.

▼ Negative transference, usually intense and pervasive. Negative feelings toward the nurse usually represent a negative attitude toward all adult authority figures. This transference is often defensive to cover feelings of shame, inadequacy, and anxiety, and it disappears as the adolescent respects the nurse's feelings. The adolescent tries to force the nurse's rejection. Open discussion to explore these feelings objectively and establish their origin is beneficial. Sometimes interpretations arouse anger toward the nurse because of the anxiety they create. These are reactions to the realities of therapy and are not to be confused with negative transference.

A true negative transference occurs when situations reactivate early experiences of negative feelings toward important others. The nurse unavoidably will frustrate the adolescent, who often has trouble delaying gratification to reach long-range goals. Negative transference, like any other resistant behavior, is dealt with through objective exploration, which includes seeking causes of anger and pointing out irrationality. This is often followed by a period of regression and depression. Empathic understanding that the adolescent is mourning a loss is helpful, but it should be emphasized that what was lost was an illusion. Another common occurrence is for an adolescent to rebel against conscience and then respond to guilt through self-destructive behaviors. Pointing out this pattern helps the adolescent to eventually become aware of this.

TERMINATION. Termination of therapy is an important part of the therapeutic process. Often, leaving therapy symbolizes the process of loosening bonds to parental images and giving up desires to be passive. One therefore expects defensive and regressive behaviors as the adolescent attempts to deal with the anxieties related to the termination process. This can mean the recurrence of emotional crises, symptoms, self-destructive fantasies, and even dependency behavior to provoke rescue.

Termination should be flexible and correctly timed. The decision should be made in line with adolescent norms, not adult ones. Often adolescents verbalize appropriate interest in termination. When this occurs, it is often helpful to open it to discussion without commitment to a set time. This implies that further work needs to be done in a definite time span, and it maintains a focus on the adolescent's responsibility to finish. Gradually supporting and approving of the adolescent's independence and mature functioning prepares for a positive termination. Some adolescents leave therapy to return later. Some can never leave forever, seeing termination as a rejection rather than a vote of confidence. Gradual reduction of sessions without pressing for final termination may help as long as the overall situation is reviewed occasionally.

Sometimes terminations occur prematurely because an alliance has not been established or some external event has occurred. Occasionally terminations are forced because of a nurse's change of location, death, or illness. The adolescent will express anger at the new therapist until the feelings about the lost therapist are accepted and resolved. In working out this attachment, a new therapeutic alliance can be established.

Medication Management

For adolescents, it is a particular challenge to determine which of the changing and often tumultuous behaviors are target symptoms for psychopharmacological interventions. This treatment strategy is more complex for this age group because of:

▼ The need for comprehensive family involvement (often optional in adults)

▼ Developmental differences that affect assessment, treatment alliance, management, compliance, and pharmacokinetics

▼ The difficulty in diagnosing emerging first episodes versus adjustment disorders in this age group

▼ The lack of controlled clinical drug trials in adolescents[9]
In terms of medication management, adolescents are

neither children nor adults. They have a metabolism more like adults than like children (who tend to require a dose higher than expected for their body weight because of their higher rate of metabolism). Thus, dosing regimens for adolescents are usually closer to those of adults. Yet research shows that, like children, adolescents have not been shown to respond better to tricyclic antidepressants (TCAs) than to placebo. Biologically, it cannot be assumed that drug response will be within the generally expected range for adults. The current state of the art in adolescent psychiatric practice is to carefully prescribe psychopharmacologic agents when they are determined to be appropriate and necessary, as part of a comprehensive treatment plan. The increased recognition of psychiatric disorders in adolescents and their resulting negative effects on social, psychological, and emotional development, the increasing efficacy and safety of these drugs in adults, and the increasing evidence of efficacy of these drugs in some adolescents have contributed to this practice.

In general, the following information may be helpful to the nurse working with adolescent patients. The use of selective serotonin reuptake inhibitors is generally preferred over TCAs in the treatment of adolescents because of their lower side effect profile and their relative safety in overdose. Additionally, there is increasing evidence that they are effective in the treatment of adolescent obsessive compulsive disorder (OCD) and some anxiety disorders, such as panic disorder. The use of benzodiazepines for anxiety is generally not recommended in this age group because of the increase in drug experimentation by adolescents and the negative effects on learning and memory that these drugs may have. Lithium is generally well tolerated in this age group and is effective in the treatment of mania, aggression, and conduct disorder. The other mood stabilizers have not been well studied in adolescents. Antipsychotics are the standard treatment for psychotic symptoms in adolescents. Although few studies exist, it appears that children and adolescents respond to lower doses of antipsychotics than adults and are more likely to experience extrapyramidal side effects, particularly teenage males when conventional rather than atypical drugs are used. Adolescents have a positive response to psychostimulants for attention deficit hyperactivity disorder, similar to that seen in younger children. Finally, of all the psychopharmacologic agents, psychostimulants are the most extensively studied in children and adolescents. Chapter 27 provides comprehensive information about psychopharmacology in general, and Chapter 36 contains tables specific for the psychopharmacological treatment of children and adolescents.

Talking with Adolescents

The following discussion focuses on some important considerations in communicating with adolescents.

SILENCE. Silence is often effective with adults but frightening to the adolescent, especially in the beginning stages of treatment or evaluation. This anxiety often reflects the adolescent's feelings of emptiness and lack of identity. Brief silences can be creative and productive when the adolescent is engaged in treatment; when the adolescent is able to tolerate them without anxiety, it indicates growth in self-confidence and acceptance of inner feelings. More often, however, silence is used defensively by adolescents to avoid discovery of hostile feelings or fantasies. Older adolescents may tolerate interpretive remarks, but with younger adolescents it is usually helpful to suggest an activity to help facilitate discussion and establish a relationship. For some adolescents, silence is a defense of inhibition and withdrawal because they have never learned to communicate in a positive way. In these cases the therapist must be responsible for dialogue.

CONFIDENTIALITY. Confidentiality is a concern to many, but especially to the adolescent who is fearful of the nurse reporting to parents. A blanket promise to tell nothing to the parents is not advised because the nurse may need to contact the parents if the adolescent reveals suicidal or homicidal behavior or the use of illegal drugs. It is usually best to tell the adolescent that the nurse will not give out any information without informing the adolescent in advance. It is also helpful to explain that feelings are confidential but that actions considered dangerous to the adolescent or others must be shared.

> **?** *You receive a call from the school guidance counselor of one of your adolescent patients asking what progress is being made in treatment. How would you respond?*

NEGATIVISM. Negative feelings are often expressed by adolescents, especially initially, because they are frightened of the implications of coming for treatment. The young adolescent's lack of objectivity and upsurge of impulses, as well as the tendency to confuse fantasy and action, make the discussion of feelings threatening. Usually, gently noting in a supportive way defensive techniques the adolescent uses during the session helps to gain cooperation.

RESISTANCE. Often adolescents begin by testing nurses to see whether they will be authoritarian figures. The rebellious adolescent may deny the need for therapy or help. If the adolescent appears anxious, it is best to be supportive and sympathetic, expressing interest in getting to know the adolescent and then discussing a neutral area. A more angry, rebellious adolescent may require a direct approach, with the nurse saying openly that the adolescent is opposing the visit because of a false belief that no help is needed. This can lead to a further discussion of feelings about the visit (such as parental coercion to come to the session) or feelings about authority. Some adolescents are just baiting and

testing to see whether the nurse is an anxious, defensive adult. If so, it is best to ignore their comments about not wanting treatment and move on. Often adolescents with an angry facade depend on their omnipotent control of the environment and are often successful in manipulating their families. They are angry at attempts to disturb this power, and the anger is expressed in their lack of cooperation in the session.

ARGUING. Adolescents often argue and, although they do not admit it, learn from arguments. Often the adolescent goes against the viewpoint of the nurse and then in the next session adopts the nurse's opinion. It is best not to comment on this and accept it as a harmless defense. If the nurse admits having areas of ignorance, it is productive to the adolescent, who may fear the need to be perfect.

TESTING. Adolescents often need and want limits. They are confused and cannot set their own limits. They experiment by trial and error to find a self-concept. Often, adolescents test nurses to see how firm and consistent they will be. Controls often are effective if there is a basic positive relationship with the nurse. Limits should be set only when they are essential for current and future well-being, and the adolescent will value the security they provide. Adolescents will dare to be independent if it is conveyed that the nurse will serve as a control against carrying independence too far.

DREAMS AND ARTISTIC CREATIONS. Adolescents are often creative, and much can be learned from studying their works. As long as the discussion is relevant, it can be a productive source for exploring inner feelings. Along with dreams, these feelings can reveal valuable information about their real concerns, even when the adolescent attempts to avoid them.

BRINGING FRIENDS. The adolescent who brings a friend to a session may be attempting to avoid therapy. There is some benefit in sharing the experiences with the peer group because this lowers anxiety. Telling the adolescent that bringing friends is not allowed may not be successful because the nurse cannot always enforce such a rule. The reason for bringing friends may vary, but it should be explored and understood. Sometimes adolescents want to refer friends. This may be positive but may also focus attention away from the original adolescent. The nurse should insist on exploring motives behind the referral before accepting the new patient because the adolescent may think the nurse's acceptance of another is a betrayal of loyalty. If the friend clearly wants and needs therapy, referral to a colleague is usually best. If a friend is brought late in therapy, it may mean that the adolescent is preparing to terminate.

EMBARRASSMENT ABOUT BEING IN THERAPY. Embarrassment may occur in any age group, but it is prominent in adolescents, especially during the early stages of treatment. It also can become an issue as therapy progresses because it often reveals the adolescent's embarrassment about a desire for dependency. Therefore, adolescents may become uncomfortable in the therapeutic relationship. This is usually dealt with by indicating that these feelings are normal. Behind the fear of accepting help is the wish for care, and this can be dealt with by pointing out the adolescent's strengths and areas of independence.

Some adolescents, by expressing embarrassment about being in therapy, are actually revealing a fear or social stigma that they have heard from their parents. The adolescent who has feelings of inferiority often focuses these on the therapeutic process, blaming therapy for discomfort. It is best to encourage and support the adolescent, gently refusing to accept blame for this discomfort.

REQUESTS FOR SPECIAL ATTENTION. Some adolescents can develop intense dependency ties to the therapist. They reflect this in requests for additional appointments, extra time in appointments, frequent telephone calls, or social contact outside the therapeutic sessions. Focus should be on the exploration of feelings of inner emptiness, deprivation, and incompleteness that are responsible for these requests.

> *Do you think adolescents can benefit from treatment if their parents deny there is a problem, refuse to be involved, or are opposed to seeking help?*

Parents of the Adolescent

If group or individual treatment is selected for the adolescent, the nurse must still consider the family. Parents cannot help the adolescent's treatment if they do not understand and accept it. The nurse can work with the parents without revealing confidential material.

Not all parents need treatment. It is helpful for parents to have treatment if the adolescent is asked to assume an inappropriate role at home because this interferes with the adolescent's adaptive responses. If the parents are resistant, the nurse must usually begin with the adolescent until the parents are more receptive.

Telephone contact is a helpful way to ensure cooperation and support by having the parent call when necessary. Parents should tell the adolescent when they call. Parents should be told of normal adolescent behavior they can expect. The nurse should avoid advising the parents about specific actions and focus on attitudes and feelings, especially concerning discipline. Parents can be helped with understanding the purpose of limit setting. Some parents exclude themselves entirely from their adolescent's life. They have brought the adolescent to treatment to ease their guilt by doing all that is possible. They may want the nurse to take over parenting functions. This should not be permitted, especially during crises. If the adolescent is suicidal or homicidal, the parents are informed and helped to take responsibility for action.

Adolescents often need help in dealing with their parents. Parents should be discussed in an open exploratory manner, with emphasis on them having their own feelings and reasons for their actions. Adolescents should be helped to see their parents realistically and to work on their own strengths and weaknesses.

Sometimes adolescents want to leave home because they hope they will feel more adult away from their parents. It is usually best to explore the wish to leave, emphasizing that it must be done in an adult way. If leaving is an impulsive thought with no feasible plan, it will ensure failure, parental rescue, and continued dependency. This is often recapitulated in termination from therapy if the adolescent quits early to avoid the pain of separation that a planned termination would bring.

EVALUATING NURSING CARE

Problems presented by adolescents, more often than those of any other group, activate the nurse's own unresolved conflicts. Thus evaluating nursing care must begin with nurses monitoring their responses, including countertransference reactions. The nurse should watch for alignment with the parents against the adolescent or the adolescent against the parents. Most adults are resistant to reexperiencing the feelings of adolescence and have repressed these experiences. As a result of anxiety, the nurse occasionally may have trouble listening or may encourage the adolescent (because of unrecognized wishes) to do what the nurse never dared do. The adolescent may be acting as the nurse did during adolescence. The nurse, in an effort to deny this, may see this adolescent behavior as nondeviant. Identification of the nurse with the adolescent can contribute to delays in exploring areas important for psychological growth. The nurse may relate well to the adolescent but because of unresolved, unrecognized conflicts or resentment toward the nurse's own parents, may be locked into adolescent rebellion. The nurse may overtly or covertly encourage adolescents to express rage toward their families. Both the adolescent and the nurse then avoid facing the reality of adult burdens.

Evaluation of psychiatric nursing care with adolescents also involves consideration of objective measurements of the adolescent's and the family's progress toward the goals of treatment. Specifically, the nurse may ask:

▼ Were the concerns of the adolescent and family addressed?

▼ Has the problematic behavior decreased and been replaced with more adaptive responses?

▼ Have the adolescent's relationships with others improved?

▼ Has school or work performance been enhanced?

▼ Are the adolescent and family satisfied with the treatment outcome?

By reviewing areas of growth and progress, the adolescent is able to integrate the learning that has been accomplished and gain from the experience a greater sense of self-efficacy and mastery.

Summary

1. Adolescence is a unique stage of development that occurs between the ages of 11 and 20 and is accompanied by a shift in development and learning.

2. Various theories explain the adolescent's resolution of tasks, including biological, psychoanalytical, psychosocial, attachment, cognitive, cultural, and multidimensional.

3. Issues that are particularly problematic for adolescents include body image, identity, independence, social role, and sexual behavior.

4. Maladaptive responses impede growth and development and require nursing intervention. These are often related to inappropriate sexual activity, unwed motherhood, suicide, running away, conduct disorders, violence, drug use, hypochondriasis, weight problems, occult involvement, and parental divorce.

5. Nursing interventions useful in working with adolescents include health education, family, group, and individual therapy, and medication management. Special attention should be given to talking with adolescents and working with their parents.

6. Evaluation of nursing care requires special focus on countertransference issues and the need for objective measurements of the adolescent's and family's progress toward the treatment goals.

COMPETENT CARING A Clinical Exemplar of a Psychiatric Nurse

Karen M. McHugh, BSN, RN, C

When I graduated with a bachelor's degree in nursing, I never imagined I would be interested in psychiatric nursing. After 1 ½ years in medical-surgical nursing, I decided I wanted more interpersonal time with my patients rather than being so skill and task oriented. One of my first experiences as a psychiatric nurse was on a 32-bed adolescent unit in North Carolina. There I encountered a 14-year-old girl, S, who was admitted to our inpatient unit for depression. At that time patients typically stayed for about 3 months, which is very different from the current length of stay for adolescents in the hospital, which is most often 5 days.

S had several problems, most occurring within the previous year. She had a history of running away, crying spells, skipping school, failing grades, and suicidal threats. She lived at home with her father and 9-year-old brother. Her mother was no longer involved in her life because she had left the family and given up custody of the children several years before.

S settled into the milieu but had a difficult time engaging with the staff. I began to spend time with her every day to establish a trusting relationship. The first few days we just sat in silence. Eventually we were able to talk about her history of oppositional behavior and low self-esteem. S trusted me more and more over time. Then, about 1 month after admission, she approached me and asked if we could talk again. S asked me if I could promise not to tell anyone (especially her father or doctors) if she confided in me about something. I knew then that something was troubling her, but I had to be honest with her. I told S that I couldn't make that promise because the treatment team works in the best interest of the patient and I would have to share pertinent information with them. She decided not to confide in me then, but the next day she approached me again.

S began to tell me that the past few months her father began to drink and had hit her several times, leaving marks on her legs and arms. She stated that one day she had to stay home from school because her legs were swollen and painful from the bruises. She said that her father always apologized once he was sober and promised that he would never hit her again. I gathered a few more details and was honest with her and informed her that I would have to collaborate with the treatment team and possibly seek help from the Department of Social Services. After meeting with the treatment team the next day, I told S that we had to report her father to Social Services. She began to yell and scream and blame me for telling everyone about her problems. Even though I had been honest with her, she couldn't understand that I was actually helping her.

At this point I had to examine my feelings, and I even questioned my judgment. I went home from work that evening quite upset. I began to ask myself, Did I do the right thing? Will S ever confide in me again or even talk with me? Despite feeling a little guilty, I knew that I had made the right decision because protecting S and her future was of utmost importance. After a few days of cooling off S approached me and was able to express her feelings of relief and even apologized to me. We began to work on identifying and expressing her feelings of guilt, relief, sadness, and concern over the situation with her father. Social Services found no evidence of abuse to her 9-year-old brother, so he remained at home with the father.

At discharge, an aunt assumed foster care of S temporarily until her father could obtain the therapy he needed. S was referred to outpatient therapy as well. Several weeks after her discharge, I saw her at the mall and she thanked me for helping and listening to her even though she didn't see it that way at first. She stated that she was happier now and was doing well in school and that she and her father were continuing therapy.

I had made the right decision. Being a child's advocate and maintaining a patient's safety during an inpatient stay and after discharge are always a nurse's first priority. As I reflected on this experience, I learned not to take things in my personal life so much for granted, such as a loving and supportive family. I also realized that psychiatric nurses do provide excellence in nursing and that we truly can make a difference.

Chapter Review Questions

1. Identify whether the following statements are true (T) or false (F).

A. ___ Brain growth ends before the beginning of adolescence.

B. ___ Chronological age is a good guide for physical maturation during adolescence.

C. ___ There is a link between an adolescent's self-concept and the use of adaptive coping responses.

D. ___ Masturbation can be an effective way for adolescents to discharge sexual tension.

E. ___ When working with adolescents it is best to have the initial contact with the family to obtain an accurate assessment of the adolescent's problem.

F. ___ Silence is a therapeutic technique that is often frightening to adolescents, especially in the beginning stages of treatment or evaluation.

2. Fill in the blanks.

A. Erikson called the task related to the stage of adolescence _____.

B. Piaget described adolescence as characterized by the cognitive functioning of _____.

C. About _____% of males and _____% of females have had sexual intercourse before age 15.

D. _____ is the second leading cause of death among adolescents.

E. When a person is overly concerned with one's body and body sensations it is called _____.

F. Two dimensions of positive mental health for adolescents are _____ and _____.

3. Provide short answers for the following questions.

A. Explain why teenagers delay seeking and using contraceptives.

B. Describe what is meant when alcohol is called a gateway drug.

C. Identify the five stages of substance abuse in adolescence.

D. Give four reasons why medication as a treatment strategy is more complex for adolescents than for adults.

REFERENCES

1. Blos P: The second individuation process of adolescence, *Psychoanal Study Child* 22:162, 1967.
2. Booth R, Zhang Y: Severe aggression and related conduct problems among runaway and homeless adolescents, *Psychiatr Serv* 47:75, 1996.
3. Brage D, Campbell-Grossman C, Dunkel J: Psychological correlates of adolescent depression, *J Child Adolesc Psychiatr Nurs* 8:23, 1995.
4. Busen N: Development of an adolescent risk taking instrument, *J Child Adolesc Psychiatr Nurs* 14:142, 1991.
5. Centers for Disease Control: Results from the national adolescent student health survey, *MMWR* 38:147, 1989.
6. DiClemente R, Hansen W, Ponton L: *Handbook of adolescent risk behavior,* New York, 1996, Plenum.
7. Erikson E: *Childhood and society,* ed 2, New York, 1963, WW Norton.
8. Galanter M: *Cults and new religious movements,* Washington, DC, 1989, American Psychiatric Press.
9. Greenhill L, Setterberg S: Pharmacotherapy of disorders of adolescents, *Psychiatr Clin North Am* 14:793, 1993.
10. Havighurst RL: *Developmental tasks and education,* ed 3, New York, 1972, David McKay.
11. Hibbs E, Jensen P: *Psychosocial treatments for child and adolescent disorders,* Washington, DC, 1996, American Psychological Association.
12. Johnson L, O'Malley P, Bachman J: *National survey results on drug use from the Monitoring the Future Study 1975-1993,* vol 1, Rockville, Md, 1994, National Institute on Drug Abuse.
13. Kalogerakis M: Emergency evaluation of adolescents, *Hosp Community Psychiatry* 43:617, 1992.
14. Ladely S, Puskar K: Adolescent suicide: behaviors, risk factors, and psychiatric nursing interventions, *Issues Ment Health Nurs* 15:497, 1994.

15. LeCroy C: *Handbook of child and adolescent treatment manuals,* New York, 1994, Lexington.

16. Lopez L, Gary F: Logical responses to youth who run away from home: implications for psychiatric mental health nursing, *J Psychosoc Nurs* 33:9, 1995.

17. Marohn R: Management of the assaultive adolescent, *Hosp Community Psychiatry* 43:622, 1992.

18. Matorin S, Greenberg L: Family therapy in the treatment of adolescents, *Hosp Community Psychiatry* 43:625, 1992.

19. McCaleb A: Global and multidimensional self concept as a predictor of healthy practices in middle adolescents, *J Child Adolesc Psychiatr Nurs* 8:18, 1995.

20. Meeks J: *The fragile alliance,* ed 4, Malabar, Fla, 1990, Robert Krieger.

21. Millstein S, Peterson A, Nightingale E: *Promoting the health of adolescents,* New York, 1993, Oxford University Press.

22. Parmelee D: *Child and adolescent psychiatry,* St Louis, 1996, Mosby.

23. Piaget J: *Six psychological studies,* New York, 1968, Vintage.

24. Powers S, Hauser S, Kilner L: Adolescent mental health, *Am Psychol* 44:200, 1989.

25. Rew L: Adolescents' perceived barriers to healthcare services, *J Child Adolesc Psychiatr Nurs* 8:5, 1995.

26. Riesch S, Forsyth D: Preparing to parent the adolescent, *J Child Adolesc Psychiatr Ment Health Nurs* 5:32, 1992.

27. Rosenstein D, Horowitz H: Adolescent attachment and psychopathology, *J Consult Clin Psychol* 64:54, 1996.

28. Savin-Williams R, Rodriguez R: A developmental, clinical perspective on lesbian, gay male and bisexual youths. In Gullotta T, Adams G, Montemayor R, editors: *Adolescent sexuality,* Newbury Park, Calif, 1993, Sage.

29. Schwartzberg A: The impact of divorce on adolescents, *Hosp Community Psychiatry* 43:634, 1992.

30. Shaffer D, Gould M, Hicks R: Worsening suicide rate in black teenagers, *Am J Psychiatry* 151:1810, 1994.

31. Stein T: Overview of new developments in understanding homosexuality. In Oldham J, Riba M, Tasman A, editors: *Review of psychiatry,* vol 12, Washington, DC, 1993, American Psychiatric Press.

32. Sullivan H: *Interpersonal theory of psychiatry,* New York, 1953, WW Norton.

33. VanderMeer J, Gabert H: Psychiatric nursing admission tool for children and adolescents, *J Child Adolesc Psychiatr Nurs* 6:15, 1993.

ANNOTATED SUGGESTED READINGS

Campbell M, Cueva J: Psychopharmacology in child and adolescent psychiatry: a review of the past seven years, *J Am Acad Child Adolesc Psychiatry* 34:1262, 1995.
  Presents a critical overview on the efficacy and safety of psychoactive agents in conduct disorder, schizophrenia, separation anxiety disorder, selective mutism, obsessive-compulsive disorder, panic disorder, depression, bipolar disorder, and sleep and eating disorders.

*Cornman J: Female adolescent response to childhood sexual abuse, *J Child Adolesc Psych Nurs* 10:17, 1997.
  Compares sexually abused adolescent females and those not sexually abused and makes the case that nurses are in a position to identify, evaluate, and treat families with adolescents who manifest a wide range of sequelae.

DiClemente R, Hansen W, Ponton L: *Handbook of adolescent risk behavior,* New York, 1996, Plenum Press.
  Describes the epidemiology of specific risk behaviors, preventive strategies, and the efficacy of treatment modalities. Excellent resource for adolescent risk behavior.

*Eggert L et al: Prevention research program: reconnecting at-risk youth, *Issues Ment Health Nurs* 15:107, 1994.
  Excellent example of nursing research directed toward preventive interventions using a multidisciplinary team.

Gordon B, Schroeder C: *Sexuality: a developmental approach to problems,* New York, 1995, Plenum Press.
  Written to inform clinicians about recent research findings, make them aware of the areas in need of more empirical work, and encourage them to rethink their approaches to the sexual problems of children and adolescents.

Hamburg D: Toward a strategy for healthy adolescent development, *Am J Psychiatry* 154(suppl):7, 1997.
  Discusses the fundamental requirements for healthy adolescent development in the context of disease prevention, sexuality, preparation for parenthood, and prevention of violence and drug abuse.

*Kendall J, Peterson G: A school-based mental health clinic for adolescent mothers, *J Child Adolesc Psych Nurs* 9:7, 1996.
  Describes a program in which a school of nursing provided services to teenage mothers and their children. Good example of nursing innovation.

LeCroy C: *Handbook of child and adolescent treatment manuals,* New York, 1994, Lexington Books.
  Practical manual of effective treatment strategies for working with adolescents. Comprehensive and filled with clear and useful examples.

Miller A et al: Dialectical behavior therapy adapted for suicidal youths, *J Pract Psychiatry Behav Health* 3:78, 1997.
  Describes the use of behavior therapy for the treatment of suicidal adolescents and is illustrated with a case study.

Newton M: *Adolescence: guiding youth through the perilous ordeal,* New York, 1995, WW Norton.
  Reviews biopsychosocial theories of adolescence and focuses on developmental "tasks" and "traps." Worthwhile reading.

Parmelee D: *Child and adolescent psychiatry,* St Louis, 1996, Mosby.
  Discusses tools for diagnosis, DSM-IV disorders, and treatments specific to children and adolescents. Easy to read, clear, and concise.

*Warren J, Gary F, Moorhead J: Runaway youths in a southern community, *J Child Adolesc Psych* 10:26, 1997.
  Nursing research on runaway youths focused into four areas of inquiry: familial abuse, school and legal conflicts, high-risk sexual behavior, and stressful life events.

*Nursing reference.

Chapter **38**

Geriatric Psychiatric Nursing

Georgia L. Stevens,
Suzanne D. Friedman,
and Beverly A. Baldwin

© 1998 M.C. Escher/Cordon Art, Baarn, Holland.

*Youth is like a fresh flower in May. Age is like a rainbow that follows the storms of life. Each has its own beauty.** **David Polis**

LEARNING OBJECTIVES

After studying this chapter the student should be able to:

▼ Identify the role and functions of the geropsychiatric nurse

▼ Compare the major biopsychosocial theories of aging

▼ Identify and describe the elements of a comprehensive geropsychiatric nursing assessment

▼ Formulate nursing diagnoses for geropsychiatric patients

▼ Analyze nursing interventions for geropsychiatric patients

▼ Evaluate nursing care of geropsychiatric patients

TOPICAL OUTLINE

Role of the Geropsychiatric Nurse
Theories of Aging
  Biological Theories
  Psychological Theories
  Sociocultural Theories
Assessing the Geriatric Patient
  The Interview
  Mental Status
  Behavioral Responses
  Functional Abilities
  Physiological Functioning
  Social Support
Diagnosis of the Geriatric Patient
  Altered Thought Processes
  Affective Responses
  Somatic Responses
  Stress Responses
  Behavioral Responses
Planning and Intervention
  Therapeutic Milieu
  Somatic Therapies
  Interpersonal Interventions
Evaluating the Care of the Geriatric Patient

People 65 years of age and older make up the fastest growing age group in the United States. One in every nine Americans, or almost 13% of the population, is 65 or older; in the first half of the twenty-first century, this will increase to one in five. Women live an average of 7 years longer than men, and more older women live alone. It is estimated that by 2030 there will be 60 million people over 65—20% of the US population. By 2050 26% of those over 65 will be members of an ethnic minority group.[26] Also, by the year 2050 nearly 1 in 4 older adults will be at least 85. This will present a tremendous challenge as the health needs of these people are the most complex and difficult to manage. Geropsychiatric nursing care must therefore address the needs of the young old (65 to 75 years of age), the middle old (75 to 85 years of age), and the old old (85 years of age and older); each group requires a different level of care.[10]

Most older adults do not have a mental disorder. In fact, it is estimated that only 22% of people 65 and older have a psychiatric illness. However, important exceptions to this general trend exist, related to type of disorder, setting, and age group. For example, older people in the United States have the highest suicide rate of any age group.[3] In addition, the prevalence of psychiatric disorders among institutionalized elderly is significant. Recent studies have suggested that 51 to 94% of residents in long-term care facilities have some type of psychiatric disorder.[5] When all types of cognitive impairment are combined, older adults have the highest prevalence rates of any age group largely because of dementias such as Alzheimer's disease. Similarly, the prevalence rate for dementias of all types varies, with approximately 30% of those over age 80 having some form of dementia. Finally, although mental disorders affect only a minority of older adults, they have a substantial impact when they occur. Nearly a quarter of hospital costs for older adults are for treatment of mental health problems. It is also known that more than half of older adults who are treated for physical disorders in hospitals, clinics, and nursing homes also have at least one mental health problem that is usually not recognized and effectively treated. Thus the economic and personal costs of mental disorders of older adults are considerable.

Helping older adults to maximize their potential can be a challenging and rewarding experience for the nurse. Stereotypes and myths often depict the elderly as a homogeneous group. On the contrary, the older adult represents a combination of multiple interpersonal, developmental, and situational experiences. The complexity and interaction of the needs and problems of old age are often understated. Mental health in late life depends on a number of factors. These include physiological and psychological status, personality, social support system, economic resources, and usual lifestyle. This chapter addresses selected aspects of the psychiatric–mental health needs of geriatric patients and their families.

ROLE OF THE GEROPSYCHIATRIC NURSE

The nurse who works with mentally ill elders is challenged to integrate psychiatric nursing skills with knowledge of physiological disorders, the normal aging process, and sociocultural influences on the elderly and their families. Many nurses who work with these patients find that it is useful to combine nurse practitioner and psychiatric nursing skills. Case management is a particularly effective approach to providing for the biopsychosocial needs of the elderly. Mental health services are provided to this population in a variety of settings including general and psychiatric hospitals, nursing homes, outpatient mental health clinics, adult day-care programs, senior centers, and the person's own home.

As a primary care provider the geropsychiatric nurse must be proficient at assessing cognitive, affective, functional, physical, and behavioral status. The nurse also needs knowledge of community resources and how to access them. Planning and nursing intervention may occur with the patient and family or other caregivers. Providing nursing care to these patients can be complex because they are often involved with a number of agencies.

As a consultant, the geropsychiatric nurse helps other providers of services to the elderly to address the behavioral and cognitive aspects of the patient's care. Often this role is assumed by nurses in their own agency. For instance, a nurse may help nursing assistants understand how to respond to a patient who wanders or one who is aggressive. Advanced practice geropsychiatric nurses who have graduate education in this specialty may be employed by agencies to help the entire staff to develop therapeutic programs for seniors with psychiatric or behavioral problems. Some nurses develop and market in-service education packages for nursing homes or other agencies that serve these patients.

Geropsychiatric nurses should be knowledgeable about the effects of psychotropic medication on elderly people. They often work closely with the physician to monitor complex medication regimens and help the patient or caregiver with medication management. They may lead a variety of groups such as orientation, remotivation, bereavement, and socialization groups, whereas nurses with advanced degrees may provide psychotherapy and medication prescriptions.

Finally, the role of patient advocate is a critical one for the nurse caring for elders with mental illnesses, particularly those concomitant with physical illness. Because of cognitive changes or symptoms of acute or chronic health problems, elders may not be able to effectively voice their wishes or concerns. Reviewing legal options such as advanced directives or a living will helps in the promotion of the elder's wishes. In cases where conflict exists regarding the elder's care, particularly in long-term care settings, an ombudsman may be contacted to help resolve these issues. Information about ombudsman or other advocacy programs for the elderly may be obtained by contacting any local office on aging.

THEORIES OF AGING

Ways of defining aging and explaining the causes and consequences of the aging process are based on two major approaches:
▼ The causes of the biological and psychological aging process
▼ The psychosocial results of aging

Gerontologists disagree about the cause and adaptation to aging. No one theory can include all the variables that influence aging and the person's response to it. It is difficult to separate the effects of stress, disease processes, and specific age-related changes. However, theories of aging may help to clarify the physical and mental changes experienced by elderly patients.

Biological Theories

BIOLOGICAL PROGRAMMING THEORY. The classic biological programming theory proposes that the life span of a cell is stored within the cell itself. Through laboratory studies, Hayflick and colleagues[19] demonstrated that normal human fibroblasts, when cultured, doubled a specific number of times and then died. The number of doublings is the same in male and female cells. This theory of a human biological clock views the decline of biological, cognitive, and psychomotor function as inevitable and irreversible, although diet changes or prolonged hypothermia may delay the process. The concept of programmed aging answers some questions about the human life span. It does not address hereditary and environmental influences on individual variations in aging.

> **?** *Give at least two examples that contradict the biological programming theory of aging. How do you feel about the idea of a biological clock determining life span?*

WEAR-AND-TEAR THEORY. The wear-and-tear theory suggests that structural and functional changes may be speeded by abuse and slowed by care. From a physiological standpoint, aging is viewed developmentally, beginning with conception and leading to decline and death. Problems associated with aging are the result of accumulated stress, trauma, injuries, infections, inadequate nutrition, metabolic and immunological disturbances, and prolonged abuse. This concept of aging is seen in widely accepted myths and stereotypes regarding the aged, as noted in such phrases as, "He's doing well for his age," or "What can you expect at that age?" Newer research on the value of exercise and cognitive stimulation in later years refutes the basic premise of this theory because both body and mind seem to benefit from use and stimulation.

> **?** *Discuss how the wear-and-tear theory of aging compares with the present emphasis on nutrition and physical fitness in American culture.*

STRESS ADAPTATION THEORY. The stress adaptation theory emphasizes the positive and negative effects of stress on biopsychosocial development. As a positive influence, stress may stimulate a person to try new, more effective ways of adapting. A negative effect of stress would be inability to function because of feeling overwhelmed. The balance of positive and negative stress experiences must be examined. Although it is often assumed that stress accelerates the aging process, there is little evidence to support that conclusion. Stress may drain a person's reserve capacity physiologically, psychologically, socially, and economically, increasing vulnerability to illness or injury.

Psychological Theories

ERIKSON'S STAGE OF EGO INTEGRITY. Erikson's[11] theory of human development identifies tasks that must be accomplished at each of the eight stages of life. The last task, related to reflection about one's life and accomplishments, is identified as ego integrity. If this is not achieved, despair results. The result of resolving the conflict between ego integrity and despair is acquired wisdom.

LIFE REVIEW THEORY. The life review was identified in 1961 by Butler.[6] In elderly people, life review is a normal process brought about by the realization of approaching death. During the life review, past experiences return to consciousness. There is also a resurgence of unresolved conflicts. The person examines and reintegrates these memories. Successful reintegration can give meaning to life and prepare the person for death by relieving anxiety and fear. According to the life review theory, this process occurs universally and is a functional preparation for the final stage of life. Although it occurs in all age groups to a certain degree, the emphasis and focused concentration are characteristic of the later stage of life. Aged people have a vivid memory for past events and can recall early life experiences with clarity and imagination. They appear to be reviewing and sorting previous life events to better understand their present circumstances.

The life review may have positive or negative consequences. Anxiety, guilt, fear, and depression may surface if the person is unable to resolve or accept old, unsolved problems. On the other hand, the righting of the earlier wrongs can help establish a sense of serenity, pride in working through old conflicts, and acceptance of mortal life. Reflection is thus seen as a positive approach to aging. Further discussion of this process is found in the section on strategies for intervening in the mental health problems of the older adult.

STABILITY OF PERSONALITY. Some gerontologists contend that personality is established by early adulthood and remains fairly stable thereafter. Stability or continuity of personality has been observed in longitudinal studies of aging people at the National Institutes of Health Gerontology Research Center in Baltimore (the intramural research center for the National Institute on Aging). Usually no decline or change in personality, compared with other cognitive changes, was evident. Radical changes in personality in older people may be indicative of brain disease. Researchers found that periods of psychological crisis in adulthood do not occur at regular intervals. This contradicts some theories such as Erikson's. However, people with a long history of emotional instability were likely to encounter more crises. Finally, the researchers noted that changes in roles, attitudes, and situational demands created the need for new behavioral responses. The majority of elderly people in these studies appeared to adapt effectively to those demands.

> **?** *Can personality traits be altered in old age? If yes, how? If no, why are we interested in intervening in nonproductive behaviors of older adults?*

Sociocultural Theories

DISENGAGEMENT THEORY. This controversial theory evolved from studies conducted by the University of Chicago Committee on Human Development.[8] It postulated that older adults and society mutually withdraw from active exchange with each other as part of the normal aging process. This was assumed to be a sign of psychological well-being and adjustment on the part of the elder. This theory did not consider the differences among the elderly and the personality variables important to coping with change. Stereotypes reinforced by this theory include the idea that older people enjoy only the company of people their own age and that retirement facilities should prohibit intergenerational living arrangements. Although many elders may desire such arrangements, others feel isolated and out of the mainstream of society.

ACTIVITY THEORY. Disputes about the reliability of the disengagement theory led to the development of the current view that activity produces the most positive psychological climate for older adults. The activity theory developed as a reaction to the negative view of disengagement. Many gerontologists support the idea that aging is a phase in the developmental process; others contend that old age is only an extension of the middle years and can be modified or abolished by increased activity levels. The activity theory maintains that the aged should remain active as long as possible. Older adults who must stop working or participating in community activities should find substitutes. This theory emphasizes the positive influence of activity on the older person's personality, mental health, and satisfaction with life.

THE FAMILY IN LATER LIFE. Whereas theorists such as Erikson consider individual development throughout the life cycle, family theorists focus on the family as the basic unit of emotional development. This framework considers the interrelated tasks, problems, and relationships of the three-generational family system. Carter and McGoldrick[7] address multigenerational patterns, myths, developmental transitions, and external stressors. They theorize that the central process of the life cycle is changing the relationship system to support the functional entry, exit, and development of family members. Each transition requires a shift in emotional attitudes to support the relationship changes. In later life the emotional process involves accepting the shifting of generational roles, and the relationship changes include:

▼ Maintaining functioning and interests during physiological decline
▼ Exploring new role options
▼ Supporting the middle generation in a more central role
▼ Making room in the system for the wisdom and experience of the older generation
▼ Supporting elderly family members without overfunctioning
▼ Dealing with the loss of significant others and preparing for death

Physical, emotional, and social symptoms are believed to reflect problems in negotiating the transitions of the family life cycle.

ASSESSING THE GERIATRIC PATIENT

Nursing assessment of the geropsychiatric patient is complex. The interplay of biological, psychological, and sociocultural factors related to aging sometimes makes it difficult to clearly identify nursing problems. For example, it can be quite difficult to sort out the behaviors related to the 4 D's of geropsychiatric assessment: depression, dementia, delirium, and delusions (see Chapter 23). Aside from major psychotic disorders, delusions are also characteristic of depression in the elderly, and those with dementia may seem delusional because of the trouble they have in interpreting the environment. Delirium may occur related to physical illness, medications, or sensory deprivation. Behaviors associated with delirium include hallucinations, delusions, confusion, disorientation, and agitation. It may be mistaken for dementia, depriving the patient of treatment that could reverse the problem. Depressed elders often appear confused and cognitively impaired because of the lethargy and psychomotor retardation related to depression. Patients with dementia may also present with anxiety, agitation, and depression, especially if they are aware of their declining mental functioning. It has also been reported that the first episode of depression in later life is associated with greater chronicity, relapse, cognitive dysfunction, and an increased rate of dementia.[2]

Behaviors have been identified that help to differentiate between depression and dementia. Depressed patients are oriented and maintain socially appropriate behaviors. They are unlikely to undress in public or be incontinent. In response to questions, patients with dementia will try to answer but have trouble with logic and relevance. Depressed patients will be annoyed and reject the questioner with silence or short, unresponsive answers. Irritability and hostility are more characteristic of the depressed person.

Careful nursing assessment can be helpful in identifying the primary disorder. Nursing diagnoses are based on observation of patient behaviors and related to current needs. Cognitive responses including Alzheimer's disease and related disorders are discussed in Chapter 23, emotional responses including depression in Chapter 19, and anxiety responses in Chapter 16.

The Interview

Establishing a supportive and trusting relationship is essential to a positive interview with the geriatric patient. The elderly person may feel uneasy, vulnerable, and confused in a new place or with strangers. Patience and attentive listening promote a sense of security. Comfortable surroundings help the patient relax and focus on the conversation.

THERAPEUTIC COMMUNICATION SKILLS. The nurse shows respect by addressing the patient by his last name: "Good morning, Mr. Smith." The nurse opens the interview by introducing herself and briefly orienting the patient to the purpose and length of the interview. Occasionally reinforcing the amount of time left may help direct a wandering discussion and give the patient the security of knowing that the nurse is in control of the situation.

Older people may respond to questions slowly because ability to respond verbally slows with age. It is important to give the patient enough time to answer. Assuming that the patient does not know the answer to a question, does not remember, or does not understand because of a slow response can lead the nurse to false conclusions.

The way the patient is interviewed is important. It may be helpful to use a life course interview format that is tied to significant historical events that occurred during the person's lifetime. Older people often are unfamiliar with new words, slang, or colloquialisms. Choice of words should also be based on knowledge of the person's sociocultural background. The nurse should avoid the use of medical abbreviations, terminology, or jargon. Questions should be short and to the point, particularly if the patient has difficulty with abstract thinking and conceptualization. Techniques such as clarification and summarization, described in Chapter 2, are important in validating information. The nurse should rephrase a question if the patient fails to answer appropriately or hesitates when answering.

Concentrated verbal interaction may be uncomfortable for the older person. The nurse can demonstrate interest and support by giving nonverbal cues and responses, such as direct eye contact, nodding, sitting close to the patient, and using touch appropriately. Touching the shoulder, arm, or hand of the patient in a firm, purposeful manner conveys support and interest. Avoid stroking or patting the patient. Cultural background and altered tactile perception may result in misinterpretation.

The nurse's ability to collect useful data depends greatly on how comfortable the nurse feels during the interview. Negative feelings toward the aged will surface in an interview. Older people are sensitive to others' lack of interest and impatience.

Although older people differ in their willingness to reveal life histories and personal experiences, most desire relationships with others and are anxious to share information with interested people. Elderly patients have much to tell and may offer more information than the nurse needs at a particular time. Older patients often reminisce. The nurse should encourage this when possible. The patient is concerned with life review. The life review may be an excellent source of data about the patient's current health problems and support resources. Reminiscence and life review may make it difficult to keep the patient focused on the topic at hand; however, they allow the nurse to assess subtle changes in long-term memory, decision-making ability, judgment-making patterns, affect, and orientation to time, place, and person.

Many geriatric patients are aware of changes in their physical or psychological functioning. They may hesitate to have their fears confirmed. They may minimize or ignore symptoms, assuming that they are age related and not related to current problems. Often these beliefs are reinforced by myths about aging and the false assumption of many health professionals that the problems of older people are irreversible or untreatable.

Contrary to popular myths, most older people do not dwell unrealistically on their health and usually have a physical problem when they say they are not well. However, some older people are preoccupied with the physical decline that occurs with age. The nurse must observe carefully for clues that help distinguish whether the patient's preoccupation reflects lifelong personality factors or current distress.

The geriatric patient may misunderstand the purpose of the nurse's questions. Questions regarding habits, previous life experience, or social supports may not seem to be related to current concerns. Careful and repeated explanations are necessary to gain the patient's cooperation. The nurse should never assume that the patient understands the purpose or protocol for the assessment interview. It is wiser to overstate than to increase the patient's anxiety and stress by omitting information. The nurse should take cues from the patient's responses by listening carefully and observing constantly.

? What special challenges might you face in obtaining informed consent for treatment from a geriatric patient? How might you deal with them?

THE INTERVIEW SETTING. The new and unfamiliar surroundings of the health-care agency may obstruct the initial interview by distracting the patient and increasing fear of the unknown. The physical environment should promote comfort. Many older people are unable to sit for long periods because of arthritis or other joint disabilities. Chairs should be comfortable. The patient should be encouraged to move about as desired. Changing positions and range-of-motion exercises stimulate circulation and prevent stiffness.

Most older people experience some form of sensory deficit, particularly diminished high-frequency hearing or changes in vision as a result of cataracts or glaucoma. The environment should be modified to decrease the impact of these deficits. The setting should be quiet and without distracting noises. A patient who is already under stress may be annoyed by these distractions. The nurse should speak slowly and in a low-pitched voice. Shouting raises the pitch of the voice and makes hearing more difficult. Because fatigue may contribute to diminished mental functioning, morning may be the best time for the interview. Patients become tired as the day progresses and cognitive ability may diminish in the late afternoon or early evening.

The reliability of the data obtained from the assessment interview should be carefully evaluated. If there are questions about some of the patient's responses, the nurse should consult family members or other people who know the patient well. The nurse should also consider the patient's physical condition at the time of the interview and other factors that may influence status, such as medications, nutrition, or anxiety level.

Mental Status

Mental status must be part of any geropsychiatric assessment for a number of reasons, including:
▼ The increasing prevalence of dementia with age
▼ The close association of clinical symptoms of confusion and depression
▼ The frequency with which physical health problems present with symptoms of confusion
▼ The need to identify specific areas of cognitive strength and limitation

An in-depth discussion of the assessment of mental status and other cognitive functioning scales used with the elderly is included in Chapter 6.

DEPRESSION. Affective status is an essential part of geropsychiatric assessment. The need to include a depression scale is based on:
▼ The prevalence of depression in the elderly
▼ The effectiveness of treatment for this disorder

▼ The potential negative outcomes of depression (such as suicide or neglect)
▼ Frequent misdiagnosis of depression as a physical problem
▼ The tendency to dismiss elders as complainers or demanding
▼ The necessity of accurately distinguishing between depressive and bipolar disorders
▼ The tendency for depression to recur with increasing age

General estimates of the prevalence of depression among the elderly are 15 to 20%. However, the estimates are higher for special populations such as elders in long-term care facilities. In general, the prevalence of depression is lower in the elderly than in younger age groups. However, there is a higher incidence of depression among people of all ages who have disabilities. Because the number of physical disabilities tends to increase with age, this may account for some of the prevalence in the elderly.[27]

Depression in the elderly differs in some ways from that in younger populations. It may begin with decreased interest in usual activities and lack of energy. There may be increased dependence on others. Conversation may focus almost entirely on the past. There may be multiple somatic complaints with no diagnosable organic cause. The person may have pain, especially in the head, neck, back, or abdomen with no history or evidence of a physical cause. Other symptoms in the elderly include weight loss, paranoia, fatigue, gastrointestinal distress, and refusal to eat or drink, with life-threatening consequences.

Physical illness can cause secondary depression (see Chapter 19). Some illnesses that tend to be associated with depression include thyroid disorders; cancer, especially lung, pancreas, and brain; Parkinson's disease; and stroke. Some medications also increase the tendency for depression, including steroids, phenothiazines, benzodiazepines, and antihypertensives.[20]

Geriatric Depression Scale. The Geriatric Depression Scale (GDS)[14] is a reliable and valid measure of depression. It was designed specifically for screening elderly people for depression. The GDS consists of 30 yes-or-no questions. It may be administered verbally or in writing. The versatility of the test makes it adaptable (for example, the verbal format can be used for an elder with visual problems). The simplicity of the answers (yes or no) and scoring is another advantage.

Anxiety. A thorough assessment of anxiety levels, coping responses, and precipitating stressors provides the nurse with information necessary for planning effective nursing care for the elderly. Anxiety disorders are a serious public health concern, lowering the quality of life for many elderly people and increasing the burden on family, care providers, and health services. Phobias, panic, obsessive compulsive disorder, and generalized anxiety disorder can all affect the elderly. When combined, their symptom prevalence among older people is estimated to be even higher than rates of depression alone. Untreated or inappropriately treated anxiety among older people can also contribute to sleep problems and cognitive impairments.[28]

Psychosis. Sometimes a nurse is confronted with an older adult with prominent psychotic features. These may take the form of delusions, hallucinations, or problems with testing reality. Being bedridden with poor caretaker relationships and being socially isolated are risk factors for psychosis among the elderly. In such cases, drug toxicity, a structural brain lesion, or a subtle seizure disorder should be considered.[15] Patients with a primary psychiatric diagnosis may respond to supportive therapy and low doses of high-potency neuroleptics. However, the nurse must keep in mind that older adults are highly sensitive to the side effects of these drugs.

Behavioral Responses

A thorough behavioral assessment is especially important as a basis for planning nursing care for an elderly person. Behavioral changes may be the first sign of many physical and mental disorders. It is important to identify who is bothered by the behavior—the patient, the family, peers, or unrelated caregivers. It is also helpful to know why the behavior is bothersome. Elders and their families may be frightened by changes in behavior because they associate them with deterioration and the possible onset of dementia. The nurse can help by explaining that behavior has many causes. Based on the assessment, the cause of the problem may be treated and the person returned to normal. For instance, a woman who is agitated because of an undiagnosed urinary tract infection returns to her normal, calm self after the infection is treated. In other cases it may not be possible to remove the cause of the behavior, but nursing intervention can help the patient and family adapt to it. For example, a man is irritable because he is becoming forgetful. Early Alzheimer's disease is diagnosed. The patient becomes less irritable after the nurse teaches him and his family ways to maximize his memory. Behavioral changes related to declining cognitive functioning are often difficult to manage and necessitate creative treatment.

If possible, initial assessment should be completed in the home environment. This will capitalize on environmental factors that reduce the elder's anxiety. It will also give the nurse a chance to observe possible triggers of disruptive behavior. Family members or other caregivers can be asked about their usual responses to the patient's behavior, especially what is helpful and unhelpful. This may provide further clues about the source of the behavior.

Behavioral assessment involves defining the behavior, its frequency, duration, and precipitating factors or triggers. When a behavioral change occurs, it is important to analyze the underlying meaning. For instance, the person may be experiencing a threat to self-esteem or a change in sensory input. A complete physical examination is needed following any abrupt behavioral change. Caregiver response to behav-

ior must also be assessed because it may reinforce or increase disturbed behavior. Common problem behaviors in the elderly are listed in Box 38-1.

> **?** *Mr. Jones, an elderly patient, strikes out at the staff every morning when he is approached to take his bath. Describe the steps you would take to assess this behavior. What questions might you ask his family? What advice would you give to the staff who work with him?*

Functional Abilities

Assessment of the geropsychiatric patient is not limited to indicators of mental health. Rather, mental status can depend greatly on the older person's overall functional ability. This discussion emphasizes the aspects of the functional assessment that have the greatest impact on mental and emotional status.

MOBILITY. Mobility and independence are important to the elder's perception of personal health. Three aspects of mobility should be assessed:

▼ Moving within the environment
▼ Participating in necessary activities
▼ Maintaining contact with others

In assessing ambulation the nurse would address motor losses, adaptations made, use of assistive devices, and the amount and type of help needed. Restriction of joints caused by degenerative diseases such as arthritis may affect ambulation. Orthostatic hypotension is possible when patients move rapidly from a lying to a standing position. The fit of footwear should be checked because gait may be unsteady. The motor ability of the arms can be tested by observing hair combing, shaving, dressing, and feeding.

In addition to altered functional ability caused by changes in physical or psychological status, many medications taken by geriatric patients alter perception, making ambulation and mobility difficult. This is particularly so with sedatives/hypnotics, antianxiety, cardiovascular, and

Box **38-1** *Problem Behaviors Observed in Geropsychiatric Patients*

Biting	Pacing
Confusion	Rapid speech
Constant talking	Refusal to eat or drink
Delusions	Repetitive movement
Fatigue	Scolding
Forgetting	Spitting
Hallucinations	Suspiciousness
Hand wringing	Swearing
Hitting	Threats of physical harm
Incontinence	Throwing things
Isolating self	Wandering
Kicking	

hypertensive drugs. Patients should be cautioned about side effects of medications and should be encouraged to take plenty of time when ambulating and moving from one position to another.

The incidence of falls and negative outcomes increases with age; 30% of people over 65 years of age fall every year, with women falling at twice the rate of men. Falls result in physical injuries such as hip fractures as well as psychological effects such as fearfulness. Risk factors must be assessed. A summary of these is presented in Table 38-1.

ACTIVITIES OF DAILY LIVING. The assessment of self-care needs and activities of daily living (ADLs) is essential for determining the patient's potential for independence. Activity may be limited because of physical dysfunction or psychosocial impairment. Although geriatric patients should be encouraged to become more independent in self-care, it is unrealistic to expect all patients to function independently. This is particularly so for people who are in a hospital or long-term care setting. Conforming

TABLE **38-1** *Assessment of Risk for Falls*

RISK FACTORS	ASSESSMENT FACTORS
Environmental hazards	Poor lighting
	Slippery or wet surfaces
	Stairs (no handrails, steep, poorly lit)
	Loose objects on the floor
	Throw rugs
	Small pets underfoot
Patient variables	History of falls
	Diurnal alertness level
	Familiarity with surroundings
	Emotional state (agitated, angry, etc.)
	Willingness to request help
	Confusion
	Usual activity level
	Type of activity
Assistive devices	Presence and adequacy of:
	Eyeglasses
	Hearing aid
	Ambulation aids (cane, tripod, walker)
	Prostheses
	Environmental aids (grab bars, hand rails)
Medications	Taking medications (prescribed or over-the-counter) that cause:
	Drowsiness
	Confusion
	Orthostatic hypotension
	Incoordination
	Decreased sensation
	Polypharmacy
Physical or mental disorders	Cardiovascular
	Orthopedic
	Neuromuscular
	Perceptual
	Cognitive
	Affective

to the routines and procedures of the institutional environment fosters dependence in the patient.

ADLs (bathing, dressing, eating, grooming, and toileting) are concrete and task oriented. They provide an opportunity for purposeful nurse-patient interaction. It is important to encourage patients to be as independent as possible in performing their own ADLs. This helps elders meet their needs for safety, security, personal space, self-esteem, autonomy, and personal identity.

The Katz Index of Activities of Daily Living. . Variations in functional status can influence the care provider's approach to the issues of daily living. The Katz Index of Activities of Daily Living provides reliable assessment of an elder's ability to care for himself or herself. With the data collected in this assessment, individualized care plans can be written. The Katz Index[21] rates dependence versus independence for each of six ADL functions: bathing, dressing, toileting, transfer, continence, and feeding. One point is assigned for each observed item of dependency. The dependent-independent categories for each function are defined in observable terms ("gets clothes from closets and drawers"). One advantage of this tool is the ability to measure change in ADL function over time, allowing evaluation of rehabilitation activities.

Physiological Functioning

Assessment of physical health is especially important with elderly patients because of the interaction of multiple chronic conditions, the presence of sensory deficits, the taking of many medications, and the behaviors presented by physical health problems. Diagnostic procedures that may be useful include the electroencephalogram, lumbar puncture, blood chemistry values, and brain visual imaging techniques such as the computed tomography scan and magnetic resonance imaging. In addition to these physiological factors, nutritional status and substance abuse must be assessed.

The latest research documents a direct relationship among stress, immune system functioning, and mood. Clinical observations have identified a failure to thrive syndrome, especially in the final phase of life. **Failure to thrive** syndrome consists of weight loss, decreased appetite, poor nutrition, and inactivity. It is often accompanied by dehydration, depressive symptoms, impaired immune functions, and low serum cholesterol. Failure to thrive in the elderly occurs in both acute and chronic forms, leading to impaired functional status, morbidity from infection, pressure sores, and increased mortality.

NUTRITION. Many elderly patients do not require help to eat or plan a nutritious diet. However, many geropsychiatric patients do have psychosocial problems that create a need for help with eating and monitoring dietary intake. These problems include:

▼ Depression or loneliness, resulting in decreased appetite
▼ Changes in cognition, such as confusion or disorientation

▼ Suicidal tendencies

▼ Removal from familiar ethnic and cultural eating patterns

▼ Fear of institutional routines or procedures

The range of physical problems varies greatly. The following areas should be assessed:

▼ Whether the patient has enough mobility and strength to open cartons of milk, cut meat, and handle utensils

▼ The presence of neurological or joint conditions that interfere with hand and arm coordination

▼ The presence of vision problems

▼ Missing teeth and other losses of chewing ability

▼ Problems in swallowing or breathing

▼ The presence of ulcerations on the tongue or elsewhere in the mouth

▼ Periodontal disease

▼ Dry mouth because of medications

The nurse should routinely evaluate the patient's dietary needs. Nutritional deficiencies are one of the most significant problems of the institutionalized elderly and can cause other problems, such as skin breakdown, inadequate absorption of medications, and impaired wound healing.

Nutritional assessment should also explore personal preferences, including prior routines (such as largest meal at lunchtime), time of day for meals, portion sizes, and food likes and dislikes. Serum cholesterol and albumin levels provide additional information about the person's nutritional status.

SUBSTANCE ABUSE. Most studies of alcoholism have focused on a younger population, so the prevalence of alcohol abuse by elders has not been well documented. There is a risk of developing alcoholism in later life if there has been habitual drinking in the past. Significant loss and role changes or increased anxiety and concern over health add to the risk. Alcohol is the most commonly abused substance by the elderly because it is readily available and not usually perceived as a drug. The abuse of prescription drugs, particularly sedative-hypnotic and antianxiety medications, is also common and may not be seen as an addiction. Alcohol and substance abuse can lead to increased morbidity and mortality. Abuse of alcohol or any substance may be a means of attaining distance from painful issues such as loss and loneliness. Assessment tools for substance abuse are presented in Chapters 6 and 24.

Social Support

Positive support systems are essential for maintaining a sense of well-being throughout life. This is especially important for the geropsychiatric patient. With age, close family members and friends are lost. As a person's significant contacts decrease in number, it is important that the remaining support systems be consistent and meaningful.

Caring behaviors among elderly nursing home residents have been found to be a major way in which residents maintain their personal identity, sense of value, and continuation of personhood. This demonstrates that support systems that develop among patients are beneficial to those who give and receive care.

The patient's ethnic and religious background may be an important factor in identifying support systems. Strong family, ethnic, and church ties promote feelings of security. Elderly people who live alone and are without family ties generally have more serious problems than those who are not isolated. These problems may affect the patient's financial stability, as well as the desire to get well, be content with life, and perform self-care whenever possible. The nurse should assess the support systems available to the patient while at home, in the hospital, or in another health-care setting. Family and friends can help reduce the shock and stress of hospitalization and offer reassurance and comfort to the distressed elder.

FAMILY-PATIENT INTERACTION. Family demographics are changing. Increased life expectancy, declining birth rate, and higher life expectancy for women all affect the availability of family to participate in caregiving and support of the elder. The majority of elders have a minimum of weekly contact with their children.

> **?** *Discuss the ways in which changing demographics in American society are affecting the social support systems of elderly people. What is the impact on their families?*

Family expectations about caring for older members vary. The decision to care for an aging member at home or to include extended family members in the household is discussed over time within the family unit. The majority of caregiving in the United States is provided by family members and three phases of caregiving have been identified (Table 38-2).

Significant issues that affect families in late adulthood are retirement, widowhood, grandparenthood, and illness. Nurses must become more comfortable and knowledgeable about dealing with issues of sexuality, marital discord, cohabitation, spousal abuse, and elder abuse. According to the Task Force on Aging Research,[26] the perception of increased abuse of elderly people is based on the escalation of combined pressures of changing cultural norms, crowded living conditions, insufficient financial support, alcohol abuse, and other disruptive behaviors. The cultural norms that previously placed elderly people in a position of respect as pivotal members of the community appear to have eroded in much of American society. Social and organizational structures have not developed supports to replace those previously available through extended family networks. There is a great deal of discussion in the literature concerning abuse of elderly people, but more research is needed to establish its prevalence and the factors related to it. The nurse should be aware of changing trends and be alert for

TABLE **38-2** *Stages of Caregiving*

STAGE	CHARACTERISTICS	NURSING ACTIVITIES
Encounter	Receiving and understanding the diagnosis Adjusting to the diagnosis Learning required caregiving skills Changing lifestyle	Provide information Teach caregiving skills Offer support and comfort Refer to support group of other new caregivers
Enduring	Heavy workloads Established routines of caregiving Little attention to personal well-being Feelings of hopelessness No planning for the future Social isolation Stress and burnout	Arrange respite care Refer to support group Encourage to pursue personal interests Focus on short-term and long-term goals Teach stress management and coping strategies Teach relaxation techniques
Exit	Decisions related to the end of caregiving Activities related to ending the role Adjustments to a changed role	Help with nursing home placement Help with grieving Discuss alternatives for activities, work, social relationships

Modified from Lindgren CL: *Image* 25:214, 1993.

TABLE **38-3** *Key Components of Geropsychiatric Nursing Assessment*

COMPONENT	KEY ELEMENTS
Interviewing	Therapeutic communication skills Comfortable, quiet setting
Mental status	Mini-Mental State Examination Mental Status Examination Depression Anxiety Psychosis
Behavioral responses	Description of behavior Assessment of behavioral change Frequently observed problem behaviors
Functional abilities	Mobility Activities of daily living Risk for falls
Physiological functioning	General health Nutrition Substance abuse
Social support	Social support systems Family-patient interaction Caregiver concerns

the possibility of elder abuse, which is addressed in more detail in Chapter 39.

When assessing the older adult, the nurse should note previous success in dealing with life issues. The elder's adjustment to losses and changes associated with aging is affected by earlier life experiences. Behavioral problems in the elderly may result from the family's inability to deal with the losses and increasing dependence of an older member.

A comprehensive nursing assessment sets the stage for the rest of the nursing process. Table 38-3 summarizes the key components of a thorough geropsychiatric nursing assessment.

DIAGNOSIS OF THE GERIATRIC PATIENT

Although older adults may experience a wide range of psychiatric problems, the nursing diagnoses of greatest significance to the nurse and patient in promoting a therapeutic outcome will be discussed.

Altered Thought Processes

MEMORY LOSS. Memory loss is one of the most distressing and frustrating aspects of aging. Although memory loss may be caused by organic brain disease or depression, it is not necessarily related to a disease process. With age, loss of short-term memory (recall of recent events) is more likely to occur than loss of long-term memory (recall of events that occurred in the distant past). The network of past thoughts, images, ideas, and experiences that makes up memory develops and matures over a lifetime. Primary memory is the conscious control system for memory. It appears to be stable over the life span. There is little difference in primary memory among people of different ages. However, speed of access appears to slow with increasing age.[1] Long-term memory (secondary memory) is the storage system for what is commonly understood as memory. Failure in retrieval, original acquisition, or learning may cause loss in secondary memory.[1]

Many factors contribute to altered memory in older adults. Stress or crisis, depression, a sense of worthlessness, loss of interest in present events, cerebrovascular changes that affect cerebral function, loss of neural cells because of disease or trauma, and sensory deprivation or social isolation may all occur with advancing age. Impaired memory for recent events may actually be a result of decreased vision or hearing. This may lead the older person to seek comfort in old memories and experiences, which replace the need to remain in touch with the present.

Institutionalized elderly people appear to have more difficulty with memory than those who live at home or in other community settings. A stimulating environment and nursing intervention can counteract and often reverse withdrawal in the psychiatric patient. As the person becomes more involved in activities, memory may improve.

CONFUSION. Confusion is a constellation of behaviors, including inattention and memory deficits, inappropriate verbalizations, disruptive behavior, noncompliance, and failure to perform ADLs. Often, *confusion* is a nonspecific term used by staff to label apathetic, withdrawn, or uncooperative patients. Several categories of patients are likely to be labeled as confused: the problem patient, the patient with communication problems (slurred speech, expressive dysphasia), the patient who challenges staff members' personal values, the depressed patient, and the patient who does not get well.

Institutionalized elders are at particular risk of confusion. From 40 to 80% suffer from some degree of organic brain disease, with disorientation to time, place, and person, remote and recent memory loss, and inability to do simple calculations. In many long-term care facilities, more than 30% of the patients have severe confusion.[9] The precipitating factors depend on both the physiological and psychological condition of the patient.

Early morning confusion, sometimes called sunrise syndrome, may result from the hangover effects of sedatives/hypnotics or other nighttime medications that interact with drugs for sleep. Sleep problems and insomnia are common in the elderly. Adverse reactions to drugs prescribed for sleep often occur. Increasing disorientation or confusion at night, resulting from loss of visual accommodation and other factors, is known as sundown syndrome. The nurse should take special precautions to prevent falls at these times.[4]

The most logical cause of sundowning is the deterioration of the suprachiasmatic nucleus in the hypothalamus. This major pacemaker of circadian rhythms regulates the sleep-wake cycle (see Chapter 5) and has been found to be deteriorated in demented people. Assessing and then minimizing or eliminating any environmental and underlying physiological causes of afternoon or evening confusion or irritability would be important activities for the nurse. These include[4]:

▼ Elimination of toxic, infectious, metabolic, or pharmacologic causes of delirium
▼ Elimination of underlying physiologic causes of agitation and confusion such as pain, febrile illnesses, and incontinence
▼ Restriction of daytime sleep
▼ At least minimal exposure to direct sunlight each day, particularly in the morning (to reset the pacemaker)
▼ Increase in mild activity, such as walking
▼ Increase in conversations and other social interactions with staff

▼ Assessing for appropriateness of short-term use of low-dose antipsychotic drugs

> **?** *A nurse's aide tells you that a patient is "wandering down the hall, staggering, pajama top unbuttoned." It is early morning, and the other patients are asleep. What would you do in this situation?*

The nurse should never assume that confusion and disorientation are natural results of changes in cognitive or physiological status. Confusion is reversible in over half the patients who experience it. It is usually transient or short term. The nurse has primary responsibility for intervening in this problem. Well-planned nursing care can be a significant factor in preventing and intervening in this distressing condition.

Although the term *disorientation* is often used interchangeably with *confusion,* they are different. A disoriented patient is not necessarily confused, and a confused patient does not necessarily experience complete disorientation. Mental status tests differentiate disorientation to place, person, and time from components of confusion, such as alterations in memory, judgment, decision making, and problem solving. Cognitive responses are discussed in detail in Chapter 23.

PARANOIA. Some older people react to loss, isolation, and loneliness with paranoia and fear. Classic paranoia, involving a well-organized and elaborate delusional system, is rare in older people. Delusions and disturbances in mood, behavior, and thinking may be temporary conditions caused by sensory deprivation or sensory loss, social isolation, or medications.

Paranoid symptoms may be general or specific. The geriatric patient may feel threatened by certain people (such as family, friends, or neighbors) or at certain times (such as night). Relocation to a new home, new room, or strange environment causes fears, anxiety, and for some, paranoid ideation.

The personality of aging paranoid patients is characterized by withdrawal, aloofness, fearfulness, oversensitivity, and often secretiveness. As long as patients do not call attention to themselves or threaten themselves or others, their paranoia may remain hidden. Once they become a potential threat to themselves or others, institutionalization may be needed. Older people who have transient or chronic paranoia are at high risk for victimization by others as well as self-neglect and abuse (such as refusal to eat, take prescribed medications, or attend to hygiene needs).

Affective Responses

Disturbances in mood, mood swings, or oversensitive emotional reactions are common to people of all ages. An older person's reaction to physical limitations or disabilities, psychological loss (particularly of a spouse or other close person), or the possibility of institutionalization depends on past coping styles, support systems (especially family), and present psychological and physiological strength.

Extreme or sudden mood changes occur in response to stress or as inadequate coping mechanisms in people facing progressive loss or dependency. When this behavior is seen in elderly people who have been content and happy, physiological factors, including side effects of medications, should be considered. Reassurance and support are given to reduce the patient's anxiety and diminish the perceived threat.

DYSFUNCTIONAL GRIEVING. Depression and sadness are sometimes viewed as a natural part of aging. In fact, depression, grief, and loss are common in later life. Prolonged grief and mourning over a real or imagined loss should be recognized and treated as depression. Common symptoms include weight loss, appetite loss, fatigue, apathy, loss of interest in friends, family, and usual activities, and psychomotor retardation. None of the symptoms are caused by increasing age; all are problems that can be effectively treated (see Chapter 19).

The person's attitude toward aging, dying, and death influences whether the depression can be treated successfully. The loss of hope expressed by some older people, particularly those with increasing disabilities, may cause or result from a depressive reaction.

Undiagnosed depression may have serious effects on the elderly because depression always causes physical symptoms. Many of the medications routinely prescribed for older people can increase depression. Examples include antianxiety drugs, neuroleptics, barbiturates, cardiotonics (digoxin), and steroids. A medication history is part of the evaluation and assessment.

It is important to understand the patient's and family's attitudes toward death and dying. The old differ from the young in their attitudes toward death in several ways: Older people tend to integrate attitudes toward death with their religious beliefs, to have experienced the death of significant others, to be more accepting of death, and to approach problems primarily from an internal focus. The state of the older person's health, in addition to what he or she has learned from seeing people die, may signal that his or her life may be ending. Awareness of the older person's "stage of dying" is important to understanding his or her needs and concerns.

RISK FOR VIOLENCE: SELF-DIRECTED. Intentional deaths among the elderly are common. Older people in the United States have the highest suicide rate of any age group. The suicide rate of white males over age 65 is more than double that of adolescents. Others at high risk include isolated elderly people who have lost family or friends through death; those with changes in body function and decreased independence because of pain, weakness, immobility, or shortness of breath; those with changes in body function because of surgery or stroke; and those who are terminally ill. Suicidal behavior is discussed in detail in Chapter 20.

Elderly suicide victims use more violent and lethal means to take their lives, resulting in a higher ratio of completed to attempted suicides. Suicide in elderly people is strongly association with depression, physical illness, loss of adaptive coping mechanisms, and neurobiologic alteration. Most sadly, the majority of elderly suicide victims have seen their primary care provider in the month before their death, but their suicidal intentions were not detected and they were not treated for their depression. Finally, other examples of intentional deaths include excessive risk taking, lack of caution in the management of ordinary affairs, refusal to eat, overuse or misuse of alcohol or drugs, and noncompliance with life-sustaining medical regimens, such as refusal to take insulin or digoxin.

> **?** *Were you surprised to learn that the elderly have the highest suicide rate? How would you increase public awareness of this important health-care problem?*

SITUATIONAL LOW SELF-ESTEEM. Low self-esteem in the elderly is often expressed through preoccupation with physical and emotional health and expression of concern through body complaints. This may be labeled hypochondriasis but really represents the person's insecurity.

As a sign of the geriatric patient's sense of deterioration, somaticism communicates the distress that accompanies decreased self-worth. The sick role is a legitimate and socially acceptable way to deal with stress and anxiety. The patient receives support, concern, and interest and experiences a sense of control.

One of the real problems encountered by elders with a history of somaticizing is health professionals' tendency to dismiss their complaints, assuming there is no real illness. All symptoms should be taken seriously and investigated thoroughly. One must never dismiss the problem as just a response to emotional distress. Whatever its cause, the problem and the patient's discomfort are real.

Somatic Responses

SLEEP PATTERN DISTURBANCE. Insomnia may be a symptom or a problem in itself for the geropsychiatric patient. Many older adults experience chronic or intermittent sleep problems. Complaints of interrupted sleep, loss of sleep, or poor sleep, with frequent awakenings and morning exhaustion, are common. Daytime napping and drowsiness add to the problem. Nonetheless, sleep disorders in the elderly can be systematically diagnosed and treated.[23]

Opinions vary regarding normal sleep patterns in older adults. Some researchers suggest that people need less sleep as they age. However, chronic fatigue, physical illness, pain, and decreased mobility may cause a need for more sleep. Geriatric patients often express distress over their inability to sleep or stay asleep. Perceived lack of sleep becomes a cyclical reaction. Worry about lack of sleep prevents falling asleep. Fatigue is the most common physical complaint of adults over the age of 75. It contributes to much of the insomnia of this age group. Lack of exercise, limited mobility, and side effects of drugs may also contribute to insomnia. It is also a symptom of depression.

ALTERED NUTRITION: LESS THAN BODY REQUIREMENTS. Appetite loss is common in patients with depression. Inadequate dietary intake also occurs in confused or disoriented patients. Forgetting to eat or being unable to prepare meals may add to the problem of appetite loss. Side effects of some drugs (such as dry mouth or change in taste) contribute to lack of interest in food. The toothless patient or someone with gum disease avoids chewing when possible. The interaction of appetite loss and emotional dysfunction should always be considered in the nutritional evaluation. Poor nutrition contributes to fatigue, listlessness, and immobility.

Stress Responses

RELOCATION STRESS SYNDROME. This condition involves physical or psychosocial disturbances related to transfer from one environment to another. Since 1950 the care of many elderly mentally ill has shifted from state psychiatric hospitals to nursing homes. In fact, the number of mentally ill elderly residing in nursing homes greatly exceeds that in state psychiatric hospitals. This shift in treatment sites drew attention to the process and consequences of relocation. Although some data on mortality have been collected, morbidity data are limited. Relocation will continue to be a fact of life, both to provide patients with less restrictive environments and to decrease the cost of long-term care of the mentally ill.

The stress of relocation should be anticipated for all geriatric patients. Intervention should be planned to reduce the impact. Allowing the patient to have personal belongings, liberal visiting hours for family or friends, and careful explanations of the purpose and routines of the institution are a few of the ways in which the stress of change can be minimized.

Establishing an effective support system within the new setting may prevent the negative behaviors often observed in isolated elders: apathy, depression, aggression, or hostility. In transfers between institutions, it may be helpful to arrange for the patient to visit the new location before the actual move. This allows the patient to meet other residents and staff, see the physical surroundings, and ask questions about the program. When possible, posttransfer visits by staff from the transferring agency also ease the transition, as well as offer staff from both agencies the opportunity to communicate about nursing approaches.

Risk factors[24] related to relocation stress syndrome include the following:

▼ Impaired psychosocial or physical health status
▼ Other recent losses

▼ Losses associated with the move
▼ Inadequate preparation for the move
▼ Feelings of powerlessness
▼ Moderate to great difference between the old and new environments
▼ Prior relocation experiences
▼ Inadequate support system

Behaviors associated with relocation stress syndrome are listed in Box 38-2.

RISK FOR CAREGIVER ROLE STRAIN. Disabled elderly people who live in the community rely on support and care from family members. As the percentage of elderly people in the population grows, family resources will be increasingly important to keep elders in the community and provide care that is less expensive than professional care. This role is stressful for people who care for frail elders. It has been well documented that providing elder care can result in emotional, physical, interpersonal, and occupational problems. Research has also demonstrated that stress to the caregiver increases over time.[29] A caregiver under stress is at risk for problems in performing the caregiver role.[24] Risk factors are listed in Table 38-4.

Behavioral Responses

SOCIAL ISOLATION. Multiple losses or fear of loss may lead to social isolation. Prolonged grief after the loss of a spouse, sibling, child, or close friend may make the elder hesitant to become involved in other close relationships. The person who has been close only to a few family members or friends will have even more difficulty with loss.

Elderly patients experiencing organic cognitive impairment (such as Alzheimer's disease and related disorders) often withdraw from social contacts, daily routines, and ADLs. They may deny having a problem or fear the consequences of memory changes. Social isolation can become a defense mechanism, reinforcing denial of perceived disability.

SELF-CARE DEFICIT. Chronic illness is one aspect of aging that may result in the inability to care for oneself.

Box **38-2** *Behaviors Associated with Relocation Stress Syndrome*

Anxiety, apprehension, restlessness, and verbalization of being concerned/upset about transfer
Vigilance, dependency, increased verbalization of needs, insecurity, and lack of trust
Increased confusion
Depression, sad affect, withdrawal, and loneliness
Sleep disturbance
Change in eating habits, gastrointestinal disturbances, and weight changes
Unfavorable comparison of posttransfer and pretransfer staff

TABLE **38-4** *Risk Factors for Caregiver Role Strain*

Category	Risk Factors
Pathophysiological	Severe illness of elder
	Unpredictable illness course
	Addiction or codependency
	Elder discharged with serious home care needs
	Caregiver health impairment
	Caregiver is female
Psychosocial	Psychosocial/cognitive problems in care receiver
	Family problems before caregiving
	Marginal caregiver coping patterns
	Poor relationship between caregiver and receiver
	Caregiver is spouse
	Care receiver has deviant or bizarre behavior
Situational	Abuse or violence
	Other sources of stress on family
	Need for long-term caregiving
	Inadequate physical environment
	Family/caregiver isolation
	Lack of caregiver respite or recreation
	Inexperience
	Competing role commitments
	Complex/demanding caregiving tasks

With increasing years comes a greater chance of multiple chronic problems. Affective illnesses such as major depression or bipolar disorder may cause psychomotor retardation, preventing elders from meeting their basic needs. Medications may cause forgetfulness, lethargy, and physical impairment. Because of increasing frailty or cognitive impairment, many elders are unable to complete basic self-care activities such as bathing, toileting, grooming, and feeding. The underlying cause of the deficit must be determined and appropriate nursing interventions planned.

PLANNING AND INTERVENTION

Expected outcomes related to the nursing care of the geropsychiatric patient must be realistically based on the person's potential to change. If the person's behavioral problems result from a treatable disorder, expected outcomes and short-term goals may reflect a return to preillness functioning. For example, a goal for a patient with depression who is neglectful of personal hygiene might be: *The patient will bathe, dress, and brush his teeth independently.*

If the condition is chronic and either no change or progressive deterioration is expected, then the outcomes of care focus on adaptation to this. For example, a goal for a patient with Alzheimer's disease who neglects personal hygiene might be: *The patient will help with bathing, dressing, and brushing one's teeth.*

If the patient's condition is not expected to improve, the expected outcomes and goals may focus on the caregiver as well as the patient. For example, a goal for a caregiver of a person with Alzheimer's disease might be: *At least once a week the caregiver will participate in a recreational activity outside of the home while the home health aide is with the patient.*

The plan of care must be developed with the active participation of the patient and the caregiver. It also must be reviewed frequently to ensure that it is relevant to the patient's current needs. Caregiver education is an important part of the plan.

Older adults respond well to both individual and group interventions. They need the opportunity to talk, be supported in their efforts to deal with day-to-day problems, and plan for a meaningful future. The type of nursing intervention selected depends on the nursing care problems identified, the interests and preferences of the elder, and the setting in which the care is to be provided. In the past most geropsychiatric care was provided in state psychiatric hospitals. Nurses will now find older patients with mental illness in these hospitals as well as in acute psychiatric units, nursing homes, emergency rooms, and increasingly in community settings. The need for a comprehensive community-based system of care has been noted in the literature.[13,33]

Nursing care for cognitively impaired patients in inpatient settings is addressed in Chapter 23, including approaches to behaviors such as wandering, aggression, agitation, falls, and confusion.

Therapeutic Milieu

Whether in a hospital, nursing home, community program, or at home, the care environment should support effective intervention. There are several basic characteristics of a therapeutic milieu.

COGNITIVE STIMULATION. Activities should be planned to maintain or improve the patients' cognitive functioning. Discussion groups help patients focus on topics of interest to them. Projects can reinforce skills and offer an opportunity for success. The nurse can collaborate with the rehabilitation therapist in planning interesting and appropriate activities.

PROMOTE A SENSE OF CALM AND QUIET. Elders often do best in a setting that is designated for their care. In particular, inpatient units that admit all age groups may be too stimulating for confused patients. In general, the geropsychiatric setting should be decorated in soft colors. If music is played, it should be soothing and preferably familiar to the elderly. Bright lights that create glare should be avoided. Although the environmental background should be subdued, planned periods of increased activity help maintain interest and alertness.

Personal belongings can offer a sense of security. For people who are not in their own home, articles such as family pictures, religious objects, favorite books, afghans, or decorative objects are reassuring (Fig. 38-1).

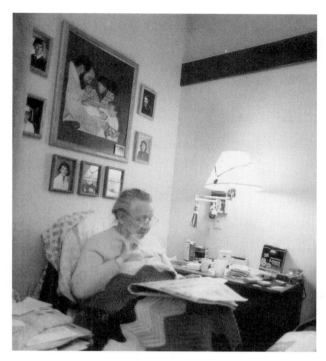

Fig. 38-1 This woman has many family pictures and other personal belongings that provide her with a sense of comfort and security.

CONSISTENT PHYSICAL LAYOUT. In residential or inpatient settings, room changes should be avoided as much as possible. Furniture arrangements should be stable; this helps disoriented people to locate themselves and adds to their security.

STRUCTURED ROUTINE. The daily schedule should be as predictable as possible. Bedtime, waking time, nap times, and mealtimes should not vary. For elders who have recently moved to a new setting, it is helpful to give them and their families copies of the weekly schedule. Time should be allowed for reviewing the schedule with patients. Periodic reinforcement of the routines may be needed until patients adjust to the environment.

FOCUS ON STRENGTHS AND ABILITIES. Most elders have strengths related to their past accomplishments. If the person is unable to communicate, family members can give information about the patient's life and suggest activities that are likely to be successful. Nursing creativity can find ways to capitalize on elders' strengths by planning opportunities for them to help staff or other patients or participate in activities based on their abilities.

MINIMIZE DISRUPTIVE BEHAVIOR. Understanding the patient's behavioral patterns can help to reduce agitation and behavioral crises. Observation reveals situations that lead to disruptions. Adhering to the person's usual lifestyle as closely as possible reduces conflicts. For instance, a person who has always taken a bath in the evening before

bed should not be forced to shower before breakfast. Patients who agitate each other should be kept apart as much as possible. Distraction can often interrupt a conflict before it gets out of control.

MINIMAL DEMANDS FOR COMPLIANT BEHAVIOR. Elders who are cognitively impaired often resist demands from others. They may not understand what is being asked of them or they may be frightened of an unexpected change in activity. Some older adults resent being under the control of others and need to assert themselves. It is best to avoid pressuring the patient to comply. Reapproaching the person after a few minutes is often successful. If the patient needs to be in control, it is helpful to negotiate a time of voluntary compliance.

> **?** *How would the therapeutic milieu differ if most patients were elderly and (a) depressed, (b) demented, or (c) delusional?*

PROVIDING SAFETY. Safety needs must be considered. The nurse should be alert for safety hazards and remove them. Because falls are a concern, floors should be free from slippery spots and obstacles. Hand rails and grab bars are helpful for frail elders. Fire is also a concern. Open flames should be avoided. If smoking is allowed, it may be necessary to provide supervision in an area of the facility that permits smoking.

In many facilities restraints are used to enhance the patient's safety. They include a variety of devices such as mitts, posey vests, and geri chairs applied with a physician's order. Although such devices may help staff to protect geropsychiatric patients, they limit freedom of choice and movement, as well as threaten dignity.[30,34] Six myths related to physical restraint of elderly patients are summarized in Table 38-5.

Somatic Therapies

ELECTROCONVULSIVE THERAPY. Electroconvulsive therapy (ECT) has been found to be very effective in the treatment of depression in the older adult. (See Chapter 28 for a detailed discussion of ECT.) Contraindications for this type of therapy are an intracranial space-occupying lesion with increased intracranial pressure, arrhythmias, and myocardial infarction within the last 3 months.

PSYCHOTROPIC MEDICATIONS. The addition of psychotropic medications to the drug regimen of elders must be approached carefully.[31] Basic guidelines for medication administration for elders include the slow initiation of medications, preferably one at a time, using lower dosages. Special consideration must be given to psychotropic medications and elders because drugs that affect behavior also affect the central nervous system. It has been documented that elderly patients are especially vulnerable to

TABLE **38-5** *Myths and Realities about Physical Restraint*

MYTHS	REALITIES
Restraints reduce the risk of injury related to falls.	Restraints do not reduce the risk of injury from falls and may increase it. Falls do increase the likelihood of future restraint.
Restraining meets the nurse's moral duty to protect the patient from harm.	Restraints may increase the risk of injury and lead to problems related to immobility, confusion, aggression, depression, and incontinence.
Failure to restrain results in legal liability.	Federal and state laws and regulations prohibit the unnecessary use of restraint.
Older people do not mind being restrained.	Older people do not wish to be restrained. They feel angry, hurt, and embarrassed by the experience.
Inadequate staffing justifies restraining patients.	Federal and state laws and regulations forbid restraining patients for staff convenience. Providing adequate nursing care to a restrained patient takes at least as much time as caring for an unrestrained one.
There are no adequate alternatives to physical restraint.	Nursing care alternatives have been identified in several categories: ▼ Physical care: comfort, relief of pain, positioning ▼ Psychosocial care: remotivation, communication, attention ▼ Activities ▼ Environmental manipulation: improved lighting, removal of restraint devices, redesigned furniture ▼ Administrative support and staff training

Modified from Evans LK, Strumpf NE: *Image* 22:124, 1990.

developing tardive dyskinesia. Table 38-6 describes recommended dosages of psychotropic medications for the elderly. (See Chapter 27 for a thorough discussion of psychopharmacology.)

Special attention must be given to the older adult when assessing medication use. Four factors place the elder at risk for drug toxicity and should be included in any assessment: age, polypharmacy, decreased medication compliance, and comorbidity. Misuse of drugs by the elderly is also a factor in the rising cost of health care for the population (Box 38-3).

Age. As a person ages, physiological responses to medications change. In the over-65 age group, drug dosages must be monitored carefully for continuing effectiveness. A medication dosage that is effective at age 65 may be toxic at age 75. Gastrointestinal absorption, hepatic blood flow and metabolism, and renal clearance may all decline. Also, the ratio of fat to lean muscle mass increases with age. Many psychoactive medications are lipophilic (attracted to fat), which increases the risk of drugs building up in fatty tissue and causing toxicity. Drug testing is often done using a younger population. This does not allow evaluation of the differing effects of new drugs on older people.

Polypharmacy. Several surveys report that older adults take an average of 8 to 10 medications daily. It is also suggested that the use of over-the-counter medicines is underreported because they are not thought to be significant. Drugs such as alcohol and acetaminophen (Tylenol) are not always reported but can be toxic in combination with other drugs.

Compliance. Many drugs take up to 6 weeks to effect a change in affective disorders. In the interim elders may see no benefit to continued compliance and may abandon their medication regimen. Education regarding the purpose,

Box **38-3** *The High Cost of Medication Misuse in the Elderly*

A study recently conducted by the US General Accounting Office reports that more than five million older Americans use medications that are inappropriate or could cause adverse interactions serious enough to warrant hospitalization.

The report, "Prescription Drugs and the Elderly," estimates that prescription misuse costs the United States approximately $120 billion each year in avoidable hospital stays plus $7 billion in hospitalizations due to noncompliance. The report was compiled from 1992 Medicare data and interviews with specialists in gerontology and elderly clinical pharmacology. The proposed solutions include:
▼ Improved communication of pertinent information between prescriber and patient, such as purpose, side effects, duration of drug therapy, and possible interactions with other drugs, foods, and alcohol.
▼ Prescriber education about the use of medication in the elderly and the complex nature of misuse in this age group.
▼ Managed care and pharmacy management programs may decrease the cost of medication treatment for the elderly. It is estimated that 25% of people cite drug cost as a factor in noncompliance with their drug therapy regimen.

therapeutic value, and side effects of medications should be provided to elders to enhance medication compliance and awareness.

Comorbidity. Acute and chronic illnesses can alter the body's response to medications. Altered response to medications may result from such illnesses as chronic renal failure, congestive heart failure, and structural and functional changes in the central nervous system. Central nervous system changes may result in heightened sensitivity to drugs such as the benzodiazepines.

TABLE **38-6** *Psychoactive Medications*

CATEGORY		RECOMMENDED DOSAGE RANGE FOR OLDER ADULTS
Selective serotonin reuptake inhibitors (SSRIs) and newer antidepressants	Fluoxetine/Prozac (SSRI)	20-80 mg/day
	Sertraline/Zoloft (SSRI)	50 mg/day
	Paroxetine/Paxil (SSRI)	20 mg/day
	Venlafaxine/Effexor (SNRI)	37.5-225 mg/day
	Nefazodone/Serzone	100 mg/day
	Mirtazapine/Remeron	15-45 mg/day
Tricyclic antidepressants (TCAs)	Amitriptyline/Elavil	10-75 mg/day
	Imipramine/Tofranil	10-75 mg/day
	Desipramine/Norpramin	10-150 mg/day
	Nortriptyline/Aventyl	10-50 mg/day
	Trazodone/Desyrel	25-150 mg/day
Monoamine oxidase inhibitors (MAOIs)	Isocarboxazid/Marplan	10-30 mg/day
	Phenelzine/Nardil	15-45 mg/day
	Tranylcypromine/Parnate	10-30 mg/day
Mood stabilizers	Lithium	300 mg tid/qid
	Carbamazepine/Tegretol	100-400 mg/day
	Valproic acid/Divalproex	125 mg bid; titrate up slowly
Anxiolytic benzodiazepines	Clonazepam/Klonopin	0.5-0.75 mg/day
	Oxazepam/Serax	10-35 mg (divided in 3-4 doses)
	Lorazepam/Ativan	0.5-1.0 mg bid to tid
Sedative/hypnotic benzodiazepines	Flurazepam/Dalmane	15-30 mg qhs
	Temazepam/Restoril	7.5-15 mg qhs
Antipsychotics	Haloperidol/Haldol	0.25-15 mg/day
	Fluphenazine/Prolixin	0.25-6.0 mg/day
	Trifluoperazine/Stelazine	2-20 mg/day
	Thioridazine/Mellaril	10-300 mg/day
	Chlorpromazine/Thorazine	10-300 mg/day
	Risperidone/Risperdal	0.25-2 mg/day
	Olanzapine/Zyprexa	5-10 mg/day

Modified from Salzman C: *Clinical geriatric psychopharmacology,* ed 2, Baltimore, 1992, Williams & Wilkins.

Interpersonal Interventions

PSYCHOTHERAPY. Elderly patients participate in both individual and group psychotherapy sessions. Nurses who have advanced degrees in psychiatric nursing are qualified to provide these services. The issue of the appropriateness of psychotherapy for this population is addressed in Critical Thinking about Contemporary Issues.

Turner[32] has identified themes that emerge during psychotherapy in this age group. They include "maintenance of self-esteem, fear of pain and suffering, helplessness and hopelessness, isolation and loneliness, physical and mental impairment, loss of competency, need to rely on those who may abandon them, and an existential perspective on death." She believes that these are important concerns that can be addressed in therapy. She also notes that transference and countertransference issues are related to the ages of the patient and therapist. Child/parent or grandchild/grandparent themes are common. Therapists often have particular difficulty responding to sexual transference with elders. This may be related to the therapist's beliefs and feelings about sexuality and aging.

Group psychotherapy is another intervention for elderly patients. Benefits of group therapy for this population include giving and receiving help, decreasing social isolation, receiving support by sharing common experiences, and improving self-esteem.[25,35] Reynolds reports that problem-solving therapy is also an effective treatment for elders with mild depression. Problem solving therapy involves helping patients in identifying issues that are critical in their lives. These issues should be described in a measurable and observable format, appropriate solutions to these issues should be devised, and possible consequences should be predicted.[27]

LIFE REVIEW THERAPY. Life review therapy was first described by Butler.[6] It has a positive psychotherapeutic function, providing an opportunity for the person to reflect on life and resolve, reorganize, and reintegrate troubling or disturbing areas. The life review works well with groups or individuals. In a group, members may positively reinforce each other and stimulate mutual learning. Developing individual autobiographies to share with the group is one way to introduce common experiences and interests among the

CRITICAL THINKING *about* Contemporary Issues

Is Psychotherapy an Appropriate Intervention for Geropsychiatric Patients?

Some believe that psychotherapy for elderly patients is inappropriate and not helpful. Psychotherapy requires confronting and working through basic personality traits. It is argued that the elderly do not have the capacity, stamina, or interest to take on such a challenging task. Is this based on an accurate estimate of the elder's cognitive ability and interpersonal potential? Psychotherapy may be a long-term process. Is it reasonable to ask a person who is nearing the end of life to make a commitment to an effort that might not be completed? People in therapy often change their relationships with others. Should the elderly be put in the position of possibly jeopardizing their support systems by changing their expectations of themselves and others?

Geropsychiatric nurse specialists have begun to document their experiences in providing psychotherapy to elders.[23,28] These nurses believe that elderly patients benefit from this intervention. They describe the elder's ability to change and grow. Psychotherapists have noted that older patients are more focused on therapeutic work, perhaps because they know they do not have unlimited time to achieve their goals. Elders have a wealth of life experiences to bring to therapy and a need to find meaning in their lives that is often aided by therapeutic intervention. In groups, they also benefit from the mutuality and cohesion they find. Thus, is it worth the investment to improve the life experience of one who may or may not have enough time left to experience long-term rewards of psychotherapy?

members and put them at ease. The group cohesion and sharing can build self-esteem and a feeling of belonging, in addition to the positive effect of the review itself.

Haight and Burnside[16] have differentiated between life review and reminiscence. Both are planned interventions that are led by a mental health professional. Reminiscence is usually a pleasant experience in which the patient reviews life events without any particular structure and talks about meanings and feelings.[17] The nurse listens and responds but does not try to interpret or probe for deeper meanings. The life review is structured, with the emphasis on analyzing life events. The nurse helps the patient to look for the meaning of experiences and to resolve conflicts and lingering feelings. Life review helps the elder to achieve the ego integrity and wisdom identified by Erikson as the goal of the last stage of life.

REALITY ORIENTATION. Both 24-hour and structured reality orientation can prevent confusion and keep patients oriented to time, place, person, and situation. The environment reinforces contact with reality, the here and now, when it is kept simple and focused. Helpful physical props include clocks, directional signs, calendars, and orientation boards (season of the year, weather, and so on).

Classroom reality orientation is an intensive small-group experience that is especially effective for the moderately to severely impaired elderly. It provides an opportunity to reinforce time, place, and person orientation with patients who have short attention spans and need extra verbal and visual stimulation. Reality orientation, along with a discussion of current events, stimulates patients to maintain contact with the real world and their place in it. Current events discussions, used alone, may be structured in various ways, such as sharing of newspaper articles or group viewing of television news programs. The scope of the group depends on the patients' abilities and the other therapeutic modalities at hand.

VALIDATION THERAPY. Although reality orientation is effective for many institutionalized and community-based elderly with confusion or disorientation, some evidence indicates that for some older adults, especially those with minimal organic impairment, disorientation may be a form of denial of unpleasant realities. These elders may become more anxious or agitated if constantly reminded of environmental realities. An alternate approach to confused and disoriented older adults was developed by Feil[12] and discussed in relation to working with the patient who does not respond to reality orientation. This approach involves searching for the emotion and meaning in the patient's disoriented or confused words and behavior (such as wandering) and validating them verbally with the patient. A series of verbal cues or steps are involved that allow the patient to focus on key words or phrases in the confused interaction and the nurse validates by asking for description, more detail, or clarification. What is sometimes identified as meaningless or incoherent conversation may often have significant meaning for the patient and can be related to current or past events. Validation is being used successfully with both mild and moderately impaired elderly and shows promise for providing an effective avenue for reaching older adults experiencing cognitive dysfunction. Little documentation is available on the use of this strategy in group settings or with severely impaired elders.

COGNITIVE TRAINING AND THERAPY. Much research is under way using cognitive training and stimulation (see Chapter 30). Problem-solving situations, formal or didactic memory training, and selected memory exercises have been effective in increasing attention span, efficiency of recall, and the ability to learn new skills (such as mathematical calculations and vocabulary). Intelligence does not decline with age but may be dulled by depression, drugs, or lack of use. Cognitive training can keep older adults active mentally, which in turn enhances emotional well-being. The "use it or lose it" adage is as true for maintenance of intelligence as it is for physical functioning.

Clinical studies and experience to date indicate that cognitive training and therapy may be especially effective for cognitively intact, motivated elderly people with minor or major depressions. Cognitive therapy supports higher-level defense mechanisms, such as rationalization and intellectualization, and encourages active participation of patients in a highly structured treatment. One positive aspect of this approach is its time-limited nature, reinforcing the goal of a positive change within a specific time period. Research has demonstrated that cognitive therapy is effective with depressed elderly patients.

Stimulating cognitive skills can challenge the nurse's creativity in relating to geropsychiatric patients. To be able to capitalize on the patient's interests and skills, the nurse must be familiar with the patient's past occupation, hobbies, and leisure activities. The nursing interview should focus on gathering as much of that information as possible on admission and adding to the database as the nurse builds a trusting relationship with the patient and family.

RELAXATION THERAPY. Besides promoting a sense of physical well-being, relaxation can release tension and reduce stress, reducing barriers to communication. Additional information about relaxation therapy is presented in Chapters 16 and 30. Relaxation, combined with mild isometric exercises, increases cardiovascular output, energy, and mobility and reduces stress. Relaxation and exercise strategies, used in group or individual contexts, do not require advanced skills of the nurse or the patient. They may begin with simple tension-releasing muscle exercises, coupled with verbal instructions about breathing and concentration.

SUPPORTIVE AND COUNSELING GROUPS. Geropsychiatric patients respond well to both supportive and counseling groups. These interventions may use either a nondirective or unstructured format or a more structured, didactic approach. Group members can ventilate feelings, try out problem-solving approaches, and resolve conflict in a rational, systematic manner. These groups may incorporate some aspects of cognitive training or reminiscence, described earlier in this chapter. Older adults respond well to a supportive group structure, which increases self-esteem, self-confidence, risk-taking, and empathy. Humor may be an effective way to reach the nonverbal or withdrawn elder. The ability to laugh at oneself and see the irony in everyday events provides an effective outlet for frustration, anger, stress, and anxiety. Promoting humor by telling jokes and stories and watching cartoons or situation comedies can be therapeutic in a group or with individual patients. Expressions of humor and active laughter allow older adults to step out of their situations, releasing some of the tension related to coping with changes accompanying aging.

PATIENT EDUCATION. Older adults often question the physiological and cognitive (memory) changes that occur naturally in aging. Slowed response time, benign memory loss, altered gait, and interrupted sleep patterns are a few of the normal changes of aging that elders may interpret as pathological. The nurse has an opportunity to teach patients about their own developmental changes during the assessment phase of the nurse-patient relationship. Dispel-

ling myths and stereotypes related to aging is a primary goal for patient education.

Depressed older adults are particularly receptive to the educative process because it is in the depressive state that they are most vulnerable and open to suggestion. Exercises for promoting positive thoughts and images, visualization, and repetitive cognitive games can be used as a basis for teaching new patterns of behavior. Cognitive training, relaxation, and life review approaches are well suited to patient education formats.

> **?** *Your friend's grandfather is 85 years old and constantly complains of feeling tired and forgetful. He has been to many physicians without feeling better. Your friend asks what she should do next. How would you respond?*

FAMILY EDUCATION AND SUPPORT. Because 80% of the elders living at home are cared for by a spouse, sibling, or adult child, family caregiver education and support groups are becoming essential. Many community agencies, clinics, and senior citizen centers are responding to the needs of this group with special activities, classes, and support groups.

Family members often view nurses as the most approachable health-care professionals for understanding family relationships, conflicts, needs, and resources. Family education related to the normal aging process, family dynamics and family systems, and stress inherent in the caregiver role can be integrated into counseling sessions with family members, referral conferences, or part of the family history on admission of the patient.

A more formal approach to family education can be developed using the numerous books now available that address caring for older adults. These materials provide practical, step-by-step guidelines to handling common problems of the frail elderly, including agitation, wandering, withdrawal, resistance, anxiety, insomnia, incontinence, anorexia, and restlessness. These books, which have been written specifically for the consumer, supply the text for nurse-family teaching sessions and are excellent resource materials for use in the home.[22]

EVALUATING THE CARE OF THE GERIATRIC PATIENT

Implementing care designed to promote optimum cognitive function and emotional well-being has been considered the role of the geropsychiatric nurse. Increasingly, research is being initiated to determine the most appropriate approach to meet the needs of the patient and the most effective intervention to use.

Evaluation of patient care should be based on a model that explains the progression of behavior from adaptive to maladaptive. The type of care and the evaluation of outcome would be directly related to the level of behavior targeted for intervention.

The goal of nursing intervention is to promote maximum independence of the older adult, based on capacity and functional abilities. Evaluation of outcomes of nursing care would not be based on reversal of behaviors or elimination of patient needs but on the change the patient demonstrates based on individual abilities. This approach reinforces the emphasis on the individual as a unit for evaluation and allows for patient differences and for the process of change over time.

Issues to be addressed in the evaluation of community geropsychiatric programs have also been identified. They include the outcome of treatment; the satisfaction of the patient, significant others, referring professionals, the community, the agency, and the staff; the expectations of those who fund the program; the compliance with accreditation and quality control standards; and cost effectiveness.[18] The nurse plays an important part in ensuring that these goals are met.

In the final analysis, the most important evaluation criterion is the feedback from the patient and caregivers that nursing care was helpful and growth producing. The challenge to the nurse is to be creative in producing a positive experience for each elderly patient.

Summary

1. The role of the geropsychiatric nurse includes providing primary mental health nursing care, including intervening with caregivers, providing case management, and consulting with other care providers. Advanced practice nurses provide individual and group psychotherapy, take leadership in program development, and prescribe medications in most states.

2. Biopsychosocial theories of aging were identified. Biological theories include biological programming, wear-and-tear, and stress adaptation. Psychological theories include Erikson's stage of ego integrity, life review, and stability of personality. Sociocultural theories include disengagement, activity, and the family in later life.

3. A comprehensive geropsychiatric nursing assessment includes application of interviewing skills. The areas to be assessed include mental status, behavioral and functional abilities, and physiological and social support.

4. NANDA nursing diagnoses related to geropsychiatric patients include altered thought processes, dysfunctional grieving, high risk for self-directed violence, situational low self-esteem, sleep pattern disturbance, altered nutrition, anxiety, relocation stress syndrome, high risk for caregiver role strain, social isolation, and self-care deficit.

5. Nursing interventions with geropsychiatric patients include creation of a therapeutic milieu, involvement in somatic therapies, and interpersonal interventions. Caregivers must be involved in planning and implementing nursing interventions.

6. Evaluation of geropsychiatric nursing care focuses on the patient's ability to reach maximum independence.

COMPETENT CARING A Clinical Exemplar of a Psychiatric Nurse

Beth Greco, MSN, RN

A frail ghost of a man sat silently in his easy chair. He did not raise his head or speak as I entered the room with his wife. He made no eye contact as I introduced myself as his new home health nurse. He simply remained quiet, barely moving even as he breathed. I was struck by his appearance. He was not the person I had expected to meet that day.

Mr. R had been reported to be "very difficult," "demanding," "noncompliant," and "an impossible patient." Emergency visits by nurses were often necessary to fix a leaky catheter, assess a drastic decrease in urinary output, unclog a clogged feeding tube, and assess reported changes in cardiac and respiratory status. His wife and primary caretaker made numerous calls to the home health office and continually asked questions about Mr. R's medicines, diet, heart problems, breathing difficulties, and overall health. After meeting Mr. R, it occurred to me that caring for this patient would involve not only extensive medical management but also intensive psychiatric nursing care for him and his family. I was very glad that I had a few years of psychiatric nursing experience before I met this family.

My immediate response in assessing Mr. R's needs was to increase the frequency of home visits to three times per week. During these visits I carefully reviewed Mr. R's medications, diet, and treatments with him and his wife at the same time. I was very careful to include Mr. R in these discussions by asking him questions and providing him opportunities to make decisions about his care. At first he was very reluctant to participate in these teaching sessions, but gradually he began to show some interest. As he became more engaged in conversations with me I began showing him how to take care of his feeding tube and catheter. I encouraged his wife to let Mr. R do his care when he felt up to it. I thought it would be very important for Mr. R to have some control over what was happening to him. I also thought it would be necessary for Mrs. R to let go of the total responsibility for her husband's care. Her anxiety level had reached almost unmanageable proportions several weeks before I had received the case.

I encouraged Mrs. R to arrange some time for herself away from the home on a regular basis. She agreed that she would have her daughter come in once a week so that she could spend time with her church friends. Mr. R stated that it would be good for his wife to get out more often and he would be all right in her absence. After a few weeks of concentrating on the tasks to be learned, Mr. R became more open to discussion of the impact of

COMPETENT CARING A Clinical Exemplar of a Psychiatric Nurse—cont'd

his illness on his life and his family. He talked about his past work and leisure activities and his disbelief over his current situation. He felt that his retirement years were supposed to be full of travel and leisure pursuits, and instead he was confined by his failing health to his home. He was very angry as he talked to me about these things, and as I glanced at a picture on his dresser of a broad-shouldered, confident military man, I better understood his anger and his pain. He had been that man in the picture, and his losses were great.

Grief work became an important focus of my nursing care in the remainder of the time that I worked with Mr. R and his family. We talked about the changes in their lives, their disappointments over missed opportunities, their anger, and their fears. We explored ways to cope with Mr. R's limitations, and I was happy to hear one day that Mr. and Mrs. R had ventured out to dinner at a restaurant. A wheelchair and some courage were the necessary ingredients for an enjoyable evening.

As time went on, Mr. R's condition stabilized and weekly maintenance visits were all that was needed. His condition re-mained acute, but he and his wife were managing his care very well at home. Emergency visits were no longer needed, and this "difficult" patient was rarely heard from between home visits.

My last visit to Mr. R's home was prompted by an early morning telephone call from my office. There was an emergency at his home on that day. When I arrived at the house I found Mr. R in bed clutching his chest. His wife explained that he had awakened with chest pain. My quick physical assessment indicated that his pulse was rapid and thready and his blood pressure was lower than his normal baseline. He was alert but looked pale and was diaphoretic. I instructed Mrs. R to call EMS, and as she did so I sat with Mr. R. I held his hand and asked him whether he was afraid. He nodded and met my eyes with his. In them I saw only his courage. He remained conscious until EMS arrived, and they promptly started an IV line and provided oxygen and whisked him off to the nearest hospital. He died later that same day, but I will always remember him for the bravery of his struggle for life.

your **INTERNET**
c o n n e c t i o n

The American Association for Geriatric Psychiatry (AAGP)
http://www.aagpgpa.org/home.html

National Institute on Aging (NIA)
http://www.nih.gov/nia

Chapter Review Questions

1. Match each term in Column A with the correct description in Column B.

Column A	Column B
___Activity theory	A. Older adults should find substitutes for work or participation in community organizations if they must stop these activities.
___Biological programming theory	
___Disengagement theory	B. The life span of a cell is stored within the cell itself.
___Life review theory	C. Older adults and society mutually withdraw from active exchange.
___Stability of personality	D. Past experiences return to consciousness and memories are examined and reintegrated.
___Stress adaptation theory	E. Personality is viewed as unchanging from early adulthood through old age.
___Wear-and-tear theory	F. Positive and negative effects of stress on biopsychosocial development.
	G. Structural and functional changes may be speeded by abuse and slowed by care.

2. Fill in the blanks.

A. Increasing disorientation or confusion at night resulting from loss of visual accommodation is called _____.

B. Mitts, posey belts, and geri chairs are examples of _____ that should be used with caution with the elderly.

C. Contraindications for _____ therapy are increased intracranial pressure, arrhythmias, and a myocardial infarction within the last 3 months.

D. When placing older patients on conventional antipsychotic medications, one must carefully assess for _____.

E. _____ orientation can prevent confusion and keep patients oriented to time, place, person, and situation.

F. Intelligence is dulled by depression, drugs, or lack of use, but is stimulated by _____ therapy.

G. Evaluation of geropsychiatric nursing care focuses on the patient's ability to reach _____.

H. Doses of psychopharmacologic drugs for older patients are usually _____.

3. Provide short answers for the following questions.

A. Highlight important communication factors to consider when interviewing older patients.

B. List the risk factors for falls with older patients.

C. Some believe that the lack of regard shown by health-care professionals for the living wills and advanced directives of the elderly is related to their high suicide rate. Explore the many aspects of this complex issue.

REFERENCES

1. Albert MS: Cognition and aging. In Hazzard WR et al, editors: *Principles of geriatric medicine and gerontology,* ed 2, New York, 1990, McGraw-Hill.
2. Alexopoulos G: Outcomes of late-life depression, *Psychiatr Ann* 26:5, 1996.
3. Buchanan D, Farran C, Clark D: Suicidal thought and self-transcendence in older adults, *J Psychosoc Nurs* 33:32, 1995.
4. Burney-Puckett M: Sundown syndrome: etiology and management, *J Psychosoc Nurs* 34:40, 1996.
5. Burns BJ et al: Mental health service use by the elderly in nursing homes, *Am J Public Health* 83:331, 1993.
6. Butler RN: Re-awakening interest, *Nurs Homes* 10:8, 1961.
7. Carter EA, McGoldrick M: *The family life cycle: a framework for family therapy,* ed 2, New York, 1989, Gardner.
8. Cumming E, Henry WE: *Growing old: the process of disengagement,* New York, 1961, Basic Books.
9. Ebersole P: *Caring for the psychogeriatric patient,* New York, 1989, Springer.
10. Ebersole P, Hess P: *Toward healthy aging—human needs and nursing response,* ed 4, St Louis, 1994, Mosby.
11. Erikson EH: *Childhood and society,* New York, 1963, WW Norton.
12. Feil N: Communicating with the confused elderly patient, *Geriatrics* 39:131, 1993.
13. Fuller K, Lillquist D: Geropsychiatric public sector nursing: placement challenges, *J Psychosoc Nurs* 33:20, 1995.
14. Gallo JJ, Reichel W, Andersen L: *Handbook of geriatric assessment,* Rockville, Md, 1988, Aspen.
15. Grossberg G, Manepalli J: The older patient with psychotic symptoms, *Psychiatr Serv* 46:55, 1995.
16. Haight BK, Burnside I: Reminiscing and life review: explaining the difference, *Arch Psychiatr Nurs* 7:91, 1993.
17. Haight B, Webster J: *The art and science of reminiscing,* Washington, DC, 1995, Taylor & Francis.
18. Harris AG, Marriott JAS, Robertson J: Issues in the evaluation of a community psychogeriatric service, *Can J Psychiatry* 35:215, 1990.
19. Hayflick L et al: The serial cultivation of human diploid cells, *Exp Cell Res* 25:585, 1961.

20. Jenkins M, Westlake R, Salloway S: The diagnosis and treatment of geriatric depression, *J Pract Psychiatry Behav Health* 2:336, 1996.
21. Katz S et al: Studies of illness in the aged: the index of ADL; a standardized measure of biological and psychosocial function, *JAMA* 185:914, 1963.
22. Mace NL, Rabins PV: *The 36-hour day,* New York, 1991, Warner Books.
23. McCall W: Management of primary sleep disorders among elderly persons, *Psychiatr Serv* 46:49, 1995.
24. North American Nursing Diagnosis Association: *NANDA nursing diagnosis: definitions and classifications 1993-1994,* Philadelphia, 1994, NANDA.
25. Pearlman IR: Group psychotherapy with the elderly, *J Psychosoc Nurs Ment Health Serv* 31:7, 1993.
26. Report of the Task Force on Aging Research: *The threshold of discovery: future directions for research on aging,* Department of Health and Human Services, Administrative Document, April 1995.
27. Reynolds C: Treatment of depression in late life, *Psychiatr Ann* 26:4, 1996.
28. Smith S, Sherrill K, Colenda C: Assessing and treating anxiety in elderly persons, *Psychiatr Serv* 46:36, 1995.
29. Stevens GL, Walsh RA, Baldwin BA: Family caregivers of institutionalized and noninstitutionalized elderly individuals, *Nurs Clin North Am* 28:349, 1993.
30. Stolley J: Freeing your patients from restraints, *Am J Nurs* 1995:27, 1995.
31. Tierney J: Practical issues in geriatric use of psychiatric medications, *Treatment Today* 3:26, 1996.
32. Turner MS: Individual psychodynamic psychotherapy with older adults: perspectives from a nurse psychotherapist, *Arch Psychiatr Nurs* 6:266, 1992.
33. Wagner B: Innovations in the geriatric continuum of care, *Continuum* 1:51, 1994.
34. Weinrich S et al: Agitation: measurement, management and intervention research, *Arch Psychiatr Nurs* 9:251, 1995.
35. Wood A, Seymour L: Psychodynamic group therapy for older adults, *J Psychosoc Nurs* 32:19, 1994.

Annotated Suggested Readings

*Bultema J et al: Geriatric patients with depression: improving outcomes using a multidisciplinary clinical path model, *J Nurs Adm* 26:31, 1996.
  Describes the development and implementation of a psychiatric clinical pathway and identifies interventions, outcomes over the course of treatment, and quality, cost, and future directions.

*Burney-Puckett M: Sundown syndrome: etiology and management, *J Psychosoc Nurs* 34:40, 1996.
  A useful review of the latest hypotheses regarding the etiology of this common problem seen in elderly patients and the research summarizing the most effective interventions.

De Leo D, Carollo G, Dello Buono M: Lower suicide rates associated with a tele-help/tele-check service for the elderly at home, *Am J Psychiatry* 152:632, 1995.
  This study of a telephone service designed to provide elderly people with home assistance was found to significantly decrease the number of suicides in the study sample with the service.

*Ferguson JS, Smith A: Aggressive behavior on an inpatient geriatric unit, *J Psychosoc Nurs* 34:27, 1996.
  Services and nursing home beds for the elderly are decreasing so

*Nursing reference.

nurses must look to the environment in which the increasing numbers of elderly patients function in order to develop strategies and techniques to maximize independence while decreasing violent behavior.

*Flowers E: Recognition and psychopharmacologic treatment of geriatric depression, *J Am Psychiatric Nurses Assoc* 3:32, 1997.
  Differential diagnostic issues in elderly depression are examined, and the pharmacokinetics, dosing strategies, and compliance issues in the elderly are outlined.

*Foreman M, Zane D: Nursing strategies for acute confusion in elders, *Am J Nurs* 96:44, 1996.
  Provides the key assessments and interventions useful in any setting in order to prevent, ease, or abbreviate the common problem of acute confusion in elders.

Haight B, Webster J: *The art and science of reminiscing: theory, research, methods, and applications,* Washington, DC, 1995, Taylor & Francis.
  Provides a valuable resource for professionals who work in the field of reminiscing, for those interested in valid forms of memory, and for a general audience interested in examining their own life histories.

*Holmberg S: Evaluation of a clinical intervention for wanderers on a geriatric nursing unit, *Arch Psychiatr Nurs* 11:21, 1997.
  Describes and evaluates a walking program for persons with severe dementia as a nursing home intervention designed to decrease unsafe wandering and reduce interpersonal tension.

Images of Aging, *Primary Psychiatry*, December, 1996.
  This issue on aging includes an overview of the newest understanding of Alzheimer's disease, practical approaches to treating behavioral symptoms, genetic epidemiology, and resources.

*Morris L: A spiritual well-being model: use with older women who experience depression, *Issues Ment Health Nurs* 17:439, 1996.
  Presents a spiritual well-being model that provides a framework to discuss the antecedents, symptoms, spiritual needs, and holistic treatment of depression experienced by older women.

*Rane-Szostak D, Herth K: A new perspective on loneliness in later life, *Issues Ment Health Nurs* 16:583, 1995.
  A better understanding of the coping strategies of elders who are not lonely yet who have experienced decreased socialization or physical function may help others with loneliness.

Reichman W, Katz P, eds: *Psychiatric care in the nursing home,* New York, 1996, Oxford University Press.
  Comprehensive and useful reference for the identification and treatment of mental health and behavioral disorders experienced by elders residing in nursing homes. State-of-the-art and highly recommended.

Report of the Task Force on Aging Research: *The threshold of discovery: future directions for research on aging,* Department of Health and Human Services, Administrative Document, April, 1995.
  Report from the task force authorized by the US Congress to assess progress in the scientific understanding of aging, advise where the search for these answers should be concentrated, and make recommendations for allocation of resources in the support of research.

Wagner B: Innovations in the geriatric continuum of care, *Continuum* 1:51, 1994.
  Excellent overview of community-based alternative treatments for the elderly that allow for maximum treatment effectiveness and efficiency within the least restrictive setting.

Care of Survivors of Abuse and Violence

Barbara Parker and
Jacqueline C. Campbell

© 1998 M.C. Escher/Cordon Art, Baarn, Holland.

When I was a laddie I lived with my granny And many a hiding my granny di'ed me.

Now I am a man and I live with my granny And do to my granny what she did to me.

Traditional rhyme, anonymous

Nurses encounter survivors of abuse and violence in many settings. However, because experiencing violence is generally devastating, survivors of abuse and violence are often seen in psychiatric settings. At times the violence is openly discussed and recognized as a precipitating factor for the current hospitalization, as when a survivor of sexual assault is treated in an emergency room.

Often, however, violence is disclosed only after the establishment of a trusting nurse-patient relationship. Although there are various forms of violence, such as gang behavior and drug-related violence, the types most often described by psychiatric patients are family violence and nonfamily rape and sexual assault. Because the dynamics of these two forms of violence are different, they are covered in two separate sections of this chapter. Rape and sexual assault also can be forms of family violence. In addition, attention is given to populations that are particularly at risk for abuse. These include children, spouses, and the elderly.

The words used to describe people who have experienced violence are important. Traditionally the word *victim* has been used, along with discussions of syndromes. These labels distance nurses from the person who has been abused as they search for differences between themselves and the victims to decrease their feelings of vulnerability. In this chapter the word *survivor* is used to emphasize that the person who has experienced abuse has many strengths and coping strategies that can be incorporated into the plan of care.

> **?** *Do you agree with the use of the word* survivor *instead of* victim *in this chapter? What do you think of when you hear the words* victim *and* survivor?

DIMENSIONS OF FAMILY VIOLENCE

Family violence is a range of behaviors occurring between family members. It includes physical and emotional abuse of children, child neglect, spouse battering, marital rape, and elder abuse. Several different issues are related to abuse within families. Although each family is unique, there appear to be characteristics common to most violent families. Furthermore, regardless of the type of abuse occurring within a family, all members, including the extended family, are affected. Family violence, although often unnoted, is at the core of many family disturbances. Violence may be a family secret and often continues through generations.

Although numerous research studies and theories have been directed toward the causes, treatment, and prevention of family violence, there are more questions unanswered than answered. Some have noted that the family is the training ground for violence and ask why the social group designated to provide love and support is also the most violent group to which most people belong. Behaviors that would be unacceptable between strangers, co-workers, or friends are often tolerated within families.

Feminist authors note that most survivors of family violence are the most vulnerable and powerless family members: women, children, and the elderly.[6,9] They propose that the root cause of violence is the abuser's need for power and control, which is acted out by violent behavior. Social norms that support or at least allow male dominance and violence are considered crucial in feminist analysis.

Violence and abuse are generally believed to be caused by an interaction of personality, demographic, situational, and societal factors. Many of the unique characteristics of the family as a social group—time spent together, emotional involvement, privacy, and in-depth knowledge of each other—can facilitate both intimacy and violence.

Thus a given family can be loving and supportive as well as violent.

To understand violence in American families, the influence of the society on the family must be examined. The United States has a high level of violence compared with other Western nations. Many believe that society's willingness to tolerate violence sets the stage for family violence. Social norms are sometimes used to justify violence to maintain the family system. For example, a husband's use of violence may be considered legitimate if the wife is having an extramarital affair. Historical attitudes toward women, children, and the elderly, economic discrimination, the nonresponsiveness of the criminal justice system, and the belief that women and children are property have been cited as factors maintaining norms allowing violence (Fig. 39-1).[6,9] Changing norms related to definitions of family privacy and when government should be allowed to intervene in family matters have also influenced the definitions and recognition of family violence.

> **?** *Why do you think more violence occurs in American society than in other Western nations? What societal factors influence the use of violence?*

Fig. 39-1 Spouse abuse is an age-old reality. This 1887 woodcut depicts wife beating in a "proper" family. (From the Bettmann Archive.)

Characteristics of Violent Families

Several factors are common to violent families. These include the multigenerational family process, social isolation, the use and abuse of power, and the effect of alcohol and drug abuse.

MULTIGENERATIONAL TRANSMISSION. Multigenerational transmission means that family violence is often perpetuated through generations by a cycle of violence. Fig. 39-2 illustrates multigenerational transmission of family violence. Several theories have been proposed regarding this phenomenon. The most enduring is social learning theory, in which violence is seen as a learned behavior.

Social learning theory related to violence states that a child learns this behavior pattern in a family setting by taking a violent parent as a role model. In this case, violence and victimization are behaviors learned through childhood experience. The child learns both the means and the approval of violence. Children who witness violence not only learn specific aggressive behaviors but also acquire the belief that violence is a legitimate way to solve problems. When frustrated or angry as an adult, the person relies on this learned behavior and responds with violence.

Social learning theory was first applied to child abuse when it was noted that many child abusers were abused as children. Many studies have suggested the multigenerational transmission of child abuse within families. However, other studies examining parental punishment history and current child abuse found no differences between abusive and nonabusive parents. Experiencing abuse as a child does not totally determine an adult's later behaviors. Many people who were abused as children are able to avoid violence with their own children. A key factor may be the age at which the child was abused or which parent was abusive. Experiencing abuse from a father at age 4 years may be totally different from experiencing abuse from a mother as an adolescent.

The incidence of violence in the families of both the survivors of wife abuse and their abusers also supports multigenerational transmission. A classic literature review by Hotaling and Sugerman[23] identified witnessing parental violence during childhood or adolescence as one of the strongest risk factors for the abuse of wives in adulthood. It is less clear that women learn to tolerate wife abuse from childhood experiences with violence.

To date, there is limited evidence of multigenerational transmission of violence in elder abuse. However, elder abuse could be the result of formerly abused children displaying both retaliatory and imitative behavior or behavior modeled by their parents with their grandparents.

Many treatment modalities, especially cognitive approaches, are based on the social learning model that violent reactions can be unlearned and replaced with constructive responses to conflict.

SOCIAL ISOLATION. It has been observed that violent families are also socially isolated. One reason may be that some types of violence are considered abnormal or illegitimate and become a family secret. Exposure of family violence can result in both formal and informal sanctions from other family members, neighbors, the police, or the judicial system; therefore, the abuser often purposely keeps the family isolated. Social isolation has been found to be a factor in elder abuse, wife abuse, and child abuse.[6]

USE AND ABUSE OF POWER. Another common factor within the various forms of family violence is the use and abuse of power. In almost all forms of family violence the abuser has some form of power or control over the victim. For example, with the sexual abuse of children, the abuser is usually a male in an authority position victimizing a child in a subordinate position.[43]

Power issues appear to be a central factor in wife abuse. Although wife abusers justify the use of violence for trivial events such as not having a meal ready or not keeping the house tidy, violence often is related to the husband's need for total domination of his wife. Wife abuse often begins or escalates when the woman behaves more independently by working or attending school. One study found that the largest category (60%) of physical abuse of the elderly was actually spouse abuse, thereby incorporating the issues of power and control central in that form of family violence.[13] Table 39-1 describes five forms of abuse within families that reflect domestic struggles for power and control.

ALCOHOL AND DRUG ABUSE. The relationship between alcohol and drug abuse and family violence has been studied extensively. Survivors of violence often report concurrent substance abuse by the abuser. However, most re-

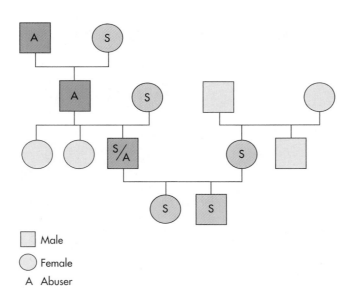

Male

Female

A   Abuser

S   Survivor

S/A   Survivor/Abuser

Fig. 39-2   Genogram demonstrates the multigenerational transmission of family violence.

searchers deny that substance abuse is a direct cause of violence because one behavior is not necessary for the other to occur. That is, people who abuse alcohol are not consistently violent, and people who are violent are not always intoxicated. Instead, it has been suggested that the person uses alcohol as a more socially acceptable explanation for the behavior. Family and friends may also attribute the conduct to the effects of alcohol, which to some extent decreases the degree of blame. The use of alcohol or drugs may also increase violent behavior by reducing fear or inhibitions and decreasing sensitivity to the impact of the behavior.

Cross-cultural studies suggest that behavior while drinking varies from culture to culture. In societies where it is believed that alcohol removes inhibitions, people become less inhibited. If they believe it is a depressant, they become depressed when drinking. If people in America believe that normal rules of behavior are suspended when one is drinking, people will behave antisocially.

Connections between drug abuse and family violence have been less well researched. Early research on aggressiveness and illicit drugs has established that marijuana and heroin use are not related to violence. In contrast, drugs such as crack cocaine, amphetamines, mescaline, "angel dust" (PCP), and steroids have been associated with increased violence, but the specific relationships with various forms of family violence are not yet established.

Nursing Attitudes toward Survivors of Violence

It can be extremely difficult and frustrating to provide nursing care for survivors of violence. The attitudes nurses bring to these situations help shape their responses. Studies of health-care professionals' attitudes indicate that myths about battered women are accepted even though there is sympathy toward the survivor. Nurses have been found not to blame rape survivors in general. However, the tendency to blame the survivor increases when a vignette describes the woman as having gone out late at night, not locked her car doors, or gone shopping for beer rather than milk for the baby.[8] Box 39-1 describes common myths about survivors of abuse.

Although most nurses do not actually blame survivors for what has happened to them, they do dislike certain behaviors. They are not happy with sexual assault survivors who do not resist "enough." They have difficulty understanding abused children who want to return to abusive parents. They especially dislike battered women who do not leave their abusers. Kurz[27] published a classic study describing the subtle blaming and distancing of battered women by emergency department personnel, including nurses. Stark and Flitcraft[40] used emergency room chart reviews to document the lack of recognition, negative labeling, and inappropriate treatment that all too often happen to battered women. One recent study of psychiatric nurses found that attitudes toward sexuality were more positive and attitudes toward sexual assault included less victim-blaming than in

TABLE **39-1** *Forms of Abuse within Families Reflecting Struggles for Power and Control*

PHYSICAL

▼ *Inflicting or attempting to inflict physical injury or illness*—for example, grabbing, pinching, shoving, slapping, hitting, hair-pulling, biting, arm-twisting, kicking, punching, hitting with blunt objects, stabbing, shooting.

▼ *Withholding access to resources necessary to maintain health*—for example, medication, medical care, wheelchair, food or fluids, sleep, hygienic assistance.

▼ *Forcing alcohol or other drug use.*

SEXUAL

▼ *Coercing or attempting to coerce any sexual contact without consent*—for example, marital rape, acquaintance rape, forced sex after physical beating, attacks on the sexual parts of the body, bestiality, forced prostitution, unprotected sex, fondling, sodomy, sex with others, use of pornography.

▼ *Attempting to undermine the victim's sexuality*—for example, treating her or him in a sexually degrading manner, criticizing sexual performance and desirability. Also, accusations of infidelity, withholding sex.

PSYCHOLOGICAL

▼ *Instilling or attempting to instill fear*—for example, intimidation, threatening physical harm to self, victim, or others, threatening to harm or kidnap children, menacing, blackmail, harassment, destruction of pets and property, mind games.

▼ *Isolating or attempting to isolate victim from friends, family, school, or work*—for example, withholding access to phone or transportation, undermining victim's personal relationships, harassing others, constant "checking up," constant accompaniment, unfounded accusations, forced imprisonment.

EMOTIONAL

▼ *Undermining or attempting to undermine victim's sense of self-worth*—for example, constant criticism, belittling victim's abilities and competency, name calling, insults, put-downs, silent treatment, manipulating victim's feelings and emotions to induce guilt, subverting a partner's relationship with the children, repeatedly making and breaking promises.

ECONOMIC

▼ *Making or attempting to make the victim financially dependent*—for example, maintaining total control over financial resources, including victim's earned income or resources received through public assistance or social security, withholding money or access to money, forbidding attendance at school, forbidding employment, on-the-job harassment, requiring accountability and justification for all money spent, forced welfare fraud, withholding information about family finances, running up bills for which the victim is responsible for payment.

From New York State Office for the Prevention of Domestic Violence.

Box **39-1** *Beyond the Myths: Recognizing Abuse Survivors*

Myth: Family violence is most common among the lower class.

Reality: Family violence occurs at all levels of society without regard to age, race, culture, status, education, or religion. It may be less evident among the affluent because they can afford private physicians, attorneys, counselors, and shelters. In contrast, people with less money must turn to public agencies for help.

Myth: Violence rarely occurs between dating partners.

Reality: Estimates vary among studies, but violence occurs in a large percentage of dating relationships.

Myth: Abused spouses can end the violence by divorcing their abuser.

Reality: According to the US Department of Justice, about 75% of all spousal attacks occur between people who are separated or divorced. In many cases, the separation process brings on an increased level of harassment and violence.

Myth: The victim can learn to stop doing things that provoke the violence.

Reality: In a battering relationship, the abuser needs no provocation to become violent. Violence is the abuser's pattern of behavior and the victim cannot learn how to control it. Even so, many victims blame themselves for the abuse, feeling guilty—even responsible—for doing or saying something that seems to trigger the abuser's behavior. Friends, family, and service providers reinforce this by laying the blame and the need to change on the shoulders of the victim.

Myth: Alcohol, stress, and mental illness are major causes of physical and verbal abuse.

Reality: Abusive people—and even their victims—often use those conditions to excuse or minimize the abuse. But abuse is a learned behavior, not an uncontrollable reaction. People are abusive because they have acquired the belief that violence and aggression are acceptable and effective responses to real or imagined threats. Fortunately, because violence is a learned behavior, abusers can benefit from counseling and professional help to alter their behavior. But dealing only with the perceived problem (for example, the alcohol, the stress, or the mental illness) will not change the abusive tendencies.

Myth: Violence occurs only between heterosexual partners.

Reality: Increasing evidence suggests that gay and lesbian partners experience violence for varied but similar reasons as heterosexual partners do.

Myth: Being pregnant protects a woman from battering.

Reality: Battering often begins or escalates during pregnancy. According to one theory, the abuser who already has low self-esteem views his wife as his property. As a result, he resents the intrusion of the fetus as well as the extra attention his wife gets from friends, family, and health-care providers.

Myth: Abused women tacitly accept the abuse by trying to conceal it, not reporting it, or failing to seek help.

Reality: Many women, when they do try to disclose their situation, are met with denial or disbelief. This only discourages them from persevering.

Modified from the Domestic Violence Training Curriculum program produced by the New York State Governor's Commission on Domestic Violence.

previously reported studies of nurses in nonpsychiatric settings. Also, the younger the psychiatric nurses were in this study, the more pronounced were the results, perhaps reflecting the societal norms in which they were raised, which have changed over time.[2]

Other studies describe how survivors find the healthcare system to be unhelpful and even traumatizing when they go for help.[1,7] King and Ryan[26] note that nurses most often use a paternalistic and individualistic model of helping battered women. The paternalistic model may be contrasted with the empowerment model. Table 39-2 compares the characteristics of these models. When the paternalistic model is used, the nurse is more likely to be frustrated because the survivor does not follow the nurse's advice. Therefore, the empowerment model is not only more helpful to the survivor but also more professionally satisfying for the nurse.

ORIGINS OF NEGATIVE ATTITUDES. Several theories can help in understanding nurses' attitudes. The just world hypothesis was first advanced by Lerner and Simmons.[30] It proposes that people believe that others generally get what they deserve: Good things happen to good people and bad things happen to bad people. This belief helps one feel safe because oneself is seen as basically good and therefore protected. When a person is victimized by violence, there is a need to make sense of this horrible idea. The easiest way is not to see it at all, which explains some of the lack of recognition. However, when family violence is unmistakable, one needs to understand why that particular person is the victim. If bad things happen to bad people, the victimized person must have done something wrong or at least something stupid, something different from what oneself would have done.

The whole process of victim blaming is easier if the survivor is of "a type" who is already the focus of bias. It is easier to blame and distance oneself from women or minority groups if there is already bias against them. Conversely, the more the person resembles oneself, the harder it is to

TABLE **39-2** *A Comparison of the Paternalistic and Empowerment Models of Intervention with Battered Women*

PATERNALISTIC MODEL	EMPOWERMENT MODEL
Nurse is perceived to be more knowledgeable than the survivor.	There is mutual sharing of knowledge and information.
Responsibility for ending the violence is placed on the survivor.	The nurse strategizes with the survivor.
	Survivors are helped to recognize societal influences.
Advice and sympathy are given rather than respect.	The survivor's competence and experience are respected.

recognize the violence at all. Thus it is not reported as often; the abuse is just not seen when the people are middle class and especially professionals. Consequently, child abuse is more likely to be reported if the family is poor and of a racial minority.

Ryan[38] discusses similar dynamics in the book *Blaming the Victim*. Ryan describes how blaming the victim helps the person avoid blaming the system in which violence is perpetuated. If the battered woman is to blame for at least not ending the violence, society is less at fault for perpetuating the notions that power, aggression, and dominance are the marks of a successful man and a successful country. Consequently, the issue is avoided. If the family who abuses elders is considered dysfunctional, others need not worry about a society that fails to provide help to the caregivers of the elderly.

As another example, consider the family member who has always been the most despised in cases of incest, the "collusive" mother. Despite the lack of evidence to support this notion, professionals are still eager to find out the mother's role in sexual abuse of her daughter. Because it is difficult to blame the child, they have shifted the blame to another female family member. Professionals should try to understand the mother's normal responses to a horrible dilemma. Even though some of the societal forces that lead to incest have been exposed, they are generally not addressed in recommendations for clinical interventions. The focus is on the "dysfunctional family unit" rather than the real issue: a criminal who has violated the safety and health of a child in a society uncomfortable with the attitudes that may encourage such behavior.

Another perspective, theories of deviance as explained by Schur,[39] is especially relevant for nursing. Deviance theory proposes that making the survivors and perpetrators of violence into objects to be studied or diagnostic categories creates further distance between them and the nurse. This is the problem with the proposed medical diagnosis of "battered woman syndrome" or a psychiatric diagnosis specific to survivors of violence. If adults receive diagnoses only because they were abused sometime in their past, the assumption of pathology becomes concrete. The survivor of family violence is officially sick and has the responsibility to become well. There is no chance that the person's responses will be seen as survival strategies or normal reactions; they become symptoms. Survivors become a "deviant group" to be studied and "fixed."

It has been suggested that more nurses have been victimized by violence than other groups, which might explain their negative attitudes toward other survivors. Research has not established whether there are more battered women among nurses than among other populations of women. In a recent study, nurses who were sexually abused as children were found to have lower self-esteem and higher present distress scores than nurses who reported no sexual abuse in childhood. Additionally, the nurses who were abused re-

ported that the abuse negatively influenced their private and professional relationships.[15] Regardless of the specific violence experience of nurses, power, control, and exploitation issues certainly have shaped the history of the nursing profession and continue to influence nurses' daily reality. Therefore, according to "oppressed group" behavior literature,[21] nurses would tend to have negative attitudes toward another oppressed group, the predominantly female survivors of family violence.

OVERCOMING NEGATIVE ATTITUDES. The first step in providing effective nursing care is exploring one's own attitudes toward survivors of family violence. Understanding the mechanisms that help create such attitudes is also helpful. It has been suggested that nurses who have had clinical experience with survivors and gotten to know them as people may be less blaming than nurses who have not.[8,14,22] Therefore, it is important to gain this experience through educational programs or as a volunteer in programs such as rape crisis centers, battered women's shelters, or child protection programs. Formal continuing and in-service education on family violence should be directed toward recognizing and changing feelings as well as learning facts about violence. Nurses can also increase their own understanding and appreciation of the experience of survivors by reading books and watching media programs about these issues.[5]

> **?** *Many television shows and movies explore the issues of family abuse and violence. Do you think they have helped to change attitudes or reinforced fears and stereotypes?*

Responses of Survivors

There is a growing body of knowledge that describes how people respond to violence from other family members. Because the definition of nursing is the diagnosis and treatment of human responses to health problems, these biopsychosocial responses to violence as a major health problem are the primary focus of nursing.

PHYSICAL RESPONSES TO BATTERING. One area of study has been the types and patterns of physical injuries received. A characteristic pattern of injuries, especially to the head, neck, face, throat, trunk, and sexual organs has been seen in all forms of family violence. For all groups experiencing family violence, sexual abuse often accompanies physical abuse. This has been best documented in battered women; several studies have found that approximately 40% were also sexually assaulted by their partners. All survivors of family violence tend to have injuries at multiple sites in various stages of healing.

Survivors of family violence often experience a range of physical symptoms not obviously related to their injuries, such as headaches, menstrual problems, chronic pain, and digestive and sleeping disturbances. Often, communicable diseases are a problem in shelters for battered women and their children.

Many characterize these symptoms as evidence of psychopathology, but similar symptoms occur after rape and other forms of violence, as well as in widows and divorcees. In addition, past injuries can cause such symptoms as headaches and other forms of chronic pain. Stress is also known to affect the immune system. Thus rather than labeling such symptoms "hysterical," "psychosomatic," or "evidence of somaticizing," such symptoms should be identified as part of a physical stress reaction. Such responses to stress are common to those who have experienced many types of emotional trauma.

BEHAVIORAL RESPONSES TO BATTERING. There have been many attempts to understand the behavior of survivors of family violence, especially their continued involvement with an abuser. This has been especially damaging in literature addressing the question of why battered women remain in the relationship. It is assumed that she should leave rather than stay. In actuality, when a battered woman leaves, she is in the most danger of being killed by a partner obsessed with power and control.[20] At the other end of the continuum, some battered women are able to end the violence but maintain their relationships using a variety of strategies.

However, family violence usually escalates in severity and frequency. In cases where the violence does not end, it is normal and healthy for a battered woman to consider her entire existence and that of her significant others for a long time before ending her most important attachment relationship.[4,28] Constraints that make it difficult to leave include cultural sanctions, an intense attachment to the man, and lack of resources. Gilligan[16,42] has observed that women usually make moral decisions by weighing the consequences to others more heavily than consequences to themselves. Thus concern for her children is a major issue in the woman's decision making.

Most battered women eventually leave a relationship that is continuously violent, but there is often a pattern of leaving and returning many times before making a final break. Rather than a sign of weakness, this can be seen as a normal behavioral pattern. It is influenced by the quality of social support and assistance to the woman and the batterer's behavior rather than the woman's psychological factors. Leaving and returning are purposeful and meant to pressure the abuser into meaningful change, test external and internal resources, or evaluate how the children react without their father.

Similar long processes of ending attachment relationships are seen with wives of alcoholics, divorced and separated women, and people experiencing anticipatory grief. In addition, grief can explain the denial that is often described in battered women.[6] Clinical reports also describe the reluctance of abused children and elderly family members to view their families as pathological rather than normal.

These responses seem more understandable and healthy if they are related to normal grief and fear of foster homes or nursing homes.

> **?** *Discuss the issue of women remaining in abusive relationships. What factors keep them in these relationships? How do health professionals usually respond to a woman who has remained in an abusive relationship? What approach would be helpful to her?*

PSYCHOLOGICAL RESPONSES TO BATTERING. More work has been done to explore psychological responses to abuse in battered women than in either child abuse or elder abuse. Most of our knowledge about the emotional responses to incest describes delayed reactions rather than immediate ones. In addition, the question of "false memories" has complicated the diagnosis and treatment process (see Critical Thinking about Contemporary Issues). Psychological responses studied most often include the cognitive responses of attribution and problem solving and the emotional responses of depression and lowered self-esteem.

Attributions. Attributions can be defined as the reasoning processes people use to explain events. A relationship to future mental health has been found in a variety of situations, including serious violence. Attributions affect how people feel about their behavior and interpret life events. It is often said that survivors of violence tend to blame themselves. Research shows that only about 20% of battered women do so. Some experts believe that internal self-blaming attributions may be adaptive for survivors of violence as a way of maintaining control over their lives. Others think that self-blame may contribute to long-term depression. To date, research has not resolved this issue for battered women or for other survivors of family violence. There is insufficient evidence to assume that self-blame is either widespread among survivors or always pathological. Nurses who work with these patients using the empowerment model will help them to identify their attributions and explore the effect on their feelings and relationships.

Problem-Solving Techniques. Several studies have found that battered women have trouble with problem solving. School problems have also been reported in abused children. In contrast, a variety of approaches are used by battered women that suggest appropriate decision making. Undoubtedly, some battered women, children, and elders are so frequently and severely beaten and controlled that their ability to solve problems is severely and chronically affected.

Extreme difficulty in problem solving could be explained by posttraumatic stress disorder, with its symptoms of memory impairment and difficulty concentrating. Problem-solving difficulties noted in widows and divorcees

CRITICAL THINKING *about* Contemporary Issues

Can Adults Remember Repressed Episodes of Child Abuse or Are These Part of a "False Memory Syndrome"?

Recently there has been considerable controversy about the validity of memories of childhood abuse. Some people have reported delayed recall of forgotten abuse that occurred during childhood, many years earlier. These reports of delayed recall of abuse have been challenged on a number of fronts, and in some cases people have retracted their allegations. Some experts claim that psychotherapists practicing "recovered memory therapy" created false memories of abuse through leading questions or excessive insisting. These therapists reportedly believe that psychopathology is related to childhood trauma and that the goal of therapy is to help patients remember incidents of previously forgotten abuse from childhood in order to get well.

The fact that many people forget episodes of childhood abuse is well established. As many as 38% of trauma survivors who experienced abuse severe enough to result in a visit to a hospital emergency room had no memory of the event 20 or more years later. At issue is the meaning of these findings. Some investigators have explained the loss of memory of abuse as secondary to "repression" or dissociative amnesia: Memories of abuse, although present in the mind, may not be available to consciousness. The opposite viewpoint holds that the loss of memories of abuse is a process of "normal forgetting," arguing that there is a popular misconception that forgotten memories exist somewhere in the brain and are only awaiting the proper stimulus to bring them to consciousness.

A recent review of this literature found that neuropeptides and neurotransmitters released during stress can modulate memory function, acting in the limbic system at the level of the hippocampus (responsible for turning short-term memory into long-term memory), amygdala (responsible for emotion), and other brain regions involved in these functions. Such release may interfere with the accurate laying down of memory traces for incidents of childhood abuse. Also, childhood abuse may result in long-term alterations in the function of these neuromodulators.[3] Nurses can help these patients by keeping up to date with the neuroscientific research in this area and the impact of these findings on the controversy surrounding these issues.

have been explained as normal responses to loss. Such problems could also be explained as one of the cognitive aspects of depression.

Depression. Depression has been noted in many research studies of battered women, adult survivors of incest, and abused children.[33,45] Depression has also been described in survivors of other forms of violence, as well as in divorcees and widows. Depression is a complex process. Detailed information about predisposing factors and precipitating stressors related to depression is discussed in Chapter 19.

Mackey and associates[33] studied depression in female survivors of sexual assault. They found that 60% were at least somewhat depressed. Factors associated with more severe depression included lack of disclosure of the assault to significant others related to stigma, having children at home, and involvement in a civil lawsuit. Women who reported being sexually active were less depressed.

Self-Esteem. Although most research has found low self-esteem in battered women and incest survivors, there have been some exceptions. One way to interpret these findings is to compare groups who are experiencing the same situational dynamics, except for the violence. Using this approach, Campbell[4] found no significant difference in self-esteem between battered women and other women considering leaving an intimate relationship, even though both groups were below norms. However, sexual abuse had a direct detrimental effect on battered women's self-esteem independent of severity and frequency of physical beatings.

In summary, responses to family violence can be interpreted as symptoms of pathology of a certain group of people. The same responses can also be interpreted as how normal people respond to incredible physical and emotional trauma and yet survive. Research regarding this latter approach is beginning to document survivor mechanisms and a recovery process from abuse.

Preventive Nursing Interventions

Preventing family violence requires the use of a variety of approaches. These include the primary prevention strategies of changing norms and values, preventive education with a variety of populations, and secondary prevention strategies of effective treatment.

PRIMARY PREVENTION. Primary prevention is an activity that stops a problem before it occurs. Changing society's acceptance of violence and abuse is an important first step in prevention. Effective primary prevention includes eliminating cultural norms and values that accept and glamorize violence.

This can begin by limiting the amount of violence permitted on television and in other media. The prevalence of violence on television plays a role in creating a social climate that says violence is exciting and appropriate. The average child watches television for 20 hours a week. It has been estimated that American children observe 18,000 killings before they graduate from high school. Video and computer games are popular with children also, and there is a great deal of concern about the violence in these games. Some manufacturers have agreed to place ratings on these games according to age appropriateness and level of violence.

A related area of primary prevention would be the elimination of pornography, especially violent pornography. Violent pornography has been particularly associated with sexual violence. However, the rate of subscription to even a mild form of pornography such as *Playboy* magazine has been positively correlated with state rape rates.

Primary prevention of abuse also includes strengthening individuals and families so they can cope more effectively with stress. Nurses can conduct programs in the schools, workplace, or community. Strategies such as nurse-developed educational programs in high school parenting classes or childbirth education classes can be used to prepare families for the stress of child rearing. Topics could include normal child development and expectations, basic skills of infant care, and means of disciplining children that do not involve physical punishment. Additional educational strategies include teaching family members that conflict resolution does not always mean one party wins while the other loses and that they should respect individual differences among family members.

Nurses can be involved in teaching family life and sex education courses in elementary and middle schools. Child sexual abuse can be prevented or detected when children are taught about inappropriate sexual contact and what they should do if it occurs. Middle school students need information about how to have relationships in which jealousy is not viewed as a sign of love and domination of one partner over the other is not expected. Peer discussions can help change the definition of manliness based on confrontation and control.

Family violence prevention also includes anticipatory guidance while working with families. For example, respite care is needed for families with chronically ill or incapacitated members, including the elderly and children. Planning in advance for relief from responsibility will prevent strained relationships and potential violence or abuse. Families also need to anticipate the difficult developmental stages of children. Parents need to know that infants are not intentionally frustrating to parents, that toddlers' obstinacy is necessary for independence in later childhood, and that bed-wetting is a signal for increased positive attention, not punishment.

A society must develop programs and policies that support families and reduce stresses and inequities. This includes adequate and appropriate day care for children and incapacitated elders, equity in salary and wages to make women less financially dependent, public education that ensures an adequate foundation for full employment of all, and sufficient financing of prevention and treatment programs.

> **?** *Go to a computer store and search for the most popular games. Evaluate them for level of violence, sexual roles, and issues related to power and control.*

SECONDARY PREVENTION. Secondary prevention of family violence is aimed at its cyclic nature. Although there

is not a perfect relationship, we do know that children raised in violent, noncaring homes are more likely to become spouse and child abusers. Therefore, one of the most effective methods of preventing violence and abuse in future generations is to stop current abuse.

Even when the violence has ended, those affected will need help. The children of battered women and siblings of abused children have witnessed violence and need help to counteract that learning. Often it is believed that abused children are "out of the woods" when they have been removed from the home or the family is no longer violent. Even if there are no identifiable long-term effects, there may have been trauma encapsulation, which may not be evident until many years afterward. In addition, these children may grow up believing that family members are normally violent to each other. Conscious resolve alone may not overcome this.

Secondary prevention also involves identification of families at risk or those who are beginning to use violence. Table 39-3 lists indicators of actual or potential abuse. These can be used for nursing assessment. Additional early indicators of families at risk include violence in the family of origin of either partner, communication problems, and excessive family stress such as an unplanned pregnancy, unemployment, or inadequate family resources. Pregnancy is an ideal time to identify women at risk to become battered or in the early stages of an abusive relationship. This is also the best time to identify the infant's risk for abuse. Pregnancy is when healthy women are most often seen in the health-care system. A comprehensive assessment should include information about relationships and child-rearing beliefs and practices. It may also be possible to identify abuse early in a relationship before abusive patterns become entrenched.[35,36] When the nurse hears an indication of risk, immediate nursing intervention is required. Taking the time to explore the risk factors, discuss perceptions and attitudes, and brainstorm with the patient about possible alternatives is time well spent.

High rates of family violence and low rates of detection, reporting, and therapeutic intervention by health-care professionals are well documented. Several authors have identified a lack of educational content on child, spouse, and elder abuse in professional training programs for physicians, nurses, psychologists, social workers, and dentists. This finding underscores the need for educators to expand curricula on family violence and for legislators to examine the ineffectiveness of current mandatory reporting laws.[32,41]

SPECIAL POPULATIONS

Child Abuse

The earliest form of family violence recognized in the health professional literature was physical abuse to children. Although violence to children was identified as a social problem in the nineteenth century, it was not until the

TABLE 39-3 *Indicators of Actual or Potential Abuse*

NURSING HISTORY

Primary Reason for Contact

Vague information about cause of problem

Discrepancy between physical findings and description of cause

Minimizing injuries

Inappropriate delay between time of injury and treatment

Inappropriate family reactions (such as lack of concern, over-concern, threatening demeanor)

Information from Family Genogram

Family violence in history (child, spouse, elder)

History of violence outside of home

Incarcerations

Violent deaths in extended family

Alcoholism/drug abuse in family history

Health History

History of traumatic injuries

Spontaneous abortions

Psychiatric hospitalizations

History of depression

Substance abuse

Sexual History

Prior sexual abuse

Use of force in sexual activities

Venereal disease

Child with sexual knowledge beyond that appropriate for age

Promiscuity

Personal/Social History

Unwanted or unplanned pregnancy

Adolescent pregnancy

Social isolation (difficulty naming people available for help in a crisis)

Lack of contact with extended family

Unrealistic expectations of relationships or age-appropriate behavior

Extreme jealousy by spouse

Rigid traditional sex-role beliefs

Verbal aggression

Belief in use of physical punishment

Difficulties in school

Truancy, running away

Psychological History

Feelings of helplessness/hopelessness

Feeling trapped

Difficulty making plans for future

Tearfulness

Chronic fatigue, apathy

Suicide attempts

Financial History

Poverty

Finances rigidly controlled by one family member

Unwillingness to spend money on health care or adequate nutrition

Complaints about spending money on family members

Unemployment

Use of elders' finances for other family members

Family Beliefs/Values

Belief in importance of physical discipline

Autocratic decision making

Intolerance of differing views among members

Mistrust of outsiders

Family Relations

Lack of visible affection or nurturing between family members

Extreme dependency between family members

Autonomy discouraged

Numerous arguments

Temporary separations

Dissatisfaction with family members

Lack of enjoyable family activities

Extramarital affairs

Role rigidity (inability of members to assume nontraditional roles)

PHYSICAL EXAMINATION

General Appearance

Fearful, anxious, hyperactive or hypoactive

Poor hygiene, careless grooming

Inappropriate dress

Increased anxiety in presence of abuser

Looking to abuser for answers to questions

Inappropriate or anxious nonverbal behavior (such as giggling at serious questions or questions related to abuse)

Flinching when touched

Vital Statistics

Overweight or underweight

Hypertension

Skin

Bruises, welts, edema

Presence of scars and indications of injuries in various stages of healing

Cigarette burns

Head

Bald patches on scalp from pulling hair

Subdural hematoma

Eyes

Subconjunctival hemorrhage

Swelling

Black eyes

Ears

Hearing loss from prior injury or untreated infections

Mouth

Bruising

Lacerations

Untreated dental caries

Venereal infection

Abdomen

Intraabdominal injuries

Abdominal injuries during pregnancy

Extremities

Bruising to forearms from attempts to protect self from blows

Broken arms

Radiological indications of previous fractures

Neurological

Developmental delays

Difficulty with speech or swallowing

Hyperactive reflex response

Continued

TABLE **39-3** *Indicators of Actual or Potential Abuse—cont'd*

Genital/Urinary	Inadequate food
Genital lacerations or bruising	Spoiled food not discarded
Urinary tract infections	**Family Communication Pattern**
Sexually transmitted disease	One parent answers all questions
Rectal	Looking for approval of other family members before answering questions
Rectal bruising	Members continually interrupt each other
Bleeding	Negative nonverbal behavior in other members when one member speaking
Edema	
Tenderness	Members do not listen to each other
Poor sphincter tone	Taboo topics (family secrets)
NURSING OBSERVATIONS	**Emotional Climate**
General Observations	Tense, secretive atmosphere
Observations that differ significantly from history	Unhappiness
Family members inadequately clothed or groomed	Lack of affection
Home Environment	Apparent fear of other family members
Inadequate heating	Verbal arguing
Inappropriate sleeping arrangements	
Total household disorganization	

1940s that it became a medical problem, even a unique "syndrome." By the end of the 1960s every state had enacted legislation mandating the report of suspected child abuse and neglect. Under current laws, nurses and any other professionals providing services to children are required to report suspected incidents of child abuse and neglect.

There are many forms of abuse to children. These include physical abuse or battering, emotional abuse, sexual abuse, and neglect. Children who witness family violence and abuse are themselves victimized,[31,37] and although they are often overlooked, they can be symptomatic as a result of this abuse (Table 39-4). Much is still unknown about the causes, treatment, or prevention of child abuse. In addition, research has failed to identify any factors that are present in all abusing and absent in all nonabusing parents.

SEXUAL ABUSE OF CHILDREN AND ADOLESCENTS. Sexual abuse is defined as the involvement of children and adolescents in sexual activities they do not fully comprehend and to which they do not freely consent.[12] Sexual abuse results in both long-term and short-term problems.[17] Physical problems include:

▼ Venereal disease or infection
▼ Vaginal or rectal bleeding, itching, or soreness
▼ Recurrent urinary tract infections
▼ Pregnancy

Emotional changes include:

▼ Sexual acting-out
▼ Physical aggression
▼ Excessive masturbation
▼ Withdrawal
▼ Low self-esteem

▼ Drop in school performance
▼ Disturbed sleep

Morris and Bihan found that physical and sexual abuse often were not considered as possible causes of these behaviors in a review of the records of 100 psychiatric hospital patients.[34]

The long-term effects of sexual abuse as a child include:

▼ Sexual problems
▼ Difficulty trusting others
▼ Anxiety and panic attacks
▼ Depression
▼ Substance abuse

A study by Feinauer[12] of adult women who had been sexually abused as children found that they experienced more emotional distress and long-term effects when the perpetrator was a person who was known and trusted by them. In addition, the kinship relationship between the victim and the abuser was less important in creating distress than the emotional bond the victim felt toward the perpetrator. Thus, a critical factor seems to be the violation of the child's trust, as well as the physical trauma.[25]

NURSING ASSESSMENT. Nursing assessment of actual or potential child abuse begins with a thorough history and physical examination. Gathering a history of child abuse can be a stressful experience for both the nurse and the family. It is essential for the nurse to examine personal values and past experiences to maintain a therapeutic and nonjudgmental clinical approach.

It is important to use an honest, open approach that is not intended to punish or shame either the child or the parent.[6,29] Most abusive parents are genuinely embarrassed about their behavior and would like help in developing al-

TABLE **39-4** *Effects of Witnessing Violence in Childhood*

INFANT	PRESCHOOL	SCHOOL-AGE	ADOLESCENT
Disrupted attachment needs	Feeling that world is not safe or stable	Greater willingness to use violence	Feelings of rage, shame, betrayal
Disrupted routines (sleeping, eating)	Yelling, irritability, hiding, stuttering; signs of terror	Holding self responsible for violence at home	School truancy, early sexual activity, substance abuse, delinquency
Risk of physical injury	Many somatic complaints and regressive behaviors	Shame and embarrassment of the family secret	Unresponsiveness
Eating and sleeping problems in 50%	Anxious attachment behaviors: whining, crying, clinging	Distracted and inattentive, labile, and hypervigilant	Little memory of childhood
Decreased responsiveness to adults, increased crying	Increased separation and stranger anxiety	Limited range of emotional responses	Defensiveness
	Insomnia, sleepwalking, nightmares, bed-wetting	Psychosomatic complaints	Short attention span
		Uncooperative, suspicious, guarded behavior	

Modified from Rhea MH: The silent victims of domestic violence: who will speak?, *JCAPN* 9:7, 1996.

ternative approaches to discipline. This knowledge can be used by the nurse to establish an environment that will facilitate honesty and sharing. The setting for the interview must be quiet, private, and uninterrupted.

In general, the child and the adults should be separated for the initial interview. However, this decision depends on the child's age and other factors. The nurse should honestly state the purpose of the interview and the type of questions being asked, and describe the subsequent physical examination. The approach must be calm and supportive because both the child and the family will be uneasy.

The interview with the parent can begin with a discussion of the problem that first brought the child to a health-care facility. During this discussion the nurse should pay particular attention to the parent's understanding of the problem, discrepancies in the stories, and the parent's emotional responses. The interview can then be expanded to discussions of how the parent "disciplines" or spanks the child. The initial interview is not the time to confront a suspected abuser directly because measures must be taken to document and report the abuse in a way that will ensure the child's safety.

NURSING INTERVENTIONS. When child abuse is suspected, the nurse must report this to protective services. An investigation by the state protective service agency is legally mandated and also reinforces to the family the seriousness of the problem. When protective services are involved, the nurse should explain to the family precisely what will happen in an investigation and the amount of time involved. The nurse should maintain frequent contact with the assigned worker to ensure a comprehensive, consistent approach. Nurses who work with violent families need to know exactly how protective services in their community operate. Ongoing professional relationships with colleagues at the agency will enable the nurse to remain informed

about policies and reporting protocols and ensure successful coordination and continuity.

Wife Abuse

The term *wife abuse* includes all forms of physical violence toward a female partner in an ongoing intimate relationship. It also refers to emotional degradation and intimidation, which almost always accompany physical abuse, of female partners, and to sexual abuse (or marital rape), which is part of the violence in about half of the cases.[4] The violence is part of a system of coercive control that may also include financial coercion, threats against children and other family members, and destruction of property. Wife abuse is the most widespread form of family violence. At least one in every six wives is hit by a husband sometime during their relationship. Although wives do hit husbands, female violence is much more likely to be in self-defense. It seldom takes the intentional repeated, serious, and controlling form characteristic of wife abuse. Therefore, using the terms *spouse abuse* and *domestic violence* obscures the gender specificity of the violence. However, the nurse must be aware that both husband abuse and homosexual partner abuse occur.

One of the most frightening realities of wife abuse is the potential for murder. The majority of female homicide victims in the United States are killed by a husband, lover, or ex-husband or ex-lover. The majority of these murders are preceded by abuse. There is evidence that a battered woman is in most danger of homicide when she leaves her abusive partner or makes it clear to him that she is ending the relationship.[20] Some battered women kill their spouses. Many of the risk factors are similar. They include having a handgun in the house, a history of suicide threats or attempts in either partner, battering during pregnancy, sexual abuse, severe substance abuse, and extreme jealousy and controlling behavior. A frequent statement heard by potentially murderous abusers is, "If I can't have you, no one can."

Stark and Flitcraft[40] assert that battering may be the most important precipitating stressor for female suicide attempts and that 10% of battered women have considered suicide. Therefore, when an abused woman is depressed, suicide potential must be carefully assessed.

 Discuss social reaction to wife abuse in relation to the Lorena Bobbitt and O.J. Simpson trials.

NURSING ASSESSMENT. It has been documented that the most prevalent cause of trauma in women treated in emergency rooms is wife abuse. It is also a common cause of female visits to psychiatric emergency departments and other mental health treatment centers. We now recognize that nursing assessment for all forms of violence is critical. Assessment for wife abuse should be mandatory in mental health settings, as well as in emergency rooms, prenatal settings, and primary care facilities.[7,35]

When there are no obvious injuries, assessment for abuse is best included with the history about the patient's primary intimate attachment relationship. Answers to general questions on the quality of that relationship should be assessed for feelings of being controlled or needing to control. A relationship characterized by excessive jealousy (of possessions, children, jobs, friends, and other family members, as well as potential sexual partners) is more likely to be violent. The patient can be asked about how the couple solves conflicts; one partner needing to have the final say or frequent and forceful verbal aggression also can be considered risk factors. Finally, the patient should be asked whether arguments ever involve "pushing or shoving." Questions about minor violence within a couple relationship help to establish the unfortunate normalcy of wife abuse and to lessen the stigma of disclosure. If the patient hesitates, looks away, displays other uncomfortable nonverbal behavior or reveals risk factors for abuse, she or he can be asked again later in the interview about physical violence.

If abuse is revealed, the nurse's first response is critical. It is important that an abused woman realize that she is not alone; important affirmation can be given with a statement about the frequency of wife abuse. The extent and types of the abuse must be identified and described in the record. Careful documentation using a body map identifying the locations of bruises, contusions, or cuts is necessary for potential legal actions, which are often child custody suits as well as criminal actions related to the violence.[35]

The woman's responses to the violence are also a critical area for mental health assessment. It is important to interpret these responses to the woman as normal within the circumstances. Signs of posttraumatic stress disorder, depres-

sion, and low self-esteem must be assessed and recorded. Attribution regarding the abuse is also important. One nursing study[4] revealed that women who blamed abuse on an unchanging personality characteristic within themselves had lower levels of self-esteem and increased depression. The nurse must carefully assess the woman's beliefs regarding the abuse and responsibility for the abuse. Because many wife abusers find an excuse for the violence, the woman may be unnecessarily accepting the blame for his actions.

If the patient is an abuser, mental state is also important and the potential for further violence must be assessed carefully. The safety of the abused partner is a concern, as is treatment for the abuser. Consultation with legal advisors about the nurse's duty to warn may be needed (see Chapter 9).[20]

NURSING INTERVENTIONS. Most communities have treatment programs for abusive men. They have been found to be most effective when the court has ordered treatment, with punishment for noncompliance. Severely abusive men seldom admit they have a problem and often need to be mandated to enter and remain in treatment. The nurse needs to confront the violence and clarify that the responsibility lies with the abuser. A combination of strategies may be needed to get the abuser into treatment if he is not involved with the court.[24]

The type of referral chosen is extremely important. Long-lasting change is more likely if the treatment combines behavioral therapy around anger control with a program designed to change attitudes toward women.[19] (Managing anger is discussed in Chapter 22 and cognitive behavioral theory in Chapter 30.) Traditional marriage therapy or couple counseling as the only treatment is potentially dangerous to the woman because of the unequal power in the relationship and the possibility of retaliatory violence.

Several investigators have identified themes expressed by women who have been in abusive relationships with men.[10,11,44] These themes, outlined in Table 39-5, can help the nurse in assessing and intervening with women who have been in abusive relationships.

To empower an abused woman, one must first make sure she has the information she needs. This includes knowledge of the related state and local laws and ordinances. She also needs to be aware of the local battered women's shelters available for advice, support, and group participation, even if she does not intend to enter the shelter yet.

Mutual goal setting is particularly important when working with abused women. Nurses can be frustrated if they impose their goals on the women, who may not be ready for drastic action. Ideally they will have an established relationship during which the nurse and patient can work through the normal denial and minimization that takes place when the primary attachment relationship is threatened. The nurse and patient can then consider all the options the woman has thought about and devise others. Dealing with an abusive situation is a recovery process that takes time and ongoing support.[28] The nurse can help the patient mobilize natural, social, and professional support so that her economic as well as emotional needs are addressed.

Evaluation of nursing interventions is based on mutual goals, not on a preconceived notion of what a battered woman should do. Because most abused women eventually leave a seriously violent situation or end the violence in some other way and seek help when the violence becomes severe,[19] the nurse can be optimistic about the eventual outcome. Interventions may not result in an immediately happy ending, but they can plant the seeds of empowerment that facilitate the woman's recovery process.

Elder Abuse

Estimates of the numbers of elderly people abused vary widely. Finkelhor and Pillemer[13] found 32 survivors of physical abuse, physical neglect, or chronic verbal aggression per 1000 elderly in Boston. However, the majority of the abuse was committed by spouses (60% of the physical abuse and 58% of the overall maltreatment). Thus, spouse abuse and elder abuse are often overlapping categories.

This also contradicts the notion that elder abuse is most likely a case of children abusing an elderly parent for whom they are providing physical care. Although caregiver stress is an important nursing concern, it may not play the central role in elder abuse that was previously assumed. In fact, one study[13] reported that an important risk factor for elder abuse was the abuser's financial dependence on the abused. Research has not found abused elders to be more functionally impaired than control groups. Rather than the condition of the elder, characteristics of the abuser, such as mental and emotional problems including substance abuse, create a family situation at risk for elder abuse.[18]

NURSING ASSESSMENT. Based on this information, it would be important to assess for elder abuse in families where a mentally ill person is financially dependent on aging parents. Consequently, family interviews would not focus exclusively on the patient but would also assess the interactions among family members for indications of verbal and physical aggression.

It is difficult for abused elders to admit being physically hurt by a child or spouse. Again, gentle inquiry about the family's usual approach to resolving interpersonal difficulties is useful. At least part of this assessment must take place with the elder alone. An elder may be reluctant to disclose abuse because of fear of being abandoned to a nursing home or a life of total isolation. Only by establishing a trusting relationship over time or using an already established relationship with someone else can the nurse explore the abusive situation completely.

Assessment is even more difficult when the elder is se-

TABLE 39-5 *Themes of Women Who Have Been in Abusive Relationships*

THEMES OF DYSFUNCTION WHILE IN THE RELATIONSHIP

▼ *Lack of relational authenticity:* The women never felt emotionally real, never established relationships with themselves as individuals, and were uncertain about their own identities. This increased their perceived threat of rejection and their efforts to please the abuser in order to maintain the relationship. Leaving the abusive relationship was seen as a threat to one's personal identity.

▼ *Immobility:* Abuse permeated every aspect of the life of women in the study. Living in constant fear for their own well-being and that of their children created an appearance to outsiders that they were scattered, incapable, and indecisive. This fear created a barrier to others that increased their sense of isolation and decreased their ability to seek help.

▼ *Emptiness:* These women experienced multiple losses in their lives, including problems maintaining relationships with others, self-esteem, pride, a sense of control, and a sense of accomplishment. They eventually escaped the pain of abuse by having no feelings, not thinking, just constantly "doing" an intense schedule of the routines of daily living. This created a numbing effect that allowed them to continue to the next day.

▼ *Disconnection:* The women's sense of sexuality was adversely affected. They equated sex with love, so being sexually active was the only way they felt connected to another person. They lacked support from extended family members, who disapproved of the relationship. The abuse created physical illnesses because of the stress of the relationship. Many had indirect self-destructive behaviors (such as alcoholism and eating disorders) and some had suicidal or homicidal ideation as a means of escaping the abuse.

THEMES OF HEALING WHILE RECOVERING

▼ *Flexibility:* Women reported a readiness to alter the course of their lives in response to changing conditions and the acquiring of new behaviors. This included an acknowledgment of the past, resiliency with everyday events, increased self-awareness, and establishment of appropriate boundaries.

▼ *Awakening:* A turning point occurred within each woman when she realized there were choices and meaning in her life. This resulted in a sense of inner strength, hope, spirituality, and inner peace.

▼ *Relationship:* Women described an integration of all aspects of self, a sense of trust and connectedness between self and others, a feeling of harmony and contentment, and a linkage between internal and external events.

▼ *Empowerment:* Women related a new ability to make choices in their lives, which resulted in a valuing of the self, self-determination, and a sense of accomplishment.

verely mentally or emotionally impaired. In those cases, physical assessment and careful attention to nonverbal behavior are critical. Bruises to the upper arms from shaking are especially common in elder abuse. Although bruises from abuse are difficult to differentiate from those normal in aging, bilateral upper outer arm bruises are definitive. Lacerations, especially to the face, are not usually caused by falls and should be regarded with suspicion. Vaginal lacerations or bruises and twisting bone fractures are particularly indicative of abuse. Signs of neglect are more common than those of physical abuse. Determining whether the neglect is intentional is the key to planning a nursing course of action.

Whenever a dependent elderly person is being cared for by another, their interaction will give important clues about the relationship. Flinching or shrinking away by the elder or rough physical treatment accompanied by verbal denigration by the caretaker are possible indicators of abuse. As with all types of family violence, the nurse needs to analyze the data from the history, physical examination, and direct observations to make an assessment of abuse. The decision to report is difficult, especially if it appears likely that the outcome will be a nursing home placement unwanted by the elder. However, most states have laws that require nurses to report suspected elder abuse.

> **?** You are providing home care services to an elderly person who shows evidence of physical abuse. The patient's caregiver handles her roughly and is impatient with her. The patient denies that she is unhappy or abused. Describe your response to this situation. What is your obligation to report your suspicions?

NURSING INTERVENTIONS. When the nurse must report elder abuse, it is usually less damaging to the therapeutic relationship to inform the family first. Deciding whether to discuss reporting beforehand is influenced by the likelihood of the abusing family member disappearing and the severity of the abuse. If the abuse is less severe or mainly a neglectful or caretaker stress situation, discussing the intent to report first makes the action seem less a condemnation, allows protective services to be perceived as a helping agency rather than a punitive one, and increases the chances that the nurse will be seen as a continuing source of help. Respite care or other stress relievers may be the key interventions for an overburdened caretaker.

In other cases the primary intervention may be therapeutic assistance for the abusers. This may include counseling, therapy for mental disorders, or substance abuse treatment. The success of various interventions for elder abuse is not yet known because research into this issue is scant. However, one should assume that the treatment will need to involve specific components aimed at the violence as well as at whatever other problems are involved.

RAPE AND SEXUAL ASSAULT

Rape and sexual assault are concerns for individuals, families, and the community. Sexual assaults against women and children (the most common survivors) result in physical trauma, psychic and spiritual disruptions, and deterioration of social relationships. In addition, fear of rape and sexual assault has major effects on women as they restrict their activities in attempts to ensure their safety. Survivors of sexual assaults include women and men of all ages, social classes, races, and occupations. Sexual assault disrupts every aspect of the survivor's life, including social activities, interpersonal relationships, employment, and career. Although males may be sexually assaulted and women sexual offenders, in this section the survivor is referred to as "she" and the offender as "he." However, it must be recognized that men and young boys are also victimized and that assessment must not be limited to women and girls.

> **?** How would you respond to a roommate who returned from a date tearful and saying that her boyfriend forced her to have sex even though she refused? Would it make any difference if she had been sexually active with him in the past? Why or why not?

Definition of Sexual Assault

Sexual assault is generally defined as forced perpetration of an act of sexual contact with another person without consent. Lack of consent could be related to the victim's cognitive or personality development, feelings of fear or coercion, or the offender's physical or verbal threats. Sexual assault is not a sexual act but is instead motivated by a desire to humiliate, defile, and dominate the victim. It has occurred for centuries but is now recognized as a social and public health problem.

Sexual consent can be conceptualized as a continuum, as seen in Box 39-2. This continuum demonstrates degrees of coercion, including bribery, taking advantage of one's position of power or trust in a relationship, or the victim's inability to consent freely.

Marital Rape

It is important to recognize that most cases of sexual assault do not occur between strangers. Marital rape has recently been recognized legally in most states. Child sexual abuse by family members, family friends, and caretakers is being reported in record numbers.

Marital rape is often reported concurrently with physical abuse. Campbell[4] found that the husbands of most of the abused women in her study believed it was their right to

Box **39-2** *Sexual Behavior: The Force Continuum*

Freely Consenting		Seduction		Bribery or Coercion		Fear Rape	
←——1———	——2———	———3———	——4———	——5———	——6———	——7———	——8——→
Economic Partnership		Psychic Rape		Acquaintance Rape		Violent Rape	

1. **Freely consenting.** Partners with equal power mutually choosing sexual activity. Equal power means each partner has equal status, knowledge, and ability to consent. This includes one partner agreeing to engage in sexual activity, even if not aroused, as an expression of love and caring for the other person.
2. **Economic partnership.** One person agrees to sexual activity as part of an economic agreement. The types of sexual behavior permitted are mutually determined as part of the economic agreement.
3. **Seduction.** One party attempts to persuade the other to engage in sexual activities.
4. **Psychic rape.** Assault to another person's dignity and self-respect, such as verbal abuse, street harassment, or the portrayal of violence or pornography in the media.

5. **Bribery or coercion.** The use of emotional or psychological force to persuade the other to take part in sexual activities. This includes situations of unequal power, especially when one person is in a position of authority.
6. **Acquaintance rape.** Sexual assault occurring when one party abuses the trust of a relationship and forces the other into sexual activities.
7. **Fear rape.** When one party engages in sexual activities out of fear of potential violence if she resists.
8. **Violent rape.** When violence is threatened or occurs. This includes forced sexual activity between spouses, acquaintances, or strangers.

have sex whenever they wanted. This included when the women were ill, had recently given birth, or were discharged from a hospital. These women described forced vaginal intercourse, anal intercourse, being hit, burned, or kicked during sex, having objects inserted into their vagina and anus, or being forced to perform sexual acts with animals or while their children were present. Many women were threatened with weapons or beaten when they refused to take part in these activities. Marital rape may be especially devastating for the survivor. She often must continue to interact with the rapist because of her dependence on him. In addition, many survivors do not seek health care or the support of family members or friends because of embarrassment or humiliation.

Rape and sexual assault are important issues for nursing because nurses treat people in the hospital and the community. Several aspects of nursing practice place nurses at an increased risk for sexual assault by strangers: hours of employment, home visiting in the community, and for some a reluctance to create a scene or defend themselves aggressively.

Nursing Care of the Sexual Assault Survivor

NURSING ASSESSMENT. The initial assessment is an important phase of the treatment of rape and sexual assault survivors. Although most nurses would quickly recognize the woman brought to the emergency department by the police following an attack by a stranger, many survivors of sexual assault are not so easily identified. Therefore, all nursing assessments must include questions to determine current or past sexual abuse. Because people have different definitions of rape, the assessment question must be

broadly stated, such as "Has anyone ever forced you into sex that you did not wish to participate in?" This question may uncover other types of sexual trauma such as incest, date rape, or childhood sexual abuse. When the answer is affirmative, it can be gently followed with broad questions, such as "Can you tell me more about it?" or "How often has it happened?" Often the response may be hesitation, questioning, or an embarrassed laugh. When this occurs, the nurse can increase the patient's comfort by explaining that the question is routine because sexual assault is common. The nurse can offer help in obtaining legal or social services.

NURSING INTERVENTIONS. When it is determined that abuse has occurred, it cannot be ignored. Disclosing sexual abuse is an indication of trust. If nurses immediately refer the patient elsewhere, they communicate that the problem is too distasteful or delicate to handle or that there are serious psychological implications. Therefore, an immediate response of nonjudgmental listening and psychological support is essential. In addition, if a recent attack is disclosed, physical evidence will be needed. Evidence collection is an appropriate nursing responsibility and requires special training. Later interventions may include referrals to survivors' groups, shelters for battered women, or legal services. The organizations listed in Box 39-3 may be useful when helping survivors of abuse organize their resources.

People respond to sexual assault differently depending on their past experiences, personal characteristics, and the amount and type of support received from significant others, health-care providers, and the criminal justice system. The acute stage, immediately after the attack, is characterized by extreme confusion, fear, disorganization, and restlessness. However, some survivors may mask these feelings and appear to be outwardly calm or subdued.

The second phase involves the long-term process of reorganization. It generally begins several weeks after the attack. This phase may include intrusive memories of the traumatic event during the day and while asleep, fears, or phobias such as extreme fears of being alone, being in a crowd, or traveling. The survivor often has a sense of living in a dangerous, unpredictable world and may become preoccupied with feelings of victimization and vulnerability. She may encounter difficulties in sexual relationships or her ability to relate comfortably to men. Some survivors develop secondary phobic reactions to people, places, or situations that remind them of the attack.

> **?** *How do you think the woman's movement and feminist thinking have influenced society's views on family violence? On rape and sexual assault? On pornography?*

Coping strategies may include changing one's phone number or residence, talking with friends or family, or taking classes in self-defense. Nursing actions to help the survivor of sexual assault include active listening, empathic responses, active concern and caring, assistance in problem solving, and referral to sexual assault crisis centers. A sample Nursing Treatment Plan for survivors of sexual assault is presented here.

Summary

1. Family violence refers to a range of behaviors occurring between family members and includes physical and

---

Box **39-3** *Hotline Numbers for Survivors of Abuse*

National Organization for Victim Assistance (NOVA): 1-800-TRY-NOVA (for community information and referrals); 202-232-6682.
National Coalition Against Domestic Violence: 202-638-6388; 303-839-1852.

 NURSING TREATMENT PLAN *Summary* **Survivors of Abuse and Violence**

Nursing Diagnosis: Rape trauma syndrome
Expected Outcome: The patient will resume his or her usual lifestyle and social relationships.

Short-term Goals	Nursing Interventions	Rationale
The patient will express feelings related to the assault, including guilt, fear, and vulnerability.	Allow patient to discuss feelings regarding assault. Communicate knowledge and understanding of emotional responses to sexual assault to help in identification of feelings. Provide anticipatory guidance regarding common physical, psychological, and social responses.	Women often experience various feelings, including guilt, shame, anger, and embarrassment. It is necessary to identify and express these feelings to develop coping skills. Knowing what to expect reassures the patient that her reactions are normal and can be managed.
The patient will identify supportive people to help in dealing with this crisis.	Explore relationships with significant others. Encourage the patient to discuss the situation with trusted and supportive people.	According to the principles of crisis intervention, it is important for the person in crisis to identify and use a social support system.
The patient will seek medical care for physical problems related to the assault.	Advise patient of the potential for sexually transmitted diseases or pregnancy. Help in identifying a medical care provider. Offer to accompany to the medical examination.	Early identification of physical problems provides the patient with the maximum number of treatment choices. Many women relive the assault during a gynecological examination. Support from a trusted person can be helpful.
The patient will be actively involved in mobilizing support systems.	Support decision making and active problem solving. Provide written information about community services and encourage use of them. Plan for a follow-up phone contact within a few days.	Active involvement in seeking resources gives the patient a sense of control over life, counteracting the helplessness related to the assault.

emotional abuse of children, child neglect, spouse battering, marital rape, and elder abuse. Characteristics of violent families include multigenerational transmission, social isolation, abuse of power, and substance abuse.

2. Many nurses have a negative response to survivors of violence. It is important to identify and overcome these attitudes.

3. Physical responses to battering include a characteristic pattern of injuries and the occurrence of a variety of stress-related symptoms. Behavioral responses to battering include reluctance to leave the violent situation. Psychological responses to violence include attributions, problem-solving techniques, and depression.

4. Nursing actions related to the prevention of family violence include strategies to change norms and values, preventive education, and secondary prevention strategies of effective treatment.

5. Nursing interventions related to special populations including children, wives, and the elderly are presented.

6. Nursing care of survivors of sexual assault include nonjudgmental listening, psychological support, evidence collection, and mobilization of community support such as shelters for battered women, survivor's groups, and legal services.

COMPETENT CARING A Clinical Exemplar of a Psychiatric Nurse

Pat Engdahl, RN, C

When thinking about how I made a difference in a patient's life, I remembered an experience I had with a young woman just over 30 years of age who was admitted in a state of extreme panic, hardly able to process a simple request such as "I need you to please move away from the door." She told me this later, saying her first memories of being on our floor included a voice saying the above words "in the kindest, firmest, most caring tones" she had ever heard—and she felt safe. She said she didn't want to move away from the locked door, but she did it anyway and she said, "I think it was your voice."

We worked very hard together. She was a survivor of childhood sexual and physical abuse and, as often happens, married to a man who also abused her. She talked; I listened. She said she had shed enough tears and wasn't going to cry anymore. I replied she needed to "cry a river" for the therapeutic process to begin. We role-played. We practiced handling verbal abuse and daring to express anger—the latter frightened her more than the former. But she was not able to deal with issues related to her abusive husband and her angry feelings of victimization in the marriage.

The night before her discharge she began to discuss these feel-

ings, as they had suddenly risen to the surface during a group meeting. In this meeting a male patient had boasted that he never struck his wife except when he was drunk, and then he "only slapped her around a few times, not enough to send her to the hospital or such—nothing like that." When my patient heard this, she got up in a rage and ran out of the group. Several hours later, during our one-on-one, she was finally able to discuss the episode. She berated herself for being "gutless" and not being able to say something right then. She paced and questioned whether she really was ready to go home and said that maybe she wasn't as strong as she thought.

We continued exploring her feelings of childhood helplessness. She talked until her rage was spent, but did not seem to reach closure in her thoughts or feelings. She was discharged the next morning before I came to work for my evening shift. However, in my mailbox, I found a powerful note in which, among other things, she simply wrote, "I was able to confront that male patient in group today. . . . I guess I was ready for discharge after all. Thanks." It was now my turn to become a little emotional as my eyes filled with tears and I whispered, "You're welcome, you'll never know how welcome."

your **INTERNET**
connection

**SafetyNet: Domestic Violence Information
and Resources**
http://www.cybergrrl.com/dv.html

Abuse Survivor's Resources
http://www.tezcat.com/~tina/psych.html

Chapter Review Questions

1. Match each term in Column A with the correct definition in Column B.

Column A

___ Attributions

___ Sexual assault

___ Multigenerational transmission

___ Myth about abuse

___ Paternalistic model of health care

___ Psychological abuse

___ The force continuum

___ Wife abuse

___ Just world view

___ Primary prevention

Column B

A. Family violence is often perpetuated from grandparents, to parents, to children.

B. Others generally get what they deserve in life.

C. Advice and sympathy are given rather than respect for a patient's competence and experience.

D. Reasoning processes people use to explain why certain events happen.

E. An intervention that stops an action before it occurs.

F. A view of sexual behavior that ranges from free consent to violent rape.

G. The victim can learn to stop doing things that provoke the violence.

H. All forms of violence toward a female partner in an ongoing intimate relationship.

I. Forced act of sexual contact with another person without consent.

J. Instilling fear or isolating victim from family, friends, school, or work.

2. Identify whether the following statements are true (T) or false (F).

A. ___ Many nurses have a negative response to survivors of violence.

B. ___ Children who only witness family violence are usually safe from its effects.

C. ___ Family violence is most prevalent among the lower class.

D. ___ Being pregnant protects a woman from battering.

E. ___ Abusive people and their victims often excuse the abuse by blaming alcohol, stress, or drugs.

3. Provide short answers for the following questions.

A. Briefly describe the four characteristics of violent families.

B. Compare the paternalistic model with the empowerment model used by nurses to help battered women.

C. Each culture and society has a different attitude toward and tolerance of violence. Compare America with another country in this regard.

References

1. Bell CC, Jenkins EJ, Kpo W, Rhodes H: Response of emergency rooms to victims of interpersonal violence, *Hosp Community Psychiatry* 45:142, 1994.
2. Boutcher F, Gallop R: Psychiatric nurses' attitudes toward sexuality, sexual assault/rape, and incest, *Arch Psychiatr Nurs* 10:184, 1996.
3. Bremner JD, Krystal JH, Charney DS, Southwick SM: Neural mechanisms in dissociative amnesia for childhood abuse: relevance to the current controversy surrounding the "false memory syndrome," *Am J Psychiatry* 153:71, 1996.
4. Campbell JC: A test of two explanatory models of women's responses to battering, *Nurs Res* 38:18, 1989.
5. Campbell JC: Ways of teaching, learning, and knowing about violence against women, *Nurs Health Care* 13:464, 1992.
6. Campbell JC, Humphreys JC: *Nursing care of survivors of family violence,* St Louis, 1993, Mosby.
7. Campbell JC, Pliska M, Taylor W, Sheridan D: Battered women's experiences in the emergency department, *J Emerg Nurs* 20:280, 1994.
8. Damrosch S et al: Nurses' attributions about rape victims, *Res Nurs Health* 10:245, 1987.
9. Dobash RE, Dobash RP: Research as social action: the struggle for battered women. In Yllo K, Bograd M, editors: *Feminist perspectives on wife abuse,* Newbury Park, Calif, 1988, Sage.
10. Farrell ML: Healing: A qualitative study of women recovering from abusive relationships with men, *Perspect Psychiatr Care* 32:23, 1996.

11. Farrell M: The sense of relationship in women who have encountered abuse, *J Am Psychiatr Nurses Assoc* 2:46, 1996.
12. Feinauer L: Comparison of long-term effects on child abuse by type of abuse and by relationship of the offender to the victim, *Am J Fam Ther* 17:48, 1989.
13. Finkelhor D, Pillemer K: The prevalence of elder abuse: a random sample survey, *Gerontol Soc Am* 28:51, 1988.
14. Fishwick N: Getting to the heart of the matter: nursing assessment and intervention with battered women in psychiatric mental health settings, *J Am Psychiatr Nurses Assoc* 1:48, 1995.
15. Gallop R, McKeever P, Toner B, Lancee W, Lueck M: The impact of childhood sexual abuse on the psychological well-being and practice of nurses, *Arch Psychiatr Nurs* 9:137, 1995.
16. Gilligan C: *In a different voice,* Cambridge, Mass, 1982, Harvard University Press.
17. Glod C: Long-term consequences of childhood physical and sexual abuse, *Arch Psychiatr Nurs* 7:163, 1993.
18. Goldstein MZ: Maltreatment of elderly persons, *Psychiatr Serv* 46:1219, 1995.
19. Gondolf EW: The effect of batterer counseling on shelter outcome, *J Interpersonal Violence* 3:275, 1988.
20. Hart B: Beyond the "duty to warn": a therapist's "duty to protect" battered women and children. In Yllo K, Bograd M, editors: *Feminist perspectives on wife abuse,* Newbury Park, Calif, 1988, Sage.
21. Hedin BA: A case study of oppressed group behavior in nurses, *Image* 18:53, 1986.
22. Henderson AD, Ericksen JR: Enhancing nurses' effectiveness with abused women: awareness, reframing, support, education, *J Psychosoc Nurs* 32:11, 1994.
23. Hotaling GT, Sugerman D: An analysis of risk markers in husband to wife violence: the current state of knowledge, *Violence Vict* 1:101, 1986.
24. Janssen E: Understanding the rapist's mind, *Perspect Psychiatr Care* 31:9, 1995.
25. Johnson L, Cheffer ND: Child sexual abuse: a case of intrafamilial abuse, *J Am Psychiatr Nurses Assoc* 2:108, 1996.
26. King MC, Ryan J: Abused women: dispelling myths and encouraging interventions, *Nurse Pract* 14:47, 1989.
27. Kurz D: Emergency department responses to battered women: resistance to medicalization, *Soc Probl* 34:501, 1987.
28. Landenburger K: A process of entrapment in and recovery from an abusive relationship, *Issues Ment Health Nurs* 10:209, 1989.
29. Ledray LE, Arndt S: Examining the sexual assault victim: a new model for nursing care, *J Psychosoc Nurs* 32:7, 1994.
30. Lerner JM, Simmons CH: Observer's reaction to the "innocent victim," *J Pers Soc Psychol* 4:203, 1966.
31. Lewin L: Child abuse: ethical and legal concerns, *J Psychosoc Nurs* 32:16, 1994.
32. Limandri BJ, Tilden VP: Nurses' reasoning in the assessment of family violence, *Image J Nurs Sch* 28:247, 1996.
33. Mackey T et al: Factors associated with long-term depressive symptoms of sexual assault victims, *Arch Psychiatr Nurs* 6:10, 1992.
34. Morris PA, Bihan SM: The prevalence of children with a history of sexual abuse hospitalized in the psychiatric setting, *J Child Psychiatr Nurs* 4:49, 1991.
35. Parker B et al: Physical and emotional abuse in pregnancy: a comparison of adult and teenaged women, *Nurs Res* 42:173, 1993.
36. Parker B, McFarlane J, Soeken K: Abuse during pregnancy: effects on maternal complications and birth weight in adult and teenage women, *Obstet Gynecol* 84:323, 1994.
37. Rhea MH, Chafey KH, Dohner VA, Terragno R: The silent victims of domestic violence: who will speak?, *J Child Adolesc Psychiatr Nurs* 9:7, 1996.
38. Ryan W: *Blaming the victim,* New York, 1976, Vintage.
39. Schur EM: *The politics of deviance: stigma contests and the uses of power,* Englewood Cliffs, NJ, 1986, Prentice Hall.
40. Stark E, Flitcraft A: Violence among intimates: an epidemiological review. In Van Hasselt VB et al, editors: *Handbook of family violence,* New York, 1988, Plenum.
41. Tilden VP, Schmidt TA, Limandri BJ, Chiodo GT, Garland MJ, Loveless PA: Factors that influence clinicians' assessment and management of family violence, *Am J Public Health* 84:628, 1994.
42. Ulrich YC: Women's reasons for leaving abusive spouses, *Health Care Women Int* 12:465, 1991.
43. Walsh D, Liddy R: *Surviving sexual abuse,* Dublin, 1989, Attic Press.
44. Weingourt R: Connection and disconnection in abuse relationships, *Perspect Psychiatr Care* 32:15, 1996.
45. Williams-Burgess C, Vines SW, Ditulio MB: The parent-baby venture program: prevention of child abuse, *J Child Adolesc Psychiatr Nurs* 8:15, 1995.

Annotated Suggested Readings

*Campbell J, Harris M, Lee R: Violence research: an overview, *Image* 9:105, 1995.

Overview of pertinent research studies on family violence and how nurses can participate in prevention approaches with policy recommendations for nursing organizations.

*Campbell J, Parker B: Clinical nursing research on battered women and their children: a review. In Hinshaw A, Shaver J, and Feetham S, eds: *Handbook on clinical nursing research,* Newbury Park, 1996, Sage.

Summarizes nursing research studies on abused women and their children. An excellent starting point for a research project.

Goldstein M: Maltreatment of elderly persons, *Psychiatr Serv* 46:1219, 1995.

Provides a historical overview of the development of legislation and other efforts to address concerns about elder abuse in the United States.

*Hattendorf J, Tollerud T: Domestic violence: counseling strategies that minimize the impact of secondary victimization, *Perspect Psychiatr Care* 33:14, 1997.

Contrasts the usefulness of several models of psychotherapy with abused women. Recommended for the advanced practice nurse.

*Johnson L, Cheffer N: Child sexual abuse: a case of intrafamilial abuse, *J Am Psychiatr Nurses Assoc* 2:108, 1996.

Presents a historic perspective of child abuse, including the existing literature, and a case study with a description of the treatment plan using the nursing process.

Kaplan S, ed: Family violence: a clinical and legal guide, Washington, DC, 1996, American Psychiatric Press.

Clearly written and excellent reference for legal and clinical issues related to family violence.

*Lynch S: Elder abuse, *Am J Nurs* 1997:27, 1997.

Concisely informs nurses on what to look for, how to intervene, and available resources for dealing with elder abuse.

*Nursing reference.

Rhea M et al: The silent victims of domestic violence—Who will speak? *J Child Adolesc Psych Nurs* 9:7, 1996.
Asserts that all mental health and school counseling interviews must incorporate standard questions about family violence because children who witness domestic violence are also victims but are often overlooked and thus do not receive adequate services.

*Shea C, Mahoney M, Lacey J: Breaking through the barriers to domestic violence intervention, *Am J Nurs* 1997:26, 1997.
Helps nurses recognize and overcome the obstacles that prevent them from helping patients who have been injured by their intimates. Highly recommended.

*Nursing reference.

*Williams-Burgess C, Vines S, Ditulio M: The parent-baby venture program: prevention of child abuse, *J Child Adolesc Psych Nurs* 8:15, 1995.
Describes an innovative, community-based program to support high-risk adolescents during the early postpartum period that severely challenges their ability to successfully achieve the maternal role.

Psychological Care of the Patient with HIV/AIDS

Paula C. LaSalle and Arthur J. LaSalle

© 1998 M.C. Escher/Cordon Art, Baarn, Holland.

While we were fearing it, it came, But came with less of fear Because that fearing it so long
Had almost made it fair. There is a fitting—dismay; A fitting—a despair.
'Tis harder knowing it is due Than knowing it is here. The trying on the utmost,
The morning it is new, Is terribler than wearing it A whole existence through.

Emily Dickinson "WHILE WE WERE FEARING IT, IT CAME"

LEARNING OBJECTIVES

After studying this chapter the student should be able to:

▼ Describe the characteristics of HIV disease
▼ Identify behaviors associated with HIV disease
▼ Discuss multidisciplinary planning and the implementation of nursing interventions related to HIV disease
▼ Evaluate nursing care related to HIV disease

TOPICAL OUTLINE

Characteristics of HIV
Assessing the Patient with HIV Disease
  Psychosocial Behaviors
  Behaviors Related to Depression
  Behaviors Related to Dementia
Planning and Implementing Care
  Service Delivery
  Medications and Treatment Issues
  Interventions Related to Risk Reduction
  Interventions Related to Changing Levels of Functioning
  Interventions Related to Changes in Body Image
  Interventions Related to AIDS Dementia Complex
  Interventions Related to Preparation for Death
  Interventions Related to Significant Others
  Response of the Nurse to the Person with HIV Disease
Evaluating Care of the Patient with HIV Disease

The term *HIV disease* describes all of the disorders resulting from infection with the human immunodeficiency virus. It includes acquired immunodeficiency syndrome (AIDS) and its associated opportunistic infections. It involves the physical, psychological, emotional, and social aspects of the patient. The psychosocial aspects of this disease are varied and complex and relate directly to the patient's health care. Knowledgeable and compassionate nurses have an opportunity to contribute greatly to the patient's quality of life.

HIV disease has become a leading killer of young adults in the United States. What started as a disease predominantly affecting homosexual men has now spread to other populations, including heterosexual men and women, intravenous drug users, children, and hemophiliacs (Fig. 40-1). The HIV virus is transmitted through direct exposure to infected blood, blood derivatives, and other body fluids. It is transmitted through various sexual behaviors with infected people, use of HIV-contaminated intravenous needles, and transfusion of infected blood or blood derivatives, and from infected mother to fetus.

As of June 1996, the Centers for Disease Control estimated that 17 million people in the world have HIV disease. In the United States there are an estimated 650,000-900,000 HIV-positive people. Exact numbers of people who are HIV positive are not available because only 27 states report HIV-positive status. However, all states report the diagnosis of AIDS. The number of reported people with AIDS is 548,102 (462,152 are men, 78,654 are women, and 7296 are children under age 13). Other trends in the data indicate that:

▼ Heterosexual transmission has increased.

▼ Homosexual transmission has decreased.

▼ 343,000 (1 in 250) people with AIDS have died since the disease was first reported in the United States in 1981.

▼ AIDS was the eighth leading cause of death in the United States for all ages in 1995.

▼ AIDS was the leading cause of death for all Americans ages 25-44 in 1995.

In the period 1992-1995, the numbers of people diagnosed with AIDS stabilized among whites and increased among blacks and Hispanics. There has also been a stabilization of the number of new HIV cases among men. Despite an increase in the number of women infected with HIV through sexual transmission, there has been a gradual decrease among children. This demonstrates the effectiveness of prenatal testing and treatment of HIV-positive pregnant women with antivirals. Thus the chances of a baby born to an HIV-positive mother also being HIV positive have been reduced from 30% to 8%.

CHARACTERISTICS OF HIV

The Centers for Disease Control and Prevention (CDC)[4] defines HIV as a retrovirus that has as its primary target the CD4+ T-lymphocyte because of the affinity of the virus for the CD4 surface marker.

> The CD4+ T-lymphocyte coordinates a number of important immunologic functions and a loss of these functions results in progressive impairment of the immune response. Studies have documented a wide spectrum of disease manifestations, ranging from asymptomatic infection to life-threatening conditions characterized by severe immunodeficiency, serious opportunistic infections, and cancers.[3]

Opportunistic infections such as toxoplasmosis and *Pneumocystis carinii* pneumonia are common. Infections can develop in the central nervous system and cause dementia. In other cases, depression related to the diagnosis of HIV may erode immunological functioning and decrease the patient's motivation to engage in health-promoting behaviors.[17]

> **?** *Have you known someone with HIV disease? What were your feelings about that person? Did you worry about becoming infected? Have your feelings changed since you began your nursing program?*

ASSESSING THE PATIENT WITH HIV DISEASE

Table 40-1 lists the major losses of people who have HIV disease.[1] Because their lives are affected in so many ways, assessment of each of these areas is an important aspect of nursing care planning. For example, a person's financial, transportation, and housing needs may directly relate to one's ability to participate in treatment.

HIV disease presents the patient and loved ones with a series of stressors, sometimes occurring simultaneously, sometimes sequentially. Nurses should pay special attention to the psychosocial needs of patients with HIV because these stressors may directly affect the patient's health and willingness and ability to fully use the health-care system.

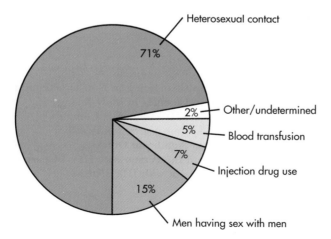

Fig. 40-1 Proportion of world AIDS cases attributable to various HIV transmission routes.

Heterosexual contact — 71%
Other/undetermined — 2%
Blood transfusion — 5%
Injection drug use — 7%
Men having sex with men — 15%

Psychosocial Behaviors

A number of social conflicts, such as fear of exposure of diagnosis and being a member of a stigmatized group, are commonly experienced by people who have HIV disease. Patients often need the nurse's support and assistance in deciding whom to tell about their status, as well as when and how. Physical changes such as Kaposi's sarcoma, wasting, or rashes may force the patient to reveal the illness before feeling prepared to do so.

Conflict regarding sexual activity may leave the person socially isolated and alone. This is especially true for people who used sex to establish interpersonal contacts. Even people in stable relationships may find their sexual relationship dramatically changed, affecting feelings of closeness and the ability to give and receive love, comfort, and affection.

Employment and insurance issues are sources of stress because patients are often rejected and stigmatized. Although employers are not legally able to fire someone because of HIV, now a legally protected disability, subtle means may be used to force the person with AIDS to leave the work setting. Reallocation of work, reassignment, poor evaluation, or redefinition of a job may result in a person with AIDS being terminated by an employer. Others have lost positions because of being physically unable to work.

Loss of a job is often associated with loss of health insurance. This is especially problematic for homosexuals because they are unable to receive health-care coverage under their partners' health benefits in most states.

Social support limitations are common especially in a mobile society in which friends and family are scattered around the world. People who have chosen to keep their lifestyle secret often move away from their family of origin and may or may not have a group in whom they confide. For many people, work colleagues make up a major portion of their social support system. When the job is lost, the isolation increases. Resources that can be used to provide social support include community agencies that offer shopping, Meals on Wheels, and housekeeping services. Some clergy and churches have become involved in transportation or other services for people with AIDS. The homosexual community has also organized support services in many areas.

Nurses can help patients with psychosocial issues if a trusting, confidential relationship is established. At times the boundaries of confidentiality are not clear (see Critical Thinking about Contemporary Issues).

STIGMA. Some of the psychosocial problems associated with HIV disease are a result of stigma. HIV stigma is closely connected to the risk behaviors that lead to infec-

---

TABLE **40-1** *Losses Associated with HIV Infection*

▼ *Employment:* Loss due to infection status, disability, stigma, or erratic work attendance related to illness or treatment requirements

▼ *Family:* Fear, stigma, inability to cope, ignorance

▼ *Friends:* Fear, stigma, inability to cope, ignorance, friends dying of AIDS

▼ *Health care:* Inability to afford care or to obtain own or partner's insurance benefits

▼ *Financial:* Cost of health care, loss of employment, cost of social resources and services, housing, food, and necessities

▼ *Social supports:* Fear, stigma, inability to cope, ignorance, easily drained due to magnitude of need

▼ *Self-esteem/pride:* Self-blame for personal infection and the epidemic in general, loss of autonomy, disfigurement, stigma, depression

▼ *Physical intimacy/sexual contact:* Irrational fears of casual transmission, stigma, shame/blame

▼ *Future goals:* Facing a life-threatening, chronic, painful, expensive illness

▼ *Physical functioning and autonomy:* Disease progression, including disability, depression, dementia, dependency, and decreased sensory, cardiac, respiratory, musculoskeletal, reproductive, cognitive, and GI functioning

▼ *Lifestyle changes:* Need to change sexual practices, improve nutrition, avoid smoking, alcohol, and other drugs, and give up pets (which may carry pathogens)

Modified from Kalichman SC: *Understanding AIDS: a guide for mental health professionals,* Washington DC, 1995, American Psychological Association.

CRITICAL THINKING *about* Contemporary Issues

Should a Person Be Obligated to Reveal HIV-Positive Status?

Harding and colleagues[9] cite conflicting opinions in the literature regarding the conditions under which confidentiality about HIV-positive status may be breached. The conflict focuses mainly on the duty to warn others who may be in danger of being infected by the patient. For example, a man who is HIV positive informs the nurse that he will not share the information with his wife and he intends to continue having sexual relations with her. The patient claims that he will protect his wife from infection but will not be specific about the method he plans to use. The nurse is caught between maintaining a confidential relationship with the patient and protecting a third party, while being unsure of the degree of danger to the wife.

A similar conflict exists regarding the responsibility of health-care workers who know that they are HIV positive to inform their patients, supervisors, and co-workers. Since several patients were believed to have been infected by a Florida dentist, there has been political pressure to require reporting. Health-care workers fear that revealing HIV disease will result in job loss. They cite evidence that HIV is not transmitted in health-care situations as long as universal precautions are observed.

Because serious consequences exist for the patient in his or her personal relationships and continued employment, there are no easy answers to this question. The nurse must consider the facts related to each situation and help the patient to consider all of the alternatives, including the likely consequences.

tion. The illness was first identified in homosexual men, an already stigmatized group. Later, it became prevalent in intravenous drug users, another stigmatized population. Because of these risk behaviors, assumptions are often made about the lifestyles of people with HIV disease. Some believe these behaviors are immoral and that the illness is a punishment for them. Stigma may inhibit people from seeking HIV testing. It also fosters reluctance to inform others of their diagnosis and to adopt risk-reduction behaviors. It is reflected in the difficulty people with HIV disease face in keeping their jobs, getting insurance, finding housing, and acquiring health care.

HIV was once thought to affect men almost exclusively, but women have shown an alarming increase in incidence. Women who live in poverty and abuse drugs are disproportionately affected by HIV.[11] These women must be more concerned with everyday survival than with a disease that may not manifest itself for many years. Additionally, indigent women who abuse drugs are often unable to negotiate safer sex practices because they are more likely to turn to prostitution. One study[19] showed that women living with HIV perceived themselves to be subjected to intense social stigma, limiting their ability to access services and support for their illness.

Interventions with HIV-positive women who continue to engage in risky sexual behaviors include education about the importance of avoiding reinfection with HIV and exposure to sexually transmitted disease, and the role of alcohol, cocaine, and other drugs in increasing the likelihood of risky sexual behaviors.[15] Impoverished populations deal on a daily basis with factors that may damage their social support systems. More research is needed about the social support network of homeless and impoverished women related to personal and behavioral variables, particularly illegal drug use, risky sexual activity, and mental health status.[21]

Stigma is very difficult to overcome, but the best way to confront it is through health education. Nurses can also model nonstigmatizing attitudes by providing sensitive and competent care to people with HIV disease. Field[7] believes that stigma contributes to the development of "AIDS phobia," a condition in which people who are not infected fear acquiring HIV and worry about it constantly. Some even become convinced they have AIDS to the extent of developing a somatoform disorder or a somatic delusion.

> **?** *Identify a situation in which you noticed stigmatizing behavior toward homosexuals, drug users, and people with HIV disease. What did you do (or could you have done) to change this behavior?*

CRISIS POINTS. Several potential crisis points occur during the course of HIV disease. The diagnosis of HIV seropositivity may be the first crisis. However, the patient may already have had a crisis based on anticipation of the poten-

TABLE **40-2** *HIV and Overlapping Symptoms of Depression and Anxiety*

HIV Symptom	Depression/Anxiety Symptom
Fatigue	Fatigue, lethargy
Muscle aches	Muscle aches, pains
Night sweats	Insomnia, increased sweating
Weight loss	Appetite and weight changes
Diarrhea	GI distress
Neurological symptoms/dementia	Neurological symptoms: headaches, poor concentration and memory, dizziness
Hopelessness, helplessness, poor self-image	Hopelessness, helplessness, poor self-image
Social isolation, stigma	Isolation, stigma
Increased suicide risk	Increased suicide risk

tial diagnosis. With the initial diagnosis the person often feels intense anxiety, fear, anger, and guilt and may act impulsively. High levels of anxiety and depression may continue for 2 to 3 months and may be exhibited in agitation, risky sexual behavior, crying, and suicidal ideation and attempts. In fact, symptoms of depression and anxiety may overlap with HIV symptoms, complicating diagnostic and treatment efforts (Table 40-2).

The patient should not be left alone or expected to make decisions immediately after learning the diagnosis. Safety precautions and taking the necessary time to allow the person to process the initial reaction are critical. The nurse should share information regarding HIV disease when the patient requests it. Helping the patient to recognize and verbalize beliefs regarding HIV may be helpful.

McCain and Gramling[16] refer to this phase of coping with HIV disease as living with dying. The person is learning to live with the knowledge of having a terminal illness. It is essential to provide structure during this time by implementing crisis intervention techniques (see Chapter 13). Medications may be indicated, but safety must be considered. Medications are not a means of suppressing the natural reactions to crisis but enable the person to function, sleep, and cope during the crisis. The following clinical example highlights some of the issues around notification of the HIV diagnosis.

Clinical Example Mr. and Ms. G are a prominent couple in the community. Mr. G was hospitalized for a severe case of herpes zoster (shingles). With his informed consent he was tested for HIV and was found to be positive. Mr. G is fearful of his wife's reaction to his diagnosis. They have been married for 24 years. He had one incident of homosexual marital infidelity 3 years ago while on a business trip. He is angry over the "unfairness" of how one experience will alter not only his health but also his relationship with his wife. He is also worried that his children will reject him and his employer will fire him. Another concern is that his high public profile will lead to negative publicity for him, his family, and the community organizations in which he has been active.

Selected Nursing Diagnoses:

▼ Anxiety related to diagnosis of AIDS, as evidenced by verbalized concerns about impact of the diagnosis on relationships

▼ Altered family processes related to changed role of husband and father, as evidenced by concern over reactions of wife and children

▼ Altered role performance related to change in health status, as evidenced by concern that job and community activities will be affected

There may be a quiet phase between the initial diagnosis and the first opportunistic infection. During this transition period the patient moves into the phase of coping identified by McCain and Gramling[16] as fighting the sickness. There is a focus on learning about HIV disease and often the adoption of a healthier lifestyle, including attention to diet, exercise, and adequate rest. Attempts to cope may include denial of the illness. However, when the first infection occurs, a crisis that is more intense than the first may be precipitated. Denial is no longer effective. The treatment phase may be characterized by alienation, depression, and discouragement. Patients may fear or experience disfigurement, pain, and loss of health. The process of treatment with medical side effects, testing, and awaiting results may cause self-absorption, frustration, and irritability. Patients with HIV may experience a loss of control, especially in dealing with the medical system. They may become fearful, demanding, and dependent on health-care providers. As treatment continues, they may be frightened to be away from the close supervision of the hospital staff or health-care provider. They may become hypervigilant and seek reassurance that they will know when to ask for help.

Finally the person enters the phase of coping called getting worn-out.[16] During this phase of preparation for death, there is a gradual decline and deterioration of the person's functional ability. Recurrence and relapse are accompanied by feelings of depression, dependency, isolation, suicidal ideation, and fear of abandonment. There is usually ambivalence, dependence, and withdrawal from the world, combined with increased self-absorption. Patients often review their lives. They may finalize their wishes related to their death and postmortem arrangements. Support and physical assistance must be given because important decisions regarding the last phases of life are being made and important goodbyes are shared.

The person who is living with HIV disease often experiences conflict about the implications of the illness. These are summarized in Fig. 40-2. Concerns related to the person's lifestyle are illustrated in the next clinical example.

Clinical Example Mr. J was diagnosed as HIV positive 4 years ago and has been asymptomatic. On his forty-fifth

Fig. 40-2 **Cycle of reactions to HIV disease.** (Modified from Kalichman SC: *Understanding AIDS: a guide for mental health professionals,* Washington, DC, 1995, American Psychological Association.)

birthday he noticed a Kaposi's sarcoma spot on his cheek and is now in a state of panic. He has not told anyone about his discovery. His parents are scheduled to arrive on the next day to celebrate his birthday. They are not aware that he is HIV positive or that he is homosexual. He knows his mother will question him about the spot. His father is vehemently antihomosexual, consistent with his religious beliefs. Mr. J is anxious about how his father would accept this information. However, Mr. J's lover is pressuring him to tell his parents so that their relationship can be open.

Selected Nursing Diagnoses:

▼ Anxiety related to parental response to sexual preference, as evidenced by secrecy about his homosexuality

▼ Body image disturbance related to discovery of facial lesion, as evidenced by not telling anyone

▼ Situational low self-esteem related to guilt about sexual preference, as evidenced by hiding relationship with lover

Behaviors Related to Depression

It has been well documented that the immune system is compromised in people with high levels of stress and with depression. In people with HIV, depression can confuse diagnostic and treatment issues of both illnesses because of the overlap between the vegetative symptoms of HIV and the neuropsychologic symptoms of depression. Depression is thought to be one of the most common psychiatric disorders in HIV-infected people, and is a potentially dangerous comorbid condition because it may hasten the course of HIV disease. It has been shown that there is a dramatic, sustained rise in depressive symptoms as AIDS develops, beginning as early as 18 months before clinical AIDS is diagnosed,[14] and that approximately 40% of hospitalized patients with HIV have clinical depression.[17]

Patients with HIV disease who are depressed experience the emotional pain and suffering common to depression, including depressed mood and decreased motivation, lowered self-esteem, guilt, increased isolation, lowered energy level, sleep disturbance, change in appetite, somatic complaints, increased sense of hopelessness, increased risk for suicide, and increased social stigma. The nurse must be careful not to normalize depression in HIV-infected people, thus depriving them of treatment that could enhance their well-being and quality of life and increase their longevity. The critical components of a successful treatment program for HIV-infected people with depression include the following[20]:

▼ *Psychotherapy:* Treatment outcome studies identify stress reduction, psychoeducation, and psychosocial support as the essential components of HIV-related psychotherapy.

▼ *Psychopharmacology:* In general, standard antidepressants are effective and usually well tolerated. HIV-positive patients may be better able to tolerate the tricyclic-induced side effects and less able to tolerate the selective serotonin reuptake inhibitor–induced sexual side effects than HIV-negative patients.[27] As with any antidepressant selection, attention to side effect profiles should be considered for individual patients. In depressed patients with HIV, low doses of the psychostimulant methylphenidate have been reported to improve the patient's well-being, reduce suicidal ideation, improve interaction with peers, and diminish vegetative symptoms. Most studies of the psychopharmacologic treatment of psychiatric symptoms in HIV-positive people were done on men because HIV-positive women have been extremely difficult to enroll and retain in placebo-controlled clinical trials.

▼ *Testosterone:* In HIV-positive patients with signs of hypogonadism, testosterone was found to improve mood and energy level.[23]

▼ *Electroconvulsive therapy (ECT):* In severe HIV-related depression, ECT has been shown to be effective and should be considered a therapeutic option.

Behaviors Related to Dementia

A major complication of HIV disease is AIDS dementia complex (ADC), a subcortical encephalopathy characterized by progressive dementia. Boccellari and Dilley[2] note that it is difficult to determine the incidence of ADC because of a lack of clear guidelines. They cite estimates ranging from 12.8% to 67% of patients with AIDS.

Although some opportunistic infections may involve the brain, ADC is believed to result primarily from direct infection with HIV.[26] The virus is believed to be transported to brain tissue by infected monocytes that cross the blood-brain barrier or by infected endothelial cells in the brain

T ABLE **40-3** *HIV Symptoms Related to Brain Structures and Functions*

BRAIN STRUCTURE	CLINICAL SYMPTOMS
Frontal lobes	Apathy, trouble concentrating and planning, loss of organizational skills, depression
Basal ganglia	Impaired movement, tremor
Limbic system	Emotional lability, memory loss, language impairment
Brain stem	Disturbances of gait, vision, and eye movement
Demyelination	Impaired fine motor skills, delayed information processing, impaired response time, incontinence

capillaries. Once the virus is in brain cells, several disruptions are believed to occur (Table 40-3).

Because ADC and depression may both present with apathy and psychomotor retardation, the nurse needs to be able to distinguish between them. Unlike demented people, depressed people typically appear sadder and express feeling hopeless and worthless. Demented people have difficulty drawing, whereas the drawing ability of depressed people is relatively unaffected. Nurses can ask patients to draw simple figures such as squares or triangles to assess whether their behavioral changes are caused by depression or dementia. Depressed people can also generate a list of words, such as a list starting with the same letter, without much difficulty. Demented people are unable to produce more than a few words. Cognitive responses are described in more detail in Chapter 23.

? *Do you believe that a person who is HIV positive should engage in sexual activity? Can any sexual activity with an HIV-positive person be safe? What types of sexual expression would you recommend? Do you feel comfortable discussing this with your patients?*

PLANNING AND IMPLEMENTING CARE

HIV disease and related opportunistic infections involving pathogens such as *Pneumocystis carinii* and *Cryptococcus,* as well as Kaposi's sarcoma, affect multiple body systems. A complete nursing assessment will result in nursing diagnoses related to all of the identified behaviors. Nursing diagnoses related to physiological disruptions are discussed in medical-surgical nursing textbooks. Box 40-1 lists NANDA nursing diagnoses that are particularly associated with the psychosocial aspects of HIV disease.

The complexity of the biopsychosocial needs of the person with HIV disease demands a team approach to health-care planning and implementation that includes the pa-

Box **40-1** *NANDA Diagnoses Related to Psychosocial Aspects of HIV Disease*

Adjustment, impaired
Anxiety
Body image disturbance
Caregiver role strain, risk for
Communication, impaired verbal
Defensive coping
Denial, ineffective
Family processes, altered
Fear
Grieving, anticipatory
Grieving, dysfunctional
Health maintenance, altered
Hopelessness
Individual coping, ineffective
Management of therapeutic regimen (individual), ineffective
Parental role conflict
Parenting, risk for altered
Powerlessness
Role performance, altered
Self-esteem, situational low
Sexual dysfunction
Sexuality patterns, altered
Social interaction, impaired
Social isolation
Spiritual distress
Thought processes, altered

From North American Nursing Diagnosis Association: *NANDA nursing diagnoses: definitions and classifications 1997-1998,* Philadelphia, 1997, The Association.

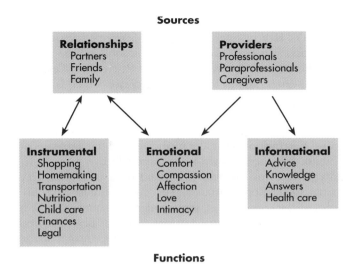

Fig. 40-3   Sources and functions of support needed by the person with HIV.

tient's entire health-care and social support system (Fig. 40-3). The physician or advanced practice registered nurse prescribes the course of medical treatment, often involving prophylactic medication or pharmacotherapy for identified physiological and psychological disorders. Occupational or physical therapy may be needed to help the patient to adjust to changing neuromuscular and cognitive functioning. Social workers help the patient and significant others to find and contact community resources. Nursing care centers around providing support and counseling while helping the patient to conserve energy and set priorities for activities. Nurses are also responsible for being sure that the patient is informed about the disease and options related to intervention.

Nurses in AIDS care have opportunities to develop close relationships with patients and their significant others. The reaction to the HIV disease process is unique to each patient. A common counseling issue is concern about the course of disease and the length of survival. This is reflected by a commonly asked question when people with HIV disease meet: "How long have you known your diagnosis?" This is a way of determining how far along the other person is in dealing with HIV. Also, there is the underlying hope that the question will identify a long-term survivor, serving

as reassurance that a person with HIV disease can live a long and fruitful life.

Service Delivery

People with HIV disease are increasingly being treated in community-based health centers and at home. Efforts at cost containment for all health-care services have resulted in more outpatient care. Community mental health centers have a wide variety of patients. Nurses must include treatment of HIV disease and the associated opportunistic infections in their patient case load and use their influence, education, and persuasion to obtain patient and family cooperation. With the increased availability of home health care, the nurse may be able to visit patients in their homes. The nurse must be skilled in dealing with family interactions and coordinating treatment with other home health-care providers.

Although many communities are attempting to organize the necessary services for people with HIV disease, services and funds are not coordinated and are often difficult to find. The person who is struggling with the HIV diagnosis has the additional burden of locating needed help. Case management by the nurse, social worker, or other professional can help to locate available services. The case manager can help in identifying medical providers, dentists, therapists, housing, and the many other resources the person with HIV will need.

Medications and Treatment Issues

Although AIDS and AIDS-related conditions are major killers, life expectancy for people with AIDS from the time of diagnosis has doubled over the last 4 years with the development of new drugs and drug combinations. Until late 1995, all drugs available on the market for treating HIV infection were **nucleoside analogs**. These drugs inhibit replication of HIV by interfering with the enzyme reverse transcriptase, which is needed for replication of the virus's genetic material. **Protease inhibitors**, a new class of antiretroviral drugs, inhibit the enzyme protease, which is necessary for the virus to get into the body's cells in order to reproduce. Protease inhibitors have lowered HIV content in blood in some patients by up to 99%. The three-drug "cocktails" that include two older medicines and one protease inhibitor have been shown to be more effective than single-drug treatments because it is more difficult for the HIV virus to develop resistance. The new cocktails have improved the condition of some patients so much that they have been able to return to work. Additionally, new **viral load tests** have been developed to help gauge how much of the virus is actually in the body. This helps the treatment team determine how effective a particular drug is and when it may be necessary to change therapy.

As of 1996, there were 122 medicines and vaccines for AIDS and AIDS-related diseases in development, in addition to 42 medicines already approved and on the market. It is estimated that the cost of the three-drug "cocktail" is $10,000 to $16,000 per year per patient, but this is much less than the $100,000 per year per patient that it costs to treat a patient with AIDS in the hospital.[22] However, many people cannot afford these new treatments. Additionally, these treatments have side effects that are not tolerated by some people. In order to inhibit resistance to these treatments from developing, patients must adhere to strict schedules of drug administration as well as rigid food guidelines, often to the exclusion of other interests and pursuits. People who have qualified for disability are concerned that their benefits will be lost as they have extended but unpredictable periods of wellness, as new treatments for HIV change it from a disease progressing quickly to death to one with a more chronic, intermittent course. Even in the face of these difficulties, the advances in AIDS research have been remarkable in a short period of time, and new studies for more effective treatments, vaccines, and testing procedures are stimulating hope for the future of HIV-positive patients, their families, the health-care community, and society in general.[25]

Interventions Related to Risk Reduction

Currently, the most effective way of combating HIV disease is by preventing it through risk reduction. Because of their credibility with the general public, nurses are in a good position to provide prevention education. Nurses should familiarize themselves with the routes of transmission of HIV (Table 40-4) and the currently recommended ways of preventing infection. Patients can be encouraged to inform sexual partners of their illness and to practice safer sex. Intravenous drug users can be referred to treatment programs, discouraged from sharing needles, and taught how to disinfect used needles. Pregnant women who are HIV positive should be helped to find obstetrical care from a

TABLE **40-4** *Routes of HIV Transmission*

RISK BEHAVIOR	TRANSMISSION MECHANISM
Anal intercourse	Infected semen or blood enters the anal/rectal mucosa or penis through absorption or micro-openings.
Vaginal intercourse	Infected vaginal fluids, semen, or blood enter the vaginal or penile mucosa or through micro-openings.
Oral-genital contact	Infected semen or vaginal fluids enter bloodstream through micro-openings in oral cavity, or infected cells enter vagina or penis through micro-openings.
Perinatal transmission	Transplacental transfer of virus during gestation, transfer of virus or maternal blood during labor/delivery, breast-feeding.
Injection drug use	Use of needles and other injection equipment previously used by an infected person; virus or infected cells directly enter blood stream.
Blood transfusion—receiving blood products	Principal risk in United States occurred before 1984 blood-screening programs; blood or blood parts from an infected person enter bloodstream.

Modified from Kalichman SC: *Understanding AIDS: a guide for mental health professionals,* Washington DC, 1995, American Psychological Association.

provider who understands the implications of the disease for the mother and infant.

People who have serious and persistent mental illnesses are often vulnerable to infection with HIV. In one study of this population,[12] many patients traded sex for money, drugs, or a place to stay, were coerced to engage in unwanted sex, had casual sexual encounters, and engaged in sexual activity after using drugs or intoxicants. These are high-risk activities. Another study[5] of high-risk activities among the seriously mentally ill found the following:

▼ There was no relationship between diagnosis and high-risk activity.

▼ Heterosexual behavior was the most common high-risk activity.

▼ Younger patients did not have more sexual activity, although they did have more partners.

Nurses need to be aware of these findings so that they can provide relevant health education to patients. Interventions may include self-esteem enhancement, assertiveness training, education about sexuality and HIV prevention, and role playing of potentially risky social situations. Condoms should be readily available to patients in all treatment settings. Graham and Cates[8] describe an educational program to inform group home residents about HIV prevention. They conducted a series of three sessions using a videotape in each, followed by a discussion period. Patients in this study responded best to a same-sex presenter. Patients with psychotic episodes sometimes incorporated the educational material into their delusional thinking. Others who tended to somaticize began to report symptoms of HIV. It was important for group home staff to be well-informed about HIV disease before the training and be prepared to respond to questions and concerns afterward.

People infected with HIV are often asymptomatic up to 10 years. Testing for the presence of HIV antibodies is the only way of determining whether a person is infected with the virus. Inferences based on sex, race, socioeconomic status, habits of cleanliness, nutrition, and sexual and drug behavior are not valid. Nurses should treat all patients as potential sources of HIV infection and protect themselves by using universal precautions.

> **?** *Describe patient behaviors related to the psychiatric diagnoses of bipolar disorder and schizophrenia that might contribute to increased risk for HIV.*

Interventions Related to Changing Levels of Functioning

The unpredictability of the course of HIV disease is itself a stressor because people with the infection cannot prepare for disease events and often feel surprised by the onset of new symptoms. They cannot determine whether a common cold is the serious *Pneumocystis carinii* pneumonia that they have heard about or whether a new mole is actually Kaposi's sarcoma. With each opportunistic infection they need to redefine what they can reasonably expect from themselves regarding energy output and physical and mental abilities.

People with HIV disease have been living longer because of medical breakthroughs and greater knowledge of the disease. This means that a person may have multiple opportunistic infections over the years. People may wonder, "Is all this worth it?" during periods of fatigue and discouragement. They may consider suicide. At this time it is helpful for nurses to listen receptively to patients' feelings and not discourage them from talking because of nurses' own discomfort or fear. Information about suicide assessment and intervention is presented in Chapter 20. Nurses can remind patients that there is no need to go through this alone because others will be there to help. The respectful and careful use of physical touch may be a powerful intervention. People with HIV disease often express the feeling of being "lepers" and may isolate themselves at times. A touch on the hand or shoulder may convey the sense of being there for the patient.

> **?** *The partner of a person who is terminally ill with AIDS asks for your opinion about assisted suicide. How would you respond?*

SUPPORT GROUPS. Nurse-led support groups may provide the patient with a safe place to express feelings regarding HIV and the physical threats that are being experienced. The patient can give and receive information and learn more effective coping strategies. The group also serves as a social network for people who are gradually losing their sociocultural roles of worker and provider. Subjects such as living wills, new medications, suicide, responses of friends and family, and the future can be discussed. Group members grieve for themselves as well as their fellow members. Lifestyle and medical questions may be asked at this time. Education about exposing others to HIV and the dangers of reexposure to themselves is important. Safer sex techniques and the responsibility to inform past sexual or needle-sharing partners must be addressed.

Some people with HIV disease strive to learn to live for today, not allowing unnecessary worry about the future to rob them of a high quality of life. One woman, who was called Amazing Grace by other support group members, was repeatedly hospitalized for opportunistic infections. Between hospitalizations, however, she sought ways to be with her children to the limits of her physical abilities. Two months before she died she drove her children on a six-state touring vacation. One week before her death, with the help of her family, she took her children to the zoo.

ENCOURAGING PRODUCTIVE ACTIVITY. The course of HIV disease is characterized by periods of relative wellness, but inconsistent health may result in unstable employment. It is important for the nurse to help patients remain contributing members of society by offering outlets for their energy and skills. Such activities could include acting as a buddy for another person with HIV disease, joining political movements to promote legislation in which they believe, volunteering at a museum or library, and expanding talents in music, poetry, and other arts.

Interventions Related to Changes in Body Image

People with HIV disease often face the impairment of disfigurement. Some examples are:

▼ Kaposi's sarcoma, which may cause large, purple, bruise-like blotches on the face, hands, and legs
▼ "AIDS hair," which resembles the thinning, fine hair of people who have received chemotherapy
▼ Wasting, during which a person continuously loses weight and becomes skeletal in appearance

The nurse should offer opportunities for the patient and significant others to talk about feelings related to body changes. Encouraging the patient to consider himself or herself as a whole person with both strong, attractive components as well as less pleasing ones may be helpful in establishing perspective. Often, the visible changes caused by HIV disease are seen as evidence of approaching death. This idea must be discussed openly and accurate information about the cause and meaning of physical symptoms should be given.

Interventions Related to AIDS Dementia Complex

Nursing interventions for the person with HIV disease must address the limitations related to AIDS dementia complex (ADC) if the patient has behaviors related to a cognitive disorder. HIV cognitive impairment is common. About one third of patients with AIDS have at least mild cognitive impairment. Up to 25% of people with AIDS have frank dementia.[10] The nursing care of patients with cognitive problems is addressed in Chapter 23. Memory problems may be especially troubling to young patients who want to remain actively involved in life, including work. The nurse may suggest ways to improve memory such as writing notes and establishing set routines for activities. Many patients are well informed about HIV disease and may worry about cognitive changes. The nurse must provide an opportunity for expression of fears and give accurate feedback about cognitive functioning. Some may interpret normal forgetfulness as a sign of pathological deterioration. Significant others should also be provided with information about this aspect of the disease.

> **?** *What is your reaction to the following statement: Patients should not be informed about potential cognitive changes related to HIV disease; because these changes cannot be prevented, they would only worry unnecessarily.*

Interventions Related to Preparation for Death

SPIRITUAL CONCERNS. Awareness of impending death often leads patients with HIV to think about the meaning of life and their spiritual belief system. For some, this means seeking comfort from a religion with which they are already connected. Others may wish to establish a connection with a member of the clergy or a lay representative of a religion. Some patients may choose not to become involved with a particular religion but may want to discuss spiritual and philosophical beliefs. The nurse should assess the patient's spiritual needs and preferences, facilitating access to the selected manner of expression. Some patients appreciate the nurse sitting quietly while they think, providing relevant reading materials or reading, and discussing religious or philosophical writings. If the nurse is comfortable with praying with the patient, this may also be helpful. If the nurse is not comfortable, it

is best to be candid and perhaps suggest a few moments of silent meditation.

ADVANCE DIRECTIVES. Taking charge of the practical aspects of their lives helps people with HIV disease feel in control. For example, making decisions about medical power of attorney, living will, and a last will helps patients in taking control during the later stages of their lives. For single parents, one of the most difficult decisions is selecting a custodian for their surviving children, as illustrated in the following clinical example.

Clinical Example Ms. B is a 30-year-old divorced woman who is the mother of a 7-year-old boy. She was diagnosed as HIV positive 2 years ago but has had a rapid progression of opportunistic infections and is now in the acute phase of her illness. As part of trying to write her durable power of attorney, living will, and last will, she is trying to decide whom she will ask to care for her son. The child's father has had no contact with them, and Ms. B believes he is unfit and probably unwilling to assume responsibility for his child. Ms. B's parents are elderly and in frail health. Her older sister is married with four children. Her older brother is unmarried and travels a great deal for business. Ms. B's best friend, who is divorced and childless, has expressed a willingness to care for her son. Ms. B is depressed about leaving her son and highly anxious regarding the best situation for him.

Selected Nursing Diagnoses:

▼ Anxiety related to conflict over arranging for son's care, as evidenced by indecision over completing will

▼ Anticipatory grieving related to expected loss of the relationship with her son, as evidenced by depressed mood

Many people wish to make decisions regarding their funeral. Some write their own obituaries; others design or even make their own quilt panel for the National AIDS Quilt. Some people prepare videotapes and letters for their family members, to be presented after their death. It is important that the nurse support these efforts to maintain control, allowing the person to live and die in his or her own style. Even though these decisions and activities may be very difficult and emotional, the patient often feels a sense of relief and completion when these tasks are accomplished.

Interventions Related to Significant Others

Families, partners, and friends of people who have HIV disease need a great deal of support to enable them to meet the needs of the patient. One nursing study of people living with HIV disease and their families revealed higher levels of psychological distress than in a nonpatient normative sample but lower than in psychiatric patients.[18] The investigators recommended the following interventions to help patients and their families:

▼ Anxiety reduction

▼ Assistance with control and appropriate expression of anger

▼ Teaching calming techniques to be used during acute distress

▼ Sleep enhancement

▼ Cognitive restructuring to develop a more realistic world view

Another nursing study[6] focused on family members, partners, and friends of young men who had HIV disease and identified their needs. When they became aware of the diagnosis, they reported feeling shocked but also needing information. The other concern at this time was related to the patient's reluctance to inform others of the diagnosis, sometimes limiting the access of significant others to their own support systems. The nurse can help by discussing the anticipated response of others to the diagnosis and supporting the patient and significant others during and after disclosure.

Significant others described the emotional stress of feeling hopeful when the patient was asymptomatic and then hopeless when an opportunistic infection occurred. Nurses must provide support and relevant information about the patient's changing condition. Interpersonal relationships often changed as a result of the HIV disease. Positive changes were related to expressions of concern and offers of help from others. Some felt increased closeness in their relationships. Negative changes were more common. Some resulted from a family member's rejection of the patient upon learning of the diagnosis. Others were related to significant others' reluctance to tell others about the diagnosis, increasing their own stress. Nurses can be very helpful by inquiring about the status of relationships with family members and others and by exploring negative responses. Family meetings may facilitate the sharing of feelings and clarification of misconceptions.

Response of the Nurse to the Person with HIV Disease

As a progressive disease is discouraging to patients, it may also be discouraging to nurses.[24] The messages people receive when first diagnosed are extremely powerful and often set the stage for the course of the illness.[1] It is essential that nurses monitor their reactions and investment in patients. Professional nurses must allow themselves the necessary time and opportunities to grieve the multiple losses their patients experience and the death of patients they know well. Nurses may confront many challenges when working with patients with HIV.

FEAR OF CONTAGION. The nurse needs to know, understand, and use universal precautions. Careful planning during procedures and taking the time for necessary steps such as gloving will eliminate most opportunities for infection from contact with a patient. Since 1978 there has been documented job-related transmission of HIV to nurses in 16 cases.[4] They were exposed to the virus via percutaneous (such as needlesticks) or mucocutaneous routes. There are 68 additional instances of possible occupationally acquired HIV infection in the United States in health-care workers such as laboratory technicians, health aides, paramedics, surgeons, and dental workers.

CULTURAL AND BEHAVIORAL DIFFERENCES. Nurses work with patients whose backgrounds and behaviors may vary markedly from their own and challenge the nurse's beliefs and values. Although a nurse is entitled to have private views, there is an obligation to provide the best nursing care available to each patient. Disapproval of the patient's past behavior is the nurse's prerogative. The challenge is to keep that view from interfering with care while accepting the patient as a person.

IDENTIFICATION. As HIV disease spreads throughout society, it will become increasingly common for the nurse to have many similarities with the patient. Patients will have more characteristics in common with the nurse, including age, lifestyle, and socioeconomic status. In some cases it is difficult for the nurse to manage the feelings aroused by patients with HIV disease and maintain an objective approach. For example, a pregnant nurse may care for a young woman who has recently delivered an HIV-infected baby. Anger, fear, confusion, disgust, and pity toward the patient are some of the reactions with which a nurse may have to cope to provide high-quality care.

Feeling emotionally involved with the patient and family, whom the nurse may know for years, may result in fatigue and diminished coping. Some signs of emotional fatigue include needing more energy than before to complete tasks, withdrawal from others, loss of humor, and feeling pressured, overwhelmed, and ineffective.

It is important that professionals be aware of their stress level and watch for signs of emotional fatigue to prevent exhaustion or burnout, allowing themselves to process the multiple losses one experiences in AIDS work. Methods of relieving or preventing stress overload include limit setting, relaxation, and exercise. The clinical example that follows illustrates this problem.

Clinical Example TJ, a 2-year-old girl, entered the hospital with a broken wrist suffered during a fall from her porch. Upon admission the treatment team is notified by her parents that she was HIV positive. She has had no opportunistic infections, has a T-cell count of 950, and is of normal weight and height for her age. She shows no symptoms of HIV disease. Ms. K, her primary nurse, has approached her senior clinical nurse with a dilemma. She believes that the only way TJ could have become infected was in utero. Ms. K is experiencing great anger toward TJ's parents, whom she believes should have taken precautions against the birth of children once they knew TJ's mother was HIV positive. Ms. K wants to be removed as TJ's primary nurse not only because of her anger against her parents, but also because Ms. K has a 2-year-old daughter and finds that she is too distressed to work with TJ.

When a nurse identifies that a patient is arousing strong feelings or if colleagues question one's objectivity, it is essential to seek out supervision or consultation from an experienced nurse.

FEAR OF DEATH AND DYING. For many nurses, dealing with death is an occasional stressor. But for the nurse caring for patients with HIV disease, death and the preparation for it are common issues. Nurses may get to know patients during the course of repeated hospitalizations or work with patients who are young and energetic but are showing signs of decreasing vitality. Unresolved grief on the nurse's part, lack of acceptance of death as an outcome, and the nurse's own religious and cultural values related to death are factors that may inhibit the nurse's ability to cope with the losses experienced while caring for patients with HIV.

> **?** *Would you apply for a nursing position in a setting that specialized in the treatment of people with HIV disease? What considerations would influence your decision?*

PSYCHIATRIC CONSULTATION LIAISON NURSING. Of special note is the role of the psychiatric consultation liaison nurse in the general hospital setting. This nurse provides consultation to, collaborates with, and educates nurses and other members of the health team in addressing the interactive effects of the biopsychosocial aspects of AIDS care. Among the services the nurse consultant can provide or coordinate are educational and informational programs on all aspects of HIV disease, consistent policies and procedures for infection control practices, postexposure education and support, institutional resources and support for patients and staff, attention to work and personal stress-reduction techniques, encouragement of supervisor and peer recognition for work well done, regular and as-needed group meetings to provide emotional support for staff, and group forums for nurses to verbalize their feelings, attitudes, values, and concerns.

It has been observed that nurses are accustomed to trying to cure, fix, and solve.[13] Nurses should recognize that complex and difficult challenges face patients and their families daily. Nurses may be burdened with their own feelings of helplessness and frustration. They do not have all the answers and may feel that they have failed the patient. It is often helpful to enlist the support of consultants who are experts at helping nurses cope with these difficult times.

EVALUATING CARE OF THE PATIENT WITH HIV DISEASE

In working with the psychosocial aspects of HIV disease, evaluation of nursing interventions focuses on the patient's reduction of maladaptive responses to the stressors associated with the disease. The primary issue for the patient is adjustment to loss. Self-esteem, social acceptance, employment and financial independence, family relationships, and future goals are all threatened by HIV disease. The nurse's assessment and counseling skills, the teaching of coping skills, and referrals to support services are appropriate areas for evaluation. Nurses also need to conduct periodic self-evaluation to prevent becoming overwhelmed by the stresses of working with patients with HIV disease.

Summary

1. HIV disease includes all of the disorders resulting from infection with the human immunodeficiency virus. It has multiple effects on all aspects of biopsychosocial functioning.
2. Behaviors related to HIV disease may be related to stigma, crisis, depression, or dementia.
3. Planning health care for the person with HIV disease must involve the multidisciplinary team. Interventions include case management, medications, risk reduction, support groups, crisis intervention, encouragement of productive activity, enhancement of self-esteem, grief counseling, support during terminal stages, and support of significant others.
4. Evaluation focuses on the patient's adjustment to the multiple losses associated with HIV disease.

COMPETENT CARING A Clinical Exemplar of a Psychiatric Nurse

Donna Green, RN

A special moment for me happened several years ago at the beginning of the AIDS epidemic. It involved a relationship I formed with a patient who was diagnosed with AIDS. I spent time with him when others stayed away, and allowed him to share his thoughts and feelings. I encouraged him to talk about his feelings concerning problems in his relationships in an atmosphere of unconditional acceptance of his sexuality. I promoted this by showing no fear of contracting the disease from him and no judgment of his life situation.

Slowly, he began to interact more on the unit by initiating conversations with the staff, although not with other patients. When he consented to a case conference, he asked that I accompany him because he felt more at ease when I was with him.

At this point I realized the time that I spent with him and the efforts I made to reach out to him had made a difference in this man's hospital stay. My efforts were also recognized by my supervisor and were a large factor in my receiving a performance award. Such are the difficult challenges and special rewards of our profession and the specialty area in which we practice.

Chapter Review Questions

1. Identify whether the following statements are true (T) or false (F).

A. ___ The AIDS virus cannot be spread through kissing, sneezing, or touching.

B. ___ A person can get AIDS by sharing kitchens and bathrooms with someone who has AIDS.

C. ___ The AIDS virus attacks the body's ability to fight off diseases.

D. ___ A person who got the AIDS virus from shooting up drugs cannot give the virus to someone by having sex.

E. ___ A pregnant woman can give the AIDS virus to her unborn baby.

F. ___ Most types of birth control also protect against getting the AIDS virus.

G. ___ Condoms make sexual intercourse completely safe from AIDS transmission.

H. ___ A person must have many different sexual partners to be at risk for AIDS.

I. ___ Donating blood carries no AIDS risk for the donor.

J. ___ Most people who have AIDS look quite ill.

2. Fill in the blanks.

A. The most common way in which HIV is transmitted is through _____.

B. Symptoms of _____ and _____ may overlap with HIV symptoms, complicating diagnostic and treatment efforts.

C. A major complication of HIV disease is subcortical encephalopathy, which results in the clinical condition of _____.

D. _____ causes large, purple, bruiselike blotches on the face, hands, and legs.

3. Provide short answers for the following questions.

A. Describe changes in the incidence of HIV in the United States over the past 10 years. Consider gender, race, age, sexual preference, and socioeconomic status.

B. Briefly describe the three medication treatments for HIV discussed in the text. Are there newer ones at this time?

C. Your classmate tells you that she saw a computer printout from the laboratory during her clinical rotation that listed your clinical supervisor as HIV positive. Discuss the issues related to this situation, including potential losses, breaches of confidentiality, and potential stigmatizing reactions. How would you respond?

REFERENCES

1. Barroso J: Focusing on living: attitudinal approaches of long-term survivors of AIDS, *Issues Ment Health Nurs* 17:395, 1996.
2. Boccellari AA, Dilley JW: Management and residual placement problems of patients with HIV-related cognitive impairment, *Hosp Community Psychiatry* 43:32, 1992.
3. Centers for Disease Control and Prevention: *1993 revised classification system for HIV infection and expanded surveillance case definition for AIDS among adolescents and adults,* Atlanta, 1992, US Department of Health and Human Services.
4. Centers for Disease Control and Prevention: *HIV/AIDS surveillance report,* Atlanta, 1996, US Department of Health and Human Services.
5. Cournos F et al: HIV risk activity among persons with severe mental illness: preliminary findings, *Hosp Community Psychiatry* 44:1104, 1993.
6. Cowles KV, Rodgers BL: When a loved one has AIDS: care for the significant other, *J Psychosoc Nurs Ment Health Serv* 29:6, 1991.
7. Field HL: Biopsychosocial aspects of AIDS, *New Dir Ment Health Serv* 57:51, 1993.
8. Graham LL, Cates JA: How to reduce the risk of HIV infection for the seriously mentally ill, *J Psychosoc Nurs Ment Health Serv* 30:9, 1992.
9. Harding AK, Gray LA, Neal M: Confidentiality limits with clients who have HIV: a review of ethical and legal guidelines and professional policies, *J Couns Dev* 71:297, 1993.
10. Heaton RK, Grant I, Butters N, et al: The HNRC 500: neuropsychology of HIV infection at different stages, *J Intern Neuropsychol Soc* 1:231, 1995.
11. Kalichman SC: *Understanding AIDS: a guide for mental health professionals,* Washington DC, 1995, American Psychological Association.
12. Kelly JA et al: AIDS/HIV risk behavior among the chronically mentally ill, *Am J Psychiatry* 149:886, 1992.

13. LaSalle AJ, LaSalle PM: Care of people living with HIV disease: counseling issues for the nurse practitioner, *Nurse Pract Forum* 2:137, 1991.

14. Lyketsos CG, Hoover DR, Guccione M, et al: Changes in depressive symptoms as AIDS develops, *Am J Psychiatry* 153:1430, 1996.

15. Malow RW, Jager KB, Ireland SJ, Penedo F: HIV infection and risky sexual behaviors among women in treatment for noninjection drug dependence, *Psychiatr Serv* 47:1197, 1996.

16. McCain NL, Gramling LF: Living with dying: coping with HIV disease, *Issues Ment Health Nurs* 13:271, 1992.

17. McEnany GW, Hughes AM, Lee KA: Depression and HIV: a nursing perspective on a complex relationship, *Nurs Clin North Am* 31:57, 1996.

18. McShane RE, Bumbalo JA, Patsdaughter CA: Psychological distress in family members living with human immunodeficiency virus/acquired immune deficiency syndrome, *Arch Psychiatr Nurs* 8:53, 1994.

19. Moneyham L, Seals B, Demi A, et al: Perceptions of stigma in women infected with HIV, *AIDS Patient Care STDs* 10:162, 1996.

20. Morris NJ: Depression and HIV disease: a critical review, *J Am Psychiatr Nurses Assoc* 2:154, 1996.

21. Nyamathi A, Flaskerud J, Leake B, Chen S: Impoverished women at risk for AIDS: social support variables, *J Psychosoc Nurs* 34:31, 1996.

22. PhRMA: *New medicines in development for AIDS,* Washington, DC, 1996, Pharmaceutical Research and Manufacturers of America.

23. Rabkin JG, Rabkin R, Wagner G: Testosterone replacement therapy in HIV illness, *Gen Hosp Psychiatry* 17:37, 1995.

24. Sherman DW: Nurses' willingness to care for AIDS patients and spirituality, social support, and death anxiety, *Image J Nurs Sch* 28:205, 1996.

25. St. Louis ME, Wasserheit JN, Gayle HD: Editorial: Janus considers the HIV pandemic: harnessing recent advances to enhance AIDS prevention, *Am J Public Health* 87:10, 1997.

26. Swanson B et al: Characterizing the neuropsychological functioning of persons with human immunodeficiency virus infection; Part 1. Acquired immunodeficiency syndrome dementia complex: a review, *Arch Psychiatr Nurs* 7:74, 1993.

27. Vitiello B, Stover ES: Psychopharmacology in HIV+ patients: research perspectives, *Psychopharmacol Bull* 32:293, 1996.

ANNOTATED SUGGESTED READINGS

Crawford I, Fishman B: *Psychosocial intervention in HIV disease,* Northvale, NJ, 1996, Baruch Aronson.

Rich descriptions of HIV and the reactions of various populations. Includes recommended therapies and a list of resources.

Kalichman S: *Understanding AIDS: a guide for mental health professionals,* Washington, DC, 1995, American Psychological Association.

A thorough and well-written book that provides the mental health professional clear and well-documented information, treatment strategies, and research directions on HIV.

*Lisanti P, Zwolski K: Understanding the devastation of AIDS, *Am J Nurs* 1997:27, 1997.

Excellent series of articles that profiles HIV, traces its destructive path through the immune system, and reviews some opportunistic illnesses that follow in its wake.

*McEnany G, Hughes A, Lee K: Depression and HIV: a nursing perspective on a complex relationship, *Nurs Clin North Am* 31:57, 1996.

A very clear yet complex review of the biological interface between depression and HIV. A "must read" for psychiatric nurses.

*Meisenhelder J: Contributing factors to fear of HIV contagion in registered nurses, *Image* 26:65, 1994.

This study found that homophobia, lack of knowledge, lack of emotional involvement, and fear of the unknown accounted for most of the fear of HIV contagion expressed by nurses.

*Morris N: Depression and HIV disease: A critical review, *J Am Psychiatr Nurses Assoc* 2:154, 1996.

A thorough review of the literature on depression and its relationship with HIV disease with implications for clinical practice.

St. Louis M, Wasserheit J, Gayle H: Janus considers the HIV pandemic: harnessing recent advances to enhance AIDS prevention, *Am J Public Health* 87:10, 1997 (editorial).

A well-written, visionary step into a future of HIV care that embraces prevention as a mandatory outcome of scientific endeavor.

*Ungvarski P: Update on HIV infection, *Am J Nurs* 1997:44, 1997.

Presents a global overview of the HIV pandemic, highlighting recent developments, and includes a list of references to further expand one's knowledge.

Vitiello B, Stover E: Psychopharmacology in HIV+ patients: research perspectives, *Psychopharmacology Bulletin* 32:293, 1996.

Provides a review of current knowledge about psychotropic drugs useful to patients with HIV and recommendations for improvement.

*Nursing reference.

Glossary

A

abreaction The release of feelings that takes place as a patient talks about emotionally charged areas.

accountability To be answerable to someone for something, focusing responsibility on the individual for personal actions or lack of actions.

action cues A category of nonverbal communication that consists of body movements and is sometimes called kinetics.

addiction The psychosocial behaviors related to substance dependence.

adolescence The period from the beginning of puberty to the attainment of maturity. The transitional stage during which the youth is becoming an adult man or woman. This period is described in terms of development in many different functions that may be reached at different times. Only conventional limits may be stated: 12 to 21 years for girls, 13 to 23 years for boys.

advanced directives Documents, written while a person is competent, that specify how decisions about treatment would be made if the person were to become incompetent.

advanced practice registered nurse (APRN) A licensed RN who has a master's degree and a depth of knowledge of psychiatric nursing theory, supervised clinical practice, and competence in advanced psychiatric nursing skills.

adventitious crisis An accidental, uncommon, and unexpected event that results in multiple losses and major environmental changes.

advocacy Helping people to receive available services and influencing providers to improve existing services and develop new ones.

affect Feeling, mood, or emotional tone.

affective Relating to a person's affect.

agnosia Difficulty recognizing well-known objects.

agonist In pharmacology, a substance that acts with, enhances, or potentiates a specific activity.

agoraphobia Fear of open spaces and the marketplace.

AIDS dementia complex Subcortical encephalopathy characterized by progressive dementia; believed to result primarily from direct infection with HIV.

akathisia A motor restlessness ranging from a feeling of inner disquiet, often localized in the muscles, to an inability to sit still or lie quietly; a side effect of some antipsychotic drugs.

alcohol hallucinosis A medical diagnosis referring to an alcohol withdrawal syndrome that is characterized by auditory hallucinations in the absence of any other psychotic symptoms.

alcohol withdrawal delirium A medical diagnosis for a serious alcohol withdrawal syndrome that is characterized by delirium and autonomic hyperactivity occurring within 1 week of reduction of alcohol intake.

alexithymia Difficulty naming and describing emotions.

altruism A concern for the welfare of others that can be expressed at the level of the individual or the larger social system.

amotivational syndrome A cluster of symptoms apparently related to prolonged marijuana use that includes apathy, lack of energy, loss of desire to work or be productive, diminished concentration, poor personal hygiene, and preoccupation with marijuana.

anaclitic depression A deprivational reaction in infants separated from their mothers in the second half of the first year of life. The reaction is characterized by apprehension, crying, withdrawal, psychomotor slowing, dejection, stupor, insomnia, anorexia, and gross retardation in growth and development.

anhedonia Inability or decreased ability to experience pleasure, joy, intimacy, and closeness.

anorexia nervosa An eating disorder in which the person experiences hunger but refuses to eat because of a distorted body image leading to a self-perception of fatness. Starvation ensues.

antecedent The stimulus or cue that occurs before behavior that leads to its occurrence.

antisocial personality disorder A disorder occurring in adult patients with a history of conduct disorder; behavior is often characterized by poor work record, disregard for social norms, aggressiveness, financial irresponsibility, impulsiveness, lying, recklessness, inability to maintain close relationships or to meet responsibilities for significant others, and a lack of remorse for harmful behavior.

anxiety A diffuse apprehension vague in nature and associated with feelings of uncertainty and helplessness. It is an emotion without a specific object, is subjectively experienced by the individual, and is communicated interpersonally. It occurs as a result of a threat to the person's being, self-esteem, or identity.

apathy Lack of feelings, emotions, interests, or concern.

aphasia Difficulty finding the right word.

appraisal of stressor An evaluation of the significance of an event for one's well-being that takes place on the cognitive, affective, physiological, behavioral, and social levels.

apraxia Inability or difficulty in performing a purposeful organized task or similar skilled activities.

assertive community treatment An intensive community intervention program, undertaken by case managers with small caseloads and 24-hour responsibility for their clients, in which a multi-disciplinary team works with patients in their homes, neighborhoods, and workplaces, providing varying intensities of services depending on patient need.

assertiveness The midpoint of a continuum that runs from passive to aggressive behavior. Assertive behavior conveys a sense of self-assurance but also communicates respect for the other person.

attention The ability to focus on one activity in a sustained, concentrated manner.

attributions Reasoning processes used to explain events.

autogenic storytelling A therapeutic version of storytelling in which the child participates in creating the story.

autonomy Self-determination that fosters independence and self-regulation; the condition that allows for definition of and control over a domain.

aversion therapy Reduces unwanted but persistent maladaptive behaviors by applying an aversive or noxious stimulus when that maladaptive behavior occurs.

axon The presynaptic cell membrane of a neuron.

B

behavior Any observable, recordable, and measurable act, movement, or response.

behavioral Relating to a person's behavior.

bibliotherapy Use of literature to help children identify and express feelings within the structure and safety of the nurse-patient relationship.

binge eating The rapid consumption of large quantities of food in a discrete period of time.

biofeedback The use of a machine to communicate physical changes; used to train a person to reduce anxiety and modify behavioral responses.

biological psychiatry A school of psychiatric thought that emphasizes physical, chemical, and neurological causes and treatment approaches.

bipolar affective disorder A subgroup of the affective disorders characterized by at least one episode of manic behavior, with or without a history of episodes of depression.

bisexuality A sexual attraction to people of both sexes and the engagement in both homosexual and heterosexual activity.

blood levels The concentration of a drug in the plasma, serum, or blood. In psychiatry the term is most often applied to levels of lithium or some tricyclic antidepressants. Maximum clinical responses to these agents have been correlated with specific ranges of blood levels.

body dysmorphic disorder A somatoform disorder characterized by a normal-appearing person's belief that he or she has a physical defect.

body image Sum of the conscious and unconscious attitudes the person has toward his or her body. It includes present and past perceptions as well as feelings about size, function, appearance, and potential.

borderline personality disorder A specific personality disorder with the essential features of unstable mood, interpersonal relationships and self-image; characteristic behaviors may include unstable relationships, exploitation of others, impulsive behavior, labile affect, problems expressing anger appropriately, self-destructive behavior, and identity disturbances.

boundary violation When a nurse goes outside the limits of the therapeutic relationship and establishes a social, economic, or personal relationship with a patient.

brain electrical activity mapping (BEAM) Images brain activity and function by using CT techniques to display data derived from EEG recordings of brain electrical activity that has been sensory evoked by specific stimuli or cognitive evoked by specific mental tasks.

bulimia nervosa An eating disorder characterized by uncontrollable binge eating alternating with vomiting or dieting.

C

capitation A funding mechanism in which all defined services for a specific period of time are provided for an agreed-upon payment, payment is tied to the care of a particular person or group, and the provider agrees to be at risk for costs exceeding the agreed-upon amount.

case management Services aimed at linking the service system to the patient and coordinating the service components so that the patient can achieve successful community living.

catatonia A stuporous state.

catharsis Release that occurs when the patient is encouraged to talk about things that bother him or her most. Fears, feelings, and experiences are brought out into the open and discussed.

certification A formal review process of clinical practice.

certified generalist A psychiatric nurse who demonstrates expertise in practice, knowledge of theories concerning personality development and behavior patterns in treating mental illness, and the relationship of such treatments to nursing care.

certified specialist A nurse showing a high degree of proficiency in interpersonal skills, the use of the nursing process, and psychological and milieu therapies.

child abuse Includes physical abuse or battering, emotional abuse, sexual abuse, and neglect. Children who witness family abuse or violence are also victimized.

circadian rhythms The correlation between human activities and behaviors and external environmental stimuli.

classical conditioning A theory describing the process by which involuntary behavior is learned, in which an event occurs when one stimulus, by being paired with another stimulus, comes to produce the same response as the other stimulus.

clinical pathway A shortened version of the plan of care for a particular patient that lists key nursing and medical processes and corresponding time lines to which the patient must adhere to achieve standard outcomes within a specified period.

cognition The mental process characterized by knowing, thinking, learning, and judging.

cognitive Relating to a person's cognition.

cognitive distortions Positive or negative distortions of reality that might include errors of logic, mistakes in reasoning, or individualized views of the world that do not reflect reality.

cohesion The strength of group members' desire to work together toward common goals.

collaboration The shared planning, decision making, problem solving, goal setting, and assumption of responsibilities by people who work together cooperatively and with open communication.

collaborative practice The diagnosis and treatment of psychiatric illness in patients with somatic complaints.

collegiality An essential aspect of professional practice that requires that nurses view their peers as collaborators in the caregiving process who are valued and respected for their unique contributions.

commitment Involuntary admission in which the request for hospitalization did not originate with the patient. When committed, the patient loses the right to leave the hospital when he or she wishes. It is usually justified on the ground that the patient is dangerous to self or others and needs treatment.

communication Process of influencing the behavior of others by sending, receiving, and interpreting messages; feedback and consideration of the context complete the cycle.

community support systems Systems developed by community mental health centers to provide patients with necessary specialized mental health service. Includes such community-based components as crisis response services, health and dental care, rehabilitation services, and protection and advocacy.

compensation Process by which a person makes up for a deficiency in self-image by strongly emphasizing some other feature that the person regards as an asset.

competence building The health education strategy of primary prevention that involves the strengthening of individuals and groups and is based on the assumption that many maladaptive responses result from a lack of competence.

compulsion A recurring irresistible impulse to perform some act.

computed tomography (CT) Depicts brain structure with a series of radiographs that is computer-constructed into "slices" of the brain that can be stacked by the computer, giving a three-dimensional view.

concreteness Use of specific terminology rather than abstractions in the discussion of the patient's feelings, experiences, and behavior.

conduct disorder Disorder with the essential feature of behavior that violates the basic rights of others or societal norms and rules.

confidentiality Disclosure of certain information to another specifically authorized person.

conflict Clashing of two opposing interests. The person experiences two competing drives and must choose between them.

confrontation An expression by the nurse of perceived discrepancies in the patient's behavior. It is an attempt by the nurse to bring to the patient's awareness the incongruence in feelings, attitudes, beliefs, and behaviors.

congruent communication A communication pattern in which the sender is communicating the same message on both the verbal and the nonverbal levels.

consequence The kind of effect (positive, negative, or neutral) the person thinks a behavior has.

consultation A specific professional process between two systems in which the consulted has a problem and requests help from an outside system, the consultant.

consultation liaison nursing care Expert psychiatric consultation provided by a psychiatric mental health nurse in various other health-care settings.

context Setting in which an event takes place.

contingency contracting A formal contract between the patient and the therapist defining what behaviors are to be changed and what consequences follow the performance of these behaviors.

conversion disorder A somatoform disorder characterized by a loss or alteration of physical functioning without evidence of organic impairment.

coping mechanism Any efforts directed at stress management. They can be problem, cognitive, or emotion focused.

coping resources Characteristics of the person, group, or environment that help people adapt to stress.

countertransference An emotional response of the nurse that is generated by the patient's qualities and is inappropriate to the content and context of the therapeutic relationship or inappropriate in the degree of emotional intensity.

crisis A disturbance caused by a stressful event or a perceived threat to self.

crisis intervention Short-term therapy focused on solving the immediate problem and allowing the patient to return to a precrisis level of function.

cultural sensitivity The ability to view each patient as a unique person, fully considering the patient's cultural experiences within the context of the common developmental challenges faced by all people.

culture-bound syndrome Recurrent, locality-specific patterns of aberrant behavior and troubling experience that may or may not be linked to a particular DSM-IV diagnostic category

cytochrome p450 inhibition SSRIs inhibit this liver enzyme, causing potentially dangerous changes in the metabolism of many drugs.

D

debriefing Therapeutic intervention that includes reviewing the facts related to an event and processing the response to them.

decatastrophizing Helping patients to evaluate whether they are overestimating the catastrophic nature of a situation.

decision making Arriving at a solution or making a choice.

defense mechanisms Coping mechanisms of the ego that attempt to protect the person from feelings of inadequacy and worthlessness and prevent awareness of anxiety. They are primarily unconscious and involve a degree of self-deception and reality distortion.

deinstitutionalization At the patient level, the transfer to a community setting of a patient hospitalized for an extended time, generally many years; at the mental health care system level, a shift in the focus of care from the large, long-term institution to the community, accomplished by discharging long-term patients and avoiding unnecessary admissions.

delinquency A minor violation of legal or moral codes, especially by children or adolescents. Juvenile delinquency is such behavior by a young person (usually younger than 16 or 18 years of age) that brings him or her to the attention of a court.

delirium The medical diagnostic term that describes an organic mental disorder characterized by a cluster of cognitive impairments with an acute onset and the identification of a specific precipitating stressor.

delirium tremens A medical diagnostic term that has been replaced with the diagnosis of alcohol withdrawal delirium.

delusion A false belief that is firmly maintained even though it is not shared by others and is contradicted by social reality.

dementia The medical diagnostic term that describes an organic mental disorder characterized by a cluster of cognitive impairments that are generally of gradual onset and irreversible. The predisposing and precipitating stressors may or may not be identifiable.

dendrite The postsynaptic membrane of a neuron.

denial Avoidance of disagreeable realities by ignoring or refusing to recognize them.

depersonalization A feeling of unreality and alienation from oneself. One has difficulty distinguishing self from others, and one's body has an unreal or strange quality about it. The subjective experience of the partial or total disruption of one's ego and the disintegration and disorganization of one's self-concept.

depression An abnormal extension or overelaboration of sadness and grief. The word *depression* can denote a variety of phenomena, a sign, symptom, syndrome, emotional state, reaction, disease, or clinical entity.

detoxification The removal of a toxic substance from the body, either naturally through physiological process, such as hepatic or renal functions, or medically by the introduction of alternative substances and gradual withdrawal.

differentiated practice Distinguishing among professionals with role descriptions and functional assignments based on education, experience, and competency; responsibilities reflect each person's unique knowledge base.

differentiation Sufficient separation between intellect and emotions so that one is not dominated by the reactive anxiety of the family's emotional system.

direct self-destructive behavior (DSDB) Suicidal behavior.

disadvantagement The lack of socioeconomic resources that are basic to biopsychosocial adaptation.

discrimination Differential treatment of individuals or groups not based on actual merit.

disengaged A transactional style in a family reflecting inappropriately rigid boundaries requiring a high level of individual stress to activate family response.

displacement Shift of an emotion from the person or object toward which it was originally directed to another, usually neutral or less dangerous person or object.

dissociation The separation of any group of mental or behavioral processes from the rest of the person's consciousness or identity.

diurnal mood variation Changes in mood that are related to the time of day.

double bind Simultaneous communication of conflicting messages in the context of a situation that does not allow escape. (See *incongruent communication*.)

drug interaction The effects of two or more drugs being taken simultaneously, producing an alteration in the usual effects of either drug taken alone. The interacting drugs may have a potentiating or additive effect, and serious side effects may result.

drug tolerance Repeated use of some substance or drug (such as narcotics) so that larger and larger doses are required to produce the same physiological or psychological effect.

drug trial The time it takes to administer a drug at adequate therapeutic doses for a long enough period to determine its efficacy for a particular patient. The trial culminates with acceptable clinical results, intolerable adverse effects, or poor response after an appropriate blood level is reached or after the drug is administered for a time specific for the illness.

DSM-IV Commonly used abbreviation for the *Diagnostic and Statistical Manual of Mental Disorders,* which contains standard nomenclature of emotional illness used by all health-care practitioners. DSM-IV is a revised version published in 1994; it updates and classifies mental illnesses and presents guidelines and diagnostic criteria for various mental disorders.

dual diagnosis Simultaneous occurrence of a mental illness and a substance abuse disorder.

dyspareunia Recurrent or persistent genital pain occurring before, during, or after intercourse (male or female).

dystonia Acute tonic muscle spasms, often of the tongue, jaw, eyes, and neck but sometimes of the whole body. Sometimes occurs during the first few days of antipsychotic drug administration.

E

echopraxia Purposeless imitation of other's movements.

ego defense mechanisms See *defense mechanisms.*

elder abuse A variety of behaviors that threaten the health, comfort, and possibly the lives of elderly people, including physical and emotional neglect, emotional abuse, violation of personal rights, financial abuse, and direct physical abuse.

electroconvulsive therapy (ECT) Artificial induction of a grand mal seizure by passing a controlled electrical current through electrodes applied to one or both temples. The patient is anesthetized and the seizure attenuated by administration of a muscle relaxant medication.

empathy Ability to view the patient's world from his or her internal frame of reference. It involves the nurse's sensitivity to the patient's current feelings and the verbal ability to communicate this understanding in a language attuned to the patient.

enabler The role that is often assumed by the significant others of substance abusers, characterized by covert support of the substance-abusing behavior.

encounter group therapy An application of the existential model of psychiatric care in a group setting. The focus is on here-and-now experience and the expression of real feelings, verbally and nonverbally, as members react to events in the group.

endogenous Developing or originating within the organism or arising from causes within the organism.

enmeshed A transactional style in a family reflecting diffuse subsystem boundaries, resulting in stress in one family member that emotionally reverberates quickly and intensely throughout the family system.

ethic A standard of behavior or a belief valued by an individual or group.

ethical dilemma Exists when moral claims conflict with one another, resulting in a difficult problem that seems to have no satisfactory solution because of the existence of a choice between equally unsatisfactory alternatives.

ethnicity A person's racial, national, tribal, linguistic, or cultural origin or background.

exhibitionism Intense sexual arousal or desire and acts, fantasies, or other stimuli involving exposing one's genitals to an unsuspecting stranger.

existential (therapy) A school of philosophical thought that focuses on the importance of experience in the present and the belief that humans find meaning in life through their experiences.

exogenous Developing or originating outside the organism.

extinction The process of eliminating the occurrence of a behavior by ignoring or not rewarding that behavior.

extrapyramidal syndrome (EPS) A variety of signs and symptoms, including muscular rigidity, tremors, drooling, shuffling gait (Parkinsonism); restlessness (akathisia); peculiar involuntary postures (dystonia); motor inertia (akinesia); and many other neurological disturbances. Results from dysfunction of the extrapyramidal system. May occur as a reversible side effect of certain psychotropic drugs, particularly antipsychotics.

F

failure to thrive A syndrome consisting of weight loss, decreased appetite, poor nutrition, and inactivity

family A group of people living in a household who are attached emotionally, interact regularly, and share concerns for the growth and development of individuals and the family.

family burden The impact of a family member's mental illness on the entire family.

family preservation Intensive home treatment modality for troubled youths and their families.

family projection process Transmission of anxiety of one or both parents onto a target child, establishing an overly protective or conflictual relationship with the child and resulting ultimately in impairment of the child.

family violence A range of behaviors occurring between family members, including physical and emotional abuse of children, child neglect, spouse battering, marital rape, and elder abuse.

fetishism Intense sexual arousal or desire and acts, fantasies, or other stimuli involving nonliving objects by themselves.

flight of ideas Overproductive speech characterized by rapid shifting from one topic to another and fragmented ideas.

flooding Exposure therapy in which the patient is immediately exposed to the most anxiety-provoking stimuli.

Food and Drug Administration (FDA) One of a number of health administrations under the assistant secretary of health of the US Department of Health, Education, and Welfare (in April 1980 Department of Health and Human Services) to set standards for, to license the sale of, and in general to safeguard the public from the use of dangerous drugs and food substances.

free association The verbalization of thoughts as they occur, without any conscious screening or censorship.

frotteurism Intense sexual arousal or desire and acts, fantasies, or other stimuli involving rubbing against a nonconsenting person.

fusion A blurring of self-boundaries in a highly reactive emotional relationship with another.

G

gender identity A person's perception of one's maleness or femaleness.

gender role The cultural role attributes attributed to one's gender, such as expectations regarding behavior, cognitions, occupations, values, and emotional responses.

genetic identity A person's chromosomal gender.

genogram A structured method of gathering information and graphically symbolizing factual and emotional relationship data.

genuineness A quality of the nurse characterized by openness, honesty, and sincerity. The nurse is self-congruent and authentic and relates to the patient without a defensive facade.

Gestalt therapy A therapeutic approach based on the existential model of psychiatric care. It was developed by Perls and focuses on the development of enhanced self-awareness.

glial cells Support cells that form myelin sheaths; thought to remove excess transmitters and ions from the extracellular spaces in the brain, provide glucose to some nerve cells, and direct the flow of blood and oxygen to various parts of the brain.

grief A person's subjective response to the loss of a person, object, or concept that is highly valued. Uncomplicated grief is a healthy, adaptive, reparative response.

H

habeas corpus A right retained by all psychiatric patients that provides for the release of a person who claims that he or she is being deprived of liberty and detained illegally. The hearing for this determination takes place in a court of law, and the patient's sanity is at issue.

half-life The amount of time it takes the body to excrete approximately half of an ingested drug; after this time the effects of the drug usually begin to deteriorate.

hallucination Perceptual distortion arising from any of the five senses.

hallucinogens A class of abused drugs that cause a psychoticlike experience.

hardiness A measurement of a person's psychological capability to resist illness when faced with a stressful life event.

health education A teaching strategy related to health issues that involves the strengthening of individuals and groups through competence building.

heterosexuality Sexual attraction to members of the opposite sex.

HIV disease Describes all of the disorders resulting from infection with the human immunodeficiency virus.

home health care Delivery of health services in the home, including mental health services.

homophobia Persistent and irrational fear of homosexuals along with a negative attitude and hostility toward them.

homosexuality Sexual attraction to members of the same sex.

hypersomnia Disorders of excessive somnolence.

hypochondriasis A somatoform disorder characterized by the belief that one is ill without evidence of organic impairment, involving somatic overconcern with and morbid attention to details of body functioning.

hypomania A clinical syndrome that is similar to but less severe than that described by the term *mania* or *manic episode*.

hypoxia Inadequate oxygen at the cellular level, characterized by cyanosis, tachycardia, hypertension, peripheral vasoconstriction, dizziness, and mental confusion.

I

ideas of reference Incorrect interpretation of casual incidents and external events as having direct personal references.

identification Process by which a person tries to become like someone else whom he or she admires by taking on the thoughts, mannerisms, or tastes of that person.

identity Organizing principle of the personality system that accounts for the unity, continuity, uniqueness, and consistency of the personality. It is the awareness of the process of being oneself that is derived from self-observation and judgment. It is the synthesis of all self-representations into an organized whole.

identity confusion Lack of clarity and consistency in one's perception of the self, resulting in a high degree of anxiety.

identity diffusion A person's failure to integrate various childhood identifications into a harmonious adult psychosocial identity.

identity foreclosure Premature adoption of an identity that is desired by significant others without coming to terms with one's own desires, aspirations, or potential.

illusions False perceptions of or false responses to a sensory stimulus.

immediacy State that occurs when the current interaction of the nurse and the patient is focused on.

impulsivity A maladaptive social behavior characterized by unpredictability, unreliability, inability to plan or learn from experience, and overall poor judgment.

incompetency A legal status that must be proved in a special court hearing. As a result of the hearing, the person can be deprived of many civil rights. Incompetency can be reversed only in another court hearing that declares the person competent.

incongruent communication A communication pattern in which the sender is communicating a different message on the verbal and nonverbal levels and the listener does not know to which level he or she should respond. (See *double bind*.)

indirect self-destructive behavior (ISDB) Any activity that is detrimental to the person's well-being and could cause death, accompanied by lack of conscious awareness of the self-destructive nature of the behavior.

informed consent Disclosure of a certain amount of information to the patient about the proposed treatment and the attainment of the patient's consent, which must be competent, understanding, and voluntary.

insanity defense Legal defense proposing that a person who has committed an act that in a usual situation would be criminal should be held not guilty by reason of "insanity."

insight The patient's understanding of the nature of the problem or illness.

insomnia Disorders of initiating or maintaining sleep.

intellectualization Excessive reasoning or logic used to avoid experiencing disturbing feelings.

interdisciplinary team A team with members of different disciplines involved in a formal arrangement to provide patient services while maximizing educational interchange.

introjection An intense type of identification in which one incorporates qualities or values of another person or group into one's own ego structure.

isolation Splitting off the emotional component of a thought. It may be temporary or long term.

K

Kaposi's sarcoma A malignant, multifocal neoplasm of reticuloendothelial cells that begins as soft, brownish or purple papules on the feet and slowly spreads in the skin; associated with AIDS.

L

learned helplessness A behavioral state and personality trait of people who believe they are ineffectual, their responses are futile, and they have lost control over the reinforcers in the environment.

lethality An estimation of the probability that a person who is threatening suicide will succeed on the basis of the method described, the specificity of the plan, and the availability of the means.

libido Freud's term for psychic energy.

life review Progressive return to consciousness of past experiences.

limbic system An area in the brain associated with the control of emotion, eating, drinking, and sexual activity.

limit setting Nonpunitive, nonmanipulative act in which the patient is told what behavior is acceptable, what is not acceptable, and the consequences of behaving unacceptably.

living will Determining in advance one's participation in heroic measures during the dying process.

logotherapy An approach to psychotherapy based on the existential model and developed by Frankl. The focus is on the search for meaning in present experiences.

loose associations Lack of a logical relationship between thoughts and ideas that renders speech and thought inexact, vague, diffuse, and unfocused.

M

magical thinking Belief that thinking equates with doing, characterized by lack of realistic understanding of cause and effect.

magnetic resonance imaging (MRI) Depicts brain structure and activity using a magnetic field that surrounds the head and induces brain tissues to emit radio waves that are then computerized for clear and detailed construction of sections of the brain.

malingering Deliberate feigning of an illness.

malpractice Failure of a professional person to give the type of proper and competent care provided by members of his or her profession. This failure causes harm to the patient.

mania A condition characterized by a mood that is elevated, expansive, or irritable.

manipulation A maladaptive social response in which people treat others as objects, enter relationships that are centered around control issues, and are self-oriented or goal oriented rather than other oriented.

masochism Intense sexual arousal or desire and acts, fantasies, or other stimuli involving being humiliated, beaten, bound, or otherwise made to suffer (real or simulated).

maturational crisis A developmental event requiring a role change.

medical diagnosis A physician's independent judgment of the patient's health problems or disease states.

memory The retention or storage of knowledge learned about the world.

mental health Indicators of mental health include positive attitudes toward self, growth, development, self-actualization, integration, autonomy, reality perception, and environmental mastery.

mental status examination Represents a cross-section of the patient's psychological life and the sum total of the nurse's observations and impressions at the moment, serving as a basis for future comparison to track the progress of the patient.

message A unit of communication.

methadone maintenance A treatment program in which methadone is given to a patient recovering from heroin abuse to prevent the characteristic withdrawal symptoms, as methadone substitutes for the heroin without causing withdrawal symptoms or impaired functioning.

modeling Strategy used to form new behavior patterns, increase existing skills, or reduce avoidance behavior in which the patient observes a person modeling adaptive behavior, and is then encouraged to imitate it.

mood The patient's self-report of prevailing emotional state and a reflection of the patient's life situation.

mourning Includes all the psychological processes set in motion by a loss. The process of mourning is resolved only when the lost object is internalized, bonds of attachment are loosened, and new object relationships are established.

multidisciplinary team A team with members of different disciplines, each providing specific services to the patient.

multigenerational transmission process The repetition of relationship patterns and anxiety associated with toxic issues passed through generations in a family.

multiple personality The existence within an individual of two or more distinct personalities or personality states, with each having its own pattern of perceiving, feeling, and thinking.

myelin sheath Provides insulation to the nervous system. (See *glial cells*.)

N

narcissism A maladaptive social response characterized by egocentric attitude, fragile self-esteem, constant seeking of praise and admiration, and envy.

narcissistic personality disorder A specific personality disorder having the essential features of a pattern of grandiosity, lack of empathy, and hypersensitivity to the evaluation of others, beginning in early adulthood; characteristic behaviors may include rageful reactions to criticism, exploitation of others, inability to recognize how others feel, sense of entitlement, envy, belief that one's problems are unique, preoccupation with grandiose fantasies, and search for constant attention and admiration.

narcolepsy A condition characterized by brief attacks of deep sleep.

National Institutes of Mental Health (NIMH) Responsible for programs dealing with mental health, NIMH is an institute within the Alcohol, Drug Abuse, and Mental Health Administration (ADAMHA). ADAMHA is an agency in the US Department of Health and Human Services that provides leadership, policies, and goals for the federal effort to ensure the treatment and rehabilitation of people with alcohol, drug abuse, and mental health problems; this agency is also responsible for administering grants to support research, training, and service programs.

negative identity Assumption of an identity that is at odds with the accepted values and expectations of society.

negative reinforcement Increases the frequency of a behavior by reinforcing the behavior's power to control an aversive stimulus.

neologisms New word or words created by the patient; often a blend of other words.

neurosis Category of health problems distinguished by the following characteristics: recognized by the person as unacceptable, reality testing is intact, behavior is overall consistent with social norms, problem is enduring or recurrent, and there is no apparent organic cause.

neurotransmission The process whereby neurons communicate with each other through chemical messengers called neurotransmitters.

neurotransmitters Chemical messengers of the nervous system, manufactured in one neuron and released from the axon into the synapse and received by the dendrite of the next neuron.

nihilistic ideas Thoughts of nonexistence and hopelessness.

noncompliance The failure of a patient to carry out the self-care activities prescribed in a health-care plan.

nonverbal communication Transmission of a message without the use of words. It involves all five senses.

norms Standards of behavior.

nuclear family emotional system Patterns of interaction between family members and the degree to which these patterns promote fusion.

nursing diagnosis A nurse's judgment of the patient's behavioral response to stress. It is a statement of the patient's problems, which may be overt, covert, existing, or potential, and includes the behavioral disruption or threatened disruption, the contributing stressors, and the adaptive or maladaptive health responses.

nursing process An interactive, problem-solving process; a systematic and individualized way to achieve the outcomes of nursing care. The phases of the nursing process as described by the *Standards of Psychiatric–Mental Health Clinical Nursing Practice* are assessment, diagnosis, outcome identification, planning, implementation, and evaluation.

O

object cues A category of nonverbal communication that includes the speaker's intentional and unintentional use of all objects, such as dress, furnishings, and possessions.

obsession An idea, emotion, or impulse that repetitively and insistently forces itself into consciousness; unwanted, but cannot be voluntarily excluded from consciousness.

operant conditioning A theory concerned with the relationship between voluntary behavior and the environment that states that behaviors are influenced by their consequences and that operant behaviors are cued by environmental stimuli.

orgasm Peaking of sexual pleasure and the release of sexual tension accompanied by rhythmic contractions of the perineal muscles and pelvic reproductive organs.

outreach clinical services Delivery of health services in which health workers reach out to patients wherever they are in the community.

P

pain disorder A preoccupation with pain in the absence of physical disease to account for its intensity.

panic An attack of extreme anxiety that involves the disorganization of the personality. Distorted perceptions, loss of rational thought, and inability to communicate and function are evident.

paraphilia Characterized by sexual arousal in response to objects or situations that are not normally arousing for affectionate sexual activities with human partners (such as pedophilia, exhibitionism, or zoophilia).

parasomnia Disorders associated with sleep stages, such as sleepwalking, night terrors, nightmares, and enuresis.

patient classification system Designed to determine the amount or intensity of nursing services needed by each patient based on patient acuity or severity of illness.

pedophilia Intense sexual arousal or desire and acts, fantasies, or other stimuli involving children 13 years of age or younger.

perception Identification and initial interpretation of a stimulus based on information received through the five senses of sight, hearing, taste, touch, and smell.

perseveration Involuntary, excessive continuation or repetition of a single response, idea, or activity; may apply to speech or movement, but most often verbal.

personality fusion A person's attempt to establish a sense of self by fusing or belonging to someone else.

pharmacokinetics The study of the process and rates of drug distribution, metabolism, and disposition in the organism.

phobia A morbid fear associated with extreme anxiety.

phototherapy Light therapy that consists of exposing patients to artificial therapeutic lights about 5 to 20 times brighter than indoor lighting.

physical abuse Harm or threatened harm to a person's health or welfare that occurs through nonaccidental physical or mental injury, sexual abuse, or maltreatment.

physical dependence A characteristic of drug addiction that is present when withdrawal of the drug results in physiological disruptions.

polypharmacy Use of combinations of psychoactive drugs in a patient at the same time; more than one drug may not be more effective than a single agent, can cause drug interactions, and may increase the incidence of adverse reactions.

positive reinforcement Increases the frequency of a behavior by reinforcing the behavior's power to achieve a rewarding stimulus.

positron emission tomography (PET) Depicts brain activity and function using an injected radioactive substance that travels to the brain and shows up as a bright spot on the scan; different substances are taken up by the brain in different amounts depending on the type of tissue and activity level.

postpartum blues Brief episodes lasting 1 to 4 days of labile mood and tearfulness that occur in about 50% to 80% of women within 1 to 5 days of delivery.

postvention Therapeutic intervention with the significant others of a person who has committed suicide.

power The member's ability to influence the group and its other members.

precipitating stressors Stimuli that the person perceives as challenging, threatening, or harmful. They require the use of excess energy and produce a state of tension and stress.

predisposing factors Conditioning factors that influence both the type and the amount of resources that the person can elicit to cope with stress. They may be biological, psychological, or sociocultural.

prejudice A preconceived, unfavorable belief about individuals or groups that disregards knowledge, thought, or reason.

premature ejaculation Ejaculation that occurs with minimal sexual stimulation or before, on, or shortly after penetration and before the person wishes it.

primary prevention Biological, social, or psychological intervention that promotes health and well-being or reduces the incidence of illness in a community by altering the causative factors before they have an opportunity to do harm.

projection Attributing one's own thoughts or impulses to another person. Through this process the person can attribute intolerable wishes, emotional feelings, or motivations to another person.

pseudodementia A depressive condition of the elderly characterized by impaired cognitive function.

psychiatric nursing An interpersonal process that strives to promote and maintain patient behavior that contributes to integrated functioning. It uses the theories of human behavior as its science and the purposeful use of self as its art. Psychiatric nursing is directed toward both preventive and corrective effects on mental disorders and their sequelae and is concerned with the promotion of optimum mental health for society, the community, and individuals.

psychoanalysis A therapeutic approach based on the belief that behavioral disorders are related to unresolved, anxiety-provoking childhood experiences that are repressed into the unconscious. The goal of psychoanalysis is to bring repressed experiences into conscious awareness and to learn healthier means of coping with the related anxiety.

psychobiological resilience A concept that proposes that there is a recurrent human need to weather periods of stress and change throughout life. The ability to weather successfully each period of disruption and reintegration leaves the person better able to deal with the next change.

psychoeducation The teaching of a patient and family about the mental illness and the coping skills that will help with successful community living.

psychoimmunology Field that explores the psychological influences on the nervous system's control of immune responsiveness.

psychological autopsy A retrospective review of the person's behavior for the time preceding death by suicide.

psychological dependence A characteristic of drug addiction that is manifested in a craving for the abused substance and a fear that it will not be available in the future.

psychological factors affecting physical condition A category of psychophysiological disruptions in which organic impairment is evident. Examples include

migraine headache, asthma, hypertension, colitis, and duodenal ulcer.

psychoneuroimmunology The scientific field exploring the relationship between psychological states and the immune response.

psychopharmacology Drugs that treat the symptoms of mental illness and whose actions in the brain provide us with models to better understand the mechanisms of mental disorders.

psychosis A category of health problems that are distinguished by regressive behavior, personality disintegration, reduced level of awareness, great difficulty in functioning adequately, and gross impairment in reality testing.

punishment Decreases the frequency of a behavior by causing an aversive stimulus to occur after that behavior.

purging A variety of maladaptive behaviors intended to prevent weight gain, including vomiting, excessive exercise, and use of diuretics, diet pills, laxatives, and steroids.

Q

quality improvement The process of evaluating treatment outcomes in inpatient settings, usually monitored by an interdisciplinary body.

R

racism The belief that inherent differences between races determine individual achievement and that one race is superior.

rational-emotive therapy (RET) A therapeutic approach based on the existential model of psychiatric care and developed by Ellis. The emphasis is on risk taking and the assumption of responsibility for one's behavior.

rationalization Offering a socially acceptable or apparently logical explanation to justify or make acceptable otherwise unacceptable impulses, feelings, behaviors, and motives.

reaction formation Development of conscious attitudes and behavior patterns that are opposite to what one really would like to do.

reality orientation Formal process of keeping a person alert to events in the here and now.

reality therapy A therapeutic approach based on the existential model of psychiatric care and developed by Glasser. The focus is on recognition and accomplishment of life goals, with emphasis on development of the capacity for caring.

receptor A specialized area on a nerve membrane, blood vessel, or muscle that receives the chemical stimulation that activates or inhibits the nerve, blood vessel, or muscle.

recurrence Return of a new episode of illness.

reframing To change the conceptual or emotional viewpoint in how a situation is experienced and to place it in a different frame that fits the "facts" of the concrete situation equally well; this changes the situation's entire meaning. Attributing positive motivations behind undesirable behavior often constitutes reframing.

regression A retreat in the face of stress to behavior that is characteristic of an earlier level of development.

rehabilitation The process of enabling a mentally ill person to return to the highest possible level of functioning.

relapse Return of symptoms.

relaxation response A protective mechanism against stress that brings about decreased heart rate, lower metabolism, and decreased respiratory rate. It is the physiological opposite of the fight-or-flight, or anxiety, response.

relaxation training Training a person to relax and thus reduce anxiety. Procedures include rhythmic breathing, reduced muscle tension, and an altered state of consciousness.

reminiscence Thinking about or relating past experiences, especially those that are personally significant.

remission Occurs when a patient is symptom-free at the end of a phase of preillness functioning, which generally lasts 6 to 12 weeks.

repression Involuntary exclusion of a painful or conflictual thought, impulse, or memory from awareness. It is the primary ego defense, and other mechanisms tend to reinforce it.

residual Remaining, or left behind; the symptoms that remain after treatment has reached its maximum effect.

resistance Attempt of the patient to remain unaware of anxiety-producing aspects within the self. Ambivalent attitudes toward self-exploration in which the patient both appreciates and avoids anxiety-producing experiences that are a normal part of the therapeutic process.

respect An attitude of the nurse that conveys caring for, liking, and valuing the patient. The nurse regards the patient as a person of worth and accepts the patient without qualification.

response Improvement with treatment.

response cost Decreases the frequency of a behavior through the experience of a loss or penalty following the behavior.

response prevention Patient is encouraged to face a particular fear or situation without engaging in the accompanying behavior.

restraint The use of mechanical or manual devices to limit the physical mobility of the patient.

reuptake The process of neurotransmitters returning to the presynaptic cell after communication with receptor cells.

risk management Assessment of activities related to situations that could result in legal action involving patients, families, the hospital, or the health-care provider.

role playing Acting out of a particular situation. It functions to increase the person's insight into human relations and can deepen one's ability to see a situation from another point of view.

role strain Stress associated with expected roles or positions and experienced as frustration.

roles Set of socially expected behavior patterns associated with one person's function in various social groups. Roles provide a means for social participation and a way to test identities for consensual validation by significant others.

room program A titration of the amount of time patients are allowed in the unit milieu, with patients asked to stay in their rooms for certain lengths of time, and conversely allowed out of their rooms for a specific amount of time.

S

sadism Intense sexual arousal or desire and acts, fantasies, or other stimuli involving the infliction of real or simulated psychological or physical suffering (including humiliation).

schizoaffective disorder Diagnosis given to a patient who meets the diagnostic criteria for schizophrenia as well as one or both of the major mood disorders of bipolar disorder and major depression.

seasonal affective disorder (SAD) Depression that comes with shortened daylight in winter and fall and that disappears during spring and summer.

seclusion Separating the patient from others in a safe, contained environment.

secondary prevention A type of prevention that seeks to reduce the prevalence of illness by interventions that provide for early detection and treatment of problems.

self-actualization Process of fulfilling one's potential.

self-concept All the notions, beliefs, and convictions that constitute a person's knowledge of self and influence relationships with others.

self-disclosure Revelation that occurs when a person reveals information about self, ideas, values, feelings, and attitudes.

self-esteem The person's judgment of personal worth obtained by analyzing how well his or her behavior conforms to self-ideal.

self-help groups Groups composed of members who organize to solve their own problems; the members share a common experience, work together toward a common goal, and use their strengths to gain control over their lives.

self-ideal The person's perception of how he or she should behave on the basis of certain personal standards. The standard may be either a carefully constructed image of the type of person one would like to be or merely various aspirations, goals, or values that one would like to achieve.

self-injury The act of deliberate harm to one's own body.

sensory integration A category of perceptual behaviors including pain recognition, stereogenesis, graphesthesia, right/left recognition, and recognition and perception of faces.

serotonin syndrome Hyperserotonergic state (confusion, autonomic dysfunction, muscle rigidity, ataxia) that occurs when SSRIs are given concurrently with other serotonin-enhancing drugs.

sexual abuse The involvement of children and adolescents in sexual activities they do not fully comprehend and to which they do not freely consent.

sexual assault Forced perpetration of an act of sexual contact with another person without consent.

sexual orientation The gender to which one is romantically attracted.

shaping Introduces new behaviors by reinforcing behaviors that approximate the desired behavior.

situational crisis Occurs when a life event upsets an individual's or group's psychological equilibrium.

sleep deprivation therapy A possible therapy for depressed and bipolar patients based on reports that as many as 60% of depressed patients improve immediately after a night of sleep deprivation.

social skills training Teaching smooth social functioning to those who do not manifest social skills, using the principles of guidance, demonstration, practice, and feedback, resulting in the acquisition of behaviors that will support community living.

somatization disorder A somatoform disorder characterized by multiple physical complaints with no evidence of organic impairment.

somatoform disorder A category of psychophysiological disruptions with no evidence of organic impairment.

splitting Viewing people and situations as either all good or all bad. Failure to integrate the positive and negative qualities of oneself and of objects.

steady state Exists when the body has reached a state of drug level equilibrium: a drug has been taken long enough that the amount of drug excreted equals the amount ingested. This occurs in approximately four to six half-lives.

stereotype A depersonalized conception of individuals within a group.

stigma An attribute or trait deemed by the person's social environment as different and diminishing.

sublimation Acceptance of a socially approved substitute goal for a drive whose normal channel of expression is blocked.

substance abuse The use of any mind-altering agent to such an extent that it interferes with the person's biological, psychological, or sociocultural integrity.

substance dependence A severe condition of addictive behaviors often resulting in physical problems as well as serious disruptions of work, family life, and social life; usually considered a disease.

subsystems Smaller components of the larger system composed of individuals or dyads, formed by generation, gender, interest, or function.

suicide Self-inflicted death.

suicide attempt A deliberate action that, if carried to completion, will result in death.

suicide gesture A suicide attempt that is planned to be discovered in an attempt to influence the behavior of others.

suicide threat A warning, direct or indirect, verbal or nonverbal, that the person plans to attempt suicide.

sundown syndrome Cognitive ability diminishing in the late afternoon or early evening.

sunrise syndrome Unstable cognitive ability upon rising in the morning.

supervision Guidance provided through a mentoring relationship between one nurse and a more experienced, skilled, and educated nurse.

suppression A process that is the conscious analogy of repression. It is the intentional exclusion of material from consciousness.

synapse The gap between the membrane of one neuron and the membrane of another. The synapse is the point at which the transmission of nerve impulses occurs.

systematic desensitization Designed to decrease avoidance behavior linked to a specific stimulus by helping the patient change the response to a threatening stimulus.

T

tardive dyskinesia Literally, "late-appearing abnormal movements," a variable complex of choreiform or athetoid movements developing in patients exposed to antipsychotic drugs. Typical movements include tongue writhing or protrusion, chewing, lip puckering, choreiform finger movements, toe and ankle movements, leg jiggling, and movements of neck, trunk, and pelvis.

target symptoms Symptoms of an illness that are most likely to respond to a specific treatment, such as a particular psychopharmacological drug.

tertiary prevention Rehabilitative measures designed to reduce the severity, disability, or residual impairment resulting from illness.

testamentary capacity Competency to make a will, which requires that people know they are making a will, the nature and extent of their property, and who their friends and relatives are.

testimonial privilege A term used in court-related proceedings to refer to the communication between two parties. The right to reveal information belongs to the person who spoke, and the listener cannot disclose the information unless the speaker gives permission. This includes communication between husband and wife, attorney and client, and clergy and church member.

themes Underlying issues or problems experienced by the patient that emerge repeatedly during the course of the nurse-patient relationship.

therapeutic community The inpatient environment described as a community with cultural norms for behaviors, values, and activity.

therapeutic impasses Roadblocks in the progress of the nurse-patient relationship. They arise for a variety of reasons and may take different forms, but they all create stalls in the therapeutic relationship.

therapeutic milieu The controlled environment of treatment facilities that shelters patients from what they perceive to be painful and frightening stressors, thus providing patients with a stable and coherent social environment that facilitates the development and implementation of treatment.

therapeutic nurse-patient relationship A mutual learning experience and corrective emotional experience for the patient in which the nurse uses self and specified clinical techniques in working with the patient to bring about behavioral change.

therapeutic touch The nurse's laying of hands on or close to the body of an ill person for the purpose of helping or healing.

thought blocking Sudden stopping in the train of thought or in the midst of a sentence.

thought stopping Teaching a patient to interrupt dysfunctional thoughts.

time-out Short-term removal of the patient from overstimulating and sometimes reinforcing situations.

token economy A form of positive reinforcement in which patients are rewarded with tokens for performing desired target behaviors.

tolerance A characteristic of drug addiction that refers to the progressive need for more of the abused substance to achieve the desired effect.

transactional analysis A model of communication developed by Eric Berne that consists of the study of the communication or transactions between people and the sometimes unconscious and destructive ways ("games") in which people relate to each other.

transference An unconscious response of patients in which they experience feelings and attitudes toward the nurse that were originally associated with significant figures in their early life.

transsexual A person who is anatomically a male or female but who expresses, with strong conviction, that he or she has the mind of the opposite sex, lives as a member of the opposite sex part-time or full-time, and seeks to change his or her sex legally and through hormonal and surgical sex reassignment.

transvestism Condition in which a male (less often a female) has a sexual obsession for or addiction to women's (men's) clothes.

triangle A predictable emotional process that takes place when there is difficulty in a relationship. Triangles represent dysfunctional efforts to reduce fusion or conflict in a relationship. The three corners of a triangle can be composed of three people, or two people and an object, group, or issue.

U

undoing An act or communication that partially negates a previous one.

unidisciplinary team A team with members of the same discipline.

utilization review A three-part process intended to ensure that resources are appropriately used. It includes a review of the initial request to hospitalize the patient, the length of the patient's stay, and a retrospective review after discharge.

V

vaginismus Recurrent or persistent involuntary spasm of the musculature of the outer third of the vagina that interferes with coitus.

validation Reflection of the content of the patient's communication back to the patient.

value clarification A method whereby a person can assess, explore, and determine personal values and what priority they hold in personal decision making.

values The concepts that a person holds worthy in personal life. They are formed as a result of one's life experiences with family, friends, culture, education, work, and relaxation.

visualization The conscious programming of desired change with positive images.

vocal communication Written or spoken transmission of a message.

vocal cues A category of nonverbal communication that includes all the noises and sounds other than speech. They are sometimes called paralinguistic cues.

voyeurism Intense sexual arousal or desire and acts, fantasies, or other stimuli involving the observation of unsuspecting people who are naked, in the act of disrobing, or engaging in sexual activity.

W

wife abuse Includes all forms of physical violence toward a female partner in an ongoing intimate relationship, as well as emotional degradation and intimidation.

word salad Series of words that seem totally unrelated.

DSM-IV Classification*

NOS = not otherwise specified.

An *x* appearing in a diagnostic code indicates that a specific code number is required.

An ellipsis (. . .) is used in the names of certain disorders to indicate that the name of a specific mental disorder or general medical condition should be inserted when recording the name (e.g., 293.0 Delirium Due to Hypothyroidism).

If criteria are currently met, one of the following severity specifiers may be noted after the diagnosis:
Mild
Moderate
Severe

If criteria are no longer met, one of the following specifiers may be noted:
In Partial Remission
In Full Remission
Prior History

Disorders Usually First Diagnosed in Infancy, Childhood, or Adolescence

MENTAL RETARDATION

Note: These are coded on Axis II.

317	Mild Mental Retardation
318.0	Moderate Retardation
318.1	Severe Mental Retardation
318.2	Profound Mental Retardation
319	Mental Retardation, Severity Unspecified

LEARNING DISORDERS

315.00	Reading Disorder
315.1	Mathematics Disorder
315.2	Disorder of Written Expression
315.9	Learning Disorder NOS

MOTOR SKILLS DISORDER

315.4	Developmental Coordination Disorder

COMMUNICATION DISORDERS

315.31	Expressive Language Disorder
315.31	Mixed Receptive-Expressive Language Disorder
315.39	Phonological Disorder
307.0	Stuttering
307.9	Communication Disorder NOS

PERVASIVE DEVELOPMENTAL DISORDERS

299.00	Autistic Disorder
299.80	Rett's Disorder
299.10	Childhood Disintegrative Disorder
299.80	Asperger's Disorder
299.80	Pervasive Developmental Disorder NOS

ATTENTION-DEFICIT AND DISRUPTIVE BEHAVIOR DISORDERS

314.xx	Attention-Deficit/Hyperactivity Disorder
.01	Combined Type
.00	Predominantly Inattentive Type
.01	Predominantly Hyperactive-Impulsive Type
314.9	Attention-Deficit/Hyperactivity Disorder NOS
312.8	Conduct Disorder *Specify type:* Childhood-Onset Type/Adolescent-Onset Type
313.81	Oppositional Defiant Disorder
312.9	Disruptive Behavior Disorder NOS

FEEDING AND EATING DISORDERS OF INFANCY OR EARLY CHILDHOOD

307.52	Pica
307.53	Rumination Disorder
307.59	Feeding Disorder of Infancy or Early Childhood

TIC DISORDERS

307.23	Tourette's Disorder
307.22	Chronic Motor or Vocal Tic Disorder
307.21	Transient Tic Disorder *Specify if:* Single Episode/Recurrent
307.20	Tic Disorder NOS

ELIMINATION DISORDERS

___.__	Encopresis
787.6	With Constipation and Overflow Incontinence
307.7	Without Constipation and Overflow Incontinence

*Reprinted with permission from the American Psychiatric Association: *Diagnostic and statistical manual of mental disorders*, ed 4, Washington, DC, 1994, American Psychiatric Association.

307.6   Enuresis (Not Due to a General Medical Condition)
Specify type: Nocturnal Only/Diurnal Only/ Nocturnal and Diurnal

OTHER DISORDERS OF INFANCY, CHILDHOOD, OR ADOLESCENCE

309.21   Separation Anxiety Disorder
Specify if: Early Onset

313.23   Selective Mutism

313.89   Reactive Attachment Disorder of Infancy or Early Childhood
Specify type: Inhibited Type/Disinhibited Type

307.3   Stereotypic Movement Disorder
Specify if: With Self-Injurious Behavior

313.9   Disorder of Infancy, Childhood, or Adolescence NOS

Delirium, Dementia, and Amnestic and Other Cognitive Disorders

DELIRIUM

293.0   Delirium Due to . . . *[Indicate the General Medical Condition]*

___.___   Substance Intoxication Delirium *(refer to Substance-Related Disorders for substance-specific codes)*

___.___   Substance Withdrawal Delirium *(refer to Substance-Related Disorders for substance-specific codes)*

___.___   Delirium Due to Multiple Etiologies *(code each of the specific etiologies)*

780.09   Delirium NOS

DEMENTIA

290.xx   Dementia of the Alzheimer's Type, with Early Onset *(also code 331.0 Alzheimer's disease on Axis III)*

.10   Uncomplicated

.11   With Delirium

.12   With Delusions

.13   With Depressed Mood
Specify if: With Behavioral Disturbance

290.xx   Dementia of the Alzheimer's Type, with Late Onset *(also code 331.0 Alzheimer's disease on Axis III)*

.0   Uncomplicated

.3   With Delirium

.20   With Delusions

.21   With Depressed Mood
Specify if: With Behavioral Disturbance

290.xx   Vascular Dementia

.40   Uncomplicated

.41   With Delirium

.42   With Delusions

.43   With Depressed Mood
Specify if: With Behavioral Disturbance

294.9   Dementia Due to HIV Disease *(also code 043.1 HIV infection affecting central nervous system on Axis III)*

294.1   Dementia Due to Head Trauma *(also code 854.00 head injury on Axis III)*

294.1   Dementia Due to Parkinson's Disease *(also code 332.0 Parkinson's disease on Axis III)*

294.1   Dementia Due to Huntington's Disease *(also code 333.4 Huntington's disease on Axis III)*

290.10   Dementia Due to Pick's Disease *(also code 331.1 Pick's disease on Axis III)*

290.10   Dementia Due to Creutzfeldt-Jakob Disease *(also code 046.1 Creutzfeldt-Jakob disease on Axis III)*

294.1   Dementia Due to . . . *[Indicate the General Medical Condition not listed above] (also code the general medical condition on Axis III)*

___.___   Substance-Induced Persisting Dementia *(refer to Substance-Related Disorders for substance-specific codes)*

___.___   Dementia Due to Multiple Etiologies *(code each of the specific etiologies)*

294.8   Dementia NOS

AMNESTIC DISORDERS

294.0   Amnestic Disorder Due to . . . *[Indicate the General Medical Condition]*
Specify if: Transient/Chronic

___.___   Substance-Induced Persisting Amnestic Disorder *(refer to Substance-Related Disorders for substance-specific codes)*

294.8   Amnestic Disorder NOS

OTHER COGNITIVE DISORDERS

294.9   Cognitive Disorder NOS

Mental Disorders Due to a General Medical Condition Not Elsewhere Classified

293.89   Catatonic Disorder Due to . . . *[Indicate the General Medical Condition]*

310.1   Personality Change Due to . . . *[Indicate the General Medical Condition]*
Specify type: Labile Type/Disinhibited Type/ Aggressive Type/Apathetic Type/Paranoid Type/Other Type/Combined Type/ Unspecified Type

293.9   Mental Disorder NOS Due to . . . *[Indicate the General Medical Condition]*

Substance-Related Disorders

[a]*The following specifiers may be applied to Substance Dependence:*

With Physiological Dependence/Without Physiological Dependence

Early Full Remission/Early Partial Remission

Sustained Full Remission/Sustained Partial Remission

On Agonist Therapy/In a Controlled Environment

The following specifiers apply to Substance-Induced Disorders as noted:

[I]With Onset During Intoxication/[W]With Onset During Withdrawal

ALCOHOL-RELATED DISORDERS

Alcohol Use Disorders

303.90   Alcohol Dependence[a]

305.00   Alcohol Abuse

Alcohol-Induced Disorders

303.00   Alcohol Intoxication

291.8   Alcohol Withdrawal
Specify if: With Perceptual Disturbances

291.0   Alcohol Intoxication Delirium

291.0   Alcohol Withdrawal Delirium

291.2   Alcohol-Induced Persisting Dementia

291.1   Alcohol-Induced Persisting Amnestic Disorder

291.x   Alcohol-Induced Psychotic Disorder
    .5   With Delusions[I,W]
    .3   With Hallucinations[I,W]

291.8   Alcohol-Induced Mood Disorder[I,W]

291.8   Alcohol-Induced Anxiety Disorder[I,W]

291.8   Alcohol-Induced Sexual Dysfunction[I]

291.8   Alcohol-Induced Sleep Disorder[I,W]

291.9   Alcohol-Related Disorder NOS

AMPHETAMINE (OR AMPHETAMINE-LIKE)-RELATED DISORDERS

Amphetamine Use Disorders

304.40   Amphetamine Dependence[a]

305.70   Amphetamine Abuse

Amphetamine-Induced Disorders

292.89   Amphetamine Intoxication
Specify if: With Perceptual Disturbances

292.0   Amphetamine Withdrawal

292.81   Amphetamine Intoxication Delirium

292.xx   Amphetamine-Induced Psychotic Disorder
    .11   With Delusions[I]
    .12   With Hallucinations[I]

292.84   Amphetamine-Induced Mood Disorder[I,W]

292.89   Amphetamine-Induced Anxiety Disorder[I]

292.89   Amphetamine-Induced Sexual Dysfunction[I]

292.89   Amphetamine-Induced Sleep Disorder[I,W]

292.9   Amphetamine-Related Disorder NOS

CAFFEINE-RELATED DISORDERS

Caffeine-Induced Disorders

305.90   Caffeine Intoxication

292.89   Caffeine-Induced Anxiety Disorder[I]

292.89   Caffeine-Induced Sleep Disorder[I]

292.9   Caffeine-Related Disorder NOS

CANNABIS-RELATED DISORDERS

Cannabis Use Disorders

304.30   Cannabis Dependence[a]

305.20   Cannabis Abuse

Cannabis-Induced Disorders

292.89   Cannabis Intoxication
Specify if: With Perceptual Disturbances

292.81   Cannabis Intoxication Delirium

292.xx   Cannabis-Induced Psychotic Disorder
    .11   With Delusions[I]
    .12   With Hallucinations[I]

292.89   Cannabis-Induced Anxiety Disorder[I]

292.9   Cannabis-Related Disorder NOS

COCAINE-RELATED DISORDERS

Cocaine Use Disorders

304.20   Cocaine Dependence[a]

305.60   Cocaine Abuse

Cocaine-Induced Disorders

292.89   Cocaine Intoxication
Specify if: With Perceptual Disturbances

292.0   Cocaine Withdrawal

292.81   Cocaine Intoxication Delirium

292.xx   Cocaine-Induced Psychotic Disorder
    .11   With Delusions[I]
    .12   With Hallucinations[I]

292.84   Cocaine-Induced Mood Disorder[I,W]

292.89   Cocaine-Induced Anxiety Disorder[I,W]

292.89   Cocaine-Induced Sexual Dysfunction[I]

292.89   Cocaine-Induced Sleep Disorder[I,W]

292.9   Cocaine-Related Disorder NOS

HALLUCINOGEN-RELATED DISORDERS

Hallucinogen Use Disorders

304.50   Hallucinogen Dependence[a]

305.30   Hallucinogen Abuse

Hallucinogen-Induced Disorders

292.89   Hallucinogen Intoxication

292.89   Hallucinogen Persisting Perception Disorder
          (Flashbacks)

292.81   Hallucinogen Intoxication Delirium

292.xx   Hallucinogen-Induced Psychotic Disorder

.11   With Delusions[I]

.12   With Hallucinations[I]

292.84   Hallucinogen-Induced Mood Disorder[I]

292.89   Hallucinogen-Induced Anxiety Disorder[I]

292.9   Hallucinogen-Related Disorder NOS

INHALANT-RELATED DISORDERS

Inhalant Use Disorders

304.60   Inhalant Dependence[a]

305.90   Inhalant Abuse

Inhalant-Induced Disorders

292.89   Inhalant Intoxication

292.81   Inhalant Intoxication Delirium

292.82   Inhalant-Induced Persisting Dementia

292.xx   Inhalant-Induced Psychotic Disorder

.11   With Delusions[I]

.12   With Hallucinations[I]

292.84   Inhalant-Induced Mood Disorder[I]

292.89   Inhalant-Induced Anxiety Disorder[I]

292.9   Inhalant-Related Disorder NOS

NICOTINE-RELATED DISORDERS

Nicotine Use Disorder

305.10   Nicotine Dependence[a]

Nicotine-Induced Disorder

292.0   Nicotine Withdrawal

292.9   Nicotine-Related Disorder NOS

OPIOID-RELATED DISORDERS

Opioid Use Disorders

304.00   Opioid Dependence[a]

305.50   Opioid Abuse

Opioid-Induced Disorders

292.89   Opioid Intoxication
          Specify if: With Perceptual Disturbances

292.0   Opioid Withdrawal

292.81   Opioid Intoxication Delirium

292.xx   Opioid-Induced Psychotic Disorder

.11   With Delusions[I]

.12   With Hallucinations[I]

292.84   Opioid-Induced Mood Disorder[I]

292.89   Opioid-Induced Sexual Dysfunction[I]

292.89   Opioid-Induced Sleep Disorder[I,W]

292.9   Opioid-Related Disorder NOS

PHENCYCLIDINE (OR PHENCYCLIDINE-LIKE)-RELATED DISORDERS

Phencyclidine Use Disorders

304.90   Phencyclidine Dependence[a]

305.90   Phencyclidine Abuse

Phencyclidine-Induced Disorders

292.89   Phencyclidine Intoxication
          Specify if: With Perceptual Disturbances

292.81   Phencyclidine Intoxication Delirium

292.xx   Phencyclidine-Induced Psychotic Disorder

.11   With Delusions[I]

.12   With Hallucinations[I]

292.84   Phencyclidine-Induced Mood Disorder[I]

292.89   Phencyclidine-Induced Anxiety Disorder[I]

292.9   Phencyclidine-Related Disorder NOS

SEDATIVE-, HYPNOTIC-, OR ANXIOLYTIC-RELATED DISORDERS

Sedative, Hypnotic, or Anxiolytic Use Disorders

304.10   Sedative, Hypnotic, or Anxiolytic Dependence[a]

305.40   Sedative, Hypnotic, or Anxiolytic Abuse

Sedative-, Hypnotic-, or Anxiolytic-Induced Disorders

292.89   Sedative, Hypnotic, or Anxiolytic Intoxication

292.0   Sedative, Hypnotic, or Anxiolytic Withdrawal
          Specify if: With Perceptual Disturbances

292.81   Sedative, Hypnotic, or Anxiolytic Intoxication
          Delirium

292.81   Sedative, Hypnotic, or Anxiolytic Withdrawal
          Delirium

292.82   Sedative-, Hypnotic-, or Anxiolytic-Induced
          Persisting Dementia

292.83   Sedative-, Hypnotic-, or Anxiolytic-Induced
          Persisting Amnestic Disorder

292.xx   Sedative-, Hypnotic-, or Anxiolytic-Induced
          Psychotic Disorder

.11   With Delusions[I,W]

.12   With Hallucinations[I,W]

292.84   Sedative-, Hypnotic-, or Anxiolytic-Induced
          Mood Disorder[I,W]

292.89   Sedative-, Hypnotic-, or Anxiolytic-Induced
          Anxiety Disorder[W]

292.89   Sedative-, Hypnotic-, or Anxiolytic-Induced
          Sexual Dysfunction[I]

292.89   Sedative-, Hypnotic-, or Anxiolytic-Induced
          Sleep Disorder[I,W]

292.9   Sedative-, Hypnotic-, or Anxiolytic-Related
          Disorder NOS

POLYSUBSTANCE-RELATED DISORDER

304.80   Polysubstance Dependence[a]

OTHER (OR UNKNOWN) SUBTANCE-RELATED DISORDERS

Other (or Unknown) Substance Use Disorders

304.90 Other (or Unknown) Substance Dependence[a]

305.90 Other (or Unknown) Substance Abuse

OTHER (OR UNKNOWN) SUBSTANCE-INDUCED DISORDERS

292.89 Other (or Unknown) Substance Intoxication
Specify if: With Perceptual Disturbances

292.0 Other (or Unknown) Substance Withdrawal
Specify if: With Perceptual Disturbances

292.81 Other (or Unknown) Substance-Induced Delirium

292.82 Other (or Unknown) Substance-Induced Persisting Dementia

292.83 Other (or Unknown) Substance-Induced Persisting Amnestic Disorder

292.xx Other (or Unknown) Substance-Induced Psychotic Disorder

  .11 With Delusions[I,W]

  .12 With Hallucinations[I,W]

292.84 Other (or Unknown) Substance-Induced Mood Disorder[I,W]

292.89 Other (or Unknown) Substance-Induced Anxiety Disorder[I,W]

292.89 Other (or Unknown) Substance-Induced Sexual Dysfunction[I]

292.89 Other (or Unknown) Substance-Induced Sleep Disorder[I,W]

292.9 Other (or Unknown) Substance-Related Disorder NOS

Schizophrenia and Other Psychotic Disorders

295.xx Schizophrenia

The following Classification of Longitudinal Course applies to all subtypes of Schizophrenia:

Episodic with Interepisode Residual Symptoms (*specify if:* With Prominent Negative Symptoms)/Episodic with No Interepisode Residual Symptoms/Continuous (*Specify if:* With Prominent Negative Symptoms)

Single Episode in Partial Remission (*specify if:* With Prominent Negative Symptoms)/Single Episode in Full Remission

Other or Unspecified Pattern

  .30 Paranoid Type

  .10 Disorganized Type

  .20 Catatonic Type

  .90 Undifferentiated Type

  .60 Residual Type

295.40 Schizophreniform Disorder
Specify if: Without Good Prognostic Features/With Good Prognostic Features

295.70 Schizoaffective Disorder
Specify type: Bipolar Type/Depressive Type

297.1 Delusional Disorder
Specify type: Erotomanic Type/Grandiose Type/Jealous Type/Persecutory Type/Somatic Type/Mixed Type/Unspecified Type

298.8 Brief Psychotic Disorder
Specify if: With Marked Stressor(s)/Without Marked Stressor(s)/With Postpartum Onset

297.3 Shared Psychotic Disorder

293.xx Psychotic Disorder Due to . . . *[Indicate the General Medical Condition]*

  .81 With Delusions

  .82 With Hallucinations

___.___ Substance-Induced Psychotic Disorder *(refer to Substance-Related Disorders for substance-specific codes)*
Specify if: With Onset during Intoxication/With Onset during Withdrawal

298.9 Psychotic Disorder NOS

Mood Disorders

Code current state of Major Depressive Disorder or Bipolar I Disorder in fifth digit:

1 = Mild

2 = Moderate

3 = Severe without Psychotic Features

4 = Severe with Psychotic Features

  Specify: Mood-Congruent Psychotic Features/Mood-Incongruent Psychotic Features

5 = In Partial Remission

6 = In Full Remission

0 = Unspecified

The following specifiers apply (for current or most recent episode) to Mood Disorders as noted:
[a]Severity/Psychotic/Remission Specifiers
[b]Chronic
[c]With Catatonic Features
[d]With Melancholic Features
[e]With Atypical Features
[f]With Postpartum Onset

The following specifiers apply to Mood Disorders as noted:
[g]With or without Full Interepisode Recovery
[h]With Seasonal Pattern
[i]With Rapid Cycling

DEPRESSIVE DISORDERS

296.xx Major Depressive Disorder,

  .2x Single Episode[a,b,c,d,e,f]

  .3x Recurrent[a,b,c,d,e,f,g,h]

300.4   Dysthymic Disorder
        Specify if: Early Onset/Late Onset
        Specify: With Atypical Features

311   Depressive Disorder NOS

BIPOLAR DISORDERS

296.xx   Bipolar I Disorder,
  .0x   Single Manic Episode[a,c,f]
        Specify if: Mixed
  .40   Most Recent Episode Hypomanic[g,h,i]
  .4x   Most Recent Episode Manic[a,c,f,g,h,i]
  .6x   Most Recent Episode Mixed[a,c,f,g,h,i]
  .5x   Most Recent Episode Depressed[a,b,c,d,e,f,g,h,i]
  .7   Most Recent Episode Unspecified[g,h,i]

296.89   Bipolar II Disorder[a,b,c,d,e,f,g,h,i]
        Specify (current or most recent episode):
        Hypomanic/Depressed

301.13   Cyclothymic Disorder

296.80   Bipolar Disorder NOS

293.83   Mood Disorder Due to . . . *[Indicate the
        General Medical Condition]*
        Specify type: With Depressive Features/With
        Major Depressive-Like Episode/With Manic
        Features/With Mixed Features

___.___   Substance-Induced Mood Disorder *(refer to
        Substance-Related Disorders for substance-
        specfic codes)*
        Specify type: With Depressive Features/With
        Manic Features/With Mixed Features
        Specify if: With Onset During Intoxication/
        With Onset During Withdrawal

296.90   Mood Disorder NOS

Anxiety Disorders

300.01   Panic Disorder without Agoraphobia

300.21   Panic Disorder with Agoraphobia

300.22   Agoraphobia without History of Panic
        Disorder

300.29   Specific Phobia
        Specify type: Animal Type/Natural
        Environment Type/Blood-Injection-Injury
        Type/Situational Type/Other Type

300.23   Social Phobia
        Specify if: Generalized

300.3   Obsessive-Compulsive Disorder
        Specify if: With Poor Insight

309.81   Post-traumatic Stress Disorder
        Specify if: Acute/Chronic
        Specify if: With Delayed Onset

308.3   Acute Stress Disorder

300.02   Generalized Anxiety Disorder

293.89   Anxiety Disorder Due to . . . *[Indicate the
        General Medical Condition]*
        Specify if: With Generalized Anxiety/With
        Panic Attacks/With Obsessive-Compulsive
        Symptoms

___.___   Substance-Induced Anxiety Disorder
        *(refer to Substance-Related Disorders
        for substance-specific codes)*
        Specify if: With Generalized Anxiety/With
        Panic Attacks/With Obsessive-Compulsive
        Symptoms/With Phobic Symptoms
        Specify if: With Onset During Intoxication/
        With Onset During Withdrawal

300.00   Anxiety Disorder NOS

Somatoform Disorders

300.81   Somatization Disorder

300.81   Undifferentiated Somatoform Disorder

300.11   Conversion Disorder
        Specify type: With Motor Symptom or Deficit/
        With Sensory Symptom or Deficit/With
        Seizures or Convulsions/With Mixed
        Presentation

307.xx   Pain Disorder
  .80   Associated with Psychologic Factors
  .89   Associated with Both Psychologic Factors
        and a General Medical Condition
        Specify if: Acute/Chronic

300.7   Hypochondriasis
        Specify if: With Poor Insight

300.7   Body Dysmorphic Disorder

300.81   Somatoform Disorder NOS

Factitious Disorders

300.xx   Factitious Disorder
  .16   With Predominantly Psychological Signs
        and Symptoms
  .19   With Predominantly Physical Signs and
        Symptoms
  .19   With Combined Psychological and Physical
        Signs and Symptoms

300.19   Factitious Disorder NOS

Dissociative Disorders

300.12   Dissociative Amnesia

300.13   Dissociative Fugue

300.14   Dissociative Identity Disorder

300.6   Depersonalization Disorder

300.15   Dissociative Disorder NOS

Sexual and Gender Identity Disorders

SEXUAL DYSFUNCTIONS

The following specifiers apply to all primary Sexual Dysfunctions:

Lifelong Type
Acquired Type
Generalized Type
Situational Type Due to Psychologic Factors
Due to Combined Factors

Sexual Desire Disorders

302.71   Hypoactive Sexual Desire Disorder

302.79   Sexual Aversion Disorder

Sexual Arousal Disorders

302.72   Female Sexual Arousal Disorder

302.72   Male Erectile Disorder

Orgasmic Disorders

302.73   Female Orgasmic Disorder

302.74   Male Orgasmic Disorder

302.75   Premature Ejaculation

Sexual Pain Disorders

302.76   Dyspareunia (Not Due to a General Medical Condition)

306.51   Vaginismus (Not Due to a General Medical Condition)

Sexual Dysfunction Due to a General Medical Condition

625.8   Female Hypoactive Sexual Desire Disorder Due to . . . *[Indicate the General Medical Condition]*

608.89   Male Hypoactive Sexual Desire Disorder Due to . . . *[Indicate the General Medical Condition]*

607.84   Male Erectile Disorder Due to . . . *[Indicate the General Medical Condition]*

625.0   Female Dyspareunia Due to . . . *[Indicate the General Medical Condition]*

608.89   Male Dyspareunia Due to . . . *[Indicate the General Medical Condition]*

625.8   Other Female Sexual Dysfunction Due to . . . *[Indicate the General Medical Condition]*

608.89   Other Male Sexual Dysfunction Due to . . . *[Indicate the General Medical Condition]*

___._   Substance-Induced Sexual Dysfunction *(refer to Substance-Related Disorders for substance-specific codes)*
Specify if: With Impaired Desired/With Impaired Arousal/With Impaired Orgasm/With Sexual Pain
Specify if: With Onset During Intoxication

302.70   Sexual Dysfunction NOS

PARAPHILIAS

302.4   Exhibitionism

302.81   Fetishism

302.89   Frotteurism

302.2   Pedophilia
Specify if: Sexually Attracted to Males/Sexually Attracted to Females/Sexually Attracted to Both
Specify if: Limited to Incest
Specify type: Exclusive Type/Nonexclusive Type

302.83   Sexual Masochism

302.84   Sexual Sadism

302.3   Transvestic Fetishism
Specify if: With Gender Dysphoria

302.82   Voyeurism

302.9   Paraphilia NOS

GENDER IDENTITY DISORDERS

302.xx   Gender Identity Disorder

   .6   in Children

   .85   in Adolescents or Adults
Specify if: Sexually Attracted to Males/Sexually Attracted to Females/Sexually Attracted to Both/Sexually Attracted to Neither

302.6   Gender Identity Disorder NOS

302.9   Sexual Disorder NOS

Eating Disorders

307.1   Anorexia Nervosa
Specify type: Restricting Type; Binge-Eating/Purging Type

307.51   Bulimia Nervosa
Specify type: Purging Type/Nonpurging Type

307.50   Eating Disorder NOS

Sleep Disorders

PRIMARY SLEEP DISORDERS

Dyssomnias

307.42   Primary Insomnia

307.44   Primary Hypersomnia
Specify if: Recurrent

347   Narcolepsy

780.59   Breathing-Related Sleep Disorder

307.45   Circadian Rhythm Sleep Disorder
Specify type: Delayed Sleep Phase Type/Jet Lag Type/Shift Work Type/Unspecified Type

307.47   Dyssomnia NOS

Parasomnias

307.47   Nightmare Disorder

307.46   Sleep Terror Disorder

307.46   Sleepwalking Disorder

307.47   Parasomnia NOS

SLEEP DISORDERS RELATED TO ANOTHER MENTAL DISORDER

307.42 Insomnia Related to . . . *[Indicate the Axis I or Axis II Disorder]*

307.44 Hypersomnia Related to . . . *[Indicate the Axis I or Axis II Disorder]*

OTHER SLEEP DISORDERS

780.xx Sleep Disorder Due to . . . *[Indicate the General Medical Condition]*

.52 Insomnia Type

.54 Hypersomnia Type

.59 Parasomnia Type

.59 Mixed type

___.__ Substance-Induced Sleep Disorder *(refer to Substance-Related Disorders for substance-specific codes)*
Specify type: Insomnia Type/Hypersomnia Type/Parasomnia Type/Mixed Type
Specify if: With Onset During Intoxication/ With Onset During Withdrawal

Impulse-Control Disorders Not Elsewhere Classified

312.34 Intermittent Explosive Disorder

312.32 Kleptomania

312.33 Pyromania

312.31 Pathological Gambling

312.39 Trichotillomania

312.30 Impulse-Control Disorder NOS

ADJUSTMENT DISORDERS

309.xx Adjustment Disorder

.0 With Depressed Mood

.24 With Anxiety

.28 With Mixed Anxiety and Depressed Mood

.3 With Disturbance of Conduct

.4 With Mixed Disturbance of Emotions and Conduct

.9 Unspecified
Specify if: Acute/Chronic

Personality Disorders

Note: These are coded on Axis II.

301.0 Paranoid Personality Disorder

301.20 Schizoid Personality Disorder

301.22 Schizotypal Personality Disorder

301.7 Antisocial Personality Disorder

301.83 Borderline Personality Disorder

301.50 Histrionic Personality Disorder

301.81 Narcissistic Personality Disorder

301.82 Avoidant Personality Disorder

301.6 Dependent Personality Disorder

301.4 Obsessive-Compulsive Personality Disorder

301.9 Personality Disorder NOS

Other Conditions That May Be a Focus of Clinical Attention

PSYCHOLOGICAL FACTORS AFFECTING MEDICAL CONDITION

316 . . . *[Specified Psychologic Factor]* Affecting . . . *[Indicate the General Medical Condition]*
Choose name based on nature of factors:
Mental Disorder Affecting Medical Condition
Psychologic Symptoms Affecting Medical Condition
Personality Traits or Coping Style Affecting Medical Condition
Maladaptive Health Behaviors Affecting Medical Condition
Stress-Related Physiologic Response Affecting Medical Condition
Other or Unspecified Psychologic Factors Affecting Medical Condition

MEDICATION-INDUCED MOVEMENT DISORDERS

332.1 Neuroleptic-Induced Parkinsonism

333.92 Neuroleptic Malignant Syndrome

333.7 Neuroleptic-Induced Acute Dystonia

333.99 Neuroleptic-Induced Acute Akathisia

333.82 Neuroleptic-Induced Tardive Dyskinesia

333.1 Medication-Induced Postural Tremor

333.90 Medication-Induced Movement Disorder NOS

OTHER MEDICATION-INDUCED DISORDER

995.2 Adverse Effects of Medication NOS

RELATIONAL PROBLEMS

V61.9 Relational Problem Related to a Mental Disorder or General Medical Condition

V61.20 Parent-Child Relational Problem

V61.1 Partner Relational Problem

V61.8 Sibling Relational Problem

V62.81 Relational Problem NOS

PROBLEMS RELATED TO ABUSE OR NEGLECT

V61.21 Physical Abuse of Child *(code 995.5 if focus of attention is on victim)*

V61.21 Sexual Abuse of Child *(code 995.5 if focus of attention is on victim)*

V61.21 Neglect of Child *(code 995.5 if focus of attention is on victim)*

V61.1 Physical Abuse of Adult *(code 995.81 if focus of attention is on victim)*

V61.1 Sexual Abuse of Adult (*code 995.81 if focus of attention is on victim*)

ADDITIONAL CONDITIONS THAT MAY BE A FOCUS OF CLINICAL ATTENTION

V15.81 Noncompliance with Treatment

V65.2 Malingering

V71.01 Adult Antisocial Behavior

V71.02 Child or Adolescent Antisocial Behavior

V62.89 Borderline Intellectual Functioning
Note: This is coded on Axis II.

780.9 Age-Related Cognitive Decline

V62.82 Bereavement

V62.3 Academic Problem

V62.2 Occupational Problem

313.82 Identity Problem

V62.89 Religious or Spiritual Problem

V62.4 Acculturation Problem

V62.89 Phase of Life Problem

Additional Codes

300.9 Unspecified Mental Disorder (nonpsychotic)

V71.09 No Diagnosis or Condition on Axis I

799.9 Diagnosis or Condition Deferred on Axis I

V71.09 No Diagnosis on Axis II

799.9 Diagnosis Deferred on Axis II

Axis II: Personality Disorders

301.0 Paranoid Personality Disorder

301.20 Schizoid Personality Disorder

301.22 Schizotypal Personality Disorder

301.7 Antisocial Personality Disorder

301.83 Borderline Personality Disorder

301.50 Histrionic Personality Disorder

301.81 Narcissistic Personality Disorder

301.82 Avoidant Personality Disorder

301.6 Dependent Personality Disorder

301.4 Obsessive-Compulsive Personality Disorder

301.9 Personality Disorder NOS

Axis III: ICD-9-CM General Medical Conditions

Infectious and Parasitic Diseases (001-139)

Neoplasms (140-239)

Endocrine, Nutritional, and Metabolic Diseases and Immunity Disorders (240-279)

Diseases of the Blood and Blood-Forming Organs (280-289)

Diseases of the Nervous and Sense Organs (320-389)

Diseases of the Circulatory System (390-459)

Diseases of the Respiratory System (460-519)

Diseases of the Digestive System (520-579)

Diseases of the Genitourinary System (580-629)

Complications of Pregnancy, Childbirth, and the Puerperium (630-676)

Diseases of the Skin and Subcutaneous Tissue (680-709)

Diseases of the Musculoskeletal System and Connective Tissue (710-739)

Congenital Anomalies (740-759)

Certain Conditions Originating in the Perinatal Period (760-779)

Symptoms, Signs, and Ill-Defined Conditions (780-799)

Injury and Poisoning (800-999)

Axis IV: Psychosocial and Environmental Problems

Problems with Primary Support Group (Childhood [V61.9], Adult [V61.9], Parent-Child [V61.2]). These include death of a family member; health problems in family; disruption of family by separation, divorce, or estrangement; removal from the home; remarriage of parent; sexual or physical abuse; parental overprotection; neglect of child; inadequate discipline; discord with siblings; birth of a sibling.

Problems Related to the Social Environment (V62.4). These include death or loss of friend, social isolation, living alone, difficulty with acculturation, discrimination, adjustment to life cycle transition (e.g., retirement).

Educational Problems (V62.3). These include illiteracy, academic problems, discord with teachers or classmates, inadequate school environment.

Occupational Problems (V62.2). These include unemployment, threat of job loss, stressful work schedule, difficult work conditions, job dissatisfaction, job change, discord with boss or coworkers.

Housing Problems (V60.9). These include homelessness, inadequate housing, unsafe neighborhood, discord with neighbors or landlord.

Economic Problems (V60.9). These include extreme poverty, inadequate finances, insufficient welfare support.

Problems with Access to Health Care Services (V63.9). These include inadequate health care services, transportation to health care facilities unavailable, inadequate health insurance.

Problems Related to Interaction with the Legal System/Crime (V62.5). These include arrest, incarceration, litigation, victim of crime.

Other Psychosocial and Environmental Problems (V62.9). These include exposure to disasters, war, other hostilities; discord with non-family caregivers (e.g., counselor, social worker, physician); unavailability of social service agencies.

Axis V: Global Assessment of Functioning (GAF) Scale*

Consider psychological, social, and occupational functioning on a hypothetical continuum of mental health–illness. Do not include impairment in functioning due to physical (or environmental) limitations.

Code (Note: Use intermediate codes when appropriate, e.g., 45, 68, 72.)

100 Superior functioning in a wide range of activities, life's problems never seem to get out of hand, is sought out by others because of his many positive qualities. No symptoms.
91

90 Absent or minimal symptoms (e.g., mild anxiety before an exam), good functioning in all areas, interested and involved in a wide range of activities, socially effective, generally satisfied with life, no more than everyday problems or concerns (e.g., an occasional argument with family members).
81

80 If symptoms are present, they are transient and expectable reactions to psychosocial stressors (e.g., difficulty concentrating after family argument); no more than slight impairment in social, occupational or school functioning (e.g., temporarily falling behind in school work).
71

70 Some mild symptoms (e.g., depressed mood and mild insomnia) OR some difficulty in social, occupational, or school functioning (e.g., occasional truancy, or theft within the household), but generally functioning pretty well, has some meaningful interpersonal relationships.
61

60 Moderate symptoms (e.g., flat affect and circumstantial speech, occasional panic attacks) OR moderate difficulty in social, occupational, or school functioning (e.g., no friends, unable to keep a job).
51

50 Serious symptoms (e.g., suicidal ideation, severe obsessional rituals, frequent shoplifting) OR any serious impairment in social, occupational, or school functioning (e.g., no friends, unable to keep a job).
41

40 Some impairment in reality testing or communication (e.g., speech is at times illogical, obscure, or irrelevant) OR major impairment in several areas, such as work or school, family relations, judgment, thinking, or mood (e.g., depressed man avoids friends, neglects family, and is unable to work; child frequently beats up younger children, is defiant at home, and is failing at school).
31

30 Behavior is considerably influenced by delusions or hallucinations OR serious impairment in communication or judgment (e.g., sometimes incoherent, acts grossly inappropriately, suicidal preoccupation) OR inability to function in almost all areas (e.g., stays in bed all day; no job, home, or friends).
21

20 Some danger of hurting self or others (e.g., suicide attempts without clear expectation of death, frequently violent, manic excitement) OR occasionally fails to maintain minimal personal hygiene (e.g., smears feces) OR gross impairment in communication (e.g., largely incoherent or mute).
11

10 Persistent danger of severely hurting self or others (e.g., recurrent violence) OR persistent inability to maintain personal hygiene OR serious suicidal act with clear expectation of death.
1

0 Inadequate information.

*The rating of overall psychological functioning on a scale of 0-100 was operationalized by Luborsky in the Health-Sickness Rating Scale (Luborsky L: Clinicians' judgments of mental health, *Arch Gen Psychiatry* 7:407-417, 1962). Spitzer and colleagues developed a revision of the Health-Sickness Rating Scale called the Global Assessment Scale (GAS) (Endicott J, Spitzer RL, Fleiss JL, Cohen J: The global assessment scale: a procedure for measuring overall severity of psychiatric disturbance, *Arch Gen Psychiatry* 33:766-771, 1976). A modified version of the GAS was included in DSM-III-R as the Global Assessment of Functioning (GAF) Scale.

Your Internet Connection

Abuse Survivor's Resources
  http://www.tezcat.com/ ~tina/psych.html

Alliance for the Mentally Ill/Friends and Advocates of the
  Mentally Ill
  http://www.schizophrenia.com/ami/

Alzheimer's Association
  http://www.alz.org

American Academy of Child and Adolescent Psychiatry
  http://www.aacap.org/web/aacap/

The American Association for Geriatric Psychiatry
  http://www.aagpgpa.org/home.html

American Association of Suicidology
  http://www.cyberpsych.org/aas.htm

American Nurses' Association: Nursing World
  http://www.ana.org

American Psychiatric Nurses Association
  http://www.apna.org

American Psychological Association PsychNET
  http://www.apa.org

Anger Management, Trauma, and Dissociation
  http://www.kumu.com/ ~grhoades/

Anorexia Nervosa and Bulimia Association
  http://qlink.queensu.ca/ ~4map/anabhome.htm

Anxiety Disorders Association of America
  http://www.adaa.org

APA Online: American Psychiatric Association
  http://www.psych.org

Association of Managed Care Providers
  http://www.comed.com/amcp

Bazelon Center for Mental Health Law
  http://www.bazelon.org/

Behavior Online
  http://www.behavior.net

Beyond Stigma: ECT and Depression
  http://www.frii.com/ ~hageseth/

Blain Nelson's Abuse Pages
  http://www.pacificrim.net/~blainn/abuse/

BPD Central: Borderline Personality Disorder
  http://members.aol.com/bpdcentral/index.html

Brainscape
  http://beast.cbmv.jhu.edu:8000/research/brain/
  brain.htm

Canadian Federation of Mental Health Nurses
  http://www.iciweb.com/cfmhn

Canadian Nurses' Association
  http://www.cna-nurses.ca

The Child Advocate
  http://itsa.ucsf.edu/ ~mww/

Community Mental Health Management Information
  Systems Resource Center
  http://www.chmis.org

Computers in Mental Health (CIMH)
  http://www.ex.ac.uk/cimh

Crisis, Grief, and Healing
  http://www.webhealing.com/

Crisis Intervention Center
  http://www.cris.com/ ~cicinc/

CYFERNet
  http://www.cyfernet.mes.umn.edu

Dual Diagnosis Web Site
  http://www.erols.com/ksciacca/

ERIC® Clearinghouse on Assessment and Evaluation
  http://ericae2.educ.cua.edu/main.htm

EthnoMed: Ethnic Medicine Guide
  http://www.hslib.washington.edu/clinical/ethnomed

Family Caregiver Alliance
  http://www.caregiver.org

Group Psychotherapy Home Page
  http://freud.tau.ac.il/ ~haimw/group2.html

Growth House, Inc., AIDS and HIV links
  http://www.growthhouse.org/hivlinks.html

Guide to Psychotherapy
  http://www.shef.ac.uk/ ~psysc/psychotherapy

Health Care Information Resources: Alternative
  Medicine
  http://www-hsl.mcmaster.ca/tomflem/altmed.html

Healthy People 2000: Mental Health and Mental
  Disorders Resource List
  http://nhic-nt.health.org/nmp/hp2kpage/
  6mental2.htm

Healthy Sexuality
  http://www.uiuc.edu/departments/mck....
  health-info/sexual/intro

Help! A Consumer's Guide to Mental Health
  Information
  http://www.iComm.ca/madmagic/help/help.html

Home Care Nurse Page
  http://junior.apk.net/ ~nurse/

Homosexuality: Common Questions and Statements Addressed
http://www.geocities.com/WestHollywood/1348/

Institute for Behavioral Health Care
http://www.ibh.com

The International Association of Group Psychotherapy
http://www.psych.mcgill.ca/labs/iagp/IAGP.html

Internet Depression Resources List
http://www.execpc.com/~corbeau/

Internet Mental Health
http://www.mentalhealth.com

Joint Commission on Accreditation of Healthcare Organizations
http://www.jcaho.org/

Life Sciences Institute of Mind-Body Health: Self-Regulation of Mind & Body
http://www.cjnetworks.com/~lifesci/

Magic Stream
http://fly.hiwaay.net/~garson

Mental Health Education Page: Removing the Stigma of Mental Illness http://www.metrolink.net/~jquimby/mh.htm

Mental Health Infosource
http://mhsource.com

Mental Health Net
http://www.cmhcsys.com

Middle Tennessee Home Health Care
http://www.medi.com/homecare/

Multiple Personality & Dissociative Disorders
http://members.tripod.com/~fsrvival

National Alliance for the Mentally Ill (NAMI)
http://www.nami.org

National Alliance for Research on Schizophrenia and Depression (NARSAD)
http://www.mhsource.com/narsad.html

National Association of Cognitive-Behavioral Therapists
http://www.nacbt.org/

National Institute on Aging (NIA)
http://www.nih.gov/nia

National Institute of Mental Health
http://www.nimh.nih.gov

National Mental Health Association
http://www.nmha.org/

Neurosciences on the Internet
http://www.lm.com/~nab

Noodles' Panic-Anxiety Page: The ANXIETY Panic Internet Resource
http://www.algy.com/anxiety

NPAD News: National Panic/Anxiety Disorder News
http://www.npadnews.com

NursingNet
http://www.nursingnet.org

ParentNews: A Unique Opportunity for Parent Information
http://parent.net

Pendulum's Bipolar Disorder/Manic-Depression Page
http://www.pendulum.org/

Personality Disorders
http://personalitydisorders.cmhc.com/

Planning and Designing Today's Mental Health Institution
http://www.tiac.net/users/hfp/mhealth/site.htm

Psychlink
http://www.psychlink.com

Psychopharmacology and Drug References on the Mental Health Net
http://www.cmhcsys.com/guide/pro22.htm#A

Psychopharmacology TIPS
http://uhs.bsd.uchicago.edu/~bhsiung/tips

Rx List: The Internet Drug Index
http://www.rxlist.com

SafetyNet: Domestic Violence Information and Resources
http://www.cybergrrl.com/dv.html

The Schizophrenia Home Page
http://www.schizophrenia.com/

The Sleep Well
http://www-leland.stanford.edu/~dement/

The Something Fishy Web Site on Eating Disorders
http://www.something-fishy.com/ed.htm

Suicide Awareness/Voices of Education (SAVE)
http://www.save.org/

WEB of Addictions
http://www.well.com/user/woa/

The WholeFamily Center
http://www.wholefamily.com

Wing of Madness: General Mental Health Sources
http://members.aol.com/depress/genment.htm

The World-Wide Web Virtual Library: AIDS
http://planetq.com/aidsvl/index.html

Appendix C

Chapter Review Questions Answer Key

Chapter 1

1. A. Linda Richards
   B. Hildegard Peplau
   C. Tertiary
   D. Direct care, communication, management
   E. Registered nurse (RN), advanced practice registered nurse (APRN)
   F. American Psychiatric Nurses Association
2. A. True
   B. True
   C. False: It is secondary prevention.
   D. False: It is primary prevention.
   E. False: It is secondary prevention.
   F. True
   G. True
   H. False: There are over 77,000 psychiatric nurses working in mental health services.
   I. False: There are few studies in this important area of psychiatric nursing.
3. A. The development of psychotropic drugs allowed patients to become more treatable and fewer environmental constraints were needed to contain patient behavior. Also, the introduction of medications gave new hope to psychiatric patients and allowed psychiatric nurses to spend more time with patients in therapeutic activities.
   B. The five core mental health disciplines are psychiatric nursing, marriage and family therapy, psychiatry, psychology, and social work.
   C. The six dimensions of the nurse-patient partnership are clinical competence, patient-family advocacy, fiscal responsibility, interdisciplinary collaboration, social accountability, and legal-ethical parameters.

Chapter 2

1. A. Preinteraction   F. Orientation
   B. Orientation   G. Preinteraction
   C. Orientation   H. Working
   D. Termination   I. Working
   E. Working   J. Termination
2. A. Incongruent   C. Empathy
   B. Validation   D. Boundary violation
3. A. Will the self-disclosure enhance the patient's (1) cooperation, (2) learning, (3) catharsis, or (4) support?

B. Names of individuals, roles of nurse and patient, responsibilities of nurse and patient, expectations of nurse and patient, purpose of the relationship, meeting location and time, conditions for termination, confidentiality

C. Purpose
   Social: Pleasure
   Therapeutic: Patient insight and behavior change
   Use of feelings
   Social: Variable
   Therapeutic: Patient encouraged to share feelings
   Content of interaction
   Social: Social and spontaneous
   Therapeutic: Goal-directed and purposeful
   Confidentiality
   Social: Not an issue
   Therapeutic: Protected for the patient
   Termination
   Social: Open-ended
   Therapeutic: Mutually predetermined and honored

4. G. Altruism   E. Resistance
   B. Catharsis   A. Transference
   F. Confrontation   C. Role-playing
   D. Countertransference

Chapter 3

1. D. Freud   C. Spitzer
   F. Rockland   B. Sullivan
   A. Rogers   E. Szasz
2. A. Difficulty in earlier stages of development
   B. Free association
   C. Faulty interpersonal relationships
   D. Satisfaction, security
   E. Social conditions that culturally define what is acceptable
   F. Social
   G. One is out of touch with one's self or the environment
   H. Existential
   I. Problems in living from biopsychosocial causes
   J. Active, partner
   K. Disorders of the central nervous system
   L. Continuous learning about the brain and nervous system using the scientific process
   M. DSM-IV

3. A. Psychoanalysis proposes that dreams provide insight into areas of unresolved conflict in thoughts or feelings. Dream analysis or dream work is a common notion in contemporary society, and dreams play an important role in the belief system of various cultures.
   B. Stranger, resource person, teacher, leader, surrogate, counselor

Chapter 4

1. A. True
   B. False: One out of every two people will do so.
   C. True
   D. False: The sympathetic division is stimulated.
   E. True
   F. True

2. A. Reality perception
   B. Psychobiological resilience
   C. Psychological
   D. Social attribution
   E. Harm/loss, threat, challenge
   F. II
   G. Culture-bound syndromes

3. A. The three parts of a hardy personality are commitment, challenge, and control. They help people cope with stress by transforming events to their advantage and reframing problems as opportunities for growth and learning.
   B. The three types of coping mechanisms are: problem-focused, cognitive-focused, and emotion-focused.
   C. Nurses assess risk factors and look for vulnerabilities; physicians assess disease states and look for causes. Nursing diagnoses focus on the adaptive-maladaptive coping continuum of human responses; medical diagnoses focus on the health-illness continuum of health problems. Nursing intervention consists of caregiving activities; medical intervention consists of curative treatments.
   D. The four stages of psychiatric treatment and related level of prevention are crisis, secondary prevention; acute, secondary prevention; maintenance, tertiary prevention; and health promotion, primary prevention.

Chapter 5

1. I. Basal ganglia   B. Kindling
   F. Challenge   E. Locus ceruleus
   L. DST   H. PET
   J. Eugenics   D. REM
   K. Hippocampus   C. Synapse
   A. Hypothalamus   G. Tryptophan

2. A. Blood-brain, blood-CSF barriers.
   B. Neurotransmission

C. Neurosciences
D. Circadian rhythms
E. Birth-cohort effect

3. A. False: Only perhaps 10% of cases.
   B. True
   C. False: This has been replaced by more complex biochemical theories.
   D. False: CT scans have found enlargement of ventricles.
   E. True

4. A. Axon: Presynaptic cell; stores and releases neurotransmitter.
      Dendrite: Post-synaptic cell; contains receptor cells.
      Receptor cell: Recognizes the neurotransmitter, receives it, and reacts to it.
      Autoregulation: Presynaptic cell assesses and regulates the amount of neurotransmitter it releases.
      Reuptake: Neurotransmitter is taken back up into the presynaptic cell.
      Enzymatic degradation: Neurotransmitter is metabolized and inactivated.
   B. It is the emotional brain, concerned with both subjective emotional experiences and body functions associated with emotional states, such as aggressive and submissive behavior, sexual behavior, pleasure, memory, learning, mood, motivation, and sensations, all central to preservation.
   C. Stage one, falling asleep; stage two, sleep (50% of sleep time); stages three and four: deep sleep (15% of sleep time); stage five, rapid eye movement (REM) sleep, or dream sleep (20 to 25% of sleep time). REM latency is the period of time (60 to 90 minutes) it usually takes the normal person to enter the first REM period. Decreased REM latency (5 to 30 minutes) is a biological marker for depression that occurs in approximately 90% of people with depression, thus indicating that there is sleep dysregulation in depression.
   D. Challenge testing is a procedure that causes panic attacks under controlled conditions to study the biology of the attack. Vulnerable people are more likely to have a panic attack when given challenges such as lactate, carbon dioxide, and caffeine than are people who do not have panic disorder. They are also less likely to have another attack when challenged again after adequate treatment with antipanic medications. PET studies show that these people also tend to have an abnormality in the parahippocampal region of the brain, an area of the cerebral cortex that is associated with the limbic system, and may be implicated in panic attacks.

Chapter 6

1. C. Affect
   A. Delusion
   E. Flight of ideas
   F. Hallucinations
   B. Illusions
   H. Insight
   D. Loose associations
   G. Mood

2. A. Flat affect
   B. Command hallucinations
   C. Sound or hearing
   D. Confabulation

3. A. The major categories of information in a mental status exam are general description, emotional state, experiences, thinking, and sensorium and cognition.
   B. Person (What is your name?), place (Where are you today?), and time (What is today's date?)
   C. To measure the extent of the patient's problem. Make an accurate diagnosis, track patient progress over time, and document the efficacy of treatment.

Chapter 7

1. A. Risk factors
   B. Ethnicity
   C. Substance abuse, antisocial personality
   D. Affective, anxiety
   E. Schizophrenia, manic depression
   F. Increase, decrease

2. F. Disadvantagement
   D. Discrimination
   G. Intolerance
   B. Prejudice
   E. Racism
   A. Stereotype
   C. Stigma

3. A. Cultural sensitivity is the ability to view each patient as a unique individual, fully considering the patient's cultural experiences within the context of the common developmental challenges faced by all people.

Chapter 8

1. A. Access
   F. Capitation
   E. Case rate
   B. Clinical appropriateness
   H. Clinical pathway
   D. Outcomes
   G. Practice guidelines
   C. Utilization review

2. A. Behavioral
   B. Person, population
   C. Quality, costs
   D. Employee assistance program
   E. Patient characteristics, nature of the therapeutic relationship, treatment intervention, placebo effect
   F. Target population, expected outcome of treatment, treatment strategies, documented variances and goal achievement
   G. Clinical, functional, satisfaction, financial

3. A. HMOs are organized delivery systems that provide care to a defined population, usually for a pre-determined fixed amount (capitation rate). Consumers enrolled in HMOs are restricted to using HMO providers.

   POSs are plans that contract with a limited number of clinicians, most often physicians, and hospitals that provide care at discounted rates.

   PPOs allow consumers to choose between delivery systems at the time they seek care.
   B. Medicare and Medicaid were designed to help those who were medically in need. The law passed in 1996 implies that chemical dependency problems are not medical conditions but rather the result of personal choice or weakness. In this way it further stigmatizes people with these debilitating conditions.

Chapter 9

1. A. True
   B. False: The police power is currently emphasized.
   C. False: The profile is that of a young, unmarried black male.
   D. False: People with mental illness are not more violent or more dangerous than people in the general population.
   E. True
   F. True
   G. False: The patient's right of confidentiality does not allow police or lawyers access to information about patients without the patient's expressed consent.
   H. True
   I. False: Patient records belong to the treatment facility or clinician, and the original should remain on file and never be given to patients.
   J. False: Back problems are the most often cited disability.
   K. False: Three states—Montana, Idaho, and Utah—have abolished the insanity defense.

2. A. 48 to 72
   B. History of violent behavior, noncompliance with medications, current substance abuse

C. Outpatient commitment

D. Competent, understanding, voluntary

E. Protection and Advocacy

F. Advanced directives

G. American Law Institute's test

3. A. Dangerous to self or others, mentally ill and in need of treatment, and unable to provide for own basic needs

B. Confidentiality involves the disclosure of certain information to another person but it is limited to authorized people. It applies to all patients at all times. Privilege or testimonial privilege applies only in court-related proceedings, and it exists only if established by law.

C. The duty to warn obliges the clinician to assess the threat of violence to another, identify the person being threatened, and implement some affirmative and preventive action.

Chapter 10

1. C. Data collection

A. Evaluation

B. Implementation

E. Nursing diagnosis

D. Outcome identification

F. Planning

2. A. Specific

B. Measurable

C. Attainable

D. Current

E. Adequate

F. Mutual

G. Psychotherapy, prescription of medications, consultation

H. Health promotion, maintenance, acute, crisis

I. Develop insight, change behavior

J. Patient

3. A. Phenomena relate to the range of actual or potential mental health problems that can be experienced by patients; theory maintains that psychiatric nurses need a theoretical base or conceptual model for their practice, action requires that the nursing process be a mutual problem-solving process, and effects identifies the need for standards of psychiatric nursing practice to evaluate the quality of care.

B. DSM-IV diagnoses are used in most mental health settings to describe and classify the symptoms of mental disorders. Nurses should use both NANDA and DSM-IV diagnoses to conceptualize patient problems, needs, and treatment strategies.

C. Goal setting with psychiatric patients can be difficult for a number of reasons, including such issues as resistance, confusion, lack of insight, de-

nial, vagueness about problem areas, and inability to articulate ideas. The nurse needs to clarify the reason and develop specific strategies to address it, which is part of the therapeutic process.

Chapter 11

1. A. True

B. False: As of 1998 a baccalaureate degree is required to become certified as a generalist in psychiatric nursing.

C. True

D. False: The statement describes utilitarianism. Fairness is based on the concept of justice and benefit to the least advantaged in society.

E. True

F. False: Much more research is needed in this area.

2. A. Accountability

B. Autonomy

C. Nurse-patient relationship

D. Internet

E. Certified generalist, certified specialist

F. Ethic

G. Interdisciplinary

3. A. The nursing process and the quality improvement process have similar steps. Each involves identifying or assessing a situation, analyzing the data to define the situation, developing a plan, implementing it, and then evaluating the results. Both of these processes are similar to the scientific process used in research.

B. The aim of supervision is to teach psychotherapeutic skills. The goal of therapy is to alter a person's patterns of coping to enable the person to function more effectively in all areas of life.

Chapter 12

1. A. Primary prevention

B. Secondary prevention

C. Tertiary prevention

2. A. Work with people to avoid or better cope with stressors; change the resources, policies, or agents of the environment to enhance individual functioning

B. Competence building

C. Healthy People 2000

D. Stigma

E. Environmental change

F. All three (primary, secondary, and tertiary)

3. A. The medical prevention model focuses on mental illness prevention and the importance of genetic and biochemical and brain research to discover the specific causes of mental illness. The nursing prevention model assumes that problems are multicausal, that everyone is vulnerable to stressful

life events, and that any disability can arise in response to them. It focuses on intervention based on stressful events and vulnerable groups with known risk factors.

B. Universal interventions are targeted to the general population without consideration of risk factors. Selective interventions are targeted to individuals or groups with a significantly higher risk of developing a particular disorder. Indicated interventions are targeted to high-risk individuals indicating a predisposition for developing the disorder.

C. Increasing a person's awareness of issues related to health and illness, increasing understanding of potential stressors and adaptive and maladaptive coping responses, increasing knowledge of where and how to acquire needed resources, and increasing the actual abilities such as the problem-solving skills, social skills, or self-esteem of the individual or group.

Chapter 13

1. G. Abreaction
   A. Clarification
   C. Exploration of solutions
   H. Manipulation
   E. Raising self-esteem
   D. Reinforcement of behavior
   F. Suggestion
   B. Support of defenses

2. A. Crisis
   B. Precipitating events
   C. Precrisis
   D. Assessment
   E. Health educator

3. A. True
   B. False: A crisis is a short-term event requiring short-term treatment.
   C. True
   D. False: The patient's perception of the precipitating event is critically important.
   E. False: The generic approach is the correct answer.

4. A. Maturational crises are social and biological developmental events requiring role changes. These types of crises can be influenced by role models, interpersonal resources, and the acceptance of others. Situational crises occur when a life event upsets an individual's or a group's psychological equilibrium. This can cause feelings of inadequacy, bereavement, role change, financial stress, fear of loss, and feelings of helplessness and guilt. Adventitious crises are accidental, uncommon, and unexpected. These crises do not occur in the lives of everyone, but they challenge every coping mechanism of the individual when they do occur because of the severity of the stress.

B. Cultural factors to be considered in crisis intervention are migration and citizen status, gender and family roles, religious belief systems, child-rearing practices, and use of extended family and support systems.

C. Identify your own behaviors, precipitating events, perception of the event, support systems and coping resources, and previous strengths and coping mechanisms.

Chapter 14

1. A. True
   B. False: The career potential of people with mental illness, as with anyone else, depends on the person's talents, abilities, experience, motivation, and health status.
   C. True
   D. False: Consumers of mental health services can be productive as providers of mental health services. They can provide positive staff-recipient relationships, good knowledge of mental health resources and ways to overcome barriers, and positive role modeling.
   E. True

2. A. Rehabilitation
   B. Family burden
   C. Deinstitutionalization
   D. Social skills training
   E. Psychoeducation

3. A. Grief, anger, powerlessness, and fear
   B. Helping people develop their strengths and potential, learn living skills, and access environmental support
   C. Ways in which nurses can share power with families include clarifying mutual goals, not expecting families to fit a specific model, acknowledging one's own limitations, pointing out family strengths, working with families as a team, learning to respond to intense feelings, encouraging family enrichment, providing psychoeducation, offering practical advice, making a personal commitment, acknowledging diverse beliefs, and developing one's own supports.

Chapter 15

1. The preventive strategies of health education, environmental change, and social support can be used with a sibling of a patient who is mentally ill.

2. Families can influence each of the following balancing factors available to a person with mental illness who is in crisis: the nature of the precipitating event or stressor, the person's perception of the event, the nature and strength of the patient's support systems and coping resources, and the patient's previous strengths and coping mechanisms.

3. Family members can work with health professionals to assist patients with mental illness by using the three basic interventions used in psychiatric rehabilitation. The interventions are helping the patient to develop strengths and potential, learn living skills, and access environmental supports.

Chapter 16

1. G. Affective responses
   A. Anxiety
   C. Cognitive responses
   I. Ego-oriented reactions
   F. Fear
   J. Moderate anxiety
   E. Neurosis
   D. Panic
   H. Psychosis
   B. Task-oriented reactions
2. A. Anxiety, depression
   B. Obsessions
   C. Emotional seduction
   D. Physical integrity and self-esteem
   E. Benzodiazepines and antidepressants
3. A. Conflict is the clashing of two opposing interests. The person experiences two competing drives and must choose between them. A reciprocal relationship exists between conflict and anxiety. Conflict produces anxiety, and anxiety increases the perception of conflict by producing feelings of helplessness.
   B. Allow the patient to determine the amount of stress he can handle at any given time. Do not force the patient into situations that he is not able to handle. Do not attack the patient's coping mechanisms or try to strip him of these. Do not ridicule the nature of his defense. Do not argue with the patient or try to talk him out of the defense. Do not reinforce the defense by focusing too much attention on it. Know when to eventually place some limits on the defense as more adaptive coping mechanisms fall into place. Assess for suicidal ideation as appropriate.

Chapter 17

1. E. Body dysmorphic disorder
   C. Conversion disorder
   H. Hypersomnia
   D. Hypochondriasis
   I. Insomnia
   F. Pain disorder
   G. Parasomnia
   J. Sleep pattern disturbance
   A. Somatization disorder
   B. Somatoform disorders

2. A. Alarm, resistance, exhaustion
   B. Repression, denial, compensation, regression
   C. Verbally, physical
   D. Conversion disorder
   E. Psychoneuroimmunology
3. A. Supportive therapy, insight therapy, group therapy, cognitive-behavioral strategies, stress reduction, relaxation training, and psychopharmacology.
   B. Secondary gain is an indirect benefit, usually obtained through an illness or disability. Such benefits may include personal attentions, release from unpleasant situations and responsibilities, or monetary and disability benefits.

Chapter 18

1. A. True
   B. False: New research indicates that self-esteem is a moderately inheritable trait.
   C. True
   D. False: The development of insight is not the desired outcome; the ultimate goal is to take action to effect lasting behavioral changes.
   E. False: Sympathetic responses by the nurse do not help patients assume responsibility for their own behavior. In fact, they can reinforce the patient's self-pity.
2. A. Self-ideal   E. Depersonalization
   B. Self-esteem   F. Child abuse
   C. Roles   G. Reminiscence
   D. Identity
3. A. Provide the child with success, instill ideas, encourage the child's aspirations, and help the child build defenses against attacks to one's self-perceptions
   B. In adolescence, the crisis of identity versus identity diffusion occurs. The task is one of self-definitions as the adolescent strives to integrate previous roles into a unique and reasonably consistent sense of self.
   C. Positive and accurate body image, realistic self-ideal, positive self-concept, high self-esteem, satisfying role performance, clear sense of identity

Chapter 19

1. C. Behaviors related to emotional responses
   A. Coping mechanisms
   D. DSM-IV diagnoses
   B. Precipitating stressors
   E. Predisposing factors
   F. Seasonal affective disorder
2. A. ECT
   B. Serotonin
   C. Bipolar, unipolar
   D. Risk

E. Prefrontal cortex

F. Anxiety disorders, substance abuse disorders

G. 75, 85

H. Response, 6, 12, remission

I. Relapse, recovery, 4, 9

J. Recurrence, indefinitely

3. A. Emotional responsiveness: The person is affected by and is an active participant in both internal and external worlds. Uncomplicated grief reaction: The person is facing the reality of the loss and is immersed in the work of grieving. Suppression of emotions: This is the denial of feelings, detachment from them, or the internalization of all aspects of one's affective world. Delayed grief reaction: This is a prolonged suppression of emotion that ultimately interferes with effective functioning. Depression/mania: The most maladaptive emotional responses, recognized by their intensity, pervasiveness, persistence, and interference with usual functioning.

B. To increase the patient's sense of control over goals and behavior, increase the patient's self-esteem, and help the patient modify negative thinking patterns

Chapter 20

1. A. False: The highest rate of suicide is among white men over age 65.

B. True

C. False: All suicidal behavior is serious and, whatever the intent, must be given full consideration.

D. True

E. True

F. False: The tricyclics have the higher rate of death by overdose.

2. A. Psychological autopsy

B. Mood disorders, substance abuse, schizophrenia

C. Serotonin (5HT)

D. Communicating hope

E. Hostility, impulsivity, depression

F. Contracting for safety

3. A. Patients often appear less depressed immediately before attempting suicide because they feel relief at having made a decision and developed a plan to do so.

B. Circumstances of the attempt, presenting symptoms, psychiatric diagnosis, personality factors, psychosocial history, family history, biochemical factors

C. Suicidal patients can be treated in a variety of settings. Factors that should be considered in deciding on the best setting relate to your assessment of overall risk and should include whether the patient is resolute or ambivalent about suicide, has impaired judgment, and has dependable social supports available in the home.

Chapter 21

1. J. Affect
   I. Anhedonia
   C. Attention
   A. Cognition
   D. Decision making
   F. Hallucinations
   B. Memory
   H. Mood
   E. Perception
   G. Soft signs

2. A. Cognition, perception, emotion, behavior, relatedness.

B. Apraxia

C. Dysregulation hypothesis

D. Symptom triggers

E. Overextension, restricted consciousness, disinhibition, psychotic disorganization, psychotic resolution

3. A. True

B. False: The majority are auditory.

C. False: Atypical antipsychotics often provide a better response, and fewer side effects should be considered first-line treatments.

D. True

E. False: It is called Journey of Hope.

4. A. Nursing interventions should address the positive symptoms of schizophrenia, which include delusions, hallucinations, thought disorders, and bizarre behaviors, as well as the negative symptoms of flat affect, alogia, avolition, anhedonia, and attentional impairment. Positive symptoms respond well to typical and atypical antipsychotic medications. Negative symptoms respond best to atypical antipsychotic medications.

B. The specific genetic defects that cause schizophrenia have not been identified yet, but family studies show increased risk for the disease and other psychiatric illnesses in people with a first-degree relative with schizophrenia. Children with a biological parent with schizophrenia have a 15% risk of developing the disorder. If both of the child's parents have schizophrenia, the risk increases up to 35%.

C. Things you may notice are facial expressions, style of dress, mannerisms, tone of voice, behaviors, use of language, and body contact with others.

Chapter 22

1. A. Cluster B
   B. Cluster C
   C. Cluster B
   D. Cluster C
   E. Cluster B
   F. Cluster B
   G. Cluster C
   H. Cluster A
   I. Cluster A
   J. Cluster A

2. A. Adolescence, adulthood

B. Borderline personality disorder

C. Serotonin
D. Splitting
E. Projective identification
F. Countertransference
G. Behavioral contract

3. A. Distinguishing characteristics of personality disorders include chronic and long-standing, not based on a sound personality structure, and difficult to change.
   B. Two levels of evaluation necessary when working with patients with personality disorders are evaluation of the nurse and the nurse's participation in the relationship and evaluation of the patient's behavior and the behavioral changes that the nurse works to facilitate.

Chapter 23

1. B. Agnosia   D. Denial
   G. Aphasia   I. Excess disability
   J. Apraxia   A. Piaget
   C. Delirium   E. Pseudodementia
   F. Dementia   H. Sundown syndrome

2. A. Neurotic plaques, neurofibrillary tangles
   B. Cognitive map
   C. Catastrophic reaction

3. A. Sensorimotor—birth to 2 years—action oriented, no language, develops awareness of body in space, develops memory for missing objects; Preoperational—2 to 5 years—symbolism appears, objects defined by function, magical thinking, imaginative play; Concrete operations—5 to 12 years—capable of relatability, syllogistic reasoning, makes and follows rules, quantifies experiences, understands conversation; Formal operations—12 and older—abstraction, development of ideals, criticism of others, self-criticism
   B. Understand the possible causes of the cognitive impairment, adjust communication approaches to the person who is cognitively impaired, assist with self-care of the individual as needed, obtain available community services, engage in stress reduction activities, use respite care, participate in a peer support group, access social supports.

Chapter 24

1. A. False: Substance abuse affects all races.
   B. False: Only 1 in 10 people progress from use to abuse to dependence.
   C. True
   D. True
   E. False: In the addicted population there is no greater prevalence of psychiatric illness than in the general population.
   F. True

G. False: Shorter half-lives result in more withdrawal.
H. True
I. False: Most people have one or more slips in their attempt at recovery.
J. True

2. A. Substitution of a medication from the same drug class for gradual tapering
   B. Dual diagnosis
   C. Gateway drugs
   D. CAGE
   E. Breathalyzer
   F. Codependence
   G. Endorphins or enkephalins
   H. CNS depressants
   I. Detoxification
   J. Antabuse, naltrexone

3. A. Patients in maintenance methadone programs may object to the following: 1) they must remain on stable doses of the drug for years—some even for the rest of their lives, and 2) they must report to the clinic daily or they may be given take-home doses for certain days if they qualify.
   B. The advantages of having treatment programs staffed by counselors who have also recovered from substance abuse include that they may have a heightened sense of empathy for the patient population, a greater understanding of the realities of the abuse, and provide positive recovery-based role modeling. There is controversy in the field, however, about what proportion of the staff should be recovered individuals. Some believe that a critical number of staff who have not been substance abusers is necessary to provide a professional balance to the treatment program. More research is needed in this area.

Chapter 25

1. A. Adaptive eating regulation responses
   C. Maladaptive eating regulation responses
   E. Predisposing factors
   B. Serotonin
   D. SSRIs

2. A. Females, 1, 4
   B. Binge eating
   C. Avoidance, intellectualization, isolation of affect, denial
   D. Anxiety, body image disturbance, fluid volume deficit, risk for self-mutilation, altered nutrition, powerlessness, self-esteem disturbance
   E. Cognitive behavioral therapy

3. A. <u>Amount of binging</u>
   Obese nonbingers: Once per month
   Obese bingers: High amount
   Nonobese bulimics: Very high amount

Purging
Obese nonbingers: Rare
Obese bingers: Infrequent
Nonobese bulimics: High level
Mood disturbance
Obese nonbingers: Same as general population
Obese bingers: One third chronic
Nonobese bulimics: One third to one half chronic
and up to 80% lifetime

B. The patient will restore healthy eating patterns
and normalize physiological parameters related to
body weight and nutrition.

Chapter 26

1. I. Bisexuality
   B. Gender identity
   J. Gender role
   A. Genetic identity
   G. Heterosexuality
   F. Homophobia
   H. Homosexuality
   E. Orgasm
   K. Sexual orientation
   C. Transsexualism
   D. Transvestism

2. A. Cognitive dissonance
   B. XX, XY
   C. Oedipus/Electra
   D. Childhood sexual abuse
   E. Education
   F. Acceptance

3. A. Between two consenting adults, mutually satisfying to both, not psychologically or physically
   harmful to either party, lacking in force or coercion, and conducted in private
   B. Safe sex practices include using condoms, reducing the number of sexual partners, and promoting
   sexual behaviors that decrease the exchange of
   body fluids.

Chapter 27

1. I. Antianxiety drugs
   L. Anti-Parkinsonian drugs
   B. Atypical antipsychotics
   J. Barbiturates
   K. Cytochrome P450 inhibition
   C. Hypertensive crisis
   F. Mood stabilizers
   D. Sedative-hypnotics
   H. Selective serotonin uptake inhibitors
   A. Serotonin syndrome
   E. Tricyclics
   G. Typical antipsychotics

2. C. 5HT reuptake inhibition
   E. $5HT_2$ receptor blockade
   B. ACh receptor blockade
   D. $Alpha_1$ receptor blockade
   F. $Alpha_2$ receptor blockade
   A. DA reuptake inhibition

H. H_1 receptor blockade
G. NE reuptake inhibition

3. A. Role of the nurse
   B. Polypharmacy
   C. Pharmacokinetics
   D. Dysregulation hypotheses
   E. Neurosciences, psychopharmacology, clinical man-
   agement

4. A. False: Serotonin syndrome is a life threatening
   emergency caused by combining 5HT-enhancing
   drugs.
   B. False: With NMS all drugs should be discontin-
   ued.
   C. True
   D. True
   E. True

5. A. Positive symptoms include delusion, hallucinations, formal thought disorder, and bizarre behavior. Negative symptoms include affective flattening, alogia, avolition/apathy/anhedonia, asoci-
   ality, and attentional impairment. These symptoms respond better to the atypical antipsychotics than they do to the typical or conventional
   antipsychotics.
   B. Reuptake inhibition occurs when drugs such as
   TCAs and SSRIs prevent the presynaptic cell from
   reabsorbing the neurotransmitter after it has been
   released into the synapse. It is thought that this
   strategy produces an antidepressant affect by
   making more neurotransmitter available to the receptors in illnesses such as depression, in which
   increasing the effects of some neurotransmitters
   appears to exert a therapeutic effect.
      Receptor blockade occurs when drugs such as
   antipsychotics prevent a receptor from receiving a
   neurotransmitter after it has been released into
   the synapse. It is thought that this strategy produces an antipsychotic effect by making less neurotransmitter available to receptors in illnesses
   such as schizophrenia, in which decreasing the effects of some neurotransmitters appears to exert a
   therapeutic effect.
   C. When receiving antidepressants for the treatment
   of depression, patients begin to look better and
   sleep and eat better, and they feel more energy
   and motivation before the remission of subjective
   depressive feelings and suicidal thoughts. Objectively, they appear to be less depressed at a time
   when their safety must still be assessed because
   they now have the energy to act on suicidal impulses that have not reponded to treatment.

Chapter 28

1.
   A. True
   B. False: ECT may be followed by antidepressant medication to prevent relapse.
   C. False: There is no evidence that ECT causes structural brain damage.
   D. True
   E. True
   F. False: The long-term efficacy of light therapy has not been fully evaluated.
   G. False: Light therapy appears to be insufficient for severely ill patients.
   H. True

2.
   A. 6, 12
   B. 20, 30
   C. Major depression
   D. 80%
   E. Surgical
   F. Headache, muscle soreness, nausea
   G. 50, 60
   H. Mania

3.
   A. ECT is a treatment in which a grand mal seizure is artificially induced in an anesthetized patient by passing an electrical current through electrodes applied to the patient's temples.
   B. Avoiding medications is often recommended for women who are in their first trimester of pregnancy. ECT allows the depression of the woman to be treated while avoiding the need to expose the fetus to antidepressant medications.

Chapter 29

1.
   A. False: Research suggests that this intervention may actually increase the patient's potential for aggressive behavior.
   B. True
   C. False: This is the premise of the behavioral view of aggression.
   D. False: A patient's diagnosis is complicated by many factors and is at best merely suggestive of potentially violent behavior.
   E. True
   F. True

2.
   A. Assertive behavior
   F. Debriefing
   B. Limit-setting
   E. Passive behavior
   G. Restraint
   D. Seclusion
   C. Token economy

3.
   A. Areas of the brain include the limbic system, frontal lobe, and temporal lobe.
   B. Preventive strategies include self-awareness, patient education, and assertiveness training. Anticipatory strategies include communication, environmental change, behavioral action, and psychopharmacology. Containment strategies include crisis management, seclusion, and restraint.
   C. You should assume a supportive stance at least one leg length or 3 feet away from the patient. You should be at an angle to the patient, with hands kept open and out of pockets.

Chapter 30

1.
   B. Behavior
   G. Biofeedback
   F. Contingency contracting
   H. Extinction
   D. Flooding
   A. Punishment
   I. Reframing
   E. Shaping
   J. Social skills training
   C. Systematic desensitization

2.
   A. Classical conditioning
   B. Operant conditioning or negative reinforcement
   C. Punishment, response cost, extinction
   D. Perception or interpretation
   E. Hierarchy
   F. Direct patient care, planning treatment programs, teaching others cognitive behavior therapy techniques

3.
   A. A cognitive behavioral assessment would include collecting data about a patient's actions, thoughts and feelings, identifying problems from the data, defining the problem behavior, deciding how to measure the problem behavior, and identifying environmental variables that influence the problem behavior. It includes a review of the patient's strengths and deficits and minimizes the use of assumptions and unvalidated inferences.
   B. The ABCs of behavior are *antecedent, behavior,* and *consequence.* The ABCs of treatment are *affective, behavioral,* and *cognitive.*
   C. Use of the form allows patients to distinguish between thoughts and feelings and to identify adaptive responses that would be alternatives to the situation.

Chapter 31

1.
   F. Complainer
   J. Encourager
   B. Facilitator
   E. Follower
   A. Gatekeeper
   I. Leader
   C. Moralist
   G. Questioner
   D. Summarizer
   H. Truant

2.
   A. Power
   B. Orientation
   C. 60-120 minutes, 20-40 minutes

D. Forming, storming, norming, performing
E. Universality, altruism
3. A. A group is a collection of individuals who have a relationship with one another, are independent, and may have common norms. Eight components of small groups are structure, size, length of sessions, communication, roles, power, norms, and cohesion.
   B. Psychoeducational groups are designed for 20 or more people who complete a series of structured educational sessions designed to teach symptom identification, symptom management, and recovery planning skills.

   Intensive problem-solving groups are designed for 6 to 10 patients, each working on the identification and resolution of specific target problems, goals, and problem-solving strategies identified in an individual treatment plan.

   Activity groups are designed to enhance the psychological and emotional well being of long-term psychiatric patients. These groups are a combination of group psychotherapy and remotivation therapy that stimulates interaction among members by focusing on simple tasks that encourage members to focus on group rather than individual goals.
   C. Group norms facilitate the accomplishment of the group's goals or tasks, control interpersonal conflict, interpret social reality, and foster group interdependence.

Chapter 32

1. A. False: It is not a problem to be in a triangle, and it is impossible to stay out of all triangles.
   B. True
   C. False: The third leg of a triangle may be a person, an issue, or an object, and they or it may not be a willing part of the emotional system of a family.
   D. False: Therapists must avoid becoming part of a triangle in a family system.
   E. True
2. A. Strengths, resources or competencies; deficits, pathologic states, and dysfunction
   B. Educate, support
   C. National Alliance for the Mentally Ill (NAMI)
   D. Bowen
   E. Thinking, feeling
   F. Ego fusion
   G. Interactional patterns
   H. Reframe
   I. Obtain a clear description of the presenting problem in specific and concrete terms
3. A. A person with high differentiation of self has personal autonomy, distinguishes between thoughts

and feelings, and retains objectivity when stressed. A person with low differentiation is fused with others, blends thoughts and feelings, and is emotionally reactive when stressed.
   B. A family genogram is a structured method of gathering information and graphically symbolizing factual and emotional relationship data related to the family.

Chapter 33

1. 1. C   6. D
   2. E   7. C
   3. D   8. E
   4. B   9. B
   5. A   10. A
2. A. Crisis, stabilization
   B. Multidisciplinary
   C. Therapeutic community
   D. Florence Nightingale
   E. JCAHO
   F. Risk management
   G. Utilization review
3. A. Crisis stabilization and intermediate-term treatment
   B. First, before admission, the patient or clinician requests approval to hospitalize the patient. This is called preauthorization. Next, concurrent review takes place after admission but before discharge. The treatment team must justify the need for continued stay or any deviations from the norm. Finally, retrospective review occurs after discharge, when the entire chart can be reviewed.

Chapter 34

1. 1. C   5. A
   2. D   6. D
   3. A   7. B
   4. C   8. B
2. A. Epidemiological
   B. Tertiary
   C. Case management
   D. Primary
   E. Assertive Community Treatment
   F. Secondary
   G. Multisystemic therapy
3. A. Common elements of ACT and MST include using a social-ecological framework, pragmatic treatment approaches, home-based interventions, individualized treatment goals, and emphasis on outcomes and innovation.

Chapter 35

1. A. True   D. False
   B. False   E. True
   C. True   F. False

2. A. Be homebound, have a diagnosed psychiatric disorder, require the skills of a psychiatric nurse
   B. Homebound
   C. Case management
   D. Medicare
   E. People more than 65 years of age who may have a history of mental illness or a newly diagnosed mental illness and, people less than 65 who qualify for Medicare because of their disabilities
   F. Standardized rating scales
   G. Clinical pathways
   H. Documentation

3. A. The advantages of home care in relationship to inpatient treatment involve its ability to serve as an alternative to hospitalization by maintaining a patient in the community, a facilitator of an impending hospital admission through preadmission assessment, an enhancement of inpatient treatment through integration of home issues in the inpatient treatment plan, a way to shorten inpatient stay while keeping the patient engaged in active treatment, and a part of the discharge planning process by assessing potential problems and issues upon discharge into the community
   B. Psychiatric nursing home care is reminiscent of the early days of public health nursing, which included home visits.

Chapter 36

1. A. False: 14 to 20% of children have some type of psychiatric disorder
   B. True
   C. True
   D. False: Young children exhibiting sexual behavior may have been abused. They should be dealt with in an open and honest way and reported to child protective services for investigation into possible abuse.
   E. False: To avoid aggression, nurses should make a consistent schedule that is developmentally based, keep staff highly visible and engaged with the children, and carefully prepare children for activities.

2. A. 1/5
   B. Handling separation and independent decision making
   C. Working for delayed gratification
   D. Bibliotherapy
   E. Autogenic storytelling
   F. Inability of the family to control the child at home
   G. Legal, ethical

3. A. Dealing with frustration and unfavorable events, celebrating good things, and feeling pleasure
   B. Parents can enhance a child's self-esteem by hav-

ing realistic caregiver expectations; demonstrating positive personal values; communicating clearly, tolerantly, and respectfully; using appropriate ways to discipline; offering guidance and support; and promoting the child's autonomy.

Chapter 37

1. A. False: Brain growth continues into adolescence, and there is also additional fine tuning of the neural system.
   B. False: Chronological age is not a good indicator of physical maturation during adolescence because growth often occurs in spurts and individual differences exist.
   C. True
   D. True
   E. False: It is best for the nurse to have the initial contact directly with the adolescent because he or she is often concerned that the nurse will be aligned with the parents rather than with the adolescent.
   F. True

2. A. Identity versus identity diffusion
   B. Formal operational thought
   C. 33, 25
   D. Suicide
   E. Hypochondriasis
   F. Coping with stress and anxiety, involvement in personally meaningful activities

3. A. Female teenagers delay seeking and using contraceptives either because they are unwilling or unable to make conscious decisions about their sexual and contraceptive behavior, or because they do not mind becoming pregnant.
   B. Alcohol is called a gateway drug because its use often precedes the use of marijuana and other illegal substances.
   C. Curiosity, experimentation, regular use, psychological or physical dependence, and using drugs to feel "normal"
   D. Medication with adolescents necessitates comprehensive family involvement; developmental differences in adolescence affect psychopharmacological assessment, treatment alliance, management, and compliance; difficulty in diagnosing emerging first episodes versus adjustment disorders in adolescents; and lack of controlled clinical drug trials in adolescents

Chapter 38

1. 1. A   5. E
   2. B   6. F
   3. C   7. G
   4. D

2. A. Sundown syndrome
   B. Physical restraints
   C. Electroconvulsive
   D. Tardive dyskinesia
   E. Reality
   F. Cognitive
   G. Maximal independence
   H. Lower than for younger patients
3. A. Show respect by addressing the patient by his or her last name, reinforce the amount of time left in the interview, give sufficient time for response, tie the interview to historic events, choose words that are based on the sociocultural background of the patient, use touch to convey support and interest, and give careful and repeated explanations to increase understanding and cooperation.
   B. Environmental hazards, patient variables, assistive devices, medications, and physical or mental disorders

Chapter 39

1. D. Attributions
   F. Force continuum
   B. Just world view
   A. Multigenerational transmission
   G. Myth about abuse
   C. Paternalistic model of health care
   E. Primary prevention
   J. Psychological abuse
   I. Sexual assault
   H. Wife abuse
2. A. True   D. False
   B. False   E. True
   C. False
3. A. Violent families have the following characteristics: multigenerational transmission (family violence is often perpetuated through generations within a family by a cycle of violence), social isolation (violent families are often isolated by the abuser to keep the "family secret," thus avoiding formal and informal sanctions from others in the community), use and abuse of power (the abuser almost always has some form of power or control over the victim), and alcohol and drug abuse (survivors often report concurrent substance abuse by the abuser, although one behavior is not necessary for the other to occur).

   B.
Paternalistic model	Empowerment model
Nurse is perceived to be more knowledgeable than the survivor.	There is mutual sharing of knowledge and information.
Responsibility for ending the violence is placed on the survivor.	The nurse strategizes with the survivor. Survivors are helped to recognize societal influences.
Advice and sympathy are given rather than respect.	The survivor's competence and experience are respected.

   C. American social norms that maintain violence include historical attitudes toward women, children, and the elderly, the belief that violence is justified to maintain the family system, economic discrimination, the nonresponsiveness of the criminal justice system, and the belief that women and children are property.

Chapter 40

1. A. True   F. False
   B. False   G. False
   C. True   H. False
   D. False   I. True
   E. True   J. False
2. A. Heterosexual contact
   B. Depression, anxiety
   C. AIDS dementia complex (ADC)
   D. Kaposi's sarcoma
3. A. The incidence of HIV infection in the United States has decreased for men in general, greatly decreased for homosexual men, and decreased for babies born to HIV-positive mothers. It has increased for women, particularly poor women, and for racial minorities.
   B. Nucleoside analogs, protease inhibitors, and a drug cocktail of two nucleoside analogs and one protease inhibitor

Index

Page numbers followed by "b" indicate boxes; "f" indicates figures;
"t" indicates tables.